OKU

10

Orthopaedic
Knowledge
Update

AAOS

AMERICAN ACADEMY OF
ORTHOPAEDIC SURGEONS

OKU
10

Orthopaedic Knowledge Update

EDITOR:
John M. Flynn, MD
Associate Chief of Orthopaedics
Children's Hospital of Philadelphia
Associate Professor of Orthopaedics
University of Pennsylvania
Philadelphia, Pennsylvania

AAOS
AMERICAN ACADEMY OF ORTHOPAEDIC SURGEONS

AAOS

AMERICAN ACADEMY OF ORTHOPAEDIC SURGEONS

The material presented in *Orthopaedic Knowledge Update 10* has been made available by the American Academy of Orthopaedic Surgeons for educational purposes only. This material is not intended to present the only, or necessarily best, methods or procedures for the medical situations discussed, but rather is intended to represent an approach, view, statement, or opinion of the author(s) or producer(s), which may be helpful to others who face similar situations.

Some drugs or medical devices demonstrated in Academy courses or described in Academy print or electronic publications have not been cleared by the Food and Drug Administration (FDA) or have been cleared for specific uses only. The FDA has stated that it is the responsibility of the physician to determine the FDA clearance status of each drug or device he or she wishes to use in clinical practice.

Furthermore, any statements about commercial products are solely the opinion(s) of the author(s) and do not represent an Academy endorsement or evaluation of these products. These statements may not be used in advertising or for any commercial purpose.

Published 2011 by the
American Academy of Orthopaedic Surgeons
6300 North River Road
Rosemont, IL 60018

Copyright 2011
by the American Academy of Orthopaedic Surgeons

ISBN 978-0-89203-736-0

Printed in the USA

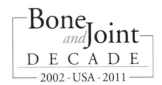

Bone *and* Joint
DECADE
2002 - USA - 2011

Acknowledgments

Editorial Board, OKU 10

John M. Flynn, MD
Associate Chief of Orthopaedics
Children's Hospital of Philadelphia
Associate Professor of Orthopaedics
University of Pennsylvania
Philadelphia, Pennsylvania

Pedro Beredjiklian, MD
Associate Professor
Chief of Hand Surgery
The Rothman Institute
Jefferson Medical College
Philadelphia, Pennsylvania

Lisa K. Cannada, MD
Associate Professor
Orthopaedic Surgery
Saint Louis University
St. Louis, Missouri

John Lawrence Marsh, MD
Professor, Carroll B. Larson Chair
Orthopaedics and Rehabilitation
The University of Iowa
Iowa City, Iowa

Kenneth J. Noonan, MD
Associate Professor
Pediatric Orthopaedics
American Family Children's Hospital
Madison, Wisconsin

R. Lor Randall, MD, FACS
Professor of Orthopaedics
Sarcoma Services
Huntsman Cancer Institute
Salt Lake City, Utah

Jeffrey C. Wang, MD
Professor, Department of Orthopaedic Surgery
and Neurosurgery
UCLA Spine Center
UCLA School of Medicine
Los Angeles, California

Contributors

JOSEPH A. ABBOUD, MD
*Clinical Assistant Professor of Orthopaedic
  Surgery*
University of Pennsylvania
Philadelphia, Pennsylvania

MICHAEL D. AIONA, MD
Chief of Staff
Shriners Hospital for Children
Portland, Oregon

TODD J. ALBERT, MD
*Richard H. Rothman Professor and Chair,
  Orthopaedics*
Professor of Neurosurgery
Thomas Jefferson University Hospitals
The Rothman Institute
Philadelphia, Pennsylvania

BENJAMIN A. ALMAN, MD, FRCSC
*A.J. Latner Professor and Chair of Orthopaedic
  Surgery*
*Vice Chair Research, Department of
  Orthopaedic Surgery*
University of Toronto
Head, Division of Orthopaedic Surgery
*Senior Scientist, Program in Developmental
  and Stem Cell Biology*
The Hospital for Sick Children
Toronto, Ontario, Canada

JEFFREY ANGLEN, MD, FACS
Professor and Chairman
Department of Orthopaedics
Indiana University
Indianapolis, Indiana

**APRIL D. ARMSTRONG, BSc(PT), MD, MSc,
  FRCS(C)**
Associate Professor
Milton S. Hershey Medical Center
Penn State University
Hershey, Pennsylvania

PETER AUGAT, PhD
Professor of Biomechanics
Institute of Biomechanics
Trauma Center Murnau
Murnau, Germany

RAHUL BANERJEE, MD
Assistant Professor
Department of Orthopaedic Surgery
*University of Texas Southwestern
  Medical Center*
Dallas, Texas

MICHAEL T. BENKE, MD
Orthopaedic Surgery
*George Washington University Medical
  Faculty Associates*
Washington, DC

MICHAEL J. BERCIK, MD
Department of Orthopaedics
Thomas Jefferson University
Philadelphia, Pennsylvania

JOSEPH BERNSTEIN, MD
Department of Orthopedic Surgery
University of Pennsylvania School of Medicine
Philadelphia, Pennsylvania

MOHIT BHANDARI, MD, MSc, FRCSC
Assistant Professor
Canada Research
*Department of Clinical Epidemiology and
  Biostatistics*
McMaster University
Hamilton, Ontario, Canada

NITIN N. BHATIA, MD
Chief, Spine Surgery
Department of Orthopaedic Surgery
University of California, Irvine
Orange, California

N. DOUGLAS BOARDMAN III, MD
Associate Professor of Orthopaedic Surgery
Medical College of Virginia
*Virginia Commonwealth University
  Medical Center*
Richmond, Virginia

MICHAEL BOTTLANG, PhD
Director, Legacy Biomechanics Laboratory
*Legacy Clinical Research and Technology
  Center*
Portland, Oregon

RICHARD J. BRANSFORD, MD
Assistant Professor
Department of Orthopaedics and Sports
    Medicine
Harborview Medical Center
University of Washington
Seattle, Washington

JOSEPH A. BUCKWALTER, MS, MD
Professor and Chair, Orthopaedics
University of Iowa
Iowa City, Iowa

LAUREN M. BURKE, MD
Orthopaedic Surgery
George Washington State University Medical
    Faculty Associates
Washington, DC

JONATHAN E. BUZZELL, MD
OrthoWest Orthopaedic and Sports Medicine
Omaha, Nebraska

MICHELLE S. CAIRD, MD
Assistant Professor of Orthopaedic Surgery
Department of Orthopaedic Surgery
University of Michigan
Ann Arbor, Michigan

PABLO CASTAÑEDA, MD
Pediatric Orthopedic Surgeon
Shriners Hospital for Children
Mexico City, Mexico

JENS R. CHAPMAN, MD
Professor and Acting Chair
Director, Spine Services
Hansjöerg Wyss Endowed Chair
Department of Orthopaedics and Sports
    Medicine
Joint Professor of Neurological Surgery
University of Washington
Seattle, Washington

NORMAN CHUTKAN, MD
Professor and Chairman
Department of Orthopaedic Surgery
Medical College of Georgia
Augusta, Georgia

CHARLES R. CLARK, MD
Dr. Michael Bonfiglio Professor of
    Orthopaedics and Rehabilitation
Department of Orthopaedics and Rehabilitation
University of Iowa Hospitals and Clinics
Iowa City, Iowa

BRETT D. CRIST, MD, FACS
Assistant Professor
Co-Director of Orthopaedic Trauma Service
Orthopaedic Surgery
University of Missouri
Columbia, Missouri

SCOTT D. DAFFNER, MD
Assistant Professor
Department of Orthopaedics
West Virginia University School of Medicine
Morgantown, West Virginia

MICHAEL D. DAUBS, MD
Assistant Professor
Department of Orthopaedic Surgery
University of Utah
Salt Lake City, Utah

MARK B. DEKUTOSKI, MD
Associate Professor of Orthopedics
Department of Orthopedic Surgery
Mayo Clinic
Rochester, Minnesota

CRAIG J. DELLA VALLE, MD
Associate Professor
Director, Adult Reconstructive Fellowship
Department of Orthopaedic Surgery
Rush University Medical Center
Chicago, Illinois

DOUGLAS A. DENNIS, MD
Adjunct Professor
Department of Biomedical Engineering
University of Tennessee
Director, Rocky Mountain Musculoskeletal
    Research Laboratory
Denver, Colorado

MATTHEW B. DOBBS, MD
Associate Professor
Department of Orthopaedic Surgery
Washington University School of Medicine
St. Louis, Missouri

GEORGES Y. EL-KHOURY, MD
Musculoskeletal Imaging
Department of Radiology
University of Iowa
Iowa City, Iowa

HOWARD R. EPPS, MD
Partner, Fondren Orthopedic Group, LLC
Texas Orthopedic Hospital
Houston, Texas

JAN PAUL ERTL, MD
Assistant Professor
Chief of Orthopaedic Surgery, Wishard Hospital
Department of Orthopaedic Surgery
Indiana University
Indianapolis, Indiana

DANIEL C. FITZPATRICK, MS, MD
Slocum Center for Orthopedics and Sports
    Medicine
Eugene, Oregon

STEVEN L. FRICK, MD
Pediatric Orthopaedic Surgeon
Orthopaedic Residency Director
Department of Orthopaedic Surgery
Carolinas Medical Center/Levine Children's
    Hospital
Charlotte, North Carolina

THEODORE J. GANLEY, MD
Sports Medicine Director
Department of Orthopaedics
The Children's Hospital of Philadelphia
Philadelphia, Pennsylvania

MICHAEL J. GARDNER, MD
Assistant Professor
Department of Orthopaedic Surgery
Washington University School of Medicine
St. Louis, Missouri

CHARLES L. GETZ, MD
Assistant Professor
Orthopaedic Surgery
The Rothman Institute
Thomas Jefferson Medical School
Philadelphia, Pennsylvania

ERIC GIZA, MD
Assistant Professor of Orthopaedics
Chief, Foot and Ankle Surgery
Orthopaedics
University of California, Davis
Sacramento, California

DAVID L. GLASER, MD
Orthopaedics
Penn Presbyterian Medical Center
Philadelphia, Pennsylvania

J. ERIC GORDON, MD
Associate Professor
Orthopaedic Surgery
Washington University School of Medicine
St. Louis, Missouri

MATT GRAVES, MD
Assistant Professor
Division of Trauma
Department of Orthopaedic Surgery and
    Rehabilitation
University of Mississippi Medical Center
Jackson, Mississippi

LAWRENCE V. GULOTTA, MD
Sports Medicine/Shoulder Service
Hospital for Special Surgery
New York, New York

RANJAN GUPTA, MD
Professor and Chair
Orthopaedic Surgery
University of California, Irvine
Irvine, California

MATTHEW A. HALANSKI, MD
Clinical Assistant Professor
Department of Surgery and Pediatrics and
    Human Development
Pediatric Orthopaedics
Helen DeVos Children's Hospital
College of Human Medicine
Michigan State University
Grand Rapids, Michigan

DANIEL HEDEQUIST, MD
Assistant Professor of Orthopedics
Department of Orthopedics
Children's Hospital
Harvard Medical School
Boston, Massachusetts

SCOTT HELMERS, MD
Staff, Orthopaedic Oncologist
Orthopedic Surgery
Naval Medical Center San Diego
San Diego, California

JOSÉ A. HERRERA-SOTO, MD
Director of Orthopedic Research
Assistant Director, Pediatric Fellowship
  Program
Orlando Health Orthopedic Department
Arnold Palmer Hospital
Orlando, Florida

WELLINGTON K. HSU, MD
Assistant Professor
Orthopaedic Surgery
Northwestern University Feinberg School
  of Medicine
Chicago, Illinois

HENRY J. IWINSKI JR, MD
Associate Professor of Orthopaedic Surgery
Assistant Chief of Staff, Shriners Hospital
University of Kentucky
Lexington, Kentucky

KEVIN B. JONES, MD
Instructor
Department of Orthopaedics
University of Utah
Salt Lake City, Utah

SCOTT G. KAAR, MD
Director of Sports Medicine and Shoulder
  Surgery
Department of Orthopaedic Surgery
Saint Louis University
St. Louis, Missouri

LEE KAPLAN, MD
Chief, Division of Sports Medicine
Associate Professor
Orthopaedics
University of Miami
Miami, Florida

LEONID I. KATOLIK, MD, FAAOS
Assistant Professor
Department of Orthopaedic Surgery
Attending Surgeon
The Philadelphia Hand Center, PC
Philadelphia, Pennsylvania

RAYMOND H. KIM, MD
Adjunct Associate Professor of Bioengineering
Department of Mechanical and Materials
  Engineering
University of Denver
Denver, Colorado

MININDER S. KOCHER, MD, MPH
Associate Director, Division of Sports Medicine
Department of Orthopaedic Surgery
Children's Hospital Boston
Associate Professor of Orthopaedic Surgery
Harvard Medical School
Boston, Massachusetts

SCOTT H. KOZIN, MD
Professor of Orthopaedic Surgery
Attending Hand Surgeon
Temple University School of Medicine
Philadelphia, Pennsylvania

SUMANT G. KRISHNAN, MD
Director, Shoulder Fellowship
Baylor University Medical Center
Shoulder Service
The Carrell Clinic
Dallas, Texas

BRIAN KWON, MD, PhD, FRCSC
Assistant Professor
Department of Orthopaedics
University of British Columbia
Vancouver, Canada

DAWN M. LaPORTE, MD
Associate Professor
Department of Orthopaedic Surgery
Johns Hopkins University School of Medicine
Baltimore, Maryland

ARABELLA I. LEET, MD
Associate Professor
Department of Orthopedics
Johns Hopkins University
Baltimore, Maryland

BRUCE A. LEVY, MD
Assistant Professor
Orthopedic Surgery and Sports Medicine
Mayo Clinic
Rochester, Minnesota

PHILIPP LICHTE, MD
Department of Orthopaedic Surgery
University of Aachen Medical Center
Aachen, Germany

TAE-HONG LIM, PhD
Professor
Biomechanical Engineering
University of Iowa
Iowa City, Iowa

FRANK A. LIPORACE, MD
Assistant Professor
Department of Orthopaedics, Trauma Division
University of Medicine and Dentistry of
   New Jersey
New Jersey Medical School
Newark, New Jersey

CHUANYONG LU, MD
Assistant Researcher
Orthopaedic Surgery
University of California, San Francisco
San Francisco, California

DOUGLAS W. LUNDY, MD, FACS
Orthopaedic Trauma Surgeon
Chair, American Academy of Orthopaedic
   Surgeons Medical Liability Committee
Resurgeons Orthopaedics
Kennestone Hospital
Atlanta, Georgia

HUE H. LUU, MD
Assistant Professor
Associate Director, Molecular Oncology
   Laboratory
Department of Surgery, Section of
   Orthopaedic Surgery
The University of Chicago
Chicago, Illinois

CRAIG R. MAHONEY, MD
Practice Management Committee, American
   Academy of Orthopaedic Surgeons
Iowa Orthopaedic Center
Mercy Medical Center
Des Moines, Iowa

STEPHEN P. MAKK, MD, MBA
Orthopaedic Surgeon – Partner
Louisville Bone and Joint Specialists
Louisville, Kentucky

ARTHUR MANOLI II, MD
Clinical Professor
Orthopaedic Surgery
Wayne State University
Detroit, Michigan
Michigan State University
East Lansing, Michigan
Michigan International Foot and Ankle Center
Pontiac, Michigan

RALPH MARCUCIO, PhD
Assistant Professor
Orthopaedic Surgery
University of California, San Francisco
San Francisco, California

JAMES A. MARTIN, PhD
Associate Research Professor
Orthopaedics and Rehabilitation
University of Iowa
Iowa City, Iowa

MICHAEL T. MAZUREK, MD
Residency Program Director
Orthopaedic Trauma
Department of Orthopaedic Surgery
Naval Medical Center San Diego
San Diego, California

JESSE A. McCARRON, MD
Associate Staff
Section Head, Shoulder Section
Department of Orthopaedics
Cleveland Clinic
Cleveland, Ohio

AMY L. MCINTOSH, MD
Assistant Professor of Orthopedics
Department of Orthopedic Surgery
Mayo Clinic
Rochester, Minnesota

EDWARD J. MCPHERSON, MD, FACS
Director
Los Angeles Orthopaedic Institute
Los Angeles, California

ERIC MEINBERG, MD
Assistant Professor
Orthopaedic Surgery
University of California, San Francisco
San Francisco, California

J. MARK MELHORN, MD
Associate Clinical Professor
University of Kansas School of Medicine,
    Wichita
The Hand Center
Wichita, Kansas

YUSUF MENDA, MD
Assistant Professor, Radiology
University of Iowa
Iowa City, Iowa

THEODORE MICLAU, MD
Professor
Orthopaedic Surgery
University of California, San Francisco
San Francisco, California

TODD MILBRANDT, MD, MS
Assistant Professor
Pediatric Orthopaedics
University of Kentucky
Lexington, Kentucky

JOSE A. MORCUENDE, MD, PhD
Associate Professor
Department of Orthopaedic Surgery and
    Rehabilitation
University of Iowa
Iowa City, Iowa

SM JAVAD MORTAZAVI, MD
Associate Professor
Orthopedic Department
Tehran University of Medical Sciences
Tehran, Iran

TAHSEEN MOZAFFAR, MD
Associate Professor, Neurology and
    Orthopedic Surgery
Director, University of California Irvine – MDA
    ALS and Neuromuscular Center
University of California, Irvine
Irvine, California

THOMAS MROZ, MD
Department of Orthopaedics
Neurological Institute
Cleveland Clinic
Cleveland, Ohio

BRIAN H. MULLIS, MD
Chief, Orthopaedic Trauma
Orthopaedic Surgery
Indiana University School of Medicine
Indianapolis, Indiana

ANAND M. MURTHI, MD
Assistant Professor
Chief, Shoulder and Elbow Service
Department of Orthopaedics
University of Maryland School of Medicine
Baltimore, Maryland

JOSEPH R. O'BRIEN, MD, MPH
Assistant Professor of Orthopaedic Surgery and
    Neurosurgery
Orthopaedic Surgery
George Washington University Medical
    Faculty Associates
Washington, DC

KENJIROU OHASHI, MD, PhD
Musculoskeletal Imaging
Department of Radiology
University of Iowa
Iowa City, Iowa

KANU OKIKE, MD, MPH
Department of Orthopaedic Surgery
Massachusetts General Hospital
Boston, Massachusetts

NORMAN Y. OTSUKA, MD
Chief of Staff
Clinical Professor, Orthopaedic Surgery
Shriners Hospital for Children
University of California, Los Angeles
Los Angeles, California

© 2011 American Academy of Orthopaedic Surgeons

HANS-CHRISTOPH PAPE, MD, FACS
Professor
Department of Orthopaedics
University of Aachen Medical Center
Aachen, Germany

BRADFORD O. PARSONS, MD
Assistant Professor
Orthopaedics
Mount Sinai
New York, New York

JAVAD PARVIZI, MD, FRCS
Professor of Orthopedic Surgery
Orthopedic Surgery
The Rothman Institute at Thomas Jefferson
University
Philadelphia, Pennsylvania

MATTHEW PEPE, MD
Assistant Professor
Department of Orthopaedic Surgery
Thomas Jefferson University School of Medicine
Philadelphia, Pennsylvania

MARK D. PERRY, MD
Professor
Department of Orthopaedic Surgery
University of South Alabama
Mobile, Alabama

CHRISTOPHER L. PETERS, MD
Professor
Chief of Adult Reconstruction
Orthopaedic Department
University of Utah
Salt Lake City, Utah

BRAD PETRISOR, MSc, MD, FRCSC
Assistant Professor
Division of Orthopaedic Surgery
Department of Surgery
McMaster University
Hamilton, Canada

PREM S. RAMAKRISHNAN, PhD
Assistant Research Scientist
Orthopaedics and Rehabilitation
University of Iowa
Iowa City, Iowa

MATTHEW L. RAMSEY, MD
Associate Professor of Orthopaedic Surgery
Shoulder and Elbow Service
Rothman Institute
Thomas Jefferson University
Philadelphia, Pennsylvania

KARL E. RATHJEN, MD
Associate Professor of Orthopaedic Surgery
Texas Scottish Rite Hospital for Children
Dallas, Texas

JOHN M. RHEE, MD
Assistant Professor
Orthopaedic Surgery
Emory Spine Center
Emory University School of Medicine
Atlanta, Georgia

K. DANIEL RIEW, MD
Mildred B. Simon Distinguished Professor
Professor of Neurological Surgery
Orthopaedic Surgery
Washington University School of Medicine
St. Louis, Missouri

SCOTT A. RODEO, MD
Co-Chief Sports Medicine
Shoulder Service
Hospital for Special Surgery
New York, New York

TAMARA D. ROZENTAL, MD
Assistant Professor
Orthopaedic Surgery
Harvard Medical School
Boston, Massachusetts

HENRY CLAUDE SAGI, MD
Director of Research and Fellowship Training
Orthopaedic Trauma Service
Tampa General Hospital
Tampa, Florida

KOICHI SAIRYO, MD, PhD
Associate Professor
Orthopedics
University of Tokushima
Tokushima, Japan

TOSHINORI SAKAI, MD, PhD
Assistant Professor
Department of Orthopedics
Institute of Health Biosciences
The University of Tokushima Graduate School
Tokushima, Japan

ANTHONY SCADUTO, MD
Charles LeRoy Lowman Professor
University of California Los Angeles
Department of Orthopaedic Surgery
Los Angeles Orthopaedic Hospital
Los Angeles, California

KEVIN SHEA, MD
Orthopaedic Surgeon
St. Luke Children's Hospital
Boise, Idaho

JODI SIEGEL, MD
Assistant Professor
University of Massachusetts
Department of Orthopaedics
University of Massachusetts Memorial
    Medical Center
Worcester, Massachusetts

RAFAEL J. SIERRA, MD
Assistant Professor
Consultant
Orthopedic Surgery
Mayo Clinic
Rochester, Minnesota

BRYAN D. SPRINGER, MD
OrthoCarolina Hip and Knee Center
Charlotte, North Carolina

MICHAEL P. STEINMETZ, MD
Assistant Professor
Center for Spine Health
Cleveland Clinic
Cleveland, Ohio

MICHAEL J. STUART, MD
Professor and Vice-Chairman
Department of Orthopedic Surgery
Mayo Clinic
Rochester, Minnesota

JAMES B. TALMAGE, MD
Occupational Health Center
Cookeville, Tennessee

VISHWAS R. TALWALKAR, MD
Associate Professor
Department of Orthopaedics
University of Kentucky
Shriners Hospital for Children
Lexington, Kentucky

VIRAK TAN, MD
Associate Professor of Orthopaedics
Department of Orthopaedics
University of Medicine and Dentistry
    New Jersey
New Jersey Medical School
Newark, New Jersey

DANIEL THEDENS, PhD
Assistant Professor
Radiology
University of Iowa
Iowa City, Iowa

JOHN R. TONGUE, MD
Clinical Assistant Professor
Department of Orthopaedic Surgery
Oregon Health Sciences University
Portland, Oregon

PAUL TORNETTA III, MD
Professor and Vice Chairman
Director of Orthopaedic Trauma
Department of Orthopaedic Surgery
Boston University Medical Center
Boston, Massachusetts

JONATHAN TUTTLE, MD
Assistant Professor
Department of Neurosurgery
Medical College of Georgia
Atlanta, Georgia

J. MICHAEL WATTENBARGER, MD
Chief, Pediatric Orthopedics
Carolinas Medical Center
OrthoCarolina
Charlotte, North Carolina

SHARON M. WEINSTEIN, MD, FAAHPM
Professor of Anesthesiology
Adjunct Associate Professor of Neurology and
*   Internal Medicine (Oncology)*
Department of Anesthesiology
University of Utah – Huntsman Cancer Institute
Salt Lake City, Utah

STUART L. WEINSTEIN, MD
Ignacio V. Ponseti Chair and Professor of
*   Orthopaedic Surgery*
University of Iowa
Iowa City, Iowa

BRAD J. YOO, MD
Assistant Professor
Department of Orthopaedics
University of California, Davis
Sacramento, California

WARREN D. YU, MD
Associate Professor of Orthopaedic Surgery
*   and Neurosurgery*
Orthopaedic Surgery
George Washington University Medical
*   Faculty Services*
Washington, DC

IRA ZALTZ, MD
Department of Orthopaedic Surgery
William Beaumont Hospital
Royal Oak, Michigan

DAN A. ZLOTOLOW, MD
Attending Physician
Shriners Hospital of Philadelphia
Philadelphia, Pennsylvania

Peer Reviewers

DONALD D. ANDERSON, PhD
Associate Professor
Department of Orthopaedics and
    Rehabilitation
The University of Iowa
Iowa City, Iowa

JEFFREY ANGLEN, MD, FACS
Professor and Chairman
Department of Orthopaedics
Indiana University
Indianapolis, Indiana

JOSEPH S. BARR JR, MD
Visiting Orthopaedic Surgeon
Orthopaedic Department
Massachusetts General Hospital
Boston, Massachusetts

ROBERT BARRACK, MD
Charles F. and Joanne Knight
    Distinguished Professor
Department of Orthopaedic Surgery
Washington University School of Medicine
St. Louis, Missouri

SIGURD H. BERVEN, MD
Associate Professor in Residence
Department of Orthopaedic Surgery
University of California, San Francisco
San Francisco, California

MATHIAS BOSTROM, MD
Professor of Orthopaedic Surgery
Hospital for Special Surgery
New York, New York

RICHARD BUCKLEY, MD, FRCSC
Head of Orthopaedic Trauma
Department of Surgery
University of Calgary
Calgary, Canada

DENIS R. CLOHISY, MD
Professor and Chairman
Department of Orthopedic Surgery
University of Minnesota
Minneapolis, Minnesota

JUDD E. CUMMINGS, MD
Assistant Professor
Department of Orthopedic Surgery
Indiana University School of Medicine
Indianapolis, Indiana

DARRYL D'LIMA, MD, PhD
Director, Musculoskeletal Research
Orthopaedics
Scripps Health
La Jolla, California

STEVEN E. FISHER, MBA
Manager, Practice Management Group
Electronic Media, Evaluation Programs, Course
    Operations and Practice Management
American Academy of Orthopaedic Surgeons
Rosemont, Illinois

CY FRANK, MD, FRCSC
Professor
Department of Surgery
University of Calgary
Calgary, Alberta, Canada

MURRAY J. GOODMAN, MD
Clinical Instructor in Orthopaedic Surgery
Salem Orthopedic Surgeons Inc.
Harvard Medical School
Boston, Massachusetts

BANG H. HOANG, MD
Assistant Professor
Orthopaedic Surgery
Univeristy of California, Irvine Medical Center
Orange, California

RAMON L. JIMENEZ, MD
Senior Consultant
Monterey Orthopaedic and Sports Medicine
    Institute
Monterey, California

WENDY LEVINSON, MD
Sir John and Lady Eaton Professor and Chair
Department of Medicine
University of Toronto
Toronto, Ontario, Canada

DOUGLAS W. MARTIN, MD, FAADEP,
   FACOEM, FAAFP
Medical Director
Center for Occupational Health Excellence
St. Luke's Regional Medical Center
Sioux City, Iowa

ROBERT G. MARX, MD
Professor of Orthopaedic Surgery
Hospital for Special Surgery
New York, New York

TIMOTHY E. MOORE, MD
Professor
Radiology
University of Nebraska Medical Center
Omaha, Nebraska

ROBERT NAMBA, MD
Attending Surgeon
Department of Orthopedics
Kaiser Permanente
Irvine, California

ANDREW T. PAVIA, MD
George and Esther Gross Presidential Professor
Department of Pediatrics
University of Utah
Salt Lake City, Utah

MICHAEL D. RIES, MD
Professor and Chief of Arthroplasty
Department of Orthopaedic Surgery
University of California, San Francisco
San Francisco, California

EMIL H. SCHEMITSCH, MD
Professor of Surgery
St. Michael's Hospital
University of Toronto
Toronto, Ontario, Canada

DAVID D. TEUSCHER, MD
Beaumont Bone and Joint Institute
Beaumont, Texas

PAUL TORNETTA III, MD
Professor and Vice Chairman
Director of Orthopaedic Trauma
Department of Orthopaedic Surgery
Boston University Medical Center
Boston, Massachusetts

ALEXANDER R. VACCARO, MD, PhD
Everrett J. and Marion Gordon Professor of
   Orthopaedic Surgery
Orthopaedic Surgery
The Rothman Institute
Jefferson Medical College
Philadelphia, Pennsylvania

DAVID VOLGAS, MD
Associate Professor
Department of Orthopaedic Surgery
University of Missouri
Columbia, Missouri

CRAIG WALKER, MD, FACR
Professor and Chairman
Howard B. Hunt Centennial Chair
Radiology Department
University of Nebraska Medical Center
Omaha, Nebraska

KEVIN WARD, MD
Chief Executive Officer
Iowa Ortho
Des Moines, Iowa

Preface

We orthopaedic surgeons face a challenging conundrum: we are driven to subspecialize because of rapid technologic advances and patients seeking very specific expertise, yet we must remain knowledgeable across the full spectrum of orthopaedics in order to deliver optimum patient care and pass certifying and recertifying examinations. We have many ways to learn: courses, textbooks, journals, weekly conferences—and now Webinars and Web-based surgical videos. Yet with all these different and evolving continuing education options, there remains a clear need for a single, rigorously peer-reviewed compendium of our entire specialty—a source that is comprehensive yet succinct, current yet founded on prior knowledge. For more than 20 years, the Orthopaedic Knowledge Update series has filled this role with great success.

The writers, section editors, and I are very proud to bring you OKU 10. In many ways, this volume builds on and improves the outstanding previous editions. The Principles of Orthopaedics and Systemic Disorders sections give the reader a basic science and medical foundation, as well as synopsis chapters on essential issues of our practice: patient safety, communication skills, evidence-based medicine, and practice management. The remaining sections--Upper Extremity, Lower Extremity, Spine, and Pediatrics-- cover the injuries and conditions we treat, each with numerically cited references and an annotated reference list. One new addition: we have incorporated the AAOS Clinical Practice Guidelines wherever appropriate. In total, OKU 10 delivers the most up-to-date, concise summary of the standard of care for orthopaedics.

"To whom much is given, much will be expected": we have all benefitted from many great surgeon-educators who trained us, and many clinical and basic science researchers who work to answer questions and advance our field. In the spirit of giving back, OKU 10 represents the culmination of an enormous volunteer effort of over 2 years. More than 100 of your colleagues have given selflessly of their time and talent to create this outstanding reference. Many of us remember reading our OKU in training until the pages were falling out. OKU 10 is our chance to give back, and perhaps inspire a future editor, perhaps of OKU 15?

During the process of creating OKU 10, one of our authors, Michael Mazurek, was killed in a tragic accident. We would like to dedicate this work in his memory. I would like to thank the incredible group of section editors and the members of the AAOS publications department, specifically, Marilyn Fox, PhD, director, and Lisa Claxton Moore, managing editor, who did the lion's share of the work. I also want to thank my wife Mary, who tolerates my academic orthopaedic hobbies. Finally, I want to thank my children Erin, Colleen, John, and Kelly. Now I appreciate them more: they have lots of homework at night, and with OKU 10, so did I.

John M. (Jack) Flynn, MD
Editor

Table of Contents

Section 6: Pediatrics

Principles of Orthopaedics

SECTION EDITOR:

JOHN LAWRENCE MARSH, MD

Chapter 1

Patient Safety and Risk Management

Douglas W. Lundy, MD   Stuart L. Weinstein, MD

Patient Safety

Overview and Joint Commission Initiatives

Patients come to orthopaedic surgeons for evaluation and treatment of their musculoskeletal conditions believing that they will hold to the Hippocratic mandate of *primum non nocere* – that is, "first, do no harm." As a leader on the health care team, the orthopaedic surgeon should partner with others to ensure that the patient's safety and best interests are held paramount. Many times, however, a more appropriate principle is *primum succurrere* – that is, "first, hasten to help." Some interventions in emergency orthopaedics may cause potential harm to the patient, but the physician should still perform certain potentially hazardous procedures to save life and limb. Nonetheless, the patient's interests are of the utmost concern, and the risks of the treatment should be managed while providing timely and appropriate care.

In 2009, The Joint Commission introduced its latest Standards Improvement Initiatives.[1] Initiatives that are of specific interest to orthopaedic surgeons include: (1) Improved accuracy of patient identification – this includes the use of two patient identifiers. (2) Improved communication between providers – this includes "read back" of orders, eliminating improper abbreviations, and improved "handoff" of patients. (3) Reducing the risk of health care–associated infections – this includes preventing multiple drug–resistant organisms and preventing surgical site infections. (4) Reconciling medications across the continuum of care. (5) Reducing the risk of falls. (6) Reducing the risk of surgical fires.

There are also three universal protocols from The Joint Commission that are germane to the orthopaedic surgeon: conducting a preprocedure verification process, marking the procedure site, and instituting a time-out.

Dr. Lundy serves as the Chair of the Medical Liability Committee of the American Academy of Orthopaedic Surgeons. Neither Dr. Weinstein nor an immediate family member has received anything of value from or owns stock in a commercial company or institution related directly or indirectly to the subject of this chapter.

"Time-Out" in the Operating Room

The purpose of the time-out is to perform a final assessment to ensure that the appropriate patient, site, procedure, position, equipment, and documentation are verified before the surgical procedure is initiated. The time-out is initiated by a designated member of the team, and this person does not necessarily need to be the surgeon. All members of the team must participate in the time-out, and all issues and questions need to be resolved before beginning the procedure.[2] The time-out needs to be done in a "fail-safe" mode – that is, no incision is made until the time-out is successfully completed. When used appropriately, the preincision time-out should eliminate wrong-site surgery in many instances.

Wrong-Site Surgery

Wrong-site surgery is a regrettable event that is of significant concern to the orthopaedic surgeon because so many of the procedures can be performed on either side of the body. Although this error appears negligent to the public, the inherent possibility of this happening to anyone at any time is clear to many conscientious orthopaedic surgeons. A retrospective closed claims study demonstrated that negligence cases involving wrong-site surgery resulted in an 84% rate of payment compared with a 30% rate of payment for other claims of medical negligence.[3]

In 1998, the American Academy of Orthopaedic Surgeons (AAOS) launched the "Sign Your Site" program. Since the program's inception, preoperative marking of the surgical site has become an essential aspect of the orthopaedic surgeon's surgical routine.[3] The Joint Commission Universal Protocol[2] has mandated several elements in preoperative site marking as outlined in **Table 1**.

The AAOS has made several recommendations to orthopaedic surgeons if they find that they have started a procedure at the wrong site.[3] The surgeon should attempt to restore the incorrectly operated site to its previous condition if at all possible. If the patient's condition will allow, the surgeon should then perform the consented procedure at the correct site. The surgeon should communicate with the patient and the patient's family (if appropriate) the occurrence of the wrong-site surgery and the consequences that may occur as a re-

Table 1

Preoperative Site Marking According to Joint Commission Universal Protocol

1. The site needs to be marked specifically in regard to laterality (left/right), level (spine), surface (volar/dorsal), digit (hand/foot), and the specific lesion if there is more than one.
2. The surgeon must mark the area before the patient enters the operating room, and the patient should be awake and alert if possible.
3. The person marking the site must be an individual licensed practitioner who is privileged by the hospital to perform that specific procedure. The person marking the patient must be involved and present during the procedure.
4. The method of marking cannot be ambiguous and must be used throughout the hospital.
5. The mark must be made at or near the incision site, and the preferred method is that the practitioner marks the site with his or her initials.
6. The mark must be visible after prepping and draping. Stick-on markers are not sufficient.
7. When operating on the spine, "special intraoperative radiographic techniques" are also used to ensure the correct site.

sult of the error. The surgeon should proceed as the patient wishes after communicating this information. If the wrong-site surgical error is discovered after the procedure is completed, the surgeon should immediately disclose the error to the patient and the patient's family (if appropriate) and determine an appropriate plan to rectify the situation.

Safety Checklists

Safety checklists are used throughout the patient care environment to improve outcomes and patient well being. When used consistently, these checklists will ensure that vital aspects of the patient's care are not accidentally overlooked. When these checklists are used in the preoperative setting, there is less chance that appropriate laboratory tests, patient risk factors, and previous anesthetic complications will be overlooked, and it will be more likely that necessary special instrumentation or implants will be available. The surgical time-out is a form of checklist in that the site and side of the procedure are verified, and the presence of preoperative antibiotics and appropriate implants, radiographs, and documents is confirmed. Postoperative checklists can also be helpful, along with standardized postoperative orders and pathways. These documents can decrease the incidence of forgotten postoperative antibiotics or thromboembolic prophylaxis. The use of electronic medical records may also facilitate the use of checklists. Discharge checklists can ensure that the patient is given appropriate follow-up information, discharge prescrip-

tions, and limitations as well as when and how to contact the physician in case there is a problem.

Communication (Handoff of Patients)

Breakdown in communication is unfortunately a significant potential cause of suboptimal patient care. Orthopaedic surgeons must ensure that appropriate information is passed and comprehended between providers during a transfer of care. This is especially true when there is an on-call physician who is temporarily covering the patient for another physician. Assumptions about what the other physician will do can easily lead to unfortunate gaps in the patient's care with potential untoward results.

Checkout lists for weekend call patients are effective in improving communication. The handoff is best done in person if possible. The AAOS also sponsors workshops that are effective in improving communication among physicians, other members of the health care team, and patients.

Retained Instruments/Sponges

Accidentally leaving sponges or instruments in a patient's body cavity is a significant concern for any surgeon. Most retained items are left in the abdomen, pelvis, or vagina. According to findings based on a review of closed claims of a large medical liability carrier, of 54 patients involved in this series, 69% had retained sponges and 31% had retained instruments.[4] Sixty-nine percent of the patients required surgery for removal of the retained instrument or sponge. Risk factors for retained foreign bodies included increased body mass index, emergency surgery, and unplanned change in the operation. Retained surgical items may cause pain, abscess formation, organ perforation, and death.

Retained surgical items are considered by the Centers for Medicare and Medicaid Services as a never event or preventable error, and this organization and private payers will not pay for the treatment required to remove a retained item or the complications arising from this event.

Fires and Burns

Fires in the operating room occur approximately 100 times per year in the United States, resulting in approximately 20 serious patient injuries.[5] The three requirements for fire (source, oxidizer, and fuel) are available and abundant in the operating room. Prevention of fires in the operating room was a focus of the Joint Commission in 2009 (standard NPSG.11.01.01).

The most common sources of ignition in the operating room are the electrocautery (68% of the time) and the laser (13% of the time) although drills and saws may also be an ignition source. Electrocautery devices should be placed in a holster when not in use. Alcohol-based preparation solutions must be allowed to dry adequately so they will not ignite. The oxygen-rich environment of the operating room makes the setting especially vulnerable to fire. The surgical team should ensure that oxygen concentration is minimized under the surgical drapes because this is a significant cause of surgical fires.[6]

Device Recalls

Implants will occasionally be found to be defective and a device recall may be initiated by the manufacturer or, less commonly, the Food and Drug Administration (FDA). The orthopaedic surgeon who implanted the device should assist in completing registry and chart documentation that will ensure patient identification in case of recall. The orthopaedic surgeon has some responsibility for the patient's safety after an implanted device has been recalled, and should assist in contacting the patients affected by a recalled device. The treating orthopaedic surgeon is in the unique position to further advance his or her role as patient advocate and help the patient in successfully navigating the issue of a potentially defective device. The patient should be carefully monitored for potential device failure and advised as to the potential risks and benefits of undertaking surgery to revise the implanted device. The AAOS strongly recommends that its members become aware of device recalls and report any information concerning defective devices to MedWatch under the auspices of the FDA.

Patients may experience a significant level of anxiety after a device recall. In many recalls, not all of the implants may be defective, and the orthopaedic surgeon may be able to alleviate the patient's fears and provide comfort. The AAOS Information Statement on implant device recalls states, "Revision surgery, in the absence of evidence of clinical failure, as a preventative measure against possible implant device malfunction is rarely, if ever, recommended."[7]

Risk Management

Communicating Adverse Events

Adverse events or disappointing outcomes may occur for a multitude of reasons and are not necessarily a result of error or negligence. It is the obligation of the treating physician to inform the patient or his or her family, as soon as possible, of any adverse event or unexpected findings at surgery and to discuss what may be perceived as a potential disappointing outcome. Good communication built on trust and honesty is a cornerstone of patient-physician relationships. Honest and open communication favorably affects not only patient satisfaction but health outcomes. It also often reduces the incidence of malpractice actions by mitigating the liability risk when patients and family members think that their surgeon is honest and caring and will not abandon them.

If the cause of the adverse event is an error, the surgeon should immediately contact the appropriate risk manager or legal counsel to determine the amount of detail that should be provided in any discussions. Some information such as root cause analysis, peer review issues, results of disciplinary actions, and legal counsel communications are privileged and should not be part of patient discussions. Careful chart documentation is an important component when dealing with medical errors.

Acknowledgment of what happened, and understanding and the assurance that steps will be taken so that the event will not occur again, and that risks of a similar occurrence will be minimized must be communicated as appropriate. An apology, if appropriate, that avoids suggestion of fault or conjecture may reduce patient anger and mistrust. Follow-up care and next steps must be addressed. An offer to transfer care to another physician may be appropriate. Comments about the reasons for the events should be made only after medical investigation is completed; the patient should be informed of the results of the completed investigation. It is best if this interaction is done in the presence of a patient liaison to not only witness the conversation but to help the patient and his or her family with needs or requests.[8]

Responding to Patient Complaints

Good communication skills are the key component of establishing the physician-patient relationship. The risk of receiving patient complaints can also be minimized by practicing patient-centered and culturally competent care and implementing a well-documented consent process.

Patient complaints are based on multiple factors. However, several common issues underlie most patient complaints, and these can be categorized into four key areas that will help minimize risk: enhance communication; provide patient-centered culturally competent care; enhance the informed consent process; and explain charges and fees up front.

Enhance Communication

Many patients have difficulty absorbing or understanding information presented to them; therefore, informational handouts are often helpful. Patients are able to take the information home, discuss it, and even do some research (the physician may suggest some "reliable" Web sites such as "Your Orthopaedic Connection" (http://orthoinfo.aaos.org) that will facilitate better understanding of the procedure and help formulate questions. Patients should be able to reach the physician (or nurse or licensed provider) for questions following his or her visit via phone or email.[9]

Practice Patient-Centered, Culturally Competent Care

A patient's cultural background and generational differences often affect how he or she relates to health care providers or processes information. In certain cultures, for example, questioning a physician may be considered rude or a challenge to authority. Therefore, important questions may go unanswered if the physician is not proactive in providing information. Enhancing cultural competency skills and developing an understanding of the predominant cultures that make up the patient base can help the physician avoid miscommunication.[10]

Enhance the Informed Consent Process

Informed consent is a process and the formal signed consent form merely documents this process, which involves explaining the nature of the problem; the proposed treatment plan; the most likely or most significant risks associated with treatment; the anticipated benefits of treatment; and reasonable alternatives to the proposed treatment, including the alternative of not proceeding with the proposed treatment. Discussion of prognosis and the duration and extent of disability following treatment compared to the same factors if treatment is not performed helps the patient make good decisions with realistic expectations.

If a procedure is recommended to a patient, the physician should distribute materials that review the basic procedure and address the risks and benefits of the procedure, important components of the informed consent process. If possible, the patient and family should be allowed time to digest the material and formulate questions. The physician should document that the patient was informed of the risks and benefits of the proposed procedure, that alternatives to the procedure were also offered, and that the risks and benefits of those alternatives were explained and understood. In addition, it should be documented that the patient had the opportunity to have his or her questions answered. The date on which the patient was first provided with this information always should be documented so that the length of time the patient was given to consider these options is clear on the record.[11]

Explain All Charges and Fees Up Front

A clear explanation of all financial considerations can help reduce complaints. All charges should be clearly explained to the patient, including the base charge for the proposed procedure and any additional charges for follow-up visits. In times of large deductibles and varying degrees of coverage it is always best to recommend that the patient check with his or her insurance company for details of coverage.

If a physician receives a patient complaint, legal assistance, preferably from an attorney who has experience working before the state board of medicine, should be sought before responding to the complaint.[12]

Saying "I'm Sorry"

Adverse events and disappointing outcomes are an unfortunate and uncomfortable aspect of an orthopaedic practice. Honest and open communication, including saying "I'm sorry" if appropriate, favorably affects not only patient satisfaction but health outcomes, and often reduces the incidence of malpractice actions. Negligence claims often occur when the patient thinks he or she has been abandoned and that there is no other recourse. Communicating with the patient and family in an honest and compassionate manner as soon as possible after an adverse event is consistent with the principles of medical ethics and professionalism. However, the thought of saying "I'm sorry" creates concern among some that an apology will be construed as an admission of guilt.

Many states have passed "I'm sorry" laws that allow physicians to express compassion to patients without this statement being construed as an admission of guilt. Senate Bill 51784 (Medic Act) was introduced in 2005 by then-Senators Clinton and Obama. One of the purposes of this act was to improve the quality of health care by encouraging open communication between patients and health care providers about medical error. Many professional liability carriers are also realizing the benefits of saying "I'm sorry" and are establishing programs to facilitate this interaction between doctors and their patients.[13,14]

Definition of Negligence

Negligence as it relates to malpractice litigation implies that an act or omission occurred in which care provided caused injury or death to the patient and deviated from the accepted standards of practice in the medical community. There are four essential elements that must be present and applicable to the defendant and the injury to establish negligence: a duty was owed; a duty was breached; the breach caused injury; and damages resulted.[15,16]

A Duty was Owed

A legal duty is established whenever a provider undertakes care or treatment of a patient. It begins with the initiation of any service to the patient (for example, emergency department encounter; clinic appointment; telephone encounter). A patient-physician relationship must be proved to demonstrate that a duty was owed.

A Duty was Breached

A Duty was Breached A breach of duty implies failure of the provider to meet the standard of care for the time and place of the alleged injury. The standard of care is established by expert testimony or in obvious errors in some jurisdictions by the doctrine of res ipsa loquitor ("the thing speaks for itself").

The Breach Caused an Injury

The claimant must demonstrate that failure to conform to the standard of care was a cause of the damages sustained.

Damages Occurred

Unless damages of some sort are sustained by the patient, there is no basis for a claim, regardless of whether or not the physician was negligent. Damages may be direct economic (measurable damages, such as lost earnings or medical expenses), indirect (subjective damages; for example, pain and suffering, loss of "consortium"), or punitive, when conduct is intentionally harmful or grossly negligent.

Analyzing a Lawsuit

The orthopaedic surgeon's first notification that there is a pending lawsuit is often only after he or she has been served with the summons. At that point, the orthopaedic surgeon should immediately notify his or her medical liability carrier, and the insurance company will assign an attorney to evaluate the case and defend the surgeon. The defendant surgeon should review the patient's medical record but it should not be altered in any way. The attorney will request all of the medical records and schedule a meeting with the orthopaedic surgeon to discuss the specifics of the case. The defense attorney will answer the summons and the period of discovery is then initiated by both sides. Expert reviewers will be selected by both sides, and the medical records will be sent to them. The opinions of the experts are of vital importance when the defense attorney evaluates a lawsuit to determine if the case can be successfully defended and at what cost. The defendant physician may also serve as expert witness in addition to his or her role as a fact witness, and their active involvement in the case often improves the chance for a successful defense.

There are many procedural and legal specifics that are of vital importance to the success or failure of a lawsuit, and these items are often beyond the knowledge of most orthopaedic surgeons. The statute of limitations is a complex doctrine that can potentially limit the period of time following treatment that the surgeon may be sued. If the alleged negligence is past the statute of limitations, the court may dismiss the case even though the defendant may have a valid complaint against the surgeon. Other procedural issues may also limit the ability of a plaintiff to sue the physician.

Interestingly, an orthopaedic surgeon may be negligent in the care of a patient, but the case may still be very defendable. Even if the plaintiff can demonstrate that there was duty and a breach of duty, the defense may win the case if damages are minimal. Some cases are delayed by the defense knowing that the patient's damages may be minimized over time, thus weakening the plaintiff's claim against the orthopaedic surgeon. The plaintiff may also have difficulty proving causation, that is, there may be a significant leap from the assumed breach of duty and the damages that occurred. The damages may have been inevitable regardless of the physician's breach of duty, and this makes the case much less attractive to effective plaintiff's attorneys.

Other variables that an attorney assesses when evaluating a lawsuit include many intangible attributes. How the plaintiff and defendant present themselves during their depositions influences both attorneys. If they appear aloof, arrogant, or unfriendly, the attorney may be concerned how the jury will view the witness whether it is the plaintiff or the defendant. Orthopaedic practice within clinical practice guidelines or definitive clinical research should produce a universally successful defense or dismissal of the case, but unfortunately the current legal system does not guarantee this outcome. The doctrine of contributory negligence exists when the patient is partially responsible for the outcome of his or her treatment. In this case, damages may be decreased because of the patient's actions, and in other instances, the patient may be barred from proceeding with the complaint.

Settling Versus Fighting

The opinions of the experts strongly affect the evaluation of whether the case can be won or lost at trial. Other parties affected by the lawsuit also contribute to the strategy of defense. Many attorneys name as many defendants as possible when filing a lawsuit to ensure both maximal recovery from the plaintiffs and that all potential parties are named within the statute of limitations. Parties may be dropped during the period of discovery if the plaintiff's attorney realizes that there is no benefit in maintaining the action against that individual. This strategy can also lead to conflicting theories and uncover facts brought to light by finger-pointing among multiple defendants.

The amount of monetary damages also affects the decision of whether to settle or continue to defend a lawsuit. If the monetary damages have the potential to be substantial, the attorney may advise the defendant in consultation with the medical liability carrier to settle the case. If the monetary damages are small, the plaintiff's attorney may decide not to pursue the case due to the lack of potential recovery. A high-low arrangement may be agreed upon by the plaintiff and defendant prior to verdict. In this arrangement, both sides agree that the defendant will pay at least the low amount but will not pay more than the high amount, thereby reducing risk for both sides. These arrangements are reportable to the National Practitioner's Data Bank (NPDB) except if the payment was at the low end, and the defendant was found to be not liable in the case.[17]

The NPDB was formed by Congress in 1986 by The Heath Care Quality Improvement Act (Title IV 99-660). Congress was concerned that "the increasing occurrence of medical malpractice and the need to improve the quality of medical care have become nationwide problems that warrant greater efforts than those that can be undertaken by any individual State." Congress was also concerned that disreputable physicians, dentists, and other health care practitioners could move from state to state without disclosing their "previous damaging or incompetent performance." The US Department of Health and Human Services is responsible for maintaining the NPDB.[18]

The NPDB is intended to be a comprehensive alert system for discreet inquiries into a physician's credentials to include loss or restriction of license, membership in professional societies, malpractice payment history, and a record of clinical privileges.[19] "Authorized NPDB queriers and reporters include state licensing boards, medical malpractice payers (authorized only to report to the NPDB), hospitals and other health care entities, professional societies, and licensed health care practitioners (self-query only)."[20] When hospitals perform a review to credential a physician for privileges, the hospital makes a confidential inquiry to the NPDB. The information in the data bank is intended to supplement a hospital's effort, not to replace credentialing. Individual practitioners may also query the database to request their own record. The information in the NPDB is not available to the general public. In the 19-year period from September 1990 to July 2009, there were 246,016 reports of physician medical malpractice made to the NPDB. The state of New York had the most reports of medical malpractice during this period (33,587).

If an orthopaedic surgeon is reported to the NPDB, the NPDB sends a report stating such to the physician. A practitioner may submit a 4,000-character response to a report on the NPDB. This response will be included when a query is made about that practitioner to the NPDB. The NPDB reports licensing and privilege issues, but in civil legal matters, the database only reports health care–related civil judgments taken in federal or state court only. As a result, if a physician has a defense verdict in a medical negligence lawsuit, there is no report made to the NPDB.

Types of Liability Insurance

Medical professionals are commonly required to maintain professional liability insurance by state regulations, hospital rules, and/or managed care organizations to offset the risk and costs of lawsuits based on medical malpractice. Sometimes, posting a bond may be done in lieu of carrying insurance. There are two basic types of professional liability insurance coverage; claims made and occurrence.[21]

Claims Made

These policies are the most common type and cover all claims made in the policy period, regardless of when the event occurred. Claims made after the policy period are not covered. When a claims-made policy expires or is cancelled, the physician no longer has coverage for events that have occurred but have not yet been reported. Because the policy covers only claims made during its term, the first few years of this type of policy typically has lower premiums while the policy reaches a steady equilibrium (maturity).

Because medical liability claims may arise many years later, special policies called tail coverage (reporting endorsement coverage) can be purchased. When a physician ceases to maintain a claims-made policy, tail coverage is purchased from the carrier at the time the claims- made policy expires. This coverage in effect converts a claims-made policy into an occurrence policy. Some carriers may waive tail coverage in the event of death, disability, or retirement or based on years of coverage.

An alternative to a reporting endorsement is prior acts coverage, commonly referred to as "nose coverage," which is purchased from the new insurance carrier. This provides coverage for future claims on acts that occurred while the previous claims-made policy was in force. When changing claims-made policies, either a tail or a nose is required to avoid a lapse in coverage.

Occurrence

This type of policy covers the insured for all claims resulting from actions occurring during the period of time covered by the policy, regardless of when the claim is made. Hence, the insured is covered for events that occur during the policy period, even if reported after the policy expires or is not renewed. The permanence of occurrence coverage generally makes it more expensive than claims-made coverage initially. Generally, a mature claims-made policy costs the same as an occurrence policy. During the early years of a claims-made policy, premiums may be less expensive but rates for occurrence policies are usually only affected by the market.

Stress of a Lawsuit

Medical negligence lawsuits can be among the most stressful crises that an orthopaedic surgeon will face in his or her professional career. Physicians often experience disbelief, anger, depression, embarrassment, and self-doubt after they have been served with a lawsuit. The stress affects not only the surgeon but also his or her family and close friends.

It is important when being sued that the physician realize that he or she is not alone. At any particular time, many competent orthopaedic surgeons are defendants in a medical negligence lawsuit, and being served with a lawsuit does not imply that the surgeon does poor-quality work. There are many programs sponsored by insurance companies and medical societies to help physicians and their families cope with the stress of a lawsuit. The AAOS offers peer counseling for fellows who have been named in a medical negligence lawsuit.

National Medical Liability Issues as They Relate to Politics, State and National Reform, and National Variation

Medical malpractice will remain a point of contention for many years to come. Although national medical negligence tort reform within the next several years is unlikely, the AAOS continues to urge the current administration to include medical liability reform in the discussions on health care reform because of the effect of lawsuits on the expense of defensive medicine. There are many different options available, including noneconomic caps, health court, early tender and affirmative defense by practicing within clinical practice guidelines.

Significant differences in medical liability reform exist between different states. Caps on noneconomic damages have been shown to effectively reduce insurance rates and limit frivolous lawsuits. States also differ in their approach to the statute of limitations, contributory negligence, joint and several liability, collateral source, and how the court deals with expert witnesses. The AAOS continues to urge the federal and state legislatures to pass effective and meaningful laws to protect the rights of patients to sue for damages from medical negligence while also protecting the rights of physicians who are named as defendants in a medical negligence lawsuit.

Summary

Patient safety and risk management are essential in the practice of orthopaedic surgery. As advocates for patient care, orthopaedic surgeons should endeavor to make the entire health care process safer so that medical errors are as infrequent as possible. Time-outs, effective handoff between providers, and safety checklists should reduce errors in patient care. Studies have demonstrated that sincere and timely apologies after complications improve the relationship between the patient and the surgeon and decrease medical negligence lawsuits. Orthopaedic surgeons are afforded significant protections if they are served with a medical negligence lawsuit, and they should be actively involved in their defense with their legal team. It is hoped that medical liability reform will expand throughout the states and eventually through federal legislation.

Annotated References

1. http://www.jointcommission.org/NR/rdonlyres/D619D05C-A682-47CB-874A-8DE16D21CE24/0/HAP_NPSG_Outline.pdf

   This Web site addresses the Standards Improvements Initiatives that the Joint Commission has established to improve the care of patients during surgery.

2. http://www.jointcommission.org/NR/rdonlyres/31666E86-E7F4-423E-9BE8-F05BD1CB0AA8/0/HAP_NPSG.pdf

   This Web site further defines the national patient safety goals established by The Joint Commission. The tables presented define specifics for each of the goals.

3. Information Statement AA: Wrong Site Surgery. http://www.aaos.org/about/papers/advistmt/1015.asp

   Wrong-site surgery is discussed, along with methods to avoid its occurrence. A safety checklist is included.

4. Gawande AA, Studdert DM, Orav EJ, Brennan TA, Zinner MJ: Risk factors for retained instruments and sponges after surgery. *N Engl J Med* 2003;348(3):229-235.

5. ECRI: A clinician's guide to surgical fires: How they occur, how to prevent them, how to put them out [guidance article]. *Health Devices* 2003;32(1):5-24.

6. http://www.jointcommission.org/SentinelEvents/SentinelEventAlert/sea_29.htm

   This is the Web site of The Joint Commission that describes standards to avoid surgical fires. A safety checklist is included.

7. AAOS: Information Statement: Implant Device Recalls. http://www.aaos.org/about/papers/advistmt/1019.asp

   This AAOS information statement discusses product recall and the implications to the orthopaedic surgeon. Patient safety and communication are emphasized.

8. AAOS Information Statement: Communicating Adverse Outcomes. http://www.aaos.org/about/papers/advistmt/1028.asp.

   This AAOS information statement describes methods for discussing adverse outcomes with patients. Disclosure with patients in addition to risk management are reviewed.

9. AAOS Communication Mentoring Skills Program. http://www3.aaos.org/education/csmp/index.cfm Accessed August 16, 2009.

   The Communication Skills Mentoring Program is described, including an overview of the program and locations at which the course is offered.

10. White AA III, Hoffman HL: Culturally competent care education: overview and perspectives. *J Am Acad Orthop Surg* 2007;15(suppl 1):S80-S85.

    This is a report of the Harvard Medical School's program to improve culturally appropriate medical care. The practices, perspectives, and experiences of this committee are portrayed.

11. Holt WJ: Informed consent: A process, not a piece of paper http://www.aaos.org/news/bulletin/sep07/managing5.asp

    The process of informed consent is described. The process, rather than the written document, is emphasized, and methods to improve consent are described.

12. Feinberg J: The Power of the Patient Complaint. http://www.aaos.org/news/aaosnow/jan08/managing8.asp.

    Four methods to decrease patient complaints are described, along with discussions on avoiding complaints and risk management.

13. Lundy DW, Cox AR: Saying "I'm Sorry" to Patients After an Adverse Outcome. http://www2.aaos.org/aaos/archives/bulletin/jun06/orm1.asp.

    The benefits of sincere apologies to patients after adverse outcomes are reviewed, along with the legal basis of the apology.

14. Clinton HR, Obama B: Making patient safety the centerpiece of medical liability reform. *N Engl J Med* 2006;354(21):2205-2208.

15. http://www.sorryworks.net/home.phtml.

    This Web site is devoted to the Sorry Works coalition, which advocates the process of complete disclosure to patients.

16. Teuscher D: Medical Legal Terms Defined: Negligence. http://www2.aaos.org/aaos/archives/bulletin/oct05/rskman3.asp.

    The definition and four elements of medical negligence are reviewed.

17. NPDB-HIPDB Data Bank News. http://www.npdb-hipdb.hrsa.gov/pubs/newsletter/January_2007_Newsletter.pdf. Accessed July 22, 2010.

    Medical malpractice payment reports submitted to NPDB were studied.

18. "The Four Elements of Medical Malpractice." Yale New Haven Medical Center: Issues in Risk Management. http://info.med.yale.edu/caim/risk/malpractice/malpractice_2.html.

The elements of negligence, along with the complaint, summons, discovery, and trial, are reviewed.

19. http://www.npdb-hipdb.hrsa.gov/npdb.html

The NPDB and why it was developed in addition to standards of confidentiality are discussed.

20. Sanbar SS, ed: *The Medical Malpractice Survival Handbook*. Philadelphia, PA, Mosby-Elsevier, 2007.

This text discusses issues related to the accused physician in a medical malpractice litigation.

21. Teuscher D: Professional Liability Insurance: A Market Overview. http://www2.aaos.org/aaos/archives/bulletin/dec05/rskman1.asp.

A broad overview of medical liability insurance and the modifications available in the market are discussed. Specifically, alternative products such as captives and risk retention groups are reviewed.

(continued back pg.)

FRACTURE HEALING

#1 factor: vascularity
#2 " : type of fx repair depends on biomechanical environ.

* throughout 4 phases, resistance @ fx ↑ thus interfragmentary strain ↓

UNSTABLE FX
- callus formation, aka indirect, 2° healing
- ↑ instability of fx, ↑ callus
- strain = $\frac{\Delta l}{l}$ under given F

interfragmentary strain = $\frac{\text{deformation @ fx site}}{\text{gap}}$

intact bone: strain tolerance of 2% before fracturing
∴ interfragmentary strain must be less than 2% for bone formation to occur

① Inflammatory
3-4 days
fx → disruption medullary vessels → ischemic, necrotic bone @ fx edges + hematoma
hematoma releases growth factors to stim. angiogenesis + bone formation
PDGF
VEGF
TGF-β
platelets, mφ, mesenchymal cells
new blood vessels form from surrounding soft tissues for transient blood supply → revascularize hypoxic fx site
mφ phagocytose necrotic bone fragments
medullary blood vessels restored

② Soft callus
primarily from periosteum & endosteum
→ mesenchymal cells + capillary ingrowth + growth factors ∴ hematoma → granulation tissue (strain tolerance of 100%)
type I, (II), III collagen, then mostly II
if unstable fx / motion ⇒ mesenchymal cells → chondrocytes for endosteal ossification
if stable fx / ∅ motion ⇒ mesenchymal cells → osteoblasts for intramembraneous ossification
by 3 wks.

③ Hard Callus
chondrocytes in fx callus produce cartilaginous matrix & differentiate into hypertrophic chondrocytes
hypertrophic chondrocytes express type X collagen, release proteases to degrade ECM, secrete VEGF
cartilage → calcified
any uncalcified cartilage degraded
new blood vessels invade
woven bone formed

④ Remodeling
70% total healing time of fx
woven bone → cortical bone
Wolff's law determines balance of osteoblastic v. osteoclastic activity (bone remodels in response to mechanical stress)
Piezoelectric changes: compression side / concave side = electronegativity → osteoblastic activity v. tension / convex side = electropositivity → osteoclastic activity

↑ instability + inadequate blood supply → atrophic nonunion
↑ instability + adequate blood supply → hypertrophic nonunion / pseudoarthrosis
e.g. braces, splints, ex-fix, bridge plating, IM nailing

1: Principles of Orthopaedics

Chapter 2

Fracture Repair and Bone Grafting

Chuanyong Lu, MD   Eric Meinberg, MD   Ralph Marcucio, PhD   Theodore Miclau, MD

1: Principles of Orthopaedics

Biology of Bone Repair

Fracture healing involves a highly integrated sequence of events through which bone is restored to its preinjured condition. The events that occur during healing have been classically divided into four phases: inflammation, soft callus, hard callus, and remodeling (**Figure 1**). Initially, during the inflammatory stage, a hematoma forms in response to the trauma, and the inflammatory cells in the hematoma débride the wound and may help recruit cells that facilitate repair. As skeletal progenitor cells are recruited and begin to differentiate into osteoblasts and chondrocytes, the hematoma is slowly transformed into a soft callus composed primar-

ily of cartilage. At this time, osteoblasts form a collar of bone adjacent to the fracture gap. After this initial period of stabilization, chondrocytes undergo a maturation process, the matrix becomes calcified, osteoclasts remove the calcified cartilage, and endothelial cells invade the cartilage. The soft callus becomes a hard callus as bone forms behind the invading vasculature. Once formed, the bone is remodeled until the skeletal injury has been completely repaired and the bone marrow cavity has been restored.

The Inflammatory Phase

Inflammation plays a key role in the initiation of fracture repair. During the inflammatory stage of repair, numerous lymphocytic cells, including macrophages, neutrophils, and degranulating platelets, infiltrate the fracture site and release cytokines, which include platelet-derived growth factor (PDGF), tumor necrosis factor ß (TGF-β), interleukins 1, 6, 10, and 12 (IL-1, IL-6, IL-10, and IL-12), and tumor necrosis factor α (TNF-α).[1-3] Some of these cytokines are detected at the fracture site as early as 24 hours postinjury and are important for the expansion of the inflammatory response by acting on a variety of cells in the bone marrow, periosteum, and fracture hematoma.[2]

Inflammatory molecules may directly regulate bone healing. In the absence of TNF-α, both endochondral and intramembranous ossification are delayed during repair, suggesting that this molecule plays an important role in the induction of osteochondro-progenitor recruitment and differentiation.[4,5] The inactivation of cyclooxygenase-2 (COX-2), the enzyme required for the production of prostaglandins, a metabolite of arachidonic acid metabolism, has been shown to delay mesenchymal cell differentiation into the osteoblastic lineage during fracture healing via the repression of *runx-2* and *osterix*, two important transcription factors for osteoblast differentiation.[6] In addition, suppression of the inflammatory response through the administration of nonsteroidal anti-inflammatory drugs (NSAIDs) has been shown to impede fracture repair by inhibiting COX enzymes.[7] Recently, leukotrienes, another metabolite of arachidonic acid, have been implicated in the repair process. Treatment of animals with either montelukast sodium or zileuton, which either block signaling or inhibit production of leukotrienes, respectively, stimulates chondrocyte proliferation during fracture healing in animal models.[8]

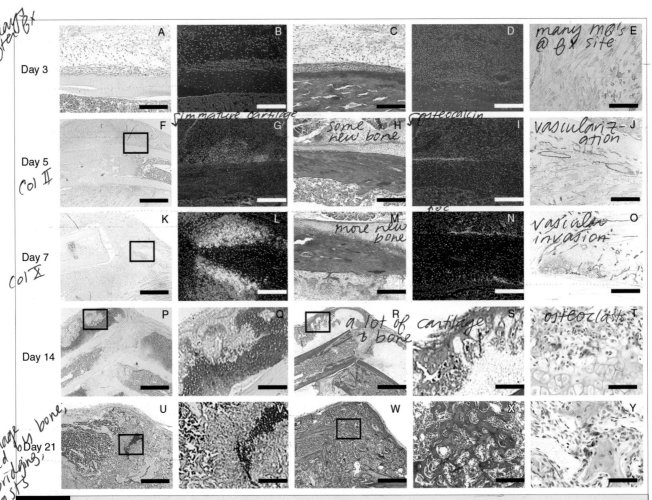

Handwritten annotations on figure:
 # day after Bx
Col II
Col X
cartilage replaced by bone; bony bridging; osteoclasts remodel callus
immature cartilage
some new bone
osteocalcin
vascularization
many mø's @ Bx site
more new bone
noc
vascular invasion
a lot of cartilage & bone
osteoclasts

Figure 1 The process of tibia fracture healing in adult mice. Tibia fractures were not stabilized. Fracture tissues were fixed, decalcified, and processed for paraffin sectioning. Safranin O/Fast Green staining (**A,F,K,P,Q,U,V**) and trichrome staining (**C,H,M,R,S,W,X**) were used to stain cartilage red and bone blue, respectively. Transcripts of collagen type II (**B,G,L,** a marker of chondrocytes), collagen type X (**L,** a marker of hypertrophic chondrocytes), and osteocalcin (OC) (**D,I,N,** a marker of osteoblasts) were detected by in situ hybridization and pseudocolored red, yellow, and green, respectively. Macrophages were stained brown via immunohistochemistry using the F4/80 antibody (**E**). Immunohistochemistry using anti-PECAM (**J,O,** platelet/endothelial cell adhesion molecule, also CD31) antibody was performed to see blood vessels in fracture calluses. Blood vessels were stained black. Osteoclasts were stained red by tartrate-resistant acid phosphatase (**T,Y**). **A,** At 3 days after fracture, no cartilage or (**B**) Col II/Col X transcripts were detected. **C,** No bone or (**D**) OC was present. **E,** A large amount of macrophages were present near the fracture site. **F,** At 5 days after fracture, immature cartilage (**G**) expressing Col II but not Col X was observed in the area of periosteal reaction. **H,** A small amount of new bone and (**I**) OC expression was apparent in the area of periosteal reaction (**J**), which is highly vascularized. **K,** At 7 days after fracture, cartilage is beginning to mature, and Col X transcripts (yellow) were apparent (**L**). **M,** More new bone and OC expression (**N**) was seen at the fracture site. **O,** Vascular invastion was observed around hypertrophic cartilage. **P** and **Q,** At day 14, a large amount of cartilage and bone (**R** and **S**) were formed. **T,** Multiple tartrate-resistant acid phosphatase positive osteoclasts were located at the front of endochondral ossification. **U** and **V,** At 21 days after fracture, cartilage has been largely replaced by bone. **W** and **X,** Fractures have healed by bony bridging. **Y,** Osteoclasts located on the surface of trabecular bone are responsible for remodeling the callus tissues. Scale bar: A-D, G-I, L-O, Q, S, V, and X, 250 μm; E, T, and Y, 60 μm; F, K, P, U, R, and W, 1 mm).

The Soft Callus Phase

Following injury, mesenchymal cells aggregate and form condensations at the site of the fracture in response to growth factors and cytokines that are present. During this early stage of repair, stem cells differentiate into chondrocytes or osteoblasts depending on the mechanical environment. In general, mechanical instability favors chondrocyte differentiation and endo- *[2° healing]* chondral ossification, whereas mechanical stabilization *[1° healing]* favors osteoblast differentiation and intramembranous ossification.[9] During endochondral ossification, cells condense and differentiate into chondrocytes. Production of cartilage provides stabilization of the fracture site, and bone eventually forms to replace the cartilage template. In contrast, during intramembranous ossification, mesenchymal cells condense and osteoblasts differentiate in these condensations in conjunction with invading endothelial cells that establish a blood supply. Clinically, the primary mode of healing is via endochondral ossification, but intramembranous ossification occurs simultaneously to varying degrees, depending on the extent of mechanical stability.

The Hard Callus Phase and Remodeling

During the healing process, the soft callus is slowly transformed into a hard callus via the process of endochondral ossification. Chondrocytes in the fracture callus produce a cartilaginous matrix and undergo a maturation process that eventually leads to their terminal differentiation into hypertrophic chondrocytes. The process of terminal differentiation is complex and involves the interplay of several signaling molecules and pathways, including Indian hedgehog (Ihh), parathyroid hormone–related peptide (PTHrP), fibroblast growth factors (FGFs), and bone morphogenetic proteins (BMPs). During development, these molecules pattern the growth plate in the developing endochondral skeleton and coordinate the timing and location of chondrocyte proliferation, maturation, hypertrophy, and terminal differentiation.[10] These molecules and pathways all are candidates for stimulating repair after injury.

Throughout the process of chondrocyte maturation, the chondrocytes begin to express collagen type X (col10), release proteases (such as mmp13) that degrade the extracellular matrix,[11] and express angiogenic factors such as vascular endothelial growth factor (VEGF).[12] Eventually the cartilage becomes calcified at the junction of the maturing chondrocytes and the newly formed bone. The chondrocytes then undergo apoptosis, the extracellular matrix is degraded, and new blood vessels invade the interface. The newly formed woven bone then undergoes remodeling through organized osteoblast and osteoclast activity, eventually forming bone that is indistinguishable from the adjacent skeletal tissues.

Source of Stem Cells During Fracture Repair

There are multiple sources of stem cells during fracture healing, which include the periosteum and endosteum, the bone marrow, the adjacent muscles, and the circulatory system. Recent evidence suggests that the major source of cells that form the cartilage and bone during fracture repair are derived from the periosteum and endosteum, with a potential contribution from the bone marrow.[13] Although bone marrow–derived mesenchymal stem cells may be an adequate source of cells for tissue engineering, the role of endogenous mesenchymal stem cells in fracture healing appears to be minimal.

Factors Affecting Bone Healing

A variety of factors must be considered when clinically treating a patient with a fracture or nonunion. Some of these factors, such as the severity of injury or patient comorbidities, cannot be altered, whereas others can be treated or manipulated to improve the rate of union and eventual outcome. Optimization of these different factors, including patient-specific factors and medications, may prove useful in achieving bone union.

Patient Factors

There are a variety of known patient-related variables that affect fracture healing. Often, multiple comorbidities are found in a single patient and may act synergistically to decrease the union rate and ultimate clinical outcome. Additionally, as the population ages, individuals are living longer and have more medical problems, which present further challenges to the treating physician.

Nutritional deficiencies, especially abnormalities in vitamin D and calcium, have long been associated with impaired fracture healing. Patients with unexplained nonunions who have undergone thorough endocrinologic assessment have been found to have associated metabolic or endocrine abnormalities that have not been previously diagnosed. In one study, 84% of patients referred for management of a nonunion were found to have a metabolic abnormality, and 68% were found to have a vitamin D deficiency.[14] Animal studies have also demonstrated the impact of protein malnutrition on fracture healing and enhancement of fracture union by means of a high-protein anabolic diet.[15] To date, the impact of protein supplementation on fracture and wound healing has been poorly studied in humans.

Gastric bypass surgery, used increasingly for the management of morbid obesity, has profound effects on bone metabolism. The Roux-en-Y procedure, the most commonly performed bariatric procedure, bypasses the duodenum, the primary site for calcium absorption. This results in calcium and vitamin D deficiency, upregulation of parathyroid hormone, and increased calcium resorption. These patients require calcium and vitamin D supplementation. Unlike those who undergo the Roux-en-Y procedure, patients who have a gastric banding procedure do not develop secondary hyperparathyroidism because the small intestine is not bypassed.[16]

Smoking has been long associated with delayed fracture union and increased risk of non-union. Nicotine inhibits tissue differentiation and the angiogenic response in early stages of fracture healing,[17] and interferes with osteoblast function.[18] In one study, grade I open tibial shaft fractures took 69% longer to heal in smokers than in nonsmokers.[19] A significantly higher rate of nonunion in Ilizarov reconstruction has also been reported.[20] Whenever practical, patients should be counseled to stop smoking to improve fracture healing.

Diabetes mellitus, in addition to its many associated complications and comorbidities such as neuropathy and peripheral vascular disease, is known to affect fracture healing. Lower extremity fractures in patients with diabetes have been shown to take approximately 1.6 times as long to heal than in control subjects who do not have diabetes,[21] whereas an ankle fracture in pa-

1: Principles of Orthopaedics

tients with Charcot arthropathy can take up to 3 months longer to heal than in those patients with protective sensation. This is thought to be caused by decreased cellularity of the fracture callus, delayed endochondral ossification, and decreased strength of the callus.[22] In animal studies, this pathway can be reversed with normalization of blood glucose with insulin,[23] suggesting the importance of careful glycemic control in clinical practice.

Because of the success of antiretroviral drugs, HIV can now be considered a chronic disease with a long-term asymptomatic phase. Patients with HIV have been noted to have a higher prevalence of osteopenia, osteonecrosis, and fragility fractures, as well as delayed bone and wound healing.[24] Many factors, including antiretroviral medications, intraosseous circulation, and derangement in cytokines such as TNF-α have been implicated. Patients also tend to have poorer nutrition and a reduced body mass index, further complicating bone healing.

Medications

The use of bisphosphonates in treatment is increasing as osteoporotic fractures are being recognized as a major public health problem. Although bisphosphonate treatment significantly decreases the incidence of osteoporotic fractures in the spine and hip, long-term bisphosphonate use may be associated with some side effects. Bisphosphonates inhibit the ostoclastic resorption of bone, therefore slowing remodeling and, possibly, bone healing.[25] Recent radiographic studies have demonstrated a longer time to union in surgically treated wrist fractures[26] and an increased rate of nonunion in humerus fractures.[27] It has been suggested that while healing time is increased, ultimate bone density and callus strength is improved. Long-term bisphosphonate use may be associated with higher risk of atypical subtrochanteric and femoral shaft fractures.[28,29] However, due to the low incidence of these atypical fractures, larger scale clinical studies are needed to further establish a causal relationship.[30]

Systemic long-term administration of corticosteroids inhibits fracture healing and callus strength in animal models.[31] Increased complications have been reported in clinical studies, including a 6.5% higher rate of nonunion of intertrochanteric hip fractures compared to that of control models.[32] In addition to steroids, NSAIDs have been associated with prolonged healing time due to their antiprostaglandin action. Animal data suggest that COX-2 selective NSAIDs have a similar negative dose-dependent effect on bone healing and should be avoided in the early stages of postfracture care.[33]

Enhancement of Fracture Healing

Many physical and biologic methods have been developed to enhance fracture healing. Some are widely used clinically, such as bone grafting and the placement of BMPs, whereas others are still in their early stages of development.

Bone Grafting
Autogenous Bone Grafts
Autogenous bone grafting continues to be the gold standard for treating osseous defects and stimulating new bone formation. Autogenous bone grafts have osteoinductive and osteoconductive properties, and can provide osteogenic cells, which are important for early bone formation. Autogenous cortical bone grafts can provide mechanical support with limited capability to supply osteoblasts. Most of the osteocytes in a cortical bone graft will die after grafting, and the nonviable bone will be slowly replaced by creeping substitution. Creeping substitution is a slow process that may take years to complete, and in many instances may never be fully accomplished. Autogenous bone grafts can be harvested from the anterior or posterior iliac crests, or local metaphyseal regions during a procedure. Harvesting of autogenous bone grafts is associated with a significant risk of complications, such as persistent pain at the surgical site; the amount of bone graft that can be harvested is limited. Therefore, efforts have been made to develop different bone graft substitutes.

Allografts
Allografts are harvested from donor cadaver tissue, thereby avoiding the complications associated with autograft harvesting. Allograft bone is available as cancellous, cancellous/cortical morcellized chips, or structural cortical grafts. Allografts have both osteoconductive and osteoinductive properties, but their osteoinductive capacity is limited in comparison with that of autografts. In addition, allografts do not provide viable osteogenic cells; therefore, their ability to form bone is not as good as that of autografts. Regular processing of allografts includes physical débridement of soft tissue, a wash with ethanol to remove blood and live cells, and gamma irradiation to sterilize the bone tissues. Processing, especially gamma irradiation, has a significant influence on the performance of allografts. High doses of irradiation, which may help kill bacteria and viruses, impair the biomechanical properties of allografts by causing splitting of polypeptide chains or radiolysis of water molecules. Irradiation may also affect the osteoconductive and osteoinductive capacities of allografts in a dose-dependent manner.[34]

Demineralized bone matrix (DBM) is a special form of allograft. It is prepared by acid extraction of allograft bone. DBM retains bone collagenous and noncollagenous proteins, including BMPs, and has both osteoinductive and osteoconductive properties. Because of demineralization, DBM has better osteoinductive capacity than regular allografts. In some reports, comparable capacity for bone formation has been observed between DBM and autogenous bone graft [35], suggesting DBM may be a suitable alternative and supplement to autogenous bone graft. There are several commercially available DBM products that are used clinically to improve spinal fusion, graft fracture nonunions, and fill bone defects. However, the efficacy of DBM varies due to different processing methods.[36] The age of the donor is not a factor that significantly affects the efficacy of DBM.[37]

Because allografts are harvested from donors, safety issues such as disease transmission are of major concern. Although harvesting techniques and thorough sterilization are important, strict donor screening is essential for reducing the risk of disease transmission. The American Association of Tissue Banks (AATB) has adopted a protocol for strict screening of tissues, and its program of accreditation has put many tissue banks under its oversight, which helps improve the safety of bone allografts. As a result, it is believed that the actual magnitude of viral transmission from allografts is very low, with estimates of less than 1 in 1 million procedures.

Synthetic Bone Substitutes *osteoconductive*
Synthetic bone substitutes were developed as an alternative to autografts and allografts. Their compositions include calcium sulfate, calcium phosphate, tricalcium phosphate, and bioglass. They are available in different forms, including powder, pellet, or putty, and can be used as implant coating or bone defect filler. Synthetic bone substitutes are osteoconductive, but not osteoinductive. Several clinical studies (level I evidence) have shown that using calcium phosphate–based bone substitutes may allow for bone defect filling, early rehabilitation, and prevention of articular subsidence in distal radius and tibial plateau fractures.[38-40] Level II evidence suggests that calcium sulfate is a safe and effective bone substitute.[41] The current trend is to develop different tissue engineering approaches and make composites from synthetic bone substitutes with collagen, DBM, growth factors, bone marrow cells, or mesenchymal stem cells to improve their osteogenic potential.

Platelet-Rich Plasma
Platelets play an important role in the inflammatory response after bone injury. Activated platelets release many growth factors, including PDGF, TGF-β, and VEGF. The effectiveness of platelet-rich plasma (PRP) in fracture healing has been tested in both animal experiments and clinical trials. In a rat diabetic fracture model, PRP improves cellular proliferation and chondrogenesis during early fracture healing and increases the mechanical strength of callus during late fracture healing.[42] The effect of PRP on fracture healing is associated with altered expression of TGF-β1 and BMP-2.[43] Clinically, the efficacy of PRP on fracture healing has not been fully confirmed. The findings of a systemic literature search showed that there is no strong evidence supporting the routine use of PRP in either acute or delayed fracture healing.[44] Further high-quality, randomized, and prospective clinical trials are required to determine whether PRP is beneficial in the treatment of fracture nonunions.

osteogenic

Bone Marrow Aspirate *autogenous; iliac crest → vertebral body*
Bone marrow aspirate has been used to enhance bone repair for more than two decades. Many clinical studies

have shown its safety and efficacy in treating fracture nonunions and bone defects.[45,46] It is well established that bone marrow contains mesenchymal stem cells, which can be expanded in culture and can differentiate into osteoblasts, chondrocytes, and other connective tissue cells in vitro under appropriate conditions. Bone marrow is also the source of circulating endothelial progenitors that can contribute to adult vasculogenesis. Therefore, some of the effects of bone marrow aspirate on fracture healing could be due to the local application of osteochondrogenic cells and/or endothelial progenitor cells during bone healing. However, there is not enough evidence showing these cells can actually differentiate into osteoblasts, chondrocytes, or endothelial cells, and further investigation is required to determine the exact role of these transplanted cells in fracture healing.

Bone Morphogenetic Proteins *osteoinductive*
BMPs were first discovered in 1965 by Urist; at least 20 different BMPs have been found thus far. All of these BMPs, except BMP-1, belong to the group of TGF-β superfamily growth factors. BMP-1 is a metalloprotease that acts on procollagen I, II, and III. Among all the BMPs, BMP-2 and BMP-7 have been extensively studied for their capacity to induce bone in a variety of conditions. BMPs are capable of recruiting stem cells from distant sites and inducing osteoblast and chondrocyte differentiation, leading to ectopic bone formation. Recent studies have shown that BMPs are involved in angiogenesis, the process of new blood vessel formation and vascular repair. BMP-7 is capable of inducing new blood vessel formation in chick chorioallantoic membranes,[47] and BMP-2, which acts in a manner similar to that of BMP-7, can increase vascularization of tumors.[48] The US Food and Drug Administration (FDA) has approved the clinical use of rhBMP-2, marketed as Infuse Bone Graft, in acute open fractures of the tibia and spinal fusion surgery, and recombinant human BMP-7 (rhBMP-7), or osteogenic protein-1 (OP-1), as an alternative to autograft in recalcitrant long bone nonunions and in compromised patients requiring revision posterolateral lumbar spinal fusion under a Humanitarian Device Exemption (HDE). Level I clinical evidence demonstrates that rhBMP-2 improves the repair of open tibia fractures.[49] Prospective case series studies have shown that rhBMP-7 is effective in treating tibial and femoral nonunions.[50,51]

Vascular Endothelial Growth Factor
Blood supply is crucial for normal fracture healing. Lack of perfusion is often associated with delayed union or nonunion. Investigators have suggested that stimulating vascular repair may represent a novel method to stimulate bone healing. Vascular repair after bone injury occurs largely through a process called angiogenesis, which is the sprouting of new blood vessels from preexisting ones. During fracture healing, angiogenesis is orchestrated by a variety of factors including VEGF, FGFs, and matrix metalloproteinases (MMPs).

1: Principles of Orthopaedics

Among these factors, VEGF is currently recognized as the most potent angiogenic factor, and it plays an important role during both skeletal development and adult bone regeneration.[52] In fracture calluses, VEGF is expressed by hypertrophic chondrocytes and may be released from cartilage matrix by matrix degradation mediated by MMP-9.[12] VEGF acts on endothelial cells and induces vascular invasion of the hypertrophic cartilage. The ability of VEGF to enhance bone regeneration has been explored in several animal models. VEGF delivered as a protein or through genetic approaches can promote healing of femoral fractures in mice,[53] radius segmental defects in rabbits,[53,54] and bone drilling defects in rats.[55] VEGF and BMPs may have synergistic effects on bone regeneration.[56] Recently, another unique approach has been developed to enhance angiogenesis during fracture healing by regulating hypoxia inducible factor-1α (HIF-1α), which is a master regulator of VEGF expression. Inhibiting HIF prolyl hydorxylase, an enzyme that deactivates HIF-1, can stabilize HIF/VEGF production, increase angiogenesis, and improve fracture healing.[57]

Fibroblast Growth Factors

FGFs are involved in bone development and fracture healing. The expression patterns of FGFs and their receptors during bone repair have been well documented.[58] In animal bone repair models, both acidic FGF and basic FGF (bFGF) stimulate cartilage formation, leading to larger fracture calluses.[59] bFGF may also increase the number of osteoclasts and accelerate remodeling of fracture calluses.[60] The effects of bFGF on bone formation are dose dependent. There is evidence showing that bFGF stimulates osteogenesis at lower doses but inhibits bone formation at high doses.[61] Clinical trials are required to establish the effectiveness of FGFs on fracture healing or repair of bone defects in patients.

Parathyroid Hormone

Parathyroid hormone (PTH) is secreted by the parathyroid glands and its normal function is to increase the calcium levels of the blood by indirectly stimulating bone resorption, increasing renal reabsorption of calcium, and increasing intestinal calcium absorption. Low-dose, intermittent administration of PTH has anabolic effects on bone metabolism, whereas continuous administration of high doses leads to catabolic effects. PTH (1-34), the 1-34 amino acid segment of recombinant human PTH, is the active form of PTH. The commercially available PTH (1-34), teriparatide, is an FDA-approved drug for postmenopausal osteoporosis and osteoporosis associated with sustained systemic glucocorticoid therapy. It can increase the bone mineral density in the lumbar spine and femoral neck in patients with osteoporosis, and reduce fracture risk.[62] Recent experimental studies have shown that PTH (1-34) is effective for enhancing fracture healing in animals.[63] PTH (1-34) treatment stimulates early bone and cartilage formation, increases callus formation, accelerates

callus remodeling, and improves the biomechanical properties of callus tissue. Further mechanistic analyses show that systemic administration of PTH (1-34) upregulates the expression of Osx and Runx2 in bone marrow–derived mesenchymal stem cells and promotes osteoblast differentiation.[64] These data suggest that PTH (1-34) is a promising treatment of fracture nonunion. However, to date there is no published clinical study on the efficacy of PTH (1-34) on fracture healing.

Wnt

Wnts are a family of extracellular cell–cell signaling molecules that regulate embryogenesis and tissue homeostasis in adults. It has been recently documented that Wnt signaling plays an important role in fracture healing. In the adult skeleton, Wnt signaling proteins are expressed by osteocytes, in the endosteum and bone marrow.[65] After bone injury, Wnt signaling is upregulated and inhibition of the Wnt pathway leads to a delay in bone regeneration.[65,66] Mutation of a Wnt coreceptor, Lrp5, results in constitutive Wnt activation. In mice that lack Lrp5, proliferation of skeletal progenitor cells at the site of bone injury is increased, but bone repair is delayed.[65] Further research has shown that Wnt signaling inhibits undifferentiated mesenchymal cells but may have positive effects on cells that have committed to the osteoblast lineage.[66] These research findings suggest that the Wnt signaling pathway is a potential target to enhance fracture healing. Indeed, lithium treatment, which activates the Wnt pathway, is found to accelerate bone formation and increase bone mass in mice.[67] However, lithium treatment should be avoided during the early stage of fracture healing because activated Wnt signaling has a negative effect on undifferentiated mesenchymal cells.[68]

Ultrasound/Electrical Stimulation

Biophysical treatments such as electrical stimulation, ultrasound, extracorporeal shock wave therapy (ESWT), and vibration can improve fracture healing. Electrical stimuli create low levels of electric currents in tissue, leading to lowered tissue Po_2, increased expression of factors such as TGF-β and BMPs, improved neovascularization, and enhanced osteogenesis. Four methods have been developed to deliver electric stimuli to the fracture site: direct current, capacitively coupled electric fields, pulsed electromagnetic fields, and combined magnetic fields.[69] These methods have been promoted as useful treatments of established nonunions and failed spinal fusion. Low-intensity pulsed ultrasound (LIPUS), as a physical method to enhance bone repair, has gained popularity recently. The exact mechanisms through which LIPUS improves fracture healing have not been well determined but could include altered gene expression, increased blood supply, and the creation of a gradient of mechanical strain. Both experimental and clinical studies have shown that LIPUS is effective in treating delayed union and nonunions, achieving healing rates at about 80%. It appears that LIPUS may work better on delayed fracture healing than nonunions and is also effective on septic fracture nonunions.[70] There are reports showing that ESWT can be used to treat delayed fracture healing and nonunions, however, its efficacy needs to be better determined. Currently, ESWT is still considered an experimental clinical procedure.[71] Additionally, providing cyclic mechanical loadings to the fracture site using low-magnitude high-frequency vibration may also stimulate bone formation.[72]

Summary

Major advancements have been achieved in the field of bone repair during the last several decades. Further discoveries in stem cell biology, molecular biology, biomaterials, and tissue engineering will continue to improve understanding of cellular and molecular factors. It is expected that orthopaedic surgeons will have more options available to stimulate and enhance bone repair.

Annotated References

1. Barnes GL, Kostenuik PJ, Gerstenfeld LC, Einhorn TA: Growth factor regulation of fracture repair. *J Bone Miner Res* 1999;14(11):1805-1815.

2. Einhorn TA, Majeska RJ, Rush EB, Levine PM, Horowitz MC: The expression of cytokine activity by fracture callus. *J Bone Miner Res* 1995;10(8):1272-1281.

3. Rundle CH, Wang H, Yu H, et al: Microarray analysis of gene expression during the inflammation and endochondral bone formation stages of rat femur fracture repair. *Bone* 2006;38(4):521-529.

4. Gerstenfeld LC, Cho TJ, Kon T, et al: Impaired fracture healing in the absence of TNF-alpha signaling: The role of TNF-alpha in endochondral cartilage resorption. *J Bone Miner Res* 2003;18(9):1584-1592.

5. Gerstenfeld LC, Cho TJ, Kon T, et al: Impaired intramembranous bone formation during bone repair in the absence of tumor necrosis factor-alpha signaling. *Cells Tissues Organs* 2001;169(3):285-294.

6. Zhang X, Schwarz EM, Young DA, Puzas JE, Rosier RN, O'Keefe RJ: Cyclooxygenase-2 regulates mesenchymal cell differentiation into the osteoblast lineage and is critically involved in bone repair. *J Clin Invest* 2002;109(11):1405-1415.

7. Gerstenfeld LC, Thiede M, Seibert K, et al: Differential inhibition of fracture healing by non-selective and cyclooxygenase-2 selective non-steroidal anti-inflammatory drugs. *J Orthop Res* 2003;21(4):670-675.

8. Wixted JJ, Fanning PJ, Gaur T, et al: Enhanced fracture repair by leukotriene antagonism is characterized by increased chondrocyte proliferation and early bone formation: A novel role of the cysteinyl LT-1 receptor.

J Cell Physiol 2009;221(1):31-39.

Mice treated with Singulair (montelukast sodium), a cysteinyl leukotriene type 1 receptor antagonist, or zileuton, a 5-lipoxygenase enzyme inhibitor, exhibit increased bone and cartilage formation during early fracture healing.

9. Thompson Z, Miclau T, Hu D, Helms JA: A model for intramembranous ossification during fracture healing. *J Orthop Res* 2002;20(5):1091-1098.

10. Kronenberg HM: PTHrP and skeletal development. *Ann N Y Acad Sci* 2006;1068:1-13.

11. Behonick DJ, Xing Z, Lieu S, et al: Role of matrix metalloproteinase 13 in both endochondral and intramembranous ossification during skeletal regeneration. *PLoS One* 2007;2(11):e1150.

Matrix metalloproteinase 13 (MMP-13) is expressed by hypertrophic chondrocytes and osteoblasts in fracture calluses. MMP-13 mutant mice exhibit delayed cartilage resorption and delayed callus remodeling.

12. Colnot C, Thompson Z, Miclau T, Werb Z, Helms JA: Altered fracture repair in the absence of MMP9. *Development* 2003;130(17):4123-4133.

13. Colnot C, Huang S, Helms J: Analyzing the cellular contribution of bone marrow to fracture healing using bone marrow transplantation in mice. *Biochem Biophys Res Commun* 2006;350(3):557-561.

14. Brinker MR, O'Connor DP, Monla YT, Earthman TP: Metabolic and endocrine abnormalities in patients with nonunions. *J Orthop Trauma* 2007;21(8):557-570.

In a selected cohort of patients with unexplained nonunions, 31 of the 37 patients were found with metabolic abnormalities including vitamin D deficiency. Level of evidence: III.

15. Hughes MS, Kazmier P, Burd TA, et al: Enhanced fracture and soft-tissue healing by means of anabolic dietary supplementation. *J Bone Joint Surg Am* 2006;88(11):2386-2394.

16. Wang A, Powell A: The effects of obesity surgery on bone metabolism: What orthopedic surgeons need to know. *Am J Orthop (Belle Mead NJ)* 2009;38(2):77-79.

This article reviews the effects of obesity surgery, including the Roux-en-Y procedure and gastric banding, on endocrine and bone metabolism.

17. Daftari TK, Whitesides TE, Heller JG, et al: Nicotine on the revascularization of bone graft: An experimental study in rabbits. *Spine (Phila Pa 1976)* 1994;19:904-911.

18. Rothem DE, Rothem L, Soudry M, Dahan A, Eliakim R: Nicotine modulates bone metabolism-associated gene expression in osteoblast cells. *J Bone Miner Metab* 2009;27(5):555-561.

Nicotine affects cultured osteoblast cells in a biphasic

manner. High levels of nicotine inhibit cell proliferation and downregulate gene expression of osteoclacin, type I collagen, and alkaline phosphatase. Low levels of nicotine have opposite effects.

19. Schmitz MA, Finnegan M, Natarajan R, Champine J: Effect of smoking on tibial shaft fracture healing. *Clin Orthop Relat Res* 1999;365:184-200.

20. McKee MD, DiPasquale DJ, Wild LM, Stephen DJ, Kreder HJ, Schemitsch EH: The effect of smoking on clinical outcome and complication rates following Ilizarov reconstruction. *J Orthop Trauma* 2003;17(10):663-667.

21. Loder RT: The influence of diabetes mellitus on the healing of closed fractures. *Clin Orthop Relat Res* 1988;232:210-216.

22. Macey LR, Kana SM, Jingushi S, Terek RM, Borretos J, Bolander ME: Defects of early fracture-healing in experimental diabetes. *J Bone Joint Surg Am* 1989;71(5):722-733.

23. Kayal RA, Alblowi J, McKenzie E, et al: Diabetes causes the accelerated loss of cartilage during fracture repair which is reversed by insulin treatment. *Bone* 2009;44(2):357-363.

    In a mouse fracture model, diabetes increases chondrocyte apoptosis and osteoclastogenesis, leading to cartilage loss and less callus formation. These effects of diabetes can be reversed by insulin.

24. Richardson J, Hill AM, Johnston CJ, et al: Fracture healing in HIV-positive populations. *J Bone Joint Surg Br* 2008;90(8):988-994.

    The authors reviewed the current evidence for an association between HIV infection and poor fracture healing.

25. Li C, Mori S, Li J, et al: Long-term effect of incadronate disodium (YM-175) on fracture healing of femoral shaft in growing rats. *J Bone Miner Res* 2001;16(3):429-436.

26. Rozental TD, Vazquez MA, Chacko AT, Ayogu N, Bouxsein ML: Comparison of radiographic fracture healing in the distal radius for patients on and off bisphosphonate therapy. *J Hand Surg Am* 2009;34(4):595-602.

    Bisphosphonate use is associated with longer times to radiographic union of distal radius fractures. However, the differences in healing times are small and not considered clinically significant. The authors concluded that bisphosphonate therapy can be continued after fracture. Level of evidence: III.

27. Solomon DH, Hochberg MC, Mogun H, Schneeweiss S: The relation between bisphosphonate use and nonunion of fractures of the humerus in older adults. *Osteoporos Int* 2009;20(6):895-901.

    In a cohort of older adults with humerus fractures, bisphosphonate use was associated with an approximate doubling of the risk of nonunion. Clinical evidence level III.

28. Lenart BA, Neviaser AS, Lyman S, et al: Association of low-energy femoral fractures with prolonged bisphosphonate use: A case control study. *Osteoporos Int* 2009;20(8):1353-1362.

    In this matched case–control study, the authors found that "prolonged bisphosphonate use is associated with low-energy subtrochanteric/shaft fractures in postmenopausal women who have no obvious secondary causes of bone loss. Furthermore, bisphosphonate use of greater than 5 years was associated with a characteristic fracture of the femur, defined as a simple transverse or oblique fracture with cortical thickening and beaking of the cortex in the subtrochanteric/shaft region. This fracture is an atypical fracture for osteoporotic women." Level of evidence: III.

29. Kwek EB, Goh SK, Koh JS, Png MA, Howe TS: An emerging pattern of subtrochanteric stress fractures: A long-term complication of alendronate therapy? *Injury* 2008; 39(2):224-231.

    In this study, the authors analyzed low-energy subtrochanteric insufficiency fractures in 17 patients who have been on alendronate therapy for an average of 4.8 years. The authors identified a characteristic fracture configuration suggestive of an insufficiency stress fracture. This consisted of (1) cortical thickening in the lateral side of the subtrochanteric region, (2) a transverse fracture, and (3) a medial cortical spike. In addition, 9 (53%) patients had bilateral findings of stress reactions or fractures. Level of evidence: III.

30. Black DM, Kelly MP, Genant HK, et al; Fracture Intervention Trial Steering Committee; HORIZON Pivotal Fracture Trial Steering Committee: Bisphosphonates and fractures of the subtrochanteric or diaphyseal femur. *N Engl J Med* 2010;362(19):1761-1771.

    The authors reviewed 284 records for hip or femur fractures among 14,195 women in three large, randomized bisphosphonate trials: the Fracture Intervention Trial (FIT), the FIT Long-Term Extension (FLEX) trial, and the Health Outcomes and Reduced Incidence with Zoledronic Acid Once Yearly (HORIZON) Pivotal Fracture Trial (PFT). The authors concluded that the occurrence of fracture of the subtrochanteric or diaphyseal femur was very rare, even among women who had been treated with bisphosphonates for as long as 10 years. There was no significant increase in risk associated with bisphosphonate use, but the study was underpowered for definitive conclusions. Level of evidence: I.

31. Waters RV, Gamradt SC, Asnis P, et al: Systemic corticosteroids inhibit bone healing in a rabbit ulnar osteotomy model. *Acta Orthop Scand* 2000;71(3):316-321.

32. Bogoch ER, Ouellette G, Hastings DE: Intertrochanteric fractures of the femur in rheumatoid arthritis patients. *Clin Orthop Relat Res* 1993;294:181-186.

33. Dimmen S, Nordsletten L, Madsen JE: Parecoxib and indomethacin delay early fracture healing: A study in rats. *Clin Orthop Relat Res* 2009;467(8):1992-1999.

Rats with tibia fractures that were treated with parecoxib or indomethacin for 7 days after injury exhibited decreased bone mineral density and biomechanical properties of fracture callus for 2 to 3 weeks.

34. Nguyen H, Morgan DA, Forwood MR: Sterilization of allograft bone: Effects of gamma irradiation on allograft biology and biomechanics. *Cell Tissue Bank* 2007;8(2): 93-105.

This article reviews the effects of gamma irradiation on the biologic and mechanical properties of allograft bone.

35. Drosos GJ, Kazakos KI, Kouzoumpasis P, Verettas DA: Safety and efficacy of commercially available demineralised bone matrix preparations: A critical review of clinical studies. *Injury* 2007;38(suppl 4):S13-S21.

The authors present a critical overview of the current clinical applications of DBM.

36. Peterson B, Whang PG, Iglesias R, Wang JC, Lieberman JR: Osteoinductivity of commercially available demineralized bone matrix. Preparations in a spine fusion model. *J Bone Joint Surg Am* 2004;86(10):2243-2250.

37. Traianedes K, Russell JL, Edwards JT, Stubbs HA, Shanahan IR, Knaack D: Donor age and gender effects on osteoinductivity of demineralized bone matrix. *J Biomed Mater Res B Appl Biomater* 2004;70(1):21-29.

38. Russell TA, Leighton RK; Alpha-BSM Tibial Plateau Fracture Study Group: Comparison of autogenous bone graft and endothermic calcium phosphate cement for defect augmentation in tibial plateau fractures: A multicenter, prospective, randomized study. *J Bone Joint Surg Am.* 2008;90(10):2057-2061.

The authors enrolled 120 acute, closed, unstable tibial plateau fractures. Subarticular defects were filled with either calcium phosphate cement or autogenous bone graft. The cement did not improve the union rates and the time to union. However, the bioresorbable calcium phosphate cement used in this study appears to be a better choice, at least in terms of the prevention of subsidence, than autogenous iliac bone graft for the treatment of subarticular defects associated with unstable tibial plateau fractures. Level of evidence: I.

39. Cassidy C, Jupiter JB, Cohen M, et al: Norian SRS cement compared with conventional fixation in distal radial fractures: A randomized study. *J Bone Joint Surg Am* 2003;85(11):2127-2137.

40. Johal HS, Buckley RE, Le IL, Leighton RK: A prospective randomized controlled trial of a bioresorbable calcium phosphate paste (alpha-BSM) in treatment of displaced intra-articular calcaneal fractures. *J Trauma* 2009;67(4):875-882.

The authors prospectively randomized 47 patients with 52 closed displaced intra-articular calcaneal fractures necessitating operative fixation to receive ORIF alone (n = 28) or ORIF plus alpha-BSM (n = 24). The results confirmed the safety of alpha-BSM–and the alpha-BSM treated fractures better retained Böhler's angle at 6 months and 1 year after surgery. Level of evidence: I.

41. Kelly CM, Wilkins RM, Gitelis S, Hartjen C, Watson JT, Kim PT: The use of a surgical grade calcium sulfate as a bone graft substitute: Results of a multicenter trial. *Clin Orthop Relat Res* 2001;(382):42-50.

42. Gandhi A, Doumas C, Dumas C, O'Connor JP, Parsons JR, Lin SS: The effects of local platelet rich plasma delivery on diabetic fracture healing. *Bone* 2006;38(4): 540-546.

43. Simman R, Hoffmann A, Bohinc RJ, Peterson WC, Russ AJ: Role of platelet-rich plasma in acceleration of bone fracture healing. *Ann Plast Surg* 2008;61(3):337-344.

In a rat femur fracture model, PRP enhances bone formation, which is associated with changes of TGF-ß1 and BMP-2 expression.

44. Griffin XL, Smith CM, Costa ML: The clinical use of platelet-rich plasma in the promotion of bone healing: A systematic review. *Injury* 2009;40(2):158-162.

This systemic literature review found limited clinical studies and no solid evidence for the efficacy of PRP in acute or delayed fracture healing.

45. Goel A, Sangwan SS, Siwach RC, Ali AM: Percutaneous bone marrow grafting for the treatment of tibial nonunion. *Injury* 2005;36(1):203-206.

46. Lokiec F, Ezra E, Khermosh O, Wientroub S: Simple bone cysts treated by percutaneous autologous marrow grafting: A preliminary report. *J Bone Joint Surg Br* 1996;78(6):934-937.

47. Ramoshebi LN, Ripamonti U: Osteogenic protein-1, a bone morphogenetic protein, induces angiogenesis in the chick chorioallantoic membrane and synergizes with basic fibroblast growth factor and transforming growth factor-beta1. *Anat Rec* 2000;259(1):97-107.

48. Raida M, Clement JH, Leek RD, et al: Bone morphogenetic protein 2 (BMP-2) and induction of tumor angiogenesis. *J Cancer Res Clin Oncol* 2005;131(11):741-750.

49. Govender S, Csimma C, Genant HK, et al: Recombinant human bone morphogenetic protein-2 for treatment of open tibial fractures: A prospective, controlled, randomized study of four hundred and fifty patients. *J Bone Joint Surg Am* 2002;84(12):2123-2134.

50. Kanakaris NK, Calori GM, Verdonk R, et al: Application of BMP-7 to tibial non-unions: A 3-year multicenter experience. *Injury* 2008;39(suppl 2):S83-S90.

The authors treated 68 patients with tibial nonunion with BMP-7. Nonunion healing was verified in 61 patients (89.7%) in a median period of 6.5 months. Level of evidence: III.

51. Kanakaris NK, Lasanianos N, Calori GM, et al: Application of bone morphogenetic proteins to femoral nonunions: A 4-year multicentre experience. *Injury* 2009;40

(suppl 3):S54-S61.

The authors treated 30 femoral nonunions with BMP-7. Nonunion healing was verified in 26 of 30 cases in a median period of 6 months. Level of evidence: III.

52. Carvalho RS, Einhorn TA, Lehmann W, et al: The role of angiogenesis in a murine tibial model of distraction osteogenesis. *Bone* 2004;34(5):849-861.

53. Street J, Bao M, deGuzman L, et al: Vascular endothelial growth factor stimulates bone repair by promoting angiogenesis and bone turnover. *Proc Natl Acad Sci U S A* 2002;99(15):9656-9661.

54. Eckardt H, Ding M, Lind M, Hansen ES, Christensen KS, Hvid I: Recombinant human vascular endothelial growth factor enhances bone healing in an experimental nonunion model. *J Bone Joint Surg Br* 2005;87(10): 1434-1438.

55. Tarkka T, Sipola A, Jämsä T, et al: Adenoviral VEGF-A gene transfer induces angiogenesis and promotes bone formation in healing osseous tissues. *J Gene Med* 2003; 5(7):560-566.

56. Kempen DH, Lu L, Heijink A, et al: Effect of local sequential VEGF and BMP-2 delivery on ectopic and orthotopic bone regeneration. *Biomaterials* 2009;30(14): 2816-2825.

Implanted ectopically, VEGF increases tissue vascularity and BMP-2 induces bone formation in rats. A combination of VEGF and BMP-2 significantly enhances ectopic bone formation compared to BMP-2 alone.

57. Shen X, Wan C, Ramaswamy G, et al: Prolyl hydroxylase inhibitors increase neoangiogenesis and callus formation following femur fracture in mice. *J Orthop Res* 2009;27(10):1298-1305.

In a mouse fracture model, prolyl hydroxylase inhibitors activate HIF-1, increase VEGF expression, increase tissue vascularity, and lead to more bone formation.

58. Schmid GJ, Kobayashi C, Sandell LJ, Ornitz DM: Fibroblast growth factor expression during skeletal fracture healing in mice. *Dev Dyn* 2009;238(3):766-774.

The authors quantitatively evaluated the temporal expression patterns of FGFs and their receptors up to 14 days after fracture in a mouse model.

59. Nakajima F, Ogasawara A, Goto K, et al: Spatial and temporal gene expression in chondrogenesis during fracture healing and the effects of basic fibroblast growth factor. *J Orthop Res* 2001;19(5):935-944.

60. Nakamura T, Hara Y, Tagawa M, et al: Recombinant human basic fibroblast growth factor accelerates fracture healing by enhancing callus remodeling in experimental dog tibial fracture. *J Bone Miner Res* 1998; 13(6):942-949.

61. Maus U, Andereya S, Ohnsorge JA, Gravius S, Siebert CH, Niedhart C: A bFGF/TCP-composite inhibits bone formation in a sheep model. *J Biomed Mater Res B Appl Biomater* 2008;85(1):87-92.

In a sheep bone defect model, the addition of 200 mg of bFGF to tricalcium phosphate (TCP) cement decreased bone ingrowth into the cement.

62. Neer RM, Arnaud CD, Zanchetta JR, et al: Effect of parathyroid hormone (1-34) on fractures and bone mineral density in postmenopausal women with osteoporosis. *N Engl J Med* 2001;344(19):1434-1441.

63. Cipriano CA, Issack PS, Shindle L, Werner CM, Helfet DL, Lane JM: Recent advances toward the clinical application of PTH (1-34) in fracture healing. *HSS J* 2009; 5(2):149-153.

This paper summarizes the experimental evidence that suggests PTH (1-34) accelerates callus formation and remodeling, and improves the biomechanical properties of the fracture callus.

64. Kaback LA, Soung do Y, Naik A, et al: Teriparatide (1-34 human PTH) regulation of osterix during fracture repair. *J Cell Biochem* 2008;105(1):219-226.

In a mouse model, teriparatide treatment increases osterix expression and improves fracture healing. Bone marrow–derived mesenchymal stem cells isolated from teriparatide-treated mice exhibit accelerated osteoblast maturation.

65. Kim JB, Leucht P, Lam K, et al: Bone regeneration is regulated by wnt signaling. *J Bone Miner Res* 2007; 22(12):1913-1923.

The authors found that Wnt signaling is activated during fracture healing. Inhibition of Wnt signaling prevents the differentiation of osteogenic progenitor cells and reduces bone regeneration.

66. Chen Y, Whetstone HC, Lin AC, et al: Beta-catenin signaling plays a disparate role in different phases of fracture repair: Implications for therapy to improve bone healing. *PLoS Med* 2007;4(7):e249.

Beta-catenin signaling is regulated by Wnt ligands. Absence of β-catenin inhibits fracture healing and activation enhances bone repair.

67. Clément-Lacroix P, Ai M, Morvan F, et al: Lrp5-independent activation of Wnt signaling by lithium chloride increases bone formation and bone mass in mice. *Proc Natl Acad Sci U S A* 2005;102(48):17406-17411.

68. Chen Y, Alman BA: Wnt pathway, an essential role in bone regeneration. *J Cell Biochem* 2009;106(3):353-362.

This comprehensive paper reviews the role of Wnt pathway in bone regeneration.

69. Karamitros AE, Kalentzos VN, Soucacos PN: Electric stimulation and hyperbaric oxygen therapy in the treatment of nonunions. *Injury* 2006;37(suppl 1):S63-S73.

70. Romano CL, Romano D, Logoluso N: Low-intensity

pulsed ultrasound for the treatment of bone delayed union or nonunion: A review. *Ultrasound Med Biol* 2009;35(4):529-536.

This article summarizes the effects of LIPUS on fracture healing, including an updated review of the basic science, animal studies, and clinical trials of LIPUS.

71. Birnbaum K, Wirtz DC, Siebert CH, Heller KD: Use of extracorporeal shock-wave therapy (ESWT) in the treatment of non-unions: A review of the literature. *Arch Orthop Trauma Surg* 2002;122(6):324-330.

72. Leung KS, Shi HF, Cheung WH, et al: Low-magnitude high-frequency vibration accelerates callus formation, mineralization, and fracture healing in rats. *J Orthop Res* 2009;27(4):458-465.

In a rat model, low-magnitude high-frequency vibration improves fracture healing through increased callus formation and accelerated remodeling.

FRACTURE HEALING CONTINUED...

RESTRICTED MOTION
combo of enchondral ossification
+ intramembranous ossification
e.g. locked plating

STABLE FX
- no callus
- akn 1° healing, direct
- combo of contact + gap

① Contact
defect of bone < 0.01 mm &
interfrag. strain < 2%
direct formation of lamellar
bone in original orientation
cutting cones across fx site
c̄ osteoclasts spearheading,
osteoblasts following to
form Haversian remodeling
& bony union
note: bone union & remodeling
occur simultaneously

② Gap
1st: lamellar bone forms
⊥ to original orientation,
but weak mechanically
2nd: @ 3-8 wks, Haversian
remodeling occurs to
form bone along
original orientation,
mechanically strong
e.g. compression plating, lag
screws

1: Principles of Orthopaedics

FRACTURE HEALING CONTINUED.

Chapter 3

Articular Cartilage and Intervertebral Disk

James A. Martin, PhD   Prem S. Ramakrishnan, PhD   Tae-Hong Lim, PhD

Daniel Thedens, PhD   Joseph A. Buckwalter, MS, MD

Articular Cartilage

Structure and Function

Articular cartilage is structurally well suited to support joint function: it provides a nearly frictionless interface between joint surfaces and protects underlying bones by redistributing loads. By bulk chemical analysis cartilage consists mainly of water (more than 70% of wet mass), proteoglycan (15% of wet mass), and collagen (15% of wet mass). More than 80% of the proteoglycan present is in the form of high-molecular-weight (more than 3.5×10^6 Da) aggregates of hyaluronic acid–linked aggrecan, a 250-kDa protein that is heavily populated with polyanionic sulfated glycosaminoglycans (keratan and chondroitin sulfate). In the matrix, aggrecan entrapment within a collagen fibril network results in densely packed negative charges, which are available to interact with water via hydrogen bonding. Electrostatic repulsion and a strong tendency to retain bound water enable cartilage to resist deformation under compression and to redistribute stresses by hydrostatic pressurization of the matrix.

Histologic analysis reveals depth-dependent variation in cartilage matrix structure; four distinct zones (superficial, transitional, radial, calcified) can be distinguished based on differences in cell morphology, matrix composition, and collagen fibril orientation. These depth-dependent variations result in marked anisotropy and, as a result, chondrocytes experience different stresses depending on their location in the depth of the matrix. The superficial zone is relatively low in proteoglycan content compared with the deeper zones and, in contrast to deeper zones where collagen fibrils run perpendicular or orthogonal to the surface, the collagen network runs parallel to the surface. Thus, this zone is specialized to resist tensile stresses. Superficial zone chondrocytes are also somewhat distinct from cells in other zones: they are comparatively flat in shape and less rigid due to the absence of vimentin filaments, which enhance the stiffness of the cytoskeleton. These features appear to be an adaptation to the relatively higher strains experienced by these cells compared with cells lodged in the deeper zones where proteoglycan is more abundant. Superficial chondrocytes also secrete a specialized glycoprotein called lubricin (also known as superficial zone protein, or PRG4), which coats cartilage surfaces and lowers surface friction. Intra-articular injection of recombinant lubricin prevented cartilage degeneration in a rat meniscal tear model of osteoarthritis (OA), indicating that friction plays a role in cartilage degeneration in OA.[1]

The cartilage extracellular matrix (ECM) is thinly populated by chondrocytes, cells of mesenchymal lineage that are adapted for life in the demanding environment of the articular surface. Despite their low tissue density, articular chondrocytes exert a profound influence on cartilage matrix stability. Chondrocyte depletion is associated with aging and OA, and the prevention of chondrocyte death blocks matrix degeneration after cartilage injury. Chondrocytes maintain the ECM by actively synthesizing its components, but also contribute to matrix degradation by synthesizing matrix proteases. Disturbance in the balance between biosynthetic and degradative activities destabilizes the ECM and is a hallmark of OA.

Cartilage is avascular and nourished only by way of synovial fluid at its surface and through subchondral bone at its base. Intratissue oxygen saturation is predictably low (2% to 10%), but chondrocytes tolerate such mild hypoxic conditions, relying for the most part on glycolysis for adenosine triphosphate (ATP) production. Presumably, in normal cartilage ATP is generated in sufficient quantity to meet demands for maintenance-level biosynthesis of proteoglycans and collagens. However, very low oxygen levels (less than 1%) inhibit glycolytic activity via negative feedback by

Dr. Buckwalter or an immediate family members serves as a paid consultant for or is an employee of ISTO and Carbylan Bioscience and is a board member, owner, officer, or committee member of the American Orthopaedic Association. None of the following authors nor any immediate family member has received anything of value from or owns stock in a commercial company or institution related directly or indirectly to the subject of this chapter: Dr. Martin, Dr. Ramakrishnan, and Dr. Thedens.

reduced intermediates such as nicotinamide adenine dinucleotide (NADH) and nicotinamide adenine dinucleotide phosphate (NADPH), which accumulate in the absence of oxidants.[2] Recent studies support earlier findings that moderate to severe intra-articular hypoxia accompanies arthritis and joint inflammation. In addition to interfering with ATP production, such severely hypoxic conditions induce chondrocytes to express vascular endothelial growth factor (VEGF), which promotes blood vessel invasion of the tidemark, a classic pathologic feature of OA.[3]

Influence of Mechanical Stresses on Matrix Composition and Cellularity

In addition to lacking blood vessels, cartilage is deprived of the neural input that drives adaptation of bone and muscle to prevailing loading conditions. Yet, numerous examples of loading effects on cartilage would seem to indicate an intrinsic capacity for load adaptation. These observations have focused attention on chondrocyte mechanoresponses, which appear to mediate many of the effects of loading on cartilage. A wealth of in vitro studies indicate that chondrocytes are sensitive to frequency, rate, and magnitude of loading. In general, physiologic cyclic stress (1 to 5 MPa) applied at moderate frequencies (0.1 to 1 Hz) and rates (less than 1,000 MPa/s) stimulate matrix synthesis and inhibit chondrolytic activity, whereas excessive stress amplitudes (more than 5 MPa), static loading (less than 0.01 Hz), or stress rates in excess of 1,000 MPa/s suppress matrix synthesis and promote chondrolytic activity. The transduction of mechanical signals resulting in changes in gene expression has long been known to involve integrins and the cytoskeleton. However, more recent findings suggest that primary cilia may act as a mechanosensory organ in chondrocytes and osteoblasts. These studies show that intracellular calcium flux, a primary effect of mechanical strain, is mediated by single cilia that protrude into the pericellular matrix and are connected to stretch-activated channels in the cell membrane.[4] The hypothesis that cilia play a role in cartilage homeostasis is supported by data from transgenic mice lacking functional cilia; signs of abnormal cartilage development and degeneration were apparent.[5]

Evidence of load adaptation in cartilage was revealed by a study in which the effects of moderate running exercise (1 hour per day 5 days per week for 15 weeks) on the stifle joints of beagle dogs were determined. The authors found that running was associated with significant gains in cartilage thickness and increased proteoglycan content in femoral condyles and patellae.[6] However, later studies showed that more strenuous long-distance running (up to 40 km per day for 40 weeks) resulted in cartilage thinning and proteoglycan loss,[7] indicating that load tolerance and adaptive capabilities of canine cartilage are limited. The relevance of the canine models to humans is uncertain. There were no substantial differences in knee MRIs between elite athletes and nonathletes, suggesting that the

capacity for human cartilage to add mass in response to increased loading is more limited than in dogs.[8] However, another study showed substantial (14%) patellar cartilage thickening in weight lifters and bobsled sprinters compared to nonathletic control subjects.[9] It remains to be seen whether human cartilage shows changes in matrix composition similar to those observed in the dog model. In a 2008 study, long-distance running effects in the human knee were tracked by serial radiography of patients over two decades (mean age = 58 years). Multivariate analysis revealed that runners (n = 45) showed no substantial increase in Kellgren-Lawrence scores compared to control subjects (n = 53), indicating that running was not associated with increased risk of OA.[10]

Habitual strenuous loading is clearly harmful to cartilage, but some form of mechanical stimulation is required for cartilage health. Atrophy in response to unloading is well documented in both animals and humans. Joint immobilization models consistently show cartilage thinning, softening, and proteoglycan loss. Recent work in a rat model revealed increases in chondrocyte apoptosis, and increased hypoxia inducible factor-α, VEGF, matrix metalloproteinase-8 (MMP-8), and MMP-13 expression.[11] This finding suggests that hypoxia may play a role in immobilization effects. MRI studies of human knees have shown progressive cartilage thinning within 2 years of spinal cord injury,[5] indicating atrophy similar to that observed in joint immobilization models. The ability of cartilage to return to a trophic state when loading is resumed is also well established. Data from immobilization models have shown varying degrees of recovery of normal cartilage thickness, stiffness, and proteoglycan (PG) content. However, in most cases, extended immobilization results in permanent deficits of up to 25% in PG content and mechanical properties. The risk of such permanent effects on cartilage in patients with extended partial weight bearing is unclear due to uncertainties regarding the time course for immobilization-induced atrophy in humans; however, a study of patients recovering from ankle fracture showed significant losses of patellar cartilage thickness (-3%) and tibial cartilage thickness (-6%) after only 7 weeks of reduced loading.[12]

Aging and Arthritis

The age-dependent incidence of OA supports the notion that age-related changes in articular cartilage are pathogenic. However, the connection of aging to OA remains unclear. Distinguishing normal age-related changes in cartilage, which do not progress to OA, from early changes that reliably progress to OA is still controversial. Therefore, longitudinal MRI studies may prove useful. In one example, MRI examination of patients with knee OA symptoms showed significant reductions in cartilage thickness over 1 year, indicating disease progression.[13] Presumably, similar studies in age-matched patients without symptomatic OA would show less progressive thinning. This coupled with an initial examination using MRI methods that are sensitive to cartilage matrix composition (delayed gadolinium-enhanced MRI of cartilage [dGEMRIC], T2, or T1ρ) could help to distinguish initial conditions that predispose patients to OA from those that do not.

Except in connection with injury, cell division is rare in mature articular cartilage, suggesting that most chondrocytes present at skeletal maturity are likely to remain in place for decades. Although their numbers remain relatively stable for most of adult life in normal cartilage, early OA is marked by increased apoptosis and, at later stages, by hypocellularity.[14] Preventing apoptosis using caspase inhibitors ameliorates the development of OA in animal models and holds great promise for the treatment of some forms of OA in humans.

Although most chondrocytes may be long-lived, several in vitro tests document age-related declines in their performance, especially after the fourth decade of life when the risk of OA increases sharply.[15] Losses in overall biosynthetic activity, particularly under growth factor stimulation, could contribute to the risk of OA by undermining matrix maintenance and repair. However, a pathogenic role for these relatively subtle cellular changes remains to be proved. Indeed, it is possible that age-related "loss" of matrix biosynthesis activity constitutes a successful metabolic adaptation to decreasing nutrition or other environmental changes, and that its association with OA is coincidental.

More obviously pertinent to OA are age-related changes in chondrocyte phenotype that lead to increased expression of catabolic cytokines and matrix proteases. Recent work suggests that dysregulation of the Wnt/β-catenin pathway, which regulates multiple genes involved in cartilage development, is strongly associated with OA. Wnt-induced signaling protein 1 (WISP-1) was found to upregulate matrix protease expression in chondrocytes.[16] Inactivating mutations in the gene encoding frizzled-related protein-3, a key negative regulator of the Wnt pathway, were found to predispose patients to OA. Moreover, transgenic mice overexpressing β-catenin, a key positive regulator of the Wnt pathway, develop osteoarthritic changes. Interestingly, β-catenin activation is regulated by mechanical stresses in chondrocytes, suggesting a role for the Wnt pathway in integrin-mediated mechanoresponses.

The cause of age-related changes in the Wnt pathway or other alterations in phenotype is uncertain. Some evidence suggests that the age-dependent accumulation of epigenetic changes alters the pattern of chondrocyte gene expression.[17] This involves altered activity of DNA methyltransferases and/or histone acetylases/deacetylases, which inappropriately silences or activates gene expression by modifying *cis*-acting sequences that control gene transcription. For example, the expression of the aggrecanase encoding gene a disintegrin and metalloproteinase with thrombospondin motif-4 (*ADAMTS-4*) in normal and osteoarthritic cartilage was analyzed, and the enzyme was found to be upregulated in superficial zone chondrocytes in OA. Further analysis revealed that increased expression in OA was related to loss of cytosine methylation at critical CpG islands in the *ADAMTS-4* gene promoter.[18] Loss of DNA methylation in a patient with developmental dysplasia of the hip was associated with increased expression of MMP-13, MMP-9, and MMP-3, all of which contribute to ECM degradation.[17] The availability of drugs targeting methylation and histone modification for cancer therapy has stirred discussion of their use in the treatment of OA.

Cell senescence, a phenomenon underlying many degenerative diseases, also occurs in articular cartilage. Senescence is defined as permanent growth arrest, but the term is also often used in connection with profound alterations in gene expression. Senescent cells can be long-lived, which might not be problematic except that they are not entirely quiescent and show abnormalities in matrix metabolism that actively disrupt tissue function.[19] Chronic oxidative damage has been shown to induce senescence in human chondrocytes and senescent cells accumulate in articular cartilage with aging. Chondrocytes generate oxidants in response to mechanical stress, suggesting a connection between mechanical factors, oxidative damage, and senescence.[20] Thus, it appears that aging changes might be slowed by avoiding stresses that result in deleterious oxidant release.

In most of the studies described above it is implicitly assumed that aging affects all cells in cartilage in the same way. However, it is increasingly apparent that cartilage harbors progenitor cells, which are distinct from normal chondrocytes in that they are highly migratory, pluripotent, and clonogenic. Progenitor cells have been identified in late-stage osteoarthritic cartilage, and may participate in the repair of damaged matrix.[21] Thus, age-related declines in this subpopulation could have a disproportionate effect on matrix stability.[22]

Injury and Repair
Biologic Responses to Mechanical Injury
Physical injury to articular cartilage surfaces can occur under a variety of circumstances, including articular fracture, ACL rupture, or simple sprains. High loading rates (>1,000 MPa/s) and high peak stress amplitudes (>20 MPa) initiate focal damage that can spread to involve even larger areas of the joint surface, leading to posttraumatic OA. Biologic responses act to repair or limit the damage inflicted by injurious stress, but progressive degeneration is a common sequela to injury, particularly in middle-aged and elderly patients. At the high loading rates characteristic of impact injuries, overall cartilage strain and water loss are minimal. However, local strains in the superficial zone during impact injuries can exceed 40%, and matrix fissuring and chondrocyte death are evident postimpact. These changes have been shown to lead to the development of OA in a rabbit model of single blunt-impact injury.[23]

Strategies to Promote Healing or Regeneration
Superficial zone chondrocyte death is strongly associated with physical injury to articular cartilage. Most of the available evidence indicates that the resulting devitalization of the cartilage matrix is permanent and de-

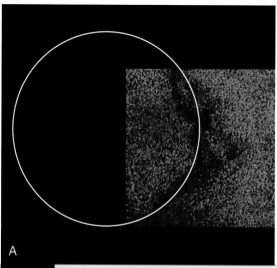
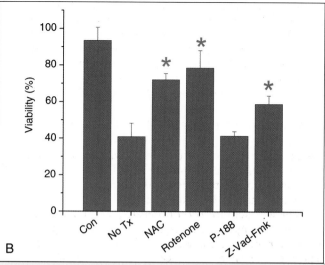

Figure 1 The effects of blunt impact injury on oxidant production and viability in osteochondral explants are shown. **A,** The confocal micrograph shows the surface of an explant stained with calcein AM for live cells (green) and dihydroethidium for superoxide production (red) 30 minutes after blunt impact with a 5-mm-diameter platen (size and placement indicated by the white circle). Note the heavy oxidant production near the periphery of the impacted site. **B,** Chondrocyte viability determined by confocal microscopy at 48 hours postimpact in the absence of treatment (No Tx) or when treated immediately with NAC, rotenone, P-188, or Z-VAD-fmk. "Con" indicates results for nonimpacted cartilage. Asterisks indicate significant improvement of viability over untreated control. Note also that viability in the group treated with rotenone, the mitochondrial electron transport inhibitor, was significantly greater than in the group treated with Z-VAD-fmk, a pan caspase inhibitor. (Data courtesy of the Iowa Orthopaedic Biology Laboratory.)

stabilizing; thus, injury-induced cell death is among the earliest pathogenic events in posttraumatic OA. Preventing cell death in the immediate aftermath of injury has become a major target of therapy for posttraumatic OA as it has for stroke and heart attack. Interestingly, neuronal death after stroke and chondrocyte death after cartilage injury both appear to involve oxidative damage associated with free radical release.

Both apoptosis and necrosis have been observed at sites of high-energy impact injury. Impact-induced chondrocyte apoptosis is a caspase-dependent process. Caspase inhibitors reduce the severity of OA in vivo. Caspase inhibitors and the surfactant P-188 were also shown to prevent nearly 50% of the chondrocyte death that occurred in human ankle cartilage subjected to a single impact.[24] P-188 is thought to prevent necrosis by restoring cell membrane integrity, which is compromised by injury. In addition, BMP-7 applied intra-articularly within 3 weeks after an experimental impact injury in the sheep stifle joint prevented apoptosis and ameliorated progressive degenerative changes in the cartilage matrix.[25]

Evidence of mitochondrial involvement in injury-induced apoptosis comes from a cartilage explant injury model, in which it was shown that a wave of calcium was released from the endoplasmic reticulum following blunt impact injury. An increase in calcium level induced permeability transition pore (PTP) formation in the inner mitochondrial membrane. The resulting depolarization was associated with cytochrome C release, Bcl-2 degradation, and caspase-dependent

apoptosis.[26] Chondrocyte apoptosis was inhibited by blocking the increase in cytoplasmic calcium or by blocking PTP formation. These results show the central role of calcium in chondrocyte responses to mechanical trauma and provide evidence that mitochondria-dependent apoptosis is a significant consequence of the disruption of calcium homeostasis.

Recent work in a bovine explant model showed that impact-induced chondrocyte death was significantly reduced by treatment with the intermediate free-radical scavenger N-acetyl cysteine (NAC),[20] and similar effects have been shown using a superoxide dismutase (SOD) mimetic. NAC applied within 2 hours of impact spared more than 75% of cells that would have otherwise died within 72 hours of injury. Moreover, impact-related decline in PG content 7 days after injury was blocked by early postimpact NAC treatment. Additional studies established that superoxide radicals are released from mitochondria in response to impact injury; blocking mitochondrial electron transport at complex I using rotenone ablated superoxide release had chondrocyte-sparing effects similar to those of NAC (**Figure 1**).

These studies demonstrate the central role of oxidative stress and mitochondrial dysfunction in acute chondrocyte death induced by articular injury. It is known that cell death under these conditions is preventable and that preserving cellularity improves tissue function and short-term matrix stability. However, the ability of such acute cytotherapies to prevent OA is not yet clear. Relieving contact stresses in injured joints via distraction offers considerable promise. This strategy, which involves external fixation and separation joint surfaces, has been applied to patients with OA of the ankle. In one study conducted 30 months after frame removal, 21 patients (91%) experienced significant improvement; only 2 of these patients had arthrodesis.[27] The mechanisms of distraction effects on articular cartilage repair and stability are still largely unknown.

Noninvasive Assessment of Cartilage Health

Novel MRI-Based Approaches

The exquisite soft-tissue contrast of MRI and the multiplicity of contrast mechanisms available in a single examination have established MRI as the method of choice for imaging articular cartilage. A typical MRI protocol will acquire proton density, T1, T2, and fat-suppressed images, which give a comprehensive picture of the morphologic changes associated with injury and subsequent degenerative processes. Ultimately, however, it is the biomechanical properties of cartilage that determine its functional state. Biomechanical properties of cartilage may in turn be assessed based on related biochemical composition of the ECM, especially in terms of PG and collagen content, the primary components responsible for the mechanical strength of healthy cartilage. Thus, the development of a noninvasive and quantitative assessment of cartilage PG content would greatly enhance the evaluation of acute injury and treatment efficacy in the clinical setting. MRI is presently the only imaging modality capable of generating this information, with four distinct techniques available to generate PG-sensitive images for interpretation and quantification. These include sodium (23Na) imaging, T2 mapping, dGEMRIC, and T1ρ imaging. Sodium nuclear magnetic resonance spectroscopy has long been applied to investigate PG depletion in cartilage. The basis for this method is that PG loss yields a reduction of fixed charge density and a loss of sodium ions (as well as a change in sodium relaxation parameters). These changes can be seen and quantified from sodium-based MRI as well and present a very direct correlation to PG loss. However, sodium MRI requires specialized hardware, and has relatively poor resolution and signal-to-noise ratio, and is unlikely to translate to standard clinical imagers. At the other end of the spectrum, T2-based MRI is a widely used and mature technique, and T2-weighted images are routinely acquired as part of musculoskeletal MRI protocols. Quantification of T2 relaxation times is also a readily available technique on most clinical scanners. Several studies have shown significant changes in T2 relaxation times in areas of cartilage degeneration, and these changes may be seen in subjects with OA in the absence of volume and thickness changes, suggesting sensitivity to biochemical changes in early OA. These changes in T2 relaxation time are relatively small, and may result from multiple mechanisms such as PG loss, water content, and collagen concentration and orientation. Thus, although T2 changes in cartilage are seen in degenerative processes and may often be diagnostically valuable, it can be unclear which of these mechanisms is the predominant cause, potentially limiting the sensitivity and specificity to PG loss.

The dGEMRIC protocol is currently the most widely used of the methods for in vivo characterization of PG loss.[28] The principle of dGEMRIC is based on the fact that glycosaminoglycans (GAGs), which are linked to core proteins to form PGs, are negatively charged. If a negatively charged MRI contrast agent such as Gd-(DPTA)2 is introduced, the distribution of this agent will be in inverse proportion to the GAG concentration. Further, the Gd(DPTA)2 concentration can be measured through measurement of T1 relaxation time through standard imaging and processing techniques, yielding a marker of GAG concentration and PG loss. Numerous in vivo and in vitro studies suggest dGEMRIC is the most specific for GAG concentrations among the described methods, demonstrating direct correlations between dGEMRIC measurements and GAG and even mechanical properties. This specificity comes at a cost of high complexity in implementing the examination. Subjects receive an intravenous injection of contrast agent, followed by a period of mild exercise to distribute the agent. Imaging then takes place 1 to 2 hours after injection. In many cases, a precontrast examination is also desirable for robust measurement of relaxation changes. Thus, while dGEMRIC shows strong abilities for accurate measurements of PG depletion, the rigors of the examination may prevent its use in clinical settings. T1ρ MRI represents a promising "middle ground" between T2 mapping and dGEMRIC. T1ρ MRI is a completely noninvasive method for quantifying cartilage PG content without the need for special hardware, contrast agents, exercise, or extended timing considerations[29] while generating information very similar to dGEMRIC.

The relaxation processes measured with T1ρ depend primarily on the exchange of protons between water and macromolecules, but are also influenced by interactions caused by collagen fibril orientation. The T1ρ technique generates images with a standard spin-echo-based pulse sequence attached to the beginning with a group of magnetization preparation pulses to set up varying amounts of T1ρ contrast, and can therefore be implemented on any clinical scanner. The image analysis required to quantify T1ρ is very similar to that required for T2 measurements. The close ties between PG content and cartilage function make T1ρ MRI a much more direct and valuable indicator of cartilage health and treatment efficacy than purely anatomic imaging. Because of the dependence on proton exchange between water and PGs, quantifying PG depletion associated with early OA development with T1ρ is a more discriminatory cartilage assessment than T2 sequences.[29] Thus, T1ρ MRI pulse sequences may be able to detect cartilage compromise occurring after catastrophic ACL ruptures. Although this dependence may not be as exclusively based on PG content as dGEMRIC, both in vitro and in vivo studies suggest that the relationship is sufficiently strong and sensitive that it may be preferred in many cases because of the considerably simpler logistical requirements. The development and validation of T1ρ MRI as an objective and quantitative measurement standard of cartilage condi-

1: Principles of Orthopaedics

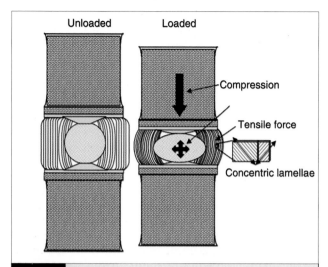

Unloaded   Loaded

Compression

Tensile force

Concentric lamellae

Figure 2 The biomechanics of an intact intervertebral disk are shown. The biomechanical functions of the intervertebral disk are directly related to the ECM components. Aggrecans present in the nucleus pulposus are highly hydrophilic, imbibing water and establishing an internal hydrostatic pressure in the intervertebral disk. This hydrostatic pressure (swelling pressure) is generated by the resistance provided by the anulus fibrosus and end plates to fluid transport. The swelling pressure in the nucleus pulposus also provides resistance to compressive forces. In addition to facilitating the maintenance of the swelling pressure, collagen fibrils run at an angle of about 60° (alternating between adjacent lamellae), ensuring tension of the anulus fibrosus structures during rotational movements. The composite nature of the end plates provides resilience and prevents fractures in the motion segment during load transmission.

tion may dramatically improve the assessment and understanding of acute injury, diagnosis, and treatment. The appearance of techniques for robust and noninvasive assessments of cartilage composition, structure, and function would be invaluable for all phases of the disease process in OA. Such information may yield detection of early OA markers before morphologic changes or physical symptoms occur. It could also direct treatment options and assess recovery in later stages of OA development. Further study is needed to validate these noninvasive techniques as clinical tools.

Biomarkers

Numerous biomarkers related to cartilage matrix metabolism have been tested for their power to predict the progression of primary arthritis. The crosslinked C-telopeptide of type II collagen (CTX-II) generated in articular cartilage by noncollagenase proteinases is a reliable urinary marker of cartilage degeneration in primary OA. Collagen type II neoepitopes resulting from collagenase activity (Col2-3/4 long, Col2-3/4 short) have also been extensively used as degenerative markers as has the aggrecan neoepitope (VDIPEN) generated by MMPs. Markers of cartilage matrix biosynthesis include the C-terminal propeptide of type II collagen (PI-ICP) and chondroitin sulfate epitopes of aggrecan (for example, 3B3). In addition to cartilage matrix markers, urinary glucosyl galactosyl pyridinoline (Glc-Gal-PYD) levels have been used to assess synovial degeneration, which is evident in OA.[30]

In general, the cartilage biomarker studies show that the levels of individual markers do not predict OA consistently, perhaps due in part to the influence of factors including age, sex, and body mass index. However, combinations of markers appear to give better results.[31] One study found that levels of CTX-II in urine correlated with multiple indices of joint degeneration in patients with hip or knee OA. High CTX-II levels and low collagen propeptide levels (PIINP) were found to be related to the rate of progression of knee OA. However, the ratio between CTX and PIINP was more strongly predictive of arthritis breakdown than either marker alone. Based on these findings, it is suggested that the calculated ratio represents disturbances in the equilibrium between collagen degradation and synthesis in osteoarthritic cartilage. The ratio of COL2-3/4 short to COL2-3/4C long was also shown to be more predictive of OA progression than the individual markers.[32] Urinary levels of the synovium-specific carbohydrate marker Glc-Gal-PYD also effectively predicted OA progression and correlated with pain and other symptoms better than cartilage matrix markers.[33]

Intervertebral Disk

Structure and Function

The intervertebral disk is a fibrocartilaginous structure that resides between adjacent vertebral bodies of the spine collectively called a motion segment (**Figure 2**). The three principal regions of the intervertebral disk, the nucleus pulposus, anulus fibrosus, and the end plates, form this specialized structure that maintains an optimal biomechanical environment in the spine. The nucleus pulposus, the central element of the intervertebral disk, has a fluidic matrix primarily composed of aggrecan and type II collagen. The cells that reside in the nucleus pulposus are originally derived from the notochord and may contain large vacuoles and prominent cytoskeletal elements in situ. Based on their biosynthetic profile and response to mechanical stimuli, nucleus pulposus cells are distinct from other cell populations in the intervertebral disk. The anulus fibrosus is composed of concentric lamellae of collagen type I fibers that circumferentially confine the fluidic nucleus pulposus. Cells of the anulus fibrosus have an ellipsoidal morphology, reside within lamellae of the anulus fibrosus, and produce both type I and type II collagen. Cells within the innermost annular regions are more rounded and sparsely distributed. By early adulthood in the human, however, the nucleus pulposus becomes populated by chondrocyte-like cells that may migrate from the adjacent end plate or inner regions of the anulus fibrosus. The vertebral bodies are separated from the nucleus pulposis superiorly and inferiorly by cartilagenous end plates.

A normal adult intervertebral disk consists of a large amount of ECM and very few viable cells (approximately 1% of total disk volume). Despite very low numbers, the resident cells are necessary for maintaining disk health, producing matrix components, and controlling matrix turnover by regulating the activation and production of extracellular and intracellular proteases. Inactive forms of growth factors such as basic fibroblast growth factor (bFGF), transforming growth factor-beta (TGF-β), and insulin-like growth factor (IGF) are normally bound by cartilage intermediate layer protein to the ECM. When chondrocytes secrete MMPs, matrix is degraded to make room for newly synthesized matrix products. Matrix-bound growth factors are released during this event that in turn stimulate the resident cells to produce more matrix, and inhibit the production of MMPs. The other factors that play important roles in maintaining tissue turnover are tissue inhibitors of metalloproteinases (TIMPs), interleukin-1 (IL-1), interferon (IFN), and tumor necrosis factor-α (TNF-α).

Due to its lack of vascularity, the intervertebral disk is deficient in nutrient supply and exchange of metabolic waste products. This deficit in solute transport manifests itself in the form of steep gradients in oxygen tension and glucose and lactic acid concentrations, which play roles in maintaining the phenotype of disk cells.

Development and Maturation

The development of the spinal column begins at the embryonic stage with the nucleus pulposus derived from the central notochord (endoderm) with the rest of the structure (vertebral bodies, cartilage, and anulus fibrosus) from the surrounding mesenchyme (mesoderm). In the embryonic disk, there is a distinct structural and compositional demarcation between the fluid-like nucleus pulposus (rich in notochordal cells and PG) and the fibrous anulus fibrosus (fibroblast-like cells and collagen). Above and below the newly forming embryonic disks, the notochord disappears and is replaced by mesenchymal cells, giving rise to the bone and cartilaginous end plates of the vertebrae. Changes in the composition of the embryonic disk begin right after birth. In the nucleus pulposus, notochordal cells are slowly replaced by chondrocyte-like cells. Complete replacement of notochordal cells occurs by 10 years after birth, leading to compositional changes and making the nucleus pulposus resemble the inner anulus fibrosus. Concurrently, the vertebral end plates decrease in thickness and diameter due to endochondral ossification. In a mature intervertebral disk, cell density is significantly low compared to its earlier stages of development, providing the rationale of decreased repair capability of a mature disk. Lack of vascularization and immune compromise limits removal of cell remnants and cellular organelles. A recent study showed that nucleus pulposus cells are capable of phagocytosis[34] and this event may be important in maintaining tissue structure and function during major cell loss. Although a mature disk is inhabited by cells of similar origin (mesenchymal), they express very distinct phenotypes depending on their location and matrix composition.

Normal Aging Compared With Degeneration

Aging causes progressive changes in disk matrix composition that resemble those of other aging collagenous tissues such as the articular cartilage. One of the earliest age-related phenomena is the fragmentation of the PGs in the nucleus. There is also a concurrent increase in collagen content (especially type I) rendering the nucleus pulposus more fibrous. Fragmented PGs degrade further and leach out of the nucleus pulposus, decreasing its capacity to imbibe water. The decrease in fluid retention results in inadequate hydrostatic pressure, a major biomechanical deficit. Because of limited repair capability, low cell density, and decreased matrix turnover, the intervertebral disk fails to recover, leading to further biologic and structural deterioration. In addition, increased crosslinking among collagen fibers and nonenzymatic glycation further inhibits matrix turnover. With exception to localized proliferation after injury, cell density and cellular function decrease with age, resulting in reduced matrix turnover. Phenotypic changes in cell populations are observed with changes in matrix composition and local stress distribution. The loss of hydrostatic pressure in the nucleus pulposus results in the anulus fibrosus sharing most of the compressive loads. These changes transform the intervertebral disk from a structure that is strong, hydrated, and flexible to one that is very stiff, desiccated, and weak. At this juncture, "normal" biomechanical forces become excessive, and lead to structural damage such as delamination and tears of the anulus fibrosus, disk prolapse, herniation, and end plate fractures. Narrowing of the disk space and radial bulging also occur because of loss of fluid pressure and end plate fractures. Age-related changes peak and signs of discogenic pain are observed as early as the third decade of life.

Degeneration and aging have similar biochemical and structural changes. However, the distinction can be made by the magnitude and mechanisms that lead to the changes in the intervertebral disk. Age-related changes that involve structural disruptions are fewer and smaller, whereas degenerative changes exhibit major structural disruptions. Aging is an inevitable process that starts soon after birth and changes are unrelated to pain in the disk, whereas degeneration is correlated to discogenic pain. Age-related changes also are common to all disks of the spine, whereas macroscopic degenerative changes occur only at levels L4-S1. Although age-related changes render the disk susceptible to further degenerative changes, intervertebral disk degeneration can be defined as a condition of structural failure and irreversible loss of biomechanical function through physical and biologic mechanisms. A degenerated disk can have accelerated and advanced signs of aging along with a possibility of pain generation. Hence, multiple factors may, in combination, incrementally predispose the intervertebral disk to degenerative disk disease.

Nutritional Deficiency

As mentioned previously, the intervertebral disk is avascular with blood vessels restricted to the outer anulus fibrosus. Most metabolite transport occurs through diffusion across end plates. Aging causes decreased metabolite transport, whereas degenerative changes and end plate disruption increase solute transport affecting intervertebral disk homeostasis. The porosity of the end plate is significantly reduced due to calcification. Periannular solute transport is minimal and occurs through microtubes, with diffusivity decreasing from the inner anulus fibrosus to its outer rims. Low oxygen tension in the center of a disk leads to anaerobic metabolism, resulting in a high concentration of lactic acid and low pH. In vitro experiments show that a chronic lack of oxygen causes nucleus pulposus cells to become quiescent, whereas a chronic lack of glucose can cause cell death.[35] Interestingly, mature nucleus pulposus cells are more tolerant to hypoxia when compared to notochordal cells, indicating that end plate porosity plays a role in regulating the phenotype of nucleus pulposus cells. Deficiencies in metabolite transport appear to limit both the density and metabolic activity of disk cells. As a result, disks have only a limited ability to recover from any metabolic or mechanical injury. Computational models developed to study solute transport in normal and degenerated disks suggest that aging, end plate calcification/disruption, and mechanical loads influence solute concentrations, affecting cell viability and activity.[36]

Nutritional deficiencies are a by-product of aging and it is unclear if improving metabolite transport would save the intervertebral disk from degenerative changes. However, there is evidence to suggest that accelerated degenerative signs may occur due to pathologic and/or environmental factors (for example, diabetes and smoking, respectively) that can affect vascular health and in turn render the metabolic status out of balance before natural aging could take its course. Tools for early detection and intervention may be beneficial to slow the process of degeneration.

Soluble Factors

The process of degeneration is manifested by a chronic imbalance in matrix turnover, with increased expression of catabolic cytokines and decreased anabolic activity. The stromelysin family of enzymes (MMPs) and ADAMTS collection are involved in matrix catabolism during intervertebral disk degeneration. MMPs-1,-3, -7, -9, -10, and -13 have been shown to be involved in degenerative activities in various studies. The ADAMTS family is composed of aggrecans that have been shown to be highly active in degenerated disks. In particular, ADAMTS-1, -4, -5, -15 are upregulated in degenerated intervertebral disks whereas endogenous TIMP-3 expression is low, affecting matrix homeostasis. TNF-α and IL-1 α and β are proinflammatory cytokines that have been studied extensively in the context of their regulation of MMPs. TNF-α has also been shown to induce sensory nerve in growth in the intervertebral disk, indicating their possible role in pain induction in degenerative disks. Upregulation of the IL-1 system is shown to induce MMPs,[37] ADAMTS, and proteinase-activated receptor-2 (PAR-2).[38] Cytokines also suppress synthesis of matrix components such as collagen type II, which is largely replaced with collagen type I in the nucleus pulposus. Cytokines mediate catabolic responses to advanced glycation end products via the advanced glycation and end products receptor (RAGE) complex.[39] Furthermore, angiogenesis, neuronogenesis and apoptosis of intervertebral disk cells depend to some extent on cytokines. The receptor antagonist of IL-1 system (IL-1Ra), which inhibits IL-1 signaling, is not upregulated in degenerated disks. Gene expression profiling of degenerated human disks suggests that TNF-α may be an early response mediator of degeneration, whereas IL-1β may be the key mediator that sustains the upregulation of matrix-degrading molecules.[37]

Recently, the presence of nerve growth factor, brain-derived neurotrophic factor (and associated receptors) and the pain-associated neuropeptide substance P were identified in human nucleus pulposus tissue along with upregulation of IL-1β, suggesting that proinflammatory cytokines can stimulate nociception and initiate pain response via nerve ingrowth. Although implicated in regulating cell proliferation, apoptosis, and senescence, elevated expression of stress proteins such as Hsp-27 and Hsp-72 in degenerated disks suggests their possible role in the degenerative catabolic process.[40] Local expression of Fas ligand (FasL) was found to be decreased in degenerated human nucleus pulposus, supporting the hypothesis that FasL may be involved in inhibiting pathologic neovasularization.[41] Increased expression of connective tissue growth factor in degenerated disks is associated with angiogenesis in intervertebral disk degeneration.[42] Angiogenesis may also be driven by overproduction of hypoxia inducible factor-1 α, which is coexpressed with VEGF in the nucleus pulposus.[43] Caveolin-1 has been shown to be increased in the nucleus pulposus of degenerated disks but not in aged normal disks, indicating its role in degenerative rather than age-induced changes in the nucleus pulposus.[44] In the same study, a positive correlation with the expression of cyclin-dependent kinase inhibitor p16[INK4a] shows that caveolin-1 may be linked to the senescent phenotype in the intervertebral disk caused by a phenomenon known as stress-induced premature senescence. These findings also support the senescence-related increased SA-βGal expression in degenerated disk.[45] The pathogenic role of reactive oxygen species and reactive nitrogen species in OA suggests they may also play a role in intervertebral disk degeneration. The presence of nitrosylation products in the degenerated nucleus pulposus and stimulation of IL expression (-1β, -6, and -8) by peroxynitrite supports this hypothesis.[46] Moreover, mechanically induced reactive oxygen species production is a phenomenon described in articular cartilage, and could also contribute to stress-induced premature senescence in cells of the intervertebral disk.

It is unclear what initiates the imbalance in cytokine profiles in intervertebral disk, but there is evidence to suggest the involvement of mechanical loading and genetic factors.

Genetic Influences

Heritable factors are linked to the risk for intervertebral disk degeneration. Based largely on studies of twins, the variance in genetic predisposition to disk degeneration has been estimated at 29% to 74%. These studies strongly implicate polymorphisms of vitamin D receptor and collagen IX to increased risk for degeneration. Other candidate degeneration-linked genes include collagen type I, IL-6, aggrecan, MMP-3, thrombospondin, TIMP-1 and cyclo-oxygenase (COX-2), cartilage intermediate layer protein, and IL-1 family members. In a recent study that involved 588 subjects, aggrecan, collagen types (COL-9A1, -9A2, -1A1, -3A1 and -11A1), and ILs (IL-1A,-18R1, and -18RAP) were found to be associated with cardinal signs of degeneration such as disk bulging and desiccation. Significant correlation between genetic influence and range of motion (in particular, flexion) was observed in patients with degeneration with an attributable variance of 64%.[47] Asporin, also known as periodontal ligament-associated protein 1, is a member of the family of small leucine-rich PG family. It is identified as a susceptibility gene in OA and was also found to be locally expressed in the outer anulus of degenerated disks among Asian and caucasian subjects.[48]

Although genetic factors associated with degeneration are significant, their mechanistic effect on the degenerative cascade in the intervertebral disk is still largely unknown. Functional analysis of genetic polymorphisms in the context of molecular pathology intervertebral disk degeneration warrants investigation.

Mechanical Influences

Computational models and in vitro biomechanical studies have previously shown that the incidence of disk degeneration and discogenic pain may be directly related to increased mechanical demands of the lumbar spine. There is increasing evidence that mechanical loads regulate solute transport and there is a physiologic range of micromechanical stimuli that may promote maximum biosynthesis, maintain cellular phenotype and cell-mediated repair.[49] Excessive spinal loading caused by environmental factors (such as heavy lifting and increased body weight), significant traumatic injury, annular injury, and scoliosis[50] can lead to the development of the radiologic and biochemical features of degeneration. Once initiated, degeneration is expected to alter the local mechanical environment[51] furthering degeneration, via further mechanical overload, structural damage, vascularization, and altered cell and matrix biology.[52] Concerted efforts are under way to understand the role of mechanical stimuli on intervertebral disk biology at the cellular level. Recently, in vivo and in vitro studies have re-emphasized existing hypotheses that dynamic loading is more tissue-friendly than static loading.[49,52] There is

also current evidence that the effect of degradative enzymes can be inhibited by mechanical stimulation,[53] providing new insights to the subject of forestalling degeneration. Disk cells are responsive to mechanical loads depending on the type, magnitude, duration, and also anatomic zone of origin.

Although cellular responses to mechanical stimuli are documented, little is known of the mechanisms that regulate these cellular changes, nor is much known regarding the precise mechanical stimuli experienced by cells during loading. Advances in the field of computational biomechanics and intervertebral disk biology may provide new insights into intervertebral disk mechanobiology. Guidelines for tissue engineering and regeneration, better management of low back health, and prevention of intervertebral disk degeneration are a few goals that are currently envisioned.

Summary

Several recent developments inspire renewed confidence that cartilage degeneration in OA may be subject to interventions that delay or even reverse its progression. This optimism is based on a more comprehensive understanding of the molecular and biomechanical mechanisms driving degeneration, which provide a wealth of potential targets for pharmacologic intervention. In that regard, BMP-7, Wnt pathway modulators, antioxidants, and caspase inhibitors all show considerable promise as disease modulators. Moreover, the further development of strategies such as joint distraction aimed at modifying mechanical conditions in vivo can only be enhanced by recent advances in understanding the mechanobiology of cartilage. The ability to quantify the effects of such treatments in vivo using MRI and molecular biomarkers provides an enormous opportunity to further accelerate progress in treatment development.

The intervertebral disk is a highly specialized tissue with a heterogeneous structure and composition. The cells residing inside the intervertebral disk are influenced by their microenvironments and exhibit unique phenotypes depending on their regional location. Based on studies to date, the cause of intervertebral disk degeneration is multifactorial. However, it is also evident that there may be a salient factor(s) that may outweigh the others during the initiation and progression of the disease. Genetic inheritance may increase predisposition to intervertebral disk degeneration. However, disk degeneration does not occur until the fourth decade of life and affects only the lower lumbar spine, indicating that environmental factors may play a greater role and genetic predisposition may only be an additive risk factor. Nutritional deficit is one of earliest changes that occurs in the intervertebral disk during maturation, with the nucleus pulposus being the most affected. However, aging changes may be the primary cause of nutritional changes and the cells seem to adapt to the environments accordingly by altering their phenotype. Numerous molecular factors have been shown to be altered in degeneration. Although of potential therapeutic value, all soluble factors identified to date are also involved in adaptive remodeling and growth. Also, cytokines and growth factor imbalance are only effects of a "cause" and not necessarily the underlying factor of degeneration. Current understanding suggests that the mechanical influence on intervertebral disk degeneration may have a greater bearing on initiation and progress of disk degeneration. Animal studies have shown that cell-mediated changes always occur following structural failure due to mechanical trauma. Hence, mechanically induced structural damage may outweigh all other factors in initiating an irreversible cell-mediated cascade leading to further degradation. Aging, genetic inheritance, nutritional deficit, and soluble factors may only predispose the disk to degeneration by weakening the structure. The role of reactive oxygen species in intervertebral disk degeneration has not received much attention in intervertebral disk biology. As in the articular cartilage, intervertebral disk may undergo similar age- and trauma-related increases in oxidative stress, weakening the tissue's metabolic system and inducing premature senescence and even cell death. There is immense therapeutic value in understanding the role of pro-oxidants in intervertebral disk degeneration and further studies are warranted. Advances in the field of intervertebral disk mechanobiology may also provide new insights in to disk pathology, facilitating development of novel interventions to prevent the initiation or forestall the progression of this debilitating disease.

Annotated References

1. Flannery CR, Zollner R, Corcoran C, et al: Prevention of cartilage degeneration in a rat model of osteoarthritis by intraarticular treatment with recombinant lubricin. *Arthritis Rheum* 2009;60(3):840-847.

   A recombinant form of lubricin (LUB1) was delivered intra-articularly one to three times per week for 4 weeks after induction of OA in a rat meniscal tear model. Compared to saline controls LUB1 treatment significantly reduced cartilage degeneration and structural damage.

2. Lee RB, Urban JP: Functional replacement of oxygen by other oxidants in articular cartilage. *Arthritis Rheum* 2002;46(12):3190-3200.

3. Murata M, Yudoh K, Masuko K: The potential role of vascular endothelial growth factor (VEGF) in cartilage: How the angiogenic factor could be involved in the pathogenesis of osteoarthritis? *Osteoarthritis Cartilage* 2008;16(3):279-286.

   Hypoxia inducible factor-1α expression induced by hypoxia in inflamed arthritic joints activates VEGF expression by chondrocytes, leading to neovascularization of cartilage. VEGF is also thought to promote the expression of catabolic factors that contribute to cartilage degeneration. This suggests that hypoxia and VEGF contribute significantly to the pathogenesis of OA.

4. Whitfield JF: The solitary (primary) cilium—a mechanosensory toggle switch in bone and cartilage cells. *Cell Signal* 2008;20(6):1019-1024.

   Articular chondrocytes sense and respond to the strains imposed on cartilage via nonmotile single cilia protruding into the pericellular matrix, which act as switches that trigger calcium release upon cartilage compression. Calcium release in turn activates intracellular signaling that results in altered gene expression, which helps cartilage to adapt to changing mechanical conditions. Moreover, the chondrocyte cilium with its Indian hedgehog-activated Smo receptor is a key player along with PTHrP in endochondral bone formation.

5. Kaushik AP, Martin JA, Zhang Q, Sheffield VC, Morcuende JA: Cartilage abnormalities associated with defects of chondrocytic primary cilia in Bardet-Biedl syndrome mutant mice. *J Orthop Res* 2009;27(8):1093-1099.

   Wild-type mice and mice bearing mutations in the ciliary proteins Bbs1, Bbs2, and Bbs6 were evaluated with respect to histologic and biochemical differences in chondrocytes from articular cartilage and xiphoid processes. The fraction of ciliated chondrocytes in cultures from mutant mice was significantly lower than in the wild-type cultures ($P < 0.05$). Bbs mutant mice showed significantly thinner articular cartilage ($P < 0.05$) and lower PG content ($P < 0.05$) than wild-type mice.

6. Kiviranta I, Tammi M, Jurvelin J, Säämänen AM, Helminen HJ: Moderate running exercise augments glycosaminoglycans and thickness of articular cartilage in the knee joint of young beagle dogs. *J Orthop Res* 1988; 6(2):188-195.

7. Arokoski J, Kiviranta I, Jurvelin J, Tammi M, Helminen HJ: Long-distance running causes site-dependent decrease of cartilage glycosaminoglycan content in the knee joints of beagle dogs. *Arthritis Rheum* 1993; 36(10):1451-1459.

8. Eckstein F, Guermazi A, Roemer FW: Quantitative MR imaging of cartilage and trabecular bone in osteoarthritis. *Radiol Clin North Am* 2009;47(4):655-673.

   Cartilage measurements at 1.5 or 3 Tesla are technically accurate, reproducible, and sensitive to change. The authors suggest that MRI of articular tissues represents a potent tool in experimental, epidemiologic, and pharmacologic intervention studies.

9. Gratzke C, Hudelmaier M, Hitzl W, Glaser C, Eckstein F: Knee cartilage morphologic characteristics and muscle status of professional weight lifters and sprinters: A magnetic resonance imaging study. *Am J Sports Med* 2007;35(8):1346-1353.

   Fourteen professional athletes (seven weight lifters and seven bobsled sprinters) were examined and compared with 14 nonathletic volunteers who had never performed strength training. Cartilage morphology was assessed with MRI. Patellar cartilage was 14% thicker in athletes than in nonathletes, but there were no significant differences in thickness in other areas of the knee.

10. Chakravarty EF, Hubert HB, Lingala VB, Zatarain E, Fries JF: Long distance running and knee osteoarthritis:

A prospective study. *Am J Prev Med* 2008;35(2):133-138.

The knees of 45 long-distance runners and 53 control subjects with a mean age of 58 years in 1984 were imaged by serial radiography through 2002. Radiographic scores showed little initial OA (6.7% of runners and 0 control subjects) and by the end of the study runners did not have more prevalent OA than did control subjects (*P* = 0.25). In contrast, higher initial body mass index and initial radiographic damage were associated with worse radiographic OA at the final assessment.

11. Sakamoto J, Origuchi T, Okita M, et al: Immobilization-induced cartilage degeneration mediated through expression of hypoxia-inducible factor-1alpha, vascular endothelial growth factor, and chondromodulin-I. *Connect Tissue Res* 2009;50(1):37-45.

    Immobilization effects on cartilage morphology and on the expression of hypoxia inducible factor-1α, VEGF, and the antiangiogenic factor, chondromodulin-I (ChM-1), were studied in ankle joints of 12-week-old rats. Significant thinning of the articular cartilage was noted in immobilized joints and vascular channels were found between calcified cartilage and subchondral bone. Hypoxia inducible factor-1α and VEGF expression increased and ChM-1 expression declined with immobilization.

12. Hinterwimmer S, Krammer M, Krötz M, et al: Cartilage atrophy in the knees of patients after seven weeks of partial load bearing. *Arthritis Rheum* 2004;50(8):2516-2520.

13. Eckstein F, Maschek S, Wirth W, et al; OAI Investigator Group: One year change of knee cartilage morphology in the first release of participants from the Osteoarthritis Initiative progression subcohort: Association with sex, body mass index, symptoms and radiographic osteoarthritis status. *Ann Rheum Dis* 2009;68(5):674-679.

    3T MRI was used to study articular cartilage thinning over 1 year in 79 women and 77 men (mean age 60.9 years) with symptomatic and radiographic knee OA. The greatest rate of cartilage loss (1.9% per year) was observed in the weight-bearing medial femoral condyle. There was a trend toward higher thinning rates in obese participants, but this was not statistically significant.

14. Del Carlo M Jr, Loeser RF: Cell death in osteoarthritis. *Curr Rheumatol Rep* 2008;10(1):37-42.

    Preclinical studies suggest that caspase inhibition, which prevents chondrocyte apoptosis, might slow OA progression. Because of the potential for unwanted systemic side effects from such agents, caspase treatments will likely need to be delivered intra-articularly. Additional interventions will be needed to reverse catabolic-anabolic imbalance in surviving cells.

15. Aigner T, Haag J, Martin J, Buckwalter J: Osteoarthritis: Aging of matrix and cells—going for a remedy. *Curr Drug Targets* 2007;8(2):325-331.

    Aging is the foremost risk factor for OA. This might be attributed to mechanical wear and tear, or the accumulation of time-related modifications of the matrix, or the loss of viable cells over time. However, recent findings support the hypothesis that stressful conditions might promote chondrocyte senescence, which might be of particular importance for the progression of OA. Senescence might someday be targeted for therapeutic intervention.

16. Blom AB, Brockbank SM, van Lent PL, et al: Involvement of the Wnt signaling pathway in experimental and human osteoarthritis: Prominent role of Wnt-induced signaling protein 1. *Arthritis Rheum* 2009;60(2):501-512.

    Wnt-induced signaling protein 1 (WISP-1) expression was strongly increased in the synovium and cartilage of mice with experimental OA. Wnt-16 and Wnt-2B were also markedly upregulated during the course of disease. Interestingly, increased WISP-1 expression was also found in human OA cartilage and synovium. Stimulation of macrophages and chondrocytes with recombinant WISP-1 resulted in IL-1–independent induction of several MMPs and aggrecanase and overexpression of WISP-1 in murine knee joints induced cartilage damage.

17. da Silva MA, Yamada N, Clarke NM, Roach HI: Cellular and epigenetic features of a young healthy and a young osteoarthritic cartilage compared with aged control and OA cartilage. *J Orthop Res* 2009;27(5):593-601.

    Epigenetic features were characterized in hip articular cartilage from patients with primary age-related OA and from a 23-year-old patient with secondary OA due to developmental hip dysplasia. MMP-3, MMP-9, MMP-13, and ADAMTS-4 were immunolocalized and the methylation status of specific promoter CpG sites was determined. Both primary and secondary OA were characterized by loss of aggrecan, formation of clones, and abnormal expression of the proteases that correlated with epigenetic DNA demethylation.

18. Cheung KS, Hashimoto K, Yamada N, Roach HI: Expression of ADAMTS-4 by chondrocytes in the surface zone of human osteoarthritic cartilage is regulated by epigenetic DNA de-methylation. *Rheumatol Int* 2009;29(5):525-534.

    ADAMTS-4, one of the major aggrecanases involved in OA, was nearly absent in control cartilage, but was expressed by numerous chondrocytes in OA cartilage and increased with disease severity. DNA methylation was lost at specific CpG sites in the ADAMTS-4 promoter in OA chondrocytes, suggesting that ADAMTS-4 is epigenetically regulated and plays a role in aggrecan degradation in human OA.

19. Loeser RF: Aging and osteoarthritis: The role of chondrocyte senescence and aging changes in the cartilage matrix. *Osteoarthritis Cartilage* 2009;17(8):971-979.

    Articular chondrocytes exhibit an age-related decline in proliferative and synthetic capacity while maintaining the ability to produce proinflammatory mediators and matrix degrading enzymes. These findings are characteristic of the senescent secretory phenotype and are most likely a consequence of extrinsic stress-induced senescence driven by oxidative stress rather than intrinsic replicative senescence.

1: Principles of Orthopaedics

20. Martin JA, McCabe D, Walter M, Buckwalter JA, McKinley TO: N-acetylcysteine inhibits post-impact chondrocyte death in osteochondral explants. *J Bone Joint Surg Am* 2009;91(8):1890-1897.

Bovine osteochondral explants subjected to a single impact load and treated thereafter with N-acetylcysteine, or a pan-caspase inhibitor, or P-188 surfactant. N-acetylcysteine doubled the number of viable chondrocytes assayed 48 hours after impact, and this effect was significantly greater than that caspase inhibitor or P-188. Moreover, N-acetylcysteine treatment significantly improved PG content at the impact sites at both 6 and 14 days after injury.

21. Khan IM, Williams R, Archer CW: One flew over the progenitor's nest: Migratory cells find a home in osteoarthritic cartilage. *Cell Stem Cell* 2009;4(4):282-284.

In this preview, the authors cite Miosge and colleagues (Koelling et al, 2009) who reported that migratory progenitor cells occupy degenerating OA tissue but that this population is not present in healthy cartilage. Better understanding of this system will enable the manipulation of chondrogenic progenitor cells to fully commit to the chondrogenic phenotype and drive the process of repair and regeneration.

22. Mimeault M, Batra SK: Aging of tissue-resident adult stem/progenitor cells and their pathological consequences. *Panminerva Med* 2009;51(2):57-79.

The fascinating discovery of tissue-resident adult stem/progenitor cells in recent years led to an explosion of interest in the development of novel stem cell–based therapies for improving the regenerative capacity of these endogenous immature cells or transplanted cells for the repair of damaged and diseased tissues. This review discusses therapeutic strategies for treating premature aging and age-related disorders including hematopoietic and immune disorders, heart failure and cardiovascular diseases, neurodegenerative, muscular, and gastrointestinal diseases, atherosclerosis, and aggressive and lethal cancers.

23. Borrelli J Jr, Silva MJ, Zaegel MA, Franz C, Sandell LJ: Single high-energy impact load causes posttraumatic OA in young rabbits via a decrease in cellular metabolism. *J Orthop Res* 2009;27(3):347-352.

A single high-energy impact blow to the medial femoral condyles of young rabbits resulted in histologic signs of articular cartilage degeneration (chondrocyte and PG depletion) at 3 and 6 months postinjury. In situ hybridization revealed that type II collagen and BMP-2 mRNA declined at injury sites at 3 months, suggesting impact-related impairment of anabolic activity.

24. Pascual Garrido C, Hakimiyan AA, Rappoport L, Oegema TR, Wimmer MA, Chubinskaya S: Anti-apoptotic treatments prevent cartilage degradation after acute trauma to human ankle cartilage. *Osteoarthritis Cartilage* 2009;17(9):1244-1251.

Histologic analysis showed that a single impact delivered to human ankle cartilage resulted in chondrocyte death, cartilage degeneration, and spread of apoptosis to areas around the impact site. Inhibitors of caspases-3 and -9 reduced death in the impact site only at early time points, but were ineffective in the area around the site, whereas P-188 prevented cell death in both the impact site and adjacent cartilage.

25. Hurtig M, Chubinskaya S, Dickey J, Rueger D: BMP-7 protects against progression of cartilage degeneration after impact injury. *J Orthop Res* 2009;27(5):602-611.

Impact injuries in sheep stifle joints were treated by two intra-articular injections of BMP-7 (OP-1) at varying times after injury and effects were evaluated after at least 97 days postinjury. Treatment within the first 21 days significantly reduced OA progression, but delaying treatment until 90 days was ineffective. Chondroprotective effects were thought to be due to enhanced chondrocyte survival.

26. Huser CA, Davies ME: Calcium signaling leads to mitochondrial depolarization in impact-induced chondrocyte death in equine articular cartilage explants. *Arthritis Rheum* 2007;56(7):2322-2334.

Transient mitochondrial depolarization was observed in equine cartilage explants subjected to impact. This leads to activation of caspase-9 and apoptosis. Blocking intracellular calcium release from the endoplasmic reticulum, or blocking activation of calcium-dependent kinase or calcium-dependent proteases, inhibited both depolarization and apoptosis.

27. Tellisi N, Fragomen AT, Kleinman D, O'Malley MJ, Rozbruch SR: Joint preservation of the osteoarthritic ankle using distraction arthroplasty. *Foot Ankle Int* 2009;30(4):318-325.

This is a retrospective review of 25 patients who underwent ankle distraction from 1999 to 2006. SF-36 scores showed modest improvement in all components. Only two of the patients in the study underwent fusion after ankle distraction. Total ankle motion was maintained in all patients, with improvement in the functional arc of motion in five patients who started with mild equinus contractures.

28. Burstein D: Tracking longitudinal changes in knee degeneration and repair. *J Bone Joint Surg Am* 2009;91(suppl 1):51-53.

MRI parameters, T2-weighted, T1rho-weighted, and dGEMRIC, enable clinicians to see OA as a regional and responsive (reversible) disease and may lead to new paradigms for developing and applying lifestyle, medical, and surgical therapeutic interventions.

29. Regatte RR, Akella SV, Lonner JH, Kneeland JB, Reddy R: T1rho relaxation mapping in human osteoarthritis (OA) cartilage: Comparison of T1rho with T2. *J Magn Reson Imaging* 2006;23(4):547-553.

30. Gineyts E, Garnero P, Delmas PD: Urinary excretion of glucosyl-galactosyl pyridinoline: A specific biochemical marker of synovium degradation. *Rheumatology (Oxford)* 2001;40(3):315-323.

31. Garnero P, Aronstein WS, Cohen SB, et al: Relationships between biochemical markers of bone and carti-

lage degradation with radiological progression in patients with knee osteoarthritis receiving risedronate: The Knee Osteoarthritis Structural Arthritis randomized clinical trial. *Osteoarthritis Cartilage* 2008;16(6):660-666.

This study (n = 2,483 patients) showed that urinary levels of CTX-II decreased with risedronate in patients with knee OA and levels reached after 6 months were associated with radiologic progression at 24 months.

32. Chu Q, Lopez M, Hayashi K, et al: Elevation of a collagenase generated type II collagen neoepitope and proteoglycan epitopes in synovial fluid following induction of joint instability in the dog. *Osteoarthritis Cartilage* 2002;10(8):662-669.

33. Jordan KM, Syddall HE, Garnero P, et al: Urinary CTX-II and glucosyl-galactosyl-pyridinoline are associated with the presence and severity of radiographic knee osteoarthritis in men. *Ann Rheum Dis* 2006;65(7):871-877.

34. Jones P, Gardner L, Menage J, Williams GT, Roberts S: Intervertebral disc cells as competent phagocytes in vitro: Implications for cell death in disc degeneration. *Arthritis Res Ther* 2008;10(4):R86.

Bovine intervertebral disk cells were competent phagocytes and worked as efficiently as dedicated phagocytes such as monocytes and macrophages in an in vitro model.

35. Jünger S, Gantenbein-Ritter B, Lezuo P, Alini M, Ferguson SJ, Ito K: Effect of limited nutrition on in situ intervertebral disc cells under simulated-physiological loading. *Spine (Phila Pa 1976)* 2009;34(12):1264-1271.

Glucose availability has implications to intervertebral disk cell viability in vitro. With limited availability, cell viability decreased and surviving cells did not compensate matrix production within the time frame studied.

36. Arun R, Freeman BJ, Scammell BE, McNally DS, Cox E, Gowland P: 2009 ISSLS Prize Winner: What influence does sustained mechanical load have on diffusion in the human intervertebral disc? An in vivo study using serial postcontrast magnetic resonance imaging. *Spine (Phila Pa 1976)* 2009;34(21):2324-2337.

Effects of sustained mechanical loading on transport of small solutes was investigated in vivo on normal human lumbar intervertebral disks using serial postcontrast MRI. The results suggested that supine creep loading (50% body weight) for 4.5 hours retards transport of small solutes into the center of human intervertebral disk, and it required 3 hours of accelerated diffusion in recovery state for loaded disks to catch up with diffusion in unloaded disks.

37. Millward-Sadler SJ, Costello PW, Freemont AJ, Hoyland JA: Regulation of catabolic gene expression in normal and degenerate human intervertebral disc cells: Implications for the pathogenesis of intervertebral disc degeneration. *Arthritis Res Ther* 2009;11(3):R65.

In vitro analysis of cells isolated from human IVDs indicated that TNF-α may be an important initiating factor in matrix degeneration, IL-1β plays a greater role in established pathologic degradation.

38. Iida R, Akeda K, Kasai Y, et al: Expression of proteinase-activated receptor-2 in the intervertebral disc. *Spine (Phila Pa 1976)* 2009;34(5):470-478.

Proteinase-activated receptor-2 (PAR-2) is a G protein-coupled receptor identified in human intervertebral disk tissues. The expression of PAR-2 is regulated by IL-1β stimulation. PAR-2 activation accelerates the expression of matrix-degrading enzymes. PAR-2 may play an important role in the cytokine-mediated catabolic cascade and consequently may be involved in intervertebral disk degeneration.

39. Yoshida T, Park JS, Yokosuka K, et al: Up-regulation in receptor for advanced glycation end-products in inflammatory circumstances in bovine coccygeal intervertebral disc specimens in vitro. *Spine (Phila Pa 1976)* 2009; 34(15):1544-1548.

Employing a bovine coccygeal intervertebral disk model, the authors demonstrate that advanced glycation end products (AGEs) and receptors of AGE were localized within the bovine intervertebral disks. AGEs significantly decreased the aggrecan expression in bovine intervertebral disk as in human intervertebral disk, and the effect was enhanced further with the presence of IL-1β.

40. Sharp CA, Roberts S, Evans H, Brown SJ: Disc cell clusters in pathological human intervertebral discs are associated with increased stress protein immunostaining. *Eur Spine J* 2009;18(11):1587-1594.

Based on increased expression of heat shock proteins hsp-27 and -72 in clustered cells of herniated disks, the authors suppose that clustered cells may be mounting a protective response to abnormal environmental factors associated with disk degeneration.

41. Kaneyama S, Nishida K, Takada T, et al: Fas ligand expression on human nucleus pulposus cells decreases with disc degeneration processes. *J Orthop Sci* 2008; 13(2):130-135.

Human nucleus pulposus cells showed strong positive staining for FasL with a significant decrease in FasL expression in the degenerated group compared with the nondegenerated group indicating a potential mechanism of protection of the intervertebral disk against degeneration.

42. Ali R, Le Maitre CL, Richardson SM, Hoyland JA, Freemont AJ: Connective tissue growth factor expression in human intervertebral disc: Implications for angiogenesis in intervertebral disc degeneration. *Biotech Histochem* 2008;83(5):239-245.

Connective tissue growth factor plays a pivotal role in angiogenesis. Increased expression of connective tissue growth factor–degenerated disks within areas of neovascularization may suggest their role in angiogenesis in the human degenerated intervertebral disk.

43. Richardson SM, Knowles R, Tyler J, Mobasheri A, Hoyland JA: Expression of glucose transporters GLUT-1, GLUT-3, GLUT-9 and HIF-1alpha in normal and degenerate human intervertebral disc. *Histochem Cell Biol* 2008;129(4):503-511.

1: Principles of Orthopaedics

Immunohistochemistry showed that human intervertebral disk cells express glucose transporters GLUT-1, -3 and -9 in both the nucleus pulposus and anulus fibrosus with hypoxia inducible factor-1α co-expression only in the nucleus pulposus. GLUT expression also changed as degeneration progressed, suggesting metabolic changes with disease pathology.

44. Heathfield SK, Le Maitre CL, Hoyland JA: Caveolin-1 expression and stress-induced premature senescence in human intervertebral disc degeneration. *Arthritis Res Ther* 2008;10(4):R87.

The expression of caveolin-1 in intervertebral disk tissue and its association with the senescent phenotype suggest that caveolin-1 and stress-induced premature senescence may play a prominent role in the pathogenesis of intervertebral disk degeneration.

45. Gruber HE, Ingram JA, Davis DE, Hanley EN Jr: Increased cell senescence is associated with decreased cell proliferation in vivo in the degenerating human anulus. *Spine J* 2009;9(3):210-215.

Asporin, also known as periodontal ligament-associated protein 1 (PLAP1), reported to have a genetic association with OA. Its D14 allele has recently been found to be associated with lumbar disk degeneration in patients of Asian descent. Immunohistochemical localization of asporin in the disk of Caucasian subjects and the sand rat showed that asporin was present in the outer anulus fibrosus, but not in the nucleus pulposus. Increased expression was observed in degenerated disks when compared to normal disks.

46. Poveda L, Hottiger M, Boos N, Wuertz K: Peroxynitrite induces gene expression in intervertebral disc cells. *Spine (Phila Pa 1976)* 2009;34(11):1127-1133.

Degenerated intervertebral disk tissue showed strong nitrosylation, especially in the nucleus pulposus. Isolated human nucleus pulposus cells showed a strong signal for nitrosylation and intracellular reactive oxygen species on stimulation with peroxynitrite or 3-morpholinosydnonimine (SIN-1), indicating that neutralizing peroxynitrite and its derivatives (for example, via the use of antioxidants) may be a novel treatment option for discogenic back pain.

47. Videman T, Saarela J, Kaprio J, et al: Associations of 25 structural, degradative, and inflammatory candidate genes with lumbar disc desiccation, bulging, and height narrowing. *Arthritis Rheum* 2009;60(2):470-481.

The authors investigated associations of 99 genetic variants with quantitative magnetic resonance imaging measurements. Twelve of the 99 variants in 25 selected candidate genes provided evidence of association ($P < 0.05$) with disk signal intensity in the upper and/or lower lumbar regions. *AGC1, COL1A1, COL9A1,* and *COL11A2* genes provided the most significant evidence of association with disk signal intensity, suggesting that genetic variants account for interindividual differences in disk matrix synthesis and degradation.

48. Gruber HE, Ingram JA, Hoelscher GL, Zinchenko N, Hanley EN Jr, Sun Y: Asporin, a susceptibility gene in osteoarthritis, is expressed at higher levels in the more degenerate human intervertebral disc. *Arthritis Res Ther* 2009;11(2):R47.

Human anulus fibrosus specimens were obtained from surgical subjects and control donors, and showed increased senescent cells with increasing grades of degeneration. A decreasing number of proliferative cells with increasing degeneration provides a rationale for increased incidence of degeneration with aging.

49. Wuertz K, Godburn K, MacLean JJ, et al: In vivo remodeling of intervertebral discs in response to short- and long-term dynamic compression. *J Orthop Res* 2009;27(9):1235-1242.

The authors demonstrate that in vivo dynamic compression maintains or promotes matrix biosynthesis without substantially disrupting disk structural integrity. Static compression, bending, or other interventions created greater structural disruption.

50. Meir A, McNally DS, Fairbank JC, Jones D, Urban JP: The internal pressure and stress environment of the scoliotic intervertebral disc—a review. *Proc Inst Mech Eng H* 2008;222(2):209-219.

With pressure profilometry, which provides stress profiles across the disk in mutually perpendicular axes, the authors show that abnormalities in high hydrostatic pressure profiles could influence both disk and end plate cellular activity directly, causing asymmetric growth and matrix changes.

51. Michalek AJ, Buckley MR, Bonassar LJ, Cohen I, Iatridis JC: Measurement of local strains in intervertebral disc anulus fibrosus tissue under dynamic shear: Contributions of matrix fiber orientation and elastin content. *J Biomech* 2009;42(14):2279-2285.

Alterations in the elastic fiber network, as found with intervertebral disk herniation and degeneration, can significantly influence the anulus fibrosus response to shear loading, making it more susceptible to micro failure under bending or torsion loading.

52. Yang F, Leung VY, Luk KD, Chan D, Cheung KM: Injury-induced sequential transformation of notochordal nucleus pulposus to chondrogenic and fibrocartilaginous phenotype in the mouse. *J Pathol* 2009;218(1):113-121.

This study is the first to use an injury-induced model to study disk degeneration in mouse. The disk degeneration induced using a needle puncture involves a transient transformation of nucleus pulposus from notochordal to chondrogenic and eventually into fibrocartilaginous phenotype, suggesting its relevance to human intervertebral disk pathology.

53. Lotz JC, Hadi T, Bratton C, Reiser KM, Hsieh AH: Anulus fibrosus tension inhibits degenerative structural changes in lamellar collagen. *Eur Spine J* 2008;17(9):1149-1159.

Annular tension is beneficial to maintain healthy lamellar appearance. Cell-mediated events and cell-independent mechanisms may contribute to the protective effect of tissue level tension in the anulus fibrosus.

Chapter 4
Muscle, Tendon, and Ligament

Lawrence V. Gulotta, MD   Scott A. Rodeo, MD

Skeletal Muscle

Structure and Function

The human body contains more than 400 skeletal muscles that comprise approximately 40% to 50% of the total body weight. Skeletal muscle serves to produce the force required for locomotion, breathing, and postural support as well as heat production during cold stress. As with most tissues, its structure is highly organized and accounts for its function. An appreciation of the structure and physiology of skeletal muscle is important because it serves as the foundation for understanding exercise physiology and muscle injuries.

All muscles have a fibrous connective tissue network within and around the muscle that is important for overall function (**Figure 1**). Tendons originate from within the muscle, or from its surface, and provide a wide area for the attachment of muscle fibers. The epimysium is connective tissue that surrounds the entire muscle. This divides the muscle from the surrounding tissues and allows it to glide freely. The perimysium surrounds bundles of muscle fibers, called fascicles, and the endomysium surrounds each individual muscle fiber. This framework is continuous within the muscle and attaches to the tendon to increase the efficiency of movement.

The microstructure of skeletal muscle is complex and accounts for the muscle's ability to contract. During development, many muscle cells, called myoblasts, fuse to form myofibrils. Because myofibrils are not made up of a single cell, the nomenclature and structure is different than that of a normal cell. As such, the plasma membrane is referred to as the sarcolemma, the endoplasmic reticulum as the sarcoplasmic reticulum, the mitochondria as the sarcosome, and the cytoplasm as the sarcoplasm. Additionally, myofibrils are made up of many nuclei. Each myofibril is made up of arrays of parallel filaments. The thick filaments are composed of the protein myosin. Thin filaments are primarily composed of the proteins actin, troponin, and tropomyosin.

The characteristic striations of skeletal muscle seen with microscopy are the result of alternating light and dark bands of the myofibril. The light band, called the I band, is made up of thin filaments. The dark band, called the A band, is made up of thick filaments.

Sarcomeres are the repeating subunit of a myofibril and are considered the smallest contractile unit of muscle. Perpendicular protein plates, called Z lines, form the boundaries of a sarcomere. From these Z lines, thin filaments extend inward toward the center of the sarcomere where they partially overlap with the thick filaments. M line proteins attach the thick myosin filaments to each other that aid in filament stabilization. Actin proteins have binding sites for a myosin crossbridge, or head. When a muscle fiber is at rest, the myosin binding sites are covered by tropomyosin proteins. These proteins are associated with troponin, another regulatory protein. When calcium is released from the sarcoplasmic reticulum in response to an action potential, it binds to troponin, causing tropomyosin to move away from the myosin binding site. This allows myosin to bind to actin at the expense of an adenosine triphosphate (ATP) molecule. Once bound to actin, the myosin head swivels and pulls the actin filament toward it, resulting in a contraction. During this process, the distance between Z lines is decreased. This process is referred to as the sliding filament model of muscle contraction.[1]

The signal for skeletal muscle contraction originates from nerves at the motor end plate. The end plate is a pocket of sarcolemma that forms around the motor neuron. The number of nerve fibers controlled by a single motor end plate is highly variable. Muscle contraction is initiated when acetylcholine is released from the motor neuron resulting in an end-plate action potential that spreads along the surface membrane (sarcolemma) and the transverse tubular system (T tubules) until it reaches the sarcoplasmic reticulum. Once stimulated by the action potential, the sarcoplasmic reticulum releases the calcium, initiating a contraction as outlined above. The greater the number of actin-myosin crossbridges that form, the greater the force of the contraction. Therefore, the peak force a muscle can generate is directly related to the physiologic cross-sectional area of all the fibers.

Muscle is made up of various types of fibers that have different functional properties, peak forces, contraction velocities, resistances to fatigue, and oxidative and glycolytic capacities. These fiber types can be

---

Dr. Rodeo or an immediate family member serves as a paid consultant to or is an employee of Wyeth. Neither Dr. Gulotta nor an immediate family member has received anything of value from or owns stock in a commercial company or institution related directly or indirectly to the subject of this chapter.

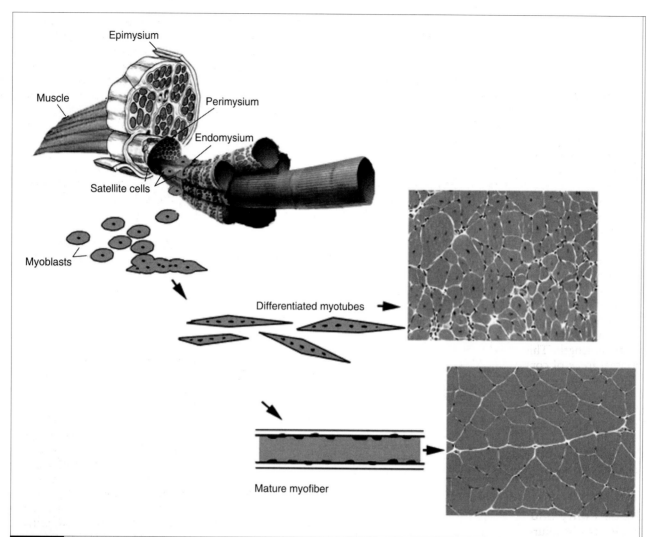

Figure 1   Schematic drawing of the structure of skeletal muscle. The endomysium is the connective tissue layer that surrounds the individual myofibers. The perimysium surrounds fascicles of myofibers. The epimysium is the outermost connective tissue layer that surrounds the entire muscle. When muscle is injured, satellite cells differentiate into myoblasts and then into differentiated myotubes and finally into mature myofibers. The histologic panels show the central location of nuclei in the immature or regenerating myotubes, but migrate to the periphery of the myofiber as it matures. (Reproduced from Beason DP, Soslowski LJ, Karthikeyan T, Huard J: Muscle, tendon, and ligament, in Fischgrund JS, ed: *Orthopaedic Knowledge Update 9*. Rosemont, IL. American Academy of Orthopaedic Surgeons, 2008, pp 35-48.)

broadly characterized into two major classes, fast twitch and slow twitch (**Table 1**). Slow-twitch fibers are also called type I fibers. They have a slow contraction velocity but are relatively fatigue resistant. They have long twitch times, low peak forces, a high concentration of oxidative enzymes and myoglobin, and a low concentration of glycolytic markers. Their high oxidative capacity makes them appear red under the microscope. Type I fibers are used for aerobic activities requiring low-level force production, such as walking or maintaining posture. Fast-twitch fibers are also called type II fibers. They have a fast contraction velocity due to a faster rate of calcium release from the sarcoplasmic reticulum and higher levels of myosin ATPase. Type II fibers can be further subclassified into two groups.

Table 1

The Three Main Types of Myofibers and Their Characteristics

Fiber Type	Contraction Velocity	Fatigue Resistance
Type I	Slow	Greatest
Type II A	Fast	Intermediate
Type II B	Fast	Least

[Handwritten margin note at top: isotonic contractions: can be either concentric or eccentric contractions, e.g. lifting & lowering dumbells. isokinetic contractions: muscle also Δ's length, but same speed, e.g. stationary bike]

Type IIA fibers have a fast contraction velocity and are moderately fatigue resistant. These fibers represent a transition between the slow type I fibers and the type IIB fibers. They are used for prolonged anaerobic activities with relatively high force output, such as a 400-m run. Type IIB fibers also have a fast contraction velocity, but they have low fatigue resistance. They are used for short, anaerobic, high-force production activities such as sprinting or lifting weights. Most muscles contain a combination of these fibers.

Muscles do not necessarily have to shorten to generate a force. Eccentric contractions occur when the muscle fibers lengthen as the muscle contracts. This occurs when the force generated by the muscle is not enough to overcome the external load. This type of contraction puts the most stress on muscles and is the most common mechanism for muscular and tendinous injuries. Isometric contractions, also called static contractions, occur when the muscle does not change length. In this case, the force generated by the muscle is equivalent to the external load. Isotonic contractions occur when the tension in the muscle remains constant despite a change in muscle length. This can occur only when a muscle's maximal force of contraction exceeds the total load on the muscle (the weight lifted). An isokinetic contraction occurs when there is a constant force applied through a full range of motion. Because velocity does not change during this contraction, kinetic energy remains constant. Muscles also undergo concentric contraction in which the muscle shortens as it contracts. In this case, the force generated by the muscle is greater than the external load.

Muscle Injury and Repair

Muscles can be injured by direct trauma, disease, medications, ischemia, and certain exercises, most notably ones that require eccentric contraction. Muscles that span two joints, such as the hamstrings and gastrocnemius, are particularly susceptible to injury. These injuries most commonly occur at the musculotendinous junction or the tendon-bone junction. Regardless of the insult, the muscle's response to injury can be broken down into four phases: necrosis, inflammation, repair, and fibrosis[2] (**Figure 2**). In the first phase, necrosis and degeneration of myofibrils occur due to breakdown of the sarcolemma, causing an ingress of calcium that results in fiber death. The injury site is then invaded by inflammatory cells, notably macrophages and T lymphocytes, that phagocytose and remove the debris created during the first phase. The inflammatory cells secrete growth factors and cytokines that promote vascularity and the migration of more inflammatory mediators. Muscle regeneration does not occur until phagocytic cells have cleared the necrotic debris. Blunting the inflammatory response (such as with nonsteroidal anti-inflammatory drugs [NSAIDs]) may have a detrimental effect on muscle healing by reducing the amount of growth factors secreted by macrophages.[3-5] These growth factors are thought to promote myoblast proliferation and regeneration and are essential for

muscle healing. Muscle regeneraion begins within 7 to 10 days from the time of injury, peaks at 2 weeks, and declines after 3 to 4 weeks. This process is mediated by several trophic substances such as insulin growth factor-I (IGF-I), basic fibroblast growth factor (bFGF), and nerve growth factor (NGF), that are released by the injured cells and stimulate differentiation, proliferation, and fusion of myoblasts from the satellite cells located between the basal lamina and the plasma membrane of individual myofibrils. At the same time as regeneration, fibrosis also occurs. Fibrosis has been shown to occur in the presence of transforming growth factor–β1 (TGF-β1). TGF-β1 promotes differentiation and proliferation of myofibroblasts that in turn produce abundant amounts of types I and III collagen. During the repair process, muscle regeneration and fibrosis compete for muscle area. Unfortunately, scar tissue, which has inferior mechanical and contractile properties than that of normal tissue, is usually predominant.

A few circumstances of muscle injury deserve special attention. Muscle lacerations heal by dense scar formation and no muscle regenerates across the injured tissue.[6] Therefore, functional continuity is not restored and the muscle lacks the ability to produce tension. Muscle contusions, which are often seen in contact sports, result in hematoma formation and inflammation. A potential complication of muscle contusions is myositis ossificans, or the calcification or ossification of tissue at the site of injury.[7] The pathogenesis is poorly understood, but may involve release of osteoblastic growth factors in the presence of muscle-derived stem cells. A major risk for the development of myositis ossificans is reinjury in the early stages of recovery. A third type of muscular injury is the fatty degeneration that occurs following tendon detachment, as seen in chronic rotator cuff tears. The exact cause is not fully appreciated, but one hypothesis is that this is caused by an increase in the space between muscle fibers that allows fat to form.[8] Regardless of the cause, fatty degeneration makes the muscle-tendon unit less compliant, thereby putting tension on repairs. This increased tension is thought to make repairs prone to failure.

New Developments in the Treatment of Muscle Injuries

The mainstay of treatment of most muscular injuries is rest, ice, compression, elevation, NSAIDs, and mobilization. However, healing occurs slowly and is often incomplete. Therapies that can augment the healing process and drive it toward regeneration and away from scar formation would improve functional outcomes.[2,9] Strategies to achieve these goals can be broadly grouped according to those that limit fibrosis and those that promote regeneration.

Antifibrotic agents such as decorin,[10] relaxin,[11] γ interferon,[12] and the antiparasitic drug suramin[13] have all been shown to limit the amount of fibrosis associated with muscle healing by inhibiting TGF-β1. However,

[Vertical text in right margin: 1: Principles of Orthopaedics]

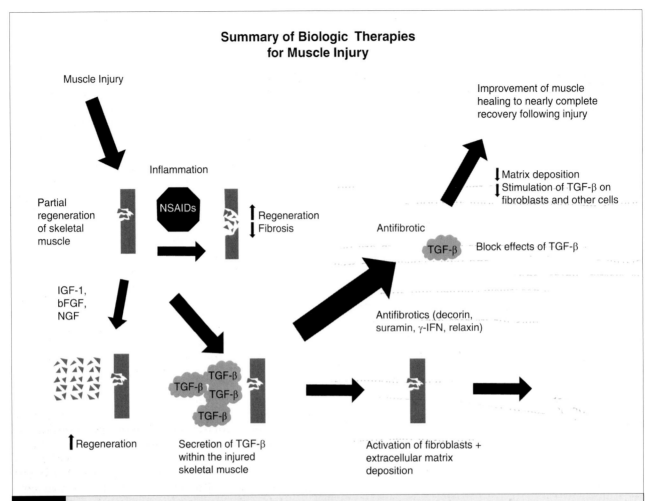

Summary of Biologic Therapies for Muscle Injury

Figure 2	Summary of biologic strategies to improve muscle healing. Following the initial injury, inflammation occurs. This appears to be a crucial step because NSAIDs appear to inhibit healing. Various growth factors such as IGF-1, bFGF, and NGF may play a role in enhancing regeneration. Following inflammation and regeneration, TGF-β1 is released that induces fibrosis. Antifibrotic factors such as decorin, relaxin, suramin, and γ-interferon (γ-IFN) may inhibit TGF-β1, thereby limiting fibrosis and improving the healing process. (Reproduced from Beason DP, Soslowski LJ, Karthikeyan T, Huard J: Muscle, tendon, and ligament, in Fischgrund JS, ed: *Orthopaedic Knowledge Update 9*. Rosemont, IL. American Academy of Orthopaedic Surgeons, 2008, pp 35-48.)

these studies have only been conducted in animal models, and each of these agents has technical obstacles or severe adverse effects that would make their application to human patients difficult. Interestingly, the antihypertensive agent losartan has been shown to have significant antifibrotic effects. Losartan is a widely used angiotensin II receptor blocker (ARB) that also inhibits TGF-β1–mediated fibrosis in vitro and in vivo. One mouse study showed that the administration of losartan immediately following gastrocnemius laceration resulted in a dose-dependent increase in the number of regenerating myofibers and a decrease in fibrosis compared to controls at 3 and 5 weeks.[14] Although these basic science studies are encouraging, trials in human patients are needed to recommend them for the augmentation of muscle healing and repair.

Exogenously administered growth factors and stem cells may be able to promote muscle regeneration. IGF-I and bFGF have both been shown to increase the number and diameter of regenerating myofibers in a mouse gastrocnemius laceration model.[15] Muscle-derived stem cells (MDSCs) are multipotent stem cells found between the basal lamina and sarcolemma that are able to double 300 times before becoming senescent (compared with embryonic stem cells that double 130 to 250 times).[9] For these reasons, they provide great promise for muscle regeneration. Applications to the musculoskeletal system have been limited to animal models that have shown improved muscle quality when administered in models with Duchenne muscular dystrophy, and better muscle integrity when given in an ischemia model.[16] Clinical studies using MDSCs have shown that they can improve the symptoms of urinary stress incontinence when implanted in the detrusor muscle in a small group of women.[17] Future studies will focus on bioengineered scaffolds that are either impregnated with MDSCs, or with factors that are capable of recruiting host MDSCs. Furthermore, these cells can be genetically modified to overexpress growth factors at the healing site.

Tendon and Ligament

Structure and Function

In the simplest sense, tendons are the connective tissue structures that serve to transmit force from skeletal muscle to bone whereas ligaments connect one bone to another. However, their function is much more complex. Ligaments help guide the three-dimensional motion of the bones during joint function and therefore carry loads during daily activities. An understanding of the structure and composition of these materials is important to understanding their function. Both are primarily composed of water and type I collagen, as well as elastin, lipids, and several types of proteoglycans. Proteoglycans are negatively charged and attract water into the structure. The accumulation of water into the tissue largely accounts for its rate-dependent response to load, or viscoelasticity.[18] However, recent evidence suggests that viscoelasticity is also dependent on the cross-sectional area of the tissue tested, whereas smaller diameter tissues exhibit a higher tensile modulus, a slower rate of relaxation, and a lower amount of relaxation in comparison to larger specimens.[19] The exact reason for this is uncertain.

Although both are similar in terms of their structure and biomechanical properties, differences between tendons and ligaments do exist. Tendons contain less elastin than ligaments. Although most ligaments contain little elastin, some, like the ligamentum flava in the spine, have a relatively high content. However, the exact elastin content in most ligaments is unknown as is its exact function within the tissue. Ligaments also contain relatively less proteoglycan matrix than tendons. Tendons are also composed primarily of densely packed collagen fibrils in cords, whereas the collagen fibrils in ligaments are slightly less in volume fraction and are less organized.

Tendons also differ from ligaments in that they are surrounded by a synovial-like membrane called the epitenon. The epitenon contains lymphatic vessels, blood vessels, and nerves. Some tendons have a loose areolar tissue around the epitenon called the paratenon, whereas in other tendons the paratenon is replaced by a bursa that is lined with synovial cells. Tendons receive nutrition through several sources such as the perimysium, periosteal attachments, and surrounding tissues. There is a distinction between vascular and relatively avascular tendons. Vascular tendons receive their blood supply directly from the vessels that run in their surrounding paratenon. Relatively avascular tendons are contained in tendinous sheaths and receive nutrition from vascular mesotenons called vincula. In addition to the vincula, these tendons receive blood from the musculotendinous and tendon-bone junctions. Tendons can also receive nutrition through diffusion from synovial fluid. Tendons that are intrasynovial, such as the flexor tendons of the hand, have different characteristics than those that are extrasynovial, such as the peroneal tendons around the ankle. Intrasynoval tendons are dependent on nutrition from the synovial fluid, and their ability to proliferate and remain metabolically active is decreased when removed from that environment. Extrasynovial tendons, on the other hand, are able to remain metabolically viable regardless of their environment.[20] Exactly what accounts for these differences is not known at this time.

The exact manner in which ligaments receive their nutrition is uncertain because most ligaments have not been studied. Some ligaments receive a direct supply from an artery, such as the anterior cruciate ligament (ACL), that receives nutrients from the middle geniculate artery. Most ligaments have an epiligament coat that is analogous to the epitenon seen in tendons. Ligaments that do not have an epiligament are usually surrounded by synovium, such as the ACL. It is thought that ligaments receive much of the nutrients needed from these surrounding structures.

Tendon and ligament insertions into bone can be classified as being either indirect (or fibrous) or direct (or fibrocartilaginous). In indirect insertion sites, the collagen fibers of the tendon or ligament enter the bone through perforating collagen fibers (called Sharpey fibers) that are oriented perpendicular to the bone. At the insertion, the endotenon becomes continuous with the periosteum. An example of an indirect insertion site is the distal insertion of the medial collateral ligament (MCL) of the knee onto the proximal tibia. In direct insertion sites, the tendon enters bone through a highly organized fibrocartilaginous transition zone that consists of four layers: tendon, unmineralized fibrocartilage, mineralized fibrocartilage, and bone. This structure allows force to be dissipated gradually as it passes from the tendon to the bone. An example of a direct insertion site is the proximal insertion of the MCL on the distal femur.

The molecular structure of tendons and ligaments is largely responsible for their biomechanical function of load transmission, as well as their characteristic response to tensile testing in the laboratory. Tendons have a stress-strain relationship similar but not identical to ligaments. They exhibit time-dependent, nonlinear viscoelastic properties such as stress relaxation (decreased stress with time under constant deformation) and creep (increased deformation with time under a constant load). Another characteristic of a viscoelastic tissue that is exhibited by ligaments and tendons is hysteresis, or energy dissipation. This means that when tissues are loaded and unloaded, the unloading curve will not follow the loading curve where the difference between the two curves is the energy that is dissipated during loading.

Structural properties of the tissue can be determined by studying the load-elongation curve. Tensile testing reveals four distinct regions on the graph that correspond to the molecular structure of the ligament (**Figure 3**). The first region is the toe region, in which there is significant deformation for a given load. In the toe

1: Principles of Orthopaedics

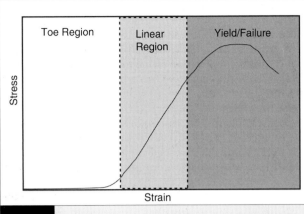

| **Figure 3** | Typical load-elongation curve for biomechanical testing of a tendon/ligament. This outlines the toe, linear, and yield/failure regions. (Reproduced from Beason DP, Soslowski LJ, Karthikeyan T, Huard J: Muscle, tendon, and ligament, in Fischgrund JS, ed: *Orthopaedic Knowledge Update 9*. Rosemont, IL. American Academy of Orthopaedic Surgeons, 2008, pp 35-48.) |

region, the crimped and relaxed fibers of the ligament are straightened and oriented to take up load. The second region is the linear region, in which the fibers are oriented longitudinal and parallel to the direction of the load. In this region, there is constant load-elongation behavior, and the tissue stiffness is represented by the slope of the load-elongation curve. The final region is nonlinear and begins at the yield point, which is the point where the tendon transitions from elastic (reversible) into plastic (irreversible) deformation. The final area of the curve is the ultimate failure of the tendon and is heralded by a steep decline in the load-deformation curve.

The material properties of the tendon are represented by the stress-strain curve. The stress on the tissue is the force per unit area, whereas strain is the change in length relative to the original length. The slope of the linear portion of this curve is the Young modulus of elasticity. The material properties of repaired ligaments and tendons are important because they signify how strong the actual tissue is. Many biologic therapies that have been investigated for their ability to improve the strength of repairs result in improved structural properties. They do this by promoting the formation of more scar tissue. However, an analysis of the material properties shows that this tissue has inferior quality.

Differences between tendons and ligaments can be seen in their stress-strain behavior, which depends on their exact physiologic roles. Tendons carry higher loads and thus recruit fibers much more quickly; therefore, they have a smaller "toe region." Ligaments, on the other hand, have a longer "toe region" in uniaxial testing because their fibers have more of a wavy, crimped pattern and are recruited more gradually. Although uniaxial testing in vitro can determine some of the characteristics of ligaments, how they respond in

vivo is unclear. This is especially true for ligaments that are composed of different bundles that take up load in various joint positions, such as the ACL and the posterior cruciate ligaments. These physiologic characteristics are important for understanding injury patterns, diagnosis, and surgical reconstruction.

Tendon Injury and Repair

Tendon ruptures or lacerations can be divided into those that require tendon-tendon healing, such as flexor tendon repairs in the hand, and those that require tendon-bone healing, such as rotator cuff repairs. Similar to muscle, both types of healing follow the stages of inflammation, cellular proliferation, matrix formation, and remodeling. During the inflammatory phase, there is an influx of neutrophils and macrophages into the zone of injury. During this phase, there is abundant production of type III collagen that is replaced over the course of a few weeks with type I collagen. Tendons are thought to be weakest between 5 to 21 days following repair that correlates with the inflammatory stage. Inflammatory cells and platelets then release several growth factors, such as TGF-β1, IGF, platelet-derived growth factor (PDGF), bone morphogenetic proteins (BMPs)-12 and -13, and bFGF, and IGF-1, for example.[21] These factors promote the differentiation and proliferation of fibroblasts that begin the reparative process. During this phase, there is a noticeable increase in cellularity and vascularity. In the final stage, remodeling, cellularity decreases and fibrosis ensues. The tissue continues to remodel over the course of 1 year or longer, but at its conclusion the tissue never assumes the preinjury appearance. In tendon-bone healing, the bone grows into the fibrovascular scar tissue over time.[22] This bone ingrowth coincides with significant increases in the strength of the healing tendon attachment. Tendons and ligaments heal with persistent scar tissue at the repair site that limits the ultimate strength of the repair and causes adhesions.

There is a fine balance between limiting load across the repair to allow healing to occur and encouraging motion to limit adhesions and fibrosis and enhance the remodeling phase of healing. Studies have shown that stress deprivation of tendons results in increases in cellular apoptosis and the presence of matrix-degrading enzymes.[23,24] Immobilization has also been shown to decrease the release of growth factors such as bFGF, NGF, and IGF-1[25] and decrease the expression of genes associated with tendon regeneration such as procollagen I, cartilage oligomeric matrix protein, tenascin-C, tenomodulin, and scleraxis.[26] Some amount of load is clearly beneficial during the healing process. These basic science studies support the early initiation of gentle range of motion following tendon repairs. However, the amount and timing of application of load that is beneficial before becoming detrimental has yet to be determined.

Several clinically relevant factors have also been shown to influence tendon and ligament healing. Smoking; NSAIDs such as indocin, celecoxib, and parecoxib;

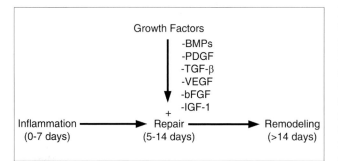

Figure 4 The stages of tendon and ligament healing involve inflammation, repair, and remodeling. Growth factors are expressed during the repair phase because they promote cell proliferation and matrix production. This timeline must be kept in mind in growth factor therapies because the addition of growth factors too early or late in the healing process may decrease their effectiveness. (Reproduced with permission from Gulotta L, Rodeo S: Growth factors for rotator cuff repair. *Clin Sports Med* 2009;28(1):13-23. http://www.sciencedirect.com/science/journal/02785919.)

diabetes; and ethanol intake all have led to adverse effects on healing following rotator cuff repairs in rats.[27-32] The effects these factors have in patients remains to be seen.

New Developments in the Treatment of Tendon and Ligament Injuries

Several biologic strategies have been used in the laboratory to augment tendon and ligament healing. These strategies include those that limit inflammation and fibrosis and those that promote regeneration[33] (**Figure 4**). Several studies have shown that blunting the immune response can actually improve tendon healing. Knockout mice for CD44, a surface receptor crucial for lymphocyte activation, experienced better healing after patellar tendon injury.[34] Interleukin-10 (IL-10) is a potent anti-inflammatory cytokine that has been shown to improve healing when applied through lentivirus to injured patellar tendons.[35] The depletion of macrophages, the main source for the profibrotic growth factor TGF-β1, resulted in improved tendon-bone healing in a rat ACL model.[36] IL-1 is another inflammatory mediator present in healing tendons and ligaments. Its blockade with an IL-1 receptor antagonist inhibited the deterioration of mechanical properties of stress-shielded patellar tendons in a rabbit model.[37] Although it appears that blunting of the inflammatory response may be beneficial for healing, it is unclear what role this strategy will play in the treatment of patients who undergo tendon or ligament repairs.

Regenerative strategies have focused on the use of mesenchymal stem cells (MSCs) to promote healing. MSCs are pluripotent cells that differentiate into muscle, adipose, tendon, ligament, bone and cartilage tissues. Studies have shown that bone, marrow–derived MSCs can improve healing of a tendon graft in a bone tunnel in rabbit and rat models based on the improved formation of the fibrocartilaginous transition zone with histology.[38-40] Another study showed that MSCs were able to promote healing of partial tears of the superficial digital flexor tendons of racehorses based on ultrasound evaluation of the tendons.[41] Although MSCs may improve tendon healing in a bone tunnel and tendon-tendon healing, these positive findings were not found in a rat model of rotator cuff repair.[42] For this instance, in which the repair site has relatively little tendon-bone surface area and is exposed to high shear stresses, MSCs alone may be insufficient. A signal, by way of a growth or differentiation factor, is most likely needed to maximize the effect.

Several growth factors have been evaluated for their ability to augment tendon and ligament healing. In an animal model of flexor tendon repair, PDGF-BB delivered in a fibrin/heparin-based carrier was able to increase cellular proliferation and activity and limit adhesions.[43] However, no improvement in tensile strength was observed. Granulocyte colony-stimulating factor improved tendon incorporation into a bone tunnel in a dog model for ACL reconstruction.[44] BMPs-2 and -12 have also shown improved healing in animal rotator cuff repair models based on structural biomechanical properties.[45,46] Although the application of various growth factors has shown improvements in the structural properties of the repairs, it has been difficult to demonstrate an increase in the material properties. These growth factors are already present during the normal healing process that results in fibrosis.[33] Therefore, it stands to reason that the exogenous application of more growth factors will result in more fibrosis. Although an increase in fibrosis does provide greater mechanical strength, it comes at the hypothetical price of increased adhesions and impingement. Therapies that exploit the biology of tendon and ligament development during embryogenesis may provide the best hope of promoting regeneration of the repaired tissue. However, research into this field is still in its infancy.

It appears that some combination of progenitor cells and growth or differentiation factors will be required to augment tendon and ligament repairs. Even when the proper combination is determined, there will be a challenge to deliver them to the repair site. Several scaffolds are currently being investigated that are designed to allow cell seeding and sustained-release growth factor delivery. One such scaffold has been used to promote primary ACL healing. The ACL has very little capacity to heal itself, which is why ligament reconstruction is the mainstay of treatment. Factors that prohibit healing are a lack of formation of a blood clot at the rupture site to serve as a scaffold for repair and its intra-articular location that contains several matrix-degrading enzymes. Research on primary ACL repair has focused on applying a scaffold with similar characteristics to the fibrin clot that normally forms to promote healing elsewhere in the body.[47] The leading scaffold is a collagen–platelet-rich plasma hydrogel. Platelets release more than 20 known cytokines in a se-

1: Principles of Orthopaedics

quential fashion to promote healing. The collagen in the system stimulates platelets.[48] Studies on the use of this scaffold in a porcine ACL transection model have shown encouraging results.[49] Although the scaffold-enhanced repairs showed improved healing over suture repair alone, the final results were far from native ACL strength.

An interesting new area of research into tendon and ligament healing has focused on the role of neuropeptides. Denervation degrades tendons and ligaments and impairs ligament healing.[50] In vitro studies have shown that the application of neuropeptides such as substance P, neuropeptide Y, and calcitonin gene-related peptide to cultured fibroblasts increased the expression of several inflammatory mediators that may be responsible for initiating the healing cascade.[51] Other studies have found that calcitonin gene-related peptide can improve healing in a medial collateral ligament transection model in a rabbit.[52] The role and extent to which these neuropeptides play in tendon and ligament healing has yet to be determined.

Tendinopathy

In patients with chronic tendon pain, the pathology is usually secondary to a degenerative process caused in part by diminished blood flow, though the exact mechanism is still unknown. A recent study has shown evidence that microscopic collagen fiber failure may lead to local stress deprivation that causes the upregulation of catabolic matrix metalloproteinases (MMPs).[53] Regardless of the cause, the formation of free radicals causes cellular apoptosis and the further release of MMPs. Histologic studies have shown the primary pathology is not inflammation. Instead of inflammatory cells, samples of diseased tendons show collagen degeneration, fiber disorientation, mucoid ground substance, hypercellularity, vascular ingrowth, and relative absence of inflammatory cells under light microscopy. Therefore, the terms tendinopathy or tendinosis have replaced tendinitis. The term angiofibroblastic hyperplasia has been used to refer to the hypercellularity and vascular ingrowth that is seen in biopsy specimens.

The mainstay of treatment of tendinopathy is NSAIDs and physical therapy.[54] Physical therapy should focus on controlled exercise with eccentric loading. Corticosteroid injections are another popular treatment option. However, studies have shown that steroid injections can decrease tenocyte proliferation, increase the amount of type III collagen present, and decrease the mechanical strength of the tendon.[55,56] Although they remain a relatively safe and effective treatment, their use should be minimized whenever possible, as there are currently few data to support corticosteroid injection for tendinopathy. Other treatments such as nitric oxide patches,[57] shock wave therapy,[58,59] the MMP inhibitor aprotinin,[60] and platelet-rich plasma injections[61,62] have all been investigated and give inconsistent results. Clearly, further study is required in this area.

Summary

Muscles, tendons, and ligaments are soft-tissue structures that work in concert to promote locomotion. Skeletal muscle is a complex tissue in which the macrostructures and microstructures reflect its specialized function. Tendons and ligaments are also specialized structures that are capable of withstanding high tensile loads from the muscle to the bone or from one bone to another, respectively. The microscopic structure of tendons and ligaments explains its response to tensile loading in the laboratory. All three tissues have a very similar response to injury. They undergo a period of degeneration and inflammation, followed by cell proliferation and matrix synthesis, remodeling, and fibrosis. Unfortunately, the end result of the healing process is predominated by fibrosis that makes the tissue weaker and less functional. Therapies that can promote the regeneration of the native tissue and limit the inflammation and resulting fibrosis would have a profound effect on the treatment of these injuries. In addition to determining the correct combination of cells and signals required to improve healing, the challenge of delivering them to the repair site remains. Bioengineered scaffolds are currently being designed to achieve this goal. However, most of the research on muscle, tendon, and ligament augmentation remains in the laboratory, with clinical application still years away.

Annotated References

1. Huxley AF: The origin of force in skeletal muscle. *Ciba Found Symp* 1975;31:271-290.

2. Huard J: Regenerative medicine based on muscle stem cells. *J Musculoskelet Neuronal Interact* 2008;8(4):337.

   This is a review paper that outlines research into the use of muscle stem cells and future directions.

3. Shen W, Prisk V, Li Y, Foster W, Huard J: Inhibited skeletal muscle healing in cyclooxygenase-2 gene-deficient mice: The role of PGE2 and PGF2alpha. *J Appl Physiol* 2006;101(4):1215-1221.

4. Shen W, Li Y, Zhu J, Schwendener R, Huard J: Interaction between macrophages, TGF-beta1, and the COX-2 pathway during the inflammatory phase of skeletal muscle healing after injury. *J Cell Physiol* 2008;214(2):405-412.

   This study showed that macrophage depletion in a muscle injury model was detrimental to healing, thereby indicating a role for macrophages in the healing process. Furthermore, it showed that prostaglandin-E$_2$ can inhibit the expression of TGF-β1 and limit that amount of fibrosis. This implies that NSAIDs may be detrimental to muscle healing by increasing the amount TGF-β1 and resulting fibrosis.

5. Shen W, Li Y, Tang Y, Cummins J, Huard J: NS-398, a cyclooxygenase-2-specific inhibitor, delays skeletal mus-

cle healing by decreasing regeneration and promoting fibrosis. *Am J Pathol* 2005;167(4):1105-1117.

6. Garrett WE Jr, Seaber AV, Boswick J, Urbaniak JR, Goldner JL: Recovery of skeletal muscle after laceration and repair. *J Hand Surg Am* 1984;9(5):683-692.

7. Jackson DW, Feagin JA: Quadriceps contusions in young athletes: Relation of severity of injury to treatment and prognosis. *J Bone Joint Surg Am* 1973;55(1): 95-105.

8. Meyer DC, Hoppeler H, von Rechenberg B, Gerber C: A pathomechanical concept explains muscle loss and fatty muscular changes following surgical tendon release. *J Orthop Res* 2004;22(5):1004-1007.

9. Quintero AJ, Wright VJ, Fu FH, Huard J: Stem cells for the treatment of skeletal muscle injury. *Clin Sports Med* 2009;28(1):1-11.

   Another review paper that nicely outlines the role of stem cells for the treatment of skeletal muscle repair.

10. Li Y, Li J, Zhu J, et al: Decorin gene transfer promotes muscle cell differentiation and muscle regeneration. *Mol Ther* 2007;15(9):1616-1622.

    This study showed that decorin gene transfer into myoblasts differentiated into myotubules at a higher rate than cells that did not undergo gene transfer. These cells displayed upregulation of myogenic genes Myf5, Myf6, MyoD, and myogenin. Therefore, decorin not only limits inflammation via inhibition of TGF-β1 but may also promote myoblast differentiation.

11. Negishi S, Li Y, Usas A, Fu FH, Huard J: The effect of relaxin treatment on skeletal muscle injuries. *Am J Sports Med* 2005;33(12):1816-1824.

12. Foster W, Li Y, Usas A, Somogyi G, Huard J: Gamma interferon as an antifibrosis agent in skeletal muscle. *J Orthop Res* 2003;21(5):798-804.

13. Nozaki M, Li Y, Zhu J, et al: Improved muscle healing after contusion injury by the inhibitory effect of suramin on myostatin, a negative regulator of muscle growth. *Am J Sports Med* 2008;36(12):2354-2362.

    Suramin was injected into the tibialis anterior muscle of mice 2 weeks following injury and was found to improve overall skeletal muscle healing. In an in vitro arm of the study, suramin enhanced myoblast and MDSC differentiation, which may explain the in vivo findings.

14. Bedair HS, Karthikeyan T, Quintero A, Li Y, Huard J: Angiotensin II receptor blockade administered after injury improves muscle regeneration and decreases fibrosis in normal skeletal muscle. *Am J Sports Med* 2008; 36(8):1548-1554.

    Mice underwent partial laceration of their gastrocnemius muscles and then were given the angiotensin II receptor blocker losartan or tap water. Those that received losartan healed with reduced fibrosis and an increased number of myofibers.

15. Menetrey J, Kasemkijwattana C, Day CS, et al: Growth factors improve muscle healing in vivo. *J Bone Joint Surg Br* 2000;82(1):131-137.

16. Bachrach E, Perez AL, Choi YH, et al: Muscle engraftment of myogenic progenitor cells following intraarterial transplantation. *Muscle Nerve* 2006;34(1):44-52.

17. Carr LK, Steele D, Steele S, et al: 1-year follow-up of autologous muscle-derived stem cell injection pilot study to treat stress urinary incontinence. *Int Urogynecol J Pelvic Floor Dysfunct* 2008;19(6):881-883.

    This is a report of 1-year follow-up of eight women who underwent injection of autologous muscle-derived stem cells into the detrusor muscle for stress incontinence. Five of eight women had improvement in symptoms.

18. Thornton GM, Shrive NG, Frank CB: Altering ligament water content affects ligament pre-stress and creep behaviour. *J Orthop Res* 2001;19(5):845-851.

19. Atkinson TS, Ewers BJ, Haut RC: The tensile and stress relaxation responses of human patellar tendon varies with specimen cross-sectional area. *J Biomech* 1999; 32(9):907-914.

20. Abrahamsson SO, Gelberman RH, Lohmander SL: Variations in cellular proliferation and matrix synthesis in intrasynovial and extrasynovial tendons: An in vitro study in dogs. *J Hand Surg [Am]* 1994;19(2):259-265.

21. Würgler-Hauri CC, Dourte LM, Baradet TC, Williams GR, Soslowsky LJ: Temporal expression of 8 growth factors in tendon-to-bone healing in a rat supraspinatus model. *J Shoulder Elbow Surg* 2007;16(5, suppl):S198-S203.

    In this study, rats underwent supraspinatus detachment and repair and were then sacrificed at 1, 2, 3, 8, and 16 weeks. Immunohistochemical staining at each timepoint outlined the expression of bFGF, BMPs-12, -13, -14, cartilage oligomeric matrix protein, connective tissue growth factor, PDGF, and TGF-β1.

22. Rodeo SA, Arnoczky SP, Torzilli PA, Hidaka C, Warren RF: Tendon-healing in a bone tunnel: A biomechanical and histological study in the dog. *J Bone Joint Surg Am* 1993;75(12):1795-1803.

23. Egerbacher M, Arnoczky SP, Caballero O, Lavagnino M, Gardner KL: Loss of homeostatic tension induces apoptosis in tendon cells: An in vitro study. *Clin Orthop Relat Res* 2008;466(7):1562-1568.

    This study showed that rat tail tendons that were stress deprived exhibited more apoptosis than those that were cyclically loaded. This highlights the need for homeostatic stress for overall tendon health.

24. Gardner K, Arnoczky SP, Caballero O, Lavagnino M: The effect of stress-deprivation and cyclic loading on the TIMP/MMP ratio in tendon cells: An in vitro experimental study. *Disabil Rehabil* 2008;30(20-22):1523-1529.

    This study shows that stress deprivation increases the

amount of MMP in rat tail tendons. This again emphasizes the idea that load is necessary to prevent tendon degeneration.

25. Bring D, Reno C, Renstrom P, Salo P, Hart D, Ackermann P: Prolonged immobilization compromises up-regulation of repair genes after tendon rupture in a rat model. *Scand J Med Sci Sports* 2009;Jul 2:[Epub ahead of print].

Rats underwent Achilles tendon rupture and then were randomized to cast immobilization or free mobilization. Those in the mobilized group had increased messenger RNA levels of brain-derived neurotrophic factor, bFGF, cyclooxygenase-1, and hypoxia-inducible factor-1α at 17 days. This led to the conclusion that mobilization responded to increased expression of regenerative growth factors and may be beneficial to healing.

26. Eliasson P, Andersson T, Aspenberg P: Rat Achilles tendon healing: Mechanical loading and gene expression. *J Appl Physiol* 2009;107(2):399-407.

Rat Achilles tendons were transected and were then randomized to receive botulinum toxin type A injections to unload the repair, or serve as a loaded control. Those that received botulinum toxin type A had less procollagen I, cartilage oligomeric matrix protein, tenascin-C, tenomodulin, and scleraxis at 14 and 21 days following injury. In the loaded samples there was increased cross-sectional area at the healing site, but the material properties were unaffected. This led to the conclusion that tendon-specific genes are upregulated with loading and may promote regeneration rather than scar formation.

27. Baumgarten KM, Gerlach D, Galatz LM, et al: Cigarette smoking increases the risk for rotator cuff tears. *Clin Orthop Relat Res* 2009;Mar 13:[Epub ahead of print].

This study showed that smoking correlated with the rotator cuff tears in a dose- and time-dependent manner.

28. Galatz LM, Silva MJ, Rothermich SY, Zaegel MA, Havlioglu N, Thomopoulos S: Nicotine delays tendon-to-bone healing in a rat shoulder model. *J Bone Joint Surg Am* 2006;88(9):2027-2034.

29. Cohen DB, Kawamura S, Ehteshami JR, Rodeo SA: Indomethacin and celecoxib impair rotator cuff tendon-to-bone healing. *Am J Sports Med* 2006;34(3):362-369.

30. Dimmen S, Engebretsen L, Nordsletten L, Madsen JE: Negative effects of parecoxib and indomethacin on tendon healing: An experimental study in rats. *Knee Surg Sports Traumatol Arthrosc* 2009;17(7):835-839.

Rats underwent Achilles tendon laceration and then were given either parecoxib, indomethacin, or saline. Those that received parecoxib and indomethacin had lower tensile strength than control subjects at 14 days.

31. Chen AL, Shapiro JA, Ahn AK, Zuckerman JD, Cuomo F: Rotator cuff repair in patients with type I diabetes mellitus. *J Shoulder Elbow Surg* 2003;12(5):416-421.

32. Hapa O, Cakici H, Gideroglu K, Ozturan K, Kükner A,

Buğdayci G: The effect of ethanol intake on tendon healing: A histological and biomechanical study in a rat model. *Arch Orthop Trauma Surg* 2009;129(12):1721-1726.

Rats were either given ethanol or served as control subjects. After 1 week, they underwent Achilles tendon laceration. At 4 weeks following injury, those that received ethanol had lower tensile strength and worse tenocyte histology scores. Therefore, ethanol has a detrimental effect on tendon healing.

33. Gulotta LV, Rodeo SA: Growth factors for rotator cuff repair. *Clin Sports Med* 2009;28(1):13-23.

The authors present a review of current research into the role of growth factors for the augmentation of rotator cuff repairs, as well as potential future directions.

34. Ansorge HL, Beredjiklian PK, Soslowsky LJ: CD44 deficiency improves healing tendon mechanics and increases matrix and cytokine expression in a mouse patellar tendon injury model. *J Orthop Res* 2009;27(10):1386-1391.

CD44 is a potent proinflammatory mediator. CD44 knockout mice showed improved healing in a mouse patellar tendon injury model. This implies that blunting the inflammatory response may improve tendon and ligament healing by reducing fibrosis and promoting regeneration.

35. Ricchetti ET, Reddy SC, Ansorge HL, et al: Effect of interleukin-10 overexpression on the properties of healing tendon in a murine patellar tendon model. *J Hand Surg Am* 2008;33(10):1843-1852.

IL-10 is an anti-inflammatory cytokine. In this study, IL-10 overexpression was able to improve healing in a mouse patellar tendon defect model. This is further evidence that reducing the inflammatory response may be beneficial to healing.

36. Hays PL, Kawamura S, Deng XH, et al: The role of macrophages in early healing of a tendon graft in a bone tunnel. *J Bone Joint Surg Am* 2008;90(3):565-579.

Macrophages produce TGF-β1 that results in fibrosis. In this study, macrophage depletion improved healing in a mouse ACL reconstruction model. Tendon grafts healed with less scar tissue and more fibrocartilage.

37. Miyatake S, Tohyama H, Kondo E, Katsura T, Onodera S, Yasuda K: Local administration of interleukin-1 receptor antagonist inhibits deterioration of mechanical properties of the stress-shielded patellar tendon. *J Biomech* 2008;41(4):884-889.

IL-1 is a potent proinflammatory mediator. In this study, application of an IL-1 receptor blocker was able to inhibit the deterioration of mechanical properties of stress-shielded patellar tendons. This signifies that inflammation is one pathway by which tendons degenerate during stress deprivation.

38. Ouyang HW, Goh JC, Lee EH: Use of bone marrow stromal cells for tendon graft-to-bone healing: Histological and immunohistochemical studies in a rabbit model. *Am J Sports Med* 2004;32(2):321-327.

39. Chong AK, Ang AD, Goh JC, et al: Bone marrow–derived mesenchymal stem cells influence early tendon-healing in a rabbit achilles tendon model. *J Bone Joint Surg Am* 2007;89(1):74-81.

In this study, autologous bone marrow–derived MSCs improved healing in a rabbit model of Achilles tendon healing.

40. Lim JK, Hui J, Li L, Thambyah A, Goh J, Lee EH: Enhancement of tendon graft osteointegration using mesenchymal stem cells in a rabbit model of anterior cruciate ligament reconstruction. *Arthroscopy* 2004;20(9):899-910.

41. Pacini S, Spinabella S, Trombi L, et al: Suspension of bone marrow-derived undifferentiated mesenchymal stromal cells for repair of superficial digital flexor tendon in race horses. *Tissue Eng* 2007;13(12):2949-2955.

Eleven racehorses received MSCs to augment partial flexor tendon laceration healing. Nine of the 11 had significant clinical recovery that allowed them to return to racing.

42. Gulotta LV, Kovacevic D, Ehteshami JR, Dagher E, Packer JD, Rodeo SA: Application of bone marrow-derived mesenchymal stem cells in a rotator cuff repair model. *Am J Sports Med* 2009;37(11):2126-2133.

Contrary to previous studies, this study failed to show improved healing in a rat rotator cuff repair model with the application of bone marrow–derived MSCs. This highlights the need to determine a combination of pluripotent stem cells and growth or differentiation factors that can be effective to augment rotator cuff repairs.

43. Thomopoulos S, Das R, Silva MJ, et al: Enhanced flexor tendon healing through controlled delivery of PDGF-BB. *J Orthop Res* 2009;27(9):1209-1215.

This study showed that PDGF-BB delivery on a fibrin/heparin-based delivery system increased tendon gliding, but failed to improve mechanical strength following flexor tendon repairs in dogs. This result occurred despite increases in cell activity, collagen crosslinks, and hyaluronic acid seen in the PDGF-BB–treated specimens.

44. Sasaki K, Kuroda R, Ishida K, et al: Enhancement of tendon-bone osteointegration of anterior cruciate ligament graft using granulocyte colony-stimulating factor. *Am J Sports Med* 2008;36(8):1519-1527.

ACL reconstruction was performed on dogs and either granulocyte colony-stimulating factor in a gelatin or the gelatin alone was applied to the tunnels. They found that bone-tendon healing strength was accelerated in specimens treated with granulocyte colony-stimulating factor by enhancing angiogenesis and osteogenesis.

45. Hashimoto Y, Yoshida G, Toyoda H, Takaoka K: Generation of tendon-to-bone interface "enthesis" with use of recombinant BMP-2 in a rabbit model. *J Orthop Res* 2007;25(11):1415-1424.

In this study, BMP-2 was injected into the flexor digitorum communis tendon of rabbits to induce ectopic ossicle formation. The resultant tendon/ossicle complex was then transferred to the tibial surface. One month follow-ing transfer, those that were originally treated with BMP-2 had histology more representative of a direct insertion site, and this histology correlated with better biomechanical properties.

46. Seeherman HJ, Archambault JM, Rodeo SA, et al: rhBMP-12 accelerates healing of rotator cuff repairs in a sheep model. *J Bone Joint Surg Am* 2008;90(10):2206-2219.

This study evaluated the ability of BMP-12 on various carriers to improve infraspinatus healing in a sheep model. They showed that BMP-12 on a collagen or hyaluronan sponge was able to accelerate healing, and resulted in maximal loads to failure that were twice that of controls.

47. Murray MM: Current status and potential of primary ACL repair. *Clin Sports Med* 2009;28(1):51-61.

This is a review of the research into developing strategies to augment primary ACL repairs.

48. Fufa D, Shealy B, Jacobson M, Kevy S, Murray MM: Activation of platelet-rich plasma using soluble type I collagen. *J Oral Maxillofac Surg* 2008;66(4):684-690.

This study showed that soluble type I collagen is necessary for the release of growth factor from platelet-rich plasma.

49. Murray MM, Spindler KP, Abreu E, et al: Collagen-platelet rich plasma hydrogel enhances primary repair of the porcine anterior cruciate ligament. *J Orthop Res* 2007;25(1):81-91.

The application of a platelet-rich plasma hydrogel was found to improve healing after primary ACL repair in a porcine model. However, the final strength of the ACL repairs was below that of the native ACL.

50. Dwyer KW, Provenzano PP, Muir P, Valhmu WB, Vanderby R Jr: Blockade of the sympathetic nervous system degrades ligament in a rat MCL model. *J Appl Physiol* 2004;96(2):711-718.

51. Salo P, Bray R, Seerattan R, Reno C, McDougall J, Hart DA: Neuropeptides regulate expression of matrix molecule, growth factor and inflammatory mediator mRNA in explants of normal and healing medial collateral ligament. *Regul Pept* 2007;142(1-2):1-6.

This study showed that the application of the neuropeptides substance P, neuropeptide Y, and calcitonin gene-related peptide to medial collateral ligaments induced several inflammatory mediators at 2 weeks. This shows that neuropeptides influence the metabolic activities on ligaments during the healing process.

52. McDougall JJ, Yeung G, Leonard CA, Bray RC: A role for calcitonin gene-related peptide in rabbit knee joint ligament healing. *Can J Physiol Pharmacol* 2000;78(7):535-540.

53. Arnoczky SP, Lavagnino M, Egerbacher M: The mechanobiological aetiopathogenesis of tendinopathy: Is it the over-stimulation or the under-stimulation of tendon cells? *Int J Exp Pathol* 2007;88(4):217-226.

The authors studied the in vitro mechanobiologic response of tendon cells in situ to various tensile loading regimes in a rat tail tendon model.

54. Andres BM, Murrell GA: Treatment of tendinopathy: What works, what does not, and what is on the horizon. *Clin Orthop Relat Res* 2008;466(7):1539-1554.

    The authors present a review article on the current status of the treatment of tendinopathy.

55. Mikolyzk DK, Wei AS, Tonino P, et al: Effect of corticosteroids on the biomechanical strength of rat rotator cuff tendon. *J Bone Joint Surg Am* 2009;91(5):1172-1180.

    This study showed that a single dose of corticosteroids significantly weakened both intact and repaired rotator cuffs in a rat model. However, the strength returned to normal in 3 weeks.

56. Wei AS, Callaci JJ, Juknelis D, et al: The effect of corticosteroid on collagen expression in injured rotator cuff tendon. *J Bone Joint Surg Am* 2006;88(6):1331-1338.

57. Murrell GA: Using nitric oxide to treat tendinopathy. *Br J Sports Med* 2007;41(4):227-231.

    The author showed that nitric oxide enhances subjective and objective recovery of patients with tendon injury in three randomized clinical trials.

58. Rompe JD, Furia J, Maffulli N: Eccentric loading compared with shock wave treatment for chronic insertional achilles tendinopathy: A randomized, controlled trial. *J Bone Joint Surg Am* 2008;90(1):52-61.

    This study showed that shock wave treatment was superior to physical therapy concentrating on eccentric loading in patients with insertional Achilles tendinopathy.

59. Rompe JD, Furia J, Maffulli N: Eccentric loading versus eccentric loading plus shock-wave treatment for midportion achilles tendinopathy: A randomized controlled trial. *Am J Sports Med* 2009;37(3):463-470.

    This study showed that shock wave treatment was superior to eccentric loading in patients with midportion Achilles tendinopathy.

60. Orchard J, Massey A, Brown R, Cardon-Dunbar A, Hofmann J: Successful management of tendinopathy with injections of the MMP-inhibitor aprotinin. *Clin Orthop Relat Res* 2008;466(7):1625-1632.

    This study showed that 76% of patients who received aprotinin injections for Achilles or patellar tendinopathy had improvement in their symptoms. The results were better for those who had Achilles tendinopathy (84% improvement) than those with patellar tendinopathy (69% improvement).

61. Mishra A, Woodall J Jr, Vieira A: Treatment of tendon and muscle using platelet-rich plasma. *Clin Sports Med* 2009;28(1):113-125.

    This is a review article outlining research into the use of platelet-rich plasma for the treatment of tendon and muscle injuries.

62. Schnabel LV, Mohammed HO, Miller BJ, et al: Platelet rich plasma (PRP) enhances anabolic gene expression patterns in flexor digitorum superficialis tendons. *J Orthop Res* 2007;25(2):230-240.

    The application of platelet-rich plasma to flexor digitorum superficialis explants resulted in higher concentrations of TGF-β1 and PDGF-BB, and higher expression of COL1A1, COL3A1, and cartilage oligomeric matrix protein.

Chapter 5

Wound Management

Jan Paul Ertl, MD   Jeffrey Anglen, MD

1: Principles of Orthopaedics

Introduction

Extremity injuries with associated soft-tissue violation present challenges to fracture stabilization and, more importantly, the initial management of the soft tissues and timing of definitive coverage. A coordinated management team is necessary to address any life-threatening injuries. Thorough débridement techniques, consisting of removal of nonviable and contaminated tissues, have been the focus of wound management.[1]

Extremity injuries should be seen as soft-tissue injuries that surround a central bone core. The soft-tissue injury in extremity trauma often dictates the outcome of fractures and takes priority in treatment to maintain a biologic barrier and blood supply to potentially exposed bone, and to avoid further tissue compromise and infection. Complications that occur during the course of fracture care ultimately increase morbidity, mortality, and treatment cost.[2] Many factors that increase the risk of further soft-tissue compromise or infection in open or closed fractures are beyond the control of the surgeon. These factors include the severity of the injury, delay in initiation of medical care, and the health status of the patient. However, some treatment decisions, including timing of surgical treatment, use of systemic and local antibiotics, wound irrigation, adequacy of surgical débridement, fracture stability, and early wound closure or flap coverage, are strongly believed to influence the incidence of infection.

The development of a wound infection is a multistage process that is the result of contamination with sufficient numbers of viable bacteria, adhesion of the bacteria to wound surfaces, proliferation of bacterial colonies on the surface, and extension of the colonies

---

Dr. Ertl or an immediate family member serves as a board member, owner, officer, or committee member of Wishard Hospital and has received research or institutional support from Amgen, Synthes, and Wyeth. Dr. Anglen or an immediate family member serves as a board member, owner, officer, or committee member of The American Board of Orthopaedic Surgery, the American College of Surgeons, and the Orthopaedic Trauma Association; has received royalties from Biomet; serves as a paid consultant to or is an employee of Stryker; and has received research or institutional support from Stryker and Wyeth.

beyond the original locations. The goals of initial wound care are to decrease the bacterial load, eliminate the devitalized tissue that serves as a medium for bacterial growth, and prevent further contamination, thereby facilitating the action of host defense systems.[3] The initial and continued management of wounds are critical in the ultimate successful outcome of fractures, and a multidisciplinary approach is usually required.

Initial Management of Open Fracture Wounds

Closed fractures with devitalized skin and all open fractures are considered contaminated. The severity of injury to the soft-tissue envelope may be difficult to assess in the emergency department, and the amount of contamination is further affected by additional factors such as patient age, energy absorbed, setting of injury (for example, barnyard), vascular disruption, and patient comorbidities. Initial wound management in the emergency department includes removal of splints and assessment of the extremity. Sterile dressings, if present, are left in place. It has been shown that redressing the wound in the emergency department causes a threefold to fourfold rise in the rate of infection.[4] The extent of soft-tissue injury is greater than is evident upon simple inspection, and is best determined in the operating room. Factors that influence the development of infection include the involved area of the body, severity of soft-tissue damage, virulence of organisms introduced into the wound, treatment regimen, presence of foreign material in the wound, and host response to both injury and wound inoculation.

Surgical wounds have been grouped into four types, based on the risk of surgical site infection: class I, clean; class II, clean-contaminated; class III, contaminated; and class IV, dirty-infected.[5] Prophylactic antibiotics are indicated for class I and II wounds. Prospective[6] and meta-analysis review have demonstrated the efficacy and benefit of prophylactic antibiotics for class I and II wounds and therapeutic antibiotics are indicated for class III and IV wounds.

Antibiotic Therapy

For patients with class III and IV wounds, antibiotics are used perioperatively not for prophylaxis but for managing a contaminated or infected wound. In open

---

Table 1

Recommendations for Intravenous Antibiotic Therapy in Open Fracture Management

Fracture Type	Clinical Infection Rates	Antibiotic Choice	Antibiotic Duration
I	1.4%	Cefazolin	every 8 h × 3 doses
II	3.6%	Piperacillin/azobactam or cefazolin and tobramycin	24 h after wound closure
IIIA	22.7%	Piperacillin/azobactam or cefazolin and tobramycin + penicillin for anaerobic, as required	3 days
IIIB	10% to 50%	Piperacillin/azobactam or Cefazolin and tobramycin + penicillin for anaerobic, as required	Continue 3 days after wound closure
IIIC	10% to 50%	Piperacillin/azobactam or cefazolin and tobramycin + penicillin for anaerobic, as required	Continue 3 days after wound closure

fractures, antibiotic therapy serves as an adjunct to surgical débridement by reducing the bacterial load in the tissue. Multiple investigators have established the role of antibiotics in treatment and confirmed their efficacy in preventing infection after treatment of open fracture in prospective, randomized, controlled trials.[7] Antibiotics should be initiated within 3 hours after injury because the risk of infection increases after that time.[8] Although the efficacy of antibiotics in the management of open fractures is clear, length of therapy and the optimal antibiotic are not. Randomized controlled trials are needed to determine these variables.

The suggested duration of antibiotic therapy is 1 to 3 days for Gustilo-Anderson grade I and II open fractures and up to 5 days for grade III wounds.[7,9-11] Antibiotic selection depends on the likely organisms contaminating the wound. For grade I and II open fractures, *Staphylococcus aureus*, streptococci, and aerobic gram-negative bacilli are the most common infecting organisms; thus, the use of a first- or second-generation cephalosporin has been proposed.[12] A quinolone (for example, ciprofloxacin) might be a reasonable alternative given its broad-spectrum coverage, bactericidal activity, good oral bioavailability, and good adverse effect profile.[13] More severe injuries should be managed with better coverage for gram-negative organisms, and the addition of an aminoglycoside to the cephalosporin is recommended.[14] Alternatives to aminoglycosides may include third-generation cephalosporins or aztreonam.[15] For severe injuries with soil contamination and tissue damage with areas of ischemia, penicillin should be added to provide coverage against anaerobes, particularly *Clostridium* species (**Table 1**).

Type of Irrigation and Volume

The optimal care of open fracture wounds involves surgical débridement and irrigation of the wound to remove the devitalized tissue, foreign material, and contaminating bacteria in an attempt to decrease the bioburden that leads to wound infection.

In a study of open fracture wounds of the lower extremity, patients were randomized to receive either bacitracin or castile soap added to the irrigation fluid.[3] The results demonstrated no significant difference in infection rate between the two groups. Problems associated with wound healing (wound dehiscence or necrosis, incision breakdown, or flap or graft failure) occurred in 9.5% of the bacitracin irrigation group and in 4% of the castile soap irrigation group. There were fewer infections and problems with fracture union in the group treated with the soap, although those differences were not significant. It was concluded that irrigation of open fracture wounds with antibiotic solution offered no advantage over the soap solution; in fact, use of the antibiotic may increase the risk of problems associated with wound healing. Irrigation of open fracture wounds with castile soap solution is advocated, particularly for the first irrigation and for wounds with gross contamination.

The authors of a 2009 study compared pulsatile (19 psi) irrigation with bulb syringe irrigation in an animal model and with multiple solutions.[16] These data suggest that use of a low-pressure device and saline solution to irrigate wounds is the best choice. It was demonstrated that bulb syringe irrigation and normal saline produced improved results, with decreased bacterial rebound at 48 hours using 6 L of solution. According to a 2006 study in a goat model, it was demonstrated that potable water can also be used to reduce bacterial counts.[17]

Timing to Irrigation and Débridement

The timing to irrigation and débridement with luminescent *Pseudomonas* bacteria was studied, and it was concluded that earlier irrigation in a contaminated wound model resulted in superior bacterial removal.[18]

A recent multicenter study concluded that the time from the injury to surgical débridement is not a significant independent predictor of the risk of infection, and instead the timing of admission to a definitive trauma treatment center had a beneficial influence (with earlier admission leading to fewer infections).[19] This finding should not be interpreted to mean that surgical débridement of open fractures should not be accomplished urgently.

Treatment

How much excisional débridement should be done is difficult to assess in most contaminated injuries. Recent consensus opinion from the Extremity War Injury Symposium was that necrotic, devitalized, and contaminated tissue must be removed but that objective assessment of completeness of débridement is difficult.[20] Contractility, color, consistency, and capacity to bleed are all important recognized indicators of viable tissue, but a great deal of experience is necessary to define nonviable tissue.[20]

The management of wounds and open fractures continues to provide challenges for the orthopaedic surgeon. Despite the improvements in technology and surgical techniques, the rates of infection and nonunion are still troublesome. Early antibiotic administration coupled with early and meticulous irrigation and débridement can lead to decreased rates of infection. Initial surgical intervention should be conducted as soon as possible, but the classic 6-hour rule does not seem to be supported in the literature.[21] All open fractures should be assessed for the risk of contamination from *Clostridium tetani*. When possible, early closure of open fracture wounds, either by primary means or with flaps, can also decrease the rate of infection, especially from nosocomial organisms. Early skeletal stabilization is necessary, which can be accomplished easily with temporary external fixation. Adhering to these principles can help surgeons provide optimal patient care and an early return to function.[20,21]

Antibiotic Bead Pouch

Beads made of polymethylmethacrylate (PMMA) containing antibiotic may be used to deliver an extremely high concentration of antibiotic to the wound, while simultaneously protecting the tissues against desiccation, contamination, and injury (**Figure 1**). Antibiotics including tobramycin, vancomycin, and cefazolin are commonly chosen because they are water soluble, heat stable, well tolerated, and broad spectrum. Vancomycin is not recommended as an initial agent because of concerns of overuse leading to development of resistant microorganisms. The wound is packed with the beads after débridement and then covered with a semipermeable membrane dressing. Rubber bands or "lacing" can be used in conjunction with beads to prevent retraction of the wounds. The bead pouch allows diffusion of an-

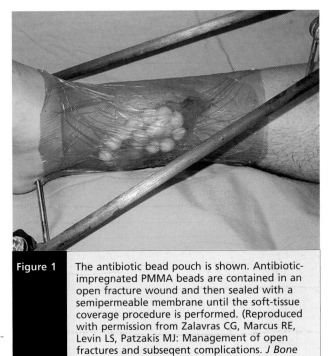

Figure 1 The antibiotic bead pouch is shown. Antibiotic-impregnated PMMA beads are contained in an open fracture wound and then sealed with a semipermeable membrane until the soft-tissue coverage procedure is performed. (Reproduced with permission from Zalavras CG, Marcus RE, Levin LS, Patzakis MJ: Management of open fractures and subseqent complications. *J Bone Joint Surg Am* 2007;89:884-895.)

tibiotic into the wound exudates. Antibiotic levels can reach very high local concentrations without systemic toxicity, even penetrating tissues with poor or absent vascularity. The bead pouch technique seals the wound from the external environment with a semipermeable barrier, thereby preventing secondary contamination by nosocomial pathogens and at the same time maintaining an aerobic wound environment.[9-11]

An infection rate of 3.7% was reported in a group of patients with open fractures who received combined treatment with both systemic antibiotics and antibiotic beads.[22] This rate was considerably lower than the 12% infection rate associated with open fractures treated with systemic antibiotics alone.

Negative Pressure Wound Therapy

Negative pressure wound therapy (NPWT) is a relatively new, commercially available treatment that has been used across many disciplines and proved beneficial in various types of complex wounds.[23-25] However, very little has been written regarding the use of NPWT in orthopaedics. Most of the articles in the literature are either case reports or small case series and many do not involve complex traumatic wounds.[26-28]

NPWT has become widely accepted in orthopaedics and used routinely in acute wound management, preoperative temporizing, complex trauma, wound bed preparation, and treatment of chronic wounds. NPWT uses micromechanisms and macromechanisms of action to increase local blood flow, reduce edema, stimulate formation of granulation tissue, stimulate cell proliferation, reduce cytokines, reduce bacterial load, and draw wounds together.[23,29] NPWT is thought to exert

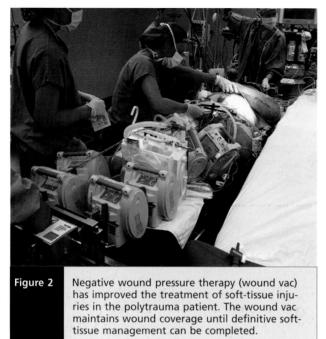

Figure 2 Negative wound pressure therapy (wound vac) has improved the treatment of soft-tissue injuries in the polytrauma patient. The wound vac maintains wound coverage until definitive soft-tissue management can be completed.

its biologic effects by first stimulating the release of local cell growth factors by induced mechanical strain similar to the mechanism of Ilizarov and then improving microcirculation by actively removing edema from injured tissue.[30,31] NPWT has been indicated in chronic, acute, traumatic, subacute, and high-risk elective surgical wounds as well as partial-thickness burns, ulcers, flaps, and skin grafts. Contraindications to treatment with NPWT include wounds with necrotic tissues, exposed vital structures, untreated osteomyelitis, unexplored fistulae, and malignant wounds. In the management of orthopaedic wounds NPWT serves as an adjunct to soft-tissue defects as a method of reducing bacterial counts in wounds, as a bridge to definitive bone coverage, treating infections, wound bed preparation for split-thickness skin grafting (STSG) dermal replacements, or flap coverage. No significant complications have been noted in reported studies to date, although there have been case reports of erosion of NPWT into vascular structures, leading to hemorrhage.[32,33]

NPWT uses application of subatmospheric pressure (less than 760 mm Hg) to the wound bed to promote healing. A range of pressures between 50 and 500 mm Hg were tested; the most efficient pressure was 125 mm Hg, which resulted in a fourfold increase in blood flow, a 63% increase in granulation tissue with continuous pressure, and a 103% increase in granulation tissue with intermittent pressure.[23,24] NPWT can be applied through both reticulated foam and gauze at the wound interface, although most published literature supports the use of reticulated foam.[31,34] Further studies are needed to compare foam and gauze dressings and the effect of each on healing.

The bacterial colonization of a wound is a recognized detrimental factor in the multifactorial process of wound healing. The harmful effects on wound healing are recognized to correspond to a level of greater than 105 colonies of bacteria per gram of tissue. NPWT has been applied to traumatic wounds for varying periods in an attempt to avoid infection and bridge the time until definitive coverage can be completed (**Figure 2**). The question of decreasing bacterial counts has been addressed in basic science animal studies and in clinical practice.[23,24] Wounds were infected with *Staphylococcus aureus* and *Staphylococcus epidermidis* and treated with foam NPWT. Sequential full-thickness punch biopsies obtained over a 2-week period demonstrated bacterial counts below 105 organisms per gram of tissue. Other investigators in a retrospective review of acute and chronic wounds did not consistently identify decreased bacterial colonization.[35] Most of the patient subgroup studied was chronic nonorthopaedic wounds; despite these findings it was concluded that most wounds healed. In a prospective randomized study, the impact of NPWT after severe open fractures on infection was evaluated.[36] Fifty-nine patients with 63 heavily contaminated types II, IIIA, IIIB, and IIIC fractures were included. All patients underwent identical treatment protocols except for the type of dressing placed over the open fracture wound. The control group received fine mesh gauze dressing and the other group received NPWT dressings. The study findings demonstrated that NPWT-treated patients were 20% less likely to develop infection in comparison with the control group.

NPWT has been used in the treatment of combat-related complex soft-tissue wounds and complex high-energy open fractures.[37,38] The isolated soft-tissue injury cohort had less débridement, faster time to closure, and no infections. NPWT was considered an important adjunct in the débridement protocols of soft-tissue injuries. The open fractures were treated aggressively with multiple débridements and NPWT was used to bridge the gap until wound closure was completed. Although there are many factors to consider, no infections were reported.

It must be emphasized that NPWT/reticulated foam is not a substitute for thorough surgical débridement of nonviable soft tissue and bony structures.[34]

NPWT and STSG

Multiple prospective, retrospective, and basic science studies have provided supporting evidence for the use of NPWT over STSG.[39,40] Application of NPWT over the skin graft is intended to minimize shear forces, pull off wound bed edema, and hinder infection. NPWT also minimizes shear forces that may be particularly advantageous in the pediatric population and other patient subgroups with limited ability to self-immobilize. The primary advantages of using reticulated foam sponges applied to STSG sites are decreased shear forces on the STSG, compression of the STSG to the recipient bed, removal of any edema, and conformance with the STSG on uneven wound surfaces. The STSG recipient site can be covered with the nonadherent/

nonpetroleum dressing stapled at the periphery to avoid unwanted tissue ingrowth. The NPWT can also be applied in a similar fashion without staples to the donor site, resulting in faster healing.[39] The literature supports removing the NPWT over the skin graft by 5 days and as early 3 days. The orthopaedic trauma patient often is in the hospital beyond the time required for NPWT, so leaving the NPWT (foam) in place for 3, 5, or even 7 days does not impede discharge from the hospital.[34,41] The use of NPWT over dermal substitutes has been used;[41] however, more clinical investigation is required.

In a study of the cost-effectiveness of NPWT, it was concluded that NPWT can reduce the need for expensive traditional soft-tissue reconstructions.[28]

NPWT is a relatively simple supplement in the treatment of complex acute and chronic wounds. Although used extensively in these wounds, NPWT does not replace the surgical principles of débridement, bony stabilization, and appropriate antibiotic therapy.

Suture for Skin Closure

The type of skin closure for compromised skin was studied in an animal model.[42] The objective of this study was to determine the effect of suture patterns on the cutaneous blood supply with increasing tension applied to the suture. A porcine model was used to measure the suture tension of simple, horizontal mattress, vertical mattress (Donati) and the Allgower modification of the Donati sutures. It was determined that the Allgower-Donati suture had the least effect on cutaneous blood flow; the Allgower-Donati suture pattern can be used for traumatized or compromised soft-tissue injuries.

Timing of Microsurgical Coverage

A coordinated effort with a microvascular surgical service is necessary to address the timely coverage of bone with soft-tissue loss. The timing of posttraumatic microsurgical lower extremity reconstruction was described in 1986, with recommendations for flap coverage of Gustilo grade IIIB and IIIC fractures within 72 hours of injury.[43] The highest risk of infection and flap loss occurred within the delayed period, defined as 72 hours to 90 days. Lower rates of flap loss and infection have been cited when repair and coverage were performed in this defined early period.[44] However, the definition of early remains vague. Many modern-day level I trauma and tertiary care centers often receive transfer patients more than 72 hours after injury, with some patients sustaining significant concomitant injury. Institutional factors also come into play, such as operating room availability and appropriate support staff, resulting in less optimal timing of immediate reconstruction of these injuries. In a 2008 retrospective study, 14 lower extremity reconstructions with free flaps were reviewed over a 4-year period.[45] All patients underwent delayed reconstruction more than 72 hours after injury.

There were no flap losses and one patient had late osteomyelitis. These results indicate that posttraumatic lower extremity reconstruction may be safely and reliably performed when the wound is adequately débrided and when the patient's other injuries have been stabilized. Reconstruction was possible an average of 22 days after injury. Aggressive débridement and liberal use of NPWT aided in decreasing the bacterial load and subsequent incidence of wound infections. It was concluded that lower extremity reconstruction can be performed safely and effectively in the delayed period (within 72 hours to 90 days of injury) to allow for wound débridement, stabilization of other injuries, and transfer to a microsurgical facility.

Newer Soft-Tissue Coverage Options

Limb replantation and free tissue flaps have been part of the limb reconstruction algorithm since the introduction of the operating room microscope in 1960. Recent developments and modifications in soft-tissue coverage include the fillet flaps, which apply a "spare parts" concept and can be customized for specific recipient sites. The so-called perforator flap makes use of feeder vessels, providing cutaneous and other composite flaps without sacrificing major vessels. The introduction of the sural flap has made it possible to avoid microsurgical reconstruction but still provide adequate, well-vascularized coverage, particularly in the distal third of the leg.[46]

By definition, fillet flaps are axial-pattern flaps harvested from amputated, discarded, or otherwise nonfunctioning or nonsalvageable tissues and body parts that can also function as composite tissue transfers. They can be used as pedicled or free flaps and are a beneficial reconstruction strategy for major defects, provided tissue adjacent to these defects is available.[47] The expanded use of the fillet flap as either pedicle flap or free tissue transfer is a method for gaining more serviceable soft-tissue coverage and for preserving length of the residual limb when amputation is required. This concept highlights the principle of stabilizing and salvaging limbs as opposed to immediate amputation, and provides the surgeon performing the eventual reconstruction or amputation with more choices for wound closure or coverage.

Another new advance for soft tissue coverage is the so-called perforator flap first described in 1987, in which the angiosomes that are distributed to skin territories can be followed to the feeder vessels, thereby increasing the armamentarium of cutaneous flaps and other composite flaps without sacrificing major vessels. These flaps based on perforating vessels, either in free or pedicled form, represent a new perspective for resolving complex wounds with lower morbidity, especially in the distal segment of the leg. The anterolateral thigh flap has become a workhorse for the treatment of upper and lower extremity defects during flap surgery. The anterolateral thigh flap is indicated for reconstruction of a diverse range of defects of various surface ar-

many ways to use antero-lateral thigh flap

eas and depths; it can be used as an ultrathin flap for resurfacing, rolled up for filling in dead space, or taken with muscle to obliterate spaces or provide bulk. The anterolateral thigh flap has been used in trauma salvage as a flow-through flap, as a tissue carrier, and to piggy-back additional flaps. The flap can be a raised pedicle (proximally or distally) or free, suprafascial or subfascial, further thinned, or harvested with muscle or additional tissue components. The anterolateral thigh flap is robust and versatile enough to fulfill a wide variety of reconstructive requirements. Harvesting these flaps requires a high level of technical skill, but increases surgeon versatility and replaces similar flaps.[48]

A distally-based fasciocutaneous flap from the sural region based on the sural artery anatomy has been described. The sural flap has progressively gained recognition as a suitable soft-tissue reconstruction alternative to microvascular free-flap transfer. The sural artery fasciocutaneous flap has become a standard for soft-tissue coverage of distal third open tibia fractures, exposed calcaneus fractures, and open wounds around the ankle when the overall wound is less than 6 cm in diameter. Most authors have described good results, with low partial and complete flap necrosis rates of between 0% and 17%.[47,49]

Summary

The philosophy of modern treatment of wounds dictates the use of methods believed to reduce the risk of complications. The adequacy of initial surgical wound care may be the most important factor under the surgeon's control and may be the difference between success and failure. Adequate sharp débridement with removal of all debris and devitalized tissue and thorough irrigation are vital. Therefore, the initial management and continued management of wounds are critical in the ultimate successful outcome of fractures and often require a multidisciplinary approach.

Annotated References

1. Bowyer G: Débridement of extremity war wounds. *J Am Acad Orthop Surg* 2006;14(10 Spec No.):S52-S56.

2. Fry DE: The economic costs of surgical site infection. *Surg Infect (Larchmt)* 2002;3(Suppl 1):S37-S43.

3. Anglen JO: Comparison of soap and antibiotic solutions for irrigation of lower-limb open fracture wounds: A prospective, randomized study. *J Bone Joint Surg Am* 2005;87(7):1415-1422.

4. Browner BD: *Skeletal Trauma: Basic Science, Management, and Reconstruction*, ed 3. Philadelphia, PA, WB Saunders, 2003.

5. Mangram AJ, Horan TC, Pearson ML, Silver LC, Jarvis WR; Hospital Infection Control Practices Advisory Committee: Guideline for prevention of surgical site infection, 1999. *Infect Control Hosp Epidemiol* 1999;20(4):250-278, quiz 279-280.

6. Boxma H, Broekhuizen T, Patka P, Oosting H: Randomised controlled trial of single-dose antibiotic prophylaxis in surgical treatment of closed fractures: The Dutch Trauma Trial. *Lancet* 1996;347(9009):1133-1137.

7. Olson SA, Finkemeier CF, Moehring HD: Open fractures, in Bucholz RW, Heckman JD (eds): *Rockwood and Green's Fractures in Adults*, ed 5. Philadelphia, PA, Lippincott-Williams & Wilkins, 2001, pp 285-318.

8. Patzakis MJ, Wilkins J: Factors influencing infection rate in open fracture wounds. *Clin Orthop Relat Res* 1989;243(243):36-40.

9. Zalavras CG, Patzakis MJ: Open fractures: Evaluation and management. *J Am Acad Orthop Surg* 2003;11(3):212-219.

10. Zalavras CG, Patzakis MJ, Holtom P: Local antibiotic therapy in the treatment of open fractures and osteomyelitis. *Clin Orthop Relat Res* 2004;427(427):86-93.

11. Zalavras CG, Marcus RE, Levin LS, Patzakis MJ: Management of open fractures and subsequent complications. *Instr Course Lect* 2008;57:51-63.

    The authors discuss the need for early, systemic, wide-spectrum antibiotic therapy in the treatment of open fractures and avoidance of certain complications.

12. Templeman DC, Gulli B, Tsukayama DT, Gustilo RB: Update on the management of open fractures of the tibial shaft. *Clin Orthop Relat Res* 1998;350(350):18-25.

13. Patzakis MJ, Bains RS, Lee J, et al: Prospective, randomized, double-blind study comparing single-agent antibiotic therapy, ciprofloxacin, to combination antibiotic therapy in open fracture wounds. *J Orthop Trauma* 2000;14(8):529-533.

14. Sanders R, Swiontkowski M, Nunley J, Spiegel P: The management of fractures with soft-tissue disruptions. *J Bone Joint Surg Am* 1993;75(5):778-789.

15. Zalavras CG, Patzakis MJ, Holtom PD, Sherman R: Management of open fractures. *Infect Dis Clin North Am* 2005;19(4):915-929.

16. Owens BD, White DW, Wenke JC: Comparison of irrigation solutions and devices in a contaminated musculoskeletal wound survival model. *J Bone Joint Surg Am* 2009;91(1):92-98.

    The authors describe an established goat model involving the creation of a reproducible complex musculoskeletal wound followed by inoculation *with Pseudomonas aeruginosa* (lux) bacteria. This genetically altered luminescent bacterium provides the ability for quantitative analysis with a photon-counting camera system. For study 1, wound irrigation was performed 6 hours after the injury and inoculation; the goats were assigned to four treatment groups: normal saline solution, bacitracin solution, castile soap, and benzalkonium chloride. All wounds received sharp débridement and irrigation with use of a pulsatile lavage device (19 psi). Images and photon counts were obtained prior to irrigation, after irrigation, and 48 hours after injury and inoculation. For study 2, the same animal model was used, and bulb syringe and pulsatile lavage irrigation was compared with saline solution. In study 1, the irrigation treatment lowered the bacterial counts in all treatment groups. The greatest reduction was seen with castile soap. In study 2, both treatment methods were effective in removing 75% of the bacteria initially.

17. Svoboda SJ, Bice TG, Gooden HA, Brooks DE, Thomas DB, Wenke JC: Comparison of bulb syringe and pulsed lavage irrigation with use of a bioluminescent musculoskeletal wound model. *J Bone Joint Surg Am* 2006; 88(10):2167-2174.

18. Owens BD, Wenke JC: Early wound irrigation improves the ability to remove bacteria. *J Bone Joint Surg Am* 2007;89(8):1723-1726.

    The authors evaluated the effect of different delays in irrigation on bacterial removal in an animal model.

19. Pollak AN, Jones AL, Castillo RC, Bosse MJ, MacKenzie EJ; LEAP Study Group: The relationship between time to surgical debridement and incidence of infection after open high-energy lower extremity trauma. *J Bone Joint Surg Am* 2010;92(1):7-15.

    The authors evaluated the relationship between the timing of the initial treatment of open fractures and the development of subsequent infection as well as assess contributing factors. Eighty-four patients (27%) had development of an infection within the first 3 months after the injury. No significant differences were found between patients who had development of an infection and those who did not when the groups were compared with regard to the time from the injury to the first débridement, the time from admission to the first débridement, or the time from the first débridement to soft-tissue coverage.

20. Ficke JR, Pollak AN: Extremity war injuries: Development of clinical treatment principles. *J Am Acad Orthop Surg* 2007;15(10):590-595.

    The authors discussed four specific areas: prehospital management of extremity wounds, initial débridement, early stabilization, and postoperative wound management during air evacuation.

21. Okike K, Bhattacharyya T: Trends in the management of open fractures: A critical analysis. *J Bone Joint Surg Am* 2006;88(12):2739-2748.

22. Ostermann PA, Seligson D, Henry SL: Local antibiotic therapy for severe open fractures: A review of 1085 consecutive cases. *J Bone Joint Surg Br* 1995;77(1):93-97.

23. Morykwas MJ, Argenta LC, Shelton-Brown EI, McGuirt W: Vacuum-assisted closure: A new method for wound control and treatment: animal studies and basic foundation. *Ann Plast Surg* 1997;38(6):553-562.

24. Argenta LC, Morykwas MJ: Vacuum-assisted closure: A new method for wound control and treatment. Clinical experience. *Ann Plast Surg* 1997;38(6):563-576, discussion 577.

25. Wongworawat MD, Schnall SB, Holtom PD, Moon C, Schiller F: Negative pressure dressings as an alternative technique for the treatment of infected wounds. *Clin Orthop Relat Res* 2003;414(414):45-48.

26. Bihariesingh VJ, Stolarczyk EM, Karim RB, van Kooten EO: Plastic solutions for orthopaedic problems. *Arch Orthop Trauma Surg* 2004;124(2):73-76.

27. Herscovici D Jr, Sanders RW, Scaduto JM, Infante A, DiPasquale T: Vacuum-assisted wound closure (VAC therapy) for the management of patients with high-energy soft tissue injuries. *J Orthop Trauma* 2003; 17(10):683-688.

28. Webb LX: New techniques in wound management: vacuum-assisted wound closure. *J Am Acad Orthop Surg* 2002;10(5):303-311.

29. Gustafsson R, Sjögren J, Ingemansson R: Understanding topical negative pressure therapy, in *European Wound Management Association Position Document Topical: Negative Pressure in Wound Management*. London, England: Medical Education Partnership Ltd, 2007, pp 2-4.

30. Webb LX, Pape HC: Current thought regarding the mechanism of action of negative pressure wound therapy with reticulated open cell foam. *J Orthop Trauma* 2008;22(10, Suppl):S135-S137.

    There are currently two main theories regarding the mechanism of action of negative pressure wound therapy with reticulated open cell foam (NPWT/ROCF). The first is based on the stimulatory effect of microstrain on cellular mitogenesis, angiogenesis, and elaboration of growth factors. This same mechanism is operational in controlled Ilizarovian distraction or in tissue expansion. The second is based on the enhancement of the dynamics of microcirculation by active evacuation of excess interstitial fluid in the form of edema. The use of NPWT/ROCF has found a place in the management of high-energy traumatic wounds and certain high-risk elective surgical wounds.

31. Saxena V, Hwang CW, Huang S, Eichbaum Q, Ingber D, Orgill DP: Vacuum-assisted closure: Microdeformations of wounds and cell proliferation. *Plast Reconstr Surg* 2004;114(5):1086-1096, discussion 1097-1098.

32. White RA, Miki RA, Kazmier P, Anglen JO: Vacuum-assisted closure complicated by erosion and hemorrhage of the anterior tibial artery. *J Orthop Trauma* 2005; 19(1):56-59.

33. Schlatterer D, Hirshorn K: Negative pressure wound therapy with reticulated open cell foam-adjunctive treatment in the management of traumatic wounds of the leg: A review of the literature. *J Orthop Trauma* 2008; 22(10, Suppl):S152-S160.

   This article reviews the evidence-based medicine in terms of NPWT/reticulated open cell foam (ROCF), as a method of reducing bacterial counts in wounds, as a bridge until definitive bony coverage, for treating infections, and as an adjunct to wound bed preparation and for bolstering split-thickness skin grafts, dermal replacement grafts, and over muscle flaps. Evidence supports a decrease in complex soft tissue procedures in grade IIIB open fractures when NPWT/ROCF is used. NPWT/ROCF appears to provide clinical benefit for the treatment of complex lower extremity wounds.

34. Flack S, Apelqvist J, Keith M, Trueman P, Williams D: An economic evaluation of VAC therapy compared with wound dressings in the treatment of diabetic foot ulcers. *J Wound Care* 2008;17(2):71-78.

   The authors evaluated the cost-effectiveness of vacuum-assisted closure therapy and found that it is less costly and more effective than both traditional and advanced dressings.

35. Weed T, Ratliff C, Drake DB: Quantifying bacterial bioburden during negative pressure wound therapy: Does the wound VAC enhance bacterial clearance? *Ann Plast Surg* 2004;52(3):276-279, discussion 279-280.

36. Stannard JP, Volgas DA, Stewart R, McGwin G Jr, Alonso JE: Negative pressure wound therapy after severe open fractures: A prospective randomized study. *J Orthop Trauma* 2009;23(8):552-557.

   The impact of NPWT after severe open fractures on deep infection was evaluated. This treatment represents a promising new therapy for severe open fractures after high-energy trauma.

37. Helgeson MD, Potter BK, Evans KN, Shawen SB: Bioartificial dermal substitute: A preliminary report on its use for the management of complex combat-related soft tissue wounds. *J Orthop Trauma* 2007;21(6):394-399.

   Bioartificial dermal substitute grafting, when coupled with subatmospheric dressing management and delayed split-thickness skin grafting, is an effective technique for managing complex combat-related soft tissue wounds with exposed tendon that can potentially lessen the need for local rotational or free flap coverage.

38. Leininger BE, Rasmussen TE, Smith DL, Jenkins DH, Coppola C: Experience with wound VAC and delayed primary closure of contaminated soft tissue injuries in Iraq. *J Trauma* 2006;61(5):1207-1211.

39. Genecov DG, Schneider AM, Morykwas MJ, Parker D, White WL, Argenta LC: A controlled subatmospheric pressure dressing increases the rate of skin graft donor site reepithelialization. *Ann Plast Surg* 1998;40(3):219-225.

40. Moisidis E, Heath T, Boorer C, Ho K, Deva AK: A pro-spective, blinded, randomized, controlled clinical trial of topical negative pressure use in skin grafting. *Plast Reconstr Surg* 2004;114(4):917-922.

41. Brandi C, Grimaldi L, Nisi G, et al: Treatment with vacuum-assisted closure and cryo-preserved homologous de-epidermalised dermis of complex traumas to the lower limbs with loss of substance, and bones and tendons exposure. *J Plast Reconstr Aesthet Surg* 2008; 61(12):1507-1511.

   The authors concluded that the combination of vacuum-assisted closure therapy and deepidermalized dermis could, in selected cases, constitute an effective treatment for complex lower limb traumatic injuries with bone and tendon exposure.

42. Sagi HC, Papp S, Dipasquale T: The effect of suture pattern and tension on cutaneous blood flow as assessed by laser Doppler flowmetry in a pig model. *J Orthop Trauma* 2008;22(3):171-175.

   The authors' objective was to determine the effects of various suture patterns on cutaneous blood flow at the wound edge as increasing tension is applied through the suture. The Allgower-Donati suture pattern had the least effect on cutaneous blood flow with increasing tension in this model.

43. Godina M: Early microsurgical reconstruction of complex trauma of the extremities. *Plast Reconstr Surg* 1986;78(3):285-292.

44. Hertel R, Lambert SM, Müller S, Ballmer FT, Ganz R: On the timing of soft-tissue reconstruction for open fractures of the lower leg. *Arch Orthop Trauma Surg* 1999;119(1-2):7-12.

45. Karanas YL, Nigriny J, Chang J: The timing of microsurgical reconstruction in lower extremity trauma. *Microsurgery* 2008;28(8):632-634.

   In a retrospective review of 14 lower extremity reconstructions with free flaps undertaken over a 4-year period, all patients underwent reconstruction in the delayed (longer than 72 hours) period. Lower extremity reconstruction can be performed safely and effectively during this "delayed" period to allow for wound débridement, stabilization of other injuries, and transfer to a microsurgical facility.

46. Levin LS: New developments in flap techniques. *J Am Acad Orthop Surg* 2006;14(10 Spec No.):S90-S93.

47. Küntscher MV, Erdmann D, Homann HH, Steinau HU, Levin SL, Germann G: The concept of fillet flaps: Classification, indications, and analysis of their clinical value. *Plast Reconstr Surg* 2001;108(4):885-896.

48. Ali RS, Bluebond-Langner R, Rodriguez ED, Cheng MH: The versatility of the anterolateral thigh flap. *Plast Reconstr Surg* 2009;124(6, Suppl):e395-e407.

   The authors discuss anatomy, planning, flap harvest, donor morbidity, and clinical applications of the anterolateral thigh flap. An algorithm is proposed that facilitates a clear, problem-based approach for the use of this versatile reconstructive option. The flap has been extremely useful in skin resurfacing and even functional reconstruction in traumatic wounds.

49. Follmar KE, Baccarani A, Baumeister SP, Levin LS, Erdmann D: The distally based sural flap. *Plast Reconstr Surg* 2007;119(6):138e-148e.

The distally based sural flap offers an alternative to free tissue transfer for reconstruction of the lower extremity. The flap's indications and composition and a variety of modifications are described. Technical aspects are discussed and clinical insight to minimize complications is provided.

1: Principles of Orthopaedics

load - F that acts on a body

σ stress = $\frac{F}{A}$ = pressure (intensity of a F)

ε strain = $\frac{\Delta l}{l}$ relative amt. of deformation of an object

stiffness = $\frac{F}{deformation}$ — rigidity of an object; extent to which an object resists deformation in response to an applied F ⟩ depends on size of material

compliance = $\frac{deformation}{F}$

E elasticity = $\frac{stress}{strain}$

$E = \frac{\sigma}{\varepsilon}$

measure of inherent stiffness of a material as a resistance to deformation under an applied load; i.e. amt. of internal F that opposes deformation in response to an external F ⟩ independent of size of material; an inherent property

Stress-Strain Curve

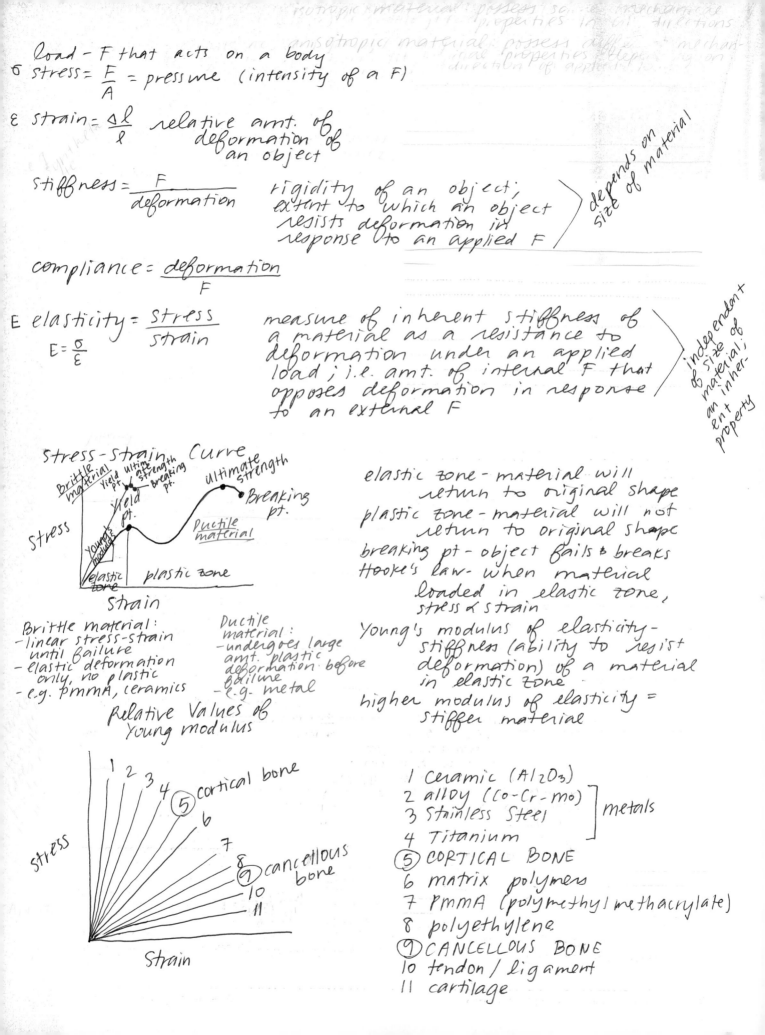

elastic zone - material will return to original shape

plastic zone - material will not return to original shape

breaking pt - object fails & breaks

Hooke's law - when material loaded in elastic zone, stress ∝ strain

Young's modulus of elasticity - stiffness (ability to resist deformation) of a material in elastic zone

higher modulus of elasticity = stiffer material

Brittle material:
- linear stress-strain until failure
- elastic deformation only, no plastic
- e.g. PMMA, ceramics

Ductile material:
- undergoes large amt. plastic deformation before failure
- e.g. metal

Relative Values of Young modulus

1 Ceramic (Al_2O_3)
2 alloy (Co-Cr-mo) ⎤
3 Stainless Steel ⎥ metals
4 Titanium ⎦
⑤ CORTICAL BONE
6 matrix polymers
7 PMMA (polymethyl methacrylate)
8 polyethylene
⑨ CANCELLOUS BONE
10 tendon/ligament
11 cartilage

Chapter 6
Musculoskeletal Biomechanics

Michael Bottlang, PhD   Daniel C. Fitzpatrick, MD   Peter Augat, PhD

1: Principles of Orthopaedics

Introduction

Biomechanics is an engineering science that describes the complex structure and function of the musculoskeletal system in terms of simplified engineering parameters. These parameters serve to quantify functional aspects of orthopaedic interventions and implants in biomechanical studies with defined, reproducible, bench-test conditions. By reducing the number of uncontrolled variables compared with clinical studies, biomechanical studies have a higher sensitivity for detecting performance differences between interventions. Conversely, simplifying and reducing variables and outcome measures too much may limit the relevance of a biomechanical study by oversimplifying the clinical scenario. Hence, the challenge both in designing and in interpreting biomechanical studies is in selecting simplified, well-defined test parameters while avoiding inappropriate oversimplification of the clinical disorder. Detailed descriptions of the many parameters and

compliance = $\frac{1}{stiffness}$ = $\frac{displacement}{F}$

principles governing orthopaedic biomechanics are available in the literature.[1] This chapter outlines principal engineering and test parameters used in current biomechanical research to aid the reader in assessing the relevance and limitations of biomechanical studies. The engineering quantities that describe the principal structures of the musculoskeletal system are defined (the properties of bones and the function of joints) and experimental and numeric test methods in biomechanical research for evaluating orthopaedic interventions are explained.

Biomechanics of Bone

Bones represent the primary load-bearing structural elements of the musculoskeletal system. Bones must be sufficiently stiff and strong to fulfill their principal function of load transmission. The stiffness and strength of bones depend on their material properties and geometric structure. *stiffness = $\frac{Force}{displacement}$*

Material Properties

Material properties characterize the mechanical function and functional limits of a material. To measure material properties, a small cube of the material in question can be gradually compressed in a controlled manner (**Figure 1**). The height of the cube will decrease with increasing amounts of compressive loading. The ratio of the applied load to the resulting compression of the cube represents the material stiffness; for a given compressive load, stiffer materials undergo less compression than more elastic materials.

For example, if a load of 10 N is required to compress the cube by 1 mm, the compressive stiffness of the cube is 10 N/mm. However, this stiffness depends not only on the material property but also on the height and cross-sectional area of the cube. To define stiffness independent of the cube size, loading is expressed in terms of stress (σ), which is calculated by dividing the load by the area the load is acting on (**Table 1**). Likewise, the resulting compression of the cube can be expressed in terms of strain (ε), which represents the amount of compression divided by the original height of the cube. Stiffness can thus be expressed in terms of the elastic modulus (E-modulus or E; E = σ/ε), which is independent of the cube size.

Assuming that the cube in the example has a side length of 10 mm (0.01 m), 10 N loading will induce a

isotropic material: possess same mechanical properties in all directions

anisotropic material: possess different mechanical properties depending on direction of applied load

compressive stress of σ = 10 N/0.0001 m² = 100,000 N/m² on the cube surface. The resulting compression by 1 mm represents a compressive strain of ε = 1 mm/10 mm = 0.1, which it typically expressed as 10%. The compressive E-modulus of the cube is expressed as

E = 100,000 N/m²/0.1 = 1,000,000 N/m². Because strain has no units, σ and E-modulus have the same units of N/m² or Pascal (Pa). These units are very small and are often expressed in MPa (10^6 Pa) and GPa (10^9 Pa).

The E-modulus for titanium (E = 110 GPa) is approximately half that of stainless steel (E = 200 GPa) (**Table 2**). Because the stiffness of these metal alloys can be sufficiently described by a single E-modulus value, they are said to have isotropic material properties. Bone tissue has anisotropic material properties, whereby the stiffness of a cortical bone cube is approximately 50% greater when loaded in the longitudinal direction (parallel to its osteon orientation) (E = 17 GPa) than in the transverse direction (E = 12 GPa). Regardless of the loading direction, stainless steel is more than 10 times stiffer than cortical bone; however, cortical bone is more than 4 times stiffer than polymethylmethacrylate bone cement (E = 3 GPa).

The E-modulus describes deformation in response to loading within the elastic "working" region of a material, where loads remain sufficiently small to allow complete elastic reversal of deformation after load removal. To determine the strength of a material, it must be loaded beyond its elastic region to induce failure. The load at which permanent plastic deformation begins to occur represents the yield strength of a material

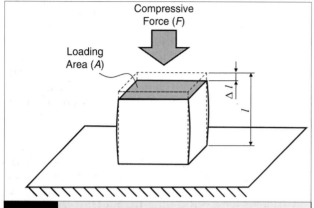

Figure 1 Illustration showing the assessment of material properties in a compression test. A compressive force is applied to a small cube of the material being tested. The height (l) of the cube decreases under the compressive loading (by Δl. The dotted lines represent the cube before compression.

Table 1

Basic Engineering Units for Material Property Characterization

Parameter	Formula	Unit	Example
Force	$F = m[kg] \times 9.81$ m/s²	[N] Newton	1-2 N ≈ force required to lift an apple
Moment	$M = F \times d$	[Nm] Newton-meter	1-2 Nm ≈ "torque" required to rotate door knob
Strain	$\varepsilon = \Delta l/l$	[unitless]; 0.01% to 1%	1% ≈ maximal cortex strain before fracture
Stress; Pressure	$\sigma = F/A$	[N/m²; Pa] Pascal	1,000 Pa ≈ pressure to push keyboard key
E-Modulus	$E = \sigma/\varepsilon =$ *stress / strain*	[Pa] 1 GPa = 1 × 10^9	110 GPa = 100 × 10^9 Pa ≈ stiffness of titanium

under compressive & tensile loading (does not include bending or torsional loading)

Table 2

Representative Values of Material Properties in Compression

amt. of stress needed to produce a specific amt. of permanent deformation

load to failure, i.e. when material fractures

	E-Modulus (GPa)	Yield Strength (MPa)	Ultimate Strength (MPa)	Failure Strain (%)
Stainless steel	200	700	820	12
Titanium alloy	110	800	860	10
Bone cortex	17	200	200	1
PMMA	3	74	74	2

← longitudinal direction of load

Tensile

PMMA = polymethylmethacrylate bone cement

Anisotropic

fatigue failure of metal implants: failure at a point below ultimate strength 2/2 repetitive loading that results in microcracks → these accumulate & eventually lead to failure   v. bone: always remodeling to repair the microcracks

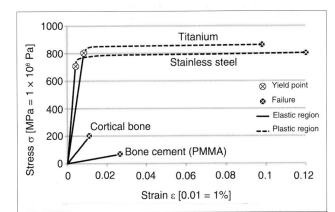

| Figure 2 | Stress-strain curves reflect the properties of representative materials in compression tests. The slope of the initial linear region of curves (continuous lines) represents stiffness (E = Δσ/Δε). Steeper slopes represent stiffer materials. Yield points indicate limits of the elastic "working" region. Brittle materials such as cortical bone fail abruptly, whereby the yield point coincides with failure. PMMA = polymethylmethacrylate. |

(**Figure 2**). The load at which the material fractures represents its ultimate strength. The ultimate strength of titanium (860 MPa) is similar to that of stainless steel (820 MPa), demonstrating that a less stiff material is not necessarily weaker than a stiffer material. Because of its anisotropic behavior, cortical bone has a higher ultimate strength when compressed in the longitudinal direction (193 MPa) than in the transverse direction (133 MPa). Additionally, cortical bone is nearly 50% stronger in compression than in tension. These values have several clinical implications. Fractures of long bones typically are initiated in the region of highest tensile stress, resulting in a predicable fracture pattern for a given loading mode. These strength values also show that the ultimate strength of stainless steel is more than four times that of cortical bone. This is important for a single peak loading event, such as a fall, which may induce a periprosthetic fracture in the bone near an implant rather than an implant fracture. Repetitive loading below the ultimate strength limit induces microcracks that can also lead to fatigue failure. In healthy bone, remodeling continuously repairs these microcracks, making bone tissue highly resistant to fatigue failure. Unlike bone, microcracks in implant materials accumulate under repetitive loading and propagate until fatigue failure occurs. For example, if a bone fracture fails to unite, the osteosynthetic construct will be subjected to prolonged loading cycles that may lead to fatigue fracture of the fixation hardware.

Analogous to the characterization of material under compressive and tensile loading, the stiffness, yield strength, and ultimate strength of a material also can be determined under bending and torsional loading to gain a comprehensive assessment of material properties specific to each principal loading mode, as described in the literature.[1]

Structural Properties

Structural properties depend not only on material properties but also on the object's size and shape. For geometrically simple structures with well-defined material properties, structural properties can be calculated without the need for mechanical testing. For example, the stiffness and strength of an osteosynthetic plate depends only on its material property and cross-sectional geometry. Assuming an osteosynthetic plate of width (w) = 15 mm and thickness (t) = 5 mm, the bending stiffness (EI) of the plate can be calculated as the product of its E-modulus and the second moment of inertia expressed by the formula (I) = (w × t^3)/12 (**Figure 3**). In this formula, bending stiffness correlates linearly with plate width but relates to the third order with plate thickness. Therefore, doubling the plate width results in twice the plate stiffness, whereas doubling the plate thickness increases plate stiffness eightfold (2^3). Similarly, the bending stiffness of a solid cylinder such as an intramedullary nail of diameter d is the product of its E-modulus and I = d^4 × π/64. Doubling the nail diameter will cause a 16-fold increase (2^4) in bending stiffness. The bending stiffness of a cylinder can be increased without increasing its cross-sectional area by introducing a hollow core while expanding the outer diameter. The resulting cylindrical tube will have gained bending stiffness while maintaining the same weight and axial stiffness and strength as a solid cylinder of equivalent cross-sectional area. This weight-optimized tubular structure represents the principal diaphyseal geometry of long bones. However, closed-form equations for calculating stiffness and strength are limited to simple and regular geometries, and such equations cannot accurately predict properties of bone structures.

Density is another important structural property of bone. Because the mineral composition of bone is fairly consistent, the stiffness and strength of an individual area of trabecular bone is within 10% to 15% of cortical bone. However, trabecular bone as a structure is far weaker than cortical bone. The three-dimensional matrix of trabecular bone has a porosity of 30% to 90%, making it much less dense than cortical bone. The stiffness and strength of trabecular bone depends primarily on its density. Osteoporosis is diagnosed by radiographically estimating bone density. The density of trabecular bone varies by approximately one order of magnitude, from approximately 0.1 g/mL to 1.0 g/mL; however, the corresponding stiffness and strength of trabecular bone varies by three orders of magnitude. Therefore, even a small decrease in density can considerably reduce the structural properties of trabecular bone. Because of variability in the geometric organization of the trabecular structure, the stiffness and strength of trabecular bone with the same apparent density can vary tenfold. The most promising approach for in vivo assessment of bone mechanical properties combines quantitative CT with microfinite element analysis, whereby quantitative CT is used to acquire high-resolution images of the trabecular structure and

1: Principles of Orthopaedics

[handwritten margin note: blt ultimate strength of stainless steel 4x greater than cortical bone]

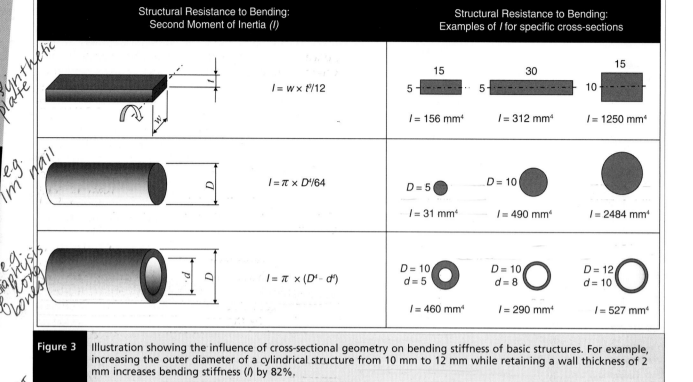

| Structural Resistance to Bending: Second Moment of Inertia (I) | | Structural Resistance to Bending: Examples of I for specific cross-sections | | |

Figure 3 Illustration showing the influence of cross-sectional geometry on bending stiffness of basic structures. For example, increasing the outer diameter of a cylindrical structure from 10 mm to 12 mm while retaining a wall thickness of 2 mm increases bending stiffness (I) by 82%.

microfinite element analysis is used to calculate bone stiffness and strength, while accounting for both density and structural organization. This microfinite element analysis approach has been shown to yield a strong correlation ($R^2 = 0.75$) between predicted and experimentally tested fracture loads, whereas strength prediction based on density alone had a considerably lower correlation ($R^2 = 0.45$).[2]

Clinical scenarios frequently involve more complex interactions between multiple structures, such as implants and bones, whereby load transfer and strength also depend on the contact interface and method of fixation between the structures. To analyze the stiffness, strength, and failure modes of these complex structures and constructs, bench-top biomechanical testing remains the gold standard. Numeric simulation by means of finite element analysis can provide distinct advantages over biomechanical testing for mechanical evaluation of structures and constructs. In most instances, these numeric approaches rely on biomechanical testing for model validation.

Clinical Correlation

Examining proximal femoral and femoral diaphyseal fracture risks in elderly individuals provides a good example of the clinical application of musculoskeletal biomechanics. Osteoporosis is a systemic disease and should affect the metaphyseal and diaphyseal bone in a similar manner. However, unlike proximal femoral fractures, an increased rate of femoral diaphyseal fractures is not observed in elderly patients. The structural properties of bone discussed in this section play a role

in the etiology of this observation. As an individual ages, the diameter of the femoral diaphysis increases and the thickness of the cortex decreases. Using the second moment of inertia principle discussed in this section, the bending stiffness of a tubular bone increases as the outer diameter increases, even as the cortical thickness and material properties of the bone decrease (**Figure 3**). The aggregate increase in strength realized by increasing the diameter of the shaft is adequate to protect elderly individuals from osteoporotic diaphyseal femoral fractures. In contrast, trabecular thinning of the metaphysis cannot be compensated by structural changes of the proximal femur, resulting in an increased risk of hip fractures in individuals with osteoporosis.

Biomechanics of Joints

Joint Loading

Joints enable functional mobility between bone segments. Joint motion is controlled by the forces and moments acting across the joint. Forces acting on a joint are typically represented by vectors, depicting the magnitude and line of action of a force. If a force vector of magnitude F is acting at a distance d from a joint, it will also create a rotational moment M around the joint. This moment has a magnitude of $M = F \times d$, whereby M linearly increases with the perpendicular distance or "lever arm" of the force vector from the joint. Unless it is counteracted by a moment of equal

Joint Reaction Force = force generated within a jt. in response to forces acting on a joint

Extension moment = Flexion moment

$$37 \text{ N} \times 0.2 \text{ m} = \text{Biceps force } (F_B) \times 0.02 \text{ m}$$
$$\rightarrow F_B = 370 \text{ N}$$

Upward forces = Downward forces

$$370 \text{ N} = 37 \text{ N} + \text{Joint force } (F_J)$$
$$\rightarrow F_J = 333 \text{ N}$$

$F_J = 333 \text{ N}$ $F_B = 370 \text{ N}$ 37 N

0.02 m

0.2 m

Figure 4	A free-body diagram of the elbow in static equilibrium while holding a gallon of milk, which exerts a downward force of 37 N. Because this force acts at a distance of 0.2 m to the elbow, it also induces an extension moment (M = 37 N × 0.2 m = 7.4 Nm) around the elbow. Assuming that the biceps is the sole elbow flexor, the biceps muscle must create a flexion moment of equal magnitude for static equilibrium to exist. Because the biceps force acts at a distance of only 0.02 m to the elbow joint, it must generate a force (F = 7.4 Nm/0.02 m = 370 N) to counteract the extension moment. To complete the free-body diagram, the sum of all forces must also be zero. Because the biceps induces an upward force of 370 N, but the gallon exerts a downward force of only 37 N, an additional downward force (F = 370 N − 37 N = 333 N) must be generated as compression at the elbow joint to equalize forces.

magnitude but opposite direction, this moment will induce rotation at the joint.

Joint forces and resulting moments are induced by external loads such as the weight of an object held in a hand, and by internal loads such as the muscle forces required to hold the object. External forces can readily be measured with scales and load sensors that determine the force acting on the body. Assessing internal loads is far more complicated because muscles cannot be instrumented with load sensors and because multiple muscles (activated to various degrees) act across the same joint. However, when a joint is at rest or in a static equilibrium, joint forces can be calculated based on the facts that the sum of all forces and the sum of all moments acting on a nonmoving joint must be zero. For this purpose, known external forces are entered into a free-body diagram along with the line of action of muscles that must generate the internal loads to achieve static equilibrium.

For example, a free-body diagram can be drawn to calculate the forces in the elbow joint while holding a gallon of milk (**Figure 4**). The free-body diagram, which illustrates the fact that holding a gallon of milk induces a force equal to approximately one half body weight of loading in the elbow joint, shows that internal forces tend to be far greater than external forces because of the small lever arms by which muscles can induce moments around joints.

In the previous example, it was necessary to assume that the biceps was the only elbow flexor. This illustrates the limitation of free-body diagram analysis; such analysis can only approximate joint forces under simplified, static loading conditions. In reality, several muscles act across the elbow joint to produce motion. Each of these muscles is activated to various degrees to produce elbow flexion. Because it is not possible to know the exact contribution that each muscle provides for elbow flexion, classic free-body diagram analysis has limited value. In this situation, optimization algorithms are used to calculate the most likely distribution of muscle forces during each instant of joint motion. Optimization is driven by the assumption that energy consumption of muscles for a given task is minimized.

In vivo assessment of joint loads and muscle forces during active motion requires a combination of five advanced biomechanical techniques. (1) In vivo instrumented implants with telemetric data transmission are used to capture joint forces and moments during typical activities of daily living. (2) Load sensors are used to assess external forces acting on the body, such as ground reaction forces during gait. (3) Video-based motion analysis is used to acquire the corresponding movement of body segments by skin marker tracking. (4) Patient-specific reconstruction of bone and muscle geometry from CT data enables translation of body segment motion into motion of bone segments around joints. (5) Synchronized data of joint loads, external loads, and skeletal motion are applied to a musculoskeletal computer model for the calculation of muscle forces and muscle activation patterns. The calculated muscle activation patterns can then be validated using electromyogram recordings. This comprehensive assessment of joint loading has been performed for the hip, knee, shoulder, and spine for a range of daily activities such as walking, running, stair climbing, sitting, and lifting.[3-7]

Using this approach, a series of clinically relevant observations on joint loading have been obtained in recent studies. In the hip, representative peak loads are 270% of body weight (body weight, approximately 700 N) during walking and 520% of body weight during running.[3] Interestingly, wearing soft-soled shoes or running on soft surfaces does not appreciably reduce peak loads; the lowest peak loads are recorded when walking barefoot. Tripping can induce peak loads of 870% of body weight. Compared with walking, stair climbing induces similar peak loads, but with more than 80% higher rotational moments. Because hips have the highest loads during walking and stair climbing, and because walking represents the most frequent

biomechan- ical techni- ques to study jt. loads + muscle F's

[Handwritten notes at top:] Compound/modified hinge - e.g. knee; bicondylar jt (condyles of tibia & condyles of femur) + saddle jt (femur c̄ patella)
Gliding - e.g. carpals, AC; only gliding/sliding mvts
Condyloid jts - e.g. radiocarpal; bones fit together c̄ an odd shape (one bone concave, one convex); flex-ext, AB & ADDuction

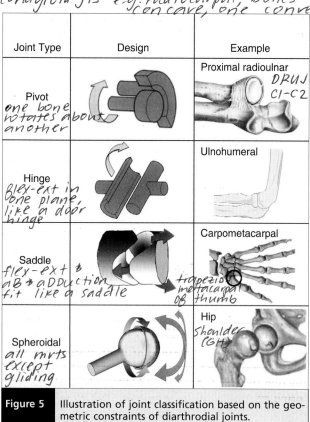

Joint Type	Design	Example
Pivot *[handwritten: one bone rotates about another]*		Proximal radioulnar *[handwritten: DRUJ C1-C2]*
Hinge *[handwritten: flex-ext in one plane, like a door hinge]*		Ulnohumeral
Saddle *[handwritten: flex-ext & aB & aDDuction fit like a saddle]*		Carpometacarpal *[handwritten: trapezio metacarpal of thumb]*
Spheroidal *[handwritten: all mvts except gliding]*		Hip *[handwritten: shoulder (GH)]*

Figure 5 Illustration of joint classification based on the geometric constraints of diarthrodial joints.

loading event (180,000 walking cycles/month),[8] implants should be tested with loading that simulates walking and stair climbing. In the shoulder, glenohumeral contact forces remain less than 100% of body weight for most daily activities but range up to 130% of body weight when lifting an object at arm's length.[6] Moments can reach up to 5.2 Nm and are attributed to friction at the bearing surface. In the knee, level walking induces peak axial forces of 280% of body weight.[5] Stair descending produces the highest forces of up to 350% of body weight in axial loading, 35% of body weight in mediolateral loading, and 36% in anteroposterior loading. It furthermore induces a considerable varus-valgus moment of 4.6% body weight x meter. This emerging body of in vivo loading data from instrumented implants provides a unique opportunity to refine and unify loading schemes in biomechanical tests for the evaluation and systematic optimization of implant performance in bench-top studies.

Joint Characterization

Joints can be characterized by the geometric and ligamentous constraints that define joint stability and by the type and range of joint motion. Geometric constraints are provided by articulating surfaces that transmit compressive forces to effect motion during load bearing. Ligaments transmit tensile loads, preventing joint dislocation while allowing a defined amount of joint laxity. As a first approximation, diarthrodial joints may be categorized by their apparent geometric

constraints into pivot joints (such as the proximal radioulnar joint), hinge joints (such as the ulnohumeral joint), saddle joints (such as the carpometacarpal joint), and spheroidal joints (such as the hip) (**Figure 5**). However, such a simplified geometry-based classification system does not reflect ligamentous constraints that are biomechanically crucial for joint function.

The hip joint resembles a ball and socket or spheroidal joint. The acetabular socket geometrically constrains translation of the femoral head in all three directions while permitting rotation (flexion-extension, internal-external, and abduction-adduction) around three axes. The high congruency of the spherical bearing interface provides load distribution over a large contact area, resulting in low contact pressure. The relatively high geometric constraint combined with a low contact pressure makes the hip joint particularly suitable for joint arthroplasty that can restore geometric constraints but not ligamentous constraints. In contrast, the bicondylar knee joint provides only modest geometric constraints of convex condyles that articulate on a substantially flat tibial plateau. The cruciate and collateral ligaments are essential stabilizers that guide knee flexion, concomitant internal-external rotation, and anteroposterior translation. These modest geometric constraints present considerable challenges for knee arthroplasty. The strong reliance on ligamentous constraints makes correct implant placement crucial to balancing tension in the medial and lateral collateral ligaments; deficient balancing may cause instability or excessive joint loading and wear. These examples show that a biomechanical analysis of joint motion and joint constraints is essential to understanding the complex function of native joints and to improving the function of joint arthroplasty.

Joint Kinematics

Joint kinematics describes the motion of one bone segment relative to the adjoining bone segment. Two adjoining bone segments exhibit six degrees of freedom—bone translation in three orthogonal directions and rotation around three orthogonal axes. To simplify the description of motion, it is usually assumed that one bone segment is fixed in space. A local reference frame is defined in the fixed segment, typically along the anatomic axes (**Figure 6**). For example, a joint coordinate system can be used to describe motion of the femur relative to a fixed tibia in terms of three translations (anteroposterior, mediolateral, and proximodistal) and three rotations (flexion-extension, internal-external, and abduction-adduction).

A variety of electromagnetic, ultrasonic, and optical motion tracking systems are available to automatically track the spatial motion of sensors or markers attached to motion segments at resolutions of better than 1 mm of translation and 1° of rotation. These systems allow convenient in vivo assessment of joint kinematics by tracking skin markers; however, accuracy is limited by skin-to-bone motion artifacts. To avoid these artifacts, in vivo joint kinematics can be directly assessed using

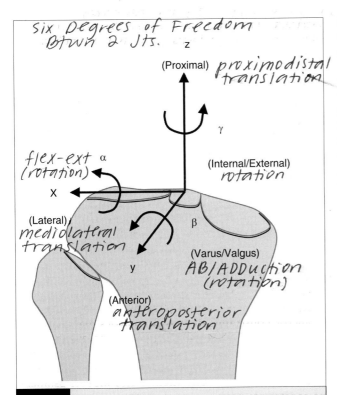

six Degrees of Freedom
Btwn 2 Jts.

proximodistal translation

flex-ext (rotation) α

mediolateral translation

anteroposterior translation

AB/ADDuction (rotation)

rotation

β

γ

Figure 6 A tibia-fixed local reference frame is centered on the tibial plateau with the orthogonal coordinate axis directed laterally (X-axis), anteriorly (Y-axis), and proximally (Z-axis). Translation of the femur relative to the tibia can now be expressed in terms of three discrete displacements along the X, Y, and Z axes. Rotation of the femur relative to the tibia can be defined by three discrete rotations α, ß, and γ around the X, Y, and Z axes, respectively.

fluoroscopy with model- or image-matching based on CT-derived models of bone segments or arthroplasty components.[9]

Analysis of the six degrees of freedom joint kinematic data can be graphically represented by six individual curves. Because of the high volume of data represented in motion curves, datasets often must be reduced to clinically relevant parameters or to a small number of joint positions to enable statistical comparison of kinematic performance between experimental groups. If the research questions seek to identify the location or axis around which motion occurs, helical axes or screw displacement axes (SDAs) can be calculated from the six degrees of freedom motion data. SDAs represent the fact that any arbitrary motion of a bone segment can be accomplished by rotation around and translation along a unique axis. For example, SDA can be calculated from the six degrees of freedom data of the ulna relative to the humerus obtained at 10° and 20° of elbow flexion. This SDA will intersect the trochlea and directly represents the axis around which ulnar rotation occurred during elbow flexion from 10° to 20°. A series of SDAs obtained from incremental joint rotations spanning the range of joint motion can provide a detailed and intuitive characterization of joint function (**Figure 7, A**). Recent SDA analysis of the knee during running showed both a translation of up to 20 mm and a change of up to 15° in inclination of the instantaneous axis of rotation during the flexion cycle, a finding that suggests a single axis knee prosthesis may oversimplify native knee motion.[10]

Joints also can be characterized in terms of their range of motion and joint laxity (**Figure 7, B**). Laxity defines the constraints to motion in response to an external load. For example, anteroposterior knee laxity

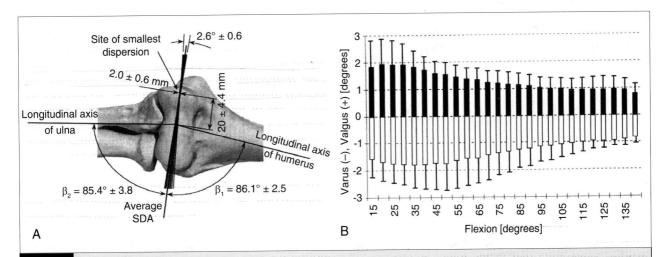

Figure 7 Illustration showing a characterization of joints. **A,** A series of SDAs obtained from incremental joint motion represents the location and dispersion of rotation axes over the elbow range of motion. The smaller the axes dispersion, the closer the joint resembles an ideal hinge joint. The angles between the average SDA and the ulnar and humeral shaft axes are denoted by ß₁ and ß₂, respectively. **B,** Graph showing joint laxity of the elbow, represented by the permissible varus-valgus rotation from a neutral motion path in response to defined varus-valgus loads over the flexion range of motion. (Reproduced with permission from Bottlang M, Madey SM, Steyers CM, Marsh JL, Brown TD: Assessment of elbow joint kinematics in passive motion by electromagnetic motion tracking. *J Orthop Res* 2000;18:197-198.)

1: Principles of Orthopaedics

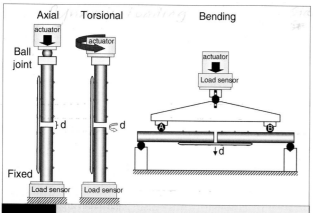

Figure 8 Illustrations showing isolated testing of a plating construct in the three principal loading modes: axial, torsional, and bending. Axial test results can considerably differ, depending on whether the specimen ends are rigidly fixed or loaded through joints. Bending is shown for a four-point-bending setup, which induces a constant bending moment between points A and B. Load-induced actuator displacements represent deformation of the entire construct and can be considerably larger than displacement (d) at the fracture zone.

represents the translation of the tibia relative to the femur in response to anteroposterior loading of the tibia, clinically known as the Lachman test. Translational laxity is measured in millimeters of translation per Newton loading, whereas rotational laxity is measured in degrees of rotation per Newton-meter torsion. If laxity is measured at joint motion increments throughout the range of motion, an envelope of joint laxity can be defined. Clinically, biomechanical measurements of joint laxity over a range of motion are important in determining safe and effective rehabilitation protocols after reconstructive surgery. For example, a recent study of medial collateral ligament sectioning suggests that after a medial collateral ligament repair at the elbow, passive range of motion with the forearm in supination is safer than passive motion with the elbow in pronation.[11]

Clinical Correlation

The interplay between geometric constraints and ligamentous stability discussed in this section is evident in the clinical case of an elbow dislocation. The elbow behaves mainly as a hinge joint with the trochlear groove and radial head providing inherent bony stability while allowing motion along the flexion-extension axis. The muscle forces acting on the elbow also provide a constant compressive force, while the medial and lateral collateral ligaments provide additional stability to the joint. After a traumatic elbow dislocation, the ligamentous constraints are disrupted. However, if the geometric (bony) constraints are intact, the elbow is stable and external splinting is not required. Conversely, if both the geometric constraints and ligamentous restraints are damaged, as occurs with a concomitant coronoid or radial head fracture, the elbow is rendered unstable and usually requires surgical repair.[12]

Bench-Top Testing

Biomechanical testing provides a time- and cost-effective strategy to analyze implant performance in a controlled bench-top environment. Different from clinical outcome studies, biomechanical testing uses simplified test conditions to describe specific aspects of implant performance. This biomechanical testing strategy relies on the definition of a specific performance criterion or a clinically relevant failure mode that will subsequently guide the experimental design and choice of outcome parameters. A clear understanding of these generally simple implant evaluation parameters is helpful in assessing the clinical relevance of results obtained in biomechanical studies.

Specimens

Implants are typically tested in either cadaver or surrogate specimens. Nonembalmed cadaver specimens realistically reflect the complex structure and material properties of bone. However, cadaver specimens can greatly vary in geometry and material properties, even when specimens of similar bone density are selected. Variability can be reduced by using paired specimens, whereby interventions are randomly assigned to either right or left specimens; however, this necessarily confines testing to a comparison between two groups. Alternatively, whole-bone synthetic surrogates of the femur, tibia, humerus, radius, and ulna are commercially available (Pacific Research Laboratories, Vashon Island, WA). These surrogate specimens, consisting of a glass fiber-reinforced epoxy cortex and cancellous bone replicated by rigid polyurethane foam, are designed to have structural properties in the physiologic range of healthy bone. Different from cadaver bone, the variability between surrogate femurs is within 2% to 10%. Polyurethane foam, however, does not replicate the density gradients and load-optimized architecture of the trabecular structure specific to cadaver bone. Also, these synthetic surrogates do not represent osteoporotic bone in which complications associated with implants are most prevalent. For this purpose, a validated surrogate of the osteoporotic femoral diaphysis has recently been introduced.[13]

Loading Mode

All bones are exposed to complex loading composed of three principal loading modes—axial, torsional, and bending. Testing implant performance individually for each of these principal loading modes simplifies the load application and enables isolation of failure mechanisms specific for each principal loading mode (**Figure 8**). To reduce the number of loading scenarios, testing is sometimes only performed in the dominant loading modes for the anatomic site being studied. For example, because the femur is loaded primarily in axial compression and bending, unicortical locked plating of femoral fractures was initially tested in axial compression and bending only, which yielded encouraging results. However, the clinically observed failure mechanism of screw

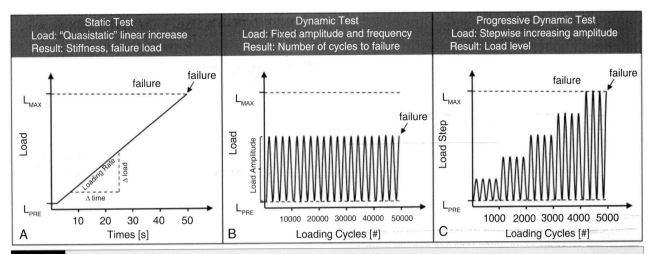

Static Test	Dynamic Test	Progressive Dynamic Test
Load: "Quasistatic" linear increase	Load: Fixed amplitude and frequency	Load: Stepwise increasing amplitude
Result: Stiffness, failure load	Result: Number of cycles to failure	Result: Load level

Figure 9 Graphs showing test load patterns. After application of a preload (L_{PRE}), testing may be conducted statically for assessing stiffness and failure load (L_{MAX}) (**A**), dynamically for assessing the number of loading cycles until fatigue failure occurs (**B**), or with progressive dynamic loading for assessing the failure load level under dynamic loading (**C**).

pullout was subsequently linked to the poor fixation strength of unicortical locking screws in torsion.[14] Therefore, results obtained in one loading mode cannot be extrapolated to alternate loading modes.

Specimen constraints highly influence the load imparted to a specimen under a principal loading mode. For example, if the ends of a plating construct are not rigidly constrained but suspended between ball joints, axial loading will primarily impart plate bending. Therefore, both the loading mode and specimen constraint must be considered when comparing results between studies.

As an alternative to simplified testing under the principal loading modes, implants may be tested under joint-specific complex loading modes representative of the activities of daily living. As previously mentioned, physiologic loading data for a range of activities have been obtained for the hip, knee, shoulder, and spine using implants instrumented with load sensors and telemetry for wireless data transfer.[4-7] For load application in biomechanical tests, these loading data can be combined into a resultant load vector that changes in magnitude and orientation throughout a specific loading task. Reproducing these physiologic transient load vectors in bench-top testing requires sophisticated joint simulators or the use of robotic equipment capable of inducing arbitrary motion and forces in space. Quasiphysiologic load application can be achieved using more standard testing systems by positioning specimens at a specific angle and offset relative to the vertical actuator of a standard material testing system to yield a specific resultant load vector and loading moment.

Physiologic loading and joint motion may also be facilitated by muscle force simulation through tendons. For this purpose, muscle force distributions and activation patterns have been computed from loading data of instrumented implants for the hip, knee, and shoulder. These recent advances in joint and muscle load assessment based on instrumented prostheses are crucial for

resolving the apparent lack of consensus on test configurations and loading conditions in biomechanical studies.

Loading Patterns

Test loads can be applied statically or dynamically. Static loading is used to assess stiffness, constraints, and load transfer but may also be used for strength assessment, whereby loading is gradually increased until failure occurs (**Figure 9, A**). However, clinical failure rarely occurs from a single loading event and most often is better simulated by dynamic loading. Traditionally, dynamic loading has been used for wear and fatigue testing of arthroplasty implants by repeating a load pattern for millions of cycles to simulate multiyear loading histories in an accelerated manner (**Figure 9, B**). Dynamic loading is increasingly being applied for testing osteosynthetic constructs to simulate fixation failure, implant migration, and fatigue. Failure may not consistently occur at a given dynamic load amplitude under a standard cyclic loading regimen. For this reason, several recent studies have applied progressive dynamic loading in which the amplitude of the dynamic load is increased in a stepwise manner to induce construct failure within a controlled number of loading cycles (**Figure 9, C**).

Testing can be conducted using displacement or load control. Displacement-controlled tests prescribe a defined linear or rotational displacement and assess the resulting forces and moments. Load controlled tests apply a force or moment and measure the resulting deformation or motion of the loaded specimen. Most biomechanical tests are conducted using load control to simulate physiologic loading regimens. However, displacement control remains an attractive alternative because of the relative simplicity of applying accurate cyclic displacements with the camshaft or screw-type actuators that are frequently used in mechanoactive tissue engineering applications.

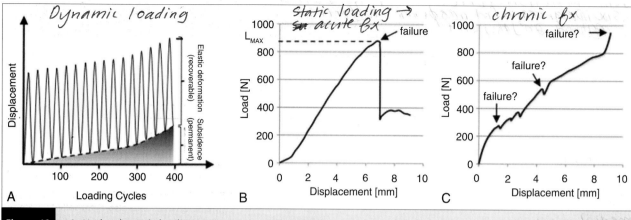

Figure 10   **A,** Under dynamic loading, specimens undergo elastic, recoverable deformation as well as subsidence or migration, which represents the accumulation of unrecoverable displacement. Progression of subsidence is indicative of failure, which can be defined by selection of an appropriate subsidence threshold. **B,** Under static loading, a sudden drop in displacement defines failure and allows identification of strength in terms of peak load (L_{MAX}). **C,** Specimens that gradually fail will complicate detection of failure for strength determination.

Outcome Parameters

Stiffness

Stiffness is frequently used to represent the deformation of a test specimen in response to loading; however, higher stiffness does not necessarily correlate with improved implant performance. Excessive stiffness can increase the risk of periprosthetic fracture because of increased stress risers at the implant-bone interface, especially in the presence of osteoporotic bone. For osteosynthetic constructs, deficient stiffness can lead to hypertrophic nonunions, whereas excessive stiffness can suppress secondary bone healing. Because bone healing depends on the stiffness at the fracture site rather than the entire testing apparatus, reports of the stiffness of osteosynthetic constructs should reflect displacement measured across the fracture site. Stiffness or degradation of stiffness under dynamic loading is sometimes used to infer strength. Although intuitive, inferring strength without testing to failure remains speculative.

Stability

Stability is not an engineering quantity but is frequently used to describe the amount of displacement across a fracture or a bone-implant interface in response to a given loading event. Subsidence or migration represents the amount of unrecovered displacement after the loading event (**Figure 10, A**). Subsidence during dynamic loading provides a sensitive parameter of implant performance. Stabilization of initial subsidence typically indicates successful settling of an implant into a stable position, whereas progression of subsidence reflects the rate of damage accumulation that eventually will lead to implant or fixation failure.

Stress

Stress (σ) in implants and bone cannot be measured directly, but is typically inferred from measurements of stress-induced material deformation and strain (ε). The resulting stress depends on the induced strain as well as on the apparent stiffness of the deforming material ($\sigma = \varepsilon \times E$). A softer material will exhibit less stress than a stiffer material for a given deformation. Strain gauges have been used since 1938 and remain the most common strain sensors because of their high sensitivity and accuracy. They are glued onto a surface of interest and contain a conductive filament that changes electrical resistance when strained. Standard strain gages measure strain in only one direction. Rosette strain gauges contain three filaments to sense the magnitude and orientation of the highest compressive and tensile strains at the strain gage location. Contemporary optical systems can capture continuous strain maps by correlating digital images of a surface obtained before and after deformation. These image correlation systems track the displacement of individual surface markers or the deformation of a speckle pattern projected by lasers onto the object surface. The high sensitivity and noncontact approach of these optical strain sensors enables acquisition of strain distributions on hard and soft tissues, reflecting load transfer mechanisms and stress concentrations.[15] However, all strain sensors are confined to measuring surface strain. Strain in structures and at interfaces can only be estimated by numeric simulation, typically with finite-element analysis.

Strength

Strength provides a clear indicator of implant performance, which correlates clinically with a reduced risk of implant failure. Although strength simply represents the ultimate load at which a structure fails, strength assessment is highly dependent on the choice of failure criterion. For a sudden catastrophic fracture of a structure, the instance of failure is defined by the fracture (**Figure 10, B**). When specimens fail gradually, the instance of failure may be less clear (**Figure 10, C**). In such cases, defining a failure criterion based on a subsidence threshold under dynamic loading can be advantageous. When strength is assessed under dynamic

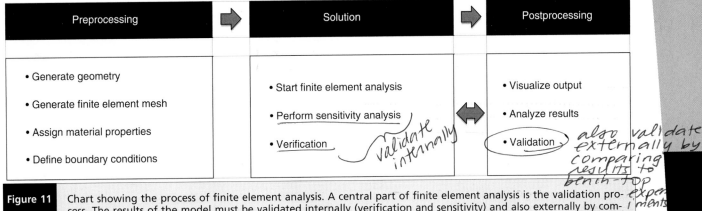

Figure 11 Chart showing the process of finite element analysis. A central part of finite element analysis is the validation process. The results of the model must be validated internally (verification and sensitivity) and also externally by comparing the computed results with bench-top experiments.

1: Principles of Orthopaedics

loading it also can be expressed in terms of fatigue strength, which represents the number of loading cycles of a given magnitude that can be sustained before failure occurs. The highest dynamic load amplitude at which no failure will occur regardless of the number of loading cycles is called the endurance limit. Most importantly, the failure modes induced in a simplified bench-top environment should correlate with clinically observed failures to support the relevance of strength results.

Kinematic Representations of Musculoskeletal Movements

Kinematic representations of musculoskeletal movements, such as displacements and rotation angles around joints, require a clearly defined, physically meaningful, and reproducible reference frame or coordinate system. For any given joint, reference frames can be aligned based on a variety of anatomic landmarks and planes, whereby kinematic representation of the same motion will differ when expressed in different reference frames. A direct comparison of kinematic results between studies is only possible when the same reference frame is used to describe motion. The effects of interventions on joint kinematics also should be evaluated for all permissible translations and rotations around a joint because an intervention may restore one particular kinematic parameter while having a detrimental effect on other kinematic parameters.

Clinical Correlation

Mechanical studies can isolate clinically relevant but rarely observed failure modes. Locked-plate constructs provide excellent fixation in osteoporotic bone; however, the difference in stiffness between the osteoporotic bone and plate is magnified in the presence of angle-stable locked screws. A recent bench-top study, which investigated the effect of a mismatch between implant and bone stiffness, reported that angle-stable, locked screws at the end of the plate increased the risk of a periprosthetic fracture relative to nonlocked screws.[16] This complication is so rare that it is unlikely to be rec-ognized in any reasonably sized clinical study. The bench-top study was valuable because it isolated and identified the problem and proposed a simple but effective solution.

Numeric Simulation

Numeric models have been developed to solve complex loading scenarios to determine stress and strain in implants and musculoskeletal structures.[17,18] Although the loading of a cantilever beam by a single force can be solved analytically, the deformation during walking of a cephalomedullary nail that fixes a subtrochanteric fracture can be considered a complex loading scenario requiring a numeric solution. Finite element analysis is the method of choice to solve these types of problems. Finite element analysis is defined as a numeric method to solve partial differential equations; practically, it is a technique to compute stress, strain, and deformation in a digitized structure (**Figure 11**). The digitized structure consists of thousands of individual elements that are connected to each other. The numeric approach is to consider each individual element and calculate its mechanical behavior as a response to all neighboring elements.

The most time-consuming aspects of a finite element analysis are correctly preprocessing the mechanical problem and verifying and validating the results. For the preprocessing of the mechanical problem, the geometry of the object (bone, implant, or device) must be provided in digital form with sufficient accuracy and spatial resolution of the locations of interest to permit visualization of the results. Mesh or element generation is strongly supported by finite element analysis software but must be tailored to the specific mechanical problem. The material properties, applied loads, and moments must be provided and often must be estimated. In the example of the cephalomedullary nail that fixes a subtrochanteric fracture (**Figure 12**), the list of boundary conditions to be described includes the external load situation, the geometry of the nail, the bone and the fracture, the contact conditions between the implants (nail, screws) and the bone, and the material

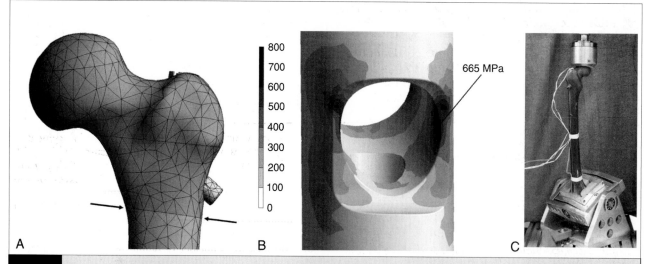

Figure 12 Finite element analysis of cephalomedullary nail fixation of a subtrochanteric fracture of the proximal femur. **A,** The bone and the implant are represented by a mesh of individual elements. Arrows point to the fracture. **B,** The model can show locations of stress concentrations in the nail depending on the type of fracture pattern. **C,** To validate the model, the results of the numeric calculations are compared with results of a biomechanical test setup, which includes strain measurements on the nail by strain gauges.

properties of the bone and the implants.

The results of a finite element analysis should not be presented before verification and validation of the model. Verification of the model requires careful examination of the procedures (such as equation solving and model building) and techniques used. It ensures that the numeric model has no technical flaws and is capable of generating reasonable results. Verification involves determining if things were done correctly. Validation by contrast challenges the model or the concept itself. To validate a numeric model, it is evaluated to determine if the theoretic model is suitable for the real-world problem. Validation involves determining if the correct things were done.

In the example of the cephalomedullary nail, the verification process would ensure the accuracy of the geometry and whether the geometric changes caused by the surgical procedure (holes, cavities, implant placement) are properly represented by the model. The constraints, the loads that act on the bone, the material properties, and the types of numeric contacts between the different parts of the assembly (such as the nail, the lag screw, and the bone fragments) would be checked for reasonableness. The final and most important part of the verification is the so-called convergence analysis. This analysis ensures that the type of finite elements and the mesh density have no influence on the results. The validation of the model would be accomplished by comparing the numeric calculations with experimentally determined measurements. In the example, the osteosynthetic stiffness measured by the testing machine and strains measured on different parts of the implant by strain gauges could be used for validation.

Although the development of a numeric model is an elaborate and time-consuming process, a valid finite element analysis model has several advantages over laboratory experiments. The finite element analysis model provides a much larger variety of results than experiments. The typical outcome measures, such as strain (ε), stress (σ), or deformation (μ), can be determined at every location in the model. For example, it is possible to find the location of the largest stress that occurs at the implant (**Figure 12, B**) or to determine the three-dimensional deformation on each aspect of the fracture gap. It also is possible to obtain measurements from the inside of the model (for example, from the nail in the medullary canal or the endosteal bone surface). Experimental measurements are restricted to limited and predefined measurement locations on the specimen surface and are often only one-dimensional. The most significant advantage of finite element analysis models is the possibility to perform parameter studies in which the model geometry, the material properties, or the boundary conditions can be iteratively changed. In the example of the cephalomedullary nail, there would be interest in determining how the outcome measurements change for different types of hip fracture, after modification of the lag screw diameter, or with the additional use of locking bolts.[17] The effects of different loading scenarios could easily be observed by changing the load direction and amplitude to account for muscle activities during different activities of daily living. Therefore, a validated finite element analysis model is perfectly suited to study the effect of parameter modifications on the mechanical performance of complex geometries and complex loading conditions.

Summary

A sound understanding of basic biomechanical principles provides a strong tool for the orthopaedic surgeon to evaluate the results of bench-top studies and to integrate this information into clinical practice. Biomechanical testing allows specific aspects of the musculoskeletal system to be evaluated in a quantitative manner, without including confounding factors that often make clinical studies difficult. Biomechanical research also enables systematic optimization of orthopaedic implants and interventions, and thereby forms the foundation for innovations that drive the biomedical device industry and that expand a surgeon's ability to improve patient care.

Annotated References

1. Mow VC, Huiskes R: *Basic Orthopaedic Biomechanics and Mechano-Biology*, ed 3. Philadelphia, PA, Lippincott Williams & Wilkins, 2005.

2. Pistoia W, van Rietbergen B, Lochmüller EM, Lill CA, Eckstein F, Rüegsegger P: Estimation of distal radius failure load with micro-finite element analysis models based on three-dimensional peripheral quantitative computed tomography images. *Bone* 2002;30(6):842-848.

3. Heller MO, Bergmann G, Deuretzbacher G, et al: Musculo-skeletal loading conditions at the hip during walking and stair climbing. *J Biomech* 2001;34(7):883-893.

4. Mündermann A, Dyrby CO, D'Lima DD, Colwell CW Jr, Andriacchi TP: In vivo knee loading characteristics during activities of daily living as measured by an instrumented total knee replacement. *J Orthop Res* 2008;26(9):1167-1172.

   An instrumented knee prosthesis was used to measure knee joint force simultaneously with motion capture during activities of daily living. The maximum total compressive load at the knee was highest during stair ascending and descending. Total compressive load exceeded 2.5 times body weight for most activities.

5. Heinlein B, Kutzner I, Graichen F, et al: ESB Clinical Biomechanics Award 2008: Complete data of total knee replacement loading for level walking and stair climbing measured in vivo with a follow-up of 6-10 months. *Clin Biomech (Bristol, Avon)* 2009;24(4):315-326.

   A telemetric tibial tray was used to measure the three forces and three moments acting on the implant, providing in vitro loading data of the knee joint for a range of activities. Stair descending was found to produce the highest loads, with peak force occurring in an axial direction, and peak moments occurring in the frontal plane.

6. Bergmann G, Graichen F, Bender A, Kääb M, Rohlmann A, Westerhoff P: In vivo glenohumeral contact forces: Measurements in the first patient 7 months postoperatively. *J Biomech* 2007;40(10):2139-2149.

   A telemetric shoulder implant was used to measure for the first time glenohumeral contact forces in vivo. Contact force remained below one body weight for most activities of daily living. Moments due to friction in the joint reached 5.2 Nm.

7. Rohlmann A, Graichen F, Bender A, Kayser R, Bergmann G: Loads on a telemeterized vertebral body replacement measured in three patients within the first postoperative month. *Clin Biomech (Bristol, Avon)* 2008;23(2):147-158.

   The forces and moments acting in the lumbar spine during activities of daily living were measured in vivo with telemeterized vertebral body replacements. Sitting or upper body flexion caused resultant forces in excess of 400 N. When working with elevated arms against the resistance of a physiotherapist, forces exceeded 700 N, and moments remained below 4 Nm.

8. Morlock M, Schneider E, Bluhm A, et al: Duration and frequency of every day activities in total hip patients. *J Biomech* 2001;34:873-881.

9. Bingham J, Li G: An optimized image matching method for determining in-vivo TKA kinematics with a dual-orthogonal fluoroscopic imaging system. *J Biomech Eng* 2006;128(4):588-595.

10. van den Bogert AJ, Reinschmidt C, Lundberg A: Helical axes of skeletal knee joint motion during running. *J Biomech* 2008;41(8):1632-1638.

    Intracortical markers were used to determine the helical axis of the knee during the stance phase of running. The axis began at the midepicondylar point at the beginning of the stance phase and moved posteriorly and distally as the knee moved into flexion.

11. Armstrong AD, Dunning CE, Faber KJ, Duck TR, Johnson JA, King GJ: Rehabilitation of the medial collateral ligament-deficient elbow: An in vitro biomechanical study. *J Hand Surg Am* 2000;25(6):1051-1057.

12. Pollock JW, Brownhill J, Ferreira L, McDonald CP, Johnson J, King G: The effect of anteromedial facet fractures of the coronoid and lateral collateral ligament injury on elbow stability and kinematics. *J Bone Joint Surg Am* 2009;91(6):1448-1458.

    Anteromedial facet coronoid fractures were simulated in cadaver elbows with and without lateral ligament repair. In the varus position, type I fractures were stable after lateral ligament repair, whereas type II and III fractures were unstable regardless of the repair status.

13. Sommers MB, Fitzpatrick DC, Madey SM, Vande Zanderschulp C, Bottlang M: A surrogate long-bone model with osteoporotic material properties for biomechanical testing of fracture implants. *J Biomech* 2007;40(15):3297-3304.

    A physical model of the osteoporotic femoral diaphysis was developed and tested to determine five key structural properties: torsional rigidity and strength, bending rigidity and strength, and screw pullout strength. Results demonstrated that all five structural properties were within the lower 16% of those reported for cadaver femurs. Therefore, the model is suitable for implant evaluation in osteoporotic bone where implant fixation is most challenging.

14. Fitzpatrick DC, Doornink J, Madey SM, Bottlang M: Relative stability of conventional and locked plating fixation in a model of the osteoporotic femoral diaphysis. *Clin Biomech (Bristol, Avon)* 2009;24(2):203-209 Epub 2008 Dec 12.

    Stiffness and strength of bridge plating with unicortical and bicortical locking plate fixation was compared with that of a nonlocked construct in a model of osteoporotic femoral diaphysis. Fixation strength was improved with the locked plate under axial loading but may be reduced in bending and torsion.

15. Bottlang M, Mohr M, Simon U, Claes L: Acquisition of full-field strain distributions on ovine fracture callus cross-sections with electronic speckle pattern interferometry. *J Biomech* 2008;41(3):701-705.

    An electronic speckle pattern interferometry system was used to evaluate the possibility of assessing continuous strain distributions on fracture callus cross-sections. Strain acquisition based on this system facilitates reproducible quantification of strain distributions on callus cross-sections.

16. Bottlang M, Doornink J, Byrd GD, Fitzpatrick DC, Madey SM: A nonlocking end screw can decrease fracture risk caused by locked plating in the osteoporotic diaphysis. *J Bone Joint Surg Am* 2009;91(3):620-627.

A locked plate with a locking screw in the last hole was compared with a locked plate with a nonlocking screw in the last hole for fixation in osteoporotic diaphyseal bone. Results showed a higher periprosthetic fracture risk in plates with a locked screw at the end.

17. Eberle S, Gerber C, von Oldenburg G, Hungerer S, Augat P: Type of hip fracture determines load share in intramedullary osteosynthesis. *Clin Orthop Relat Res* 2009;467(8):1972-1980.

    A finite element model of a pertrochanteric fracture, a femoral neck fracture, and a subtrochanteric fracture all fixed with a cephalomedullary nail was developed to evaluate the mechanical performance of the nail. Results showed similar construct stiffness with the lowest peak stress in the fixed femoral neck fracture.

18. Li W, Anderson DD, Goldsworthy JK, Marsh JL, Brown TD: Patient-specific finite element analysis of chronic contact stress exposure after intraarticular fracture of the tibial plafond. *J Orthop Res* 2008;26(8): 1039-1045.

    Patient-specific finite element analysis models of fractured ankle and the uninjured contralateral ankle were developed. Results showed areas of chronic stress overload in the fractured ankles relative to the uninjured ankles.

Chapter 7

Bearing Surface Materials for Hip, Knee, and Spinal Disk Replacement

Javad Parvizi, MD, FRCS   Michael Bercik, MD   Todd Albert, MD

Introduction

Total joint arthroplasty represents one of the most successful surgical procedures in orthopaedics. Joint replacement surgery, especially total hip arthroplasty (THA) and total knee arthroplasty (TKA), often enable patients who were limited by pain and decreased range of motion to return to higher states of function. In the past, total joint arthroplasty was generally indicated for geriatric patients with low activity demands; however, its success has recently expanded its use into treatment plans for more active patients younger than 65 years.[1] The acceptance of more liberal indications for total joint arthroplasty also has highlighted the complication of prosthetic failure. Aseptic loosening and osteolysis secondary to wear has been identified as the primary

cause of prosthetic failure.[2] Much research currently is focused on increasing the longevity of prostheses by increasing wear resistance, which then reduces the overall rate of prosthetic failure and the need for revision surgery. Attempts at wear reduction have involved altering the structure of polyethylene, primarily through the process of cross-linking. Another strategy avoids the use of polyethylene and instead uses bearing surface materials, such as metal and ceramic, which are intrinsically more resistant to wear. This chapter will discuss the basic principles of bearing surfaces and wear; the advantages and disadvantages of the bearing surfaces used in THA and TKA (**Table 1**); and total disk arthroplasty (TDA), a relatively new tool in the orthopaedic repertoire.

Bearing Surfaces

In engineering terms, a bearing surface represents the area of contact between two objects. In total joint arthroplasty, bearing surfaces are the areas on the prosthesis that articulate within the joint. In THA, the femoral head and the acetabular component are the primary bearing surfaces, whereas modular junctions represent secondary bearing surfaces. In TKA, the femoral component, the tibial base plate, and the polyethylene insert are all areas of contact. In TDA, the core replacing the disk and the end plates are the articulating contact areas. These surfaces lie perpendicular to the force transmitted through the joint and are subject to relative motion; consequently, these bearing surfaces are subject to wear.

Wear Defined

Wear Mechanisms

Wear is the removal of material from opposing surfaces under an applied load that occurs when they are put into relative motion. The primary mechanisms of wear that occur with total joint arthroplasty are abrasion,

Dr. Parvizi or an immediate family member serves as a board member, owner, officer, or committee member of the American Association of Hip and Knee Surgeons, American Board of Orthopaedic Surgery, British Orthopaedic Association, Orthopaedic Research and Education Foundation, and SmartTech; serves as a paid consultant to or is an employee of Stryker; and has received research or institutional support from KCI, Medtronic, the Musculoskeletal Transplant Foundation, Smith & Nephew, and Stryker. Dr. Bercik or an immediate family member is a board member, owner, officer, or committee member of the American Academy of Orthopaedic Surgeons. Dr. Albert or an immediate family member serves as a board member, owner, officer, or committee member of the Cervical Spine Research Society and Scoliosis Research Society; has received royalties from DePuy; is a member of a speakers' bureau or has made paid presentations on behalf of DePuy and Biomet; serves as a paid consultant to or is an employee of DePuy; has received research or institutional support from DePuy, AO, Biomet, Medtronic Sofamor Danek, and Synthes; and has stock or stock options held in K2M, Gentis, In Vivo Therapeutics, Vertech, Biomerix, Breakaway Imaging, Paradigm Spine, Pioneer, Invuity, and Crosstree Medical.

Table 1

Summary of Bearing Surfaces Available for THA and TKA

Bearing Surface	Advantages	Disadvantages
Conventional polyethylene	Nontoxic Lower cost Multiple liner options Better fatigue resistance than cross-linked polyethylene	Most bioactivity and osteolysis Not suitable for long-term use or active patients
Highly cross-linked polyethylene	High wear resistance Nontoxic Lower cost Multiple liner options Proven history	Reduced fatigue resistance Increased bioactivity and osteolysis compared with metal and ceramic
Ceramic on ceramic	Highest wear resistance Bioinert Long in vivo experience Wettability Decreased surface roughness Resistance to oxidative wear	Acetabular liner chipping Fracture risk Squeaking Increased cost Limited neck lengths
Metal on metal	Very high wear resistance Larger head diameters Long invivo experience	Increased ion levels Delayed-type hypersensitivity response Corrosion at metal junctions Precise machining required Potential carcinogen
Oxidized zirconium on polyethylene	Wear resistance similar to ceramic Fatigue resistance similar to metal	Limited clinical data to support use Susceptible to damage after dislocation and closed reduction attempts
Ceramic on metal	Reduced wear Reduced friction Less metal ion release	Limited clinical data to support use

adhesion, fatigue, and third-body wear. Abrasion is a mechanical process in which asperities of a harder surface remove material from a softer surface by cutting into and driving through that surface. Adhesion occurs when two materials are pressed against one another, resulting in a bond. When the surfaces are subsequently separated, material is pulled from the softer surface. Fatigue is the progressive local damage inflicted on a material after repeated cyclic loadings. Material is released from a surface when local stresses exceed the fatigue strength of the material.[3] Fatigue damage can range from microscopic pitting to large areas of delamination. Third-body wear is a form of abrasive wear that occurs when particulates such as cement and bone become entrapped in an articular surface and act as asperities. The microscopic materials released from bearing surfaces through the aforementioned mechanisms of wear are called wear particles.

Wear Modes

Wear modes describe the conditions under which the prosthesis is functioning when wear occurs.[4] Mode 1 occurs when two articulating surfaces move relative to each other. This is the primary source of wear in a well-functioning prosthesis. Mode 2 describes wear that occurs when a primary bearing surface moves relative to a secondary surface that was not intended to be part of the articulation. Mode 3 wear occurs when third-party bodies interpose between the primary surfaces. Mode 4 wear describes the relative motion between two secondary bearing surfaces, such as the motion that occurs between the tibial base plate and the undersurface on the polyethylene insert in a TKA prosthesis.

Differences Between Hip, Knee, and Spine Wear Characteristics

The biomechanics and kinematics differ between the hip, the knee, and the spine because of differences in anatomy and movement. Consequently, the bearing surfaces in knee, hip, and spinal disk prostheses are subject to a different milieu of forces and motions that lead to wear. These variations are clinically important because properties of bearing surfaces necessary for function and longevity in one prosthesis may not be as applicable in another prosthesis.

The hip is a congruent ball-in-socket joint, with surface motion primarily occurring as the femoral head slides within the acetabulum. In THA, this sliding movement at the articulation of components produces microabrasion and microadhesion of the bearing surfaces.[5] Although most wear particles arise from the articulating surface, unintentional impingement and motion at the modular junctions also contribute to wear. Currently, the leading cause of THA failure is aseptic loosening and osteolysis that develops secondary to the release of wear particles.[6]

The knee is a complex pivotal hinge joint that allows flexion and extension as well as some internal and external rotation. As with THA, osteolytic loosening of components secondary to the host response to wear particles is one of the leading causes of prosthetic failure. There are two type of bearing surface wear in TKA: articular wear and undersurface wear. Articular wear occurs secondary to contact stresses at the primary bearing surfaces coupled with movement at the articulation. Undersurface wear occurs in knee prostheses between the tibial insert and the tibial base plate. When inserted onto the tibial base plate, current tibial inserts used in fixed-bearing knee prostheses incorporate some type of locking mechanism to prevent motion; however, no system can completely diminish movement between these two components. The resultant micromotion between the insert and the base plate produces some polyethylene particles, which may then contribute to an inflammatory osteolytic response.[7] Mobile-bearing prostheses, which allow free movement between the tibial insert and the base plate, seek to reduce undersurface wear by reducing joint loads. Also, mobile-bearing prostheses permit the use of highly polished cobalt-chromium baseplates, which, because of manufacturing constraints, are more difficult to produce with suitable intraoperative locking mechanisms for standard polyethylene inserts.[8]

In addition to aseptic loosening, TKA may also fail because of fatigue damage and gross fracture. This complication occurs more commonly in TKA than in THA. Because of the hinge-like nature of the knee, contact zones move with respect to the polyethylene component during knee flexion and extension. At one point during gait an area of contact may be under compression, whereas the same area may be under tension at another point during gait. This alternation of forces produces cyclic loading, fatigue, and ultimately, delamination at the bearing surface. Gross failure and fracture of the bearing surface may develop as the end point of this process.[9]

TDA is a relatively recent procedure that was developed to relieve pain associated with degenerative diseases of the spine. Although degrees of motion in vertebral disks are relatively small compared with those seen in knee and hip joints, vertebral disks are subject to axial loads and relative movement during rotation, flexion, and extension of the spine. At the central bearing surface of the polyethylene core, microabrasion and microadhesion are the primary mechanisms of wear. At the rims, fatigue and gross fracture predominate.[10] Interestingly, the components used in TDA incorporated features of both THA and TKA. Under neutral alignment, the axial load is distributed mainly across the central region of the core, and the sliding motion of the disk is similar to that of the hip. During bending movements, compression and tension forces act primarily along the edges of the artificial disk, producing fatigue and failure. Currently, much less is known about the clinical importance of wear in TDA than is understood about the role of this factor in THA and TKA.

Tribology

Tribology is the science of interactive surfaces in relative motion. It incorporates the concepts of wear, friction, and lubrication. Wear is the removal of material from a surface through the mechanisms of adhesion, abrasion, and fatigue. Friction is the force that resists the relative motion of two surfaces in contact; it is described by the coefficient of friction. The coefficient of friction in the native joint is 0.008 to 0.02. Prostheses are designed to replicate (or better) this value to reduce frictional forces across the joint. Lubricant interposed between two opposing surfaces helps carry the existing load between those surfaces. The lambda (λ) ratio describes the ratio of fluid-film thickness to surface roughness. A higher λ ratio is desirable because it translates into reduced friction and wear. A λ ratio greater than 3 is ideal because it represents fluid-film lubrication; in this setting, asperities of opposing surfaces are completely separated and the load is entirely carried by the lubricant. In vivo, mixed film lubrication (defined by a λ ratio between 1 and 3) predominates, and the surfaces are only partially separated.[3]

Biomechanical studies attempt to explore tribology by in vitro simulation of movement at a joint in its natural environment. To better understand and predict wear mechanisms in hip prostheses, hip joint simulators have been used to mimic both the movements of the hip and the lubrication of synovial fluid. Physiologic knee simulators attempt to closely mimic the natural movement and lubrication of a knee over the course of several million cycles to simulate the in vivo wear that occurs in knee prostheses. Unidirectional and multidirectional disk movement simulators have been used to predict wear patterns in vivo. Multidirectional methods appear to more closely reflect the activities of daily living.[11] A variety of methods can be used to analyze wear, including measuring the weight loss of the component, deviation from a reference geometry, and visualization with an electron microscope.

Polyethylene

History and Structure

Polyethylene is a viscoelastic and thermoplastic polymer consisting of long chains of the monomer ethylene. It is composed of the repeating unit $(C_2H_4)_n$, in which all carbon-carbon and carbon-hydrogen bonds are single. First discovered in a reproducible set of chemical conditions in 1935, polyethylene has since become one of the most commercially used plastics in the world. Depending on its density and the branching of its chains, polyethylene can be classified into several different categories. High-density polyethylene is defined by a density greater than 0.941 g/cm^3 and is used in packaging (such as detergent bottles). Low-density polyethylene is defined by a density of 0.910 to 0.940 g/cm^3 and is more suited for the production of plastic bags and film. These two examples hint at the applicability of polyethylene to biologic engineering. Polyethylene has the capacity to be both a sturdy, tough solid that is resistant to wear as well as a material that is ductile and conformable into appropriate geometries. Both properties have clear benefit in the design of replacement components for the complex movements and anatomy of human joints. Sterilization was historically performed with gamma radiation. This also produced free radicals that could participate in cross-linking or oxidation. In an attempt to avoid oxidative damage, sterilization in an oxygen-free environment, usually with ethylene oxide or gas plasma, was performed. Polyethylene components sterilized in this manner showed increased wear by avoiding cross-linking.

Ultra-High–Molecular–Weight Polyethylene

Ultra-high–molecular–weight polyethylene (UHMWPE) is the product of polyethylene catalyzation and is defined by an average molecular weight of greater than 3 million g/mol. It has been the preferred bearing material in orthopaedic joint arthroplasty for more than 40 years. UHMWPE consists of extremely long chains of polyethylene. Its microstructure consists of crystalline domains embedded within an amorphous matrix. The crystalline phase is created by rows of folded carbon chains, whereas the amorphous surrounding is a randomly oriented and entangled environment of polymer chains. Tie molecules connect these sets of chains, providing resistance to mechanical deformation.[12] Despite favorable properties for use in bioengineering, polyethylene remains an imperfect product for bearing surfaces because it is not impervious to wear and inevitably fails after repeated use. This limitation has motivated the search for other materials that produce better clinical results via improved wear resistance. Alternative bearing surfaces with better wear resistance, such as metal and ceramic bearing surfaces, have their own advantages and disadvantages.

Alternative Bearing Surfaces

Bearing Surface Problems

The primary cause of failure in THA and TKA is aseptic loosening secondary to osteolysis. At one time, periprosthetic weakening of the bone and its associated finding on radiographic imaging (such as lytic lesions around the prosthesis) were considered a response to the cement used in implantation. Referred to as cement disease, this process is now better understood and attributed to wear particles. These particles incite a complex inflammatory response in the body involving cytokines, chemokines, and multiple cell types. Although the steps have not been entirely elucidated, osteoclastic maturation in response to the presence of wear particles is known to lead to resorption of the bone surrounding the prosthesis. All wear particles are not equally responsible for inciting an inflammatory response. In THA, macrophages appear most sensitive to submicron-sized particles.[13] Different bearing surfaces produce different ratios in the sizes of created microscopic wear particles. Polyethylene bearing surfaces produce wear particles within the size ranges that are ideal for inciting an inflammatory response. Metals and ceramics produce particles in the less active ranges of inflammatory incitation, which should result in less osteolysis.[14]

The search for clinically superior alternative bearing surfaces has intensified because the proportion of patients younger than 65 years (and perhaps even those as younger than 45 years) who are being treated with joint replacement surgery is increasing.[1] In THA, metal on polyethylene remains the most common type of implant. The realization that polyethylene wear and subsequent osteolysis is the leading cause of prosthetic failure has encouraged some surgeons to use alternative bearing surfaces, most notably metal-on-metal and ceramic-on-ceramic implants, which currently are the second and third most commonly used bearing surfaces, respectively.[15] These bearing surfaces have their own limitations; however, both are more wear resistant than polyethylene.

Metal-on-Metal Prostheses

Metal-on-metal hip prostheses have been in clinical use longer than any bearing surface. In 1938, an entire hip was replaced with stainless steel components. Improvements were made on this initial design because stainless steel is not optimal for use in an articular surface. In the 1960s, the McKee-Farrar metal-on-metal prosthesis was introduced using a cobalt-chromium alloy. Metal-on-metal hip prostheses were the most commonly used hip replacement option until the 1970s, when the Charnley polyethylene-on-metal hip prosthesis almost universally supplanted their use. The Charnley model gained favor for several reasons, including the early success of the Charnley prosthesis, known failures of metal prostheses, and concerns regarding metal sensitivity and carcinogenesis.[16] As the role of polyethylene wear in prosthetic failure became better understood, the search for clinically superior alternative bearing surfaces rejuvenated the use of metal-on-metal prostheses. Recent retrieval analyses have shown that the metal-on-metal prostheses achieve excellent long-term results.[17] Long-term survivorship of metal-on-metal prostheses compare favorably with the Charnley and other metal-on-polyethylene prostheses.[18] The Metasul (Zimmer, Warsaw, IN) hip replacement, a cobalt-alloy bearing reintroduced in the 1980s, is still a commonly used metal-on-metal prosthesis. The Metasul incorporates a polyethylene acetabular cup with a metal inlay that directly articulates with the metallic alloy of the femoral head. Other improvements on first-generation metal-on-metal prostheses include better bearing geometry and an enhanced surface finish.

The most apparent advantage of the metal-on-metal hip prosthesis is its greater resistance to wear compared with polyethylene. Run-in wear represents a period of increased wear, usually during the first million cycles, which is followed by a longer period with a lower rate of consistent wear (steady-state wear). Modern metal-on-metal prostheses have shown a yearly run-in wear rate of approximately 25 µm, and steady-state wear of 3 to 7 µm. This rate represents only 2% of the wear rate typically seen in historic (such as non–cross-linked) polyethylene.[19] Metal-on-metal prostheses also have shown a unique ability to "self-polish." Given the ductility of metal components, larger scratches on the component surface may be polished down to smaller scratches with continued use.[20] Reducing wear increases the potential longevity of a prosthesis by keeping the wear particle concentration and size below the threshold for osteolysis.[11] Theoretically, a metal-on-metal prosthesis should last the lifetime of a patient, even a younger and more active patient.

Another advantage of the metal-on-metal prosthesis is its tolerance of larger femoral heads. This factor is clinically important because larger diameter articulating couples are more stable and allow greater range of motion. With polyethylene components, larger femoral heads lead to increased wear rates; therefore, to optimize wear resistance and longevity, overall stability is compromised with the use of a smaller femoral head. In contrast, metal-on-metal femoral heads allow for less exclusivity between wear resistance and stability because metal-on-metal components have reduced wear with larger femoral heads.[21] A larger femoral head pulls more fluid into the articulation, leading to an increased state of fluid-film lubrication and a reduction of frictional forces in the prosthesis.

Concerns remain regarding the long-term biologic effects of metal ions released from metal-on-metal prostheses. For example, elevated levels of chromium have been found in patients with metal-on-metal implants, with the prosthetic component indicated as the primary source of the ions.[22] Theoretically, increased metal ions carry risks for carcinogenesis, delayed hypersensitivity reactions, and organ toxicity. In the local periprosthetic tissue, evidence of hypersensitivity and unusual lymphocytic aggregates have been reported. The term acute lymphocytic vasculitis associated lesions (ALVAL) has been used to describe the lymphocyte proliferation and associated vasculitis that occur in response to the release of metal particles.[23] One study evaluating metal-on-metal prostheses reported a unique perivascular lymphocytic infiltrate.[23] Although an immunologic response was evident, it was unlike that seen with macrophagic response to polyethylene debris, which is characterized by a foreign body response and granuloma formation. Rather, this response was more indicative of a type IV delayed hypersensitivity reaction. Notably, osteolysis was reported as a cause of implant failure; replacement with more inert metals was required for successful revision. Similar cases of metallic hypersensitivity necessitating revision have been reported, including a case report of two revisions that describe a similar type IV hypersensitivity reaction as well as tissue hyperreactivity caused by gross wear.[24]

Another concern with the use of a metal-on-metal bearing surface has been the development of joint effusion and local soft-tissue reaction (pseudotumor) that is known to occur independent of failure or loosening of the components. In most instances, the patient is asymptomatic. Pseudotumors are thought to occur with greater wear and in the presence of higher concentrations of metal ions. A recent study investigating the wear characteristics of implants revised for the presence of pseudotumors, as compared with a control group revised for other reasons, showed increased wear associated with the presence of pseudotumors. Edge loading and its associated loss of fluid-film lubrication appeared to be the dominant mechanism of wear. The authors of this study suggest that inadequate coverage of the femoral head component from the outset may have led to increased wear and subsequent pseudotumor formation.[25]

Perhaps more concerning is the systemic distribution of metal ions in the body. Increased levels of metal ions, particularly cobalt and chromium, have been observed in the blood and urine of patients treated with metal-on-metal hip prostheses. Postoperatively, these ions can increase in concentration fivefold to tenfold.[26] As metal-on-metal prostheses are more often considered for younger and more active patients because of their resistance to wear and potential longevity, the relationship between activity level and metal ion release is becoming more important. Unfortunately, a definitive answer regarding this relationship has not been determined. One study showed little variability in metal ion levels over the course of 2 weeks with varying amounts of activity,[27] whereas a later study reported a direct relationship between increased ion levels after short periods of activity.[28] Current studies, however, have not proven a direct relationship between ion levels and primary malignancies.[29]

Because the implantation of metal-on-metal prostheses is a relatively recent trend, there are few long-term studies showing efficacy. Two recent studies have shown survivorship rates of 93% to 98% after 10 years of implantation.[29,30] This remains an area of active investigation.

Ceramic-on-Ceramic Prostheses

Alumina ceramic-on-ceramic prostheses have been in use since the early 1970s. Historically, ceramic-on-ceramic prostheses did not fare as well initially as their counterparts. The underperformance of first-generation ceramic prostheses was associated with the complications of excessive wear, fracture, and migration.[31] These complications were attributed to the inadequate production of materials and poor surgical technique. To increase fracture resistance and overall strength, material was inserted into second-generation ceramics to limit grain size, thereby reducing cracking and fracture propagation. Ceramic-on-ceramic prostheses, now in their third generation of production, have continued to improve. Proof testing, the process by which ceramics are subjected to stresses greater than those expected in their routine use, helps ensure quality; weaker components are removed from circulation prior to distribution and clinical implementation.

Advantageous properties of third-generation ceramics and better clinical results can be primarily attributed

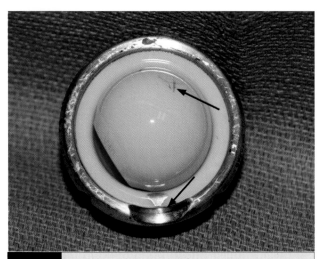

Figure 1 The impingement between the femoral neck and the acetabular rim is believed to lead to metal transfer and patch wear that, when combined with other factors (such as the type and position of components), may lead to squeaking.

to improvements in purity, grain microstructure, and strength. Advances in ceramic manufacturing include the ability to produce very pure, fully dense ceramics with a small grain size; this reduces crack propagation and fracture. Third-generation ceramics have the lowest wear rates of all the currently used bearing surfaces and produce low rates of osteolysis.[32] Given their hardness, ceramics can maintain polish in the presence of third body particles. Ceramics also are hydrophilic, which leads to higher wettability of the surface and better lubrication within the joint. Ceramics, unlike metal prostheses, are biologically inert. They are fully oxidized and thus do not release ions or further oxidize in vivo.[18] Of the two most commonly used ceramics, zirconia and alumina, zirconia appears to be harder and stronger but may be less thermostable. Reports of phase transformation of zirconia have been reported.[33]

Ceramic-on-ceramic prostheses also have limitations. To prevent excessive wear and fracture, ceramics must be inserted with optimal positioning, which can be complicated by the reduced head size options for ceramic prostheses. Wear, surface damage, and rarely, fracture can occur. When gross fracture occurs, total revision with removal of all components is often necessary.[34] The most unusual complication of ceramic-on-ceramic prostheses is squeaking. Reports of squeaking rates vary from less than 3% to more than 10%.[35] Currently, the etiology of squeaking remains unclear, but a multifactorial cause is likely.[36] It is believed that a contact (impingement) between the femoral neck and the metal rim of the acetabulum may lead to generation of metal particles, which if transmitted into the bearing surface, may result in squeaking (**Figure 1**). The latter may explain why the incidence of squeaking is much higher with a particular ceramic-on-ceramic prosthetic design that encases the ceramic bearing in a metal housing on the acetabular side. Other factors are be-

lieved to play a role in noise generation with ceramic-on-ceramic bearing surfaces, including component positions, which increases the likelihood of impingement; the type of components (a specific design of femoral stem made of titanium, molybdenum, zirconium, and ferrous alloy [TMZF; Stryker, Kalamazoo, MI] is currently implicated); and possibly, the thickness of the acetabular shell. It is important to note that the etiology of squeaking associated with a ceramic-on-ceramic bearing surface remains unknown and the aforementioned factors are mere speculations. The problem of squeaking is generally a curious annoyance for most patients, but for some it may necessitate revision. Ceramic components also are notably more expensive than are their polyethylene counterparts.

Clinical results of modern ceramic-on-ceramic prostheses are generally encouraging. In comparison with metal-on-polyethylene hip replacements, ceramics have shown no significant difference in patient satisfaction but have resulted in fewer revisions and less evidence of osteolysis.[37] Fracture rates have generally been reported as very low, although one recent study showed a 1.7% rate of alumina bearing surface failure caused mainly by impingement and acetabular cup chipping.[38] The extrapolation of these numbers to other alumina prostheses is uncertain.

Highly Cross-Linked Polyethylene

UHMWPE has been the most commonly used acetabular component in hip prostheses for the past 30 years. UHMWPE is less suitable for younger, active patients because component wear causes failure secondary to osteolysis and loosening around the prosthesis. In an effort to improve the wear properties of polyethylene cups, highly cross-linked UHMWPE was introduced in the 1990s.

Cross-linking is performed via a series of steps that includes irradiation, thermal processing, and sterilization. Radiation breaks carbon-hydrogen bonds in polyethylene chains, creating free radicals that then participate in covalent bonds. Formation of these covalent bonds makes polyethylene more resistant to wear and deformation. A relationship between dose irradiation, cross-linking, and wear resistance has been reported.[39] The most rapid decrease in wear rate occurs with irradiation of 0 to 5 mrad, and then further decreases, becoming too small to measure after 10 mrad. Although the created free radicals may form covalent bonds, they may also react with oxygen if they remain in the plastic. Oxidation weakens the plastic and can be viewed as an opposing force to cross-linking. Thermal processing of irradiated polyethylene reduces the amount of free radicals present. This can be accomplished via remelting (heating to a point above the melting point of the plastic) or annealing (heating to a point just below the melting point). Remelting completely removes the free radicals from the plastic but in doing so changes the crystalline structure and consequently reduces its mechanical and fatigue properties. Annealing does not change mechanical properties but leaves free radicals available for oxidation. Another strategy to reduce oxidation is the addition of antioxidant agents, such as vitamin E, to the polyethylene; these agents appear to "quench" the free radicals.

Attempts to resolve these problems has led to the current process of polyethylene manufacturing. Polyethylene is initially cross-linked via irradiation, then thermally processed to remove remaining free radicals, then sterilized in a nonoxidative environment to avoid reintroducing free radicals and subsequent oxidation.[40]

In vitro studies have shown the increased wear resistance of highly cross-linked polyethylene cups.[41] When this wear resistance is considered along with the established benefits of polyethylene—a proven history of clinical satisfaction, nontoxicity, affordable cost, and multiple liner options providing increased flexibility—highly cross-linked polyethylene continues to be a popular bearing surface option. Clinical studies have shown no significant clinical differences in early and intermediate follow-up periods but have supported laboratory data showing increased wear resistance as compared with conventional polyethylene.[42] It is hoped that longer-term studies will show an extrapolation of these positive results, with clinically superior end results.

Increasing wear resistance via cross-linking weakens fatigue strength. This compromise in mechanical properties has been verified as a potential factor leading to fatigue failure in highly cross-linked components.[43] The clinical success of UHMWPE components will depend on striking a balance between wear, fatigue, and fracture resistance.

Other Options

A ceramic-on-metal combination prosthesis has been developed to incorporate the benefits of hard bearing surfaces while reducing the risks associated with both metal and ceramic components. More specifically, ceramic-on-metal prostheses reduce metal ion release and ceramic fracture. Comparisons of tribology and ion release of ceramic-on-metal THAs compared with ceramic-on-ceramic and metal-on-metal THAs showed reduced friction, wear, and metal ion release in laboratory studies, and a reduction of ion release in early clinical studies.[44] Oxidized zirconium represents another attempt to create the ideal bearing surface. These surfaces are derived from a zirconium base that is heated and then infused with oxygen, transforming the outermost layer into a ceramic shell. This surface essentially combines the fracture resistance of metal with the wear resistance of ceramics. The major advantage of oxidized zirconium is its apparent capacity for reduced wear when coupled as a femoral head component to a polyethylene cup.[45] No clinical studies to date have identified any clinical benefit. There is a case report describing damage to the oxidized zirconium head after recurrent dislocations.[46] Although the oxidized zirconium shell is strong, the zirconium base may be less suitable as a bearing surface based on the reported femoral head damage.

Total Disk Arthroplasty

TDA began in the 1960s.[47] Although the original TDA prosthesis ultimately failed, newer models have been developed as alternatives to fusion for alleviating back pain. Although lumbar fusion has been successful in treating back pain, it has been associated with complications such as pseudarthrosis and adjacent-level disk disease (the exact etiology of the latter is not yet fully understood, but altered biomechanics after fusion are thought to play a role). TDA is based on the theory of replacing the diseased disk, thereby relieving pain and reproducing functional movement. This would have two advantages over fusion: removing the need for fusion and the risk of pseudarthrosis, and possibly reducing adjacent-level disk disease. There are three categories of disk replacements currently in use in lumbar TDA: unconstrained, semiconstrained, and constrained prostheses. The Charité prosthesis (DePuy Spine, Raynham, MA) is composed of cobalt-chromium-molybdenum alloy end plates and a polyethylene core (**Figure 2, A**). This unconstrained model theoretically parallels the natural motion of a native disk. The ProDisc-L (Synthes, West Chester, PA) prosthesis is a semiconstrained model (**Figure 2, B**). The core is locked into the inferior end plate, reducing the risk of extrusion, but perhaps at the cost of a decreased range of motion. The ProDisc-L contains a polyethylene core. The constrained FlexiCore (Stryker) represents the newest TDA implant.[47]

Much less is known concerning the in vivo biomechanics of the spine than is known about the in vivo biomechanics of the hip and the knee. As TDA is a relatively young science, the tribologic behavior of disk prostheses requires further investigation. In vitro studies simulating multidirectional wear seem to more accurately reflect the activities of daily living and induce more profound wear than unidirectional studies.[11] Despite the finding of a higher proportion of wear than originally anticipated, osteolysis does not seem to be as serious a concern in TDA as it is in THA and TKA. In one study, periprosthetic tissue inflammation and activated macrophages were observed; however, osteolysis was not evident in 96.6% of the revisions.[48] For the all-metal disk replacements, there is concern regarding metal ion release locally and systemically. Cobalt and chromium metal ion release in TDA may be similar to that which occurs in THA.[49]

The primary cause of failure in THA and TKA, aseptic loosening, is rare in TDA. As mentioned, osteolysis seems to be a much more rare complication in TDA. In one study of 18 patients treated with TDA revision surgery, osteolysis was reported in only 1 patient.[10] Subsidence was the most common complication. Anterior migration, core dislocation, and subluxation also were more common than osteolysis in this study. This study involved only short- and medium-term follow-up. With longer follow-up, the prevalence of osteolysis may become more frequent. Also, because TDA is still a very new procedure, inadequate surgical technique and infe-

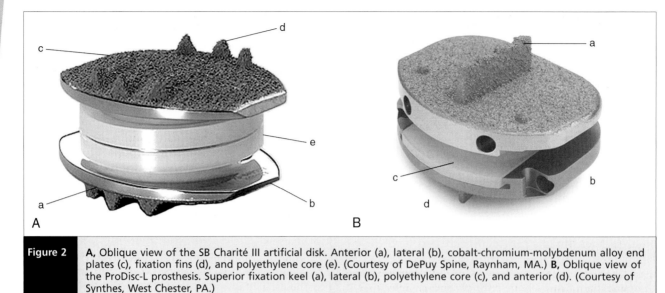

Figure 2 **A,** Oblique view of the SB Charité III artificial disk. Anterior (a), lateral (b), cobalt-chromium-molybdenum alloy end plates (c), fixation fins (d), and polyethylene core (e). (Courtesy of DePuy Spine, Raynham, MA.) **B,** Oblique view of the ProDisc-L prosthesis. Superior fixation keel (a), lateral (b), polyethylene core (c), and anterior (d). (Courtesy of Synthes, West Chester, PA.)

rior products are almost certainly more ubiquitous and clinically relevant than in THA or TKA. As TDA evolves and surgeon familiarity increases, the current leading complications may become more infrequent and osteolysis more prominent. It also must be noted that because of the proximity of the disk prosthesis to the spine and the more invasive surgical approach necessary to reach the spine, TDA failure may induce more morbidity than THA or TKA.

There is a dearth of clinical data supporting TDA. One study found lumbar TDA to be more efficacious and superior to fusion in certain patients.[50] Similar conclusions have been reached in trials of cervical TDA.[51] These studies have not yet provided long-term data. Other TDA procedures that initially were deemed successful have produced poor results when observed over longer periods. One study reported good clinical short-term results; however, longer follow-up showed that the patient ultimately required revision secondary to massive osteolysis.[52] Further investigation into the long-term clinical results of lumbar and cervical TDA are necessary before definitive statements can be made regarding their efficacy.

Future Directions

The quest continues for optimal bearing surfaces for total joint arthroplasty. The evolution of bearing surfaces in the hip, the knee, and for disk replacement surgery will strive to develop components with more resistant surfaces and improved fatigue strength. For polyethylene components, alternative mechanisms for neutralizing free radicals, including vitamin E quenching and multistage annealing, are being incorporated. More studies are needed to follow up on the long-term clinical results of metal and ceramic components and the frequency and outcomes of potential complications. Indications and contraindications for TDA must be better defined. More extensive investigations into the biologic and tribologic properties of disk prostheses are under way; findings from these studies will help predict and build on in vivo outcomes.

Annotated References

1. Kurtz SM, Lau E, Ong K, Zhao K, Kelly M, Bozic KJ: Future young patient demand for primary and revision joint replacement: National projections from 2010 to 2030. *Clin Orthop Relat Res* 2009;467(10):2606-2612.

   The authors used the Nationwide Inpatient Sample between 1993 and 2006 to project the upcoming demands for total joint replacement. They predict that younger populations (younger than 65 years) will exceed 50% of all total hip replacements and total knee replacements by 2011.

2. Clohisy JC, Calvert G, Tull F, McDonald D, Maloney WJ: Reasons for revision hip surgery: a retrospective review. *Clin Orthop Relat Res* 2004;429(429):188-192.

3. Heisel C, Silva M, Schmalzried TP: Bearing surface options for total hip replacement in young patients. *Instr Course Lect* 2004;53:49-65.

4. McKellop HA: The lexicon of polyethylene wear in artificial joints. *Biomaterials* 2007;28(34):5049-5057.

   The author defines the vocabulary pertaining to polyethylene wear in artificial joints. Broad categories include modes, mechanisms, damage, and debris.

5. McKellop HA, Campbell P, Park SH, et al: The origin of submicron polyethylene wear debris in total hip arthroplasty. *Clin Orthop Relat Res* 1995;311(311):3-20.

6. Ulrich SD, Seyler TM, Bennett D, et al: Total hip arthroplasties: what are the reasons for revision? *Int Orthop* 2008;32(5):597-604.

This study evaluated the indications for revision hip arthroplasty in patients requiring revision surgery less than 5 years after the index THA and more than 5 years after the index THA.

7. Wasielewski RC, Parks N, Williams I, Surprenant H, Collier JP, Engh G: Tibial insert undersurface as a contributing source of polyethylene wear debris. *Clin Orthop Relat Res* 1997;345:53-59.

8. Callaghan JJ, Insall JN, Greenwald S, et al: Mobile-bearing knee replacement. *J Bone Joint Surg Am* 2000; 82:1020-1041.

9. Wright TM, Bartel DL: The problem of surface damage in polyethylene total knee components. *Clin Orthop Relat Res* 1986;205:67-74.

10. Kurtz SM, van Ooij A, Ross R, et al: Polyethylene wear and rim fracture in total disc arthroplasty. *Spine J* 2007; 7(1):12-21.

    The authors analyzed 21 implants from 18 patients treated with TDA to evaluate the magnitude and rate of polyethylene wear and surface damage.

11. Grupp TM, Yue JJ, Garcia R Jr, et al: Biotribological evaluation of artificial disc arthroplasty devices: influence of loading and kinematic patterns during in vitro wear simulation. *Eur Spine J* 2009;18(1):98-108.

    The authors of this study reported in vitro wear differences in total disk prostheses with multidirectional versus unidirectional moving patterns. There was increased wear associated with the multidirectional group. The authors suggest that in vivo loading likely follows a multidirectional path.

12. Kurtz SM, Muratoglu OK, Evans M, Edidin AA: Advances in the processing, sterilization, and crosslinking of ultra-high molecular weight polyethylene for total joint arthroplasty. *Biomaterials* 1999;20(18):1659-1688.

13. Holt G, Murnaghan C, Reilly J, Meek RM: The biology of aseptic osteolysis. *Clin Orthop Relat Res* 2007;460: 240-252.

    This literature review describes the biochemical processes leading to aseptic osteolysis, with emphasis on the receptor activator of nuclear factor-kappa β ligand (RANKL)–receptor activator of nuclear factor (RANK)-kappa β pathway.

14. Campbell P, Shen FW, McKellop H: Biologic and tribologic considerations of alternative bearing surfaces. *Clin Orthop Relat Res* 2004;418(418):98-111.

15. Bozic KJ, Kurtz S, Lau E, et al: The epidemiology of bearing surface usage in total hip arthroplasty in the United States. *J Bone Joint Surg Am* 2009;91(7):1614-1620.

    The authors reviewed the Nationwide Inpatient Sample database to determine the prevalence of each type of hip replacement in 112,095 primary THAs.

16. Amstutz HC, Grigoris P: Metal on metal bearings in hip arthroplasty. *Clin Orthop Relat Res* 1996;329(suppl): S11-S34.

17. Brown SR, Davies WA, DeHeer DH, Swanson AB: Long-term survival of McKee-Farrar total hip prostheses. *Clin Orthop Relat Res* 2002;402:157-163.

18. Jacobson SA, Djerf K, Wahlström O: Twenty-year results of McKee-Farrar versus Charnley prosthesis. *Clin Orthop Relat Res* 1996;329(suppl):S60-S68.

19. Dumbleton JH, Manley MT: Metal-on-Metal total hip replacement: What does the literature say? *J Arthroplasty* 2005;20(2):174-188.

20. Sieber HP, Rieker CB, Kottig P: Analysis of 118 second-generation metal-on-metal retrieved hip implants. *J Bone Joint Surg Br* 1999;81:46-50.

21. Dowson D, Hardaker C, Flett M, Isaac GH: A hip joint simulator study of the performance of metal-on-metal joints: Part I: the role of materials. *J Arthroplasty* 2004; 19(8, suppl 3):118-123.

22. Maezawa K, Nozawa M, Matsuda K, Sugimoto M, Shitoto K, Kurosawa H: Serum chromium levels before and after revision surgery for loosened metal-on-metal total hip arthroplasty. *J Arthroplasty* 2009;24(4):549-553.

    The authors analyzed the serum chromium levels in 10 patients with metal-on-metal articulations before and after revision surgery. Mean serum chromium levels decreased from 2.53 µg/L to 0.46 µg/L in patients with no residual metal articulations, and decreased from 2.85 µg/L and 1.90 µg/L in patients with retained metal articulations on the contralateral side.

23. Willert HG, Buchhorn GH, Fayyazi A, et al: Metal-on-metal bearings and hypersensitivity in patients with artificial hip joints. A clinical and histomorphological study. *J Bone Joint Surg Am* 2005;87(1):28-36.

24. Mikhael MM, Hanssen AD, Sierra RJ: Failure of metal-on-metal total hip arthroplasty mimicking hip infection. A report of two cases. *J Bone Joint Surg Am* 2009; 91(2):443-446.

    The authors describe a case report of prosthetic failure secondary to metal hypersensitivity reactions in two patients with similar clinical presentations that were suggestive of periprosthetic infection.

25. Kwon YM, Glyn-Jones S, Simpson DJ, et al: Analysis of wear of retrieved metal-on-metal hip resurfacing implants revised due to pseudotumours. *J Bone Joint Surg Br* 2010;92(3):356-361.

    The authors quantified the wear in vivo of implants revised for pseudotumors and for those revised for other reasons. They found a significantly higher rate of median linear wear in both the femoral and acetabular components of implants revised for pseudotumors.

26. MacDonald SJ: Metal-on-metal total hip arthroplasty: The concerns. *Clin Orthop Relat Res* 2004;429:86-93.

1: Principles of Orthopaedics

27. Heisel C, Silva M, Skipor AK, Jacobs JJ, Schmalzried TP: The relationship between activity and ions in patients with metal-on-metal bearing hip prostheses. *J Bone Joint Surg Am* 2005;87(4):781-787.

28. Khan M, Takahaski T, Kuiper JH, Sieniawska CE, Takagi K, Richardson JB: Current in vivo wear of metal-on-metal bearings assessed by exercise-related rise in plasma cobalt level. *J Orthop Res* 2006;24(11):2029-2035.

29. Grübl A, Marker M, Brodner W, et al: Long-term follow-up of metal-on-metal total hip replacement. *J Orthop Res* 2007;25(7):841-848.

    The authors investigated the rate of primary malignancies in 98 patients with 105 metal-on-metal primary THAs over a 10-year period. Malignancies did not occur at a greater rate than seen in the general population.

30. Neumann DR, Thaler C, Hitzl W, Huber M, Hofstadter T, Dorn U: Long-term results of a contemporary metal-on-metal total hip arthroplasty: A 10-year follow-up study. *J Arthroplasty* 2009; Jul 10. [Epub ahead of print]

    One hundred metal-on-metal prostheses were prospectively analyzed up to 126 months postoperatively. Implant survivorship was measured using component removal secondary to aseptic loosening as the end point.

31. Winter M, Griss P, Scheller G, Moser T: Ten- to 14-year results of a ceramic hip prosthesis. *Clin Orthop Relat Res* 1992;282:73-80.

32. Lusty PJ, Tai CC, Sew-Hoy RP, Walter WL, Walter WK, Zicat BA: Third-generation alumina-on-alumina ceramic bearings in cementless total hip arthroplasty. *J Bone Joint Surg Am* 2007;89(12):2676-2683.

    The authors report on a 5-year study investigating the rates of wear and osteolysis associated with modern ceramic hip prostheses; 301 third-generation alumina-on-alumina cementless primary hip replacements in 283 patients performed at one center using the same surgical technique and implant were investigated.

33. Kim YH, Kim JS: Tribological and material analyses of retrieved alumina and zirconia ceramic heads correlated with polyethylene wear after total hip replacement. *J Bone Joint Surg Br* 2008;90(6):731-737.

    The surface characteristics and penetration rates of alumina versus zirconia ceramic heads were compared with ceramic-on-polyethylene components. Phase transformation in the zirconia heads was also examined.

34. Barrack RL, Burak C, Skinner HB: Concerns about ceramics in THA. *Clin Orthop Relat Res* 2004;429:73-79.

35. Jarrett CA, Ranawat AS, Bruzzone M, Blum YC, Rodriguez JA, Ranawat CS: The squeaking hip: a phenomenon of ceramic-on-ceramic total hip arthroplasty. *J Bone Joint Surg Am* 2009;91(6):1344-1349.

    The authors reviewed 149 ceramic-on-ceramic hips in 131 patients at a minimum 1-year follow-up. Fourteen patients described a squeaking noise, squeaking was reproducible in four patients, and one patient reported squeaking before prompting by the questionnaire. Level of evidence: Therapeutic level IV.

36. Restrepo C, Parvizi J, Kurtz SM, Sharkey PF, Hozack WJ, Rothman RH: The noisy ceramic hip: is component malpositioning the cause? *J Arthroplasty* 2008;23(5):643-649.

    In 999 patients treated with THA, 28 reported squeaking postoperatively. Radiographic analyses of acetabular positioning in squeaking and nonsqueaking prostheses were compared. No significant difference was found in cup inclination. Four retrieved components were analyzed for stripe wear.

37. Capello WN, D'Antonio JA, Feinberg JR, Manley MT, Naughton M: Ceramic-on-ceramic total hip arthroplasty: Update. *J Arthroplasty* 2008;23(7, suppl)S39-S43.

    The authors report on a prospective, randomized, multicenter study of alumina-on-alumina hip prostheses that included 475 hips in 452 patients. The authors suggest clinically superior results compared with conventional polyethylene-on-metal bearings.

38. Park YS, Hwang SK, Choy WS, Kim YS, Moon YW, Lim SJ: Ceramic failure after total hip arthroplasty with an alumina-on-alumina bearing. *J Bone Joint Surg Am* 2006;88(4):780-787.

39. Ries MD, Pruitt L: Effect of cross-linking on the microstructure and mechanical properties of ultra-high molecular weight polyethylene. *Clin Orthop Relat Res* 2005;440:149-156.

40. Jacobs CA, Christensen CP, Greenwald AS, McKellop H: Clinical performance of highly cross-linked polyethylenes in total hip arthroplasty. *J Bone Joint Surg Am* 2007;89(12):2779-2786.

    The authors present a review of the clinical performance of highly cross-linked polyethylene and summarize information on the manufacturing processes and other influences on clinical performance.

41. McKellop H, Shen F, Lu B, Campbell P, Salovey R: Effect of sterilization method and other modifications on the wear resistance of acetabular cups made of ultra-high molecular weight polyethylene. A hip-simulator study. *J Bone Joint Surg Am* 2000;82-A(12):1708-1725.

42. McCalden RW, MacDonald SJ, Rorabeck CH, Bourne RB, Chess DG, Charron KD: Wear rate of highly cross-linked polyethylene in total hip arthroplasty. A randomized controlled trial. *J Bone Joint Surg Am* 2009;91(4):773-782.

    This prospective, randomized controlled study compared clinical outcomes and head penetration in 50 patients with highly cross-linked polyethylene prostheses and 50 patients with conventional polyethylene. Level of evidence: Therapeutic level I.

43. Tower SS, Currier BH, Lyford KA, Van Citters DW, Mayor MB: Rim cracking of the cross-linked longevity

polyethylene acetabular liner after total hip arthroplasty. *J Bone Joint Surg Am* 2007;89(10):2212-2217.

Four fractured highly cross-linked polyethylene acetabular liners were examined to determine the factors that played a role in their failure. The authors suggest that material properties of the acetabular liners were partly responsible for fractures.

44. Williams S, Schepers A, Isaac G, et al: The 2007 Otto Aufranc Award: Ceramic-on-metal hip arthroplasties. A comparative in vitro and in vivo study. *Clin Orthop Relat Res* 2007;465:23-32.

An in vitro and in vivo comparison of ceramic-on-metal bearing couples with metal-on-metal and ceramic-on-ceramic bearing couples is presented. Thirty-one patients were analyzed for metal ion levels at 6-month follow-up. Level of evidence: Therapeutic level II.

45. Bourne RB, Barrack R, Rorabeck CH, Salehi A, Good V: Arthroplasty options for the young patient: Oxinium on cross-linked polyethylene. *Clin Orthop Relat Res* 2005;441:159-167.

46. Kop AM, Whitewood C, Johnston DJ: Damage of oxinium femoral heads subsequent to hip arthroplasty dislocation: Three retrieval case studies. *J Arthroplasty* 2007; 22(5):775-779.

The authors highlight the relative softness of the zirconium base beneath the oxidized zirconium femoral head. Significant damage after hip dislocation and subsequent reduction was reported in three retrieval case studies.

47. Lin EL, Wang JC: Total disk arthroplasty. *J Am Acad Orthop Surg* 2006;14(13):705-714.

48. Punt IM, Cleutjens JP, de Bruin T, et al: Periprosthetic tissue reactions observed at revision of total intervertebral disc arthroplasty. *Biomaterials* 2009;30(11):2079-2084.

Periprosthetic tissue samples were obtained during revision of TDAs in 16 patients; osteolysis was observed in 1 patient.

49. Zeh A, Becker C, Planert M, Lattke P, Wohlrab D: Time-dependent release of cobalt and chromium ions into the serum following implantation of the metal-on-metal Maverick type artificial lumbar disc (Medtronic Sofamor Danek). *Arch Orthop Trauma Surg* 2009; 129(6):741-746.

The authors measured the serum cobalt and chromium concentrations in 15 patients after lumbar metal-on-metal TDA and reported concentrations similar to those seen with THA and TKA. First and second follow-ups occurred at an average of 14.8 and 36.7 months, respectively.

50. Zigler J, Delamarter R, Spivak JM, et al: Results of the prospective, randomized, multicenter Food and Drug Administration investigational device exemption study of the ProDisc-L total disc replacement versus circumferential fusion for the treatment of 1-level degenerative disc disease. *Spine (Phila Pa 1976)* 2007;32(11):1155-1162, discussion 1163.

This prospective, randomized, multicenter clinical trial evaluated 286 patients at 6 weeks and 3, 6, 12, 18, and 24 months to compare lumbar disk replacement and circumferential spinal fusion for treating discogenic pain at one vertebral level between L3 and S1.

51. Nunley P, Gordon C, Jawahar A, et al: Total disc arthroplasty affords quicker recovery in one-level degenerative disc disease of cervical spine: Preliminary results of a prospective randomized trial. *Spine J* 2008;8:17S.

The authors present clinical data from a prospective, randomized, multicenter trial comparing cervical TDA with anterior cervical diskectomy and fusion for treating single-level degenerative disk disease. Fifty-one patients were evaluated at an average follow-up of 13 months.

52. Devin CJ, Myers TG, Kang JD: Chronic failure of a lumbar total disc replacement with osteolysis. Report of a case with nineteen-year follow-up. *J Bone Joint Surg Am* 2008;90(10):2230-2234.

This case report describes a patient treated in 1993 with an L3-L4 TDA that was determined to have good results. Revision was required 19 years later. Significant osteolysis led to biomechanical failure of the TDA.

Chapter 8

Musculoskeletal Imaging

Kenjirou Ohashi, MD, PhD   Georges Y. El-Khoury, MD   Yusuf Menda, MD

Introduction

Imaging studies are an integral part of orthopaedic practices. As the availability of imaging modalities increases, having a working knowledge and understanding of the indications of each modality is becoming increasingly important for orthopaedic surgeons. Recent advances in technology, indications for each imaging test, and imaging features of common pathologies will be discussed in this chapter.

Radiography

Advances in Technology

Since the discovery of x-rays in 1895, images have been captured and reviewed on silver halide–based hard films. Although digital image acquisition began in the mid 1980s, filmless methodology became available in the early 1990s with the advent of picture archiving and communication systems. Computed radiography, a cassette-based photostimulable phosphor and plate reading storage system, initially replaced the analog screen film system. Alternate (cassetteless) technologies for digital imaging, historically categorized as digital radiography, appeared in the mid 1990s. The digital radiography system reads the x-ray signal immediately after exposure with the detector in place.

Currently, the term digital radiography is used to refer to all types of digital radiographic systems for both cassette and cassetteless operations. The efficiency of digital radiography has markedly improved; however, without constant quality control there is a potential risk of a gradual increase in patient radiation dose (dose creep). Digital radiography systems must provide quality imaging services and protect patients from unnecessary radiation.[1,2]

Dr. Menda or an immediate family member has received research or institutional support from Siemens Medical Solutions. Neither of the following authors or a member of their immediate families has received anything of value from or owns stock in a commercial company or institution related directly or indirectly to the subject of this chapter: Dr. Ohashi and Dr. El-Khoury.

Fracture Imaging

Spine Fractures

Although cervical spine radiography is limited in visualizing ligamentous injuries, quality radiographs can exclude unstable cervical spinal injuries in a high percentage of patients.

Cervical spine radiography is no longer used to rule out injuries to the cervical spine in high-risk multitrauma patients when CT of the head or other body parts is performed. For patients with more than a 5% risk of a cervical spine fracture, CT of the cervical spine is more efficient than obtaining multiple radiographic views.[3,4] In patients with traumatic injuries, radiographic studies often require several exposures and may not detect up to 61% of cervical spine fractures.[5] CT screening is also a cost-effective modality in patients at high or moderate risk for cervical spine fracture.[6]

Patients 65 years or older with blunt trauma have characteristic injury patterns and require special diagnostic strategies. Approximately two thirds of the fractures involve the upper cervical spine (level C0-C2) and can be caused by low-energy mechanisms such as a fall from standing[7] (**Figure 1**). A retrospective analysis of cervical spine injuries in elderly patients (age 65 to 75 years compared with those older than 75 years) suggested that CT may be appropriate as the primary modality for all trauma patients older than 75 years because of increased incidence of injuries in low-energy mechanisms.[7] For these patients, radiographic detection of cervical spine fractures is often difficult due to degenerative changes.

AP, lateral, open-mouth, and swimmer's views are often used in imaging of the cervical spine. The lateral view should include the C7-T1 junction (**Figure 2**). Quality radiography remains a valuable screening test for thoracic and lumbar spinal fractures. Because the shoulders overlap on lateral views, visualization of the upper thoracic spine is often limited. CT is increasingly being used to diagnose or exclude thoracic and lumbar spine fractures, especially in patients with multiple traumatic injuries.

Fractures of the Extremities

The diagnosis and assessment of extremity fractures are the most common indications for radiography. At least two orthogonal views should be obtained because the fractures may not be seen on a single view. Additional and/or special views are commonly used for the wrist, elbow, shoulder, and ankle. The cross-table lateral view

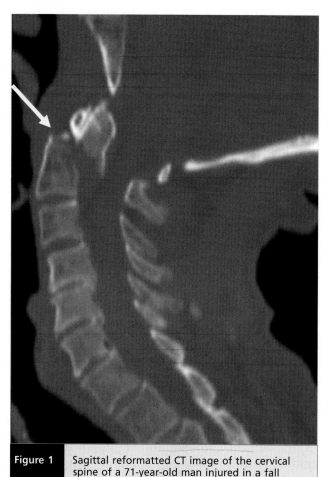

Figure 1 Sagittal reformatted CT image of the cervical spine of a 71-year-old man injured in a fall shows a type II odontoid fracture (*arrow*) with posterior subluxation of C1 on C2.

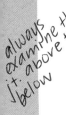

always examine the it above & below

can be used to detect fluid-fluid levels (lipohemarthrosis) in the knee. Adjacent joints should be examined separately if there is a clinical suspicion of injury. Radiography can detect radiopaque foreign bodies; however, ultrasound has higher sensitivity for detecting foreign bodies. Radiographs are less sensitive for detecting fractures in severely osteopenic patients. Certain fractures, such as scaphoid, radial head and/or neck, and proximal femoral fractures are easily missed by radiography.

Scaphoid Fractures
The scaphoid is the most commonly fractured bone in the wrist. Early diagnosis is important because immediate treatment minimizes the risks of nonunion and osteonecrosis. Standard radiographic imaging includes PA, oblique, lateral, and scaphoid (ulnar flexion) views. Imaging protocols, including the indications for advanced techniques such as MRI, may vary from hospital to hospital.

Radial Head and/or Neck Fractures
The radial head capitellar view (oblique lateral) may be added to AP and lateral views of the elbow to detect subtle fractures of the radial head and/or neck. The fat pad sign (capsular distention), even without obvious

fracture, is highly predictive of an occult intra-articular fracture (**Figure 3**).

Proximal Femoral Fractures
Nondisplaced fractures of the femoral neck or intertrochanteric region may be missed on standard radiographs in patients with osteopenia. Because of the serious consequences of a delayed diagnosis, limited MRI (coronal images through both hips) may be indicated for early diagnosis or to exclude the presence of a fracture.

Arthritis
The diagnosis of arthritis is primarily based on radiographic findings. Radiography is not sensitive for detecting early soft-tissue changes; however, characteristic bony changes often lead to a specific diagnosis.[8,9] Classic radiographic assessment for arthritis includes evaluation of joint alignment, bone mineral status (osteopenia), cartilage (joint space, erosion), and distribution of the affected joints. A weight-bearing study is necessary to assess joint-space narrowing in the hip, knee, and ankle joints.

Rheumatoid Arthritis
Proximal joints of the hand and foot are typically affected by rheumatoid arthritis. Periarticular soft-tissue swelling, osteopenia, marginal erosion, and uniform joint-space narrowing are characteristic radiographic findings. A semisupinated oblique view of the hand and wrist (so-called ball-catcher view) will better show metacarpophalangeal and pisotriquetral joint erosions.

Osteoarthritis
Osteoarthritis (OA) affects the cartilage in weight-bearing joints of the hip and knee and is characterized by increased bone mineralization (subchondral sclerosis), osteophyte formation, and nonuniform joint-space narrowing. Identical radiographic findings in the distal joints of the hand and foot, which typically occur in women 50 years or older, are referred to as idiopathic OA. Radiographic findings of OA in the hands may be associated with central erosive changes and typically occur along the articular surfaces. This variant is called erosive OA. The erosive changes may be accompanied by osteopenia or proliferative changes.

Pyrophosphate Arthropathy
Calcium pyrophosphate dihydrate crystal deposition occurs in the soft tissues in and around a joint and may cause synovitis. Pyrophosphate arthropathy typically affects elderly patients but can affect relatively young adults.[10] Chondrocalcinosis (calcification of cartilage) may be present. The knee (meniscus), symphysis pubis (disk), and wrist (triangular fibrocartilage) are common locations for chondrocalcinosis. Bone minerals are typically preserved. Large osteophytes and uniform joint-space narrowing can be observed. Findings of large osteophytes in non–weight-bearing joints, such as the glenohumeral and patellofemoral joints, should raise the possibility of pyrophosphate arthropathy.

1: Principles of Orthopaedics

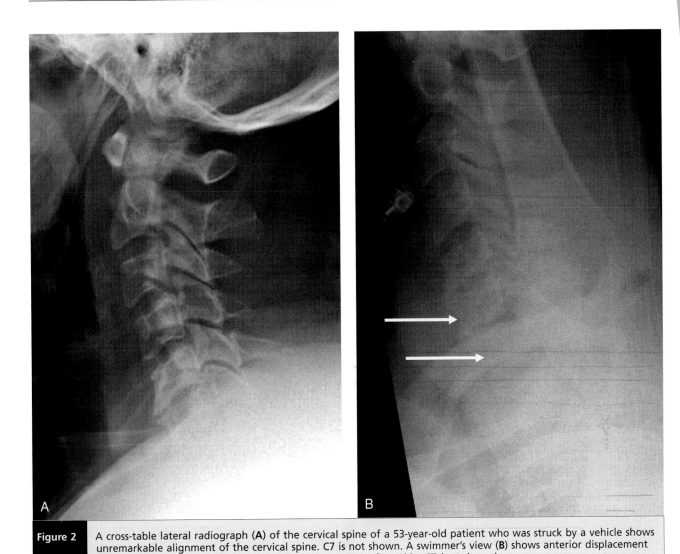

| **Figure 2** | A cross-table lateral radiograph (**A**) of the cervical spine of a 53-year-old patient who was struck by a vehicle shows unremarkable alignment of the cervical spine. C7 is not shown. A swimmer's view (**B**) shows anterior displacement of C6 on C7 (*arrows*). Unilateral facet dislocation was confirmed by CT (not shown). |

Seronegative Spondyloarthropathies

Seronegative arthropathies include ankylosing spondylitis, sacroiliitis associated with inflammatory bowel disease, psoriatic arthritis, and reactive arthritis. The unifying radiographic manifestation is enthesitis—chronic inflammation at the tendon/ligament insertion. Erosions initially occur at the capsular insertion followed by bony proliferation (sclerosis and bony outgrowth) (**Figure 4**). Ankylosis may eventually occur.

Neuropathic Arthropathy

Chronic repetitive trauma in a joint with poor sensibility may explain some of the radiographic changes of neuropathic arthropathy, but the exact pathogenesis is not clear. The radiographic changes include the wide spectrum of bony changes from total bony resorption (an atrophic neuropathic joint) to excessive repair (a hypertrophic neuropathic joint). The hypertrophic changes show the classic pattern of joint destruction, dislocation, debris, and excessive bone formation. In the foot and ankle, diabetes mellitus is the most common cause of neuropathic arthropathy, typically involving the midfoot and forefoot. Septic joint and osteomyelitis are often difficult to exclude in patients with a neuropathic joint.

Neoplasms

Diagnosing bone tumors is primarily based on the patient's history (age and symptoms) and the radiographic findings. The tumor location, border (for lytic lesions), periosteal reaction, and matrix calcifications should be evaluated. Cross-sectional imaging with CT and MRI may be used to confirm the radiographic findings and provide additional information such as the cystic nature of the lesion (fluid-fluid levels or peripheral enhancement after intravenous contrast) and the extent of the tumor. Clinically important distinctions between benign and malignant tumors rely mainly on radiographic findings. Without radiographic correlation, MRI findings alone can be misleading in diagnosing certain benign lesions such as osteoid osteoma, osteoblastoma, chondroblastoma, and eosinophilic granuloma. In such instances, the appearance of the lesion on MRI scans may suggest an aggressive tumor.

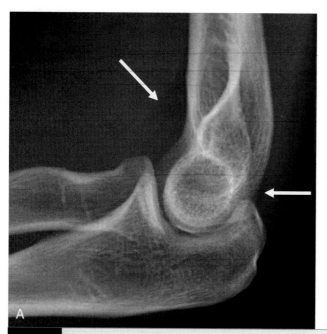

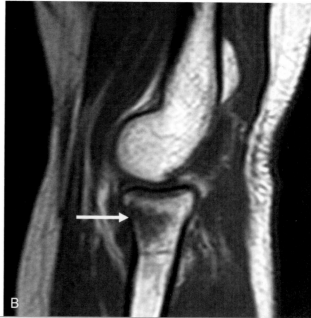

Figure 3 **A,** Lateral radiograph of the elbow of a 26-year-old man with an impacted posterior aspect of the elbow after a fall shows no acute fracture. Moderate capsular distention is noted with displaced fat pads (*arrows*). **B,** Sagittal T1-weighted MRI scan shows a linear low signal (*arrow*) along the radial head-neck junction consistent with a nondisplaced fracture.

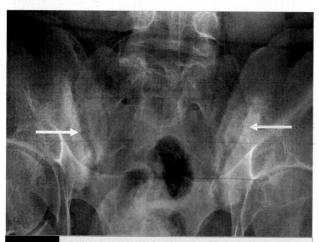

Figure 4 Ferguson radiographic view shows extensive bony erosion along the sacroiliac joint with proliferative sclerotic changes especially along the iliac side bilaterally (*arrows*) in a 29-year-old man with a stiff neck and back pain. The radiographic findings are consistent with sacroiliitis. The patient was diagnosed with ankylosing spondylitis.

Radiography is generally not helpful in diagnosing soft-tissue tumors. Radiography may detect calcification (for example, in synovial cell sarcomas), phleboliths (for example, in hemangiomas), and hyperostosis at the adjacent bone (associated with benign soft-tissue lesions). Cross-sectional images provide information about the location and size of a lesion and its relationship to the adjacent structures, especially neurovascular structures. Additional advantages of cross-sectional images include evaluation of fat content and cystic or solid nature of the lesions.

Infections

Radiography is less sensitive than other imaging modalities, such as bone scanning and MRI, for the early detection of acute osteomyelitis; however, radiography may show focal osteolysis and periosteal reaction in patients with acute osteomyelitis. A comparison with previous radiographs is important, especially for patients with diabetic foot infections in whom it can be difficult to differentiate between neuropathic osteoarthropathy and infection. Radiography is sensitive for detecting soft-tissue emphysema (**Figure 5**), which can be caused by a life-threatening infection.

Metabolic Diseases

Digital radiography automatically adjusts the amount of radiation in the field of view. Because a wide range of settings is available to review the digital images on the display monitor, the bone density, which is subjectively estimated by a digital system, can be misleading. Cortical thinning and accentuation of trabeculae can be assessed when considering the diagnosis of osteoporosis. Characteristic radiographic findings of rickets are often seen on a chest radiograph (**Figure 6**). Enlargement of the rib ends (rachitic rosary), widening of the proximal humeral physes, and subcortical bone resorption at the inferior scapular angles can be detected. Fragile osteopenic bones in patients with osteogenesis imperfecta usually lead to multiple fractures. Radio-

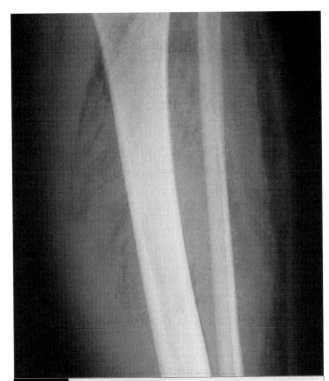

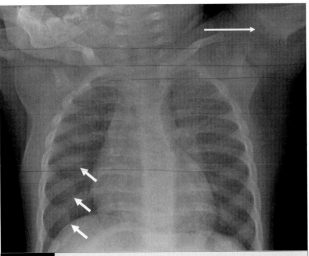

Figure 6   Chest radiograph of a 13-month-old boy with failure to thrive shows enlargement of rib ends (rachitic rosary) (*short arrows*) and widening of the physis of the proximal humerus (*long arrow*) consistent with rickets.

Figure 5   AP radiograph of the tibia and fibula shows extensive air lucencies in the soft tissue (subcutaneous emphysema) consistent with gas gangrene. ← *most commonly*
↳ *clostridium perfringens*
medical emergency

graphic features of rickets and osteogenesis imperfecta may overlap with those of child abuse.

Congenital Anomalies

Radiography can be used in the diagnosis of certain congenital bony anomalies. Congenital dislocation of the radial head may be an isolated abnormality or may be associated with other conditions such as scoliosis or Klippel-Feil and nail-patella syndromes. Radial head dislocation is associated with a small, dome-shaped radial head and hypoplastic capitellum (**Figure 7**). Congenital pseudarthrosis of the clavicle almost always occurs in the right clavicle. Radiographically, the middle segment is partially missing with tapering of the medial segment (**Figure 8**). These congenital anomalies can potentially be misdiagnosed as a posttraumatic condition. A standing PA view of the entire spine is obtained on a single image for the evaluation of scoliosis. The PA projection reduces radiation exposure to the breast and thyroid by threefold to sevenfold compared with the AP projection. Lateral radiographs may be obtained after scoliosis is diagnosed to assess sagittal alignment.

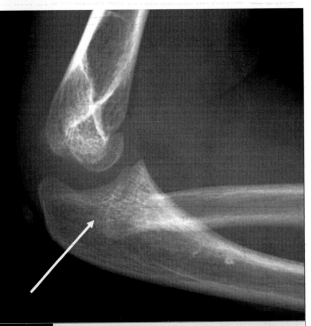

Figure 7   Lateral radiograph of the elbow of a 6-year-old girl shows congenital posterior dislocation of the radial head, which is dome-shaped (*arrow*). The capitellum is hypoplastic. No capsular distention is seen.

Computed Tomography

Recent Advances in Technology

Substantial advances in CT technologies have occurred in the past two decades. Helical CT was commercially introduced in 1988 and multidetector CT (MDCT) technologies were introduced in 1992. In a single-detector helical CT, detectors are aligned along the patient's axial plane (x-y plane). With MDCT, detectors are also stacked along the long axis (z-axis), enabling collection of large amounts of data per each x-ray tube rotation. Increasing the speed of the x-ray tube rotation (to 0.5 to 0.35 seconds/rotation) contributed to further reduction of total scanning time. CT scanners with 64 detectors have been installed in many facilities, and scanners with 320 detectors became commercially available in 2008. With MDCT, the emitted x-ray beam is more efficiently used than before, thus contributing to a reduction in the radiation dose.

MDCT is capable of generating multiple thin slice images (reconstructed images) from large volumetric data sets. With this technology, hundreds of axial images are usually generated with each study. The images are reviewed as a volume rather than as individual axial images. Three-dimensional workstations are necessary for viewing these large image data sets from which

multiplanar reformatted images can be interactively reviewed in any chosen plane and are not limited to sagittal or coronal planes (**Figure 9**). Internet-based three-dimensional software can be easily accessed by multiple readers and may eventually replace three-dimensional workstations.

Fracture Imaging

Spine Fractures

The increased availability of CT has contributed to the recent change in indications for CT of cervical spine fractures in the emergency department. Because the time required to reach a correct diagnosis is a critical factor for managing multitrauma patients, CT has become an essential tool for ruling out or diagnosing cervical spine fractures. A recent survey has shown that 40% of emergency departments in the United States have CT scanners.[11] Indications for cervical spine CT in high-risk patients were previously discussed in this chapter.

CT is recommended to assess spine trauma in patients with ankylosing spondylitis or diffuse idiopathic skeletal hyperostosis whose spines are rigid because of bony fusion.[12] In patients with advanced ankylosing spondylitis, severe osteoporosis makes radiographic detection of a fracture less reliable (**Figure 10**). Fractures in an ankylosed spine are typically oriented transversely and affect all three columns. Multiplanar reformatted images clearly delineate such fractures, which are difficult to detect on axial images.

Because CT allows poor visualization of ligaments compared with MRI, it is debated whether CT alone

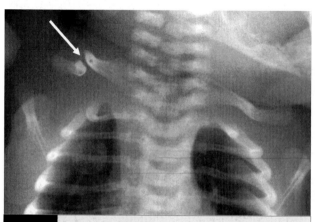

Figure 8   Chest radiograph of a 4-day-old girl shows pseudarthrosis of the right clavicle (*arrow*). Opposing midclavicular ends are corticated and no callus formation is seen.

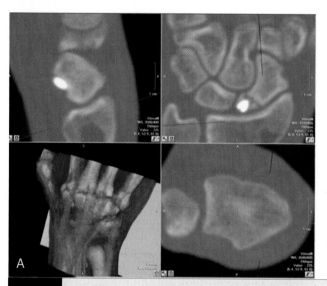 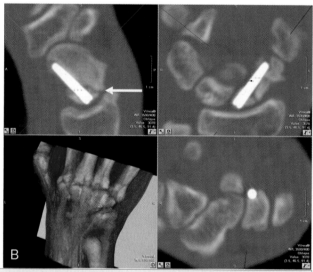

Figure 9   A: Orthogonal three-plane (sagittal [*upper left*], coronal [*upper right*], and axial [*bottom right*]) CT images of the wrist of a 20-year-old man with a scaphoid fracture show screw placement. Color three-dimensional volume-rendered CT image showing bone and tendon (*lower left*). The color lines represent the location and orientation of the slices seen in the other boxes. **B,** Double oblique CT images along the screw show the long axis of the scaphoid to a better advantage (*upper right* and *left*). Screw displacement and angular deformity of the scaphoid (*arrow; upper left*) is noted. The short axis (transverse plane) of the scaphoid is shown in the lower right image. The lower left image is a color three-dimensional volume-rendered CT image showing bone and tendon. The color lines represent the location and orientation of the slices seen in the other boxes.

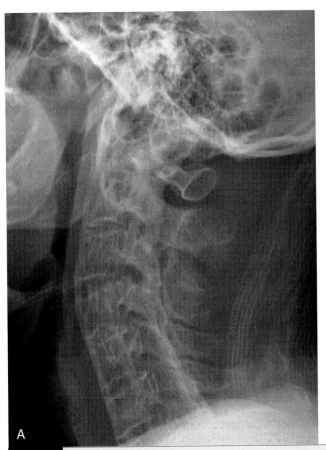
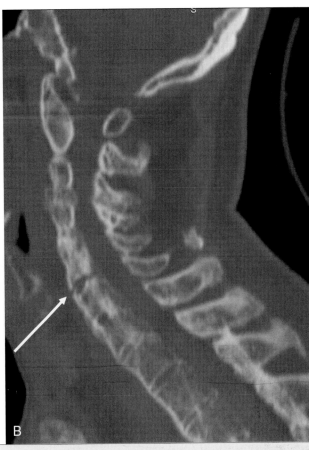

Figure 10	**A,** Cross-table lateral radiograph of the cervical spine of a 49-year-old man with known ankylosing spondylitis who was involved in a motor vehicle crash shows extensive bony fusion of the spine. No fracture is seen. **B,** Sagittal reformatted CT image shows a nondisplaced fracture at the C5-C6 level (*arrow*).

can be used to exclude cervical spine injuries. However, studies have shown that pure ligamentous injuries without fractures are uncommon.[13] Studies on ruling out cervical spinal injuries in obtunded patients have shown that CT, in comparison with a composite reference standard (subsequent imaging and clinical examinations) or with MRI, has a 99% negative predictive value for ruling out ligamentous injuries and a 100% negative predictive value for ruling out unstable cervical spine injuries.[14,15]

In the thoracic and lumbar areas of the spine, most fractures occur at the fulcrum of motion between T11 and L2. These fractures account for approximately 50% of all spinal fractures. In multitrauma patients imaged with MDCT of the chest, abdomen, and pelvis, spine CT images can be reconstructed without additional scanning. CT body studies using a 2.5-mm detector collimation and reconstructed spinal CT images have shown high accuracy in depicting thoracic and lumbar spine fractures.[16,17] Single-pass, whole-body scanning can be used to cover an extended area from the head to the pelvis. This method contrasts with the segmented approach in which each body region is scanned separately. The single-pass, whole-body approach exposes the patient to 17% less radiation than the segmented approach because there is no overlap between the irradiated fields.[18,19]

Pelvic and Acetabular Fractures

Because of the complex anatomy of the pelvis, conventional radiography often fails to show the full extent of a fracture, the spatial relationship of the major fracture fragments, and the intra-articular bony fragments. Specific indications for CT include acetabular fractures, sacroiliac joint involvement, and sacral and lumbosacral junction injuries.[20]

Approximately 30% to 40% of pelvic injuries involve the acetabulum.[21,22] The Letournel classification is based on AP and oblique (Judet) pelvic radiographs. CT is routinely performed to aid preoperative planning. Standard pelvic radiographs add little information to CT scans in classifying acetabular fractures;[23] however, standard radiographs are still important for intraoperative assessment and follow-up evaluation.

Fractures of the Extremities

Wrist Fractures

Traditionally, clinically suspected scaphoid fractures are treated with immobilization and followed clinically and radiographically regardless of the initial radio-

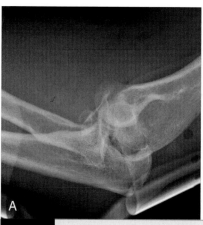
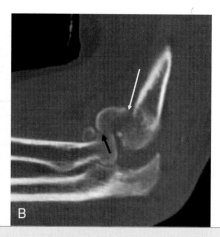
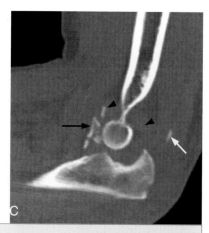

Figure 11 **A,** Lateral radiograph of the elbow of a 51-year-old man shows a right elbow fracture-dislocation. **B,** Sagittal CT image through the radius shows a radial head fracture (*black arrow*) and a coronally oriented lateral condyle fracture of the humerus (*white arrow*). **C,** Sagittal CT image through the ulna shows a comminuted coronoid fracture (*black arrow*) and a proximally displaced small avulsion fracture of the olecranon (*white arrow*). Displaced anterior and posterior fat pads are noted (*arrowheads*).

graphic findings. To improve cost-effectiveness and speed a patient's return to function, more sensitive imaging modalities such as bone scans, MRIs, and high-spatial-resolution ultrasound studies are now commonly used.[24-30] CT has been used to detect occult fractures of the wrist when radiographs are negative.[25,31] There have been case reports of scaphoid fractures diagnosed by bone scanning and/or MRI but missed by CT.[32,33]

Elbow Fractures

Complex fractures or fracture-dislocations of the elbow can be difficult to characterize by radiography alone, especially after cast immobilization. CT can clearly show the relationship between multiple bony fragments when reviewed on multiplanar reformatted images along the humerus, radius, and ulna and on three-dimensional images (**Figure 11**).

Tibial Plateau Fractures

Studies of CT using multiplanar reformatted or three-dimensional imaging have shown that using CT scans in addition to radiographs changes an observer's classification of a tibial plateau fracture in 12% to 55% of cases compared with using radiographs alone; the use of both imaging modalities also results in treatment modifications in 26% to 60% of patients.[34-37] CT is an excellent modality for assessing comminution in a tibial plateau fracture and the amount of depression of the articular fragments, and is helpful in preoperative planning.

Ankle Fractures

Radiographic studies may underestimate the size and displacement of a posterior malleolar fracture. A report of 57 surgically treated patients with a posterior malleolar fracture showed a wide variation in fracture orientation and that approximately 20% of the fractures extended to the medial malleolus.[38]

Calcaneal Fractures

In the mid 1990s, CT was shown to allow excellent visualization and evaluation of the pathoanatomy of intra-articular calcaneus fractures with direct axial and coronal scans.[39] Since that time, CT with multiplanar reformatted imaging and three-dimensional imaging has become the standard investigative modality to guide the treatment of intra-articular fractures of the calcaneus.[40] Using isotropic imaging, single scanning through the calcaneus is sufficient to evaluate the integrity of subtalar and calcaneocuboid joints. Volume rendering to visualize tendon-bone relationships has been introduced and clinically applied to evaluate the tendons in the ankle and foot[41] (**Figure 12**).

Postoperative Complications

The use of CT in patients with orthopaedic hardware can be hampered by severe metal artifacts. Metal artifacts are displayed on CT scans as streak or sunburst artifacts, which degrade the image quality. With proper data acquisition, image reconstruction, and image reformatting, diagnostic CT scans can be obtained for most patients. Prostheses made of a cobalt-chromium alloy cause substantial artifacts, whereas titanium implants produce less significant metal artifacts. The use of multiplanar reformatted imaging helps to decrease the adverse effects of metal artifacts on image quality. Three-dimensional volume rendering is also helpful in reducing streak artifacts associated with hardware.[42,43]

Postoperative CT may be performed to evaluate intra-articular fracture reduction and hardware placement. In the spine, pedicle screw misplacement can be associated with neurologic complications. CT has been reported to be 10 times more sensitive than radiography for detecting medial pedicle cortex violations.[44] Recently developed three-dimensional C-arm CT scanning with flat-panel detectors has been introduced into orthopaedic practices.[45] C-arm CT has been used to intra-

CT often changes management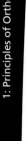

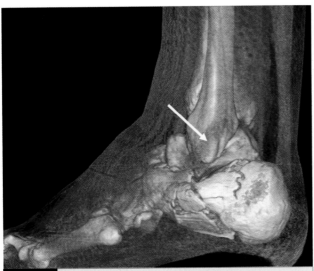

Figure 12 Three-dimensional color volume-rendered CT image of the ankle (tendon and bone) of a 35-year-old man with a closed calcaneal fracture shows dislocation of the peroneal tendons (*arrow*) and a comminuted fracture of the calcaneus.

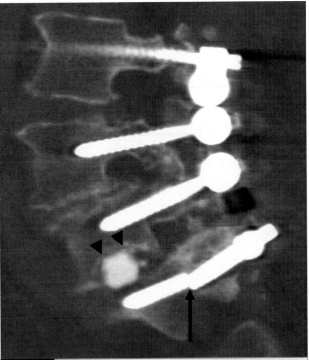

Figure 13 Sagittal reformatted CT image of the lumbar spine of a 61-year-old woman shows fracture of S1 pedicle screw (*arrow*) associated with marginal lucency around the screw and sagging of L5 inferior end plate (*arrowheads*) at the bone graft.

operatively assess spinal fusion and pedicle screw placement.

Failure of Bony Fusion

Radiography is inaccurate in assessing bony fusion when compared with CT.[46] Radiography may underestimate or overestimate bony fusion in patients with fracture fixation or arthrodesis.[46] In a recent investigation, CT was reported to be useful in predicting stability for patients with ankle or subtalar arthrodesis.[47]

Following surgery for spinal fusion, the assessment of the bony fusion with flexion and extension lateral radiographic views may be useful for the gross evaluation of instability. Sagittal and coronal reformatted CT images through the fusion site are best for evaluating bone bridging and the integrity of the fusion mass.[48]

Osteolysis

Radiographic detection of osteolysis can be influenced by the patient's body habitus, the position of the hardware, and the location of the lesion. Radiography can provide limited information, even with multiple projections, on the location and amount of osteolysis. Fluoroscopically guided radiographs may be indicated to obtain true tangential views of components in total knee replacements.[49] CT may be indicated not only for the detection of osteolysis but also for the evaluation of bone loss before surgery.[50-52]

Hardware Problems

Hardware fractures may be detected on CT scans and are usually associated with other complications such as nonunion and osteolysis (**Figure 13**). The position of the component, subsidence of the component, and polyethylene wear following hip or knee arthroplasty are usually assessed on radiographs. CT can be used to detect polyethylene liner dislocations. Patellofemoral symptoms may be associated with component malrotation. CT is the study of choice to evaluate rotational malalignment of the femoral and tibial components in total knee arthroplasty.[53,54]

The efficacy of CT in detecting hardware complications has not been well investigated. One study of 114 CT imaging studies from 109 patients used clinical or surgical outcomes as the reference standard and measured sensitivity, specificity, and positive and negative predictive values of CT (74%, 95%, 88%, and 88%, respectively).[55] Radiography alone was less sensitive in detecting hardware complications such as nonunion and osteolysis than was CT alone.

Magnetic Resonance Imaging

Advantages and Limitations

Because of its excellent soft-tissue contrast, MRI has become the diagnostic modality of choice for evaluating bone marrow, cartilage, and soft tissues; the absence of ionizing radiation also makes it an ideal mo-

1: Principles of Orthopaedics

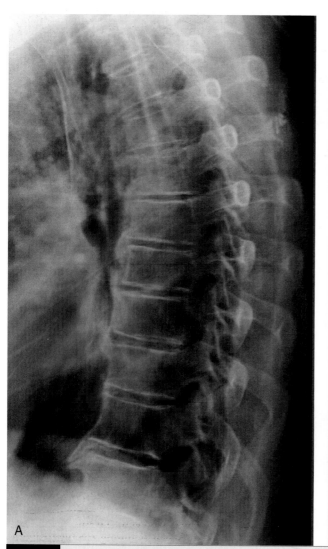
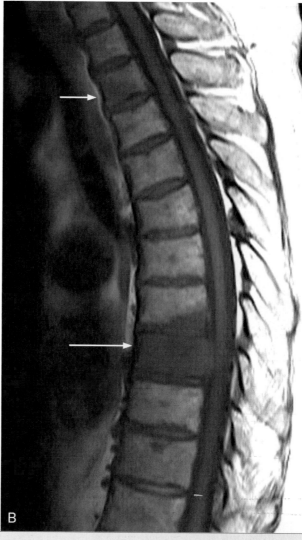

Figure 14   A lung tumor in a 66-year-old man metastasized to the thoracic spine. **A,** Lateral radiograph of the thoracic spine is unremarkable except for some degenerative changes. **B,** Sagittal T1-weighted MRI of the thoracic spine shows an infiltrative process involving the entire vertebral body of T10 with extension into the body of T9 (*long arrow*). Early involvement of the body of T3 was also suspected (*short arrow*).

dality for imaging in children. Limitations of MRI include the relatively long scanning time, which necessitates the use of sedation or general anesthesia in young children and uncooperative adults. MRI cannot be used in patients with cochlear implants or a pacemaker, and may not be useable in some patients with certain orthopaedic metal implants that are located in close proximity to the area being scanned. Fortunately, most modern orthopaedic implants are nonferromagnetic and will not displace when the patient is within a strong magnetic field. When an implant is suspected of being ferromagnetic, an identical implant can be tested with a horseshoe magnet before MRI. In practice, most radiology departments try to obtain the specific manufacturer's part number and check for magnetic resonance compatibility. Specific absorption rate (SAR) is related to the amount of tissue heating resulting from radiofrequency pulses. Modern scanners typically esti-

mate the SAR values and will suggest protocol changes to reduce SAR values to safe levels. SAR increases at higher field strengths, which may require adjustments to the imaging protocol such as increasing the repetition time or reducing the number of slices. Most metal implants produce susceptibility artifacts, rendering the images nondiagnostic for abnormalities close to the metal implants. Ideally, the radiologist should be notified in advance about the presence of a metal implant in the area of interest; a special MRI sequence can then be prescribed that can reduce, but not completely eliminate, metal artifacts.[56]

MRI Sequences

Orthopaedic surgeons should be familiar with the capabilities of commonly used MRI sequences. T1-weighted sequences take a short time to acquire and are excellent for the initial investigation of any disease process in

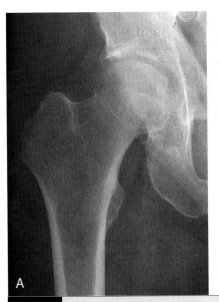
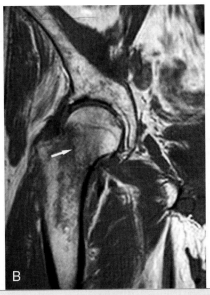
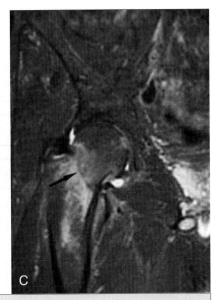

Figure 15   A 73-year-old man presented to the emergency department with right hip pain and inability to bear weight on the right hip. **A,** AP radiograph of the right hip was unremarkable. **B,** Coronal T1-weighted MRI of the pelvis shows a fracture line in the right femoral neck (*arrow*) surrounded by an area of low signal, which represents marrow edema. **C,** Coronal fat-suppressed T2-weighted image of the pelvis shows the fracture in the right femoral neck (*arrow*) surrounded by bright signals, which represent marrow edema.

bones, joints, or soft tissues. T1-weighted sequences show good anatomic detail and are highly sensitive for detecting marrow abnormalities such as infiltrative processes, metastases, or infections[57] (**Figure 14**). A T1-weighted sequence is often the only sequence needed to diagnose an occult fracture of the hip in elderly patients or metastases in the spine. Most abnormalities have low signal intensity on a T1-weighted sequence.[58]

T2-weighted sequences are ideally suited for diagnosing pathologic processes. When fat suppression is added to T2-weighted sequences, all fat-containing tissues appear black. Fat suppression is useful in accentuating the difference in contrast between normal and abnormal tissues. T2-weighted sequences are water sensitive; therefore, a bright signal is displayed for lesions containing water, such as bone marrow edema (**Figure 15**), soft-tissue edema, tumors, infections, abscesses, and acute fractures.

Proton density-weighted sequences (also known as intermediate-weighted sequences) have a high signal-to-noise ratio and reveal exquisite anatomic detail. Fat-suppressed proton density sequences have been used, with excellent results, for imaging articular cartilage.

A short-tau inversion recovery (STIR) sequence is also a water-sensitive sequence. This sequence suppresses the signals from fat much like the fat-suppressed T2-weighted sequences; however, it has two advantages over the fat-suppressed T2-weighted sequences. STIR sequences uniformly suppress fat over a large field of view, which is often not the case with fat-suppressed T2-weighted sequences. Metal artifacts are significantly less pronounced with a STIR sequence than with other sequences, although STIR imaging has

a lower signal-to-noise ratio than the fat-suppressed sequences.

Gradient-echo sequences also have advantages for some applications, and typically a short acquisition time. Some gradient-echo sequences are good for imaging articular cartilage because articular cartilage can be distinguished from intra-articular fluid by assigning slightly different signal intensity to each. Gradient-echo sequences also are useful when scanning for hemosiderin in lesions such as pigmented villonodular synovitis. The three-dimensional fat-suppressed spoiled gradient-echo sequence in the steady state and the three-dimensional gradient-echo double excitation sequence in the steady state have been successfully used for cartilage imaging[59] (**Figure 16**).

Contrast Agents for MRI

Gadolinium compounds have been used in musculoskeletal imaging for approximately 20 years and can be used intravenously to evaluate synovial inflammation, vascular lesions, neoplasms, and abscesses. Gadolinium is useful in differentiating a neoplasm from a cyst because the neoplasm enhances after an intravenous injection of gadolinium, whereas the cyst does not enhance. This contrast agent can be used to differentiate a drainable abscess from a phlegmon because pus within the abscess will not enhance, whereas the entire phlegmon will enhance (**Figure 17**). It also can be used to assess the extent of necrosis within a tumor. Such information is helpful in planning a biopsy because the necrotic tissue can be avoided and the biopsy needle can be directed at the enhancing tissue. The recommended dose for gadolinium is 0.1 mmol per kg of body weight. Re-

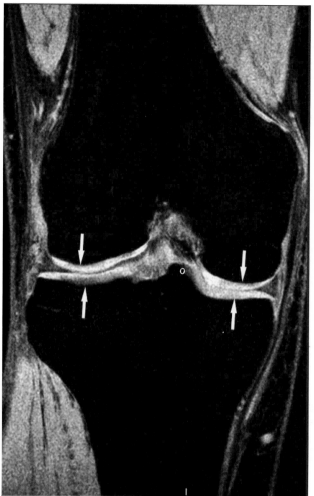

Figure 16 Coronal fat-suppressed gradient-echo MRI sequence of the knee on a normal individual shows normal articular cartilage, which appears bright on this sequence (*arrows*).

cently, gadolinium was shown to cause serious adverse effects in patients with impaired renal function; a potentially lethal disease known as nephrogenic systemic fibrosis developed in some patients.[60]

Diluted gadolinium (1:100) is frequently used as an intra-articular contrast agent before magnetic resonance arthrography. It clearly delineates intra-articular abnormalities such as labral tears, recurrent meniscal tears, and cartilage defects. Despite the widespread use of gadolinium as an intra-articular contrast agent, the FDA has not approved its use for this purpose.

Recent Advances in Technology

In 2003, 3-Tesla (3-T) MRI began to achieve more widespread use as a clinical tool for musculoskeletal imaging. Because of the delay in creating dedicated coils for the different joints, the impact of the 3-T magnet on musculoskeletal imaging has been less dramatic than in other systems, such as the nervous system. The advantage of the 3-T magnet is in its high signal-to-

noise ratio, which provides the potential for improved diagnostic confidence. There is little evidence, however, to show that 3-T MRI provides better diagnostic accuracy compared with 1.5-T MRI in diagnosing anterior cruciate ligament tears, meniscal tears, or shoulder abnormalities. Current clinical experience suggests that the higher signal-to-noise ratio enhances the visualization of ligaments and articular cartilage in small structures such as the hand and wrist.[61]

Isotropic data sets on 100 consecutive shoulder examinations were acquired after the injection of diluted gadolinium into the joint.[62] An isotropic gradient-echo sequence and thin sections (0.4 mm) were used. With arthroscopy as the reference standard, 3-T MRI was reported to be accurate in assessing rotator cuff tears and labral tears.[62] The authors of another study used isotropic MRI to study internal derangement of the knee with a three-dimensional fast spin-echo sequence.[63] Initial results from this study on knees of healthy volunteers were promising.

Occult Fractures

The most common lawsuit filed against emergency department physicians involves missed orthopaedic injuries. In the past two decades, MRI has become an important tool for diagnosing injury in trauma patients in the emergency department. MRI is particularly useful in evaluating suspected occult fractures (those not initially seen on radiographs) and for ruling out ligamentous injuries in the cervical spine of obtunded patients. Common sites for occult fractures are the femoral neck, scaphoid bone, tibial plateau, and talar neck.

Hip radiography has more than a 90% sensitivity for detecting fractures; however, approximately 3% to 4% of patients present with occult hip fractures. Current evidence favors MRI as the best modality for detecting these occult fractures. Coronal T1-weighted images of the hip typically show a dark line at the fracture site (**Figure 15**). Studies have reported that a T1-weighted sequence is sufficient for diagnosing occult hip fractures.[64]

Occult scaphoid fractures can be challenging to diagnose, and delayed treatment increases the risk of complications. There is mounting evidence to suggest that MRI is the modality of choice for detecting occult scaphoid fractures.[65]

Cervical Spine Injuries

Cervical spine injuries occur in approximately 2% to 6% of patients with blunt trauma; there is a real potential for a catastrophic neurologic deficit if such injuries are undiagnosed. In an alert trauma patient without a distracting injury, the cervical spine can be clinically cleared provided the neurologic examination is negative and the cervical spine has full range of motion and is without pain or tenderness. In the obtunded or unreliable patient, the optimal approach for ruling out cervical spinal injury has not yet been determined. The possibility of an unstable ligamentous injury is a troubling consideration in the obtunded patient and is the reason

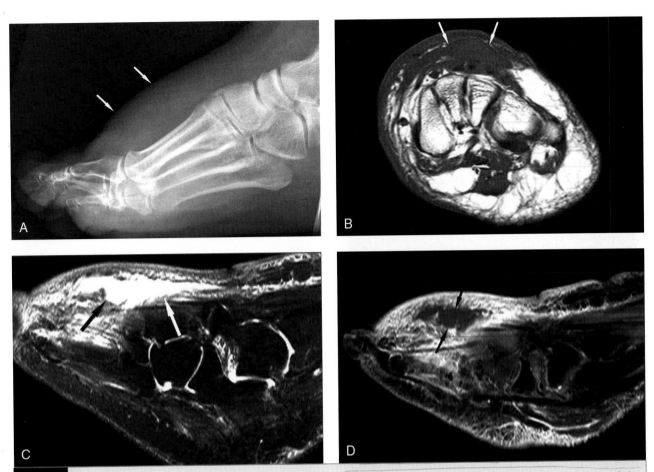

| **Figure 17** | A 57-year-old man with type II diabetes mellitus presented with pain and soft-tissue swelling on the dorsum of the left forefoot. **A,** Lateral radiograph shows significant soft-tissue swelling on the dorsum of the forefoot (arrows). **B,** Axial T1-weighted MRI shows an area of low signal in the subcutaneous fat on the dorsum of the foot (*arrows*). **C,** Sagittal fat-suppressed T2-weighted image shows bright signals (*arrows*) corresponding to the dark area in **B. D,** Sagittal fat-suppressed T1-weighted image after an intravenous gadolinium injection shows a central dark area (*arrows*) surrounded by a bright zone. This appearance is characteristic of a soft-tissue abscess. |

for further imaging after a negative CT examination to confirm intact ligamentous structures. The use of lateral flexion and extension views with fluoroscopy was briefly advocated, but was judged too hazardous and has been replaced with MRI. Recently, several investigators have reported that MDCT alone is sufficient for clearing the cervical spine.[14] Because MDCT cannot be used to image spinal ligaments or the spinal cord, MRI continues to be recommended by some authors to rule out unstable ligamentous injuries of the cervical spine in obtunded patients.[66] However, transporting an obtunded patient from the intensive care unit to the MRI suite is a difficult task and involves risks for the patient.

A retrospective review of 366 obtunded patients whose cervical spines were evaluated with both CT and MRI showed that 12 patients (3.3%) had cervical spine injuries that were not detected by MDCT; however, none of the injuries were unstable and none of the patients required surgery. It was concluded that MDCT has negative predictive values of 98.9% for detecting ligamentous injuries and 100% for detecting unstable injuries.[14] Another review of 202 patients initially eval-

uated with CT followed by MRI showed that MDCT continues to miss both stable and unstable cervical spinal injuries.[66] Of 18 patients (8.9%) who had abnormal MRI examinations, 2 required surgical spinal repairs, 14 required extended use of a cervical collar, and the cervical collar was removed in 2 patients at the discretion of the attending surgeon. It was concluded that MRI changed treatment management in 7.9% of patients with negative MDCT examinations. The continued use of MRI for cervical spine clearance in the obtunded or unreliable patient was recommended by the study authors. However, recent evidence supports the belief that MRI is unlikely to uncover unstable cervical spine injuries in obtunded patients when a late-generation MDCT examination is negative.[67]

Spinal Cord Injury Without Radiographic Abnormalities
The acronym SCIWORA was coined in 1982 for describing the presence of spinal cord injury without radiographic abnormality in children. After MRI became widely available for assessing spinal cord injuries, the term SCIWORA became somewhat ambiguous.[68] In a

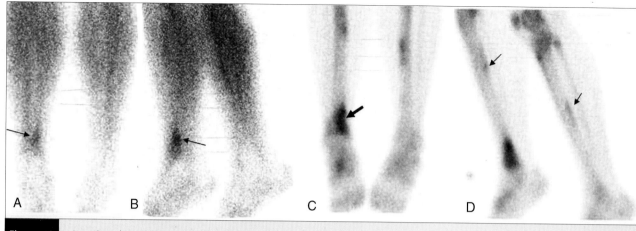

Figure 18 Imaging showing a stress fracture. **A** and **B,** Blood pool images of the bone scan show focal hyperemia (*arrows*) in the right distal tibia. **C** and **D,** Delayed bone scan images show intense uptake of the bone tracer involving the entire cortical thickness of the right distal tibia (*arrow* in **C**), consistent with an advanced stress fracture. There is also mild superficial uptake in the right proximal and left midfemur (*arrows* in **D**), consistent with early stress fractures.

2008 literature review performed to clarify this ambiguity, it was recommended that if any pathology is detected on MRI, with or without radiographic abnormality, the classification of SCIWORA should not be used for the patient.[68] It was also recommended that the label and meaning of SCIWORA be changed to reflect the concept of spinal cord injury without neuroimaging abnormality. A 2004 study also recommended the importance of considering MRI findings before using the SCIWORA classification for a patient.[69]

Nuclear Medicine

The most common radionuclide studies in musculoskeletal imaging are bone scans and positron emission tomography (PET) scans. Bone scans are performed using technetium-Tc 99m-labeled phosphonates (Tc-99m methylene diphosphonate [MDP], Tc-99m hydroxyethylidene diphosphonate). After intravenous injection, approximately one third of the injected dose of Tc-99m MDP localizes in the bone within 2 to 4 hours. Tc-99m emits gamma photons with a half-life of 6 hours. The gamma photons are detected by a gamma camera to produce images reflecting the distribution of the radiopharmaceutical. Tc-99m—labeled phosphonates accumulate preferentially in areas of active bone formation. As a result, areas of increased bone remodeling caused by tumor, infection, trauma, or metabolic bone disease appear "hot" on a bone scan. Therefore, bone scan abnormalities may not be specific for a disease process and should be interpreted in conjunction with the clinical history and other imaging modalities. Bone scans are routinely done 2 to 4 hours after injection of the radiopharmaceutical. Whole-body bone scans are used for screening the entire skeleton for metastatic bone disease. Single photon emission CT (SPECT) provides imaging in transaxial, coronal, and sagittal tomographic scans and is particularly helpful for evaluating the spine.

PET uses radiopharmaceuticals that are labeled with positron emitters. The most commonly used radiopharmaceutical in clinical PET is fluorine-18 deoxyglucose (FDG), which is a glucose analog labeled with fluoride-18, with a half-life of 110 minutes. FDG-PET is primarily used in staging and restaging of malignancies. FDG shows increased accumulation in cancer cells because of enhanced transport of glucose and an increased rate of glycolysis in tumors. Most PET imaging currently is done on integrated PET-CT scanners. The CT portion of PET-CT is used for localization of metabolically active lesions but also may be used to obtain diagnostic-quality CT scans. FDG-PET scans are performed 60 to 90 minutes after injection of the radiopharmaceutical. FDG-PET scans should not be obtained in patients with uncontrolled diabetes because high glucose levels reduce the uptake of FDG in tumors.

Occult Fractures and Stress Fractures

Bone scans are highly sensitive for diagnosing occult fractures in symptomatic patients with negative radiographs. Bone scans are most often done to evaluate fractures in the wrist, hips, and spine; the scans are positive in 90% to 95% of fractures within 24 hours of the traumatic event. In elderly patients, bone scans may be negative in the initial 24 hours; therefore, repeated imaging at 72 hours is recommended if the initial bone scan is negative.[70] Bone scans may remain positive for up to 3 years after a fracture because of persistent bone remodeling.[71]

Bone scans also can be helpful in diagnosing stress fractures. These fractures may not be initially identified on plain radiographs. A negative bone scan excludes the presence of a stress fracture.[72] A long-bone stress fracture on a bone scan shows focal fusiform increased uptake at the site of injury (**Figure 18**). Bone scintigraphy also is useful in differentiating stress fractures from shin splints. Shin splints typically refer to tibial perios-

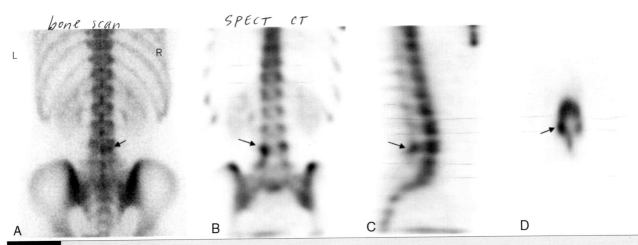

bone scan   SPECT CT

L   R

A   B   C   D

Figure 19 Imaging showing spondylolysis. **A,** Planar posterior bone scan image shows subtle uptake at L5 vertebra (*arrow*). Tracer uptake is clearly visualized on SPECT coronal (**B**), sagittal (**C**), and transaxial (**D**) bone scans, which localize the focus in the right pars region (*arrows*) of the L5 vertebra, consistent with a pars fracture.

titis and usually require a shorter recovery period than stress fractures.[73] The typical appearance of shin splints is linear uptake along the posteromedial aspect of the middle third of the involved tibia.

Spondylolysis refers to a bone defect in the pars interarticularis of a vertebra, most commonly at L4 or L5, and is believed to occur as a result of a stress fracture. Patients with spondylolysis may be asymptomatic; in such instances, the condition may be diagnosed as an incidental imaging finding. However, in some patients, spondylolysis causes severe low back pain. A positive bone scan with focal uptake in the pars region indicates that the spondylolysis may be the cause of low back pain and correlates with a good outcome after fusion surgery.[74] SPECT images of the lumbar spine always should be obtained because more than 50% of active spondylolysis may not be detected with routine planar bone scans[75] (**Figure 19**). Bone scans should be interpreted in correlation with radiographs and/or CT scans because other conditions such as infections, osteoid osteomas, and tumors may also be positive on bone scintigraphy.

Infection

After a negative radiograph, a three-phase bone scan is considered a good choice for diagnosing osteomyelitis. The typical findings of acute osteomyelitis on a bone scan are focal increased flow and focal increased uptake of the tracer on the delayed bone scan phase. In patients with no prior fracture or hardware, a three-phase bone scan is highly accurate for diagnosing osteomyelitis, with a sensitivity and specificity of more than 90%.[76] Increased bone tracer uptake may be seen after a fracture, surgery, or hardware placement. In these patients, labeled white blood cell (WBC) scans are needed to complement the bone scans for diagnosis of osteomyelitis.

Labeled WBC scans are considered the primary imaging modality for assessing osteomyelitis in trauma patients with metallic implants or in patients with pros-

thetic joints. WBC scans can be labeled with indium-111 (In-111) or Tc-99m. Labeled WBCs do not show significant accumulation at surgical sites or fractures in the absence of infection. Labeled WBCs, however, accumulate in the bone marrow. Therefore, WBC scans need to be complemented with bone marrow scans if active marrow distribution is altered as a result of surgery, hardware, or diabetic osteoarthropathy. In osteomyelitis, there is an increased accumulation of labeled WBCs, which is incongruent with the bone marrow distribution delineated on Tc-99m sulfur colloid bone marrow scans[77] (**Figure 20**). The sensitivity and specificity of labeled WBC scans for osteomyelitis in the peripheral skeleton and prosthetic joints is between 83% and 89%.[78]

Labeled WBC scans are less accurate for diagnosing spinal osteomyelitis because of intense uptake of labeled WBCs in normal bone marrow, and possibly because of the reduced delivery of labeled WBCs. Vertebral osteomyelitis may show decreased uptake of labeled WBCs (cold vertebra); however, this pattern is nonspecific and may also be seen with tumors, infarcts, compression fractures, and in Paget disease.[77] MRI is the modality of choice for imaging spinal infections. If MRI cannot be used or is inconclusive, radionuclide studies, including gallium-67 and FDG-PET scans, may be helpful. The exact mechanism of gallium-67 accumulation in inflammation is not known but appears to be related to the increased vascular permeability and presence of iron-binding proteins such as lactoferrin and siderophores in inflammatory lesions.[79] Gallium-67 is taken up in areas of both bone remodeling and inflammation and may be inconclusive in a substantial group of patients.[80] Although FDG-PET is primarily used in malignancy workup, substantial accumulation of FDG is also observed in infections because of increased glucose metabolism in activated neutrophils and macrophages.[81] Experience using FDG-PET to diagnose infections is limited; however, the available data are encouraging, particularly as an alternative imaging

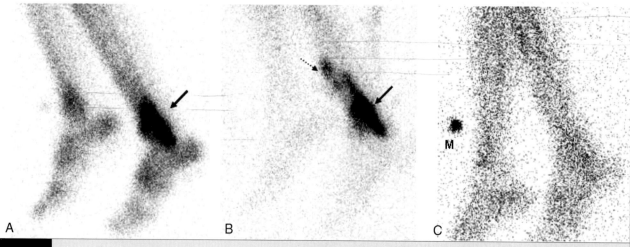

Figure 20 Osteomyelitis in a patient with screw fixation for a tibial fracture. **A,** Bone scan of the ankle shows intense uptake in the left distal tibia (*arrow*). **B,** Labeled WBC scan shows increased accumulation of labeled WBCs in the left distal tibia (*bold arrow*) and in the soft tissue superficially (*dashed arrow*). **C,** Bone marrow scan of the ankles shows symmetric uptake. The radioactive marker (M) indicates the right side. The WBC accumulation in the bone is incongruent with the marrow distribution, which is consistent with osteomyelitis.

modality in chronic osteomyelitis. In a recent meta-analysis that included four studies with FDG-PET, the sensitivity and specificity for diagnosing osteomyelitis was 96% and 91%, respectively.[82] FDG-PET is promising in diagnosing spinal infections, with a reported sensitivity of 100% and specificity of 88%.[78]

Tumors

Whole-body bone scans are routinely used for surveillance of metastatic bone disease. The typical pattern of osseous metastasis is the presence of multiple focal areas of increased tracer uptake predominantly in the axial skeleton. Bone scanning is more sensitive than radiography for detecting metastatic bone disease. A notable exception is multiple myeloma, which does not induce a significant osteoblastic response and is better detected on radiographs. Osteosarcomas and Ewing sarcomas show intense tracer uptake on bone scans. The primary use of bone scans in osteosarcoma and Ewing sarcoma is for initial staging and follow-up of the disease. Many benign bone tumors and tumor-like lesions may also show intense tracer uptake on bone scans. Therefore, bone scans cannot be used to differentiate between benign and malignant lesions. Bone scans can be used to screen for polyostotic disease in fibrous dysplasia, enchondroma, and Paget disease. Bone scans are also highly sensitive for diagnosing osteoid osteoma in patients with chronic pain and negative radiographic results.[83]

FDG-PET is increasingly being used in sarcoma workups. In a recent study that included 160 soft-tissue sarcomas and 52 osseous sarcomas, the sensitivity of FDG PET was 94% for detecting soft-tissue sarcomas and 95% for osseous sarcomas.[84] The sensitivity was 80% or greater for all histologic types, with false negative lesions seen in synovial sarcoma, liposarcoma, chondrosarcoma, and osteosarcomas. High-grade sar-

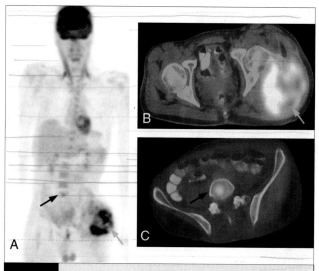

Figure 21 Imaging studies of a patient with gluteal metastatic sarcoma. **A,** Maximum-projection whole-body image shows normal distribution of FDG in the brain, myocardium, liver, spleen, kidneys, bone marrow, and neck muscles. **B** and **C,** Representative transaxial PET CT images of the sarcoma. There is intense uptake of FDG in the high-grade left gluteal sarcoma (orange arrow in **A** and **B**), which also includes areas of decreased uptake in the center of the tumor, consistent with central necrosis. There is also a focus of increased uptake at the L5 vertebra (*black arrow* in **A** and **C**) with an underlying small lytic lesion on CT, which is consistent with metastasis.

comas generally have more intense FDG uptake than low-grade lesions; however, because of significant overlap, FDG-PET cannot be used to reliably grade sarcomas.[85] False-positive PET scans can occur in several benign bone lesions, including giant cell tumors, fibrous

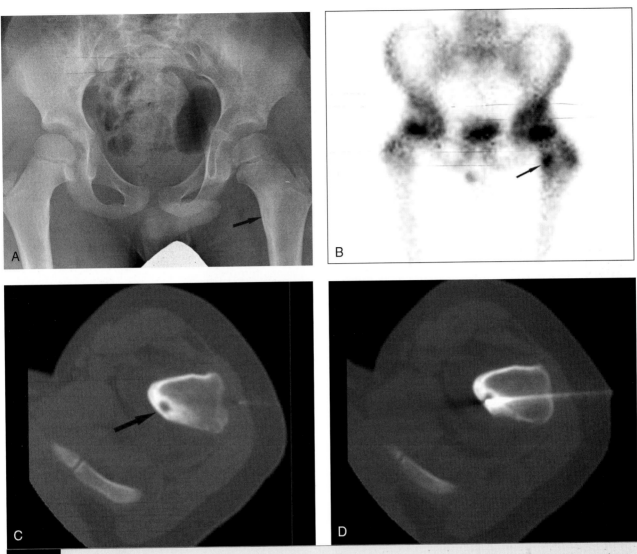

Figure 22 A 10-year-old boy presented with left hip pain of 4 months' duration. **A,** AP radiograph of the pelvis shows sclerosis and thickening of the medial cortex in the left femoral neck (*arrow*). **B,** Bone scan with Tc-99m MDP shows focal increase in uptake of the radiotracer at the medial aspect of the left femoral neck (*arrow*). **C,** Axial CT section through the left femoral neck shows a small lucent nidus surrounded by a sclerotic reaction (*arrow*). The appearance is characteristic of an osteoid osteoma. **D,** Axial CT section shows the tip of the RFA needle within the nidus.

dysplasias, eosinophilic granulomas, chondroblastomas, aneurysmal bone cysts, and nonossifying fibromas.[86] FDG-PET can be helpful in guiding the biopsy to sample the metabolically active part of the tumor.

FDG-PET CT is highly accurate in staging sarcomas (**Figure 21**). An 88% sensitivity was reported for PET CT in nodal staging of 117 patients with sarcoma compared with a 53% sensitivity for conventional imaging, which included MRI, chest radiographs, whole-body contrast-enhanced CT, and bone scans.[87] PET CT was also more sensitive for detecting distant metastases, with a sensitivity of 92% compared with 65% for conventional imaging.[87] These findings were confirmed in a multicenter prospective study, which included 46 pediatric patients with osteosarcoma, Ewing sarcoma, or rhabdomyosarcoma.[88] The sensitivity of PET is limited in diagnosing lung metastases, particularly for lesions smaller than 1 cm;[89] however, those lesions can be diagnosed on the CT component of the PET CT scan. FDG-PET CT was also found to be useful in detecting recurrent metastatic disease after therapy.[90]

The use of FDG-PET CT also has been investigated as a tool in evaluating the chemotherapy response in patients with sarcomas. In one study, the change in FDG uptake between baseline and post therapy PET scans was found to be a significantly better predictor for evaluating the response to neoadjuvant therapy than the change in lesion size.[91] Large multicenter trials are needed to further define the role and criteria for PET in assessing responses to chemotherapy in sarcoma patients.

Interventional Procedures

Needle Biopsy

Percutaneous needle biopsies have been a safe and accurate procedure for more than 70 years. For primary bone tumors and soft-tissue sarcomas, a core needle biopsy is preferred over fine-needle aspiration. Core needle biopsy is better for determining the cell type and tumor grade.[92] For metastatic lesions and round cell sarcomas, fine-needle aspiration can suffice. Currently, most bone biopsies are performed with CT guidance, whereas soft-tissue tumors are biopsied with ultrasound guidance. In the past decade, CT fluoroscopy was introduced to assist in real-time positioning of the needle; its value has been documented in thoracic and abdominal lesions. Using CT fluoroscopy in the biopsy of musculoskeletal lesions achieved similar or better results than conventional CT. However, the high ionizing radiation exposure to both the patient and operator are an important risk factor in using this technique.

Recently, MRI-guided percutaneous biopsies for musculoskeletal lesions have been attempted.[93] Indications include the need to improve the lesion conspicuity when it is not well seen by other imaging techniques or when the lesion is adjacent to critical structures that are better visualized with MRI. The open-configuration magnet has been recommended for interventional procedures because it provides better access to the patient. Results in one study ranged from very good for bone lesions to moderate and fair for soft-tissue lesions.[93]

Three to four biopsy cores are usually sufficient for arriving at a pathologic diagnosis. Most biopsies are performed under local anesthesia. Less than one third of adult patients require conscious sedation. General anesthesia is reserved for young children and uncooperative adults. For primary bone tumors, it is recommended that the approach and needle route be discussed with the orthopaedic tumor surgeon. If the tumor has a necrotic center, it should be avoided and the biopsy cores should be cut from the periphery of the lesion. The main drawback of a needle biopsy is the possibility of a false-negative result because the accuracy of a negative result can be established only by follow-up or by open biopsy. The diagnostic yield is higher in lytic than in sclerotic lesions, in larger lesions, and in those with increased core length. Nondiagnostic cores tend to occur with benign lesion.

Percutaneous Radiofrequency Ablation for Osteoid Osteoma

Osteoid osteoma accounts for about 12% of all benign bone tumors. Although spontaneous resolution has been reported, pain may persist for years and patients often seek definitive treatment. Over the past decade, radiofrequency ablation (RFA) has become the treatment of choice for osteoid osteomas. The technique involves the introduction of an electrode through a biopsy needle into the lesion to heat the abnormal tissue and produce cell death. The tip of the electrode is heated to approximately 90°C for 4 minutes. Most of the experience with RFA is in the lower extremity where most osteoid osteomas occur (**Figure 22**). Lesions that do not allow a safe distance between the electrode tip and a major neurovascular structure may require surgical excision. This is true for the spine, hand, and carpus. However, some investigators have found RFA for spinal lesions to be safe and effective.[94] The cost of RFA is estimated to be approximately 25% of the cost of open surgery.

Summary

Current imaging techniques and the indications for various orthopaedic conditions have been discussed along with characteristic imaging features. Working knowledge of imaging studies is important for orthopaedic surgeons to provide quality patient care.

Annotated References

1. Williams MB, Krupinski EA, Strauss KJ, et al: Digital radiography image quality: Image acquisition. *J Am Coll Radiol* 2007;4(6):371-388.

   The authors describe current technologies of digital radiography compared with conventional screen-film systems. Image acquisition to establish image quality standards is discussed.

2. Krupinski EA, Williams MB, Andriole K, et al; ACR; AAPM; Society for Imaging Informatics in Medicine: Digital radiography image quality: Image processing and display. *J Am Coll Radiol* 2007;4(6):389-400.

   The authors describe current technologies of digital radiography to provide high-quality radiologic care. Image processing and display are discussed. The management of data may have a great impact on the quality of patient care.

3. Hanson JA, Blackmore CC, Mann FA, Wilson AJ: Cervical spine injury: A clinical decision rule to identify high-risk patients for helical CT screening. *AJR Am J Roentgenol* 2000;174(3):713-717.

4. Daffner RH: Helical CT of the cervical spine for trauma patients: A time study. *AJR Am J Roentgenol* 2001; 177(3):677-679.

5. Woodring JH, Lee C: Limitations of cervical radiography in the evaluation of acute cervical trauma. *J Trauma* 1993;34(1):32-39.

6. Blackmore CC, Ramsey SD, Mann FA, Deyo RA: Cervical spine screening with CT in trauma patients: A cost-effectiveness analysis. *Radiology* 1999;212(1):117-125.

7. Lomoschitz FM, Blackmore CC, Mirza SK, Mann FA: Cervical spine injuries in patients 65 years old and older: Epidemiologic analysis regarding the effects of age

and injury mechanism on distribution, type, and stability of injuries. *AJR Am J Roentgenol* 2002;178(3):573-577.

8. Jacobson JA, Girish G, Jiang Y, Sabb BJ: Radiographic evaluation of arthritis: Degenerative joint disease and variations. *Radiology* 2008;248(3):737-747.

   The authors review radiographic features of several types of arthritis emphasizing the radiographic differentials in degenerative joint disease and its variations.

9. Jacobson JA, Girish G, Jiang Y, Resnick D: Radiographic evaluation of arthritis: Inflammatory conditions. *Radiology* 2008;248(2):378-389.

   The authors review the radiographic features of several types of arthritis emphasizing the radiographic differentials in inflammatory conditions.

10. Hayashi M, Matsunaga T, Tanikawa H: Idiopathic widespread calcium pyrophosphate dihydrate crystal deposition disease in a young patient. *Skeletal Radiol* 2002;31(4):246-250.

11. Thomas J, Rideau AM, Paulson EK, Bisset GS III: Emergency department imaging: Current practice. *J Am Coll Radiol* 2008;5(7):811-816, e2.

    A snapshot of the demographics of current imaging practices in emergency departments in the United States is presented. The study is based on the responses to an e-mail survey from 192 (28%) of contacted radiology groups.

12. Whang PG, Goldberg G, Lawrence JP, et al: The management of spinal injuries in patients with ankylosing spondylitis or diffuse idiopathic skeletal hyperostosis: A comparison of treatment methods and clinical outcomes. *J Spinal Disord Tech* 2009;22(2):77-85.

    A retrospective review of 12 patients with ankylosing spondylitis and 18 patients with diffuse idiopathic skeletal hyperostosis reported complete neurologic deficits in 41% of patients with ankylosing spondylitis and 28% of those with hyperostosis. Level of evidence: III.

13. Chiu WC, Haan JM, Cushing BM, Kramer ME, Scalea TM: Ligamentous injuries of the cervical spine in unreliable blunt trauma patients: Incidence, evaluation, and outcome. *J Trauma* 2001;50(3):457-463, discussion 464.

14. Hogan GJ, Mirvis SE, Shanmuganathan K, Scalea TM: Exclusion of unstable cervical spine injury in obtunded patients with blunt trauma: Is MR imaging needed when multi-detector row CT findings are normal? *Radiology* 2005;237(1):106-113.

15. Harris TJ, Blackmore CC, Mirza SK, Jurkovich GJ: Clearing the cervical spine in obtunded patients. *Spine (Phila Pa 1976)* 2008;33(14):1547-1553.

    Based on this retrospective cohort study of 367 obtunded patients, initial cervical CT failed to identify an injury in one patient, resulting in a false-negative rate of 0.3%. The upright radiographs did not show any additional injuries for all study patients. Level of evidence: II.

16. Wintermark M, Mouhsine E, Theumann N, et al: Thoracolumbar spine fractures in patients who have sustained severe trauma: Depiction with multi-detector row CT. *Radiology* 2003;227(3):681-689.

17. Roos JE, Hilfiker P, Platz A, et al: MDCT in emergency radiology: Is a standardized chest or abdominal protocol sufficient for evaluation of thoracic and lumbar spine trauma? *AJR Am J Roentgenol* 2004;183(4):959-968.

18. Ptak T, Rhea JT, Novelline RA: Radiation dose is reduced with a single-pass whole-body multi-detector row CT trauma protocol compared with a conventional segmented method: Initial experience. *Radiology* 2003;229(3):902-905.

19. Fanucci E, Fiaschetti V, Rotili A, Floris R, Simonetti G: Whole body 16-row multislice CT in emergency room: Effects of different protocols on scanning time, image quality and radiation exposure. *Emerg Radiol* 2007;13(5):251-257.

    For multitrauma patients, whole-body, single-pass CT protocol in 26 patients was compared with conventional segmented protocol in 20 patients to define scanning time, image quality, and radiation dose. The whole-body protocol showed a reduced total radiation dose with no relevant loss of diagnostic image quality.

20. Leone A, Cerase A, Priolo F, Marano P: Lumbosacral junction injury associated with unstable pelvic fracture: Classification and diagnosis. *Radiology* 1997;205(1):253-259.

21. Gansslen A, Pohlemann T, Paul C, Lobenhoffer P, Tscherne H: Epidemiology of pelvic ring injuries. *Injury* 1996;27(suppl 1):S-A13-S-A20.

22. Tibbs BM, Kopar P, Dente CJ, Rozycki GS, Feliciano DV: Acetabular and isolated pelvic ring fractures: A comparison of initial assessment and outcome. *Am Surg* 2008;74(6):538-541.

    The authors retrospectively reviewed and compared the outcomes among the patients with acetabular and pelvic ring fractures (1,334 patients with 320 acetabular, 826 pelvic ring, and 188 combination fractures). Level of evidence: II.

23. Ohashi K, El-Khoury GY, Abu-Zahra KW, Berbaum KS: Interobserver agreement for Letournel acetabular fracture classification with multidetector CT: Are standard Judet radiographs necessary? *Radiology* 2006;241(2):386-391.

24. Dorsay TA, Major NM, Helms CA: Cost-effectiveness of immediate MR imaging versus traditional follow-up for revealing radiographically occult scaphoid fractures. *AJR Am J Roentgenol* 2001;177(6):1257-1263.

25. Groves AM, Kayani I, Syed R, et al: An international

1: Principles of Orthopaedics

survey of hospital practice in the imaging of acute scaphoid trauma. *AJR Am J Roentgenol* 2006;187(6): 1453-1456.

26. Tiel-van Buul MM, van Beek EJ, Broekhuizen AH, Bakker AJ, Bos KE, van Royen EA: Radiography and scintigraphy of suspected scaphoid fracture: A long-term study in 160 patients. *J Bone Joint Surg Br* 1993;75(1): 61-65.

27. Tiel-van Buul MM, Broekhuizen TH, van Beek EJ, Bossuyt PM: Choosing a strategy for the diagnostic management of suspected scaphoid fracture: A cost-effectiveness analysis. *J Nucl Med* 1995;36(1):45-48.

28. Gaebler C, Kukla C, Breitenseher M, Trattnig S, Mittlboeck M, Vécsei V: Magnetic resonance imaging of occult scaphoid fractures. *J Trauma* 1996;41(1):73-76.

29. Breitenseher MJ, Metz VM, Gilula LA, et al: Radiographically occult scaphoid fractures: Value of MR imaging in detection. *Radiology* 1997;203(1):245-250.

30. Herneth AM, Siegmeth A, Bader TR, et al: Scaphoid fractures: Evaluation with high-spatial-resolution US initial results. *Radiology* 2001;220(1):231-235.

31. Welling RD, Jacobson JA, Jamadar DA, Chong S, Caoili EM, Jebson PJ: MDCT and radiography of wrist fractures: Radiographic sensitivity and fracture patterns. *AJR Am J Roentgenol* 2008;190(1):10-16.

    Radiographic and CT studies of 103 consecutive patients who were suspected of having wrist fractures were reviewed in this retrospective study. Thirty percent of wrist fractures were not prospectively diagnosed on radiography. Level of evidence: II.

32. Tiel-van Buul MM, van Beek EJ, Dijkstra PF, Bakker AJ, Broekhuizen TH, van Royen EA: Significance of a hot spot on the bone scan after carpal injury: Evaluation by computed tomography. *Eur J Nucl Med* 1993; 20(2):159-164.

33. Groves AM, Cheow H, Balan K, Courtney H, Bearcroft P, Dixon A: 16-MDCT in the detection of occult wrist fractures: A comparison with skeletal scintigraphy. *AJR Am J Roentgenol* 2005;184(5):1470-1474.

34. Chan PS, Klimkiewicz JJ, Luchetti WT, et al: Impact of CT scan on treatment plan and fracture classification of tibial plateau fractures. *J Orthop Trauma* 1997;11(7): 484-489.

35. Liow RY, Birdsall PD, Mucci B, Greiss ME: Spiral computed tomography with two- and three-dimensional reconstruction in the management of tibial plateau fractures. *Orthopedics* 1999;22(10):929-932.

36. Wicky S, Blaser PF, Blanc CH, Leyvraz PF, Schnyder P, Meuli RA: Comparison between standard radiography and spiral CT with 3D reconstruction in the evaluation, classification and management of tibial plateau fractures. *Eur Radiol* 2000;10(8):1227-1232.

37. Macarini L, Murrone M, Marini S, Calbi R, Solarino M, Moretti B: Tibial plateau fractures: Evaluation with multidetector-CT. *Radiol Med* 2004;108(5-6):503-514.

38. Haraguchi N, Haruyama H, Toga H, Kato F: Pathoanatomy of posterior malleolar fractures of the ankle. *J Bone Joint Surg Am* 2006;88(5):1085-1092.

39. Sanders R, Gregory P: Operative treatment of intra-articular fractures of the calcaneus. *Orthop Clin North Am* 1995;26(2):203-214.

40. Prasartritha T, Sethavanitch C: Three-dimensional and two-dimensional computerized tomographic demonstration of calcaneus fractures. *Foot Ankle Int* 2004;25(4): 262-273.

41. Ohashi K, Restrepo JM, El-Khoury GY, Berbaum KS: Peroneal tendon subluxation and dislocation: Detection on volume-rendered images. Initial experience. *Radiology* 2007;242(1):252-257.

    A preliminary study consisting of 32 patients with acute calcaneal fractures showed that viewing three-dimensional volume-rendered images is more time-efficient compared with reviewing multiplanar reformatted images for detecting peroneal tendon dislocation. Level of evidence: III.

42. Calhoun PS, Kuszyk BS, Heath DG, Carley JC, Fishman EK: Three-dimensional volume rendering of spiral CT data: Theory and method. *Radiographics* 1999;19(3): 745-764.

43. White LM, Buckwalter KA: Technical considerations: CT and MR imaging in the postoperative orthopedic patient. *Semin Musculoskelet Radiol* 2002;6(1):5-17.

44. Farber GL, Place HM, Mazur RA, Jones DE, Damiano TR: Accuracy of pedicle screw placement in lumbar fusions by plain radiographs and computed tomography. *Spine (Phila Pa 1976)* 1995;20(13):1494-1499.

45. Linsenmaier U, Rock C, Euler E, et al: Three-dimensional CT with a modified C-arm image intensifier: Feasibility. *Radiology* 2002;224(1):286-292.

46. Krestan CR, Noske H, Vasilevska V, et al: MDCT versus digital radiography in the evaluation of bone healing in orthopedic patients. *AJR Am J Roentgenol* 2006; 186(6):1754-1760.

47. Dorsey ML, Liu PT, Roberts CC, Kile TA: Correlation of arthrodesis stability with degree of joint fusion on MDCT. *AJR Am J Roentgenol* 2009;192(2):496-499.

    The authors of this study, based on the retrospective review of 42 consecutive CT studies from 29 patients, reported that ankle or subtalar fusion is likely stable if more than 33% of the joint has bone fusion on sagittal CT images. Level of evidence: III.

48. Shah RR, Mohammed S, Saifuddin A, Taylor BA: Comparison of plain radiographs with CT scan to evaluate interbody fusion following the use of titanium interbody

cages and transpedicular instrumentation. *Eur Spine J* 2003;12(4):378-385.

49. Fehring TK, McAvoy G: Fluoroscopic evaluation of the painful total knee arthroplasty. *Clin Orthop Relat Res* 1996;331:226-233.

50. Chiang PP, Burke DW, Freiberg AA, Rubash HE: Osteolysis of the pelvis: Evaluation and treatment. *Clin Orthop Relat Res* 2003;417:164-174.

51. Berry DJ: Recognizing and identifying osteolysis around total knee arthroplasty. *Instr Course Lect* 2004;53:261-264.

52. Claus AM, Totterman SM, Sychterz CJ, Tamez-Peña JG, Looney RJ, Engh CA Sr: Computed tomography to assess pelvic lysis after total hip replacement. *Clin Orthop Relat Res* 2004;422:167-174.

53. Jazrawi LM, Birdzell L, Kummer FJ, Di Cesare PE: The accuracy of computed tomography for determining femoral and tibial total knee arthroplasty component rotation. *J Arthroplasty* 2000;15(6):761-766.

54. Scuderi GR, Komistek RD, Dennis DA, Insall JN: The impact of femoral component rotational alignment on condylar lift-off. *Clin Orthop Relat Res* 2003;410:148-154.

55. Ohashi K, El-Khoury GY, Bennett DL, Restrepo JM, Berbaum KS: Orthopedic hardware complications diagnosed with multi-detector row CT. *Radiology* 2005;237(2):570-577.

56. Olsen RV, Munk PL, Lee MJ, et al: Metal artifact reduction sequence: Early clinical applications. *Radiographics* 2000;20(3):699-712.

57. Ruzal-Shapiro C, Berdon WE, Cohen MD, Abramson SJ: MR imaging of diffuse bone marrow replacement in pediatric patients with cancer. *Radiology* 1991;181(2):587-589.

58. Carmody RF, Yang PJ, Seeley GW, Seeger JF, Unger EC, Johnson JE: Spinal cord compression due to metastatic disease: Diagnosis with MR imaging versus myelography. *Radiology* 1989;173(1):225-229.

59. Murphy BJ: Evaluation of grades 3 and 4 chondromalacia of the knee using T2-weighted 3D gradient-echo articular cartilage imaging. *Skeletal Radiol* 2001;30(6):305-311.

60. Wiginton CD, Kelly B, Oto A, et al: Gadolinium-based contrast exposure, nephrogenic systemic fibrosis, and gadolinium detection in tissue. *AJR Am J Roentgenol* 2008;190(4):1060-1068.

    A retrospective review of seven patients with nephrogenic systemic fibrosis showed that symptoms of the condition developed in all of the patients after receiving gadolinium and all had renal failure. The authors found an association between the use of gadolinium in patients with renal failure and the development of nephrogenic systemic fibrosis.

61. Goncalves-Matoso V, Guntern D, Gray A, Schnyder P, Picht C, Theumann N: Optimal 3-T MRI for depiction of the finger A2 pulley: Comparison between T1-weighted, fat-saturated T2-weighted and gadolinium-enhanced fat-saturated T1-weighted sequences. *Skeletal Radiol* 2008;37(4):307-312.

    The authors used a 3.0-T magnet with three different spin-echo sequences to study the visualization of normal and abnormal finger A2 pulley. They found that transverse fat-saturated T1-weighted gadolinium-enhancement sequences are best for depicting an abnormal A2 pulley.

62. Magee T: Can isotropic fast gradient echo imaging be substituted for conventional T1 weighted sequences in shoulder MR arthrography at 3 Tesla? *J Magn Reson Imaging* 2007;26(1):118-122.

    The author presents the results of a retrospective review of 100 consecutive shoulder MR arthrograms studied by standard T1-weighted spin-echo sequences and by isotropic gradient-echo imaging using 0.4-mm thin sections. The author found that isotropic imaging provides the same clinical information as conventional imaging and can be acquired in less than 3 minutes.

63. Gold GE, Busse RF, Beehler C, et al: Isotropic MRI of the knee with 3D fast spin-echo extended echo-train acquisition (XETA): Initial experience. *AJR Am J Roentgenol* 2007;188(5):1287-1293.

    In this prospective study, the authors compared isotropic three-dimensional fast spin-echo extended echo-train acquisition with two-dimensional fast spin-echo and two-dimensional fast recovery fast spin-echo for MRI of the knee. The authors reported that the three-dimensional fast spin-echo extended echo-train acquisition method acquires high-resolution isotropic data with intermediate- and T2-weighting that may be reformatted in arbitrary planes.

64. Haramati N, Staron RB, Barax C, Feldman F: Magnetic resonance imaging of occult fractures of the proximal femur. *Skeletal Radiol* 1994;23(1):19-22.

65. Nikken JJ, Oei EH, Ginai AZ, et al: Acute wrist trauma: Value of a short dedicated extremity MR imaging examination in prediction of need for treatment. *Radiology* 2005;234(1):116-124.

66. Menaker J, Philp A, Boswell S, Scalea TM: Computed tomography alone for cervical spine clearance in the unreliable patient: Are we there yet? *J Trauma* 2008;64(4):898-903, discussion 903-904.

    The authors report on a retrospective review of patients with blunt trauma who had cervical spine imaging with CT and MRI in the acute phase. Newer generation CT missed cervical spine injuries in unreliable patients. MRI findings changed treatment in 7.9% of patients. Two patients required surgical repair. The authors recommend using MRI for clearing the cervical spine in unreliable patients.

67. Tomycz ND, Chew BG, Chang YF, et al: MRI is unnecessary to clear the cervical spine in obtunded/comatose trauma patients: The four-year experience of a level I trauma center. *J Trauma* 2008;64(5):1258-1263.

The authors report on a retrospective review of 180 trauma patients who had a normal CT examination on admission along with a cervical spine MRI. In 38 patients (21.1%), the MRI showed acute traumatic findings; however, surgery was not needed and delayed instability did not develop. The authors concluded that MRI is unlikely to detect unstable cervical spine injuries when the CT examination is normal.

68. Yucesoy K, Yuksel KZ: SCIWORA in MRI era. *Clin Neurol Neurosurg* 2008;110(5):429-433.

A literature review was undertaken to investigate whether the meaning of SCIWORA had changed after the advent of MRI. The authors found that SCIWORA had an ambiguous meaning in the literature. They recommended that spines with MRI abnormalities, with or without radiographic abnormalities, should not be classified as SCIWORA.

69. Pang D: Spinal cord injury without radiographic abnormality in children, 2 decades later. *Neurosurgery* 2004; 55(6):1325-1342, discussion 1342-1343.

70. Holder LE, Schwarz C, Wernicke PG, Michael RH: Radionuclide bone imaging in the early detection of fractures of the proximal femur (hip): Multifactorial analysis. *Radiology* 1990;174(2):509-515.

71. Matin P: The appearance of bone scans following fractures, including immediate and long-term studies. *J Nucl Med* 1979;20(12):1227-1231.

72. Zwas ST, Elkanovitch R, Frank G: Interpretation and classification of bone scintigraphic findings in stress fractures. *J Nucl Med* 1987;28(4):452-457.

73. Minoves M: Bone and joint sports injuries: The role of bone scintigraphy. *Nucl Med Commun* 2003;24(1):3-10.

74. Raby N, Mathews S: Symptomatic spondylolysis: Correlation of CT and SPECT with clinical outcome. *Clin Radiol* 1993;48(2):97-99.

75. Bellah RD, Summerville DA, Treves ST, Micheli LJ: Low-back pain in adolescent athletes: Detection of stress injury to the pars interarticularis with SPECT. *Radiology* 1991;180(2):509-512.

76. Maurer AH, Chen DC, Camargo EE, Wong DF, Wagner HN Jr, Alderson PO: Utility of three-phase skeletal scintigraphy in suspected osteomyelitis: Concise communication. *J Nucl Med* 1981;22(11):941-949.

77. Palestro CJ, Torres MA: Radionuclide imaging in orthopedic infections. *Semin Nucl Med* 1997;27(4):334-345.

78. Prandini N, Lazzeri E, Rossi B, Erba P, Parisella MG, Signore A: Nuclear medicine imaging of bone infections. *Nucl Med Commun* 2006;27(8):633-644.

79. Love C, Palestro CJ: Radionuclide imaging of infection. *J Nucl Med Technol* 2004;32(2):47-57, quiz 58-59.

80. Schauwecker DS, Park HM, Mock BH, et al: Evaluation of complicating osteomyelitis with Tc-99m MDP, In-111 granulocytes, and Ga-67 citrate. *J Nucl Med* 1984; 25(8):849-853.

81. Kaim AH, Weber B, Kurrer MO, Gottschalk J, Von Schulthess GK, Buck A: Autoradiographic quantification of 18F-FDG uptake in experimental soft-tissue abscesses in rats. *Radiology* 2002;223(2):446-451.

82. Termaat MF, Raijmakers PG, Scholten HJ, Bakker FC, Patka P, Haarman HJ: The accuracy of diagnostic imaging for the assessment of chronic osteomyelitis: A systematic review and meta-analysis. *J Bone Joint Surg Am* 2005;87(11):2464-2471.

83. Lisbona R, Rosenthall L: Role of radionuclide imaging in osteoid osteoma. *AJR Am J Roentgenol* 1979;132(1): 77-80.

84. Charest M, Hickeson M, Lisbona R, Novales-Diaz JA, Derbekyan V, Turcotte RE: FDG PET/CT imaging in primary osseous and soft tissue sarcomas: A retrospective review of 212 cases. *Eur J Nucl Med Mol Imaging* 2009;Jul 11:[Epub ahead of print].

This large study evaluates the sensitivity of FDG-PET for detecting osseous and soft-tissue sarcomas with different histologies.

85. Folpe AL, Lyles RH, Sprouse JT, Conrad EU III, Eary JF: (F-18) fluorodeoxyglucose positron emission tomography as a predictor of pathologic grade and other prognostic variables in bone and soft tissue sarcoma. *Clin Cancer Res* 2000;6(4):1279-1287.

86. Schulte M, Brecht-Krauss D, Heymer B, et al: Grading of tumors and tumorlike lesions of bone: Evaluation by FDG PET. *J Nucl Med* 2000;41(10):1695-1701.

87. Tateishi U, Yamaguchi U, Seki K, Terauchi T, Arai Y, Kim EE: Bone and soft-tissue sarcoma: Preoperative staging with fluorine 18 fluorodeoxyglucose PET/CT and conventional imaging. *Radiology* 2007;245(3):839-847.

This retrospective study compares PET-CT with CT, MRI, and bone scans in staging osseous and soft-tissue sarcomas.

88. Völker T, Denecke T, Steffen I, et al: Positron emission tomography for staging of pediatric sarcoma patients: Results of a prospective multicenter trial. *J Clin Oncol* 2007;25(34):5435-5441.

This prospective study evaluates the role of FDG-PET CT and its added value to conventional imaging in staging pediatric sarcomas.

89. Franzius C, Daldrup-Link HE, Sciuk J, et al: FDG-PET

for detection of pulmonary metastases from malignant primary bone tumors: Comparison with spiral CT. *Ann Oncol* 2001;12(4):479-486.

90. Arush MW, Israel O, Postovsky S, et al: Positron emission tomography/computed tomography with 18fluorodeoxyglucose in the detection of local recurrence and distant metastases of pediatric sarcoma. *Pediatr Blood Cancer* 2007;49(7):901-905.

    The authors report on the role of FDG-PET CT in evaluating local recurrence at the primary site and distant disease in children with sarcoma.

91. Evilevitch V, Weber WA, Tap WD, et al: Reduction of glucose metabolic activity is more accurate than change in size at predicting histopathologic response to neoadjuvant therapy in high-grade soft-tissue sarcomas. *Clin Cancer Res* 2008;14(3):715-720.

    The authors compare the change of FDG uptake (measured in standarized uptake value) with the change in tumor size in predicting the response of sarcomas to chemotherapy.

92. Espinosa LA, Jamadar DA, Jacobson JA, et al: CT-guided biopsy of bone: A radiologist's perspective. *AJR Am J Roentgenol* 2008;190(5):W283-W289.

The authors present an overview of approaches to bone biopsies intended to minimize potential tumor seeding into the soft tissues. They also discuss safe approaches related to specific anatomic parts.

93. Carrino JA, Khurana B, Ready JE, Silverman SG, Winalski CS: Magnetic resonance imaging-guided percutaneous biopsy of musculoskeletal lesions. *J Bone Joint Surg Am* 2007;89(10):2179-2187.

    In a retrospective case series of 45 biopsies performed with magnetic resonance guidance, the authors reported very good results for bone lesions, moderate results for extra-articular soft-tissue lesions, and fair results for intra-articular soft-tissue lesions.

94. Vanderschueren GM, Obermann WR, Dijkstra SP, Taminiau AH, Bloem JL, van Erkel AR: Radiofrequency ablation of spinal osteoid osteoma: Clinical outcome. *Spine (Phila Pa 1976)* 2009;34(9):901-904.

    The authors present the findings of a prospective study of 24 patients with spinal osteoid osteoma treated with RFA. The authors concluded that RFA is a safe and effective treatment for spinal osteoid osteoma. Surgery should be reserved for lesions causing nerve root compression.

1: Principles of Orthopaedics

Chapter 9

Patient-Centered Care: Communication Skills and Cultural Competence

John R. Tongue, MD   Norman Y. Otsuka, MD

Introduction

The concept of patient-centered care compels physicians to treat patients as partners, involving them in decision making and enlisting a sense of self-responsibility for their care, while respecting their individual values and concerns.[1] Specifically, this process includes striving to maintain eye contact; leaning forward; remaining physically calm; avoiding jargon and interruptions; validating the patient's emotions; learning about the patient's lifestyle; checking for understanding; and offering support.[2] Effective communication skills allow for more accurate diagnoses, better adherence to treatment plans, decreased medical liability, and better patient outcomes.[1]

Orthopaedic surgeons have tended to focus primarily on the technical aspects of caregiving;[3,4] however, there is a need to improve communication skills as well as surgical skills. Good interviewing skills allow a surgeon to assess the level of a patient's understanding and permit successful engagement to meet the patient's expectations. The challenges of effective communication are driven by the increasing complexity of health care, the shifting demands of health care reform, and the progressively diversifying patient language and cultural barriers. To provide culturally competent care, orthopaedic surgeons must do their best to understand each patient's cultural background, belief systems, and perception of their illness.

Patient-centered care also requires knowledge of the

Dr. Tongue or an immediate family member serves as a board member, owner, officer, or committee member of the Western Orthopaedic Association. Dr. Otsuka or an immediate family member serves as a board member, owner, officer, or committee member of the American Academy of Orthopaedic Surgeons, California Orthopaedic Association, and Pediatric Orthopaedic Society of North America; and has received research or institutional support from the National Institutes of Health and Shriners Hospitals for Children.

patient's experiences and lifestyle, which then allows blending of these factors with the biomedical elements of patient care. This psychosocial information is best obtained with an interviewing style that actively seeks the patient's input, and is facilitated through open-ended questions, expressions of concern, checks for understanding, and requests for opinions and expectations. The result is a more effective medical intervention, resulting in both increased patient and physician satisfaction.[5] Nearly 70% of the variance in patient satisfaction scores has been attributed to communication, including nonverbal communication, attitude, information giving, and the style of decision making.[6]

There is increasing interest and regard for the process of informed consent. Physicians are concerned about their ability to effectively complete the requirements of informed consent while efficiently managing their time. Surgeons who do well at fostering informed consent do not have substantially longer patient interviews than their colleagues.[7] Recent court rulings set a high standard for achieving informed consent, and have stated that it "... is a health care provider's duty to communicate information to enable a patient to make an intelligent and informed choice" and that "the law does not allow a physician to substitute his judgment for that of the patient."[8] An open, patient-centered, interview approach can achieve timely informed patient consent, meeting both medical and legal standards, while uncovering relevant information that may otherwise be withheld by the patient.[9]

Medical students are often drawn to careers in orthopaedic surgery because of their attraction to biomedical technology and scientific method. Medical school studies of the doctor-patient relationship are sometimes dismissed as an unscientific and low priority. There is often a striking decline in the attitudes of medical students toward the emotional and interpersonal dimensions of patient care as they seek to apply an overwhelming array of "hard science." In this stressful environment, avoiding emotional situations with patients and the need to comfort them are common coping mechanisms. Emotional encounters with patients

Table 1

Interpersonal Skills Evaluation by Consumers and Orthopaedic Surgeons[a]

	Skills Important to Consumers (2008)	Skills That Orthopaedic Surgeons Believe Are Important to Patients (2008)
Highly trained	82%	71%
Listens	83%	53%
Successful results	84%	89%
Caring/compassionate	74%	55%
Spends time with patient	74%	39%
Value/cost	73%	44%
Easy appointment scheduling	65%	24%

[a]Orthopaedic surgeons undervalue the interpersonal skills of listening, demonstrating compassion, and spending time with patients compared with patients' ratings of these characteristics. Questions were developed on a scale from 1 to 5, with a higher number representing an increasing level of favorability. In analyzing this type of question, it is customary to combine 4 and 5 rating responses as a strong measure of agreement or performance and are valid at approximately ± 3.5% at a 95% confidence level. The table information is based on an AAOS 2008 Tracking Survey.[12]

are often viewed as onerous and time consuming. When teachers exhibit dehumanizing patterns of communication, students imitate these patterns of dealing with patients.[10] This hidden curriculum may also be evident as attending surgeons and senior residents are observed dealing with patients from multicultural backgrounds, with those observed interactions having a significant impact on how younger residents will relate to patients when they have their own practices.[11]

Background

Most practicing orthopaedic surgeons receive limited formal education in the communication skills necessary for patient-centered care; however, a substantial amount of time is spent talking with patients (approximately 160,000 interviews during a typical career).[1] Comparable surveys in 1998 and 2008 by the American Academy of Orthopaedic Surgeons (AAOS) showed that surgeons continue to believe that they have high technical and high interpersonal skills. However, orthopaedic surgeons also continue to view their colleagues as having much lower communication skills. The public believes that orthopaedic surgeons have low communication skills.[12] Also, both surveys strongly indicate that orthopaedic surgeons do not value interpersonal skills as strongly as the public views such skills (**Table 1**).

The AAOS 2008 Tracking Survey highlights the variance among the consumers' stated beliefs on the importance of physician rating factors and the surgeons' self-perceptions of their performance.[12] Consumers favorably rate orthopaedic surgeons on successful medical results, which is the most important factor. However, the interpersonal skills of listening, demonstrating compassion, and spending time with patients also rank very high with patients but much lower with orthopaedic surgeons.

The most common deficiency in daily interviews with patients is the consistent failure of the orthopaedic surgeons to offer empathic responses.[13] Social science research clearly indicates that doctors trained in empathy can improve their ability to make eye contact, appear more attentive, reflect understanding, and express feelings that encourage patients to talk openly.[14]

Another challenge for surgeons is to complete effective, informed decision-making interviews within the time constraints of a busy office practice. A concern, which is often raised, is that proposed models of excellent communication may not be feasible in the time-pressured setting of an orthopaedic surgeon's practice. Research, however, indicates that a few additional minutes during an initial patient visit saves time later, while developing mutual trust, understanding, and satisfaction.[14]

Among surgical specialty physician groups, orthopaedic surgeons have been reported to be both more satisfied and more dissatisfied than any other specialty groups, indicating a divided workforce.[15] Possible explanations include variance in the ability to cope with losses in income and autonomy, the constraints of managed care, and differing communication skill sets for both residents and practicing orthopaedic surgeons. A recent report by the American Orthopaedic Association states, "Residents reported a significant burnout, showing a high level of emotional exhaustion and depersonalization." The report adds, "... excellent communication skills contribute to effective prevention stress management," and that "... preventive stress management skills help avert burnout, emotional exhaustion, and even surgical errors."[16]

Skilled medical interviews also reduce the risk of lawsuits. The burden of the protracted legal process involved in defending a malpractice suit adds considerable stress to the day-to-day practice of orthopaedic surgery. Malpractice lawsuits are frequently initiated because of a difference in expectations between the

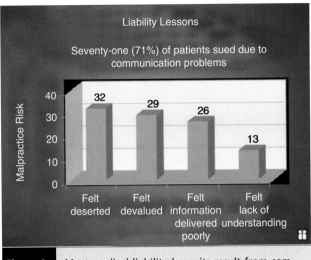

Figure 1 Most medical liability lawsuits result from communication problems in the doctor-patient relationship. A 1994 study showed that 71% of patients sue because of communication problems. The number at the top of the bars represents the percentage of patients who answered questions affirmatively. The numbers on the Y axis represent the percentage of patients in the study who sued. (Reproduced with permission from Beckman HB, Markakis KM, Suchman AL, Frankel RM: The doctor-patient relationship and malpractice: Lessons from plaintiff depositions. *Arch Intern Med* 1994;154(12):1365-1370.)

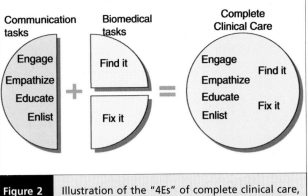

Figure 2 Illustration of the "4Es" of complete clinical care, which represent a model for physician-patient communication. (Reproduced with permission from Tongue JR, Epps HR, Forese LL: Communication skills for patient-centered care: Research-based, easily learned techniques for medical interviews that benefit orthopaedic surgeons and their patients. *J Bone Joint Surg Am* 2005;87:652-658.)

physician and the patient. The tipping point for most medical liability suits in the United States has been attributed primarily to breakdowns in communication. Better communication reduces potential misunderstandings and unmet expectations[17] (**Figure 1**).

Good patient interviews have been shown to foster stronger patient-physician relationships while gathering superior qualitative and quantitative information that improves diagnostic accuracy, reduces medical errors, improves patient outcomes, and makes the practice of orthopaedic surgery less stressful and more enjoyable.[1]

Communication Skills Techniques

The "4Es" educational model for communication is particularly useful for orthopaedic practices. Excellent orthopaedic care requires a high level of patient cooperation and adherence to treatment protocols to achieve the best possible outcomes. The "4Es" of critical communication tasks, to engage, empathize, educate, and enlist patients have been proposed.[18] These communication tasks are considered to be of equal importance to the biomedical tasks, or the "2Fs," of finding the problem (diagnosis) and fixing the problem (treatment) (**Figure 2**).

Engagement

Engagement establishes an interpersonal connection that sets the stage for the patient-physician interaction, drawing the patient in. The patient will respond to the doctor who smiles; maintains eye contact; has a relaxed body posture; speaks with a calm consistent tone of voice; and sits, leaning forward with arms opened. Open-ended questions allow patients to tell their story and avoid possible false assumptions regarding the patient's agenda.[19,20] For example, the physician can begin with, "How can I help you today?" The question should be spoken with a combination of a smile, calm voice, handshake, and eye contact. By contrast, asking a vulnerable patient, "How ya doing today?" can create conflict for patients who feel compelled to answer "fine" to this typical American greeting, just before explaining why they have come to see a doctor. Unfortunately, doctors interrupt patients in most interviews within 23 seconds, and once interrupted, patients finish their comments in only 8% of interviews.[21] Older patients report higher satisfaction rates when accompanied by a family member, friend, or advocate.[22]

Empathy

Empathy allows physicians to demonstrate an understanding of and concern for the patient's thoughts and feelings. The patient is seen, heard, and understood. Audiotaped interviews have shown that expressions of empathy by orthopaedic surgeons are rare.[9,11] It is possible that surgeons feel uncomfortable showing empathy, fearing that statements of compassion will lead to time-consuming conversation, unpleasant emotional scenes, and the need to comfort patients.[23] Empathy is the surgeon's most powerful and underused tool. A true expression of empathy, such as "that must have been painful/frustrating/frightening," spoken with a concerned tone and facial expression that models that of the patient can quickly establish a trusting relationship.

Empathy, contrary to popular belief, actually saves time. Showing compassion with empathic comments encourages patients to express their true agenda and hidden concerns.[24] Time-saving techniques include prioritizing discussion topics by inquiring about the patient's primary concerns early, keeping any personal physician disclosures brief, and using scenarios during informed consent.[8] Acknowledging a patient's emotions and values recognizes their individuality.

Education

Educational information, when successfully communicated, enhances the patient's knowledge and increases his or her capacity to deal with treatment options while decreasing anxiety. Patients generally prefer detailed and extensive disclosure of alternative therapies; however, only 50% of physicians believe that patients want information about alternative treatments.[25] Patients also prefer information regarding risks (even those that are rare), whereas physicians often believe that such detailed information regarding drugs will decrease the placebo effect, increase adverse effects, and decrease compliance. Patients express the opposite view. For example, explaining the potential benefits and adverse effects of a nonsteroidal anti-inflammatory drug will increase rather than decrease adherence to the treatment plan.

Patients often lack the skill to ask appropriate questions during an interview.[26] Inquiring about the patient's primary concerns at the beginning of the educational phase of a new patient interview will both open a focused discussion and save time. Patients should be encouraged to ask questions at any time. Physicians may mistake a patient's respect or reserve as a lack of interest. Conversely, assertive patients who push for detailed information may be perceived as litigation risks.[27]

Physicians should avoid long educational monologues. Stopping to check the patient's verbal understanding (not just their nonverbal expressions) is important, but rare. For example, the physician can say, "I have given you one explanation, so how does this fit with what you've been thinking?" The physician also can inquire about the patient's concerns about a planned surgery. It should be recognized that every patient presents with a self-diagnosis. The physician should be wary of patients who do not engage in open discussion; those patients may later complain that important information was not provided.[1]

Enlistment

Enlistment extends an offer to the patient to actively participate in decision making. Enlistment acknowledges that patients control much of their treatment plan. To achieve successful outcomes, orthopaedic patients must be confident that their treatment will help them and must be convinced that they can achieve treatment plan goals in the face of competing interests for their time and energy.[23] A perfect flexor tendon repair or knee replacement will stiffen and fail without the cooperation of a well-informed and motivated patient.

Missed clues by patients regarding possible barriers to treatment often lead to misunderstandings and

wasted time during interviews.[24] Older patients, especially African Americans, are quite selective in disclosing important information during interviews with orthopaedic surgeons. A 2008 study reported that orthopaedic surgeons responded inadequately to 29% of patient concerns (23 of 80)[9] (**Table 2**). A "minimal acknowledgment" was the most common response to the concerns of patients about their ability to meet the challenges of surgery.

A 2001 study showed that patients do not adhere to treatment plans when they disagree with the physician (37%), are concerned about cost (27%), find the instructions too difficult to follow (25%), think the recommendations are in conflict with their personal beliefs (20%), or do not understand the plan (7%).[28] Patients can help to reduce medical errors in the hospital when they are fully informed of their treatment plan on a daily basis during the physician's morning rounds.[29]

Communicating Bad News

Specific techniques are useful in communicating adverse events.[30] A physician may feel defensive when an unexpected complication or medical error occurs, resulting in the patient not being fully informed. Discussions between team members will help prepare an appropriate response, thereby reducing the possible perception by the patient and family members that the event has been handled insensitively. Apologies without accepting blame should be offered. The focus should be on the disease, not the team members. Adequate time should be allowed for difficult and often emotional discussions. The physician should listen carefully, avoid interruptions, and frequently check for understanding. A proactive, timely plan with clear statements and documentation should be presented. The physician should remain hopeful, regroup before moving on to other tasks, and follow up on the announced plan in a timely manner. Patients who receive full disclosure are reported to have more trust and a more positive emotional response.[31] Patients were more likely to litigate following errors if there was not full disclosure.[32]

Culture

Definition

At its most basic, culture is defined as a combination of acquired beliefs and behaviors that are shared among a particular group or groups. The culture of medicine often clashes with that of patient groups, resulting in disparities of care. The National Center for Cultural Competence defines culture as "an integrated pattern of human behavior that includes thoughts, communications, languages, practices, beliefs, values, customs, courtesies, rituals, manners of interacting, roles, relationships, and expected behaviors of a racial, ethnic, religious, or social group."[33] Six realities of cultural programming that should be considered by clinicians in

Table 2	

Orthopaedic Surgeon Responses to 80 Concerns Expressed by Older Patients[a]

Positive Acknowledgment by the Surgeon	Surgeon Responses to Patient Concerns
Reassurance	40
With explanation	27
Without explanation	13
Supportive/accommodating	12
Empathy	1
Inadequate Acknowledgment by the Surgeon	
Minimal acknowledgment	13
Failure to address concern	8
Premature acknowledgment	2
Negative Response by the Surgeon	
Inappropriate humor	3
Denial	0
Termination of conversation	1

[a] Older patient concerns about surgery (80) were separated from a total of 155 concerns identified. (Reproduced with permission from Hudak PL, Armstrong K, Braddock C III, Frankel RM, Levinson W: Older patients' unexpressed concerns about orthopaedic surgery. *J Bone Joint Surg Am* 2008;90(7):1427-1435.)

Table 3	

Six Realties of Cultural Programming

Culture is not obvious

We all think that our own culture is best

We misinterpret the actions of others if we do not understand their interpretations of their own observations

We may not know when we are offending others

Awareness of difference and possible barriers improves our chances for successful interactions

Understanding our own "software" or value system is a crucial step in providing culturally competent care

(Adapted with permission from from Tongue JR, Epps HR, Forese LL: Communication skills for patient-centered care: Research-based, easily learned techniques for medical interviews that benefit orthopaedic surgeons and their patients. *J Bone Joint Surg Am* 2005;87:652-658.)

managing their patients are summarized in **Table 3**.

Culture is very dynamic and includes many characteristics, such as education, socioeconomic class, sexual orientation, and sex. These characteristics combine and react with the life experiences of an individual to form that person's identity and current cultural perspective.[34,35] It has been argued that culture must be defined and explored in light of these influences to get a true picture of the individual and their perceptions, preferences, and needs.[36] For example, an African-American female cardiac surgeon has life experiences that are multifaceted. To classify her within the boundaries of a stereotypic definition of African-American women would be incomplete. She is African American, female, her socioeconomic class is high, she is well educated, and non–African-American men dominate her medical specialty. Her culture has many influences.

Culture is not only an integrated pattern of learned beliefs and behaviors that can be shared among groups, but it is also thought processes, communication styles, views on roles and relationships, values, practices, customs, and methods of interacting. Many factors, including ethnicity, race, nationality, language, sex, socioeconomic status, physical and mental ability, sexual orientation, and occupation, influence culture. These influences work together to shape values, to help form belief systems, and to motivate the behavior of an individual.[35]

The Culture of Medicine

Using the definition of culture, it can be shown that medicine has attributes and characteristics of a unique, distinct, fluid group with its own language, thought processes, styles of communication, customs, and beliefs; therefore, medicine has its own culture.[34]

The language of medicine is characterized by statistical facts, probability, gradations of severity, and the use of acronyms and medical terminology, which are frequently not understood by people outside the field. It is important to use language that is understood by patients.[34,37]

Medicine has its own way of speaking and its own mannerisms of discussion. For example, physicians often discuss a case rather than a person or a patient. Patients are often considered to be separate from the disease process. When a patient describes his or her symptoms, physicians describe this information as subjective rather than factual. To the patient, however, the information is very factual.[37]

The manner in which physicians conceptualize health (the explanatory model) is another example of the culture of medicine. A physician's explanatory model of a disease process is derived from the perception of its etiology, onset, pathophysiology, course, and treatment—a biomedical model. This model is derived from the medical school curriculum and environment along with interactions with peers and mentors. A patient's explanatory model of disease is obtained from social network experiences and may determine if treatment is sought. A patient's explanatory model of a disease process may be very different from that of the physician. It is, therefore, very important for the physician to understand these differences when planning a course of therapy that is mutually agreeable.[37,38]

Medicine also has its own dress and rituals. The white coat has been the traditional attire associated with medicine. Doctors began wearing white coats in the 19th century and it became a symbol of science and the art of healing. The white coat has been shown to foster confidence and trust in patients. Students entering medical school attend the "white coat ceremony." This ceremony is an example of a cultural ritual of medicine.[37-40]

The culture of medicine lacks ethnic and sex diversity. For example, 80% of orthopaedic surgeons are white males.[41]

Culturally Diverse Patient Populations

Physicians and staff need to be educated regarding certain cultural norms in the diverse populations they serve. Educating medical staff regarding cultural diversity increases the health care provider's own comfort level with diverse populations and increases patient satisfaction and positive outcomes of treatment.[42] When studying traditional cultural values, ideas, and beliefs of the many diverse populations in this nation, it is important to remember that a group of people may share traditional values, beliefs, and behaviors, but they are also influenced by their current environment, socioeconomic status, age, sex, sexual orientation, and level of education. Every man, woman, and child is a unique individual and must be approached as such.

For example, Latinos or Hispanic Americans are a diverse community. Although Spanish is the main language spoken, as in any language, there are many dialects. Among Latino/Hispanic Americans, the family bond is very strong. The decision maker is the male head of the family. Many Hispanic/Latino patients have traditional beliefs about what makes them sick and what can heal them. Negative emotions, natural phenomena, magic, and an imbalance between hot and cold are often believed to be causative factors in disease.[43] Fatalismo, the belief in fate, may also have an important role in attitudes about illness and treatment.[44]

The Muslim community is composed of people who follow the religion of Islam (the second largest religion in the world) and live in at least 184 different countries. Doctors should not shake hands or hug unless such an action is initiated by the Muslim patient. Some Muslim people avoid prolonged eye contact out of respect.[45] Traditionally, the Muslim faith does not allow the ingestion of pork or alcohol, which can be problematic if a medication contains alcohol or is derived from pork, such as porcine heparin. Exceptions are often made for life-saving emergency treatment. It is important for the medical provider to be aware of and sensitive to this issue. While fasting during the month of Ramadan, the Muslim faith technically does not allow the use of intravenous drugs and pharmaceutical agents. Consultation with an imam, a Muslim religious leader in the community, may be needed to allow medications during Ramadan.[45]

Asian American is a term that also includes a wide variety of cultures, ethnic groups, and countries. According to a 2002 estimate from the Census Bureau, more than 13 million Asian people live in the United States. Asians make up 4.5% of the population and are the fastest-growing racial group in America. Saving face is very important in Asian culture. If an Asian patient is asked if he or she understands something, many patients will answer in the affirmative out of respect for the physician. It is better to ask open-ended questions such as, "please explain to me your understanding of this." Asian patients may also hesitate to make eye contact, out of respect for the physician. Asian families may use traditional Asian and herbal remedies before using Western medicine. Physicians need to be aware of potential interactions of prescribed medications with these herbal remedies.[46,47]

Each cultural group has its beliefs, traditions, and values. The AAOS has published a guidebook that contains tip sheets with information regarding different cultures and ethnic groups.[44] This book is a good reference tool and can help increase the cultural competency of orthopaedic surgeons.

Language Divides

How can language be divisive? Studies have shown that patients with limited English proficiency feel less satisfied with their health care, often receive insufficient health education, and have increased problems with medication errors. It has been shown that the children of non–English-speaking families do not receive the same access to health care nor do they receive equal medical and dental care compared to children from English-speaking families.[48]

When translators are available, words may get translated but often subtle nuances or cultural variables can be missed if the translator is not aware of or trained to recognize these factors. The literature refers to these subtle nuances and cultural variables as "the shared meaning" of words. Everyone involved must use words with the same meaning when discussing the care of a patient.

Miscommunication can cause patient dissatisfaction, potential errors, and negative outcomes. People of diverse cultural and language backgrounds require not only an exchange of words but also an exchange of shared meanings, which can be difficult to achieve in a clinical encounter. Effective translators and bilingual office staff members must have the skill to translate words along with the cultural knowledge and the ability to relate subtle cultural nuances in communication.[49]

Language barriers are divisive. Language and/or culture can prevent adequate communication among health care providers and patients, which has been shown to result in patient dissatisfaction and less than desirable outcomes. Even with the help of an interpreter, patients with language barriers require more time for visits with the physician and may require more visits.[50,51] In the absence of a professional interpreter or bilingual physician, decision making may become more cautious, resulting in an increase in diagnostic testing.[52]

Health Disparities

Health disparities are defined as gaps in the quality of health and health care in certain racial, ethnic, and other minority groups.[53] A 1985 study reported that people in racial and ethnic minority groups were dying at a faster rate than the average for the population as a whole.[54] The fatal diseases were curable and controllable. Subsequently, research requested by Congress resulted in the widely read *Unequal Treatment: Confronting Racial and Ethnic Disparities in Health Care* published by the Institute of Medicine.[55] This report documented racial, cultural, and language disparities in health care. The study recommended including cross-cultural education for health care professionals. Health disparities currently are well recognized as a reality in the United States and the world.[56]

Ninety-eight percent of leaders in the health care industry are white. Minorities represent 28% of the US population but represent only 3% of medical school faculties. Minorities make up 16% of public health officials and 17% of city and county health officers. More diversity in health care system leadership would make it easier to teach cultural competency. Minorities also make up a small number of the health care workforce. Patient satisfaction and the perception of the quality of care are greater when patients are treated by health care providers of a similar race or ethnicity.[54]

In the United States, it is now well documented that African Americans, Asian Americans, Latino/Hispanic Americans, and Native Americans have a higher incidence of mortality and chronic disease. These groups have higher rates of cardiovascular disease, human immunodeficiency virus, acquired immunodeficiency virus, and infant mortality.[56] The incidence of cancer among African Americans is 10% higher than that for whites.[57] African Americans and Latino/Hispanic Americans have almost twice the incidence of diabetes.[58] African American and Hispanic women in the United States are underdiagnosed for osteoporosis.[59,60]

Surveys have shown that most Americans, including physicians, do not believe that there are ethnic and racial disparities in health care despite strong evidence to the contrary. A survey published in the 2003 Harvard Forum on Health reported that only 22% of white Americans believed that minorities received lower-quality health care based on race or ethnicity; however, 65% of African Americans and 41% of Hispanics believed that there were racial disparities in health care.[61,62] National studies have consistently found a lower rate of hip and knee joint surgeries for arthritis in older black adults than white adults. Further investigation of this disparity is necessary, but access to medical care may be a factor.[63,64]

Many organizations and academic departments are now including the study of cross-cultural education and health disparities in their mission statements. The Johns Hopkins School of Public Health Primary Care Policy Center for Underserved Populations mission includes: "research, analysis, and education concerning the organization, financing, and mode of delivery for primary care to underserved and vulnerable populations."[65]

The National Medical Association (NMA), which was established in 1895, is the oldest and largest organization in the United States representing the interests of physicians of African descent and their patients. A strategic goal of the NMA is the elimination of health disparities. In 2004, the NMA launched the W. Montague Cobb/NMA Health Institute (Cobb Institute) to focus on the strategic goal of eliminating health disparities.[53]

Cultural Competency

What does it mean to be culturally competent? Such competency starts with an understanding of the communities and cultures of the region served by the physician. It is the knowledge that a person's ethnicity, race, or culture forms an important part of who that person is and a recognition that current environment, educational level, socioeconomic status, sex, sexual orientation, and age also influence how a person thinks and formulates ideas and beliefs.

To provide culturally competent care, physicians must bring to each patient encounter an understanding of varied cultural backgrounds and belief systems and their effect on the perception of health, illness, treatment, and diagnosis.[44] These cultural differences influence a patient's understanding and willingness or preparedness to follow a treatment regimen. A clinician who lacks awareness and understanding of cultural norms can easily evoke mistrust.

Stereotyping can be avoided by considering the patient's cultural background and his or her current social situation. A clinician who assumes that a person has certain cultural norms based solely on his or her race or ethnicity can be stereotyping the patient and thereby creating miscommunication and a sense of unease with the patient. Current social influences must always be a part of the process of understanding the needs of the patient. Physicians must also reflect on their own culture, values, and beliefs that influence their interactions with patients. Respect for the patient's needs, preferences, and sensitivity to nonmedical and spiritual dimensions are also important components of culturally competent care.

Summary

Patient-centered care recognizes and enhances the necessary trust between patients and their doctors and depends on quality communications as well as the assumption that physicians will strive to give equal care to all patients. Communication skills should be taught with the same rigor as other core clinical skills; however, like all skills, communication skills can be retained or lost over time. Current role models in orthopaedic training are not effective in encouraging patient-centered care. Experience alone rarely causes a change in behavior.

Physicians must treat some patients differently to offer them equal treatment. Unconscious stereotypical views regarding race, class, or age tear at the fabric of the unique patient-physician relationship. Culturally competent care requires physicians to be aware, understanding, and inclusive. A physician does not need to know or understand every nuance about every culture because this is impossible. Physicians must bring four things to the physician-patient encounter: a heightened awareness, sensitivity, and curiosity; compassion; communication skills; and an open accepting mind. Physicians must recognize and accept the increased time and cost required to provide equal care for patients of a different culture, ethnicity, or language.

Annotated References

1. Tongue JR, Epps HR, Forese LL: Communication skills for patient-centered care: Research-based, easily learned techniques for medical interviews that benefit orthopaedic surgeons and their patients. *J Bone Joint Surg Am* 2005;87:652-658.

2. Epstein RM, Street RL: Patient-centered communication in cancer care. National Cancer Institute. http://www.outcomes.cancer.gov/areas/pcc/communication/pccm_ch1.pdf. Accessed July 19, 2010.

   The authors present a detailed review of patient-centered care.

3. Lundine K, Buckley R, Hutchison C, Lockyer J: Communication skills training in orthopaedics. *J Bone Joint Surg Am* 2008;90(6):1393-1400.

   Communication skills should be taught with the same rigor as other core clinical skills and can be taught, retained over time, and lost. Current role models are not effective. Experience alone rarely causes a change in behavior.

4. Frymoyer JW, Frymoyer NP: Physician-patient communication: A lost art? *J Am Acad Orthop Surg* 2002; 10(2):95-105.

5. Roter DL, Stewart M, Putnam SM, Lipkin M Jr, Stiles W, Inui TS: Communication patterns of primary care physicians. *JAMA* 1997;277(4):350-356.

6. Clark PA: Return on Investment in Satisfaction Measurement and Improvement: Working Paper from Press Ganey Associates, vol 1, edition 1, August 31, 2005. http://www.pressganey.com/files/roi1.pdf. Accessed February 25, 2010.

7. Braddock C III, Hudak PL, Feldman JJ, Bereknyei S, Frankel RM, Levinson W: "Surgery is certainly one good option": Quality and time-efficiency of informed decision-making in surgery. *J Bone Joint Surg Am* 2008; 90(9):1830-1838.

   Time-efficient strategies for informed surgical decision making include using scenarios to illustrate choices, encouraging patient input, and addressing primary patient concerns. In more than 140 consent interviews, none received perfect scores. The surgeon should prioritize to save time.

8. Sorrel AL: Two state courts, same ruling: Informed consent must include all options. Posted August 24, 2009. Dylan McQuitty vs. Donald Spangler, MD, Maryland Court of Appeals. American Medical News Web site. http://www.ama-assn.org/amednews/2009/08/24/prl20824.htm#s1. Accessed February 25, 2010.

   These court decisions set a high standard for informed consent for all relevant treatment alternatives and risks.

9. Hudak PL, Armstrong K, Braddock C III, Frankel RM, Levinson W: Older patients' unexpressed concerns about orthopaedic surgery. *J Bone Joint Surg Am* 2008; 90(7):1427-1435.

   The Levinson group reviewed the patient audiotapes of 900 Chicago-area orthopaedic surgeons. Patients raised only 50% of their concerns and were more likely to raise concerns during a discussion rather than in response to an inquiry. A patient's limited capacity to meet the demands of surgery may impinge on their willingness to agree to treatment.

10. Kramer D, Ber R, Moore M: Impact of workshop on students' and physicians' rejecting behaviors in patient interviews. *J Med Educ* 1987;62(11):904-910.

11. Jimenez RL, Lewis VO, Frick SL: Residency training programs, in Jimenez RL, Lewis VO, eds: *The AAOS Culturally Competent Care Guidebook.* Rosemont, IL, American Academy of Orthopaedic Surgeons, 2007, pp 7-8.

    Written by orthopaedic surgeons, this guidebook discusses residency training, ethnic and racial patient groups, and issues related to sex and faith.

12. Tongue JR, Jenkins L, Wade A: Low-touch surgeons in a high-touch world. American Academy of Orthopaedic Surgeons Web site. http://www.aaos.org/news/aaosnow/may09/cover1.asp. Accessed February 25, 2010.

    A 10-year tracking study by the AAOS showed the changing image of orthopaedic surgeons, who are now better known and more highly valued by the public. The surgeon's self-image is now more modest; however, interpersonal skills are undervalued by orthopaedic surgeons but rate highly with patients.

13. Levinson W, Roter DL, Mullooly JP, Dull VT, Frankel RM: Physician-patient communication: The relationship with malpractice claims among primary care physicians and surgeons. *JAMA* 1997;277(7):553-559.

14. Fine VK, Therrien ME: Empathy in the doctor-patient relationship: Skill training for medical students. *J Med Educ* 1977;52(9):752-757.

15. Leigh JP, Kravitz RL, Schembri M, Samuels SJ, Mobley S: Physician career satisfaction across specialties. *Arch Intern Med* 2002;162(14):1577-1584.

16. Quick JC, Saleh KJ, Sime WE, et al: Symposium: Stress management skills for strong leadership. Is it worth dying for? *J Bone Joint Surg Am* 2006;88(1):217-225.

17. Beckman HB, Markakis KM, Suchman AL, Frankel RM: The doctor-patient relationship and malpractice: Lessons from plaintiff depositions. *Arch Intern Med* 1994;154(12):1365-1370.

18. Keller VF, Carroll JG: A new model for physician-patient communication. *Patient Educ Couns* 1994;23: 131-140.

19. Tongue JR. Approaching new orthopaedic patients *AAOS Bulletin*. 2003;51(4):31-32.

20. Tongue JR: Communication skills mentoring program: Patient encounter tips. AAOS Web site. http://www3.aaos.org/education/csmp/InitialMedEncounter.cfm. Accessed February 25, 2010.

    The information is presented as an outline of interview tips and pitfalls specific to orthopaedic patient needs.

21. Marvel MK, Epstein RM, Flowers K, Beckman HB: Soliciting the patient's agenda: Have we improved? *JAMA* 1999;281(3):283-287.

22. Wolff JL, Roter DL: Hidden in plain sight: Medical visit companions as a resource for vulnerable older adults. *Arch Intern Med* 2008;168(13):1409-1415.

    Sick patients benefit most when accompanied by companions who record instructions, ask questions, provide information, and explain physician instructions.

23. Keller V, White M: Choices and changes: A new model for influencing patient health behavior. *J Clin Outcomes Manag* 1997;4(6):33-36.

24. Levinson W, Gorawara-Bhat R, Lamb J: A study of patient clues and physician responses in primary care and surgical settings. *JAMA* 2000;284(8):1021-1027.

25. Faden RR, Becker C, Lewis C, Freeman J, Faden AI: Disclosure of information to patients in medical care. *Med Care* 1981;19(7):718-733.

26. Hughes D: Control in medical consultation: Organizing talk in a situation where co-participants have differential competence. *Sociology* 1982;16(3):359-376.

27. Studdert DM, Mello MM, Sage WM, et al: Defensive medicine among high-risk specialist physicians in a volatile malpractice environment. *JAMA* 2005;293(21):2609-2617.

28. 2001 Commonwealth Fund Health Care Quality Survey. The Commonwealth Fund Web site. http://www.commonwealthfund.org/Contents/Surveys/2001/2001-Health-Care-Quality-Survey.aspx. Accessed February 25, 2010.

29. Levin PE, Levin EJ: The experience of an orthopaedic traumatologist when the trauma hits home: Observations and suggestions. *J Bone Joint Surg Am* 2008;90(9): 2026-2036.

    This personal essay explores the psychosocial upheaval that accompanies major physical trauma. The authors report that breakdowns in communication cause misunderstandings and medical errors. The authors also discuss the appropriate role of the orthopaedic trauma surgeon in providing the emotional support and hope necessary for healing.

30. Epps HR, Tongue JR. Communicating adverse outcomes. *AAOS Bulletin*. 2003;51(2):29, 33.

31. Mazor KM, Simon SR, Yood RA, et al: Health plan members' views about disclosure of medical errors. *Ann Intern Med* 2004;140(6):409-418.

32. Wu AW, Cavanaugh TA, McPhee SJ, Lo B, Micco GP: To tell the truth: Ethical and practical issues in disclosing medical mistakes to patients. *J Gen Intern Med* 1997;12(12):770-775.

33. Georgetown University Center for Child and Human Development Web site. National Center for Cultural Competence: Curricula Enhancement Module Series. http://www.nccccurricula.info/glossary.html. Accessed February 25, 2010.

    An online resource for accessing organizations to teach interested parties about cultural competence is presented.

34. Boutin-Foster C, Foster JC, Konopasek L: Viewpoint: Physician, know thyself. The professional culture of medicine as a framework for teaching cultural competence. *Acad Med* 2008;83(1):106-111.

35. Betancourt JR, Green AR, Carrillo JE: Cultural competence in health care: Emerging frameworks and practical approaches. The Commonwealth Fund. October 2002. http://www.commonwealthfund.org/usr_doc/betancourt_culturalcompetence_576.pdf. Accessed February 25, 2010.

36. Green AR, Betancourt JR, Carrillo JE: Integrating social factors into cross-cultural medical education. *Acad Med* 2002;77(3):193-197.

37. The Culture of Medicine. January 5, 2009. Science Daily Web site. http://www.sciencedaily.com/releases/2008/12/081231182014.htm. Accessed August 2, 2009.

    A brief review of a study dealing with the environment of American academic medicine from the perspective of faculty is presented.

38. Lerner EB, Jehle DV, Janicke DM, Moscati RM: Medical communication: Do our patients understand? *Am J Emerg Med* 2000;18(7):764-766.

39. Rehman SU, Nietert PJ, Cope DW, Kilpatrick AO: What to wear today? Effect of doctor's attire on the trust and confidence of patients. *Am J Med* 2005;118(11):1279-1286.

40. Van Der Weyden MB: White coats and the medical profession. *Med J Aust* 2001;174(7):324-325.

41. Jimenez RL: Current activities in orthopaedic culturally competent care education. *J Am Acad Orthop Surg* 2007;15(suppl 1):S76-S79.

    Legislation for culturally competent care has been passed in California and New Jersey, and legislation is pending in Arizona, Illinois, New York, and Texas. The Diversity Advisory Board of the AAOS has advanced the education of diversity for orthopaedic surgeons.

42. National Institute for Children's Health: Improving

1: Principles of Orthopaedics

cultural competency in children's health care. Expanding perspectives. http://www.nichq.org/pdf/NICHQ_CulturalCompetencyFINAL.pdf. Accessed February 25, 2010.

An extensive reference aimed at reducing disparities in health care for children is presented.

43. Weiss B: Caring for Latino patients. *Med Econ* 2004; 81(8):34-40.

44. Jimenez RL, Lewis VO, eds: *Culturally Competent Care Guidebook: Companion to the Cultural Competency Challenge CD-ROM.* Rosemont, IL, American Academy of Orthopaedic Surgeons, 2007.

The guidebook was developed by the AAOS to help educate orthopaedic surgeons on culturally competent care.

45. Pennachio DL: Caring for your Muslim patients: Stereotypes and misunderstandings affect the care of patients from the Middle East and other parts of the Islamic world. *Med Econ* 2005;82(9):46-50.

46. Pennachio DL: Caring for Chinese, Japanese, and Korean patients. *Med Econ* 2004;81(13):54-59.

47. Pennachio DL: Cultural competence: Caring for your Filipino, Southeast Asian and Indian patients. Modern Medicine Web site. October 22, 2004. http://www.modernmedicine.com/modernmedicine/Medical+Practice+Management%3A+Patient+Relations/Cultural-Competence-Caring-for-your-Filipino-South/ArticleStandard/Article/detail/128909. Accessed February 25, 2010.

48. Flores G, Tomany-Korman SC: The language spoken at home and disparities in medical and dental health, access to care, and use of services in US children. *Pediatrics* 2008;121(6):e1703-e1714.

This multivariable analysis of children in non-English primary language households reports specific disparities in medical health and in access and use of medical services.

49. Johnstone MJ, Kanitsaki O: Culture, language, and patient safety: Making the link. *Int J Qual Health Care* 2006;18(5):383-388.

50. Kravitz RL, Helms LJ, Azari R, Antonius D, Melnikow J: Comparing the use of physician time and health care resources among patients speaking English, Spanish, and Russian. *Med Care* 2000;38(7):728-738.

51. Derose KP, Baker DW: Limited English proficiency and Latinos' use of physician services. *Med Care Res Rev* 2000;57(1):76-91.

52. Hampers LC, McNulty JE: Professional interpreters and bilingual physicians in a pediatric emergency department: Effect on resource utilization. *Arch Pediatr Adolesc Med* 2002;156(11):1108-1113.

53. Morgan RC Jr, Davis SJ: Cobb Institute strategies for the elimination of health disparities. *J Am Acad Orthop Surg* 2007;15(suppl 1):S59-S63.

The W. Montague Cobb/NMA Health Institute studies and provides solutions to eliminate health disparities in African Americans and other underserved populations. The Cobb Institute provides information regarding the health of African Americans.

54. Secretary's Task Force on Black and Minority Health: *Report of the Secretary's Task Force on Black and Minority Health.* Washington, DC, US Department of Health and Human Services, 1985.

55. Smedley BD, Stith AY, Nelson AR: *Unequal Treatment: Confronting Racial and Ethnic Disparities in Health Care.* Washington, DC, National Academies Press, 2002.

56. Centers for Disease Control and Prevention: *Disease Burden & Risk Factors.* Washington, DC, Office of Minority Health, 2007.

The CDC has published exhaustive data of deaths and disease rates by religion and ethinc/racial patient groups.

57. National Cancer Institute: Cancer health disparities: A fact sheet. *Benchmarks* 2005;5:2.

58. Centers for Disease Control and Prevention: *National Diabetes Fact Sheet: United States 2005.* Atlanta, GA, Centers for Disease Control and Prevention, 2005.

59. Thomas PA: Racial and ethnic differences in osteoporosis. *J Am Acad Orthop Surg* 2007;15(suppl 1):S26-S30.

In the United States, osteoporosis is underdiagnosed in women in minority racial groups. Disparities exist for diagnosing osteoporosis based on racial and ethnic lines.

60. National Osteoporosis Foundation: *Fast Facts.* Washington, DC, National Osteoporosis Foundation, 2006.

61. Harvard Forums on Health: *Americans Speak Out on Disparities in Health Care.* Boston, MA, Harvard School of Public Health, 2003.

62. Nelson CL: Disparities in orthopaedic surgical intervention. *J Am Acad Orthop Surg* 2007;15(suppl 1):S13-S17.

Research in health care has shown the existence of disparities in orthopaedic care. The disparities in total hip and knee replacement have been the most studied.

63. Dunlop DD, Manheim LM, Song J, et al: Age and racial/ethnic disparities in arthritis-related hip and knee surgeries. *Med Care* 2008;46(2):200-208.

Black adults younger than 65 years self-report similar rates of hip/knee arthritis surgeries, yet national data document lower rates of arthritis-related hip/knee surgeries for older black adults compared with those for white adults age 65 years or older.

64. Manheim LM, Chang RW: Racial disparities in joint replacement use among older adults. *Med Care* 2003; 41(2):288-298.

65. The Johns Hopkins School of Public Health Primary Care Policy Center for Underserved Populations: Mission statement. http://www.jhsph.edu/pcpc/.
    This federally-funded academic program has produced evidence of the importance of primary care, including musculoskeletal conditions.

Chapter 10

Practice Management

Craig R. Mahoney, MD   Stephen P. Makk, MD, MBA

Introduction

The volume of information required to successfully practice orthopaedics in America continues to expand. Diagnostic and therapeutic breakthroughs are reported daily, and those breakthroughs allow orthopaedic surgeons to improve patient care and the quality of life.

More than 60% of orthopaedic surgeons in the United States own their practices. Therefore, they must not only be clinically competent, but must also understand the basic principles required to manage the business aspect of their practice. Given the recent political landscape, the physician must keep informed of issues that will change the economics of health care and affect income. In this ever-changing environment, information addressing practice management is critical in ensuring the success of the physician and the practice itself (**Figure 1**).

The number of orthopaedic surgeons working for hospitals as employees has steadily risen. It is important to study ownership trends in orthopaedics, specifically comparing physician-owned practices with hospital-owned practices and examining the concept of concierge medical practice. The management strategy used by a medical practice is vital to the success of the business, along with practice governance, a topic that is often overlooked. The chapter will also address the advantages and disadvantages of using electronic medical records (EMRs).

Ownership Trends of Orthopaedic Practices

Currently there is a move by nonprofit, community-based hospitals to buy orthopaedic practices and hire orthopaedic surgeons as employees. This trend, however, is not unique to orthopaedics. In 2007 and 2008, approximately 50 large cardiology practices were purchased by nonprofit hospitals. There have also been other large cardiology groups that have entered into close relationships with hospitals, avoiding direct employment but integrating management and sharing of services and revenue using existing models.[1]

Over the past 20 years, hospitals have been active in purchasing primary care practices. These purchases were thought to aid hospitals in supplying themselves with a steady stream of patients through referrals from their employed physicians. By controlling referral patterns through employment of the referring physician, it was thought that hospitals could more efficiently organize the delivery of care and ancillary services. Utilization of inpatient and outpatient services increases with a rise in referrals. Further, it was thought that a larger number of patients being integrated into a health sys-

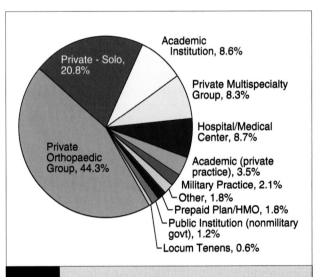

| Figure 1 | Orthopaedic surgeon practice setting. (Reproduced from the American Academy of Orthopaedic Surgeons Research and Scientific Affairs: Orthopaedic Practice in the US 2008. Rosemont, IL, 2008. Http://www3.aaos.org/research/opus/2008CensusMembers.cfm.) |

1: Principles of Orthopaedics

tem would improve negotiating strategies when dealing with managed care payers. In many instances, physicians joined hospitals because of incentives offered by the hospitals (capital expenditures for physician practices, reduced overhead because of economies of scale, and enhanced ability to negotiate with insurers due to size).[2]

Unfortunately, many hospital-owned primary care practices were not successful. In 1997, Coopers and Lybrand, Ltd., reported mean losses for acquired practices of $97,000 per physician per year. Because of this perceived failure, hospital ownership of physician offices has decreased.[3]

Changes in how health care is delivered and recognized financially have increased interest in hospital practice ownership. However, this is now occurring on the subspecialty side. Medicare and private insurance companies are now placing more emphasis on bundling of payments for related services and payment for disease management rather than reimbursing for individual procedures. The Medicare Payment Advisory Commission (MedPAC) is an independent congressional agency established by the Balanced Budget Act of 1997 (P.L. 105-33) to advise the US Congress on issues affecting the Medicare program.[4] MedPAC has proposed merging Part A and Part B of Medicare in a bundled fashion whereby both the hospital payment and professional component would be grouped together when delivering services. The Centers for Medicare and Medicaid Services has piloted this bundling in 28 inpatient cardiac surgery centers.[1]

Hospitals continue to perceive the need to be closely aligned with medical staff, specifically to ensure loyalty, to align incentives when delivering care, and to control costs in delivering care. Recognizing physician effort in a direct employment environment is easier when trying to avoid violation of Stark regulation in a hospital situation. In an effort to enhance employment packages, hospitals have divided revenues from professional services with employed physicians. This process is still under some legal scrutiny, and some nonprofit hospitals have also been challenged because of potential conflicts.[5]

Physicians have been motivated to pursue employment with the hospital for several reasons. Currently, there is great economic uncertainty in the practice of medicine. Incomes in many surgical subspecialties have decreased over the past 5 years. Reimbursement for many services provided by physicians' offices, such as imaging, has decreased.[6] There continues to be a large number of regulations regarding physician self-referral and in-office imaging. Office overhead for many orthopaedic offices has increased steadily, but there has been no consistent increase in fees received through delivery of services. The threat of further increases in overhead exists because of implementation of newer technology, such as the EMR, and compliance with governmental and private insurance quality initiatives.

Physician-Owned Medical Practice

When considering hospital employment, several different issues need to be considered. Maintaining a level of autonomy and control of his or her practice is important to many orthopaedic surgeons. Regardless of the location or scope of a particular practice, there will need to be involvement with a hospital in most instances. When the physician owns his or her practice, he or she can determine the level of involvement with the hospital and the extent to which patients are committed to using the services provided by the hospital. As an employee of a hospital there may be contractual obligations that encourage patients to use a particular hospital, a practice that can alienate patients from physicians.

Maintaining financial independence offers huge advantages for most independent orthopaedic groups. There have been changes in the tax law recently that have motivated practices to reevaluate their ownership structure in response to those tax law changes.[7] It is also easier to maintain a level of transparency in an orthopaedic practice when it is not involved with a hospital. Nonprofit hospitals purchasing orthopaedic practices are large organizations with many layers of bureaucracy. Obtaining accurate and up-to-date financial records and benchmarking production levels with income is much easier in a physician-owned practice than a hospital-owned practice. Maintaining ancillary income is also an advantage for the physician-owned practice. Because of declining reimbursement for many procedures, passive income sources continue to be stressed in most practices. Passive income sources and ancillary income sources include ownership in ambulatory surgery centers, employing physician extenders such as physician assistants and nurse practitioners, ownership of imaging modalities, durable medical equipment, and ownership of physical therapy and occupational therapy services. Many orthopaedic practices remain profitable because of the existence of these passive income sources. Ownership in surgery centers has been reported to generate close to $170,000 per physician, ownership in MRI up to $66,000 per physician, ownership in physical therapy or occupational therapy services up to $67,000, and durable medical equipment can generate up to $25,000.[8]

There are many inherent risks to private ownership. An owner employs many people to assist in the delivery of care. Management of those employees is vital to the success of the practice. As the size of the group expands, there is increased need to hire managers to appropriately guide employees. These layers of management increase overhead costs for physicians without a direct return on investment. Further, the cost of employing managers, nurses, and radiology technicians continues to outpace increases in reimbursement seen for procedures.

Although there are many opportunities to earn money through ancillary sources, current proposed legislation could place this opportunity at risk. HR 2962 is the Integrity in Medicare Advanced Diagnostic Imaging Act of 2009. The bill would close the in-office ancillary service exemption for MRI, CT and positron-emission tomography currently allowed under the Stark self-referral law and end the practice of self-referral for those modalities under Medicare.[9] If this legislation were to pass, then the income provided by those ancillary services would be eliminated.

Hospital Employment

In many instances, medical practices and orthopaedic practices consider selling to a hospital because of the great economic uncertainty of the current environment. Some practices have seen their incomes fall over the past 5 to 10 years, in part because of increasing overhead and decreasing fees received for services provided. There is a threat that with the implementation of EMRs and further compliance issues, practice expenses could rapidly increase in the near future, adding to the stress of running an orthopaedic office. Orthopaedic surgeons also list lifestyle concerns as a primary reason for making a transition to a hospital practice. Most think that a hospital-based practice would decrease the administrative duties required by physicians.[8]

The relationship that exists between the hospital and the physician is critical to successful employment, and this includes the ability for both parties to fairly negotiate contracts. The contracts drafted would need to clearly outline work expectations and the salary that will be paid if those expectations are met. Further, a bonus structure will need to be outlined for physicians who are motivated to do "extra work." On-call requirements and pay for call will also need to be outlined in initial contract negotiation. Despite the perception that administrative issues may lessen in a hospital-based practice, there will certainly be administrative responsibilities and staff support issues that continue to arise regardless of practice setting. Clear delineation of these administrative responsibilities and financial recognition for fulfilling those responsibilities also need to be included in the contract. Benefit packages and support for continuing medical education (CME) also need to be clearly delineated in any hospital-based practice situation.

There are many risks associated with being employed by a hospital; the first and most important issue is loss of autonomy and control. Any physician who moves into a hospital-based situation will be moving into an employee/employer relationship. With this relationship comes a decrease in leverage/bargaining power for the physician. In a hospital with other subspecialty employees, there's a possibility that the orthopaedic surgeon could be "subsidizing" physicians who do not produce similar revenue. Currently, orthopaedics is an integral part of most hospitals' income streams, and yet the number of orthopaedic surgeons who are required to create this income stream are far outnumbered by the rest of the medical staff. There is risk that the orthopaedic surgeons could be marginalized by the medical staff. As an employee, the orthopaedic surgeon would need to be comfortable with the hospital form of management and with having a limited view of all things financial. Most hospitals are large organizations that cannot act as quickly as smaller physician organizations.

The Internal Revenue Service has looked closely at nonprofit hospitals and their benefit to the community. Specifically, the tax-exempt status and executive compensation practices have been scrutinized. This is an important consideration for physicians who are considering hospital employment, as the tax-exempt status of the hospital allows greater latitude in subsidizing employee-physician salaries. Without this exemption, a theoretic reduction in physician salaries in employed situations could occur.[10]

Other Options

One possible hybrid employment option available to physicians involves contracting with a hospital to provide orthopaedic care while maintaining physician ownership of the medical practice. This scenario could exist under many forms, with the most common being a management services agreement.

A management services agreement is a business agreement that outlines services provided by a physician group, and then that group is paid directly by the hospital. This would be similar to using consultants or outside managers in private business where those personnel are not employees of a business, but rather work for a business for a given amount of time with a well-defined reimbursement schedule. Businesses can experience cost savings when using consultants in a way that decreases the number of full-time employees that they use. Expenses for recruitment benefits and bonuses can be theoretically bypassed in a management services agreement.

Hospitals are also exposed to these expenses and would be in a situation where physicians are hired to work at the hospital as an employee. By contracting with the physician group for specific medical services or service lines, there would be a theoretic reduction in cost. Other advantages would include defining the length of the contract rather than creating an employment agreement between the hospital and the physician. This would allow the contract to be reworked on a periodic basis and avoid the process of hiring and firing.

From a physician standpoint, working under a management services agreement is attractive. Physicians can negotiate on the front end with the hospital regarding the amount of work they provide and the reimbursement per work unit used (relative value units could be used as quantification for work in many instances). This process would allow the physician to skip the process of billing and submitting claims and would decrease the physician's overhead by decreasing the need for billing and coding staff.

Another benefit to physicians would be negotiating a base salary that would be paid on a monthly or quarterly basis. This guarantee would allow a consistent in-

1: Principles of Orthopaedics

come for the physician and also create an alliance between the hospital and the physician group. Both entities would have the same incentive to recruit patients to be served by the physicians under the management services agreement. The hospital could use this as leverage for the physician group when discussing referrals with other employed or engaged physician groups, such as a primary care. As a part of a management services agreement, clinical comanagement agreements could be drafted. Physicians and hospitals have been asked by the Centers for Medicare and Medicaid Services to launch focused quality initiatives. A clinical comanagement agreement could be a model used for integration of hospital services. In the arrangement, physicians will provide management of medical services with the hospital at a level that would exceed conventional medical director agreements. These arrangements typically occur between an organized group of physicians and a health care system. The physicians are then empowered to improve care, making a specific service line competitive in a targeted market but are also recognized financially for their efforts. The physicians would be charged with day-to-day management of hospital processes. It can benefit the hospital by engaging physicians in direct participation in design and oversight of a specific service line but also in capital and operating budgets. Physicians can also be engaged in assisting quality initiatives by setting up audit programs monitoring outcomes.

A clinical comanagement arrangement can compensate physicians either on an hourly or annual basis with bonuses based on performance, clinical outcomes, patient satisfaction, or improved operating efficiencies. Compensation can also be awarded based on a predetermined, negotiated sum regardless of method of payment. Both parties are well served under the clinical comanagement model.

Finally, physician groups can also pursue affiliations with hospitals through outpatient joint ventures. This involves capital investment on behalf of both the hospital and the physician group. This again aligns the hospital and the physician group in increasing the likelihood of success of the specific venture.

Regardless of who owns a practice, physicians need to maintain a very active role in the management and direction of whatever practice situation they choose. Physicians who do not stay involved risk losing autonomy and the ability to direct the group in ways they deem appropriate.

Concierge Medicine

Concierge medicine is a term used to describe a personal relationship that a physician has with a patient, whereby the patient pays a retainer or an annual fee to maintain the relationship with the physician. Most concierge medicine relationships involve an enhanced form of care for the patient.

Because of the personal attention provided by the physician and the extra time physicians take in admin-

istering care, concierge medical practices often maintain a smaller number of patients in comparison with a conventional physician practice. The annual fees required vary widely based on the type of medicine practiced, the geographic region, and the exclusivity of the services being provided to the individual. More exclusive relationships have required up to $25,000 per year from a family to a specific physician.[11]

The fee does not substitute for insurance and does not cover patients for consultations that would fall outside of the typical scope of the practice engaged. This means that outside of the care provided by the concierge medical specialists, and the access provided by the relationship, insurance typically is still purchased by the involved patients to cover medical costs that fall outside of the concierge's relationship. This includes further laboratory procedures, medications, hospitalizations, and emergency care from other providers.

Dr. Howard Maron is thought to be the first physician to offer concierge medicine as formal practice. He initially founded a company called MD^2 International in 1996. His company currently charges patients up to $20,000 per year for exclusive primary care services. He reports that he has fewer than 100 patients in his practice and in an average day may be required to see only one or two patients. Prior to moving to a concierge situation, his patient roster numbered greater than 4,000. Many physicians employed in concierge situations are able to increase their yearly salary and also spend more time on their patients. One physician practicing in Boca Raton, FL, stated, "It's allowed me to focus on being a doctor again."[12]

Reported advantages include spending more time with each patient and having the time to research each individual complaint that a patient brings to the physician. Physicians also report less stress regarding financial concerns due to declining reimbursements. Many physicians report increased patient compliance and better outcomes when their concierge patients are compared with those in a more conventional practice.

Orthopaedic applications in a concierge medicine situation could include a conventional model, which would provide exclusive orthopaedic care for an individual or an individual's family. This is not attractive to most patients, though, because of the limited frequency with which most visit the orthopaedic surgeon.

Another possibility would include increased patient access and timeliness of that access with a physician or group in return for an upfront annual retainer fee. This retainer would ensure that the patients would receive timely consultations with physicians of their choice. Other services that could be provided would include orthopaedic screening, house calls, or even emergency department visits in some situations. The concept of access is important to consider. The average age of the United States population is rising, and that population will require more orthopaedic care. There is a relatively static number of US orthopaedic surgeons, so providing care when the patient requests it may hold real value.[13] Assuring access in an environment of scarcity may ultimately be the key when the concept of concierge medicine is considered.

Concerns with concierge medicine include abandonment of existing patients, care for indigent or uninsured patients, and the perception that only the rich could afford this type of care. The current economic and political climate also does not easily lend itself to a concierge situation.

A more likely scenario in the field of orthopaedics would be up-front guarantees for patients to ensure access to their orthopaedic surgeon of choice. Current legislation regarding health care reform will in all likelihood determine future directions for concierge medicine.

Governance

One of the most critical aspects of running a successful medical practice or business involves setting up a successful management structure. Many practices do not have a formal outline of their management practices but rather settle into a method of governance based on past history or ease of administration.

Successful forms of management in a medical practice have key characteristics in common.[14] First, forms of governance within a practice need to allow the practice principals or shareholders to make decisions on major issues impacting the business. There has to be shared acceptance of responsibility by the principals in a group for the decisions they make. If no one in the group is ultimately held accountable for the decisions, then key decision makers would never be rewarded for good decisions and bad decision makers would never be educated. Shareholders need adequate clerical and administrative support provided by their staff to run day-to-day activities so the shareholders can focus on the major issues impacting the business. If the shareholders are required to address day-to-day activities that would otherwise keep them from efficiently and effectively seeing patients, then the income stream of the medical practice may suffer. Efficient and cost-effective support provided by clerical and administrative staff is key in the overall management of a medical practice.

A commonly overlooked characteristic of a successful practice is having a well-thought-out mission statement.[14] A mission statement should define the services that are provided by the group and the geographic region where those services are provided. It should also address why those services are being provided in a specific geographic region and when the services are available. If the mission statement is not given the attention that it deserves, it will be poorly done and not beneficial to the practice.

Medical practices need legal agreements that document practice structure. Articles of Incorporation or Ownership, such as exist with S Corps, C Corps, partnerships, and LLCs, need to be documented and easily accessible for the group. Along with those documents, bylaws of the group are also critical to maintain. This would include documents outlining buying into a practice and exiting a practice, employment contracts, and standards of care and professionalism. Effective forms of governance provide a framework for good professional relations between practice principals and support staff. Behavior of the principals needs to be assessed and monitored, and standards need to be placed on this behavior. Well-outlined standards allow the principals themselves to assess their own behavior and set or modify standards as appropriate. A standard for work quality also needs to be outlined, specifically regarding patient care. From a quality standpoint, the group is benefitted not only by the improved outcomes but also by having a quality assurance program in place. When obtaining professional liability insurance, a quality assurance process often is necessary and in some instances can lower rates.

Work expectations such as time off, on-call responsibilities, and day-to-day responsibilities need to be documented and well outlined, especially within a larger group. Including the shareholders in the formulation of these work expectations engenders a sense of ownership from the members of the group, and also decreases the risk of having a disgruntled member failing to uphold his or her end of the bargain when it comes to work effort. Organizational structure needs to be formally defined, providing all the employees with a role and a template defining who they report to and who they are responsible for.

Finally, the way that the group financially rewards work needs to be well defined and easy to follow for the owners and employees of the group. Compensation formulas need to recognize not only work effort but also the ability to gather revenue. Compensation formulas may need to be modified on a periodic basis; however, it is imperative that all the partners are included in the process of computing the compensation formula.

Work plans outline pathways to achieve short- and long-term goals, and should be updated on at least an annual basis to reflect the mission of the group but also reflect the individual needs of group members. A lack of planning can contribute to financial instability, high turnover, and high levels of dissatisfaction. The plan should address the description and intensity of the services that will be provided by the group, the supporting activities involved in maintaining those services, any marketing initiatives that will be instituted to support the group, the anticipated staffing requirements to support the group, planning in terms of physical facility, and investments in practice infrastructure.

A good governance strategy is important to medical groups in several different ways. Consistent management strategies will improve efficiency, allowing workers to maximize their potential. This improved efficiency will often translate into increased revenues and/or decreased expenses. In the event of an audit, a consistent, well-documented governance system will allow information to be easily obtained by an outside auditing firm. More favorable audits typically will result in lower penalties in the event of a problem being discovered.

Consistent, well-planned governance can also lower the group's risk of litigation. Intraoffice relationships between personnel and physicians are always well-defined within a well-run group. People who understand and accept their roles are happier in their jobs, and happy employees and partners would be less apt to sue based on personnel decisions. A satisfied workforce also relates better to customers. Patients and payers who sense a satisfied workforce will likely have a better interaction during their exposure to the group and are less likely to sue.

When examining the organizational structure of a group, there are signs of organizational dysfunction to look for. Inability to obtain or out-of-date corporate documents often signal a lack of organizational control within a group. Physician contract disputes may indicate a dysfunctional organizational structure. Employees in a dysfunctional organization can exhibit a disdain for authority. Principals of the group may exhibit inappropriate, selfish behavior or act in a unilateral fashion while not risking their personal position within the group. Many times, selfish or inappropriate behavior may involve the management of money. Many times the shareholders themselves will exhibit selfish behavior, specifically as it relates to money. In addition, principals of the group may commonly exhibit inappropriate behavior, and are sometimes disrespectful toward staff. They may actively act in a unilateral fashion and will not risk their personal position in the group to stop illegal or immoral behavior.

Strategies to improve governance within a group include engaging the support of the practice administrator. Many of the issues determining successful governance need the full support of the administrator. The administrator has a very large stake in this and is critical to the development and success of a governance strategy.

Principals within the group need to be educated regarding the importance of governance. Unless there is buy-in to a governance strategy, it is doomed to fail. One way to educate partners is to discuss governance-related issues at business meetings and continue to update members when changes occur in governance strategies. Meetings need to be held at least on an annual basis and effectively run. Protocols should be established to manage disagreements that may arise and should be followed when other techniques of conflict resolution fail.

Corporate documents should be reviewed annually to make sure they remain relevant. Changes to these documents need to be recommended after their review. If specific documents that have been mentioned above do not exist, then they need to be created, and the principals of the group should be engaged in this process.

It is important to remember that governance does not happen on its own. It is a learned behavior that will not improve overnight. When good governance is absent, there will be resistance to change, but over time, most principals will realize the benefits of having a stable governance strategy in place.

Electronic Medical Records

As of 2009, EMRs are at the forefront of medicine. Currently less than 10% of orthopaedic practices use a full EMR technology or technologies; however, the current US government's proposed stimulus package offers up to $44,000 per physician (up to $65,000 in some underserved areas) to be used to adopt EMRs with a national standard. Costs for EMR adoption have been estimated to be $44,000 per physician, with $8,500 for annual maintenance. There are annual hardware costs and also interest costs to consider if these systems are financed.[15] The thought is that EMRs can create efficiencies and savings in medicine as well as high-quality recordkeeping and the avoidance of errors.[8] It is difficult to measure the return on investment in smaller to medium-sized practices, especially when considering the cost of these systems and the verification of real or perceived quality improvement. Nonetheless, most agree that using EMRs will change future practice patterns. It should be noted that there are challenges in adopting EMRs and that failure rates exist.

A full EMR helps document pertinent patient demographic data, the patient encounter, and the physician's actions so that he or she gets paid. Advantages of a full EMR include the establishment of a database that uses medical terms for storing medical records, laboratory and imaging results, findings, and treatment actions. Additionally, a properly implemented EMR can facilitate patient interaction and speed office work flow in comparison with traditional paper charts. Ultimately, it is hoped that the EMR will decrease practice operating costs (overhead), including those associated with paper charts, issues with evaluation and management coding compliance, real-time notes, and transcription. Disadvantages include implementation and a learning curve, procedural changes that affect office work flow, and high start-up costs.

EMR implementation challenges involve creating templates, installing and maintaining workstations, and changing physician behavior pertaining to the entry of clinical information. Clinical information can be input by "point and click," which is the preferred route by surgeons; voice recognition; keyboarding; and scanning.

Work flow requires new processes and physician and staff training, and the dynamic of the physician/patient encounter is changed. It is important to have physician leaders in this regard in order to obtain successful results. EMRs interface with other technologies, including billing systems and picture archiving and communication systems.

The US government currently is developing the Health Information Technology for Economic and Clinical Health (HITECH) Act, better known as part of the stimulus package of President Obama's administration. Final regulations are forthcoming. Terms that need to be defined in this Act include "meaningful use" and "reporting requirements." Implementation of the EMR mandate will begin in 2011, with $18 billion earmarked for funding. Funds are to be paid over 5 years. The take-home message is that the physician has time to do his or her homework and evaluate how to best implement these developments in his or her practice. Other considerations would be whether or not the physician has a current EMR. If so, it may not meet the certification requirements, which are yet to be defined.

As for EMR standards, few systems have orthopaedic-specific modules or templates, although some exist. There is also no defined set of requirements for an orthopaedic practice or for EMR system service. Defined training programs are lacking, although these are likely to arise in the next several years. Current concerns and also part of the HITECH Act are that there is interoperability between EMR systems. The current Health Level-7 standards are generally met by most EMRs; however, there is little or no interoperability between systems. Stimulus legislation required for formal certification, currently a certifying body, the Certification Commission for Healthcare Information Technology, deals with interoperability, date of security, privacy, and compliance in prescribing health information networks and ambulatory and hospital EMRs.

Failure rates are a concern; learning and adoption curves are not underestimated. Challenges include the integrity of the clinical information, usability, quality of care, and work flow guided by the record and malpractice protection, sometimes with a lack of complete documentation. All information needs to be checked for evaluation management compliance.

The Practice Management Committee created in February 2007 "The Electronic Medical Record: A Primer for Orthopaedic Surgeons." This document is free to members and can be accessed at www.aaos.org. The document explains the economics of EMRs, lessons learned, standards, data file security, and the political landscape.

Summary

The technical aspects of running an orthopaedic practice continue to become increasingly more complex. Remaining informed and engaged is key to making decisions that benefit the individual and the practice. Questions regarding practice ownership will continue to be discussed in the foreseeable future. Although there may be some short-term benefits related to hospital ownership, surgeons need to be cognizant of the loss of autonomy this situation brings. As health care reform evolves, new business relationships between doctors and hospitals will also develop. The successful business will be one that can maintain income streams while limiting overhead growth.

Concierge medicine allows the orthopaedic practice an opportunity to continue to provide care to everyone in addition to a level of care that is perceived as enhanced by some. A guarantee of prompt, efficient, and patient-centered service may allow surgeons to market themselves to patients outside of the current practice model. Governance will continue to be important in the

management of the successful practice. Having a successful business is difficult, and organized, well-documented governance will put orthopaedic surgeons in the best position to succeed.

Annotated References

1. Wann S: Nonprofit hospitals buying up cardiology practices. *Cardiology Today*. http://www.cardiologytoday.com/view.aspx?rid=33243. Published December 1, 2008. Accessed August, 29 2009.

   The author discusses the relationship between cardiology groups and nonprofit hospitals. Specifically, the risks and benefits of hospital ownership are outlined.

2. Boblitz MC, Thompson JM: 7 steps for evaluating primary care practice ownership: Burned by physician practice ownership in the past? Chances are your strategy was ill-fated from the start. BNET. http://findarticles.com/p/articles/mi_m3257/is_11_58/ai_n7069413/. Published November 2004. Accessed August 29, 2009.

   The authors examine practice ownership from the hospital perspective. A seven-step approach is offered to analyze primary practice ownership.

3. Bakhtiari E: Facilities learn from physician management and compensation mistakes. *HealthLeaders Media*. http://www.healthleadersmedia.com/content/92849/topic/WS_HLM2_HOM/Facilities-learn-from-physician-management-and-compensation-mistakes.html. Published October 4, 2007. Accessed August 29, 2009.

   The author outlines the risks and benefits of physician hospital employment.

4. About MedPAC. *MedPAC*. http://www.medpac.gov/about.cfm. Accessed August 29, 2009.

   The Medicare Payment Advisory Commission (MedPAC) is a congressional agency established by the Balanced Budget Act of 1997 (P.L. 105-33) that advises Congress on issues affecting Medicare.

5. Leys T: Waterloo hospital pays feds $4.5 million. *Des Moines Register*. http://www.desmoinesregister.com/apps/pbcs.dll/article?AID=2009908260358. Published August 26, 2009. Accessed August 30, 2009.

   The author reports on a hospital being fined by the US attorney's office for reportedly overpaying physicians in an alleged scheme to boost its business.

6. Ross JR: Radiology practices fight declining technical revenues. http://www.imagingbiz.com/articles/view/radiology-practices-fight-declining-technical-revenues/. Published February 15, 2010. Accessed August 19, 2010.

   This article outlines declining technical revenues for radiology procedures.

CHI: brain loses ability to autoregulate BF in areas of _____ also requires ↑ amt. of glucose → BF-metabolism mismatch → highly susceptible to ischemic injury, esp (if ↓) 12-24 hrs. intraop hypotension ↑ risk of ↑↑ ARDS → brain injury

7. 5-Year Carryback of 2008 and 2009 Net Operating Losses (NOLs) for Eligible Small Businesses. http://www.irs.gov/formspubs/article/0,,id=207330,00.html. Accessed August 19, 2010.

   This Web site describes two laws that can affect businesses with net operating losses.

8. American Association of Orthopaedic Executives (AAOE): 2008 Orthopaedic Benchmark Survey, 2009.

   A survey comparing financial information from multiple orthopaedic practices is presented.

9. ACR Action Alert: Congressmen Anthony Weiner (D-NY) and Bruce Braley (D-IA) to Offer Self-Referral Amendment to House Health Care Reform Package. *RadRounds* http://www.radrounds.com/profiles/blogs/acr-action-alert-congressmen. Published July 20, 2009. Accessed August 29, 2009.

   This radiology Web site encourages congressional support of HR 2962, a bill designed to close in-office ancillary service exemptions for MRI, CT and positron emission tomography.

10. Internal Revenue Service. http://www.irs.gov/pub/irs-tege/execsum_hospprojrept.pdf.

    An IRS study of nonprofit hospitals was conducted for the IRS and other stakeholders to better understand nonprofit hospitals and their community benefit and executive compensation practices.

11. Sack K: Despite Recession, Personalized Health Care Remains in Demand. *New York Times*. http://www.nytimes.com/2009/05/11/health/policy/11concierge.html. Published May 10, 2009. Accessed August 30, 2009.

    The author describes concierge medicine and its appeal despite the recent downturn in the economy.

12. O'Shaughnessy P: Michael Jackson's death puts 'concierge doctors' in the spotlight. *NY Daily News*. http://www.nydailynews.com/entertainment/michael_jackson/2009/07/05/2009-07-05_concierge_doctors_for_the_rich__famous.html#ixzz0Le1XQWMl). Published July 5, 2009. Accessed August 30, 2009.

    The author outlines the risks associated with the practice of concierge medicine.

13. Medscape. http://www.medscape.com/viewarticle/588854. Accessed August 30, 2010.

    This article outlines anticipated shortages in the orthopaedic workforce.

14. Fisher SE: Six steps to effective group practice governance. http://www2.aaos.org/aaos/archives/bulletin/aug05/fline9.asp. Accessed August 19, 2010.

    The development of effective governance is discussed.

15. Miller RH, West C, Brown TM, Sim I, Ganchoff C: The value of electronic health records in solo or small group practices. *Health Aff (Millwood)* 2005;24(5):1127-1137.

ARDS

1. Definition & Pathogenesis
   - inflamm. of pulm. parenchyma → cytokines & fluid extravasation → PMN & lymphocytes also extravasate → leaky capillaries...
   - ptns. extravasate too, around alveoli, form hyaline membranes within alveolar walls, causing diffuse alveolar disease...
   - impaired gas exchange & collapse of alveoli → hypoxemia

2. Diagnostic Criteria
   1) Acute onset
   2) CXR: diffuse Ⓑ patchy infiltrates (v. pulm. edema: homogenous)
   3) ratio $\frac{PaO_2}{FiO_2} < 200$

   PaO_2 = partial P. of arterial O_2 (60-100 = good)

   FiO_2 = fraction of inspired O_2; % of O_2 participating in gas exchange

   $\frac{PaO_2}{FiO_2}$ → demonstrates how well lungs are fxning to deliver inspired O_2 to blood → the lower the ratio the less inspired O_2 getting to blood

   ratio < 300 = acute lung injury
   < 200 = ARDS
   300-500 = normal

3. Causes
   1) sepsis
   2) polytrauma
   3) aspiration
   4) large vol. resuscitation
   * mortality rate ~50-60%

4. Treatment
   - mechanical ventilation in ICU
   - 60% pts. have nosocomial PNA assoc. c̄ ARDS → ABx
   - ARDSnet: improved mortality when vent. @ TV 6 mL/kg (v. 12)
   - IVF: diuresis helps ↓ pulm. fxn
   * ARDS can lead to MODS → ± fatal

Chapter 11

Polytrauma Care

Hans-Christoph Pape, MD, FACS   Philipp Lichte, MD

1: Principles of Orthopaedics

Handwritten margin notes (top):
younger trauma pts:
1. cap refill
2. UOP
3. pH, base excess, lactate
→ pulse & BP are late signs

Initial Assessment

In patients with severe injuries, fatal outcome continues to be a major concern.[1] The trimodal pattern of death described by Trunkey is a valuable tool to assess the treatable conditions. Death occurring within the first hours after trauma is usually due to severe hemorrhage or head trauma. In patients who succumb within several hours, death is usually a result of airway, breathing, or cardiovascular issues and has been identified to be potentially preventable. The third mortality peak is caused by sepsis and multisystem organ failure and appears more than 1 week after trauma.

Polytrauma may be defined as injuries to at least two organ systems associated with a potentially life-threatening condition. To quantify the severity of multiple injuries, several trauma scores have been described. The most common ones are the Injury Severity Score (ISS) and the New Injury Severity score, both of which are based on the Abbreviated Injury Scale (AIS). Injuries of six body regions (head, face, chest, abdomen, extremities [including pelvis], and external structures) are classified from 1 (mild) to 6 (usually fatal).[2] Based on the ISS, a polytrauma is considered if the ISS exceeds 16 points. To achieve reliable data, clinical and radiologic assessment should be completed. During the ongoing process of achieving reliable patient information, the clinical scenario can change. Hemorrhage can become more severe, or improvement can be achieved by volume therapy. In addition to the extent of the anatomic injuries, assessment of the pulmonary and hemodynamic status is required as described in the Advanced Trauma Life Support (ATLS) algorithm. ATLS requires ruling out other causes of acute decompensation such as tension pneumothorax, cardiac tamponade, and herniation.

Hemorrhagic Shock, Volume Treatment, and Fracture Care

From the orthopaedic point of view it is understood that early fracture stabilization is a major goal. Prior to clearing a patient for an orthopaedic procedure, severe

hemorrhage should be identified and controlled. Ongoing hemorrhagic shock has to be ruled out, and it is important to recognize that alterations in pulse and blood pressure are late signs, especially among patients younger than 40 years. Due to the cardiovascular reserve of younger patients, the extent of hypovolemia can be underestimated in adolescents and young adults. In these patients, capillary refill is a valid clinical parameter. Another secondary parameter is urine output, along with arterial pH, base excess, and plasma lactate levels. The plasma lactate levels may serve for assessment of the end points of volume therapy. The four major sources of bleeding are usually external, thoracic, abdominal, and pelvic.

Handwritten margin note (right): use these parameters in younger pts.

External blood loss is usually apparent. The exact quantity of blood loss may be difficult to assess, especially in cases of prolonged extrication. Initial treatment before rushing the patient to the operating room may be the use of a compressing towel or a tourniquet. Internal sources of hemorrhage can be identified by clinical examination, abdominal ultrasound, or CT scan. Unstable pelvic fractures can also be a source of massive hemorrhage, requiring acute external tamponade by pelvic sheets or binders, or internal tamponade during surgery. Some centers apply an external fixator or a pelvic clamp. Selective angiography and embolization of the source of bleeding is becoming more common.

Handwritten margin note (right): lactate levels indicative of vol. status & perfusion

Principles of Stabilizing the Cardiovascular Status of a Multiply Injured Patient

Volume therapy should be administered using several large-bore intravenous lines. Although some controversy remains, crystalloid fluids are widely used. The use of hypertonic saline for small-bolus infusions seems to be beneficial for those with intracranial injuries but not for polytraumatized patients without brain injury. In severe hemorrhage, replacement of red blood cells is necessary to improve oxygen-carrying capacity. If there is no improvement with volume treatment, other causes such as pneumothorax should be considered and the indications for chest drains should be evaluated.

Recent data confirm that concentrated amounts of hemoglobin, 5 g/L, may be acceptable for normovolemic volunteers. In trauma patients, concentrations between 7 and 9 g/L appear to be sufficient. Dilution effects and depletion of components of the coagulation cascades represent one aspect of posttraumatic coagulopathy. Hypothermia and acidosis can cause further

CHI: brain loses ability to autoregulate BF in areas of injury but also requires ↑ amts. of glucose → BF-metabolism mismatch → highly susceptible to ischemic injury esp. in first 12-24 hrs.; intraop hypotension is risk factor for 2° brain injury,: don't fix fx until cerebral perfusion is OK

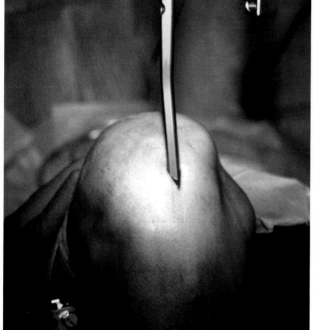

Figure 1 Approach for ipsilateral femur and tibia fractures, treated by initial retrograde femoral and antegrade tibial nailing in a stable patient.

Table 1

Criteria to Diagnose a Borderline Condition
ie. patients at risk

ISS > 40

Body temperature below 95°F = hypothermia

Multiple injuries (ISS > 20) in combination with thorax trauma

Multiple injuries in combination with severe abdominal or pelvic injury and hemorrhagic shock on admission — initial SBP < 90

Radiographic evidence of pulmonary contusion

Bilateral femur fractures

Moderate or severe head trauma in addition to other major fractures *(above)*

(Adapted with permission from Pape HC, Giannoudis P, Krettek C. The timing of fracture treatment in polytrauma patients: Relevance of damage control orthopaedic surgery. Am J Surg 2002;183:622-629.)

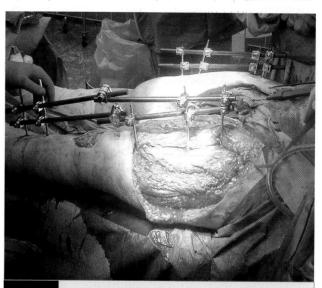

Figure 2 Extremity of an unstable patient with bilateral open femur fractures, liver laceration, and lung contusions. The external fixator is placed anteriorly to allow treatment in the rotatory bed (RotoRest, Kinetic Concepts, San Antonio, TX).

deterioration and should be avoided or corrected in a timely fashion. Replacement of blood products and alternate strategies such as recombinant factor VII in selected cases may be of value.

Grading of the Patient Condition

Completion of the initial assessment implies the diagnosis of major fractures and the cardiovascular, pulmonary, and inflammatory status as a decision guide for surgical therapy. Four categories have been identified: stable, borderline, unstable, and in extremis.[3]

1 — **Stable Condition** → early total care c̄ definitive fx fixation
Stable patients have no immediate life-threatening injuries, respond to initial interventions, and are hemodynamically stable. They are normothermic and show no physiologic abnormalities. These patients should undergo initial surgical fixation of their major fractures[4] (**Figure 1**).

2 — **Borderline Condition** → ETC v. DCO
Patients in this category respond to resuscitation but may have a delayed response to resuscitation and can have other sources of occult bleeding.[5] The criteria listed in **Table 1** have proved useful to classify a patient as borderline. In these patients, a higher possibility of deterioration of the patient's condition has to be considered. If these patients are stabilized appropriately, early definitive care can be used safely in the treatment of their major fractures.[6] In case of deterioration, conversion to damage-control techniques should be considered. Some authors consider damage-control nailing to

minimize the duration of initial surgery. In these cases, an unreamed, unlocked nail is used initially and locking and/or further reduction is performed secondarily.

3 — **Unstable Condition** → ETC v. DCO
If patients do not respond to initial resuscitation and remain hemodynamically unstable, a rapid deterioration in the patient's condition can occur. Surgical treatment consists of lifesaving surgery followed by temporary stabilization of major fractures[7] (**Figure 2**). The patient should then be monitored in the intensive care unit. Complex reconstruction procedures should be postponed several days until the patient is stable and the acute immunoinflammatory response has subsided.

2&3 — borderline & unstable → after resuscitation, stable? meeting endpoints? of lactate, UOP, BP, oxygenation, temp, coags → if so, early total care, but if not, damage control orthopedics c̄ ex-fix

in process of dying

4 — In Extremis Condition → *damage control ortho*

In these patients, uncontrolled bleeding occurs and the response to resuscitation is inadequate. Hypothermia, acidosis, and coagulopathy are present, thus allowing lifesaving procedures only. Reconstructive surgical procedures can be done in course, if the patient survives.[8]

Interactions Between Hemorrhage, Coagulation, Hypothermia, and Inflammation

Various interactions induced by hemorrhage occur that affect the cascade systems of coagulation, hypothermia, and inflammation. Ongoing hemorrhage can cause sustained coagulopathy and disseminated intravascular coagulation. Also, hypothermia can induce a coagulopathic state. Both systems also interfere with inflammation. Thus, all four systems can interfere with each other and cause another system to deteriorate. The assessment of just a single parameter or end point of resuscitation is not sufficient. **Table 2** summarizes various staging systems of patients with multiple injuries and reflects the four different systems and patient status. *all systems are interrelated*

Management of Extremity Injuries

Fracture stabilization is important to reduce pain, minimize fat embolization, and allow for early patient mobilization. Primary definitive osteosynthesis is the best way to achieve this goal. Usually, temporary external fixation, splints, or casts should be avoided. Exceptions may apply according to the status of the patient (**Tables 2 and 3**).

Grading of Local Injury Severity in Closed Fractures

The assessment of true soft-tissue damage in closed fractures may be difficult immediately after injury. Both a puncture wound in an open fracture and a skin contusion can represent similar damage to the skin barrier. The result can be skin necrosis, resulting in increased risk of infection. Early quantification of the soft-tissue injury should be attempted by using scoring systems, as shown in **Table 4**.

Special Situations: Crush Injury

In the presence of severe soft-tissue injuries, complete débridement of necrotic tissue is crucial. In a polytrauma situation, amputation is the treatment of choice more frequently than in isolated fracture management. Antibiotic coverage should be instituted, and some centers advocate the use of hyperbaric oxygen therapy. The most important focus of therapy should be to minimize tissue necrosis and the risk of secondary infection. Repeated revisions and staged surgical débridements are required to achieve this goal.

Management of Open Fractures

Primary surgical therapy in open fractures implies débridement, extensive irrigation, assessment of the dam-

age, and fixation of the fracture. The first careful assessment is an important step for planning the therapeutic strategy. Knowledge of the extent of the vascular and nerve damage is essential in order to decide whether to reconstruct or amputate a severely injured limb. Other important factors include the time and mechanism of injury, energy of causative force, and severity of the fracture. Open fractures following low-energy trauma produce soft-tissue damage that often is minor. These fractures usually can be treated in a manner similar to that of closed fractures after the initial débridement.

Many fracture types in polytraumatized patients can be handled in a manner similar to that of isolated injuries. Intra-articular open fractures require special treatment strategies. Usually, a two-step strategy consisting of initial débridement followed by reconstruction of the joint surface is advised. Often, the joint surface is reduced by temporary fixation with Kirschner wires followed by fixation with lag screws and adjusting screws. After consolidation of the soft tissue, definitive osteosynthesis is achieved. Some authors favor the use of a hybrid fixator system.

Management of Bilateral Fractures and Fracture Combinations

Simultaneous treatment can be a useful concept for the treatment of bilateral fractures. In bilateral tibia fractures, both legs can be prepped and draped simultaneously. Because of the handling of the fluoroscope, fixation should be performed sequentially. The same process applies for bilateral femur fractures. In these injuries, a higher kinetic energy has occurred and additional injuries imply a higher risk of acute respiratory distress syndrome (ARDS) and multiple organ dysfunction syndrome (MODS).[9,10] If the condition of the patient deteriorates, external fixation should be considered. For the management of ipsilateral femoral and tibia fractures, a staged management is advised, as shown in **Table 3**.

Unstable Pelvic Injuries

Clinical and radiologic examination of the pelvis are part of the initial assessment. Pelvic injuries can be classified on the basis of the examination results considering the history of the trauma.[11] Type A fractures include stable fractures of the anterior pelvic ring that do not require surgical treatment. Type B injuries are characterized by partially intact posterior structures. Rotational instability may be possible. Open-book fractures with externally rotated alae have an increased risk of hemorrhage complications and urogenital lesions. However, type B injuries may initially be in internal rotation, which results in bony compression and self-stabilization of the pelvis. Type B injuries require osteosynthesis of the anterior pelvic ring only.[12]

The differentiation of type B and C fractures may be difficult.[11] A CT scan can give important additional information on stable patients. If a CT scan is not available, inlet and outlet radiographic views should be ob-

unlike other injuries with pelvic fx, autotamponade does not occur. retroperitoneal bleeding can mimic intraabdom. injury note: chest injuries usually involve rib Bxs or pulm. contusion; pulm. contusion → pulm. edema → ARDS

Table 2

Criteria Used to Facilitate Determination of the Clinical Condition of Multiple-Trauma Patients[a]

Factor	Parameter	Patient Status			
		Stable	Borderline	Unstable	In extremis
① Shock	Blood pressure (mm Hg)	≥100	80-100	<80	70
	Blood units given in a 2-h period	0-2	2-8	5-15	>15
	Lactate levels (mg/dL)	Normal range according to local laboratory	≈2.5	>2.5	Severe acidosis
	Base deficit level (mmol/L)	Normal range according to local laboratory	No data	No data	>6-8
	ATLS classification	I (normovolemia)	II-III (slight shock)	III-IV (severe shock)	IV (life-threatening shock)
② Coagulation	Platelet count (/mm³)	>110,000	90,000-110,000	<70,000-90,000	<70,000
	Factor II and V (%)	90-100	71-89	50-70	<50
	Fibrinogen (g/dL)	>1	≈1	<1	Disseminated intravascular coagulation
	D-dimer (μg/mL)	Normal range according to local laboratory	Abnormal	Abnormal	Disseminated intravascular coagulation
③ Temperature	°C (°F)	<33	33-35	30-32	≤30
④ Soft-tissue injuries	Lung function; Pao₂/Fio₂ (mm Hg)	350-400	300-350	200-300 ALI	<200 ARDS
	Chest trauma scores; AIS	AIS I or II (eg, abrasion)	AIS ≥2 (eg, 2-3 rib fractures)	AIS ≥3 (eg, serial rib fixation >3)	AIS ≥3 (eg, unstable chest)
	Chest trauma score; TTS	0 concussion	I-II slight thoracic trauma	II-III moderate	IV severe
No, slight, moderate, severe	Abdominal trauma (Moore)	≤ grade II	≤ grade III	Grade III	≥ Grade III
No, slight, moderate, severe	Pelvic trauma (AO classification)	A type	B or C type	C type	C type (crush, rollover abd.
No, slight, moderate, severe	External	AIS I-II (eg, abrasion)	AIS II-III (eg, multiple tears >20 cm)	AIS III-IV (eg, <30% burn)	Crush injury (>30% burn)

[a]Three of the four criteria should be met to classify for a certain grade. Patients who respond to resuscitation qualify for early definitive fracture care provided that prolonged surgeries are avoided. ATLS = Advanced Trauma Life Support; AIS = Abbreviated Injury Scale; PaO₂ = partial pressure of oxygen in arterial blood; FiO₂ = Fraction of inspired oxygen; TTS = thoracic trauma score.

It is of note that the clinical status can change rapidly. The initial assessment therefore can change during the first hours. Also, the existing scores have not necessarily been designed to differentiate between borderline, stable, and unstable patients nor has this table been validated prospectively. Nevertheless, it may be helpful to facilitate an overview of several clinical conditions and may be a guide to treatment.

(Adapted with permission from Pape HC, Giannoudis P, Krettek C, Trentz O: Timing of fixation of major fractures in blunt polytrauma: Role of conventional indicators in clinical decision making. *J Orthop Trauma* 2005;19:551-562.)

note: pt ③ with a chest inj. why? AIS (abbreviated injury scale ≥2) + femoral Bx = "patient at risk"

if lung injury + femur fx, can do EDT if oxygenating well → can mobilize earlier → be in upright position → better oxygena-tion or ventila-tion

unstable + not oxygenating well, DCO to avoid 2nd hit phenomenon

tained. Type C fractures are characterized by translational instability of the dorsal pelvis, which results in separation of one or both pelvic halves from the trunk. These injuries are associated with a high risk of hemorrhagic complications and concomitant injuries of intrapelvic organs. Type C injuries require stabilization of the anterior and posterior pelvic ring.

More than 80% of all unstable pelvic injuries are associated with multiple injuries. The goal of initial treatment of unstable pelvic injuries in multiply injured pa-

Table 3

Management of Ipsilateral Femur and Tibial Shaft Fractures

	Stable	Borderline	Unstable	In extremis
Initial treatment				
	Femur: nail	Femur: resuscitation successful; nail resuscitation difficult: traction consider damage control nailing	Femur: external fixation/traction	Femur: traction
	Tibia: nail	Tibia: nail	Tibia: external fixation/traction	Tibia: traction
Staged treatment				
	N/A	Femur: nail	Femur: nail	Femur: nail
	N/A		Tibia: nail	Tibia: nail

note: Ⓑ femur fxs have high morbidity & mortality → if treated with Ⓑ IM nailing, ↑↑ fat embolization, ↑ risk fat embolus, ARDS, overal mortality → considered life-threatening injury

Table 4

Soft-Tissue Injury Classification

	Soft-tissue injury	Type of fracture
Closed fracture G0	No or very minor	Simple fractures, ie, caused by indirect trauma
Closed fracture G1	Superficial abrasions or contusions from internal fragment pressure	Simple to moderate
Closed fracture G2	Deep, contaminated abrasions or local dermal and muscular contusions due to tangential forces Compartment syndrome	Moderate to severe, usually caused by direct forces
Closed fracture G3	Extensive skin contusion or muscular destruction, subcutaneous decollement Obvious compartment syndrome	Severe and comminuted
Closed fracture G4	Same injury as G3 with significant vascular damage	Severe and comminuted

tients is adequate stabilization and bony compression of the pelvis to avoid massive bleeding. Therefore, stabilization techniques with the patient supine are preferred during this primary period.

Unstable Injuries of the Spine

In all cases, the spine should be assessed with radiographs or CT scans. To rule out the presence of fragments in the spinal canal, further diagnostic procedures (MRI) are required.

Surgical treatment of unstable spine injuries is mandatory. The length of immobilization and intensive care unit stay are significantly reduced due to internal fixation of the spine. Internal stabilization of spinal fractures (even without neurologic symptoms) has been advocated more commonly in the last few years.

Closed reduction of unstable spine injuries without neurologic symptoms is performed in fractures of the cervical spine and rotational injuries of the lower thoracic or lumbar spine. In multiply injured patients, closed reduction may be difficult because of injuries of the extremities. In these cases, surgery is required for proper correction of rotation and axis.

If bony fragments or an intervertebral disk are interposed or displaced into the spinal canal, open reduction and extraction of the fragment should be performed to avoid spinal cord injury.

The standard approach to surgical management of the cervical spine is the ventral approach. Injuries of the thoracic or lumbar spine requiring dorsal and ventral stabilization should be treated in a two-stage fashion. Despite the presence of thoracic or intra-abdominal injuries, prone positioning can be done if performed carefully.

Intensive Care Unit Aspects

One of the challenges in intensive care therapy is the management of ARDS and multiple organ failure. In polytraumatized patients a pulmonary parenchymal lesion (lung contusion) can alter pulmonary function di-

1: Principles of Orthopaedics

Table 5

Criteria for Patient Assessment on the Intensive Care Unit

Input/output ratio	Negative (> 500 mL) for 2 consecutive days *no more capillary leak*
Lung function	$PaO_2 / FiO_2 > 250$ *no ARDS* No chest radiograph infiltrates
Coagulation	Platelet count 90,000/mm³ and rising, or no requirement for replacement of blood products *no DIC*
Acid / base status	Normal values for pH and base excess
Hepatic function	Hepatic malperfusion should be ruled out
Cardiac function	Vasopressors: none or minimal
Inflammation	Decreasing interleukin values (IL-6 < 500 and dropping)

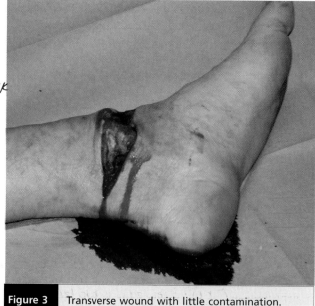

Figure 3 | Transverse wound with little contamination. Initial closure can be performed.

rectly. In addition, vascular and endothelial permeability is increased in the entire body secondary to hemorrhagic shock. Increased water content in all organs occurs and in the lung it increases the risk of ARDS.

Pulmonary failure usually develops first in MODS, the most severe complication after severe trauma. One-phase MODS is characterized by rapid failure of all organs, whereas in two-phase MOF, lung dysfunction is followed by cardiovascular and renal failure. To avoid two-phase MODS, ventilation strategies help decrease mortality. Once the full-blown syndrome of MODS has developed, treatment is based on the patient's symptoms.

Distinct criteria are known to be important when assessing a patient during the course of intensive care. First, hypothermia has to be normalized because it is known to interfere with coagulopathy induced by platelet loss and loss of coagulatory factors due to the initial hemorrhage. Second, the capillary leak caused by ischemia and blood loss is known to last for several days and usually peaks around day 3 or 4 after the initial injury. A positive input/output ratio usually is indicative of an ongoing capillary leak. A negative fluid balance of 500 mL or more should be present for a day or two before taking a patient to the operating room for a prolonged procedure. Third, coagulation factors should be normalized and platelet count exceeding 90,000/mm³ or rising for 2 consecutive days is a good parameter. Fourth, the chest radiograph should not show signs of edema or infiltration. Fifth, inflammatory parameters, such as proinflammatory cytokines (IL-6, IL-8) may be helpful, if available. Likewise, the systemic inflammatory response syndrome score can be counted to assess the inflammatory status as it has been shown to correlate with IL-6 levels. An overview of the intensive care unit assessment criteria is presented in **Table 5**. Usually, days 2 through 4 are difficult in terms of ongoing edema, coagulopathy, and inflammation, whereas after day 6 the inflammatory status usually has normalized.

Soft-Tissue Reconstruction

Wound healing of multiply injured patients is complicated by the relative hypoxia of the tissues, which raises the risk of delayed wound healing and wound infections. Therefore, forced primary wound closure should not be performed.

Small wounds can be closed (**Figure 3**) or covered with artificial skin replacements, or negative pressure used until the swelling decreases. Definitive closure of the wound or mesh graft transplantation is an option. For the past decade, the vacuum-assisted closure has been increasingly used for temporary closure of soft-tissue injuries and to prepare the wound for definitive closure. Advantages include low infection rates and proper granulation of the wound.

If implants, bones, joints, or tendons are visible on the ground of the wound, every attempt should be undertaken to cover them rapidly with vital and well-perfused soft tissue (**Figure 4**). If wound coverage is not achieved within a few days, there is a sustained risk of infection and nonunions. Close cooperation between the orthopaedic surgeon and plastic surgery services is recommended for an optimal overall result.

Medium-sized wounds can often be closed by local transposition of the surrounding tissue after mobilization. This secondary covering procedure should be performed in the period of 72 hours after trauma. Rotational flaps consist of different combinations of muscle, fascia, and skin and should be fit in the defect without tension. Among multiply injured patients it can be difficult to find enough healthy tissue to perform a local

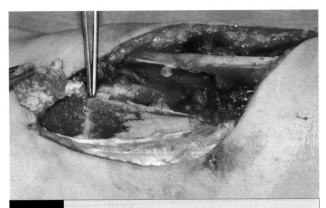

Figure 4 Tendons are visible. Coverage should be achieved as soon as possible.

flap due to serial injuries. Distant flaps are often required in the treatment of these patients. Distant flaps are also indicated if the defect zone is too large to be covered with a rotational flap. Free microvascular flaps are usually preferred by plastic surgeons. However, it has to be kept in mind that prolonged surgical procedures stress the general condition of the patient. If a distant flap is required, the general condition should be kept in mind for this prolonged operation. Yet, coverage of the defect continues to be an urgent issue.

Rehabilitation

Mobilization of all major joints should be initiated during the course of the intensive care treatment. This may imply continuous passive motion therapy. Delayed and aggressive mobilization has been shown to increase the risk of heterotopic ossifications and should be avoided. On the ward these measures usually are accompanied by active exercises performed under supervision of a physical therapist. Mobilization should occur several times a day. Weight bearing is determined according to the combination of fractures and the fracture type.
mobilization & PT are important!

Summary

Polytrauma may be defined as injuries to at least two organ systems associated with a potentially life-threatening condition or an ISS higher than 16 points. The initial assessment should detect at first acute life-threatening injuries. In patients with multiple injuries the clinical condition can change rapidly within the first hours after trauma. Next to severe head trauma, ongoing or uncontrolled hemorrhage is the major reason for the development of a life-threatening condition. The four sources of major bleeding usually derive from an extremity (vascular tear), thoracic, abdominal, and pelvic trauma. Four categories have been identified: stable, borderline, unstable, and in extremis. These four categories can help the surgeon decide whether the patient's condition allows early definitive care of major

fractures or if temporary stabilization by external fixation is advised. The assessment to categorize these patients includes the volume status, pulmonary and renal function, body temperature, coagulation and acid-base status. The decision whether the patient is cleared for definitive surgery can be made on the basis of these parameters.

From the orthopaedic point of view, stabilization of major extremity fractures is an important goal. The time points of stabilization are control of major, life-threatening bleeding (minutes to hours); stabilization of major fractures (first day of surgery); planned revisions and complex fixations (fourth day after surgery and afterward); and late reconstruction (after the second week for example, maxillofacial).

Annotated References

1. Rotondo MF, Esposito TJ, Reilly PM, et al: The position of the Eastern Association for the Surgery of Trauma on the future of trauma surgery. *J Trauma* 2005;59(1): 77-79.

2. Baker SP, O'Neill B, Haddon W Jr, Long WB: The injury severity score: a method for describing patients with multiple injuries and evaluating emergency care. *J Trauma* 1974;14(3):187-196.

3. Pape HC, Giannoudis PV, Krettek C, Trentz O: Timing of fixation of major fractures in blunt polytrauma: Role of conventional indicators in clinical decision making. *J Orthop Trauma* 2005;19(8):551-562.

4. Canadian Orthopaedic Trauma Society: Reamed versus unreamed intramedullary nailing of the femur: Comparison of the rate of ARDS in multiple injured patients. *J Orthop Trauma* 2006;20(6):384-387.

5. Pape HC, Rixen D, Morley J, et al: Impact of the method of initial stabilization for femoral fractures in patients with multiple injuries at risk for complications (borderline patients). *Ann Surg* 2007;246(3):491-499.

   This was a prospective randomized study that eliminated patients at high risk for ARDS and multiple organ failure. Patients were randomized to acute intramedullary nailing of the femur versus external fixation. The authors separated stable from borderline multiple trauma patients and looked at the incidence of acute lung injuries that developed postoperatively. In stable patients, early definitive fixation of the femur was associated with a shorter ventilation time. In borderline patients, early definitive fixation was associated with a higher incidence of acute lung injury. The authors conclude that the indication for initial definitive fixation should be selected according to the condition of the patient.

6. Pape HC, Giannoudis P, Krettek C: The timing of fracture treatment in polytrauma patients: Relevance of damage control orthopedic surgery. *Am J Surg* 2002; 183(6):622-629.

1: Principles of Orthopaedics

7. Scalea TM, Boswell SA, Scott JD, Mitchell KA, Kramer ME, Pollak AN: External fixation as a bridge to intramedullary nailing for patients with multiple injuries and with femur fractures: damage control orthopedics. *J Trauma* 2000;48(4):613-621, discussion 621-623.

8. Morshed S, Miclau T III, Bembom O, Cohen M, Knudson MM, Colford JM Jr: Delayed internal fixation of femoral shaft fracture reduces mortality among patients with multisystem trauma. *J Bone Joint Surg Am* 2009; 91(1):3-13.

   The study used the US National Trauma Databank and included fractures of the femoral shaft; an ISS of greater than or equal to 15; and internal fixation of the femur. Five time periods were selected a priori. The authors used an inverse-probability-of-treatment-weighted analysis to estimate the risk of mortality for a defined treatment time. Their results document that definitive fixation in all but one (24 – 48 hours) of the four delayed treatment categories was associated with a significantly lower risk of mortality to about 50% of that expected with early treatment (< 12 hours). Also, patients with serious associated injuries demonstrated greater risk reductions from delayed fixation when compared with those with less serious or no abdominal injury. The authors conclude from this study that a cautious approach to early definitive femoral shaft fracture fixation among multisystem trauma patients should be performed, and reinforce this for patients who present with serious associated abdominal injuries.

9. Nork SE, Agel J, Russell GV, Mills WJ, Holt S, Routt ML Jr: Mortality after reamed intramedullary nailing of bilateral femur fractures. *Clin Orthop Relat Res* 2003; 415(415):272-278.

10. Copeland CE, Mitchell KA, Brumback RJ, Gens DR, Burgess AR: Mortality in patients with bilateral femoral fractures. *J Orthop Trauma* 1998;12(5):315-319.

11. Olson SA, Burgess A: Classification and initial management of patients with unstable pelvic ring injuries. *Instr Course Lect* 2005;54:383-393.

12. Cothren CC, Osborn PM, Moore EE, Morgan SJ, Johnson JL, Smith WR: Preperitonal pelvic packing for hemodynamically unstable pelvic fractures: A paradigm shift. *J Trauma* 2007;62(4):834-839, discussion 839-842.

   The authors describe a close cooperative effort between orthopaedic surgeons and general surgeons to perform initial surgical fixation of patients with unstable pelvic ring fractures. They brought them to the operating room and performed external or internal fixation and initial packing of major intrapelvic bleedings. Their results are in favor of this management plan. It is understood that the usage of pelvic binders also provides hemorrhage control temporarily, although it does not reduce the pelvic fracture anatomically.

Fat Embolism (esp. femur)

- most common after long bone fx or pelvic fx, also pts. c̄ sickle cell disease
- after long bone or pelvic fx, incidence 10%, but serious clinical manifestations 1-3%
- traumatic pathophysiology: fx → fat into pulm. vasculature → pulm. lipase hydrolyzes fat → release of toxic FFA → cause endothelial injury
- clinical manifestations: injury, latent 12-72 hr. period; primarily lung findings - dyspnea, hypoxemia, diffuse lung lesion; neuro findings 2/2 cerebral fat embolism - confusion, obtundation, coma; derm - petechiae on chest, neck, face; heme - thrombocytopenia, anemia → clinical dx
- early fixation of fxs ↓ incidence
- tx: same as ARDS → PEEP↑ oxygenation via mechanical ventilation ± corticosteroids

Chapter 12

Coagulation, Thromboembolism, and Blood Management in Orthopaedic Surgery

Charles R. Clark, MD

Coagulation and Thromboembolism

Venous thromboembolic disease and prophylaxis are subjects of controversy in orthopaedic surgery. Venous thromboembolism is a major risk in patients undergoing total hip and knee arthroplasty as well as repair of a hip fracture. In addition, patients sustaining major orthopaedic trauma including spinal cord injury as well as patients undergoing treatment of various other musculoskeletal conditions are at potential risk for thromboembolism. Morbidity and mortality are associated with both thromboembolic disease and prophylaxis.

Various forms of pharmacologic and mechanical prophylaxis are available and are presented in the American Academy of Orthopaedic Surgeons' guideline on prevention of pulmonary embolism.[1] This clinical practice guideline was based on a systematic review of published studies of patients undergoing total hip and total knee arthroplasty to prevent pulmonary embolism.[2] The guideline found no difference in the pulmonary embolism rate, death rate, or death related to bleeding from prophylaxis among different thromboembolic prophylactic measures[1] (Table 1).

The Surgical Care Improvement Program (SCIP) of the Centers for Medicare and Medicaid Services (CMS) was initiated in an attempt to minimize venous thromboembolic disease and includes pay-for performance programs. This program has focused additional attention on thromboembolic disease. Specifics of the basic guidelines will be presented later in this chapter. A 2008 study determined the incidence, risk factors, and long-term sequelae of postoperative hematomas requiring surgical evacuation after primary total knee arthro-

Dr. Clark or an immediate family member serves as a board member, owner, officer, or committee member of University of Iowa Hospitals and Clinics; has received royalties from DePuy; serves as a paid consultant to or is an employee of DePuy and Smith & Nephew; and has received research or institutional support from DePuy and Smith & Nephew.

plasty and pointed out the potential for adverse sequela of anticoagulation.[3] The authors found a significantly increased risk of the development of deep infection and/or subsequent major surgery in patients who returned to the operating room within 30 days after the index total knee arthroplasty for evacuation of a postoperative hematoma. The authors concluded that these results support all efforts to minimize the risk of postoperative hematoma formation. Consequently, when patients are managed with pharmacologic prophylaxis it is important to prevent the development of a postoperative hematoma, to monitor for the development of a hematoma, and to practice techniques that will minimize its occurrence.

One study found that patients treated with aspirin or warfarin were somewhat less likely to have associated bleeding complications than were patients treated with low-molecular-weight heparin (LMWH) or subcutaneous heparin.[4]

Pharmacologic Prophylaxis

The ideal prophylactic agent should be effective, have minimal adverse effects, not require monitoring, be administered orally, and be cost-effective.[5] Of all of the interventions (reviewed by the Agency for Healthcare Research and Quality [AHRQ]) in terms of the ability to reduce adverse events while decreasing overall costs, prophylaxis for deep venous thrombosis has received the highest safety rating.[5]

The four most common pharmacologic prophylaxis agents used in the United States are warfarin, LMWH, pentasaccharide, and aspirin (acetylsalicylic acid). It is important to appreciate the evidence supporting the use of the various pharmacologic prophylactic agents. Evidence-based medicine typically includes a level of evidence as well as an indication of the strength of a recommendation. Table 2 describes the levels of evidence commonly cited in the medical literature, including *The Journal of Bone and Joint Surgery*. The levels range from level I, which includes a high-quality randomized trial, to level V, expert opinion. Strengths of recommendation (Table 3) range from grade A, which

Table 1

American Academy of Orthopaedic Surgeons Clinical Practice Guideline on the Prevention of Symptomatic Pulmonary Embolism in Patients Undergoing Total Hip or Knee Arthroplasty: Summary of Recommendations

Recommendation 3.3

Chemoprophylaxis of patients undergoing hip or knee replacement

Recommendation 3.3.1

Patients at standard risk for both PE and major bleeding should be considered for one of the chemoprophylactic agents evaluated in this guideline, including, in alphabetical order: aspirin, LMWH, synthetic pentasaccharides, and warfarin, (Level III, Grade B [choice of prophylactic agent], Grade C [dosage and timing])

Note: The grade of recommendation was reduced from B to C for dosage and timing because of the lack of consistent evidence in the literature defining a clearly superior regimen.

Recommendation 3.3.2

Patients at elevated (above standard) risk for PE and at standard risk for major bleeding should be considered for one of the chemoprophylactic agents evaluated in this guideline, including, in alphabetical order: LMWH, synthetic pentasaccharides, and warfarin, (Level III, Grade B [choice of prophylactic agent], Grade C [dosage and timing]) *NOT aspirin*

Note: The grade of recommendation was reduced from B to C for dosage and timing because of the lack of consistent evidence in the literature on risk stratification of patient populations.

Recommendation 3.3.3

Patients at standard risk for PE and at elevated (above standard) risk for major bleeding should be considered for one of the chemoprophylactic agents evaluated in this guideline, including, in alphabetical order: aspirin, warfarin, or none. (Level III, Grade C) *NOT lovenox or synthetic pentasaccharides*

Note: The grade of recommendation was reduced from B to C for dosage and timing because of the lack of consistent evidence in the literature on risk stratification of patient populations.

Recommendation 3.3.4

Patients at elevated (above standard) risk for both PE and major bleeding should be considered for one of the chemoprophylactic agents evaluated in this guideline, including, in alphabetical order: aspirin, warfarin, or none. (Level III, Grade C) *NOT lovenox or synthetic pentasaccharides*

Note: The grade of recommendation was reduced from B to C for dosage and timing because of the lack of consistent evidence in the literature on risk stratification of patient populations. No studies currently include patients at elevated risk for major bleeding and/or pulmonary embolism (PE) in study groups.

(Reproduced from the American Academy of Orthopaedic Surgeons: Clinical Practice Guideline on the Prevention of Pulmonary Embolism. Rosemont, IL, American Academy of Orthopaedic Surgeons, May 2007. Http://www.aaos.org/Research/guidelines/PEguide.asp.)

Table 2

Levels of Evidence

I	High-quality randomized trial
II	Cohort study (good control)
III	Case-control study
IV	Uncontrolled case series
V	Expert opinion

(Reproduced with permission from Haas SB, Barrack RL, Westrich G, Lachiewicz PF: Venous thromboembolic disease after total hip and total knee arthroplasty: An instructional course lecture, American Academy of Orthopaedic Surgeons. *J Bone Joint Surg Am* 2008;90:2764-2780.)

Table 3

Strengths of Recommendation

A	Good evidence: level I studies with consistent findings (adequate quality and applicability)
B	Fair evidence: level II or III studies with consistent findings (adequate quality and applicability)
C	Poor evidence: level IV or V studies with consistent findings
D	Insufficient or conflicting evidence not allowing a recommendation

(Reproduced with permission from Haas SB, Barrack RL, Westrich G, Lachiewicz PF: Venous thromboembolic disease after total hip and total knee arthroplasty: An instructional course lecture, American Academy of Orthopaedic Surgeons. *J Bone Joint Surg Am* 2008;90:2764-2780.)

consists of good evidence based on level I studies with consistent findings that have adequate quality, to grade D, in which there is insufficient or conflicting evidence that precludes a recommendation.

Warfarin

Warfarin is a vitamin K antagonist that is attractive because it is an oral agent. Based on the American College of Chest Physicians (ACCP) Guidelines[6] there is grade IA data supporting its use in prophylaxis in patients undergoing elective hip replacement and elective knee replacement, with an international normalized ratio (INR) target of 2.5 and a range from 2.0 to 3.0. It is also effective in the prophylaxis of patients undergoing hip fracture surgery with a grade of IB when the INR range is 2.0 to 3.0 with a target of 2.5. Limitations of warfarin include the need for monitoring, interaction with other drugs, and variable metabolism based on a genetic basis; it has a long half-life and its effects are difficult to reverse.

rivaroxaban = Xarelto : direct factor Xa inhibitor (no reversal)

Low-Molecular-Weight Heparin *(lovenox)*

LMWH is attractive because it has rapid antithrombotic activity[5] and a half-life of approximately 4.5 hours. LMWH does not require regular monitoring; however, it is associated with increased cost and a risk of bleeding. All heparin agents have some risk of heparin-induced thrombocytopenia as well as a higher risk of postoperative drainage. According to one study, there was a significantly increased risk of "minor" bleeding events in patients undergoing total hip replacement in comparison with patients who received warfarin prophylaxis.[7] According to the ACCP guidelines[6] there is grade IA data for prophylaxis with LMWH for patients undergoing elective hip replacement, elective knee replacement, and hip fracture surgery. However, one study showed both low efficacy and a high complication rate with the enoxaparin protocol.[8]

Pentasaccharide *Fondaparinux = Arixtra*

Fondaparinux is a synthetic pentasaccharide and an inhibitor of factor Xa. In a study of patients undergoing elective major knee surgery, a significantly decreased rate of thromboembolic complications ($P < 0.001$) was reported, but the rate of bleeding was significantly increased ($P < 0.006$) when compared with that of patients treated with enoxaparin.[9]

← related to heparin, but ↓ risk of HIT (v. heparin)

Aspirin *+ SCDs*

Aspirin is a safe, inexpensive oral agent that does not require monitoring. However, it is less effective in terms of prophylaxis when used alone. A prospective randomized study was conducted comparing treatment with LMWH and a calf mechanical compression device along with aspirin.[10] The rates of deep venous thrombosis were assessed with ultrasonography and there were no significant differences between the two groups, showing that aspirin in combination with mechanical compression may be as effective as and safer than more aggressive anticoagulant therapy.

Mechanical Prophylaxis

Mechanical prophylaxis primarily consists of compressive devices that provide prophylaxis by decreasing venous stasis and increasing fibrinolysis. One of the major drawbacks of compression devices is compliance, not only in terms of the amount of time in which the patient is in the device, but also how effectively the device is applied to the extremity. A 2006 study of 275 patients undergoing unilateral total knee replacement evaluated the use of a mechanical compression device and aspirin compared with enoxaparin for prophylaxis following total knee replacement and found that when used in combination with pneumatic compression, enoxaparin was not superior to aspirin in preventing deep venous thrombosis.[10]

Inferior Vena Cava Filter

An inferior vena cava (IVC) filter functions by preventing a pulmonary embolus as opposed to preventing a deep venous thrombosis. Typically, this device is indicated for patients with a previous history of deep venous thrombosis and/or pulmonary embolism as well as those who sustain major trauma and in whom pharmacologic prophylaxis is contraindicated. IVC devices are expensive. Retrievable devices are now available.

Thromboembolic Disease After Total Hip and Knee Arthroplasty

Many orthopaedic surgeons have taken issue with whether deep venous thrombosis should be the surrogate marker for pulmonary embolism or death in thromboembolic disease.[5,11] Based on an AAOS systematic review, the rate of deep venous thrombosis does not correlate with pulmonary embolism or death following total hip and total knee arthroplasty. This view is not shared by the ACCP. The rate of deep venous thrombosis is two to three times greater in patients undergoing total knee arthroplasty compared with patients undergoing total hip arthroplasty; however, the pulmonary embolism rate is equivalent.[11] As previously noted, a 2007 study reported poor results with the ACCP 1A protocol using enoxaparin.[8] These authors found that patients were returned to the operating room for wound care three times more frequently when the ACCP protocol was followed compared to a previous group of patients in whom the authors used a non-ACCP protocol with warfarin.

Thromboembolic Disease After Spine Surgery

An evidence-based analysis of thromboprophylaxis in patients with acute spinal injuries was performed.[12] The authors studied patients who underwent surgery following spinal injury and compared the groups with and without spinal cord injury. The authors found an increased incidence of deep venous thrombosis in patients with spinal cord injury compared to those without. They recommended that prophylaxis begin as soon as possible once it is deemed safe in terms of bleeding potential. Further, the authors found that the use of LMWH was more effective with respect to deep venous thrombosis prophylaxis than unfractionated heparin with less bleeding. In addition, it was concluded that prevention of pulmonary embolism appeared successful with the use of vitamin K antagonists.

The American Academy of Orthopaedic Surgeons Clinical Guideline on Prevention of Symptomatic Pulmonary Embolism in Patients Undergoing Total Hip or Knee Arthroplasty[1] recommendations are based on an assessment of the patient risk for pulmonary embolism and the risk for major bleeding. The guideline stratified patients into one of four categories based on whether the patient has a standard or elevated risk of pulmonary embolism and a standard or elevated risk of major bleeding, hence the recommendations are patient specific (**Table 4**). Patients at standard risk for both pulmonary embolism and major bleeding should be considered for treatment with one of the following chemoprophylactic agents, listed in alphabetical order: aspirin, LMWH, synthetic pentasaccharide, and warfarin. Patients at an elevated risk for pulmonary embo-

Table 4

General Recommendations Derived With the Consensus Process

Recommendation	Level of Evidence/ Strength of Recommendation[a]
Assess all patients preoperatively to determine whether risk of pulmonary embolism is standard or high	III/B
Assess all patients preoperatively to determine whether risk of bleeding complications is standard or high	III/C
Consider use of vena cava filter in patients who have contraindications to anticoagulation	V/C
Consider intraoperative and/or immediate postoperative mechanical compression	III/B
Consider regional anesthesia for the procedure (in consultation with anesthesiologist)	IV/C
Consider continued use of mechanical prophylaxis postoperatively	IV/C
Rapid patient mobilization	V/C
Routine screening for thromboembolism is not recommended	III/B
Educate patient about symptoms of thromboembolism after discharge	V/B

[a]See Tables 2 and 3
(Reproduced with permission from Haas SB, Barrack RL, Westrich G, Lachiewicz PF: Venous thromboembolic disease after total hip and total knee arthroplasty: An instructional course lecture, American Academy of Orthopaedic Surgeons. *J Bone Joint Surg Am* 2008;90:2764-2780.)

lism and at standard risk for major bleeding should be considered for treatment with LMWH, a synthetic pentasaccharide, and warfarin. Patients at standard risk pulmonary embolism and at an elevated risk for major bleeding should be considered for treatment with aspirin, warfarin, or neither agent. Patients at an elevated

risk for both pulmonary embolism and major bleeding should be considered for prophylaxis with aspirin, warfarin, or neither agent. In addition, patients should be considered for intraoperative and postoperative mechanical compression. Patients with known contraindications to anticoagulation should be considered for vena cava filter placement.

The AAOS clinical guideline provides additional recommendations based on the results of the objective AAOS Consensus Process in which the work group members participated, and these recommendations are provided in **Table 5**. General recommendations include use of an IVC filter in patients who have contraindications for anticoagulation, rapid patient mobilization, and educating patients about symptoms of thromboembolism after discharge.

A risk assessment was performed for patients undergoing total hip and knee arthroplasties, and a multimodal protocol for thromboprophylaxis was developed.[13] Patients were divided into two groups based on low or high risk. Low risk factors are cardiac disease (congestive heart failure) classified as class I (according to the system of the New York Heart Association),[14] prior deep venous thrombosis that occurred more than 5 years previously, inactive malignant disease, current use of hormone replacement therapy (HRT), chronic tobacco use, and blood disorders consisting of sickle cell trait, polycythemia vera, or thrombocytopenia. Some patients had a combination of these risk factors. High risk factors are a history of a venous thromboembolic event that occurred within the previous 5 years, congestive heart failure classified as class II or III according to the system of the New York Heart Association, atrial fibrillation with cardiac disease and the use of warfarin, recent surgery for the treatment of malignant disease, or current adjuvant drug therapy and thrombophilia, including factor V Leiden, prothrombin disorders, protein-S deficiency, antithrombin disorders, or hypercoagulability states. In addition, some patients had a combination of these factors. Low-risk patients were managed with aspirin, dipyridamole, or clopidogrel bisulfate as well as intermittent pneumatic calf compression devices. High-risk patients were managed with LMWH or warfarin and intermittent calf compression. The authors concluded that a multimodal thromboembolic prophylactic regimen is consistent with protecting patients while limiting adverse clinical outcomes secondary to thromboembolic, vascular, and bleeding complications. The level of evidence was therapeutic level III.

Blood Management in Orthopaedic Surgery

Rather than relying on an automatic transfusion trigger, the surgeon should identify patient-specific risk factors such as the anticipated difficulty of the proposed surgical procedure, the preoperative hemoglobin level, and comorbidities and develop a plan for blood management.[15] Medical errors in orthopaedic surgery were examined in a recent study, and 5.5% of errors were re-

Table 5

Recommendations for Medication Derived From Literature Review and Analysis Process

Risk	Agents[a]	Level of Evidence/Strength of Recommendation[b]
Standard risk of pulmonary embolism and major bleeding	Aspirin, LMWH, pentasaccharide, warfarin (INR ≤2)	III/B (C for dosing and timing)
Elevated risk of pulmonary embolism; standard risk of bleeding	LMWH, pentasaccharide, warfarin (INR <2)	III/B (C for dosing and timing)
Standard risk of pulmonary embolism; elevated risk of bleeding	Aspirin, warfarin, (INR <2), no prophylaxis	III/C
Elevated risk of pulmonary embolism and bleeding	Aspirin, warfarin (INR ≤2), no prophylaxis	III/C

[a]The agents in each row are given in alphabetical order.
[b]See Tables 2 and 3
(Reproduced with permission from Haas SB, Barrack RL, Westrich G, Lachiewicz PF: Venous thromboembolic disease after total hip and total knee arthroplasty: An instructional course lecture, American Academy of Orthopaedic Surgeons. *J Bone Joint Surg Am* 2008;90:2764-2780.)

lated to a blood or tissue event.[16] An algorithm of blood management was developed based on anticipated blood loss in patients undergoing total hip and total knee arthroplasty.[17] When the algorithm was followed the transfusion rate with allogeneic blood was 2.1%, which was significantly lower (*P* < 0.001) than a transfusion rate of 16.4% when the algorithm was not followed (**Figure 1**).

Preoperative Blood Management

It has been reported in patients undergoing lower extremity total joint arthroplasty that if the preoperative hemoglobin level was less than 13 g/dL, the risk of requiring an allogeneic blood transfusion was four times greater compared with a hemoglobin level of 13 to 15 g/dL and was 15.3 times greater compared to patients with a preoperative hemoglobin level of greater than 15 g/dL.[18] These data indicate that preoperative hemoglobin levels can be used to dictate the need for different blood management strategies. It has been recommended that preoperative anemia be corrected with oral iron supplementation.[19] Preoperative medical conditions can influence risks, including the need for transfusions. A 2009 study found that uncontrolled diabetes mellitus, whether type I or type II, was significantly associated with additional surgical and systemic complications including postoperative hematoma, transfusion risk, and infections following lower extremity total joint arthroplasty.[20] Patient-specific factors such as age, sex, whether or not the patient was hypertensive, and body mass index were evaluated.[21] The authors found that when a patient had two or more of these factors, there was a significantly increased risk of allogeneic blood transfusion (*P* < 0.02).

Autologous Donation

A snapshot assessment of 9,482 patients undergoing lower extremity total joint arthroplasties was performed and the then-current blood usage was described.[22] Sixty-one percent of patients predonated autologous blood. However, 45% of the predonated autologous blood was not used. Nine percent of patients required allogeneic blood despite predonated autologous blood. For each unit of donated blood, the hemoglobin level is decreased approximately 1.2 to 1.5 g/dL. Autologous donation is an option that the surgeon should consider for the patient, bearing in mind concerns regarding wasted donated units and the resultant associated preoperative decrease in hemoglobin.

Donor-Directed Donation

The risk of hepatitis B and C transmission as well as the risk of human immunodeficiency virus (HIV) transmission is increased in patients who received donor-directed donations as opposed to autologous blood.[15] This increased risk is possibly because directed donations are from family members or friends who often may be reluctant to disclose risk factors for viruses such as hepatitis and/or HIV. Donor-directed donation is rarely used because of these concerns.

Erythropoietin is effective for rapidly increasing the hemoglobin level and is indicated for patients with a hemoglobin level of 10 to 13 g/dL. Further, erythropoietin is an important component of the blood conservation algorithm shown in **Figure 1**; in that study, patients who followed the algorithm and were given erythropoietin if the anticipated hemoglobin was below a certain level had a reduced need for blood transfusion following total hip and total knee arthroplasty.[17]

1: Principles of Orthopaedics

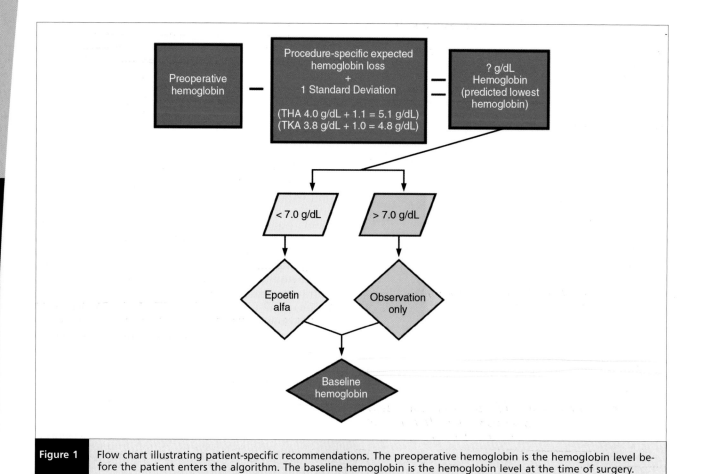

Figure 1 Flow chart illustrating patient-specific recommendations. The preoperative hemoglobin is the hemoglobin level before the patient enters the algorithm. The baseline hemoglobin is the hemoglobin level at the time of surgery.

Intraoperative Blood Management

Methods for intraoperative blood management include effective anesthetic techniques, intraoperative blood salvage, acute normovolemic hemodilution, the use of antifibrinolytic agents, the use of a bipolar ceiling device, perioperative injections, and topical agents. Patients undergoing total knee arthroplasty were compared using a computer-assisted minimally invasive technique with a standard technique in a prospective randomized study.[23] The authors found that despite increased duration of surgery, patients treated with the computer-assisted minimally invasive technique had a decreased length of hospital stay and decreased blood loss.

A meta-analysis of the use of antifibrinolytic agents in spine surgery found that aprotinin, tranexamic acid, and epsilon-aminocaproic acid were effective in reducing blood loss and transfusions.[24] These agents were particularly effective in patients undergoing correction of spinal deformities and in patients with long arthrodesis constructs. However, at the present time, these agents are not approved by the United States Food and Drug Administration for these indications. The use of tranexamic acid in patients undergoing total hip replacement was evaluated in a 2009 study. Intravenous administration of 1 g of tranexamic acid during induction resulted in decreased early postoperative blood loss and total blood loss, but intraoperative blood loss was not affected.[25] Tranexamic acid acts during the early phase of the fibrinolytic cascade. Concerns about the use of antifibrinolytic agents include an increased risk of thrombosis; however, an increased incidence of deep venous thrombosis was not found. Concern has also been expressed about the cost of these agents; however, tranexamic acid was cost-effective in reducing blood loss and transfusion requirements after total hip replacement, especially in women, in the 2009 study.

Topical agents such as a fibrin sealant have been studied in patients undergoing total knee arthroplasty. According to results from a prospective randomized trial, the use of the fibrin sealant safely decreased blood drainage while maintaining higher hemoglobin levels.[26] Fibrin sealant should be considered as part of a blood management strategy, particularly in patients undergoing total knee arthroplasty and especially in those who have an inflamed synovium.

Postoperative Blood Management

Patients undergoing total hip and total knee replacement who preoperatively had mild anemia and hemoglobin levels ranging from 10 to 13 g/dL were studied.[27] Treatment of patients with preoperative erythropoietin injections was found to be more effective but more costly in reducing the need for allogeneic blood transfusion in mildly anemic patients than the use of postoperative reinfusion of autologous shed blood. In a randomized controlled trial of patients undergoing total knee replacement, the use of autologous retransfusion was evaluated.[28] No adverse reactions associated with retransfusion of autologous blood were found. This study confirmed the safety of reinfusion drains in total knee arthroplasty but casts doubt regarding their efficacy in reducing the need for allogeneic transfusion compared with standard suction drainage after total knee arthroplasty.

The use of allogeneic blood transfusion is part of the strategy for blood management and is an option that should be considered. Allogeneic blood is currently safer than ever before because blood can be screened for various viruses. However, a risk of viral transmission as well as bacterial contamination of the blood exists but has greatly decreased. In 1984 the risk of HIV transmission was greater than 1 per 1,000, and in 2001 it was less than 1 per 1 million.[29] Further, administrative errors persist.[19]

Summary

Coagulation, thromboembolism, and blood management are important topics related to patient management, particularly for those patients undergoing total hip or total knee arthroplasty. The AAOS clinical guideline on the prevention of symptomatic pulmonary embolism in these patients is based on a systematic review of the literature and is evidence based. This guideline provides useful information related to patient management regarding pulmonary embolism prophylaxis. In addition, ACCP provides evidence-based guidelines, which include deep venous thrombosis and pulmonary embolism. Prevention of deep venous thrombosis is important; however, orthopaedic surgeons are most concerned with prevention of pulmonary embolism, which can be fatal. A patient-specific plan for blood management should be developed based on factors including preoperative hemoglobin level and anticipated blood loss of the proposed surgical intervention. Patients undergoing a particularly difficult revision will more urgently need multiple blood management strategies than the patient undergoing an anticipated straightforward unilateral primary joint arthroplasty.

Annotated References

1. American Academy of Orthopaedic Surgeons: *American Academy of Orthopaedic Surgeons Clinical Guideline on Prevention of Symptomatic Pulmonary Embolism in Patients Undergoing Total Hip or Knee Arthroplasty: Summary of Recommendations.* Rosemont, IL, American Academy of Orthopaedic Surgeons, 2007, pp 1-63.

   This is an executive summary of the recommendations of the AAOS clinical guideline on prevention of pulmonary embolism in patients undergoing total hip or knee arthroplasty.

2. Johanson NA, Lachiewicz PF, Lieberman JR, et al: Prevention of symptomatic pulmonary embolism in patients undergoing total hip or knee arthroplasty. *J Am Acad Orthop Surg* 2009;17(3):183-196.

   This is a summary of the AAOS clinical practice guideline on the prevention of symptomatic pulmonary embolism in patients undergoing total hip or knee arthroplasty.

3. Galat DD, McGovern SC, Hanssen AD, Larson DR, Harrington JR, Clarke HD: Early return to surgery for evacuation of a postoperative hematoma after primary total knee arthroplasty. *J Bone Joint Surg Am* 2008; 90(11):2331-2336.

   The authors found that patients who returned to the operating room within 30 days following a primary total knee arthroplasty for evacuation of a hematoma were at significantly increased risk for the development of deep infection and are undergoing subsequent major surgery.

4. Brookenthal KR, Freedman KB, Lotke PA, Fitzgerald RH, Lonner JH: A meta-analysis of thromboembolic prophylaxis in total knee arthroplasty. *J Arthroplasty* 2001;16(3):293-300.

5. Haas SB, Barrack RL, Westrich G, Lachiewicz PF: Venous thromboembolic disease after total hip and knee arthroplasty. *J Bone Joint Surg Am* 2008;90(12):2764-2780.

   A summary of venous thromboembolic disease after total hip and knee arthroplasty is presented.

6. Hirsh J, Guyatt G, Albers GW, Harrington R, Schünemann HJ; American College of Chest Physicians: Executive summary: American College of Chest Physicians Evidence-Based Clinical Practice Guidelines (8th Edition). *Chest* 2008;133(6, Suppl):71S-109S.

   This is an executive summary of the 2008 ACCP evidence-based clinical guidelines.

7. Colwell CW Jr, Collis DK, Paulson R, et al: Comparison of enoxaparin and warfarin for the prevention of venous thromboembolic disease after total hip arthroplasty. Evaluation during hospitalization and three months after discharge. *J Bone Joint Surg Am* 1999; 81(7):932-940.

8. Burnett RS, Clohisy JC, Wright RW, et al: Failure of the American College of Chest Physicians-1A protocol for lovenox in clinical outcomes for thromboembolic prophylaxis. *J Arthroplasty* 2007;22(3):317-324.

   The authors compared their results of prophylaxis following an ACCP 1A protocol using Lovenox and found that returning to the operating room for wound complications occurred three times more frequently with the use of Lovenox than a previous study using warfarin.

9. Bauer KA, Eriksson BI, Lassen MR, Turpie AG; Steering Committee of the Pentasaccharide in Major Knee Surgery Study: Fondaparinux compared with enoxaparin for the prevention of venous thromboembolism after elective major knee surgery. *N Engl J Med* 2001; 345(18):1305-1310.

10. Westrich GH, Bottner F, Windsor RE, Laskin RS, Haas SB, Sculco TP: VenaFlow plus Lovenox vs Vena-Flow plus aspirin for thromboembolic disease prophylaxis in total knee arthroplasty. *J Arthroplasty* 2006; 21(6, Suppl 2):139-143.

11. Callaghan JJ, Dorr LD, Engh GA, et al; American College of Chest Physicians: Prophylaxis for thromboembolic disease: Recommendations from the American College of Chest Physicians—are they appropriate for orthopaedic surgery? *J Arthroplasty* 2005;20(3): 273-274.

12. Ploumis A, Ponnappan RK, Maltenfort MG, et al: Thromboprophylaxis in patients with acute spinal injuries: An evidence-based analysis. *J Bone Joint Surg Am* 2009;91(11):2568-2576.

    The incidence of deep venous thrombosis is higher in spinal cord injury patients undergoing spine surgery than in patients without spinal cord injury. LMWH was more effective for the prevention of deep venous thrombosis with less bleeding complications than on fractionated heparin. Prevention of pulmonary embolism appeared to be successful with the use of vitamin K antagonists.

13. Dorr LD, Gendelman V, Maheshwari AV, Boutary M, Wan Z, Long WT: Multimodal thromboprophylaxis for total hip and knee arthroplasty based on risk assessment. *J Bone Joint Surg Am* 2007;89(12):2648-2657.

    A multimodal thromboembolic prophylactic regimen was consistent with protecting patients while limiting adverse clinical outcome secondary to thromboembolic, vascular, and bleeding complications.

14. Hunt SA, Baker DW, Chin MH, et al; American College of Cardiology/American Heart Association: ACC/AHA guidelines for the evaluation and management of chronic heart failure in the adult: Executive summary. A report of the American College of Cardiology/American Heart Association Task Force on Practice Guidelines (committee to revise the 1995 guidelines for the evaluation and management of heart failure). *J Am Coll Cardiol* 2001;38(7):2101-2113.

15. Clark CR: Perioperative blood management in total hip arthroplasty. *Instr Course Lect* 2009;58:167-172.

    Patient-specific risk factors such as the anticipated difficulty of the procedure, preoperative hemoglobin level, and comorbidities should be identified and the surgeon should develop a plan for blood management.

16. Wong DA, Herndon JH, Canale ST, et al: Medical errors in orthopaedics: Results of an AAOS member survey. *J Bone Joint Surg Am* 2009;91(3):547-557.

    This review of medical errors in orthopaedics based on an AAOS survey revealed that 5.5% of the events were a blood or tissue event.

17. Pierson JL, Hannon TJ, Earles DR: A blood-conservation algorithm to reduce blood transfusions after total hip and knee arthroplasty. *J Bone Joint Surg Am* 2004;86(7):1512-1518.

18. Salido JA, Marin LA, Gómez LA, Zorrilla P, Martínez C: Preoperative hemoglobin levels and the need for transfusion after prosthetic hip and knee surgery: Analysis of predictive factors. *J Bone Joint Surg Am* 2002; 84(2):216-220.

19. Lemaire R: Strategies for blood management in orthopaedic and trauma surgery. *J Bone Joint Surg Br* 2008; 90(9):1128-1136.

    This paper considers the various strategies available for the management of blood loss in patients undergoing orthopaedic and trauma surgery.

20. Marchant MH Jr, Viens NA, Cook C, Vail TP, Bolognesi MP: The impact of glycemic control and diabetes mellitus on perioperative outcomes after total joint arthroplasty. *J Bone Joint Surg Am* 2009;91(7):1621-1629.

    Regardless of diabetes type, patients with uncontrolled diabetes mellitus exhibited significantly increased odds of surgical and systemic complications including postoperative hemorrhage during their index hospitalization following lower extremity total joint arthroplasty.

21. Pola E, Papaleo P, Santoliquido A, Gasparini G, Aulisa L, De Santis E: Clinical factors associated with an increased risk of perioperative blood transfusion in nonanemic patients undergoing total hip arthroplasty. *J Bone Joint Surg Am* 2004;86(1):57-61.

22. Bierbaum BE, Callaghan JJ, Galante JO, Rubash HE, Tooms RE, Welch RB: An analysis of blood management in patients having a total hip or knee arthroplasty. *J Bone Joint Surg Am* 1999;81(1):2-10.

23. Dutton A, Yeo SJ, Yang KY, Lo NN, Chia KU, Chong HC: Computer-assisted minimally invasive total knee arthroplasty compared with standard total knee arthroplasty: A prospective, randomized study. *J Bone Joint Surg Am* 2008;90(1):2-9.

    The authors found there was less blood loss and no increase in the rate of short-term complications in the group undergoing computer-assisted, minimally invasive total knee arthroplasty compared with standard total knee arthroplasty.

24. Gill JB, Chin Y, Levin A, Feng D: The use of antifibrinolytic agents in spine surgery: A meta-analysis. *J Bone Joint Surg Am* 2008;90(11):2399-2407.

    The authors performed a meta-analysis of antifibrinolytic agents in spine surgery and found that they were effective for reducing blood loss in transfusions. The use of these agents, which include aprotinin, tranexamic acid, and epsilon-aminocaproic acid, is not an FDA approved indication for these agents.

25. Rajesparan K, Biant LC, Ahmad M, Field RE: The effect of an intravenous bolus of tranexamic acid on blood loss in total hip replacement. *J Bone Joint Surg Br* 2009;91(6):776-783.

    The authors found that a preoperative bolus of 1 g of tranexamic acid was cost-effective in reducing blood loss in transfusion requirements after total hip replace-

*note: IVC filters can be placed in multi-trauma pts., esp. c̄ long bone fx, S.C. injury, or pelvic fx to prevent massive PE

ment especially in women. The results suggest that fibrin sealant can safely reduce blood drainage following total knee arthroplasty while maintaining higher hemoglobin levels.

26. Wang GJ, Hungerford DS, Savory CG, et al: Use of fibrin sealant to reduce bloody drainage and hemoglobin loss after total knee arthroplasty: A brief note on a randomized prospective trial. *J Bone Joint Surg Am* 2001; 83(10):1503-1505.

27. Moonen AF, Thomassen BJ, Knoors NT, van Os JJ, Verburg AD, Pilot P: Pre-operative injections of epoetin-alpha versus post-operative retransfusion of autologous shed blood in total hip and knee replacement: A prospective randomised clinical trial. *J Bone Joint Surg Br* 2008;90(8):1079-1083.

Preoperative epoetin injections were more effective but more costly in reducing the need for allogeneic blood

transfusions in mildly anemic patients who had postoperative retransfusion of autologous blood.

28. Amin A, Watson A, Mangwani J, Nawabi D, Ahluwalia R, Loeffler M: A prospective randomised controlled trial of autologous retransfusion in total knee replacement. *J Bone Joint Surg Br* 2008;90(4):451-454.

The authors concluded the cost-effectiveness and continued use of autologous drains in total knee replacement should be questioned.

29. Vamvakas EC, Blajchman MA: Transfusion-related mortality: The ongoing risks of allogenic blood transfusion and the available strategies for their prevention. *Blood* 2009;113(15):3406-3417.

This article reports that levels of allogenic blood transfusion-transmitted virus in the United States are exceedingly low.

1: Principles of Orthopaedics

Pulmonary Embolism in Ortho Pts: Dx & Tx

- DVT occurs more frequently in prox. v. distal LE fx
- tachycardia, O_2 desat, SOB = most common presentation
- many PE's are silent
- risk factors include h/o DVT/PE, high BMI, cancer, OCP's, immobilization
- Dx: Wells score + D-dimer = useful; CTA best imaging test
- ↑ incidence PE α ↑ incidence subsegmental/non-central PE, no Δ in fatal PE's or central PE's, ∴ m/l 2/2 ↑ sensitivity of tests
- these clinically silent, incidental (non-central) PE's often do not need tx c̄ anticoag. b/c anticoag. carries own risks, esp. in postop pts. → risks include bleeding primarily, which can lead to: 1) ↑ pain, 2) ↑ rehab. duration, 3) compartment syndrome, 4) return to OR, 5) anemia & transfusion, 6) wound infection
- anticoag. tx for confirmed PE: 1) LMWH, 2) IV or SQ unfractionated heparin, 3) SQ fondaparinux x 5d c̄ coumadin until INR ≥ 2 → if transient risk factors, 3 mo. v. no risk factors, 3 mo. + eval for lifetime tx
- downside: coumadin requires monitoring, heparin & fondaparinux are non-oral
- anticoag. can be dangerous in spine pts., definitely in NSGY pts.
- tricky b/c pts. at greatest risk for PE in 1st 2 wks. postop, and early recurrent PE have high mortality rate, but this is also when anticoag. most dangerous in surgical pt.
- may not want to do bolus of heparin in surgical pts.
- IVC filters to prevent LE DVT from entering pulm. circuit is option for pts. c̄ PE & high bleeding risk for cannot toler- ate anticoag.

note: IVC filters can be placed in multi-trauma pts, esp. long bone fx, S.C. injury, or pelvic fx to prevent massive PE

(central PE), no Δ in ...

titrate / continue monitoring, repair

Work-Related Illness, Cumulative Trauma, and Compensation

J. Mark Melhorn, MD, FAAOS, FAADEP, FACOEM, FACS   James B. Talmage, MD, FAADEP, FACOEM

Introduction

All states in the United States have a workers' compensation system. Each state's system is unique, but they all have some common features. Workers' compensation injuries or illnesses represent a significant percentage of case volume in some orthopaedic practices. Physicians should learn the state's rules that are applicable to a given case. At times, such as in cases in which an employee lives in one state, works for a company located in a different state, and is injured in a third state, it can be challenging to determine which rules apply.

History

Workers' compensation pays for medical care for work-related injuries or illnesses beginning immediately after the injury occurs, pays temporary disability benefits (partial wage replacement) after a waiting period of 3 to 7 days, pays permanent partial and permanent total disability benefits to workers who have lasting consequences from injuries caused on the job, pays rehabilitation and training benefits for those unable to return to preinjury careers (in some states); and pays benefits to the survivors of workers who die of work-related causes. One program under the Social Security Admin-

istration, in contrast, pays benefits to workers with long-term disabilities resulting from any cause, but only when the disabilities preclude any type of work and usually only after the individual is off work for more than 1 year.

Although there is considerable variation in rules from state to state, workers' compensation is designed to function as a "no-fault" system involving numerous parties, including the worker, the physician, the employer, the employer's insurance carrier, case managers, and others. Even though workers' compensation systems are designed to be "no fault," many injured workers hire legal counsel. Although the goal should be to return the injured worker to maximal function in the shortest period of time with the least residual disability and the shortest absence from work, there are often conflicting goals among the involved parties. Most patients want to receive care and get better; however, some noninjury-related issues or barriers are often involved. On occasion, patients may not want to return to work because of issues as far ranging as a hostile work environment to possible secondary monetary gain. In some systems, injured workers who do not return to work receive greater financial compensation. In all systems it is probable that the injured worker's lawyer will receive more income if the worker cannot return to work. Attorney involvement typically delays claim closure and increases costs.[1] Most treating physicians prefer to administer care as expeditiously as possible. Employers generally want employees to receive as little sick or compensable time away from work as possible, and insurance carriers want to resolve cases with as little expense as possible.

Costs

The medical cost of treating workers' injuries and illnesses can be considered from the standpoint of the total medical cost for these patients or from the standpoint of the practice overhead experienced by the physician who treats these patients. The most recent review from the National Council on Compensation Insurance[2] determined a number of relevant findings. Workers' compensation pays more than group health insurance to treat comparable injuries. The differences

Table 1

Odds of Worse Results in Workers' Compensation Patients for Conditions Commonly Treated by Orthopaedic Surgeons

Procedure	Number of Studies	Odds Ratio	95% Confidence Interval
Shoulder acromioplasty	13	4.48	2.71 – 7.40
Lumbar fusion	19	4.33	2.81 – 6.62
Lumbar diskectomy	24	4.77	3.51 – 6.50
Lumbar intradiskal chymopapain	9	3.67	2.45 – 5.51
Carpal tunnel release	10	4.24	2.43 – 7.40

in the utilization of medical services dominate price differences and explain 80% of the difference in overall treatment costs. Utilization of services varies principally based on the type of injury, with all the injuries considered showing higher medical service utilization for workers' compensation patients than for group health insurance patients. Traumatic injuries to arms or legs consistently have smaller cost and utilization differences, whereas chronic pain-related injuries such as bursitis, back pain, and carpal tunnel syndrome have larger differences. Differences in payment between workers' compensation and group health insurance depend on the type of service provided. Evaluation, management, and physical therapy costs are higher in workers' compensation cases because of greater use of those medical services. Radiology costs are higher in workers' compensation cases than in group health insurance cases because of higher prices and greater utilization. Greater use of physical therapy services is more prominent for workers' compensation patients with acute traumas than for those with other injuries. Greater use of office visits and radiology services is more prominent for workers' compensation patients with chronic pain-related injuries than for patients with other injuries.

The overhead expenses of the physician's practice are substantially higher for treating workers' compensation patients than for treating patients with other forms of payment or insurance.[3] For example, in one practice the total orthopaedic expense per episode of care in 2000 for patients was $123 for self-payers, $195 for those with an indemnity plan, $148 for Medicare patients, $178 for those with preferred provider organizations, $208 for patients with health maintenance organizations/point-of-service plans, and $299 for workers' compensation patients. These differences among payer types persisted even after accounting for patient age, sex, treatment type (nonsurgical versus surgical), and the number of office visits.

According to 2007 data published by the Bureau of Labor Statistics, the employers' costs of workers' compensation vary among industries and occupations, depending on the number of workers employed. Costs also vary if an employer is union or nonunion and by geographic location within the United States.[4] Statistics also showed that litigation results in an increased number of subjective patient complaints, poorer medical outcomes, increased patient use of health care, and increased physician workloads.[5]

Many states have workers' compensation fee schedules and most pay physicians somewhat more than the rate paid by Medicare for the same current procedural terminology (CPT) code, which is reasonable because these cases generate increased practice overhead. Despite slightly higher rates of pay for office visits, procedures, and other medical care, the main reason for the increased cost in workers' compensation cases is overutilization of medical services.

Documented overutilization of services and societal concern for controlling costs in the workers' compensation system to promote US competitiveness in the global marketplace have led an increasing number of states to impose utilization review requirements that approve or deny requested care using evidence-based treatment guidelines. The trend of using evidence-based treatment guidelines to determine authorized care is expected to increase over the next decade for both workers' compensation and health insurance patients, regardless of the outcome of government health care reform.

The "human cost" of workers' compensation injuries is related to medical outcomes and residual impairment and/or disability. Results of a meta-analysis of 211 studies found that the same injury or condition treated in a compensation setting (usually workers' compensation) was much more likely to have a poorer outcome than if the injury or illness had been treated under personal health insurance.[6] In the 211 reviewed studies, 175 showed worse outcomes with workers' compensation when compared with noncompensation patients, 35 found no difference, and 1 study found improved outcomes in workers' compensation patients. Table 1 summarizes the odds of worse results in workers' compensation patients for conditions commonly treated by orthopaedic surgeons.

The poorer outcomes were not determined by objectively measurable outcomes such as range of motion or neurologic deficit but were based on outcome assessments by validated questionnaires that recorded self-reported symptoms and descriptions of functional ability. If two seemingly identical injuries are treated in a workers' compensation patient and a patient with a health insurance payer, the patient treated under the workers' compensation system would be expected to receive more medical treatments, have higher medical costs, and have a much poorer outcome than the patient with the health insurance payer. Therefore, the treating physician's initial decision on causation (determining if a given injury or illness is related to work) is not only a matter of cost allocation and ethical fairness but a potential determinant of the patient's outcome. A similar relationship between compensation status and increasing disability has been reported.[7]

Causation

Many physicians make causation determinations based on their understanding of tradition (for example, prior training, prior experience, or consensus among other doctors in the community) rather than based on science. This reasoning leads to anecdotal determinations, such as attributing nonspecific back pain with the teaching occupation because the teacher either sits or stands all day, or attributing limping from a meniscal tear in one knee as the causative factor in a meniscal tear in the contralateral knee and nonspecific back pain.

Causation determinations are complicated because legal causation is not medical causation. States differ in the percentage of the cause that must be attributed to a work-related injury or exposure for the patient to qualify for coverage in the workers' compensation system under the legal theory of aggravation of a preexisting condition. This area of understanding is critical. The concept that causation does not equal compensability is poorly understood by both physicians and patients. Physicians need to understand the "rules of the system" when asked to provide an opinion about causation because many believe that when asked about medical causation that this will automatically be applied to the legal issue of compensability, and this is not necessarily the case. Several states, such as Kansas and Tennessee, have very liberal rules allowing almost any change in a condition imagined by a physician to qualify a worker for treatment in the workers' compensation system. California has a 1% rule (1% or more of the causation must be from the industrial injury or exposure). Texas has a 3% threshold, whereas states such as Arkansas, Florida, and Missouri require more than a 50% threshold. Consequently, the statutory or case-law basis that defines aggravation of the patient's condition for each state will tremendously impact the number of cases treated in the workers' compensation system and the costs to industry and society. These rules make the physician's causation decisions problematic because there is no scientific literature to determine, for example, if walking at work may play a less than 1% role or a more than 3% role in knee osteoarthritis. For many of the causation questions that arise in cases with potential compensation for injury or illness, the only science

available is case-control studies, which can provide hypotheses for testing, but which cannot establish causation.[8,9] Physicians are forced to use their own understanding of the legal standard of causation in a state, even if there is no scientific support for the interpretation. This factor explains why two apparently equally well-trained, competent physicians can testify in a case, agreeing completely on the diagnosis and treatment, and yet have opposite opinions on causation and whether the case should be treated in the workers' compensation system.

The literature on the epidemiology of occupational musculoskeletal disorders is often confusing because of conflicting evidence on the importance of various potential risks or causal factors. Occupational exposures and their association with, or causation of, injuries and illnesses are often debated. Because a determination for association or causation is required to establish eligibility for compensation and financial responsibility for workers' compensation or tort cases, debates and disputed legal cases often ensue.[10] The significance of such disputes is underscored by the reported direct health care costs for the nation's workforce of more than $418 billion and indirect costs of more than $837 billion.[11]

It is important that common perceptions or popular opinions of causation be based on the best available scientific evidence. For example, the speculation that carpal tunnel syndrome is related to arm use is widely accepted, but is unproven.[9] Because this proposed linkage is appealing and pervasive and seems to make sense, the lay press has advanced this association despite quality scientific investigations that have found little or no relationship between carpal tunnel syndrome and occupation or hand use.[12,13]

Recent studies on causation indicate that many conditions that have been routinely accepted as work-related by workers' compensation systems are actually not scientifically caused by work. For example, a 2006 study reported that most of the minor common injuries of life do not cause episodes of chronic significant back pain, unless those episodes of pain occur in a compensation setting, in which case they are often erroneously attributed to minor trauma.[14] In a different study, the authors obtained "preinjury" (baseline) lumbar MRIs, in an attempt to document which MRI finding commonly seen in asymptomatic individuals is the "weak link in the chain" that "breaks" when chronic back pain subsequently develops.[15] The authors reported that none of the preexisting changes on MRI correlated with the subsequent development of adult chronic back pain; follow-up MRIs after the onset of low back pain were typically unchanged from the baseline MRIs. It was concluded that in the cohort study, minor trauma did not appear to increase the risk of serious low back pain episodes or disability and that most incident-adverse low back pain events can be predicted by a small set of demographic and behavioral variables rather than by structural findings or minor trauma.

A 2009 systematic review of methodologically sound studies on spinal mechanical loading as a risk factor for low back pain reported conflicting evidence that leisure

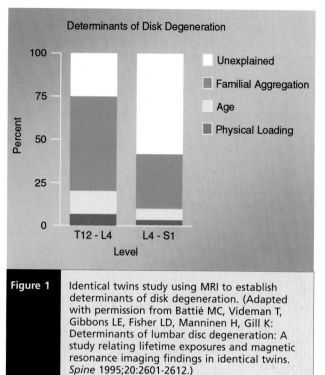

Figure 1 Identical twins study using MRI to establish determinants of disk degeneration. (Adapted with permission from Battié MC, Videman T, Gibbons LE, Fisher LD, Manninen H, Gill K: Determinants of lumbar disc degeneration: A study relating lifetime exposures and magnetic resonance imaging findings in identical twins. *Spine* 1995;20:2601-2612.)

activities, whole-body vibration, and the performance of nursing tasks, heavy physical work, and working with the trunk in a bent or twisted position were associated with adult low back pain, whereas sitting, prolonged standing and/or walking, and participation in leisure sports activities were not associated with low back pain.[16]

In a study of pairs of identical twins from the Finnish Twin Registry, the authors found a substantial genetic influence in degenerative back disorders and provided a list of the genes associated with the disorders.[17] Despite an extraordinary discordance between twin siblings in occupational and leisure time physical loading conditions on the spine throughout adulthood, surprisingly little effect on disk degeneration was observed. No evidence was found to suggest that exposure to whole-body vibration in motor vehicles leads to accelerated degenerative changes. Some evidence was found that routine spinal loading was actually beneficial to lumbar disks. The effects of personal physical factors such as body weight and muscle strength on disk degeneration were modest, and much greater than the minimal effect of occupational physical demands. The most striking visual evidence in this article, and in prior publications from the same study group, is the series of MRIs that show identical lumbar MRIs in identical twins regardless of the physical loading. The authors found that familial aggregation (heredity) was the best predictor of lumbar disk degeneration as seen in **Figure 1**.

Thus, the idea that repetitive activity, minor trauma, or lifting is actually the cause of low back disorders in adults of working age is being seriously questioned in

scientific studies, despite compensation systems accepting these long-held beliefs.

The decision on causation in cases of potentially compensable injuries is further confounded by the patient history. In many instances, the key piece of evidence alleging that a spinal disorder should be considered work-related or compensable is the patient's own reported history of no prior spinal pain or problems before the onset of pain at work, and of no potential confounders such as substance abuse or psychiatric disorders. In a 2009 study, 335 adults who reported back pain after a motor vehicle crash were randomly selected from the outpatient clinics of five spine specialists.[18] The authors correlated information retrieved from a search of prior medical records with the patients' self-reported history. They found that approximately 50% of the patients had previously reported axial pain based on the medical record audit; however, none had reported the prior pain to the spine specialist after their motor vehicle crash. The medical record audit also showed that approximately 75% of the patients had one or more preexisting comorbid conditions (alcohol abuse, illicit drug use, and psychological diagnosis) that were not reported to the spine specialist. In the patients who perceived that the crash was the fault of another person, the rate of documented previous back and neck pain based on the past medical records was more than twice the self-reported rate ($P < 0.01$). The rate of documented preexisting psychological disorders in the past medical records was more than seven times the rate of self-reported psychological problems ($P < 0.001$). In patients who perceived that the crash was their own fault or no one's fault, a decreased rate of underreporting of axial pain and comorbid conditions was found. Therefore, if a physician bases causation decisions solely on the alleged temporality of a condition without a review of prior medical records, causation conclusions may be flawed.

The physician must understand that occupational causation involves medical and legal requirements.[19] Medical causation deals with scientific cause and effect. Legal causation arises from a desire for social justice, not science, and requires two separate and distinct components: cause in fact and proximate (or legal) cause.[9] Proximate cause is the defendant's (employer's) alleged action that started the chain of events that led to the injury, whereas cause in fact is typically the actual traumatic event (for example, the proximate cause could be a defective warning signal at a railroad crossing, and the cause in fact could be the train striking the car crossing the railroad tracks).

A systematic approach for assessing epidemiologic studies and their application for determining work-relatedness (occupational causation) is in the public domain and is available on the Internet[20] and in the published literature.[21] This approach is consistent with the principles of using evidence-based medicine for establishing clinical treatment guidelines.

Return to Work

Why is staying at work or returning to work in the patient's best interest? For most people, work plays an important role in giving meaning and purpose to life as well as providing income for life's necessities.[22] Being unemployed when young or old enough to be working actually causes physical disease, premature mortality, and emotional problems.[22] Consensus statements by the Canadian Medical Association,[23] the American College of Occupational and Environmental Medicine,[24] the American Academy of Orthopaedic Surgeons,[25] and the American Medical Association (AMA)[26] all support and strongly recommend that physicians return patients to their usual work roles as soon as possible. Another view of the importance of staying at work or returning to work is a 2008 study that showed that inactivity was the only modifiable factor found to be predictive of total health care costs; this factor also appears to have an increasing effect with advancing age.[27]

Assessing the Patient's Risk, Capacity, and Tolerance for Work

Physicians are often asked for medical information and work status certification. In other words, "How do I fill out the return-to-work forms indicating what a patient should be safely able to do at work?" The key concepts for the physician to understand are risk, capacity, and tolerance.[28]

Risk refers to the chance of harm to the patient or to the general public if the patient engages in specific work activities. Risk is the basis for physician-imposed work restrictions, which are requested on many return-to-work forms. The physician should consider risk as two parts. First is the concept of risk reduction, which involves preventing a patient from doing something that the patient may be able to do but might cause harm. The second concept involves having the physician avoid preventing a patient from doing something that they are otherwise capable of doing (avoiding iatrogenic disability behavior). Unfortunately, there is little scientific literature on the entailed risks of working for employees with known medical conditions. For example, patients with osteonecrosis of the femoral head may be restricted from medium, heavy, or very heavy labor to minimize the progressive collapse of the femoral head. Although such a restriction would appear to be based on common sense, there are no published studies to indicate exactly how much weight an employee with femoral head osteonecrosis can safely handle.

Capacity refers to the ability to perform a task and is usually measured by strength, flexibility, and endurance. Capacity implies that the individual is already maximally trained and fully acclimated to the job or activity in question. Current ability can often be increased toward achieving maximum capacity by conditioning, which can either be accomplished with formal physical therapy or by work restrictions that progressively decrease over time. Capacity is the basis for physician-described work limitations. Many return-to-work forms ask the physician to provide work limitations for the patient based on the concept of capacity or ability. For example, if after a rotator cuff repair, a patient lacks the shoulder motion to reach an overhead control of a factory punch press, the patient lacks the capacity (has a work limitation) to do this task. The physician's work guideline describes what the patient is not physically able to do.

Tolerance refers to the biopsychosocial aspect of the patient. Tolerance is the basis for a patient's decision if the rewards of work (such as money and self-esteem) exceed the cost of work (such as pain and fatigue). The tolerance level is one of the factors that makes a person unique and involves how each person deals with other people, stress, pain, and impairment. Tolerance is often affected by motivation and rewards and is not scientifically measurable or verifiable. Tolerance is frequently less than either capacity or current ability in a compensated population, although tolerance may be higher than capacity if there is high incentive or personal motivation. Shortly after a significant injury or surgery, tolerance for pain may be a basis for a physician to certify that a patient should not work; however, many return-to-work forms do not ask that a physician list tolerance issues. Thus, after a rotator cuff repair, a physician may certify a work absence of a few days for a patient who performs sedentary desk work that can be done with one hand. For chronic conditions, tolerance is the basis by which the patient (not the physician) decides if the rewards of the job exceed the costs (symptoms). If there is no significant risk, and the patient can do the task despite symptoms, the decision to work, to change careers, or to apply for disability should be the patient's decision. In these cases, the physician should not impose restrictions or claim limitations but should indicate on evaluation forms that the patient may choose to work.

Studies have been conducted with physicians in many specialties using return-to-work vignettes to elicit ideal responses. Results show a striking lack of consistency among different physicians in determining work guidelines and restrictions; however, there is less variability in the decisions of an individual physician in implementing similar guidelines on different occasions for patients with similar cases.[29]

Point of View

The biologic model of disease used by Western culture has typically focused on the physical aspects of illness; the nonphysical suffering associated with disease and injury are often ignored. With this disease model, a physician may be inclined to misinterpret a patient's distress or anxiety about a medical condition as indicative of a more serious physical condition, requiring more elaborate treatment or diagnostic testing, rather than understanding the distress as an indication that

1: Principles of Orthopaedics

the patient is having difficulty coping because of psychosocial or other extraneous stressors. It is precisely this inability to differentiate, by some clinicians, between a patient's pain and/or distress and the underlying pathology that becomes an obstacle to improving management of many disorders, especially in workers' compensation cases.

Perhaps in part because of personal experience or medical school training, physicians have a bias against the importance of initially approaching the injury care of a patient using a biopsychosocial model of disease rather than the purely biologic approach. The initial treating physician can and should address the psychosocial issues that play such a large role in cases in which the injured worker is not recovering as expected.

When injured, the patient does not necessarily deal with the injury in an appropriate or inappropriate (dysfunctional) manner. Most patients deal with injury in stages. Understanding these stages allows for better treatment and appropriate intervention. In the acute injury stage, the degree of physical impairment usually correlates with identifiable physical and pathologic impairments that are expected with a given type of injury. The transition stage is the critical stage at which a physician should identify the patient in whom a chronic pain state or a dysfunctional attitude may develop. Often, such a patient will not be recovering as expected. The patient's subjective complaints exceed objective findings. The longer dysfunctional behaviors continue, the more entrenched the behaviors become. It is important for the physician to change management strategies to reduce the dysfunctional behavior. Physicians may administer a questionnaire such as the Fear Avoidance Belief Questionnaire and/or the Distress and Risk Assessment Method, which is a simple patient classification to identify distress and evaluate the risk of a poor outcome.[30,31] More complete guidance in using the biopsychosocial model is available in the literature.[32]

The learned stage of injury occurs when additional impairments and disabilities result from drug misuse, inactivity, and deconditioning. The patient becomes a professional patient and incorporates the sick patient role into all activities. Avoiding this stage is the key to good outcomes. The "Ds" is a memory device for physicians to aid awareness of the observable factors that may result in chronic preventable disability.[33,34] These factors include: (1) Dramatization—the patient's report of vague, diffuse, nonanatomic pain and the use of emotionally charged words to describe pain and suffering. Patients exhibit exaggerated histrionic behavior and a theatrical display of pain. (2) Drugs—the misuse of habit-forming pain medications or alcohol. (3) Dysfunction—stated bodily impairments related to various physical and emotional factors and a withdrawal from the fabric of life. Patients disengage from work and recreation and alienate friends, family, employers, and health care providers. (4) Dependency—the patient exhibits passivity, depression, and helplessness. (5) Disability—the patient's pain is contingent on financial compensation and pending litigation claims. (6) Duration—the pain persists long after tissue damage should

have healed and the disability persists long after impairments should have resolved. (7) Despair—patients become embittered, defensive, and rigid. The four manifestations of despair are depression, apprehension, irritability, and hostility. (8) Disuse—prolonged immobilization occurs. Pain is aggravated with attempts to resume normal activities.

To deal effectively with patients who are at risk for chronic preventable disability, the physician and employer must be actively involved in the patient's care. The physician must listen attentively to the patient and have a desire for the patient to get better. The physician must attempt to understand the patient's method of dealing with injury and pain, and should help the patient to become a more active and useful participant in life activities, including work. The physician needs to become a facilitator or rehabilitator by focusing on the patient's ability to function rather than on his or her pain. These patients are stuck, and the physician's challenge is to get them moving again. This concept has been paraphrased in Martin's Law of Return to Work Decision Making Entrophy: A Corollary to the Laws of Motion and Dynamics. Things at rest stay at rest, things in motion stay in motion unless acted upon by an outside force. Workers' compensation patients who are actively managed and allowed to return to normal continue to improve whereas patients left alone without proactive management tend to assume a disorganized state.

Impairment

Accurate and consistent impairment ratings continue to be a concern for the employee, employer, and rating physician. In an attempt to standardize and classify impairments, the AMA publishes the *Guides to the Evaluation of Permanent Impairment* (*Guides*). The workers' compensation systems of many states mandate the use of a specific edition of the *Guides* to determine an impairment percentage, or a number that attempts to quantify how serious the residual problems are after a compensable injury or illness. This often results in attempts to convert impairment (defined in the *Guides* as "a significant deviation, loss, or loss of use of any body structure or function in an individual with a health condition, disorder or disease") to disability (an umbrella term for activity limitations and/or participation restrictions in an individual with a health condition, disorder, or disease). The number (impairment percentage) is used in various ways by various jurisdictions to determine a financial award for the worker's injuries. Traditionally, physicians rate impairment (medical disorders) and the judicial system determines disability (how the impairment translates into an employment handicap). Understanding the differences between impairment and disability is crucial. There is no correlation between impairment and disability except in cases with extreme injury. Some physicians develop a reputation as being "friendly" to injured workers in rating impairments, whereas others develop a reputation as being "friendly" to employers. All physicians should be neutral and apply the *Guides* impartially. Differences in opinion about impairment ratings may result in extended litigation, which usually impacts treatment outcomes.

The first five editions of the *Guides*, published by the AMA from 1972 to 2000, used the same concept of medical impairment and basically the same methodology. In the sixth edition of the *Guides*, published in late 2007, the AMA used an entirely new conceptual model of impairment and disability created by the World Health Organization and adopted by 192 countries, including the United States. The new methodology is used to determine impairment. Physicians who provide patient ratings based on the *Guides* new model of impairment and disability will find it a more diagnosis-based model; however, it is less intuitive to use. Future refinement of the *Guides* should include reduced complexity, improved intrarater and interrater reliability, an evidence-based approach when available, and a rating more reflective of the loss of function.

Clinical Treatment Guidelines

The trend in workers' compensation is toward legislated clinical guidelines, which have the presumption of being correct for determining authorization for treatment. Some clinical guidelines are well developed using strict criteria and established levels of evidence. Such guidelines result in summarized consensus statements that often include discussions of prevention; diagnosis; prognosis; therapy, including dosage of medications; indications for tests and invasive treatment; risks and benefits; and cost-effectiveness. Additional objectives of clinical guidelines are to standardize medical care, to raise the quality of care, to reduce risks, and to achieve the best balance between cost and medical treatment.

Independent Medical Evaluations

An independent medical evaluation (IME) is a medical evaluation conducted by a physician who is not involved in the treatment of the individual being examined. Within the context of workers' compensation, an IME typically documents the worker's condition by addressing diagnosis, causation, functional status, treatment needs, maximum medical improvement determination, and impairment.[35] This information helps to determine appropriate assistance for the individual and aids in making a fair decision on the claim. A 2009 search of "independent medical examinations" using an Internet search engine returned 2,850,000 sites. Most of the sites were associated with personal injury attorneys with specific instructions (coaching) as to what IME examiners are expected to ask and with information on responding to their questions. Unfortunately, such coaching may inject disinformation into the evaluation.[36,37]

Ergonomics

Ergonomics is the science of fitting the job to the worker. Ergonomics is designed to consider the worker's physical capability, anatomy, and physiology (risk, capacity, and tolerance) and match these factors to the job requirements. Strategies for preventing workplace injuries can begin with epidemiologically-based recommendations regarding relative risks.[38,39] Reducing workplace risks should logically be balanced with reducing individual risks, such as reducing obesity and smoking.[40]

Summary

The treatment of workers' compensation injury patients is a significant part of many orthopaedic practices. Most orthopaedic residencies prepare their graduates to provide excellent biomedical care but may not provide training in the biopsychosocial and legal issues that orthopaedic surgeons confront daily when caring for workers' compensation patients. Recently, important research has been published to help orthopaedic surgeons understand the complex issues of medical-legal causation and the biopsychosocial treatment of work-related injuries and illnesses.

Annotated References

1. Bernacki EJ, Tao XG: The relationship between attorney involvement, claim duration, and workers' compensation costs. *J Occup Environ Med* 2008;50(9):1013-1018.

   A review of 738 claims with attorney involvement and 6,191 claims without attorney involvement paid by the Louisiana Workers' Compensation Corporation showed that attorney involvement resulted in increased claim duration and workers' compensation costs.

2. Robertson J, Corro D: Workers Compensation vs. Group Health: A Comparison of Utilization. NCCI Research Brief, November, 2006. http://www.ncci.com/documents/research-wc-vs-group-health.pdf. Accessed March 31, 2010.

3. Brinker MR, O'Connor DP, Woods GW, Pierce P, Peck B: The effect of payer type on orthopaedic practice expenses. *J Bone Joint Surg Am* 2002;84A(10):1816-1822.

4. Blum F, Burton JF Jr: Workers' compensation costs in 2007: Regional, industrial, and other variations. Workers Compensation Policy Review, 2008. John Burton's Workers' Compensation Resources Web site. http://www.workerscompresources.com/WCPR_Public/WCPR%20PDFs/MA08.pdf. Accessed March 31, 2010.

   The four types of workers' compensation cash benefits are examined. The concept of operational versus purpose of benefits is discussed.

1: Principles of Orthopaedics

5. Kasdan ML, Vender MI, Lewis K, Stallings SP, Melhorn JM: Carpal tunnel syndrome: Effects of litigation on utilization of health care and physician workload. *J Ky Med Assoc* 1996;94(7):287-290.

6. Harris I, Mulford J, Solomon M, van Gelder JM, Young J: Association between compensation status and outcome after surgery: A meta-analysis. *JAMA* 2005; 293(13):1644-1652.

7. Sander RA, Meyers JE: The relationship of disability to compensation status in railroad workers. *Spine (Phila Pa 1976)* 1986;11(2):141-143.

8. Genovese E: Causality, in Demeter SL, Andersson GBJ, eds: *Disability Evaluations*. Chicago, IL, American Medical Association, 2003, pp 95-100.

9. Melhorn JM, Ackerman WE, Glass LS, Deitz DC: Understanding work-relatedness, in Melhorn JM, Ackerman WE, eds: *Guides to the Evaluation of Disease and Injury Causation*. Chicago, IL, American Medical Association Press, 2008, pp 13-32.

   The authors discuss work-related issues with regard to causation of diseases and injuries using an evidence-based medicine approach.

10. Melhorn JM, Ackerman WE: Introduction, in Melhorn JM, Ackerman WE, eds: *Guides to the Evaluation of Disease and Injury Causation*. Chicago, IL, American Medical Association Press, 2008, pp 1-12.

    The authors discuss the methodology for determining causation of diseases and injuries using an evidence-based medicine approach.

11. Brady W, Bass J, Moser R Jr , Anstadt GW, Loeppke RR, Leopold R: Defining total corporate health and safety costs: Significance and impact. Review and recommendations. *J Occup Environ Med* 1997;39(3):224-231.

12. Lozano-Calderón S, Anthony S, Ring D: The quality and strength of evidence for etiology: Example of carpal tunnel syndrome. *J Hand Surg Am* 2008;33(4):525-538.

    A quantitative scoring system was developed to review the literature for quality and strength based on Bradford Hill criteria for causal association between carpal tunnel syndrome and physical activities. The etiology of carpal tunnel syndrome is largely structural, genetic, and biologic, with environmental and occupational factors such as repetitive hand use playing a minor and more debatable role.

13. Fisher B, Gorsche R: *Diagnosis, Causation and Treatment of Carpal Tunnel Syndrome: An Evidence-Based Assessment*. Alberta, CA, Workers' Compensation Board, 2006, pp 1-153.

14. Carragee E, Alamin T, Cheng I, Franklin T, Hurwitz E: Does minor trauma cause serious low back illness? *Spine (Phila Pa 1976)* 2006;31(25):2942-2949.

15. Carragee E, Alamin T, Cheng I, Franklin T, van den Haak E, Hurwitz E: Are first-time episodes of serious LBP associated with new MRI findings? *Spine J* 2006; 6(6):624-635.

16. Bakker EW, Verhagen AP, van Trijffel E, Lucas C, Koes BW: Spinal mechanical load as a risk factor for low back pain: A systematic review of prospective cohort studies. *Spine (Phila Pa 1976)* 2009;34(8):E281-E293.

    A meta-analysis was performed to review the past literature for spinal mechanical loading as a risk factor for low back pain. The authors found 18 high-quality methodological articles, which allowed the review of 24,315 subjects. The authors reported that the evidence for associations was conflicting.

17. Battié MC, Videman T, Kaprio J, et al: The Twin Spine Study: Contributions to a changing view of disc degeneration. *Spine J* 2009;9(1):47-59.

    A multicenter study of twins reported that the once commonly held view that disk degeneration is primarily a result of aging and mechanical insults and injuries is not supported by evidence from this study.

18. Don AS, Carragee EJ: Is the self-reported history accurate in patients with persistent axial pain after a motor vehicle accident? *Spine J* 2009;9(1):4-12.

    A multicenter validation study of 702 patients found that the accuracy of a self-reported history for persistent axial back pain after a motor vehicle crash was poor; results were worse in patients who perceived that another person was at fault for the crash.

19. Hegmann KT, Oostema SJ: Causal associations and determination of work-relatedness, in Melhorn JM, Ackerman WE, eds: *Guides to the Evaluation of Disease and Injury Causation*. Chicago, IL, American Medical Association Press, 2006, pp 33-46.

20. Causation methodology procedure: The approach on how to determine causation. Download 8504. CtdMAP Web site. http://www.ctdmap.com/DownLoadsInfo/default.aspx. Accessed April 2, 2010.

    A method for determining work-relatedness was created for evaluating the scientific evidence using standardized quality scoring processes. The framework for how to determine causation for specific activities, conditions, or events is presented. This methodology was placed into the public domain and may be freely copied or reprinted if the reference source is appropriately acknowledged.

21. Melhorn JM, Ackerman WE, eds: *Guides to the Evaluation of Disease and Injury Causation*. Chicago, IL, American Medical Association Press, 2008.

    This textbook presents a review and detailed discussion of the medical literature regarding causation of diseases and injuries.

22. Waddell G, Burton AK: *Is Work Good for Your Health and Well-Being?* Norwich, England, Stationery Office, 2006.

23. Canadian Medical Association: The physician's role in helping patients return to work after an illness or injury. *CMAJ* 1997;156(5):680A-680F.

24. The Personal Physician's Role in Helping Patients with Medical Conditions Stay at Work or Return to Work, 2008. American College of Occupational and Environmental Medicine Web site. http://www.acoem.org/guidelines.aspx?id=5460. Accessed March 31, 2010.

   The American College of Occupational and Environmental Medicine provides their position statement on the benefits of returning to work after illness or injury.

25. Position statement: Early return to work programs. American Academy of Orthopaedic Surgeons Web site. http://www.aaos.org/about/papers/position/1150.asp. Accessed March 31, 2010.

   AAOS supports safe and early return-to-work programs and believes that these programs are in the best interest of patients in an effort to help the injured workers improve performance, regain functionality, and enhance quality of life. The success of an early return-to-work program is dependent on appropriate planning as well as attention to a host of physical, psychological, and environmental factors.

26. Report 12 of the Council on Scientific Affairs: Physician Guidelines for Return to Work After Injury or Illness. 2004. American Medical Association Web site. http://www.ama-assn.org/ama/no-index/about-ama/13609.shtml. Accessed March 31, 2010.

27. Wilkerson GB, Boer NF, Smith CB, Heath GW: Health-related factors associated with the healthcare costs of office workers. *J Occup Environ Med* 2008;50(5):593-601.

   A study of 214 employees found that inactivity was the only modifiable factor predictive of total health care costs among officer workers.

28. Talmage JB, Melhorn JM: How to think about work ability and work restrictions: Capacity, tolerance, and risk, in Talmage JB, Melhorn JM, eds: *A Physician's Guide to Return to Work*. Chicago, IL, American Medical Association, 2005, pp 7-18.

29. Rainville J, Pransky GS, Indahl A, Mayer EK: The physician as disability advisor for patients with musculoskeletal complaints. *Spine (Phila Pa 1976)* 2005;30(22):2579-2584.

30. Waddell G, Newton M, Henderson I, Somerville D, Main CJ: A Fear-Avoidance Beliefs Questionnaire (FABQ) and the role of fear-avoidance beliefs in chronic low back pain and disability. *Pain* 1993;52(2):157-168.

31. Main CJ, Wood PL, Hollis S, Spanswick CC, Waddell G: The distress and risk assessment method: A simple patient classification to identify distress and evaluate the risk of poor outcome. *Spine (Phila Pa 1976)* 1992;17(1):42-52.

32. Kendall NA, Burton AK: *Tracking Musculoskeletal Problems: The Psychosocial Flags Framework: A Guide for Clinic and Workplace*. London, England, The Stationery Office, 2009.

   This textbook helps treating physicians to better understand the psychosocial impact of musculoskeletal pain and the patient's ability to perform work tasks.

33. Brena SF, Champman SL: Pain and litigation, in Wall PD, Melzack R, eds: *Textbook of Pain*. New York, NY, Churchill Livingstone, 1984, pp 832-839.

34. Melhorn JM: Stay at work and return to work for upper limb conditions, in Melhorn JM, Yodlowski ML, eds: *10th Annual AAOS Occupational Orthopaedics and Workers' Compensation: A Multidisciplinary Perspective*. Rosemont, IL, American Academy of Orthopaedic Surgeons, 2008, pp 103-120.

   The author presents a review of factors that predict disability and details information on returning the patient to work.

35. Melhorn JM: Forward, in Grace TG, ed: *Independent Medical Evaluations*. Rosemont, IL, American Academy of Orthopaedic Surgeons, 2001, pp vii-viii.

36. Barth RJ: Observation compromises the credibility of an evaluation. *American Medical Association Guides Newsletter*, July-August 2007, pp 1-5.

   A review of the impact of having an observer present during the completion of an independent medical evaluation is presented.

37. Cain DM, Detsky AS: Everyone's a little bit biased (even physicians). *JAMA* 2008;299(24):2893-2895.

   This commentary reviews biases in the developed policies and guidelines in response to increasing concerns over potential conflicts of interest.

38. Melhorn JM, Wilkinson LK, O'Malley MD: Successful management of musculoskeletal disorders. *J Hum Ecolog Risk Assessment* 2001;7:1801-1810.

39. Kasdan ML: Upper-extremity cumulative trauma disorders of workers in aircraft manufacturing. *J Occup Environ Med* 1998;40(1):12-15.

40. Amadio PC: Work-related illness, cumulative trauma, and compensation, in Koval KJ, ed: *Orthopaedic Knowledge Update 7*. Rosemont, IL, American Academy of Orthopaedic Surgeons, 2002, pp 121-125.

Chapter 14

Evidence-Based Orthopaedics: Levels of Evidence and Guidelines in Orthopaedic Surgery

Kanu Okike, MD, MPH   Mininder S. Kocher, MD, MPH

Introduction

Evidence-based medicine is "the conscientious, explicit, and judicious use of current best evidence in making decisions about the care of individual patients."[1] Although this form of medical practice is often contrasted with decision making on the basis of opinion and experience (a phenomenon sometimes termed "eminence-based medicine"[2]), it is important to note that the ideal practice of evidence-based medicine involves "integrating individual clinical expertise with the best available external clinical evidence from systematic research."[1]

Although the term "evidence-based medicine" did not appear in the medical literature until 1992,[3] it has since become the dominant paradigm in the practice of clinical medicine. Orthopaedic surgery has been no exception,[4-6] as evidence-based medicine has generally been welcomed by practicing orthopaedists.[7]

Along with this increased emphasis on evidence in clinical decision making, there has developed a need for the critical analysis of scientific research. Studies may be subject to bias, confounding, and other shortcomings, which may limit the extent to which the data may be used to guide the clinical care of patients. Therefore, hierarchical level of evidence classification systems have been developed to aid in the assessment of research quality.

The movement toward evidence-based medicine has also created a need for mechanisms to synthesize the available evidence and distill it into a form that can be used effectively by practicing physicians. The sheer volume of the scientific literature, coupled with ever-present time constraints, means that it is no longer feasible for physicians to critically review all studies published in one's field.[8] Clinical practice guidelines, which provide recommendations for the management of specific conditions based on a systematic review of the best available evidence, are well placed to satisfy this growing need.

Levels of Evidence

History and Purpose

The concept of grading studies on the basis of their methodology was first proposed in a 1986 article on the use of antithrombotic agents.[9] The Journal of Bone and Joint Surgery: American volume was the first orthopaedic publication to adopt the classification system, as it began assigning levels of evidence to all clinical studies published in the Journal in 2003.[10] In the adoption of this classification system, the Journal's goals were threefold: to familiarize authors, reviewers, and readers with the concept of levels of evidence; to improve orthopaedic studies via the explicit articulation of a primary research question; and to place clinical research studies into context for the reader.[10]

Over the past few years, several other orthopaedic journals have adopted similar level of evidence classification systems, including Clinical Orthopaedics and Related Research, Arthroscopy, The American Journal of Sports Medicine, and The Journal of Hand Surgery.[11-13] The American Academy of Orthopaedic Surgeons (AAOS) followed suit by adopting its own level of evidence classification system in 2005[14] (**Table 1**).

Assigning Levels of Evidence

There are three basic steps in the assignment of a level of evidence to a particular clinical study: determine the primary research question, establish the study type, and assign a level of evidence.[15]

Dr. Kocher or an immediate family member serves as a board member, owner, officer, or committee member of The American Orthopaedic Society for Sports Medicine, The Arthritis Foundation, and The Pediatric Orthopaedic Society of North America; serves as a paid consultant to or is an employee of Biomet, CONMED Linvatec, Smith & Nephew, Covidien, OrthoPediatrics, and Gerson Lehrman Group; and has received research or institutional support from CONMED Linvatec. Dr Okike has received research or institutional support from Depuy Orthopaedics.

Table 1

Levels of Evidence for Primary Research Question

Types of Studies[a]

	Therapeutic Studies Investigating the results of treatment	Prognostic Studies Investigating the effect of a patient characteristic on the outcome of disease	Diagnostic Studies Investigating a diagnostic test	Economic and Decision Analyses Developing an economic model or decision model
Level I	High-quality randomized trial with statistically significant difference but narrow CIs Systematic review[b] of level I RCTs (and study results were homogeneous[c])	High-quality prospective study[d] (all patients were enrolled at the same point in their disease with ≥ 80% follow-up of enrolled patients) Systematic review[b] of level I studies	Testing of previously developed diagnostic criteria on consecutive patients (with universally applied reference "gold" standard) Systematic review[b] of level II studies	Sensible costs and alternatives; values obtained from many studies; with multiway sensitivity analyses Systematic review[b] of level I studies
Level II	Lesser-quality RCT (eg, < 80% follow-up, no blinding, or improper randomization) Prospective[d] comparative study[e] Systematic review[b] of level II studies or level I studies with inconsistent results	Retrospective[f] study Untreated controls from an RCT Lesser-quality prospective study (eg, patients enrolled at different points in their disease or < 80% follow-up)	Development of diagnostic criteria on consecutive patients (with universally applied reference "gold" standard) Systematic review[b] of level II studies	Sensible costs and alternatives; values obtained from limited studies; with multiway sensitivity review Systematic review[b] of level II studies
Level III	Case-control study[g] Retrospective[f] comparative study[e] Systematic review[b] of level III studies	Case-control study[g]	Study of nonconsecutive patients; without consistently applied reference "gold" standard Systematic review[b] of level III studies	Analyses based on limited alternatives and costs; poor estimates Systematic review[b] of level II studies
Level IV	Case series[h]	Case series	Case-control study Poor reference standard	Analyses with no sensitivity analyses
Level V	Expert opinion	Expert opinion	Expert opinion	Expert opinion

RCT = randomized controlled trial; CI = confidence interval
[a] A complete assessment of quality of individual studies requires critical appraisal of all aspects of the study design.
[b] A combination of results from two or more prior studies.
[c] Studies provided consistent results.
[d] Study was started before the first patient enrolled.
[e] Patients treated one way (eg, cemented hip arthroplasty) compared with a group of patients treated another way (eg, uncemented hip arthroplasty) at the same institution.
[f] The study was started after the first patient enrolled.
[g] Patients identified for the study based on their outcome, called "cases" (eg, failed total arthroplasty), are compared with those patients who did not have outcome, called "controls" (eg, successful total hip arthroplasty).
[h] Patients treated one way with no comparison group of patients treated another way.
Reproduced from American Academy of Orthopaedic Surgeons: Levels of evidence for primary research question. Available at: http://www.aaos.org/Research/Committee/Evidence/loetable1.pdf. Accessed July 23, 2010.

It is important to note that levels of evidence are applied to the primary research question of a given study only. Although a study may have multiple research questions, only one should be designated as primary. The primary research question of a given study should be specified by the authors, preferably at the time of study inception.

Once the primary research question has been determined, the study type must be established. In the clas-

sification scheme used by the AAOS as well as several orthopaedic journals, including *The Journal of Bone and Joint Surgery*, studies are categorized as therapeutic, prognostic, diagnostic, or economic/decision analysis (discussed in detail in the next sections). Although nearly all clinical studies can be placed into one of these categories, the categorization scheme is not exhaustive and it is possible for a particular study to not fit neatly into any one of the above categories. Only after the primary research question has been determined and the study type has been established can a specific level of evidence be assigned (**Table 1**).

Therapeutic Studies

Therapeutic studies investigate the effect of treatment on the outcome of disease and represent the most common type of study in the orthopaedic literature.[16-18]

Level I therapeutic studies are high-quality randomized controlled trials (RCTs), which are generally considered to represent the best possible evidence available. To be considered a high-quality study, an RCT must satisfy several criteria. It must be appropriately powered, either by detecting a significant difference (in the case of a "positive" trial) or documenting sufficient power (in the case of a "negative" trial). High-quality RCTs must use an appropriate randomization technique, in which allocation of the next study participant cannot be determined by members of the research team before the patient receives his or her treatment allocation. Rates of follow-up must be high – generally above 80%. Whenever possible, patients, caregivers, and researchers should be blinded to the treatment assignment. This is by no means an exhaustive list, and there are several other characteristics that must be fulfilled for a trial to be considered of high quality. However, one can reliably assume that studies not fulfilling the above criteria will generally not be considered level I evidence.

Level II therapeutic studies include lesser-quality RCTs (as previously discussed), as well as prospective comparative studies. Comparative studies (also known as cohort studies) involve the comparison of one group of patients treated in a particular way with another group of patients treated in another way. For example, a study comparing the outcomes of patients with intertrochanteric hip fractures treated with a sliding hip screw or a cephalomedullary device would be considered a comparative (or cohort) study. Although the distinction between prospective and retrospective can sometimes be confusing,[15] AAOS considers prospective investigations to be those in which the study was initiated (the research question was posed) before the first patient was enrolled or treated.

Level III therapeutic studies include retrospective comparative studies (as previously discussed), as well as case-control studies. Case-control studies, which are retrospective, involve the comparison of one group of patients who have a particular outcome with another group of patients who do not have the outcome of interest. These "case" and "control" groups are compared to each other on the basis of characteristics plausibly associated with the outcome of interest. For example, a comparison of children who developed slipped capital femoral epiphysis to a similar group of children who did not develop this condition would be considered to be a case-control study. Such a comparison could be made on the basis of risk factors, such as obesity or sex.

Level IV therapeutic studies, which represent the most common type of study in the orthopaedic

literature,[16-19] are case series of patients treated in one way without any comparison group of patients treated in another way. Although the evidence provided by this type of study is relatively low in the level of evidence hierarchy, it is important to emphasize that these studies do have their place in the orthopaedic literature. If a level IV case series is well executed, it can provide important information to guide patient care. A well-designed case series is one that has 100% of patients with the same diagnosis, strict inclusion and exclusion criteria, a standard treatment protocol, patient follow-up at specified time intervals, well-defined outcome measures that include clinical parameters, and validated patient-derived instruments for functional assessment.[17]

Expert opinion, without the support of clinical data, is considered to be level V evidence. This is true for all study types, including therapeutic studies.

The terms "systematic review" and "meta-analysis" are often assumed to be interchangeable, but their definitions do differ slightly. Whereas a systematic review is a comprehensive literature search to identify studies appropriate for answering a particular clinical question, a meta-analysis is a statistical method of combining the data provided by these studies. Combining multiple studies into a single meta-analysis may address problems of small sample size and insufficient power, but it will not alter the level of evidence because meta-analyses are assigned levels of evidence based on the quality of the studies used in the meta-analysis.

Nontherapeutic Studies

Prognostic studies, which represent the second most common type of study in the orthopaedic literature,[16-18] investigate the effect of a patient characteristic on the outcome of disease. Differentiating between therapeutic and prognostic studies can be difficult because both examine the effects of factors with the potential to influence the outcome of disease. James Wright, MD, MPH, Associate Editor for Evidence-Based Orthopaedics at *The Journal of Bone and Joint Surgery: American volume*, suggests considering whether the factor of interest can be randomized or not: "If [a factor] can be randomly allocated, one is dealing with a therapeutic study."[15] For example, an investigation of physical therapy on outcome after proximal humerus fracture would be considered a therapeutic study, whereas an investigation of the effect of age following this same injury would be considered to be a prognostic study. The criteria for assigning levels of evidence to prognostic studies are detailed in **Table 1**.

Diagnostic studies are the third most common type of study in the orthopaedic literature[16-18] and evaluate the performance of tests designed to detect the presence or absence of a particular condition. Of central importance in the evaluation of a diagnostic test is the "gold standard," a second diagnostic test generally regarded to provide the most definitive evidence for or against the presence of a particular condition. For example, a study evaluating the ability of physical examination to

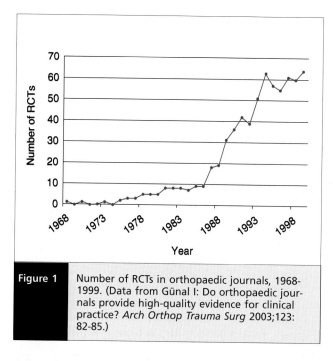

Figure 1 Number of RCTs in orthopaedic journals, 1968-1999. (Data from Günal I: Do orthopaedic journals provide high-quality evidence for clinical practice? *Arch Orthop Trauma Surg* 2003;123: 82-85.)

detect a meniscal tear could use arthroscopy as the gold standard. For a diagnostic study to be considered of high quality, there must be a gold standard that is universally applied to all cases. (In the previous example, all study participants would have to undergo arthroscopy for it to be considered a high-quality diagnostic study.) Another feature of high-quality diagnostic studies is the inclusion of consecutive patients, as detailed in **Table 1**.

The final study type included in the AAOS level of evidence classification system is economic and decision analyses. This study type is relatively uncommon in the orthopaedic literature, as it has been found to represent less than 1% of clinical studies published in orthopaedic journals.[16-18] Details on the criteria used to assign levels of evidence to these types of studies are described in **Table 1**.

Interrater Reliability in the Assignment of Levels of Evidence

For the level of evidence classification system to be most useful, there must be consistency of grade assignment between different raters. Recently, there have been several studies assessing interrater agreement in the assignment of levels of evidence to orthopaedic research, and interrater reliability has been found to range widely.[16-18,20,21]

One of the factors that appears to influence interrater reliability is the training and experience of the raters who are submitting level of evidence grades. For example, in a study of individuals reviewing manuscripts for *The Journal of Bone and Joint Surgery: American volume*, the authors found that reviewers with training in epidemiology demonstrated near-perfect agreement (intraclass correlation coefficient [ICC] of 0.99 to 1.00, versus 0.61

to 0.75 for reviewers not trained in epidemiology).[16] Similarly, the authors of another study found that agreement in the assignment of level of evidence was higher among experienced reviewers (practicing orthopaedic surgeons) than between experienced and inexperienced reviewers (orthopaedic residents and medical students) (kappa 0.75 versus 0.62).[17] In addition, the ability of orthopaedic residents to identify the level of evidence of 10 blinded articles from *The Journal of Bone and Joint Surgery: American volume*, was assessed. The mean percentage correct was found to be only 29.5% (41.3% after an educational intervention).[21]

Most recently, the feasibility of assigning levels of evidence to abstracts presented at the AAOS Annual Meeting was examined. In particular, the levels of evidence assigned by authors, volunteer graders (with access to the abstract only), and session moderators (with access to the full paper) were examined. Agreement ranged from slight to moderate (kappa 0.16 to 0.46).[20] However, this study did not consider the experience or epidemiologic training of the raters in question. The study also found that authors tended to grade the level of evidence of their own work more favorably than did other graders,[20] which is a finding deserving of further investigation.

Current Levels of Evidence in the Orthopaedic Literature

Recent studies have been fairly consistent in describing the current status of the orthopaedic literature. The most common study type is therapeutic (69% to 71%), followed by prognostic (20% to 25%), diagnostic (6% to 9%), and economic/decision analysis (0% to 0.5%).[16,17] With regard to level of evidence, level IV studies comprise 54% to 58% of the orthopaedic literature, whereas level I evidence accounts for only 11% to 16%.[16-18] Upon closer examination of the level I data, many of these studies appear to have shortcomings.[22,23]

However, recent studies provide reason to be optimistic regarding levels of evidence in the orthopaedic literature. In a 2009 study, 551 articles in *The Journal of Bone and Joint Surgery: American volume* published over the past 30 years were examined. The percentage of clinical studies providing level I evidence increased from 4% to 21% between 1975 and 2005, while the percentage of level IV studies decreased from 81% to 48% over this same period.[24] An earlier study found that the number of randomized trials published in orthopaedic journals increased substantially between 1968 and 1999[25] (**Figure 1**). Similar trends have been observed within the subspecialty field of sports medicine, as a 2005 study documented significant increases in the number of randomized controlled trials and prospective cohort studies coupled with a significant decrease in the number of case series and descriptive studies between 1991-1993 and 2001-2003.[26]

In recent years, some researchers have sought to investigate the relationship between levels of evidence and other factors in orthopaedic research. Manuscripts

Table 2

Grades of Recommendation

Grade	Overall Quality of Evidence	Description of Evidence
A	Good-quality evidence	More than one level I study with consistent findings for or against recommending intervention
B	Fair-quality evidence	More than one level II or III study with consistent findings or a single Level I study for or against recommending intervention.
C	Poor-quality evidence	More than one level IV or V study or a single level II or III study for or against recommending intervention
I	No evidence or conflicting evidence	There is insufficient or conflicting evidence not allowing a recommendation for or against intervention.

Data from Grades of Recommendation for Summaries or Reviews of Orthopaedic Surgical Studies. Rosemont, IL, American Academy of Orthopaedic Surgeons. Http://www.aaos.org/research/evidence/gradesofrec.asp. Accessed Nov. 10, 2010.

submitted to *The Journal of Bone and Joint Surgery: American volume* were studied; studies with a higher level of evidence were more likely to be accepted for publication.[19] Articles published in three prominent general orthopaedics journals also were examined, and it was found that studies with a higher level of evidence were also more likely to be cited following publication.[27] The relationship between level of evidence and declared funding support was examined in a recent study. It was determined that industry-funded studies were more likely to provide level IV evidence than were studies funded by not-for-profit sources.[28] This last association has not been documented previously and is certainly deserving of further investigation.

Using Levels of Evidence in Orthopaedic Practice

The levels of evidence classification system provides a rapid assessment of study quality, which may help readers to quickly place studies into context. Because studies of higher level of evidence have greater methodologic safeguards against bias, they may provide better information to guide physicians in their care of patients.

However, it is important to emphasize that a level of evidence rating does not tell the whole story with regard to a particular study. Assignment of a particular level of evidence represents an assessment of the study design as reported by the authors but does not address other factors such as quality of data gathering or interpretation.[16] This is emphasized in the first footnote in **Table 1**, which states that "a complete assessment of [the] quality of individual studies requires critical appraisal of all aspects of the study design."[29] Levels of evidence cannot be used in a blind manner; orthopaedic surgeons must always consider all aspects of a given study, and integrate these data with their individual clinical expertise.

Clinical Practice Guidelines

History and Purpose

When medical decision making is based largely on opinion, wide variation in clinical practice is expected. Although variability certainly persists within the evidence-based model, large discrepancies in practice patterns invite investigation. It was in this context that the Institute of Medicine first proposed clinical practice guidelines, defined as "systematically developed statements to assist practitioner and patient decisions about appropriate health care for specific clinical circumstances."[30]

Since they were first proposed in 1990,[30] the number of such guidelines has grown rapidly. By August of 2010, for example, there were nearly 2,500 guidelines listed in the National Guideline Clearinghouse.[31]

Over the past few years, AAOS has begun to publish clinical practice guidelines on a variety of topics within orthopaedic surgery.[32] As of August 2010 there were nine such guidelines that had been approved by AAOS, with several more in various stages of the development process.

Developing Clinical Practice Guidelines

In the selection of topics for guideline development, ideal candidates include common conditions with a solid evidence base but wide variation in practice patterns. In these cases, clinical practice guidelines have the best opportunity to achieve their objectives of decreasing practice variability, optimizing clinical outcomes, and promoting cost efficiency.

The backbone of any clinical practice guideline is the literature review, which proceeds in a systematic and carefully considered manner. Retrospective case reviews are excluded, and underpowered studies are not considered (unless used as part of a de novo meta-analysis).

1: Principles of Orthopaedics

Table 3		

Sample of Recommendations From a Recent AAOS Clinical Practice Guideline on the Treatment of Pediatric Diaphyseal Femur Fractures

	Level of Evidence	Grade of Recommendation
1. We recommend that children younger than 36 months with a diaphyseal femur fracture be evaluated for child abuse.	II	A
2. Treatment with a Pavlik harness or a spica cast are options for infants 6 months and younger with a diaphyseal femur fracture.	IV	C
3. We suggest early spica casting or traction with delayed spica casting for children age 6 months to 5 years with a diaphyseal femur fracture with less than 2 cm of shortening.	II	B
8. It is an option for physicians to use flexible intramedullary nailing to treat children age 5 to 11 years diagnosed with diaphyseal femur fractures.	III	C
9. Rigid trochanteric entry nailing, submuscular plating, and flexible intramedullary nailing are treatment options for children age 11 years to skeletal maturity diagnosed with diaphyseal femur fractures, but piriformis or near piriformis entry rigid nailing are not treatment options.	IV	C
10. We are unable to recommend for or against removal of surgical implants from asymptomatic patients after treatment of diaphyseal femur fractures.	IV	Inconclusive

Adapted from American Academy of Orthopaedic Surgeons: *Treatment of Pediatric Diaphyseal Femur Fractures: Guideline and Evidence Report.* Rosemont, IL, American Academy of Orthopaedic Surgeons, 2009.

On the basis of the best available evidence, recommendations are made regarding the management of patients. Each recommendation carries a level of evidence derived from the data underlying the recommendation, as well as a grade of recommendation (**Table 2**). **Table 3** presents a sample of recommendations from a recent AAOS Clinical Practice Guideline on the management of pediatric diaphyseal femur fractures. Once a guideline has been created, it must undergo peer review and finally a thorough approval process. The entire process of developing an AAOS clinical practice guideline is quite extensive and usually takes 12 to 18 months to complete.

Concerns Regarding Clinical Practice Guidelines

Although clinical practice guidelines have generally been welcomed by the evidence-based medicine community, this reception has not been universal. Some argue, for example, that clinical practice guidelines erode physician autonomy and run the risk of transforming clinical practice into "cookbook medicine." Others complain that existing guidelines are too comprehensive or too narrowly focused, and quickly become outdated. Still others voice fears that guidelines will be used to critique the treatment decisions of physicians in legal and pay-for-performance settings.[33]

More recently, critics have pointed to the potential for bias in the recommendations made by clinical practice guideline authors. In a recent study of physicians who authored 44 clinical practice guidelines on common adult diseases, it was found that 87% of the au-

thors had some form of interaction with the pharmaceutical industry, including 59% who had relationships with companies whose products were considered in the guideline they authored. However, in only two cases were these personal financial interactions specifically disclosed in the final published guideline.[34] Although clinical practice guidelines are meant to be completely objective, the development process does involve subjective judgments where competing interests could come into play. AAOS has taken several steps to combat bias in the development of clinical practice guidelines, including requiring full conflict of interest disclosure from all authors and using well-defined, systematic processes that are transparent and reproducible.[35]

Using Clinical Practice Guidelines in Orthopaedic Practice

Like levels of evidence, clinical practice guidelines are not instruments to be used blindly. Guidelines provide recommendations that are to be carefully evaluated by each physician and integrated with his or her clinical expertise.[36] The Evidence-Based Medicine Working Group, writing in the *Journal of the American Medical Association (JAMA)* in 1995, proposed several questions that physicians should consider when using a particular clinical practice guideline.[37] In particular, clinicians are urged to evaluate the validity and content of the guideline recommendations, as well as their applicability to the patient in question. By following the steps outlined in this article, physicians have the best opportunity to use clinical practice guidelines in a manner that will provide the greatest benefit for their patients.

Summary

Levels of evidence and clinical practice guidelines are tools of the evidence-based medicine movement that can help physicians provide better care for their patients. They do not represent "cookbook" instructions to be followed blindly, but rather instruments to be carefully evaluated and integrated with clinical expertise.

There is reason to be optimistic regarding evidence-based practice in the field of orthopaedic surgery. Levels of evidence are steadily increasing in the orthopaedic literature, and randomized trials are becoming more common. Several carefully researched clinical practice guidelines have recently been approved by AAOS, and others are under development. These advances have the potential to not only enhance the orthopaedic evidence base but also improve patient care.

Annotated References

1. Sackett DL, Rosenberg WM, Gray JA, Haynes RB, Richardson WS: Evidence based medicine: What it is and what it isn't. *BMJ* 1996;312(7023):71-72.

2. Isaacs D, Fitzgerald D: Seven alternatives to evidence based medicine. *BMJ* 1999;319(7225):1618.

3. Evidence-Based Medicine Working Group: Evidence-based medicine: A new approach to teaching the practice of medicine. *JAMA* 1992;268(17):2420-2425.

4. Bernstein J: Evidence-based medicine. *J Am Acad Orthop Surg* 2004;12(2):80-88.

5. Schünemann HJ, Bone L: Evidence-based orthopaedics: a primer. *Clin Orthop Relat Res* 2003;413:117-132.

6. Bhandari M, Tornetta P III: Evidence-based orthopaedics: A paradigm shift. *Clin Orthop Relat Res* 2003;413: 9-10.

7. Poolman RW, Sierevelt IN, Farrokhyar F, Mazel JA, Blankevoort L, Bhandari M: Perceptions and competence in evidence-based medicine: Are surgeons getting better? A questionnaire survey of members of the Dutch Orthopaedic Association. *J Bone Joint Surg Am* 2007; 89(1):206-215.

   In this survey of Dutch orthopaedic surgeons, evidence-based medicine was welcomed and clinical practice guidelines were perceived as the best means of proceeding from opinion-based medicine to evidence-based practice.

8. Davidoff F, Haynes B, Sackett D, Smith R: Evidence based medicine. *BMJ* 1995;310(6987):1085-1086.

9. Sackett DL: Rules of evidence and clinical recommendations on the use of antithrombotic agents. *Chest* 1986; 89(2, Suppl):2S-3S.

10. Wright JG, Swiontkowski MF, Heckman JD: Introducing levels of evidence to the journal. *J Bone Joint Surg Am* 2003;85(1):1-3.

11. Lubowitz JH: Understanding evidence-based arthroscopy. *Arthroscopy* 2004;20(1):1-3.

12. Reider B: Read early and often. *Am J Sports Med* 2005; 33(1):21-22.

13. Hentz RV, Meals RA, Stern P, Manske PR: Levels of evidence and the Journal of Hand Surgery. *J Hand Surg Am* 2005;30(5):891-892.

14. Wright JG. Levels of evidence and grades of recommendation. *AAOS Bulletin* 2005;53(2).

15. Wright JG: A practical guide to assigning levels of evidence. *J Bone Joint Surg Am* 2007;89(5):1128-1130.

    Practical tips for assigning levels of evidence to orthopaedic articles are provided.

16. Bhandari M, Swiontkowski MF, Einhorn TA, et al: Interobserver agreement in the application of levels of evidence to scientific papers in the American volume of the Journal of Bone and Joint Surgery. *J Bone Joint Surg Am* 2004;86(8):1717-1720.

17. Obremskey WT, Pappas N, Attallah-Wasif E, Tornetta P III, Bhandari M: Level of evidence in orthopaedic journals. *J Bone Joint Surg Am* 2005;87(12):2632-2638.

18. Wupperman R, Davis R, Obremskey WT: Level of evidence in *Spine* compared to other orthopedic journals. *Spine (Phila Pa 1976)* 2007;32(3):388-393.

    In this study of articles published in *Spine* between January and June 2003, 16.1% were level I, 22.3% level II, 8.0% level III, and 53.6% level IV. With regard to study type, 43.8% were therapeutic, 37.5% prognostic, 17.9% diagnostic, and 0.9% economic.

19. Okike K, Kocher MS, Mehlman CT, Heckman JD, Bhandari M: Publication bias in orthopaedic research: An analysis of scientific factors associated with publication in the Journal of Bone and Joint Surgery (American Volume). *J Bone Joint Surg Am* 2008;90(3):595-601.

    In this study of manuscripts submitted to *The Journal of Bone and Joint Surgery: American volume*, studies of higher level of evidence were more likely to be accepted for publication.

1: Principles of Orthopaedics

20. Schmidt AH, Zhao G, Turkelson C: Levels of evidence at the AAOS meeting: Can authors rate their own submissions, and do other raters agree? *J Bone Joint Surg Am* 2009;91(4):867-873.

In this study of abstracts accepted for presentation at the 2007 AAOS Annual Meeting, interrater reliability ranged from slight to moderate, and authors were found to grade the level of evidence of their own work more favorably than did others who graded the abstract.

21. Wolf JM, Athwal GS, Hoang BH, Mehta S, Williams AE, Owens BD: Knowledge of levels of evidence criteria in orthopedic residents. *Orthopedics* 2009;32(7):494.

In this study, orthopaedic residents were able to identify the level of evidence of blinded studies only 29.5% of the time before an educational intervention, and just 41.3% of the time posteducation.

22. Bhandari M, Richards RR, Sprague S, Schemitsch EH: The quality of reporting of randomized trials in the Journal of Bone and Joint Surgery from 1988 through 2000. *J Bone Joint Surg Am* 2002;84(3):388-396.

23. Poolman RW, Struijs PA, Krips R, Sierevelt IN, Lutz KH, Bhandari M: Does a "Level I Evidence" rating imply high quality of reporting in orthopaedic randomised controlled trials? *BMC Med Res Methodol* 2006;6:44.

24. Hanzlik S, Mahabir RC, Baynosa RC, Khiabani KT: Levels of evidence in research published in The Journal of Bone and Joint Surgery (American Volume) over the last thirty years. *J Bone Joint Surg Am* 2009;91(2):425-428.

In this study of articles published in *The Journal of Bone and Joint Surgery: American volume* between 1975 and 2005, the percentage of level I studies increased from 4% to 21% while the percentage of level IV studies decreased from 81% to 48%.

25. Kiter E, Karatosun V, Günal I: Do orthopaedic journals provide high-quality evidence for clinical practice? *Arch Orthop Trauma Surg* 2003;123(2-3):82-85.

26. Brophy RH, Gardner MJ, Saleem O, Marx RG: An assessment of the methodological quality of research published in The American Journal of Sports Medicine. *Am J Sports Med* 2005;33(12):1812-1815.

27. Okike K, Kocher MS, Torpey JL, Nwachukwu BU, Mehlman CT, Bhandari M: Level of evidence and conflict of interest disclosure associated with higher citation rates in orthopedics. *J Clin Epidemiol* 2010 Oct 12. Epub ahead of print.

In this study of articles published in three general orthopaedics journals in 2002-2003, factors associated with an increased number of citations at 5 years were high level of evidence, large sample size, representation from multiple institutions, and self-reported disclosure of a conflict of interest.

28. Noordin S, Wright JG, Howard A: Relationship between declared funding support and level of evidence. *J Bone Joint Surg Am* 2010;92(7):1647-1651.

In this study of articles published in *J Bone Joint Surg Am* between 2003 and 2007, studies funded by industry were significantly more likely to report level IV evidence as compared to studies funded by governments, foundations, or universities.

29. The American Academy of Orthopaedic Surgeons: Levels of evidence for primary research question. http://www.aaos.org/Research/Committee/Evidence/loetable1.pdf. Accessed August 29, 2010.

A table summarizing the characteristics of each level of evidence as it applies to therapeutic, prognostic, diagnostic, and economic / decision analysis studies is presented.

30. Committee to Advise the Public Health Service on Clinical Practice Guidelines / Institute of Medicine: *Clinical Practice Guidelines: Directions for a New Program.* Washington, DC: National Academy Press, 1990.

31. The National Guideline Clearinghouse: The National Guideline Clearinghouse. http://www.guideline.gov. Accessed August 29, 2010.

The National Guideline Clearinghouse is a repository of Clinical Practice Guidelines maintained by the Agency for Healthcare Research and Quality (AHRQ), a branch of the United States Department of Health and Human Services. Its stated mission is to "provide physicians and other health professionals, health care providers, health plans, integrated delivery systems, purchasers, and others an accessible mechanism for obtaining objective, detailed information on clinical practice guidelines and to further their dissemination, implementation, and use."

32. The American Academy of Orthopaedic Surgeons: AAOS Evidence-based Clinical Practice Guidelines. http://www.aaos.org/research/guidelines/guide.asp. Accessed August 29, 2010.

A repository of clinical practice guidelines developed by the AAOS is presented.

33. Shaneyfelt TM, Centor RM: Reassessment of clinical practice guidelines: Go gently into that good night. *JAMA* 2009;301(8):868-869.

The authors describe the shortcomings of clinical practice guidelines as they currently exist and argue that they should undergo major changes or be abandoned.

34. Choudhry NK, Stelfox HT, Detsky AS: Relationships between authors of clinical practice guidelines and the pharmaceutical industry. *JAMA* 2002;287(5):612-617.

35. The American Academy of Orthopaedic Surgeons: AAOS Evidence-based Clinical Practice Guidelines - Frequently Asked Questions. http://www.aaos.org/research/guidelines/Guideline_FAQ.asp. Accessed August 29, 2009.

A summary of answers to frequently asked questions regarding clinical practice guidelines in orthopaedics.

36. American Academy of Orthopaedic Surgeons: *Treatment of Pediatric Diaphyseal Femur Fractures: Guideline and Evidence Report*. Rosemont, IL, American Academy of Orthopaedic Surgeons, 2009.

   This document, which makes recommendations regarding the management of pediatric diaphyseal femur fractures, represents a typical example of a Clinical Practice Guideline.

37. Hayward RS, Wilson MC, Tunis SR, Bass EB, Guyatt G: Users' guides to the medical literature: VIII. How to use clinical practice guidelines: A. Are the recommendations valid? The Evidence-Based Medicine Working Group. *JAMA* 1995;274(7):570-574.

Orthopaedic Research: Health Research Methodology

Brad A. Petrisor, MSc, MD, FRCSC   Mohit Bhandari, MD, MSc, FRCSC

Introduction

The paradigm of evidence-based surgical practice requires a clear delineation of clinical questions and actions based on the best available evidence. Proficiency in health research methods is needed to identify and appraise the best available surgical literature. Surgeons must be able to categorize clinical research into a hierarchy of evidence, identify pitfalls in the conduct of clinical research, and understand fundamental 'practical' statistics.

The Language of Research: Common Terms to Relay a Treatment's Effect

Surgeons, in general, are interested in the results of high-quality clinical studies such as randomized trials. These results guide clinical practitioners in making treatment decisions and communicating the risks and benefits of these treatments to their patients. Results of trials are based on the occurrence or nonoccurrence of an outcome event. The two main categories of outcomes are dichotomous outcomes and continuous outcomes (or continuous variables).[1-3] Dichotomous outcomes (such as death, nonunion, infection, or revision surgery) either occur or do not occur. Continuous outcomes can take the form of a scale of values such as health outcome scores, laboratory values, or range of motion measurements. For the purposes of this discussion, the focus will be on dichotomous outcome variables.

Results of dichotomous outcomes are commonly expressed in the language of proportions (such as relative risk, relative risk reduction, or odds ratios) or in terms of absolute differences between risks, the absolute risk reduction, risk difference, or the number needed to treat.[1,4] The relative risk is defined as the "ratio of the risk of an event among an exposed population to the risk among an unexposed population"[1,3] (**Table 1**). If the relative risk is equal to 1, there is no difference between the exposed or unexposed (or experimental and control, respectively) populations. If the relative risk is

Dr. Petrisor or an immediate family member is a member of a speakers' bureau or has made paid presentations on behalf of Stryker, Smith & Nephew, and AO; serves as a paid consultant to or is a paid employee of Stryker; and has received research or institutional support from Synthes and Stryker. Dr. Bhandari or an immediate family member is a member of a speakers' bureau or has made paid presentations on behalf of Stryker, Smith & Nephew, and Amgen; serves as a paid consultant to or is an employee of Amgen, Pfizer, Baxter, King Pharmaceuticals, Wyeth, Smith & Nephew, and Stryker; and has received research or institutional support from Canadian Institutes of Health Research (CIHR), Canadian Orthopedic Foundation, AO, DePuy, National Institutes of Health (NIAMS & NICHD), Smith & Nephew, and Stryker.

Table 1

Table of Events for a Fictitious Trial With an Experimental Group and a Control Group Illustrating the Calculation of Different Measures of Treatment Effect

	Outcome Event	No Outcome Event
Experimental group N = 100	10	90
Control group N = 100	20	80
Relative risk		10/100 20/100 = 0.5
Relative risk reduction		1 – RR =50%
Odds ratio		10/90 20/80 = 0.44
Absolute risk reduction		10% - 20% = 10%
Number needed to treat		1/ARR = 10

RR = relative risk, ARR = absolute risk reduction

less than 1, then risk is, by convention, given in terms of the relative risk reduction or 1 minus the relative risk (1 − RR). For example, in a hypothetical experiment with treatment A versus a control group receiving no treatment, if the relative risk of infection with treatment A is 0.5, then an individual is 50% as likely to get an infection with treatment A compared with the control. Similarly the relative risk reduction would then be 1 − 0.5, or 50%; that is, an individual is 50% less likely to have an infection with treatment A compared with the control.

Odds ratios are another way of expressing treatment effects. In general, odds ratios are used to approximate relative risk in retrospective study designs in which the baseline risk or incidence rates are unknown or when event rates are very low.[1,3] Some researchers believe that odds ratios may overestimate or underestimate treatment effects if event rates are high, and that clinicians intuitively understand relative risks better than odds ratios.[5-7] An odds ratio by definition is "the ratio of the odds of having an event in an exposed group to the odds of having an event in a group that is not exposed"[1] (**Table 1**). Odds themselves are the ratio of events to nonevents.

Relative risk is a common way to report the treatment effect based on a dichotomous outcome variable; however, it can at times be misleading. For instance, in the aforementioned example, if treatment A reduces the risk of infection by 50% then it stands to reason that most people would choose treatment A over control (receiving no treatment). However, if the baseline risk of infection is 1%, then treatment A would reduce the risk of infection to 0.5%, a potentially clinically meaningless reduction in risk. Thus, relative risks do not take into account baseline risks. To be truly meaningful, relative risks should be presented along with baseline risks.[5,6,8,9] It has been shown that patients prefer to have relative risks and baseline risks presented during discussions with their physicians.[9]

The absolute risk reduction is defined as "the absolute difference in the rate of harmful outcomes between experimental groups and control groups"[1,3] (**Table 1**). Thus, if the infection rate in treatment A is 20% and the infection rate in the control group is 10%, then the absolute risk difference would be 10%. For every 100 patients treated with treatment A, 10 patients will not get an infection. Stated another way, for every 10 patients treated with treatment A, one infection can be prevented. This is the "number needed to treat" and is given by 1 divided by the absolute risk reduction (1/ARR).[1,3,10,11] This is arguably a powerful number to clinicians because it helps them to understand the potential clinical relevance of an intervention. Confidence intervals should also be provided for all of these results to help clinicians understand the precision of the measure of treatment effect. Accuracy can be defined as how close the measure of treatment effect is to the truth; precision can be defined as how close repeated measures of effect are to each other.

Randomized Controlled Trials

Within the hierarchy of evidence, randomized controlled trials are considered by many researchers and clinicians to provide the highest-quality evidence.[4,12] Randomized controlled trials are experimental study designs. In simple terms, patients are randomly allocated to either an experimental group or a control group. This study design is considered by many researchers to be the best study design to determine therapeutic efficacy or effectiveness.[13,14] The strength of randomization, or random allocation, is that patients in the study groups are "balanced at baseline."[1,3,13] That is, both the known and unknown prognostic or confounding factors are balanced between groups. Although it is easy to balance for known confounding factors or prognostic factors, such as age, sex, or comorbidities, it is not possible to balance for unknown prognostic factors except through the act of randomization. Even though randomization is considered the best method to evaluate a therapy, this study design presents several challenges, especially within the field of orthopaedic surgery. Medical randomized trials often compare drug A against placebo, or drug A against drug B, looking for either superiority or at least equivalence or noninferiority. In surgical situations, sham surgery would be equivalent to placebo. However, inducing anesthesia in patients, cutting skin, and not providing treatment presents many ethical issues. Although sham surgery has been used successfully in orthopaedic trials in the past,[15] the significant ethical concerns with respect to both the patient and the surgeon can severely limit patient recruitment and a surgeon's willingness to participate. Indeed, it would be difficult to obtain the consent of institutional research ethics boards. For this reason, randomized trials in orthopaedic surgery tend to assess two different treatments of a particular condition, such as total hip implant A compared with total hip implant B, and sometimes surgical versus nonsurgical treatment.

There are several potential barriers to conducting randomized controlled trials in orthopaedic surgery. Such trials can be very costly to manage and coordinate. A well-managed randomized trial includes a steering committee to oversees the overall conduct of the study, an outcome adjudication committee to assess all outcome events, a data safety and monitoring committee, a methods center with its associated staff, and individual site investigators.[11,16] Because it is often necessary to collaborate with numerous medical centers, many surgeons with different levels of expertise in particular procedures must be asked to recruit patients. There are also ethical concerns regarding the use of new implants or devices. Because surgeons often have a preferred technique or their own nuances for a common technique, they may be reluctant to participate in a trial or to recruit patients for a trial that uses a different technique. Although such issues are challenging, they are not insurmountable. Many randomized trials have been conducted and published in the orthopaedic

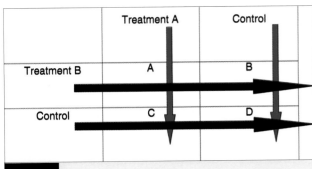

	Treatment A	Control
Treatment B	A	B
Control	C	D

Illustration of a factorial trial design. Patients are randomized to either treatment A, treatment B, or control. The red arrows denote analysis 1: treatment A versus control. The blue arrows denote analysis 2: Treatment B versus control. With this trial design, the same study population is used for two interventions and analyses.

literature, although there have been far fewer randomized trials compared with the number of observational trials.[17,18]

Although randomization can balance both known and unknown prognostic variables, the prognostic balance can be threatened in several ways. If patient allocation to treatment groups is not concealed, patients can be differentially excluded; this leads to prognostically uneven treatment groups. If investigators and outcomes assessors know to which group a patient has been allocated (that is, they were not blinded or masked), they can affect the way the patient is treated throughout the trial. The lack of concealment in allocation and blinding can affect the validity of the trial.[13,19,20] It has been shown that trials with inadequate concealment of allocation may overestimate the effect of interventions by as much as 40%.[21,22] In the orthopaedic literature, the lack of blinding may be associated with an overestimation of the benefit of some treatment effects.[19]

Sample size is another important factor in surgical trials. Surgical trials are typically significantly smaller than trials in other medical specialties such as cardiology. When trials have fewer participants, imbalances within groups can occur through random chance. In trials with fewer patients, the prognostic balance between groups can be achieved in several ways, including the use of stratified randomization. For example, a trial is designed to compare the outcomes of using a new type of plate to fix tibial plafond fractures with two centers selected to enroll patients. One center is a high-volume trauma center and the other is a community hospital in a small town. It is likely that the patients from the trauma center will differ prognostically (more high-energy fractures and open wounds) than the patients at the community hospital. If the randomization is stratified by center, then the centers will contribute patients to both arms of the study on a fairly equal basis. This method will balance the groups for the potential prognostic differences of patients in the two cen-

ters. However, when stratification is used, blocked randomization also should be incorporated into the randomization scheme. Blocking ensures that the groups are similar with respect to the number of patients in each group and aids in concealing the randomization scheme. For example, if the block size is four, and three patients have been randomized to treatment groups (A, A, and B) then the next patient will be randomized to group B. The block sizes can be changed from two to four or six (or any size); usually blocks will alternate from four to six or eight and back.

Randomized controlled trials can take several different designs, including the parallel design, crossover design, factorial design, or the expertise-based design.

Parallel Design

The parallel design trial is the simplest and most classic design for a randomized controlled trial. In this trial design, participants are randomized to two or more groups of different treatments and each group is exposed to a different intervention and only that intervention.[11,13] In medical parallel design trials, one group is often given a treatment or an experimental drug and the other group receives no treatment or a placebo. In an orthopaedic surgical parallel trial, one group may receive one type of treatment and the other group a different type of treatment. For example, in a parallel design trial of fracture fixation, one group may be treated with intramedullary nail fixation and the other with extramedullary fixation. This trial design produces between-group or -participant comparisons. Multiple comparisons and interventions can be made depending on the number of groups to which patients are randomized. However, increasing the number of groups (or arms) in the trial requires a larger sample size to permit statistically and clinically meaningful comparisons.

Crossover Design

In the crossover design trial, both groups receive both interventions over a randomly allocated time period.[11,13] This design is easier to implement in medical trials. Group A can receive the treatment, and after a suitable washout period, can receive the placebo. Group B can receive the placebo and later can receive the treatment; this produces within-participant comparisons.[13] The advantage of a crossover design trial is that fewer participants may be needed to produce both statistically and clinically meaningful results compared with parallel design trials.[13] The crossover design trial has a limited role in surgical interventions because it is difficult or impossible for patients to receive both treatment interventions, such as plate and nail fixation, or a cemented versus an uncemented total hip replacement.

Factorial Design

Factorial design trials allow for two interventions to be compared within the same study group[23] (**Figure 1**). For example, a participant can be randomized to receive treatment A, treatment B, or control. This design is more easily represented in a two-by-two table with

1: Principles of Orthopaedics

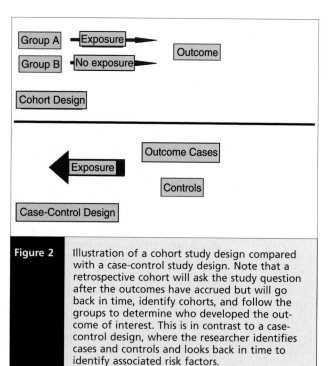

Figure 2 Illustration of a cohort study design compared with a case-control study design. Note that a retrospective cohort will ask the study question after the outcomes have accrued but will go back in time, identify cohorts, and follow the groups to determine who developed the outcome of interest. This is in contrast to a case-control design, where the researcher identifies cases and controls and looks back in time to identify associated risk factors.

those receiving or not receiving treatment A being analyzed, and those receiving treatment B or not receiving treatment B being analyzed. Practically, patients are randomized to either treatment A and B, treatment A or control, treatment B or control, or no treatment. The strength of this trial design is that two interventions can be assessed with the same study population. Also, any interaction between the treatments can be determined[11] (for example, does treatment A work differentially when combined with treatment B?)

Expertise-Based Design

Another type of randomized controlled trial design is the expertise-based trial, or randomizing to a particular surgeon with expertise in the treatment.[23,24] If the use of an intramedullary nail for proximal tibia fractures is to be compared with a proximal minimally invasive locking plate, the non–expertise-based trial would randomize the patients to treatment A or treatment B, and the surgeon would perform either treatment A or treatment B based on this randomization. The problem with this trial design is that the participating surgeons may not have equal expertise in performing both types of procedures. A surgeon who does not have significant expertise with intramedullary nailing could choose to use a minimally invasive plate, thus creating a protocol deviation that could potentially affect the outcome. Alternatively, the surgeon may elect not to participate in the trial. In expertise-based trials, a patient would be randomized to treatment A and surgeon A, who would be an expert in intervention A; another patient may be randomized to treatment B and surgeon B, an expert in the B procedure. This trial design ensures that the intervention is done by the requisite expert in the interven-

tion. However, the expertise-based design may affect the generalizability of the results.[24] For example, if outcomes are better with treatment A, is it because of the treatment or because patients were treated by experts in that treatment? How would the results apply to patient care for a surgeon who in the past had primarily used treatment B? The outcome would mean that a surgeon would either need to obtain training in treatment A or should refer patients to another surgeon who is an expert in treatment A.

Conclusion

Randomized controlled trials are not appropriate for all research questions. Some situations make it unethical to randomize patients for treatment. For example, to determine how smoking affects fracture healing or bone ingrowth on an implant, it is not ethical to randomize one group of patients to smoking and the other group to nonsmoking. In other situations, a condition may be too rare to perform a randomized controlled trial. For example, without substantial collaboration, it would be difficult to randomize patients with infected tibial nonunions to treatment with an Ilizarov one-stage reconstruction or a two-stage reconstruction because it would take many years to perform such a study. For these reasons, it may be necessary to use observational studies.[11,25]

Observational Studies

Observational studies necessarily observe participants in groups within the study; these groups are not randomized. There are three main types of observational study designs: the cohort study, the case-control study, and the case series.

Cohort Studies

The cohort study can be done prospectively or retrospectively[26] (**Figure 2**). By nature, the prospective study design produces higher-quality evidence than the retrospective design and it is considered level I evidence, or the highest level of evidence in studies of a prognostic nature.[4,27] The prospective cohort study design would be similar in every respect to a randomized controlled design except that the patients are not randomized to the study groups. Patient groups are determined on the basis of having received a specific "exposure" or not having received the "exposure." For example, in a study to determine the effect of smoking on fracture nonunion, a prospective cohort design could include one group of patients with fractures who smoke and one group with fractures who do not smoke. The groups can be matched by age, sex, and medical comorbidities. The only known difference between groups then would be smoking (the exposure). Thus, the prospective cohort design attempts to match the groups for known prognostic variables; however, it is not known if unrecognized prognostic variables have also been matched. In the analysis of results, researchers must be cognizant of any confounding variables that may as yet be unknown. Prospective cohort designs can be powerful studies. They should have strict inclusion and exclusion criteria, validated outcomes that use outcome assessors and data analysts, and high follow-up rates.[26]

A retrospective cohort study also can be done using a database of information that allows a question in the present to be answered by using an already established database to identify two cohorts of patients, who are followed to determine an outcome of interest. The problem with the retrospective study design is that not all of the requisite data points may have been determined, treatments could have changed over the course of the database, and not all of the important outcomes may have been assessed.

Case-Control Studies

The case-control study design is often confused with a retrospective cohort design; however, in the case-control design, the patients who have an outcome of interest are identified and then matched to a control group who did not have the outcome of interest. The researcher then proceeds backward in time to identify the factors potentially associated with the outcome of interest.[28,29] The case-control design is necessarily a retrospective study. Although this design produces a lower level of evidence, the case-control design can be useful for evaluating rare outcomes or diseases.[28] Case-control studies are often far less expensive to conduct than prospective trials, and are useful for generating a hypothesis. Case-control studies allow the calculation of incidence rates and odds ratios to potentially approximate the relative risk.

Case Series

A case series is a study of patients receiving a particular treatment, often by a single surgeon or at a single institution. The case series can be prospective or retrospective and can be used to determine important information such as the natural history of a disease and possible complications of a particular treatment. This study design can be used to generate hypotheses for further research. The hallmarks of a well-designed case series include prospective data collection, inclusion of each patient who received the treatment, validated outcome measures, the use of independent outcomes assessors and data analysts, and a high follow-up rate.

Conclusion

Within the orthopaedic literature, observational studies—case series, case-control designs, and cohort designs—have provided most of the information that guides clinical practices. Only a small number of orthopaedic studies are randomized controlled trials.[17]

There is controversy concerning the relative merits of observational study designs versus experimental designs. Some authors have suggested that observational studies overestimate or underestimate treatment effects or relative risks.[25,30] In moving along the hierarchy of evidence from cases series to randomized controlled tri-

als, increasing safeguards against bias are introduced. It can be argued, however, that methodologically superior observational trials can result in estimates of effect with more accuracy and precision than methodologically flawed randomized controlled trials; therefore, it is important to determine the validity of the trial based on its methodology.

Limiting Bias in Clinical Research

Bias is often defined as a systematic tendency or deviation from the truth, which is different than deviations from the truth caused by chance.[1,11] The fundamental difference between randomized trials and observational studies is that observational studies are more prone to bias. If a randomized trial was repeated 100 times, the results would vary to some degree based on random chance. Biases that can encroach on the validity of a study include selection, ascertainment, observational, and measurement biases.

In randomized controlled trials, selection bias can occur, especially if randomization has not been concealed to the enrolling investigator. However, even if randomization is concealed, some patients could be excluded systematically from the trial. Selection bias is more readily apparent in an observational trial.

Ascertainment bias occurs when the outcomes or conclusions of a trial are systematically distorted by the knowledge of which intervention each participant received.[13] This type of bias is combated by the act of blinding or masking information from those involved in the trial. Blinding differs from concealment of allocation in that blinding attempts to keep those involved in the trial unaware of the intervention to which the patient has been randomized. The importance of blinding is that it preserves randomization because those involved in the trial (such as surgeons, nurses, physiotherapists, outcomes assessors, data analysts, and patients) can affect and influence how someone is treated if they have knowledge of the group to which the patient was randomized. From a surgical point of view, it is obviously not possible to blind a surgeon to the treatment allocated to a patient, nor is it possible to blind the surgical team (residents, fellows, and nursing staff). In some instances, however, it may be possible to blind the patient, clinic staff, outcomes assessors, and data analysts to the allocated treatment. Trials where outcome assessors were unblinded had significantly greater treatment effects than in those trials where outcomes assessors were blinded.[19]

Observational and measurement biases can be introduced by those collecting outcome data and, in part, by the outcome instruments used. Independent outcomes assessors, a team of independent blinded outcomes adjudicators, and valid and reliable outcome measures help to limit this type of bias. Biases can result in systematic deviations from the "truth" that are different than deviations resulting from random chance.

Conducting Subgroup Analyses

Subgroup analyses are performed to look for important differences in treatment effects.[11,31] These differences can be related to different characteristics of the patients (such as older versus younger, male versus female) or to aspects of the treatment (such as reaming versus nonreaming of tibial nails, open versus closed fractures, or cemented versus uncemented implants). To determine when a subgroup effect is believable, certain information must be determined.[1,3,32] It is necessary to know if the subgroup was determined before or after the study began. For example, in a 2008 study to prospectively evaluate patients with tibial fractures treated with reamed intramedullary nails, the investigators noted a potential subgroup effect of open versus closed fractures.[33] This factor was discussed as an important subgroup effect before patients were enrolled and before the trial started. Investigators who argue against post hoc subgroup analyses suggest that this may be a form of "data dredging" and that multiple statistical analyses will by chance alone find a statistically significant result.[1] Some guidelines have been developed to determine if an identified potential subgroup effect is real and some relevant questions have been formulated.[1,3,34] (1) Did the hypothesis precede, rather than follow, the analysis? (2) Was the subgroup difference one of the small number of hypothesized effects? (3) Is the magnitude of the subgroup difference large? (4) Is the subgroup difference consistent? (5) Was the subgroup difference statistically significant? (6) Does external evidence support the hypothesized subgroup difference?

It is sometimes difficult to determine true and statistically significant subgroup effects in small trials, especially if these trials are underpowered to detect differences in even the primary outcome. Hence, the practice of multiple statistical testing on limited data can result in spurious-false positive findings of subgroup effects.

Practical Statistics for Surgeons

In statistical testing for experimental studies, the initial hypothesis must be determined by the investigators. For statistical testing, the null hypothesis, which states that there is no difference between the two groups being studied, is used. In comparison, the alternate hypothesis is that there is a difference between the two groups being studied. Two main types of error can occur when testing these hypotheses. The first type of error is known as the type I error, or α error, or a false positive.[35-37] In statistical terms, this is the rejection of the null hypothesis when the hypothesis is true. A difference between study groups is found when there is no difference. The second type of error in hypothesis testing is the type II error, or the β error, or a false negative, which is the acceptance of the null hypothesis when the hypothesis is false. No difference between treatment groups is found when there is an actual difference between the groups. The term α is given to the probability of committing an α error, or type I error, and is represented by the P value (often set by convention at 0.05). The term β represents the probability of committing a type II error and is related to the power of the trial. The power of a study is the ability of a trial to detect a difference when in fact a true difference exists between groups; the power of the test is designated as $1 - β$. This is the probability that the study will detect a true difference when one actually exists.

P Values and Confidence Intervals

As was previously mentioned, the P value (or α) is the probability of committing a type I error, or stated another way, it is the probability of finding a difference between groups in a trial when in fact there is no difference. By convention, the P value is set at 0.05. The P value by itself indicates if groups in a trial are statistically significantly different. If the P value is less than 0.05, there is less than a 5% chance that the difference between groups is caused by chance. A P value does not provide information about the size of the treatment effect or whether the observed effect is clinically significant.[38,39] In contrast, confidence intervals (CIs) indicate the probability of committing a type I error and provide information on the clinical significance of the results, the precision of the results, and the magnitude of the treatment effect.[1,35,40,41] By convention, a 95% CI is used. This means that if a trial is repeated 100 times, 95 of 100 times the result will fall within the 95% CI. Thus, 5% of the time the result would fall outside of the 95% CI and it would erroneously be concluded that there was a difference between groups when in fact there was no difference. CIs can be used around any measure of treatment effect, including relative risk, odds ratio, absolute risk reduction, and the number needed to treat. The treatment effect of a main study outcome is termed a point estimate or the point estimate of effect (that is, the relative risk, odds ratio, or risk reduction). With a 95% CI around the point estimate of effect, it would depict the true result 95% of the time. The CI determines the precision of the estimate of effect; the wider the CI, the less precise is the measure of effect.[1,40] Several factors, including sample size, determine the width of the CI in clinical trials. The smaller the sample size, the lower the event rate and the more imprecise the measure of effect. A small sample size results in a large or wide CI. The size of the CI (90%, 95%, or 99%) also affects the CI width. Another factor affecting the size of the CI width is the actual level of variability within the study population. Increasing variability will increase the size of the CIs because increasing variability is associated with less precision. While indicating the precision around the estimate of effect, the CI also represents the spread of possible treatment effects. This information helps to determine the clinical significance of the treatment effect as well as the statistical significance (**Figure 3**).

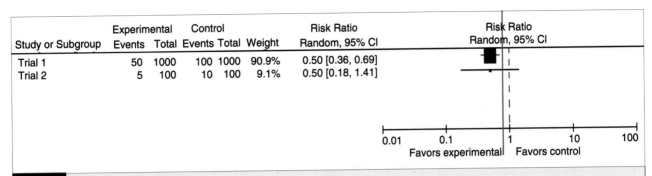

Study or Subgroup	Experimental Events	Total	Control Events	Total	Weight	Risk Ratio Random, 95% CI
Trial 1	50	1000	100	1000	90.9%	0.50 [0.36, 0.69]
Trial 2	5	100	10	100	9.1%	0.50 [0.18, 1.41]

Figure 3 A forest plot showing two fictitious trials. Both have relative risk reductions of 50% in favor of the experimental group. Trial 1 denotes a larger trial with a more precise estimate of treatment effect (the 95% CIs are narrow). Trial 2 has fewer patients, fewer events, and is less precise in its measure of treatment effect. The solid vertical line denotes a fictitious level of clinical significance (this level can be based on clinical judgment and what surgeons believe is a clinically important result). Trial 1 is both clinically and statistically significant. That is, the CI does not include either the line indicating clinical significance or 1 (the line of no effect). Trial 2, however, is neither statistically nor clinically significant.

Study Power

Study power, as previously mentioned, relates to the ability of the study to find a difference between groups if one really exists; study power is given by $1 - \beta$. The larger the sample size for a clinical trial (and some argue, the higher the outcome event rate), the more ability the trial has to determine statistically and clinically important differences between groups. The power of the study is set conventionally at 0.8, or 80%, meaning that there would be an 80% chance that the study would detect true differences between groups if there was a difference to be found. Consequently, there is a 20% chance (β) that the study would find no difference if in fact there was a true difference. Study power is typically determined before the study begins and in the trial design phase.

Sample Size

The sample size calculation is an important component of the study design. It is suggested that a statistician be consulted when calculating the sample size for a study. Internet search engines also can help in identifying Web sites that provide assistance with sample size calculations.[42] The general reasons for doing a sample size calculation relate to issues of hypothesis testing. That is, investigators do not want to erroneously say there is a difference between study groups when there is no difference (α or type 1 error), nor do they want to say there is no difference between study groups when in fact there is a difference (β or type 2 error). Thus, sample size helps determine the power ($1 - \beta$) of the study (accurately identifying a difference in groups when in fact there is one). Sample size calculations need to take into account α (usually set at 0.05), β (usually set at 0.2), and the power (usually 0.8). Other factors to consider when calculating sample size are the potential effect size as well as the dropout rate of the trial. Although researchers should strive for 100% follow-up, it is not always attainable. Convention suggests that 80% follow-up is good; sample size calculations should take this into account. The potential effect size should be approximated from previous research or a pilot trial. The clinically significant effect size, which can be determined from previous literature as well as survey data (such as clinical information gathered from other surgeons), also should be incorporated.

The Era of Evidence-Based Orthopaedics: Critical Appraisal

The description of evidence-based medicine has evolved like medicine itself. In 1991, it was initially described as a shift in the medical paradigm, and placed a higher value on evidence derived from clinical research and a lower value on authority.[2] More recent descriptions of evidence-based medicine express not only the need for a hierarchy of evidence with an understanding of the best available evidence, but also the need to combine this evidence with discussions of patients' values and preferences, the pros and cons of particular treatments, and clinical experience and acumen.[1,14,43,44] The combination of this triumvirate—best available evidence, patients' values and preferences, and clinical expertise—encompasses what is construed by many physicians as evidence-based practice.[1,3,12]

The object of critical appraisal is not to deconstruct every study so severely that the study must be completely disregarded, but to understand how well the study was constructed methodologically to determine its validity (does it answer the question or questions it seeks to answer?) and to understand its methodological limitations, which can introduce bias into the trial, thus systematically deviating the results from the truth. Critical appraisal also aids in understanding the results of a particular trial and in applying (if possible) those results to the specific patients who a surgeon is treating. When assessing an article on therapy, the surgeon should ask several questions (**Table 2**). (1) Are the results valid? (2) What are the results? (3) How can I apply the results to patient care? For the purposes of explanation, the following discussion focuses on the

1: Principles of Orthopaedics

Table 2

Questions for Assessing a Therapy Trial

Are the Results Valid?

Did experimental and control groups begin the study with a similar prognosis?

Were patients randomized?

Was randomization concealed?

Were patients analyzed in the groups to which they were randomized?

Were patients in the treatment and control groups similar with respect to known prognostic factors?

Did experimental and control groups retain a similar prognosis after the study started?

Were five important groups (patients, caregivers, collectors of outcome data, adjudicators of outcome, data analysts) aware of group allocation?

Aside from the experimental intervention, were groups treated equally?

Was follow-up complete?

What Are the Results?

How large was the treatment effect?

How precise was the treatment effect?

How Can I Apply the Results to My Patient's Care?

Were the study patients similar to my patient?

Were all patient-important outcomes considered?

Can the worth of likely treatment benefits be favorably balanced against any potential harms and costs?

(Reproduced with permission from Guyatt GH, Rennie D: American Medical Association: *User's Guides to the Medical Literature: A Manual for Evidence-Based Clinical Practice*, ed 2. Chicago, IL, American Medical Association Press, 2001.)

critical appraisal of a therapeutic randomized controlled trial.

Are the Results Valid?

In assessing the validity of results, it is first necessary to ascertain if the patients start out the trial with the same prognosis. It should then be determined if the patients were randomized. Randomization can be achieved through the generation of random number tables or through the use of computer programs that generate a randomization sequence. Randomization is the only method to obtain balance in prognostic factors, both known and unknown. As an extreme example of the pitfall of nonrandomization is a trial evaluating the efficacy of intramedullary nail fixation versus plate fixation for a long-bone fracture in which only patients with open fractures are placed in the intramedullary nail group and only those with closed fractures are assigned to the plate fixation group. This lack of randomization creates a severe prognostic imbalance from the trial's inception. Because open fractures have a worse

prognosis, the intramedullary nail group would presumably have significantly poorer outcomes than the plate group because of the initial prognostic imbalance rather than the treatment. This example, illustrates the significance of prognostic balance at the beginning of trials. Observational studies that are not randomized risk creating prognostic imbalance based not necessarily on the known prognostic variables, which can be addressed, but on any potential unknown variables.

Next, it should be determined if randomization was concealed. This is a pivotal factor because a trial investigator may exclude a patient from the trial if it is known to which group the patient will be randomized. Unconcealed randomization can introduce bias such as a selection bias. Some examples of unconcealed randomization include studies using hospital admissions on even or odd days, or sealing hospital records in opaque envelopes, which can sometimes be "brightlighted" or opened and resealed.[1,45] Clinical trial centers commonly use a remote telephone call-in or Internet-based randomization method to preclude the possibility of predicting in which group the patient will be placed.[11]

A third factor in assessing the validity of results is to determine if the patients in the study group were similar with respect to known prognostic factors. This typically includes an assessment of patient demographic data within each group. This demographic assessment will let the reader know how well randomization was working. If there are significant imbalances in known prognostic factors, such as age, sex, or medical comorbidities, it may indicate that randomization was not working properly.

Next, it should be determined if prognostic balance was maintained as the study progressed. The best method to maintain prognostic balance and maintain randomization is to blind as many people as possible to study information that may lead to bias; therefore, it is important to determine who was blinded in the trial (investigators, patients, outcomes assessors, research associates, data analysts, the writing committee). Individual subjective biases can be introduced throughout the course of the trial if it is known to which group the patients have been randomized. Treatment effects can be underestimated or overestimated in unblinded trials compared with those that are blinded.[19] It is important not to think of randomized trials based on terms such as double-blinded or triple-blinded, but to consider the principle that everyone should be blinded who can possibly be blinded.

Maintaining prognostic balance at the study's completion is another important consideration. It is necessary to determine if follow-up was complete, if the patients were analyzed in the groups to which they were randomized, and if the trial was stopped early. Follow-up is clearly important because a differential loss to follow-up between groups can lead to biased results. For example, the end-of-study prognostic balance can be affected if a group of patients with specific prognostic characteristics dropped out of one arm of a study. Although 80% follow-up is considered good, researchers should strive for 100% follow-up. To help determine if the loss to follow-up is significant, a "worst-case scenario" can be calculated. If all patients who are lost to follow-up in each group are assigned a poor outcome or a worst-case outcome and the results do not change significantly, follow-up can be considered sufficient. Several strategies have been devised for researchers to obtain follow-up goals, including collecting information on the patient's family, obtaining multiple contact numbers, obtaining contact information for the patient's family doctors, and confirming future follow-up commitments at each visit.

Analyzing patients in the groups to which they were randomized is termed an intention-to-treat analysis. If two groups receive different treatments, it is intuitive to believe that a patient who crossed over to another group should be analyzed in the group to which they crossed over. Analyzing patients based on the treatment they received is called a per-protocol analysis. The power of intention-to-treat analysis is that it preserves randomization. If there were several patients who crossed over in a particular trial, there may be some prognostic difference between those patients and the other patients in the trial; therefore, the prognostic balance can be affected at the completion if the trial. Some trials will conduct both an intention-to-treat analysis and a per-protocol analysis, presenting both analyses in the trial write-up.

After the methodology of a particular therapeutic randomized trial has been discussed, it is often a good exercise for those involved in the critical appraisal to rate the validity of the trial. This rating sets the stage for further discussions of the results as well as the application of the results. If the methodology of the trial is significantly weak, caution would be appropriate when discussing the applicability of the trial to patient care.

What Are the Results?

The discussion of the results should ascertain the size and precision of the treatment effect. The presentation of treatment effects has been previously described in this chapter as well as the estimation of the precision around this effect (CIs). Treatment effects for continuous variables, such as those for outcome scores, can be presented as mean differences or standardized mean differences between groups. CIs around this estimate also can be presented.

How Can the Results Be Applied to Particular Patients?

The final aspect in the critical appraisal of a trial is the determination of the applicability of the therapy to particular patients. Physicians must determine if the study patients are similar to their own patients, if all important patient outcomes were considered, and if the worth of likely treatment benefits can be favorably balanced against any potential harms and costs. The methodology of the trial write-up refers to its internal validity, whereas extrapolating or generalizing the results to

patient care refers to the external validity of the trial.

One method that physicians can use to assess the generalizability of a trial is to determine if their patients would have been included in the study. Evaluating inclusion and exclusion criteria is important in determining the applicability of the results. Physicians also can assess if described outcomes of the trial would be important to their patients. For example, if a randomized controlled trial on hip implant A versus hip implant B reports on surgical time, this arguably is less important to the patient than the risk of infection, the need for transfusion, or the functional outcome following the treatment. If a trial does not report important outcomes, it is difficult to apply the results to a patient. If the trial results are discussed, described, and found to be applicable to a patient, it is necessary to determine if the recommended treatment fits with a particular patient's values and preferences. What are the pros and cons and the risks and benefits for the patient? For example, in a trial of treatment A compared with treatment B for femoral shaft fractures, treatment A results in quicker weight bearing but treatment B has a decreased transfusion requirement; both result in good function. Some patients may value quicker weight bearing whereas others may chose delayed weight bearing with a decreased risk of a blood transfusion.

Summary

Evidence-based medicine requires a knowledge and appraisal of the literature, sound clinical judgment, and a discussion with patients to incorporate their values and preferences when making treatment decisions. This necessarily entails obtaining information from the patient, obtaining relevant treatment data, and assessing evidence and results to formulate a plan that will achieve an optimal outcome for the patient. Thus, evidence-based medicine begins and ends with the patient.

Annotated References

1. Guyatt GH, Rennie D: *American Medical Association: User's Guides to the Medical Literature: A Manual for Evidence-Based Clinical Practice*, ed 2. Chicago, IL, American Medical Association Press, 2001.

2. Haynes B, Sackett DL, Guyatt GH, Tugwell P: *Clinical Epidemiology: How to Do Clinical Practice Research*. Philadelphia, PA, Lippincott Williams and Wilkins, 2006.

3. Guyatt GH, Rennie D, Meade M, Cook DJ: *American Medical Association: User's Guides to the Medical Literature: A Manual for Evidence-Based Clinical Practice*, ed 2. Chicago, IL, American Medical Association Press, 2008.

   This book highlights critical appraisal of study designs and how to incorporate evidence-based medicine into practice.

4. Sackett DL, Haynes RB, Guyatt GH, Tugwell P: *Clinical Epidemiology: A Basic Science for Clinical Medicine*, ed 2. Boston, MA, Little, Brown, and Company, 1991.

5. Gigerenzer G, Edwards A: Simple tools for understanding risks: From innumeracy to insight. *BMJ* 2003; 327(7417):741-744.

6. Gigerenzer G, Hertwig R, van den Broek E, Fasolo B, Katsikopoulos KV: "A 30% chance of rain tomorrow": How does the public understand probabilistic weather forecasts? *Risk Anal* 2005;25(3):623-629.

7. Grimes DA, Schulz KF: Making sense of odds and odds ratios. *Obstet Gynecol* 2008;111(2 Pt 1):423-426.

This article discusses the advantages and disadvantages of using odds ratios.

8. Citrome L: Relative vs. absolute measures of benefit and risk: What's the difference? *Acta Psychiatr Scand* 2010; 121(2):94-102.

This article provides a review of relative measures of effect in comparison with absolute measures of effect.

9. Edwards AG, Evans R, Dundon J, Haigh S, Hood K, Elwyn GJ: Personalised risk communication for informed decision making about taking screening tests. *Cochrane Database Syst Rev* 2006;4:CD001865.

10. Cook RJ, Sackett DL: The number needed to treat: A clinically useful measure of treatment effect. *BMJ* 1995; 310(6977):452-454.

11. Bhandari M, Joensson A: *Clinical Research for Surgeons*. Stuttgart, Germany, Georg Thieme Verlag, 2009.

This book highlights theoretical and practical techniques for designing and understanding clinical trials.

12. Sackett DL, Rosenberg WM, Gray JA, Haynes RB, Richardson WS: Evidence based medicine: What it is and what it isn't. *BMJ* 1996;312(7023):71-72.

13. Jadad AR, Enkin MW: *Randomized Controlled Trials: Questions, Answers and Musings*. Malden, MA, Blackwell Publishing, 2007.

This book provides an excellent discussion of the different types of randomized trials, methodology, critical appraisal, and interpretation of results.

14. Bhandari M, Guyatt GH, Swiontkowski MF: User's guide to the orthopaedic literature: How to use an article about a surgical therapy. *J Bone Joint Surg Am* 2001;83(6):916-926.

15. Moseley JB, O'Malley K, Petersen NJ, et al: A controlled trial of arthroscopic surgery for osteoarthritis of the knee. *N Engl J Med* 2002;347(2):81-88.

16. Hulley SB, Cummings S, Browner WS, Grady DG, Newman T: *Designing Clinical Research*, ed 3. Philadelphia, PA, Lippincott Williams and Wilkins, 2006.

17. Poolman RW, Struijs PA, Krips R, Sierevelt IN, Lutz KH, Bhandari M: Does a "Level I Evidence" rating imply high quality of reporting in orthopaedic randomised controlled trials? *BMC Med Res Methodol* 2006;6:44.

18. Bhandari M, Richards RR, Sprague S, Schemitsch EH: The quality of reporting of randomized trials in the Journal of Bone and Joint Surgery from 1988 through 2000. *J Bone Joint Surg Am* 2002;84(3):388-396.

19. Poolman RW, Struijs PA, Krips R, et al: Reporting of outcomes in orthopaedic randomized trials: Does blinding of outcome assessors matter? *J Bone Joint Surg Am* 2007;89(3):550-558.

This study highlights the differences in treatment effects seen in unblinded and blinded trials.

20. Jadad AR, Moore RA, Carroll D, et al: Assessing the quality of reports of randomized clinical trials: Is blinding necessary? *Control Clin Trials* 1996;17(1):1-12.

21. Schulz KF: Subverting randomization in controlled trials. *JAMA* 1995;274(18):1456-1458.

22. Schulz KF, Chalmers I, Hayes RJ, Altman DG: Empirical evidence of bias. Dimensions of methodological quality associated with estimates of treatment effects in controlled trials. *JAMA* 1995;273(5):408-412.

23. Bhandari M, Pape HC, Giannoudis PV: Issues in the planning and conduct of randomised trials. *Injury* 2006; 37(4):349-354.

24. Devereaux PJ, Bhandari M, Clarke M, et al: Need for expertise based randomised controlled trials. *BMJ* 2005; 330(7482):88.

25. Hoppe DJ, Schemitsch EH, Morshed S, Tornetta P III, Bhandari M: Hierarchy of evidence: Where observational studies fit in and why we need them. *J Bone Joint Surg Am* 2009;91(Suppl 3): 2-9.

This study provides a review of observational studies.

26. Grimes DA, Schulz KF: Cohort studies: Marching towards outcomes. *Lancet* 2002;359(9303):341-345.

27. Sackett DL: Rules of evidence and clinical recommendations on the use of antithrombotic agents. *Chest* 1986; 89(2, suppl)2S-3S.

28. Grimes DA, Schulz KF: Compared to what? Finding controls for case-control studies. *Lancet* 2005; 365(9468):1429-1433.

29. Schulz KF, Grimes DA: Case-control studies: Research in reverse. *Lancet* 2002;359(9304):431-434.

30. Grimes DA, Schulz KF: Bias and causal associations in observational research. *Lancet* 2002;359(9302):248-252.

31. Schulz KF, Grimes DA: Multiplicity in randomised trials II: Subgroup and interim analyses. *Lancet* 2005; 365(9471):1657-1661.

32. Bhandari M, Devereaux PJ, Li P, et al: Misuse of baseline comparison tests and subgroup analyses in surgical trials. *Clin Orthop Relat Res* 2006;447:247-251.

33. Bjandari M, Guyatt G, Tornetta P III, et al; SPRINT Investigators: Study to prospectively evaluate reamed intramedually nails in patients with tibial fractures (S.P.R.I.N.T.): Study rationale and design. *BMC Musculoskelet Disord* 2008;9:91.

    This study is the largest orthopaedic randomized controlled trial comparing reamed and unreamed intramedullary tibial nails.

34. Bhandari M, Whang W, Kuo JC, Devereaux PJ, Sprague S, Tornetta P III: The risk of false-positive results in orthopaedic surgical trials. *Clin Orthop Relat Res* 2003; 413:63-69.

35. Lang TA, Secic M: *How to Report Statistics in Medicine,* ed 2. Philadelphia, PA, American College of Physicians, 2006.

36. Altman DG: *Practical Statistics for Medical Research.* London, England, Chapman and Hall, 1991.

37. Petrie A: Statistics in orthopaedic papers. *J Bone Joint Surg Br* 2006;88(9):1121-1136.

38. Goodman SN: Toward evidence-based medical statistics. 1: The P value fallacy. *Ann Intern Med* 1999; 130(12):995-1004.

39. Hoffrage U, Lindsey S, Hertwig R, Gigerenzer G: Medicine. Communicating statistical information. *Science* 2000;290(5500):2261-2262.

40. Altman DG: Why we need confidence intervals. *World J Surg* 2005;29(5):554-556.

41. Grimes DA, Schulz KF: An overview of clinical research: The lay of the land. *Lancet* 2002;359(9300):57-61.

42. Power and sample size programs. University of California, San Francisco, Web site. http://www.epibiostat. ucsf.edu/biostat/sampsize.html. Accessed March 4, 2010.

    A program used to calculate treatment effects is presented.

43. Haynes RB, Sackett DL, Gray JM, Cook DJ, Guyatt GH: Transferring evidence from research into practice: 1. The role of clinical care research evidence in clinical decisions. *ACP J Club* 1996;125(3):A14-A16.

44. Haynes RB, Sackett DL, Gray JA, Cook DL, Guyatt GH: Transferring evidence from research into practice: 2. Getting the evidence straight. *ACP J Club* 1997; 126(1):A14-A16.

45. Schulz KF, Grimes DA: Allocation concealment in randomised trials: Defending against deciphering. *Lancet* 2002;359(9306):614-618.

1: Principles of Orthopaedics

Systemic Disorders

SECTION EDITOR:

R. LOR RANDALL, MD

Chapter 16

Bone Metabolism and Metabolic Bone Disease

Hue H. Luu, MD

Introduction

The skeleton is one of a few organs with tremendous regenerative capacity. For bone formation, a complex and regulated series of events is needed that leads to the net result of a structure that has the ability to continually repair and remodel throughout life. The human skeleton has multiple functions aside from providing structural support. These functions often include other organ systems such as the hematopoietic and endocrine systems. Fundamental in the cascade of bone formation is the highly controlled process of osteoblastic differentiation. This process is essential for the normal development of bone, physiologic remodeling, and fracture repair. Over the past 5 to 10 years, researchers have begun to understand the important regulatory elements of osteoblastic differentiation and bone formation. These key factors include morphogens, signal transduction proteins, and transcription factors. Mutations and/or deletions in key regulatory genes lead to several musculoskeletal disorders. As a better understanding is gained concerning the normal processes of osteogenesis and bone metabolism, researchers may potentially identify new therapies for regeneration of injured or diseased bone and bone loss caused by aging.

Osteoblastogenesis and Bone Formation

Osteoblastic Differentiation

Bone formation is a complex sequence of events that begins with the stimulation of mesenchymal stem cells to differentiate into mature osteoblasts, and eventually osteocytes. The mesenchymal stem cells have the capacity to differentiate into multiple lineages, including osteoblastic, myogenic, adipogenic, and chondrogenic lines (**Figure 1**). The lineage down which mesenchymal stem cells differentiate depends on the stimuli received. In osteoblastic differentiation, for example, the mesenchymal stem cells receive stimuli to become

osteoprogenitor cells. Several transcription factors are turned on, differentiating the cells into preosteoblasts and eventually mature osteoblasts. Some of the osteo-

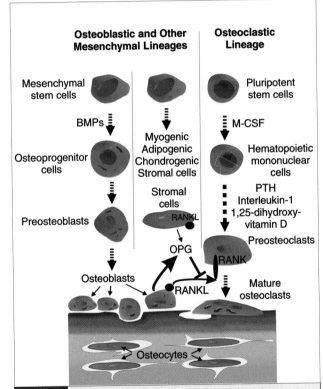

Figure 1 Diagram showing osteoblastic and osteoclastic differentiation. Osteoblasts and other mesenchymal lineages are derived from mesenchymal stem cells. BMPs are potent stimulators of osteoblastic differentiation. Osteoclasts are derived from pluripotent stem cells that have been stimulated by M-CSF to become hematopoietic mononuclear cells and subsequently into preosteoclasts. The preosteoclasts differentiate into mature osteoclasts when activated by the RANKL pathway. OPG is secreted by osteoblasts and stromal cells to inhibit osteoclastic maturation. BMP=bone morphogenetic protein; OPG=osteoprotegerin; M-CFS=macrophage-colony-stimulating factor; PTH = parathyroid hormone; RANKL=receptor activator of nuclear factor κ-B ligand.

The University of Chicago Section of Orthopaedic Surgery has received royalties from Biomet.

2: Systemic Disorders

blasts become osteocytes within a bony matrix; these ostecytes serve as mechanoreceptors and regulate calcium homeostasis.

Many growth factors, transcription factors, and sex hormones that stimulate osteoblastic differentiation have been identified. Among these, bone morphogenetic proteins (BMPs) have been intensely studied and clinically applied during the past decade. BMPs are potent osteoinductive factors that promote osteoblastic differentiation and eventual bone formation. BMPs are secreted proteins, are found abundantly in bone, and are part of the transforming growth factor-beta (TGF-β) superfamily.[1] The discovery of these proteins was first reported in the 1960s when the introduction of demineralized bone matrix was observed to be capable of inducing bone formation in animal models. From the demineralized bone matrix, BMPS were purified and identified.[2] Although not all BMPs are osteogenic, at least 20 members of this protein family have been identified. Both BMP-2 and BMP-7 are used clinically to promote bone formation in procedures such as spinal fusions, fracture care, and maxillofacial reconstructions.

Both BMPs and TGF-β are potent stimulators of osteoblastic differentiation and share a common signaling pathway. The BMP and TGF-β ligands bind to their respective tetrameric receptor complexes of two pairs of transmembrane proteins. Upon binding, the activated receptors phosphorylate the receptor-regulated SMADs (R-SMADs). SMADs are intracellular proteins that help in transduction of the BMP or TGF-β signal to the nucleus. The R-SMADs then dimerize with SMAD-4, also known as co-SMAD, and the dimer translocates into the nucleus. Once in the nucleus, the SMAD complex acts as a transcription factor to regulate several downstream genes, such as *RUNX2*. These genes then stimulate the mesenchymal stem cells down a path of differentiation toward mature osteoblasts. The osteoblasts then secrete an osteoid matrix that eventually becomes mature bone.

As with any signaling pathway, BMP signaling can be modulated at multiple levels. Bone formation involves the balanced coordination of stimulus signals, such as BMPs and BMP antagonists. In the extracellular compartment, several BMP antagonists, such as noggin, have been identified. Many of these antagonists work by binding to the BMP ligand to prevent the binding of the BMPs to their receptors. In the cytoplasmic compartment, inhibitor-SMADs (I-SMADs) are inhibitors of BMP and TGF-β signaling and compete with the R-SMADs for binding to the type I BMP receptor, thereby inhibiting transduction of the BMP signal.[1] Several human skeletal diseases have been linked to defects in the signaling pathway for osteoblastic differentiation. These diseases include fibrodysplasia ossificans progressiva (FOP), which is linked to mutations in the BMP receptor; cleidocranial dysplasia, which is linked to mutations in *RUNX2*; and Camurati-Engelmann disease, which is linked to mutations in *TGFB1*.

Diseases Caused by Defects in Osteoblastic Function

Fibrodysplasia Ossificans Progressiva

Fibrodysplasia Ossificans Progressiva is a rare disabling genetic disease that results in multiple skeletal malformations with progressive heterotopic ossification. The prevalence of FOP is approximately 1 in 2 million individuals worldwide, with no apparent ethnic, racial, sex, or geographic predisposition.[3] Recently, the etiology of this disease has been associated with abnormal BMP signaling and has been specifically linked to the type I BMP receptor (activin receptor 1A [ACVR1], also known as activin-like kinase 2 [ALK2]).[4] The molecular pathogenesis is an activating mutation of the type I BMP receptors on the cell membrane. Although BMP-4 has been shown to bind to this receptor and have increased signaling in patients with FOP, other BMPs also have the potential to bind to this receptor. The net result is hyperactivation of the BMP signaling pathway. There are two clinical hallmarks of this disease—progressively extensive heterotopic bone formation throughout the body (**Figure 2, *A***) and deformities of the great toes bilaterally (**Figure 2, *B***).

During the first decade of life, areas of painful and highly inflammatory swelling develop in patients with FOP; heterotopic bone may eventually form at these sites.[3] Minor traumas, such as falls, intramuscular injections for immunization, or nerve blocks for procedures, can lead to heterotopic bone formation. Systemic illness such as influenza can trigger a flare-up and also lead to progressive systemic heterotopic bone formation. The heterotopic bone can form in skeletal muscles and other connective tissue, such as fascia, ligaments, tendons, and aponeuroses. There is a characteristic spatial and temporal pattern of heterotopic bone formation that mimics the pattern of normal embryonic skeletal formation. Contracted joints often develop in the extremities.

Interestingly, several skeletal muscles, such as the diaphragm, tongue, and extraocular muscles, are spared.[3] Cardiac and smooth muscles also are spared. Most patients are confined to a wheelchair by the third decade of life and die at a median age of 45 years. Death is typically caused by pulmonary complications related to thoracic insufficiency syndrome.

Treatment for these patients involves management of symptoms. Surgical releases of joint contractures are usually unsuccessful and can induce formation of more heterotopic bone.[3] General anesthesia in a patient with FOP is challenging; awake, fiberoptic intubation is often required because of ankylosis of the temporomandibular joints. Fall prevention is essential. Anecdotal use of corticosteroids, cyclooxygenase-2 inhibitors, leukotriene inhibitors, and mast cell stabilizers has been reported.[3] To date, there is no proven therapy that will halt or reverse the natural progression of FOP. Bone marrow transplant has been investigated as an option for treatment, but results have not been promising.

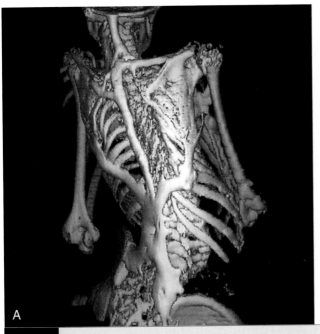
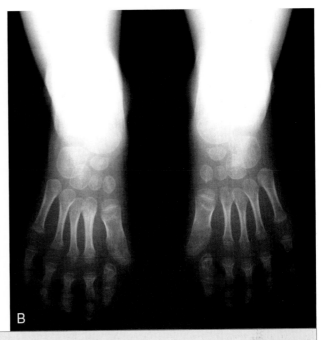

Figure 2 The characteristic features of FOP are diffuse heterotopic bone formation and great toe deformities. **A**, CT scan with three-dimensional reconstruction shows diffuse heterotopic bone in the soft tissues in a patient with FOP. **B**, AP radiograph of the feet shows bilateral great toe deformities. (Reproduced with permission from Shore EM, Xu M, Feldman GJ, et al: A recurrent mutation in the BMP type I receptor ACVR1 causes inherited and sporadic fibrodysplasia ossificans progressiva. *Nat Genet* 2006;38(5):525-527.)

Cleidocranial Dysplasia

Cleidocranial dysplasia is an autosomal dominant skeletal disorder resulting from a mutation in the *RUNX2* gene.[5] *RUNX2* (also known as *CBFA1* or *OSF2*) is a transcription factor and master regulator of osteoblastic differentiation. *RUNX2* is one of several key genes that is turned on with BMP stimulation of mesenchymal stem cells into mature osteoblasts. The estimated prevalence of cleidocranial dysplasia is approximately 1 in 1 million individuals; however, the disease may be more common and underdiagnosed because of the relatively low rate of musculoskeletal symptoms occurring in patients with mild forms of the disease.[6] Cleidocranial dysplasia has been reported in all ethnic groups and has no sex predilection. Patients with cleidocranial dysplasia have several craniofacial abnormalities, including frontal bossing, wormian bones (extra bones within cranial sutures), delayed ossification of the fontanelle caused by delayed closure of the sutures, depression at the base of the nose, and supernumerary and late erupting teeth (**Figure 3, A**). Other radiographic findings include hypoplasia of the sphenoid and maxilla, as well as delayed closure of the mandibular symphysis.

In addition to the craniofacial abnormalities, patients with cleidocranial dysplasia often have several orthopaedic abnormalities, including short stature, rudimentary or absent clavicles, a wide pubic symphysis, peripheral joint laxity, progressive coxa vara, joint dislocations, scoliosis, and kyphosis.[6] Although the severity of the disease varies widely, the characteristic feature of this disease is the hypoplastic or absent clavicles. Absence of the clavicle allows for hypermobility of the shoulders; the patient can bring the two humeral heads in near contact with each other anteriorly (**Figure 3, B**). Treatment is primarily symptomatic. Coxa vara may develop in up to 50% of patients but often resolves spontaneously with growth and may not require surgery. In rare cases, coxa valga can develop. The femoral head has been described as having a "chef's hat" appearance in patients with cleidocranial dysplasia.[7] Osteotomy is not recommended until the Hilgenreiner epiphyseal angle exceeds 60°.[8] In a study with few patients, it was reported that a femoral valgus derotational osteotomy resulted in good outcomes with no recurrences.[8]

Osteoclastogenesis and Bone Turnover

Osteoclastic Differentiation

Bone resorption is an essential step in the normal repair and remodeling of the skeleton. Osteoclasts are responsible for the degradation of bone in the Howship lacunae. Osteoclasts are derived from pluripotent stem cells that have differentiated into hematopoietic monocytes and eventually into multinucleated osteoclasts[9] (**Figure 1**). The initial stimulus for pluripotent stem cells to expand and differentiate into hematopoietic monocytes is mediated by macrophage-colony stimulating factor (M-CSF). Hematopoietic monocytes are stimulated directly or indirectly to differentiate into osteoclast precursor cells by several factors, including interleukin-1, para-

2: Systemic Disorders

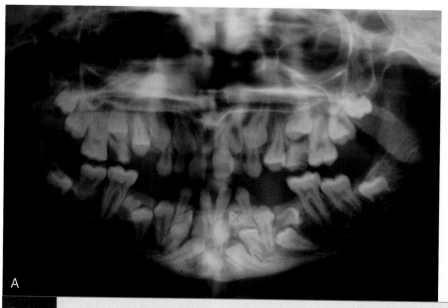
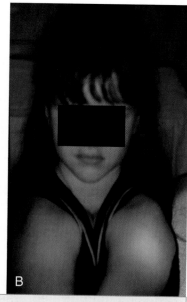

Figure 3 Patients with cleidocranial dysplasia characteristically have hypoplastic or absent clavicles as well as several craniofacial abnormalities. **A,** Supernumerary teeth and tooth germs are commonly present. **B,** Absence of the clavicle allows for hypermobility of the shoulders. (Reproduced with permission from Suba Z, Balaton G, Gyulai-Gaál S, Balaton P, Barabás J, Tarján I: Cleidocranial dysplasia: Diagnostic criteria and combined treatment. *J Craniofac Surg* 2005;16(6):1122-1126.)

thyroid hormone (PTH), and 1,25-dihydroxyvitamin D. Essential to the terminal differentiation of osteoclasts is the stimulation by receptor activator of nuclear factor-κ B ligand (RANKL). The preosteoclasts express receptor activator of nuclear factor-κ B (RANK) on their cell surfaces. This stimulation is antagonized by osteoprotegerin (OPG), which is secreted by stromal cells and osteoblasts. OPG is a decoy receptor that binds RANKL and prevents its binding to RANK on preosteoclasts. This pathway is the target of many investigational drugs for several human conditions, including osteoporosis, osteolysis, and other metabolic disorders.

When stimulated, osteoclasts secrete enzymes from their lysosomes into the extracellular matrix. The cells form the distinctive ruffled border at the interface between themselves and the bone matrix. In this low pH environment, the calcium of mineralized bone is hydrolyzed to essentially dissolve the bone matrix. The acidic environment is mediated by the combined functions of several proteins, including carbonic anhydrase II, vacuolar H+-adenosine triphosphatase, and chloride channel ion pumps.[10] The degraded bone matrix undergoes endocytosis by the osteoclasts, is transported to the opposite membrane, and released. This allows the osteoclasts to continually remove bone degradation products without releasing the sealing zone on the bone. This sealing zone is dynamic, mediated by cell adhesion molecules, and moves with the cell as the osteoclasts migrate along the bone surface. Dysfunction of this low pH microenvironment, as well as other osteoclastic functions, can lead to several human diseases.

Diseases Caused by Defects in Osteoclastic Function

Osteopetrosis

Osteopetrosis is a rare metabolic bone disease in which there is inadequate bone resorption and the continual accumulation of bone deposition by osteoblasts. The clinical course of osteopetrosis can range from mild with no symptoms to severe. Even within the same family, there is heterogeneity of manifestations, which suggests that the disease exhibits variable penetrance. Several genetic defects have been identified in osteopetrosis (**Table 1**), and many involve the inability to resorb bone at the ruffled border. Some of the described examples include *CAII* (carbonic anhydrase II) mutations, *RANKL* loss of function, *CLCN7* (chloride channel 7) loss of function, and *OSTM1* (a protein associated with the chloride channel) loss of function.[10,11]

The genetic inheritance of osteopetrosis includes autosomal dominant osteopetrosis (ADO), autosomal recessive osteopetrosis, and X-linked osteopetrosis.[10] The prevalence of osteopetrosis is variable and depends on the type.[12] For example, one form of the autosomal dominant variant of osteopetrosis (ADO II) has a prevalence of 5.5 per 100,000 individuals, whereas the second autosomal dominant variant (ADO I) has been reported only in three families. The autosomal recessive variant is estimated to occur in 1 in 200,000 individuals. The severity of the disease can be variable and can include diffuse sclerosis in nearly all bones, as seen in the severe forms of the disease. The characteristic radiographic feature of osteopetrosis is the alternating pattern of lucent bands with denser bands. This feature is commonly de-

Table 1

Known Mutations in Osteopetrosis

Inheritance Pattern	Gene	Severity
Autosomal dominant	CLCN7 (dominant negative)	Ranges from asymptomatic to lethal
	LRP5 (N-term mutation)	Mild
	PLEHKM1 (missense mutation)	Mild
Autosomal recessive	Carbonic anhydrase II (loss of function)	Intermediate with brain calcifications
	TCIRG1 (several mutations)	Severe with replacement of marrow
	OSTM1 (loss of function)	Severe with neural and eye involvement
	RANKL (loss of function)	Severe
	ITGB3	Severe with Glanzmann thrombasthenia
	PLEHKM1 (loss of function)	Intermediate
	CLCN7 (missense mutation)	Severe with retinal and optic nerve involvement
X-linked	NEMO	Severe with immunodeficiency and lymphedema

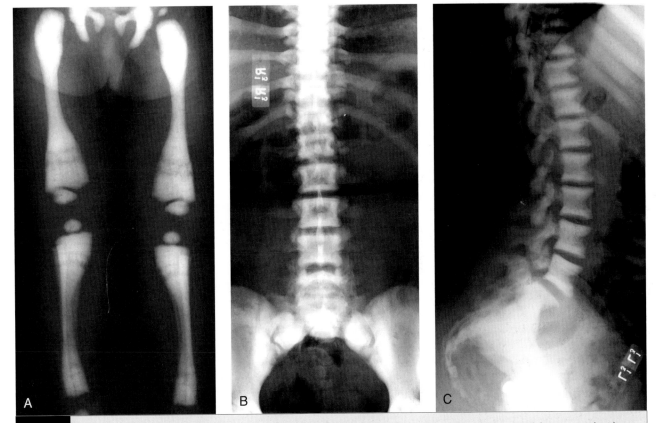

Figure 4 **A,** Sclerosis in nearly all bones with the characteristic Erlenmeyer flask appearance of the distal femur can develop in patients with osteopetrosis. **B** and **C,** Radiographs of the spine often demonstrate a rugger jersey appearance.

scribed as a "bone in bone" pattern. Radiographs of the patient's spine can show the rugger jersey spine sign resulting from focal sclerosis; the characteristic Erlenmeyer flask appearance often develops in the distal femur (**Figure 4**). Although there is increased bone mineral density (BMD), the bone is prone to fracture because of the fragile and poorly organized bone matrix that is commonly described as "brittle marble bones."

In patients with severe osteopetrosis, sclerotic bone can replace normal marrow; life-threatening disorders such as anemia and pancytopenia can develop. Osteomyelitis and sepsis may also occur because of poorly developed bone marrow and an impaired hematopoietic system. In these patients, secondary hematopoiesis in the spleen and liver occurs with resultant hypertrophy in these organs. Blindness and deafness also may develop as a result of nerve compression by the rapidly growing sclerotic bone. Patients with osteopetrosis may also have tooth eruption defects and severe dental caries.

The treatment of patients with osteopetrosis centers on managing disorders resulting from the bone fragility. Patients often require multiple open reduction and internal fixation procedures for recurrent fractures and deformity correction. Some patients eventually are treated with joint arthroplasties. Patients with osteopetrosis have a high rate of surgical complications, including iatrogenic fractures, infection, implant loosening, and nonunions.

Paget Disease

Paget disease of bone was first described in 1877. This bone disorder is believed to be an osteoclastic disease and is marked by focally increased skeletal remodeling within the axial or appendicular skeleton. There is an initial wave of osteoclast-mediated bone resorption, followed by the second phase of disorganized skeletal repair. This process leads to excessively disorganized woven bone and lamellar bone, characterized by osteosclerosis and hyperostosis, respectively, and results in the characteristic findings of cement lines seen histologically. The disorganized bone is weaker and prone to fractures. The final phase of the disease is the quiescent phase in which there is little bone turnover. Radiographically, Paget disease can involve only one bone or multiple bones, and is further characterized by coarse trabeculae. The risk of malignant degeneration to Paget sarcoma of bone is rare but has been well described.

Although the etiology of Paget disease remains uncertain, there is increasing evidence of a genetic cause. Many scientists believe that Paget disease is caused, in part, by a paramyxoviral infection due to the presence of inclusion bodies seen microscopically. However, to date, no intact virus has ever been recovered from patients with this disease. It is unknown why people from certain geographic origins, such as northern Europeans, are more likely to have Paget disease, because paramyxoviral infections (such as measles) are common worldwide. This factor leads scientists to believe that genetic factors play an important role in the etiology of or susceptibility to Paget disease of bone.

Recent studies have strengthened the theory of a genetic etiology for Paget disease.[13,14] Four genes (*SQSTM1, RANK, OPG,* and *VCP*) have been associated with Paget disease.[13] Recent studies have linked a subset of patients with Paget disease to mutations on the *SQSTM1* gene located on chromosome 5. Approximately 26% of familial and 9% of sporadic Paget cases were linked to *SQSTM1* mutations.[14] The *SQSTM1* gene product (also known as p62) binds indirectly to the cytoplasmic portion of *RANK* in the nuclear factor κB signaling pathway. The differentiation of osteoclasts relies on *RANK,* which is expressed on preosteoclasts. Similarly, mutations in *VCP* (also known as p97) have also been linked to Paget disease. Like *SQSTM1, VCP* indirectly binds to the cytoplasmic portion of *RANK* to regulate osteoclastic differentiation.[13]

Additionally, the early onset form of Paget disease has been linked to an activating mutation in *RANK* itself. Mutations in the *OPG* gene have recently been identified as a cause of the rare juvenile form of Paget disease. *OPG* is a decoy ligand to *RANK* and acts to inhibit osteoclastic differentiation. Taken together, there is increasing evidence that at least one third of Paget disease cases may be caused by mutations in genes important in osteoclastic differentiation. Although other regulatory genes for osteoclastic differentiation may be involved, they remain to be identified.

The treatment of Paget disease has changed significantly with the advent of bisphosphonates (such as pamidronate, alendronate, and zoledronic acid).[13] Bisphosphonates act to inhibit osteoclasts at the ruffled border where active bone resorption occurs. The bisphosphonates serve to prevent complications (such as fracture) caused by the disease. Bisphosphonates are commonly used to treat postmenopausal osteoporosis and Paget disease. Calcitonin also is used to treat Paget disease. Nonsteroidal anti-inflammatory medications can help relieve pain related to active Paget disease. In some instances, patients are treated with orthopaedic procedures such as fracture care and joint arthroplasty. Operating on pagetoid bone is associated with increased bleeding and a longer time to union in patients treated with osteotomies or fracture care.[13] Knee replacement in patients with pagetoid bone is characteristically challenging, with a greater incidence of suboptimal alignment.

Hormonal and Steroid Regulation of Bone

Bone serves as a major reservoir for calcium. The release of calcium from bone is highly regulated by several hormones and steroid derivatives. Calcium has many important roles in the human body, such as functioning as a second messenger for cell signaling and nerve conduction and as a mediator of muscle cell contraction. Calcium in the serum exists in three separate fractions: 45% protein bound, 45% ionized, and 10% complex calcium bound to various anions.[15] The serum level of calcium (ranging from 8.5 to 10 mg/dL) is fairly stable and relies on tight hormonal regulation.

Each day, approximately 200 to 300 mg of calcium is absorbed in the adult digestive tract based on the recommended daily intake of 1,000 mg for middle-aged adults.[15] Most of the calcium is absorbed by active transport in the duodenum and jejunum. The recommended intake of calcium varies with age and depends on the relative need for calcium for skeletal maintenance and growth (**Table 2**). Calcium intake should be higher during periods of growth, lactation in women, and in older individuals because of increased bone resorption. The excretion of calcium is approximately 150 to 200 mg/day through renal and fecal losses. The absorption of calcium from the digestive tract, resorption from bone, and excretion of calcium is well controlled by several hormones.

PTH and Parathyroid Hormone-Related Protein

PTH regulates the serum levels of calcium and phosphate in the body by altering the resorption of bone by osteoclasts and the excretion of calcium and phosphate in the kidneys. There are receptors for PTH on osteoblasts and stromal cells, which stimulate the expression of osteoclastic stimulatory factors, such as M-CSF and RANKL, to induce preosteoclasts to terminally differentiate and resorb bone.[14] PTH acts to stimulate the reabsorption of calcium and inhibit the reabsorption of phosphate in the glomerular filtrate. PTH indirectly stimulates the intestinal absorption of calcium by stimulating the production of 1,25-dihydroxyvitamin D in the kidney. The net effect of PTH stimulation is to increase serum calcium and decrease serum phosphate levels. As a feedback loop, elevated levels of calcium will inhibit the secretion of PTH by the parathyroid cells.

Although the net effect of PTH on bone is an increase in osteoclast number and activity, osteoclasts paradoxically do not express the receptor for PTH. Stimulation through the osteoblasts or stromal cells drives the mononuclear osteoclast precursors to mature into multinucleated osteoclasts. This functional linkage of osteoblasts and osteoclasts explains the abundance of both cell types in the brown tumor in hyperparathyroidism. As will be described later in the chapter, PTH is the target of recent novel therapies in osteoporosis and fracture prevention.

Parathyroid hormone-related protein (PTHrP) is a recently discovered second member of the PTH family.[15] PTHrP was first identified as the cause of hypercalcemia in malignancy. This disorder is characterized by both hypercalcemia and hypophosphatemia. Interestingly, because PTH levels were noted to be low in these cancer patients, this finding led to the search for and identification of PTHrP. This protein has since been found in normal physiologic conditions. There is high sequence homology in the N-terminal region of PTHrP and PTH. PTHrP binds to the same receptor as PTH on osteoblasts and renal cells. The effects of PTHrP are similar to those of PTH in that preosteoclasts are stimulated to differentiate, and the production of 1,25-dihydroxyvitamin D is accelerated in the kidneys. The serum level of PTHrP is considerably lower than PTH and likely has a less significant role in regulating calcium.

Calcitonin

Calcitonin is a 32–amino-acid hormone that is primarily secreted by C cells in the thyroid gland. The effect of calcitonin on bone is to inhibit osteoclasts. Within minutes of calcitonin administration, osteoclasts begin to shrink in size and decrease their bone resorptive activity.[15] Recombinant calcitonin is approved by the Food and Drug Administration (FDA) for use in subcutaneous, intramuscular, and nasal spray formulations. Calcitonin is used to treat Paget disease, osteoporosis, and hypercalcemia in malignancy. Clearance of calcitonin

Table 2

Recommended Daily Calcium Intake

Age	Amount (mg/day)
Up to 6 months	210
6 to 12 months	270
1 to 3 years	500
4 to 8 years	800
9 to 18 years	1,300
19 to 50 years	1,000
Older than 50 years	1,200
Pregnant and Lactating Women	
14 to 18 years	1,300
19 to 50 years	1,000

(Data from the Office of Dietary Supplements, Bethesda, MD, National Institutes of Health. http://ods.od.nih.gov/.)

occurs within minutes and is primarily mediated by the kidneys. Calcitonin also can be secreted by medullary thyroid carcinoma and multiple endocrine neoplasia type II tumors.

Sex Hormones and Steroids

Both estrogen and testosterone have anabolic effects on bone. It is evident that women begin to have dramatic bone loss after menopause. This is caused by the decrease in estrogen levels and the fact that there are estrogen receptors on osteoblasts and osteoclasts. The net effect of estrogen is to stimulate bone production. Soon after menopause, annual bone loss is 2% to 3% for the first 6 to 8 years as a result of the abrupt drop in estrogen levels.[15]

It has been well recognized that glucocorticoids induce bone loss since Cushing described the effects of hypercortisolism on the human skeleton. Systemic corticosteroids are currently used to treat several human diseases, such as autoimmune disease and asthma. Interestingly, glucocorticoids have a greater effect on trabecular bone than cortical bone. Therefore, fractures are more likely to occur in vertebrae, ribs, and the metaphyseal regions of long bones. Bone loss, as determined by BMD, is very rapid in the first year of high-dose steroid treatment.[15] For example, the administration of prednisolone exceeding 2.5 mg/day can cause significant trabecular bone loss and increase the risk of vertebral fractures. Glucocorticoids appear to have an inhibitory effect on osteoblastic proliferation and differentiation. A much lower physiologic concentration of glucocorticoid is essential for terminal differentiation of osteoblasts; however, the doses used to treat several human conditions far exceed these physiologic requirements. Glucocorticoids inhibit pituitary secretion of gonadotropins, which stimulate the production of sex hormones. This further promotes accelerated bone loss because of the loss of the anabolic effects of the sex hormones.

2: Systemic Disorders

Table 3

Criteria for Osteoporosis

Normal	BMD within 1 SD of the young adult reference mean
Osteopenia	BMD between –1.0 to –2.5 SD of the young adult reference mean
Osteoporosis	BMD ≥ –2.5 SD below the young adult reference mean

BMD = bone mineral density; SD = standard deviation
(Data from the World Health Organization, Geneva, Switzerland. http://www.who.int.)

Vitamin D

Vitamin D is a secosteroid that is made by the skin when exposed to sunlight. The active metabolite, 1,25-dihydroxyvitamin D, is formed by two successive hydroxylations in the liver and in the kidney, respectively.[15] The major role of 1,25-dihydroxyvitamin D is to maintain a normal serum calcium level. Although 1,25-dihydroxyvitamin D stimulates the terminal differentiation of osteoclasts, it also stimulates the intestinal absorption of calcium. When osteoclasts have matured, however, they lose their ability to respond to 1,25-dihydroxyvitamin D and rely on osteoblasts to release cytokines for stimulation. Important to the skeleton, 1,25-dihydroxyvitamin D promotes the mineralization of osteoid matrix laid down by osteoblasts. This is done by maintaining the extracellular calcium and phosphate concentrations within normal limits, which helps in the deposition of calcium hydroxyapatite in the bone matrix.

Recently, there has been an increase in the number of patients with vitamin D deficiency.[16] This is believed to be caused by less time spent outside in the sun. Vitamin D deficiency is on the rise in all children because of less time playing outdoors; however, it is particularly prevalent in black children because darker skin blocks much of the ultraviolet light necessary for the production of vitamin D. The amount of time outside needed to maintain normal vitamin D levels depends on the geographic latitude because latitude determines the intensity of sunlight. Sun exposure through glass or Plexiglas is ineffective because the light does not contain the ultraviolet band that is necessary for the production of vitamin D.

Osteoporosis

There are two broad categories of metabolic bone disease: (1) osteoporosis, in which there is decreased bone mass; and (2) osteomalacia or rickets, in which there are defects in mineralization of bone. Osteoporosis is the most common metabolic bone disease and is highly prevalent in postmenopausal women. Osteoporosis is characterized by decreased bone mass, with loss of the microarchitecture of bone, leading to increased fragility and an increased risk of fractures. Osteoporosis is de-

fined by a BMD that is 2.5 or more standard deviations below that of normal young adults (**Table 3**). In the United States, an estimated 4 to 6 million women and 1 to 2 million men older than 50 years have osteoporosis, whereas an additional 13 to 17 million women and 8 to 13 million men have osteopenia.[17] Osteopenia is defined by a BMD between 1.0 up to 2.5 standard deviations below the mean of normal young adults. The etiology of osteoporosis is multifactorial, and several medical conditions are associated with an increased risk of osteoporosis.

In 2005, the cost for treating osteoporotic fractures in the United States was $17 billion, and it is expected to increase by 50% by 2025.[17] Therefore, screening for and treating osteoporosis is essential for decreasing the overall cost of health care. Most osteoporotic fractures involve cancellous bone and often occur in vertebrae, ribs, the distal radius, and the proximal femur. The treatment of long-bone osteoporotic fractures follows principles similar to the treatment of fractures resulting from trauma. However, it is essential that orthopaedic surgeons refer patients with osteoporosis to specialists who will initiate laboratory tests and medical therapies to prevent future fractures. Often, presentation to an orthopaedic surgeon for treatment of a fracture is the first indication that a patient has osteoporosis.

Novel Treatments

Recently, there has been controversy regarding the surgical treatment of vertebral compression fractures in patients with osteoporosis. Vertebroplasty and kyphoplasty have gained popularity over the past decade, with the principal goal of more rapid pain reduction. However, two recent randomized controlled trials comparing vertebroplasty to placebo demonstrated no improvement in reducing overall pain or activity-related pain in patients with osteoporotic vertebral compression fractures.[18,19] However, the authors of a recent randomized controlled trial reported improvement in pain and function in patients with vertebral compression fractures treated with kyphoplasty compared with nonsurgical treatment.[20] The advantage of kyphoplasty is that it has the potential to correct kyphotic deformities caused by a compression fracture. Theoretically, this is only possible if the kyphoplasty is performed relatively soon after the fracture occurs and before bone healing.

Pharmacologic Treatment

The development of bisphosphonates has revolutionized the treatment of osteoporosis. In addition to calcium and vitamin D, a few antiresorptive agents, such as bisphosphonates, calcitonin, estrogen, and teriparatide (PTH peptide), have been used to treat osteoporosis.

Bisphosphonates

Bisphosphonates have gained popularity in part because of their ease of administration and favorable tolerability. There are several different bisphosphonates with varying dosing regimens. A relatively new bisphosphonate, zoledronic acid, is appealing to patients because it is administered intravenously only once every 12 months. Bisphosphonates decrease osteoclast-mediated bone resorption by promoting apoptosis and inhibiting enzymes in the cholesterol synthesis (mevalonate) pathway. The molecular mechanism of bisphosphonates depends on the presence of a nitrogen atom on the alkyl chain.[15] Non–nitrogen-containing bisphosphonates (such as etidronate, clodronate, and tiludronate) are taken up by the osteoclasts and cause the production of toxic adenosine triphosphate analogues that lead to premature death in these cells. Nitrogen-containing bisphosphonates (such as pamidronate, alendronate, risedronate, and zoledronate) are taken up by osteoclasts and inhibit farnesyl pyrophosphate synthase, an enzyme in the mevalonate pathway.[15] Exposure of osteoclasts to bisphosphonates results in the loss of cytoskeletal integrity at the ruffled border. This leads to reduced resorptive activity and accelerated apoptosis of osteoclasts. Bisphosphonates also have been shown to inhibit the maturation of osteoclasts. Interestingly, bisphosphonate therapy has been linked to osteonecrosis of the jaw and subtrochanteric stress fractures in rare instances.

Estrogen

Estrogen therapy is also classified as an antiresorptive agent because it inhibits bone resorption by decreasing the frequency of activation of the bone remodeling cycle. There are estrogen receptors in both osteoclasts and osteoblasts.[15] The ability of estrogen to affect gains in bone mass is limited to an annual increase of approximately 2% to 4% for the first 2 years of therapy. Estrogen therapy has several important disadvantages, including increased risk of endometrial hyperplasia, breast cancer, and thromboembolic events.

Calcitonin

Calcitonin, like estrogen, inhibits bone resorption, decreases the rate of bone loss, and is used as another mode of therapy for osteoporosis. The beneficial effect of calcitonin is observed as long as it is given in intermittent pulse regimens. Calcitonin also has analgesic properties, likely related to its concomitant function as a neurotransmitter. The main adverse effects are flushing, nausea, vomiting, and diarrhea. These adverse effects are virtually eliminated with the nasal spray formulation.

Teriparatide (PTH Peptide)

Over the past few years, there has been an increase in the use of human recombinant PTH peptide (teriparatide) in the treatment of osteoporosis. Teriparatide is a recombinant peptide that contains the first 34 amino acids of PTH, and was approved by the FDA in 2002. Although continuous administration of teriparatide leads to net bone loss, intermittent administration of teriparatide has an anabolic effect on bone and stimulates bone formation. A strong positive effect of teriparatide has been demonstrated in postmenopausal women and osteoporotic men in randomized controlled studies.[21,22] In postmenopausal women, there was an increase in BMD and a reduction in vertebral and nonvertebral fractures. In men, there was an increase in BMD in the spine and hip and a trend toward fracture reduction.[22] Combination treatment with bisphosphonates and teriparatide also has been shown to have a strong positive effect in both men and women.[23] A second recombinant PTH protein, hrPTH 1-84 (H05AA03 or preotact), has been reported to have positive results in Europe but has not yet received FDA approval in the United States.

Although the anabolic effects of teriparatide have been beneficial, there is a potential risk for the development of osteosarcoma based on the observation that osteosarcoma developed in approximately 45% of rats who received the highest tested dose of teriparatide.[24] As a result, the FDA has mandated a "black-box" warning and a company-sponsored surveillance program. Since its approval in 2002 by the FDA, more than 430,000 patients have received teriparatide; osteosarcoma developed in 2 patients. It is noteworthy that both of these patients also received radiation for the local treatment of breast or prostate cancer. After teriparatide, osteosarcoma developed in the rib and pubic ramus (the radiated fields), respectively. It remains uncertain whether osteosarcoma was caused by the radiation, teriparatide, or both. Clinicians must consider this risk when contemplating the use of teriparatide.

Rickets and Osteomalacia

In addition to osteoporosis, rickets and osteomalacia combined are the second broad category of metabolic bone disease. The principal abnormality in both rickets and osteomalacia is a defect in the mineralization of the osteoid matrix. The difference between the two diseases is that rickets is used to describe the condition before closure of the physis, whereas osteomalacia occurs after physeal closure. The mineralization defect is caused by inadequate calcium and phosphate deposition in the matrix. Deficiencies in vitamin D, calcium, or phosphorus caused by inadequate intake or malabsorption can result in rickets or osteomalacia. Additionally, drugs resulting in hypocalcemia or hypophosphatemia can lead to rickets or osteomalacia (**Table 4**).

Several genetic disorders result in rickets, including vitamin D-dependent rickets and hypophosphatemic vitamin D-resistant rickets.[15] Vitamin D-dependent rickets is caused by a mutation in the renal tubular 25-hydroxyvitamin D_1 hydrolase. This enzyme is required for the second of the two successive hydroxylations of vitamin D to form the active metabolite 1,25-dihydroxyvitamin D. These patients are easily treated with 1,25-dihydroxyvitamin D or 1-alphahydroxy-vitamin D_3. In hypophosphatemic vitamin D-resistant rickets there is a mutation in the *PEX* gene, which codes for a membrane bound endopeptidase. This gene is located on the X chromosome and, to date, there have been more than 180 different mutations identified on

2: Systemic Disorders

Table 4

Factors Causing Osteomalacia or Rickets

Substances Associated With Vitamin D Deficiency

Cadmium

Cholestyramine

Glucocorticoids

Phenobarbital

Phenytoin

Rifampin

Sunscreen

Substances Affecting Phosphate Homeostasis

Aluminum-based antacids

Cadmium

Ifosfamide

Saccharated ferric oxide

Substances Affecting Bone Mineralization

Aluminum

Etidronate

Fluoride

this gene. *PEX* is needed for phosphate transport in the proximal renal tubules. Patients with X-linked hypophosphatemic vitamin D-resistant rickets are treated with high doses of 1,25-dihydroxyvitamin D.

In rare circumstances, certain tumorous conditions, ranging from benign tumors (such as a nonossifying fibroma) to malignant tumors (such as an osteosarcoma) can induce rickets or osteomalacia.[15] These tumors are not restricted to bone but also can be soft-tissue tumors or carcinomas. The pathophysiology of tumor-induced osteomalacia remains unknown; however, it is speculated that it may result from humoral factors that may affect multiple functions of the proximal renal tubules.

Summary

At the core of bone metabolism are the steps in bone formation and the sequence necessary for bone resorption. Bone formation and regeneration is a complex and well-regulated cascade of events involving cells of mesodermal origin. The mesenchymal stem cells are recruited and stimulated to differentiate by several secreted factors such as BMPs. Defects in this highly controlled process can lead to several human diseases. Once bone has formed, it is continually remodeled and regulated by several hormones and metabolites, including sex hormones, PTH, PTHrP, calcitonin, corticosteroids, and vitamin D.

Bone resorption also involves the well-coordinated stimulation of pluripotent stem cells to differentiate into monocytes and eventually into osteoclasts. Critical in this process is the RANKL pathway in the terminal

differentiation of osteoclasts. Activation and function of osteoclasts is an important aspect of osteoporosis and is also the target of novel therapies. As the complex mechanism of bone metabolism is further studied and understood, new strategies or therapies to treat bone-related diseases may emerge along with new techniques to stimulate bone regeneration.

Annotated References

1. Deng ZL, Sharff KA, Tang N, et al: Regulation of osteogenic differentiation during skeletal development. *Front Biosci* 2008;13:2001-2021.

   Osteoblastic differentiation is a complex cascade of events controlled by multiple genes. This article reviews the highly regulated process of osteoblastic differentiation and bone formation.

2. Urist MR: Bone: formation by autoinduction. *Science* 1965;150(698):893-899.

3. Kaplan FS, Le Merrer M, Glaser DL, et al: Fibrodysplasia ossificans progressiva. *Best Pract Res Clin Rheumatol* 2008;22(1):191-205.

   The authors review the clinical findings and treatment options for patients with FOP.

4. Shore EM, Xu M, Feldman GJ, et al: A recurrent mutation in the BMP type I receptor ACVR1 causes inherited and sporadic fibrodysplasia ossificans progressiva. *Nat Genet* 2006;38(5):525-527.

5. Cohen MM Jr: The new bone biology: pathologic, molecular, and clinical correlates. *Am J Med Genet A* 2006;140(23):2646-2706.

6. Cooper SC, Flaitz CM, Johnston DA, Lee B, Hecht JT: A natural history of cleidocranial dysplasia. *Am J Med Genet* 2001;104(1):1-6.

7. Aktas S, Wheeler D, Sussman MD: The 'chef's hat' appearance of the femoral head in cleidocranial dysplasia. *J Bone Joint Surg Br* 2000;82(3):404-408.

8. Trigui M, Pannier S, Finidori G, Padovani JP, Glorion C: Coxa vara in chondrodysplasia: Prognosis study of 35 hips in 19 children. *J Pediatr Orthop* 2008;28(6):599-606.

   The authors report on the results of a retrospective study examining 35 surgically treated hips in patients with coxa vara secondary to chondrodysplasia. Some patients in the study had cleidocranial dysplasia. Those patients were treated with femoral varus derotational osteotomies and had excellent outcomes and no recurrences.

9. Duplomb L, Dagouassat M, Jourdon P, Heymann D: Concise review: Embryonic stem cells: A new tool to study osteoblast and osteoclast differentiation. *Stem Cells* 2007;25(3):544-552.

The development of osteoblasts and osteoclasts from stem cells is reviewed in this article, along with a discussion of the conditions needed for differentiation of stem cells into osteoblasts and osteoclasts in vitro.

10. Del Fattore A, Cappariello A, Teti A: Genetics, pathogenesis and complications of osteopetrosis. *Bone* 2008; 42(1):19-29.

The authors present a comprehensive review of genetic mutations that lead to the development of osteopetrosis. There are multiple mutations that can lead to osteopetrosis, and many are discussed in this article. The clinical manifestations of osteopetrosis also are reviewed.

11. Pangrazio A, Poliani PL, Megarbane A, et al: Mutations in OSTM1 (grey lethal) define a particularly severe form of autosomal recessive osteopetrosis with neural involvement. *J Bone Miner Res* 2006;21(7):1098-1105.

12. Helfrich MH: Osteoclast diseases. *Microsc Res Tech* 2003;61(6):514-532.

13. Ralston SH, Langston AL, Reid IR: Pathogenesis and management of Paget's disease of bone. *Lancet* 2008; 372(9633):155-163.

Mutations in *SQSTM1*, *RANK*, *OPG*, and *VCP* have been linked to Paget disease. This article reviews the mechanistic consequences of these mutations as well as the clinical management of Paget disease.

14. Hocking LJ, Lucas GJ, Daroszewska A, et al: Domain-specific mutations in sequestosome 1 (SQSTM1) cause familial and sporadic Paget's disease. *Hum Mol Genet* 2002;11(22):2735-2739.

15. Rosen CJ, ed: *Primer on the Metabolic Bone Diseases and Disorders of Mineral Metabolism*, ed 7. Washington, DC, American Society for Bone and Mineral Research, 2008.

This textbook, written by experts in the field, presents an overview of bone metabolism and metabolic bone diseases.

16. Prentice A: Vitamin D deficiency: A global perspective. *Nutr Rev* 2008;66(10, Suppl 2):S153-S164.

Vitamin D deficiency is common in many parts of the world, and recently there has been a resurgence of rickets in children. This article reviews the risk and prevalence of vitamin D deficiency in different ethnic groups globally.

17. Lim LS, Horksema LJ, Sherin K; ACPM Prevention Practice Committee: Screening for osteoporosis in the adult U.S. population: ACPM position statement on preventive practice. *Am J Prev Med* 2009;36(4):366-375.

Osteoporosis is the most common metabolic bone disease. This article reviews the prevalence of osteoporosis in the United States and discusses the role of screening. Risk assessment tools to identify patients who may have osteoporosis are also discussed.

18. Buchbinder R, Osborne RH, Ebeling PR, et al: A randomized trial of vertebroplasty for painful osteoporotic vertebral fractures. *N Engl J Med* 2009;361(6): 557-568.

The authors present the findings of a multicenter, randomized, double-blind, placebo-controlled trial examining the role of vertebroplasty in the treatment of vertebral compression fractures. The study did not show any benefit of vertebroplasty with respect to pain relief, functional benefits, quality of life, and perceived improvement. Level of evidence: I.

19. Kallmes DF, Comstock BA, Heagerty PJ, et al: A randomized trial of vertebroplasty for osteoporotic spinal fractures. *N Engl J Med* 2009;361(6):569-579.

This multicenter, randomized, placebo-controlled trial examined the benefit of vertebroplasty in patients with osteoporotic vertebral fractures. The authors concluded there are no benefits of vertebroplasty with respect to pain and pain-related disabilities. Level of evidence: I.

20. Wardlaw D, Cummings SR, Van Meirhaeghe J, et al: Efficacy and safety of balloon kyphoplasty compared with non-surgical care for vertebral compression fracture (FREE): a randomised controlled trial. *Lancet* 2009; 373(9668):1016-1024.

The authors present the findings of a randomized controlled trial examining the efficacy and safety of balloon kyphoplasty versus nonsurgical care in 300 patients. There was a significant difference in the Medical Outcomes Study 36-Item Short Form scores between the two groups, with no difference in adverse events. The authors concluded that kyphoplasty is safe and effective in treating acute vertebral compression fractures. Level of evidence: I.

21. Bouxsein ML, Chen P, Glass EV, Kallmes DF, Delmas PD, Mitlak BH: Teriparatide and raloxifene reduce the risk of new adjacent vertebral fractures in postmenopausal women with osteoporosis. Results from two randomized controlled trials. *J Bone Joint Surg Am* 2009; 91(6):1329-1338.

The findings of a randomized, controlled, double-blind trial examining the effects of teriparatide and raloxifene on the risk of subsequent vertebral fractures are presented. Both teriparatide and raloxifene can reduce the risks of new vertebral fractures. Level of evidence: I.

22. Geusens P, Sambrook P, Lems W: Fracture prevention in men. *Nat Rev Rheumatol* 2009;5(9):497-504.

Although there is substantial literature on osteoporosis in women, much less is written about osteoporosis in men. This article reviews epidemiology, the differences in the pathophysiology of bone loss between men and women, fracture prevention, and treatment options for men with osteoporosis.

23. Pleiner-Duxneuner J, Zwettler E, Paschalis E, Roschger P, Nell-Duxneuner V, Klaushofer K: Treatment of osteoporosis with parathyroid hormone and teriparatide. *Calcif Tissue Int* 2009;84(3):159-170.

Teriparatide has recently emerged as a treatment option for osteoporosis in the United States. The authors review the pharmacokinetic and clinical experience in us-

2: Systemic Disorders

ing PTH and teriparatide to treat patients with osteoporosis.

24. Subbiah V, Madsen VS, Raymond AK, Benjamin RS, Ludwig JA: Of mice and men: Divergent risks of teriparatide-induced osteosarcoma [published online ahead of print July 14, 2009]. *Osteoporos Int.* PMID: 19597911.

This article analyzed the risk of osteosarcoma in rats that received the highest tested dose of teriparatide in preclinical studies. Additionally, surveillance data on 430,000 patients who received teriparatide revealed that osteosarcoma developed in 2 patients. Both patients had received radiation for cancer treatment in the area where the osteosarcoma developed.

Chapter 17

Musculoskeletal Oncology

Kevin B. Jones, MD

Basic Principles

Population Science

Cancer is a common disease, newly affecting more than 1 million Americans each year; however, neoplasms that primarily affect musculoskeletal tissues are relatively rare. According to the Surveillance, Epidemiology, and End Results (SEER) database, an estimated 2,570 individuals were diagnosed with bone sarcomas, with 1,470 deaths in 2008. Soft-tissue sarcomas were more common, with 10,660 diagnoses and 3,820 deaths in 2008.[1]

Recent reviews of the SEER database have elucidated several epidemiologic facts about specific sarcoma subtypes. Osteosarcoma was confirmed to have a bimodal distribution in age of onset, arising as a primary malignancy in adolescents and young adults but as a secondary cancer or complication of Paget disease of bone in elderly patients.[2] Osteosarcoma survival rates have not improved over the past 20 years. Anatomic location, age, and stage at presentation are each critical for prognosis.

Ewing sarcoma was found to be more prevalent in Caucasians than in persons of African or Asian descent.[3] It also was found that chondrosarcoma survival rates have not improved; tumor grade and stage of disease remain the only independent predictors of survival.[4] For soft-tissue sarcomas in general, age, surgical resection, use of radiation, and tumor grade and size each correlated with survival.[5] Synovial sarcomas present across a range of ages but have a better prognosis in younger patients.[6] For patients with clear cell sarcomas, nodal as opposed to distant metastasis results in a dramatically better prognosis.[7] Age younger than 16 years and disease that is localized, surgically resectable, and does not involve the lymph nodes are predictive factors of long-term survival in patients with epithelioid sarcomas.[8]

Molecular Biology

Sarcomas can be grouped into those with abundant cytogenetic and genetic perturbations and those with balanced, reciprocal translocations. The biologic understanding of representative tumors in each group is progressing rapidly but has produced only minimal impact on therapeutic treatments.

Osteosarcoma and pleomorphic soft-tissue sarcomas are prototype, complex, genotype sarcomas. Insights into their pathophysiology have arisen from their increased incidence in hereditary cancer syndromes such as Li Fraumeni (from *p53* disrupting mutations), congenital retinoblastoma, and Rothmund-Thomson syndrome (from truncating mutations in the *RECQL4* helicase.) Mouse models of these sarcomas, using targeted disruption of varied tumor suppressor genes, have recently been described. Combined disruption of both *p53* and *pRb* in preosteoblasts generated osteosarcomas that mimic the human disease.[9] Disruption of *Kras* and either *Ink4a-Arf* or *p53* in the muscles of limbs generated pleomorphic soft-tissue sarcomas.[10]

Subtype-specific diagnoses have improved dramatically for translocation-associated sarcomas (**Table 1**). Molecular methods, such as spectral karyotyping, fluorescent in situ hybridization, and real-time reverse transcription polymerase chain reaction for fusion transcripts are becoming more widely available to diagnostic laboratories. Mouse models have confirmed the causative relationship between the translocation-generated fusion protein and the sarcoma for three specific types: myxoid liposarcoma, alveolar rhabdomyosarcoma, and synovial sarcoma.[11-13]

Other sarcomas also have discernible genetic backgrounds (**Table 2**). Patients with neurofibromatosis type I, from inherited mutation in the *NF1* gene, are predisposed to the development of malignant peripheral nerve sheath tumors. Patients with Ollier disease or Maffucci syndrome have multiple enchondromas with a high rate of malignant transformation to chondrosarcomas. Mouse models of Ollier disease, which use a variety of genetic derangements to effect increased Indian hedgehog signaling, have been used to study the progression to chondrosarcoma.[14] Patients with multiple osteochondromas, bearing germline mutations in *EXT1* or *EXT2*, develop numerous metaphyseal osteochondromas and rarely a surface chondrosarcoma (1% to 3% lifetime risk per patient).[15]

The neoplastic character of two lesions, whose clonality has long been questioned, has recently been settled. Pigmented villonodular synovitis and aneurysmal bone cysts both share a unique pathophysiology characterized by a small amount (usually less than 10%) of

---

Neither Dr. Jones nor any immediate family member has received anything of value from or owns stock in a commercial company or institution related directly or indirectly to the subject of this chapter.

Table 1

Sarcoma Translocations

Sarcoma	Chromosome Translocation	Fusion Gene
Alveolar rhabdomyosarcoma	t(2;13)(q35;q14)	PAX3-FKHR
	t(1;13)(q36;q14)	PAX7-FKHR
Alveolar soft-part sarcoma	t(X;17)(p11;q25)	TFE3-ASPL
Aneurysmal bone cyst	17p3 rearrangement	USP6 increase
Clear cell sarcoma	t(12;22)(q13;q12)	EWS-ATF1
Congenital fibrosarcoma	t(12;15)(p13;q25)	ETV6-NTRK3
Dermatofibrosarcoma protuberans	t(17;22)(q22;q13)	COL1A1-PDGFB
Desmoplastic small round cell tumor	t(11;22)(p13;q11)	EWS-WT1
Extraskeletal myxoid chondrosarcoma	t(9;22)(q22;q12)	EWS-CHN
	t(9;17)(q22;q11)	TAF2N-CHN
Ewing sarcoma family of tumors	t(11;22)(q24;q12)	EWS-FLI1
	t(21;22)(q22;q12)	EWS-ERG
	t(7;22)(p22;q12)	EWS-ETV1
	t(2;22)(q33;q12)	EWS-E1AF
	t(17;22)(q12;q12)	EWS-FEV
Fibromyxoid sarcoma, low-grade	t(7;16)(q33;p11)	FUS-CREB3L2
	t(11;16)(p11;p11)	FUS-CREB3L1
Inflammatory myofibroblastic tumor	t(1;2)(q22;p23)	TPM3-ALK
	t(2;19)(p23;p13)	TPM4-ALK
Myxoid liposarcoma	t(12;16)(q13;p11)	FUS-DDIT3
	t(12;22)(q13;q12)	EWS-DDIT3
Pigmented villonodular synovitis	5q33 rearrangement	CSF1 increase
Synovial sarcoma	t(X;18)(p11;q11)	SYT-SSX1
		SYT-SSX2
		SYT-SSX4

Table 2

Sarcomas Associated With Genetic Predispositions to Cancer

Heritable Syndrome	Gene(s) Involved	Associated Musculoskeletal Neoplasm
Li Fraumeni	p53	Osteosarcoma, pleiomorphic rhabdomyosarcoma, pleiomorphic undifferentiated sarcoma
Congenital bilateral retinoblastoma	RB1	Osteosarcoma
Rothmund-Thomson	RECQL4	Osteosarcoma
Multiple hereditary exostoses	EXT1, EXT2	Osteochondroma, secondary chondrosarcoma
Neurofibromatosis (type I)	NF1	Neurofibroma, malignant peripheral nerve sheath tumor
McCune-Albright	GNAS1	Fibrous dysplasia
Ollier disease	PTHR1 in minority	Enchondromas

cells in the tumor volume composed of neoplastic cells bearing specific chromosomal translocations: *CSF-1* gene rearrangements[16] and chromosome 17p3, *USP6* gene rearrangements,[17] respectively. The remaining cells in the lesion are not neoplastic, but are recruited to the neoplasm to create what is termed a landscape effect.

Clinical Research Paradigms

Surgically-related clinical research is focused on improving the quality and longevity of functional outcomes following limb-sparing resection of tumors. The previous standard outcomes instruments were the 1987 and 1993 Musculoskeletal Tumor Society outcome scores. Often, both scores are used in tandem. The former score is joint specific and the latter score is more generalized. Both instruments use a physician-focused rather than a patient-focused approach. The Toronto Extremity Salvage Score is a patient- and function-focused outcome score that also is generalized and is not joint or limb specific.

Most surgical studies in the literature related to sarcoma come from single centers or ad hoc collaborations between a few centers. There have been a few cross-Canadian and cross-European collaborative studies, but more are needed. The study of sarcoma began with one of the first national collaborative registries, called the Bone Tumor Registry, which focused on musculoskeletal neoplasms. This registry was in operation from the 1920s through 1953, when data collection ceased. The current medicolegal environment and requirements of the Health Insurance Portability and Accountability Act (HIPAA) make it very unlikely that a similar contemporary registry will be established in the United States.

There are collaborative groups that continue to study sarcoma, including the Children's Oncology Group, Sarcoma Alliance for Research through Collaboration, and the Radiation Therapy Oncology Group; however, these groups rarely conduct studies regarding surgical techniques or outcomes.

Bone Lesions

Patient Presentations

Musculoskeletal neoplasms and lesions that mimic such neoplasms come to the attention of medical caregivers when a patient presents for treatment because of pain, a detected mass, a fracture, or when an imaging abnormality is noted during the evaluation for an unrelated disorder. This last group of incidentally noted lesions requires diligent management; however patience and serial imaging may confirm the latency of such lesions without the anxiety or expense created by investigations using more complex modalities. Each of these four categoric presentations can overlap. Even incidentally noted lesions may be found to be symptomatic when the patient is probed with specific questions. These overlaps in the reason the patient seeks treatment can guide the development of a differential diagnosis.

For example, a patient who presents with a fracture through a lesion who had experienced antecedent pain raises suspicion of different diagnoses than a patient whose fracture occurred through a previously asymptomatic lesion.

Clinical Evaluation

When taking the patient's history, there should be a critical focus on discerning the patterns of typical orthopaedic diagnoses. Specifically, the history of pain over time is crucial. Pain at rest or at night is indicative of biologic pain from the growth of a lesion in a bone. Pain with weight bearing or activity raises the suspicion of mechanical pain from poor structural integrity in the bone. Pain after activity is more indicative of an inflammatory phenomenon than a neoplasm. The pace of disease over time also can be informative. A mass that is present for years is unlikely to be an aggressive malignancy unless there has been a recent change in the pace of the disease process. A lytic lesion causing bone pain that evolves over hours or days is more likely infectious than neoplastic, whereas lesional pain evolving over weeks or months is more likely to indicate a neoplasm.

The physical examination should be focused on ruling out alternate orthopaedic diagnoses. Identifying the precise location of the pain is critical. If pain does not colocalize with the mass or bone lesion identified with imaging, it should be determined if the pain fits typical referred pain locations, a radicular distribution, or a peripheral nerve distribution.

Few laboratory tests provide useful diagnostic information. Important exceptions are inflammatory markers in the setting of possible infections, lactate dehydrogenase in the setting of possible lymphoma of bone, serum and urine protein electrophoreses when there is concern about myeloma, alkaline phosphatase as a prognosticator for osteosarcoma, and specific tumor markers in the workup of metastatic carcinoma such as prostate-specific antigen.

Imaging

Plain radiography remains the diagnostic imaging modality of choice for nearly all skeletal neoplasia. For lesions located in areas that would be difficult to visualize with plain radiography, such as the sacrum and the scapulae, CT is the first alternative. These x-ray–based modalities demonstrate the matrix formed by the lesion and the zone of transition between the lesional tissue and host bone. Matrix types include bone (appearing as smooth mineralization), cartilage (appearing as stippled mineralization in rings and arcs), and fibro-osseous matrix (ground-glass appearance).

The classic categorization of zones of transition between lesion and host tissue was first described in 1980.[18] Three such categories are in current use: latent lesions surrounded by a reactive cortical rim; active lesions with an abrupt, easily discernible transition but no reactive rind (**Figure 1**); and aggressive lesions, with a broad, infiltrating border with the host. These classifications reflect the lesion's presumed activity over

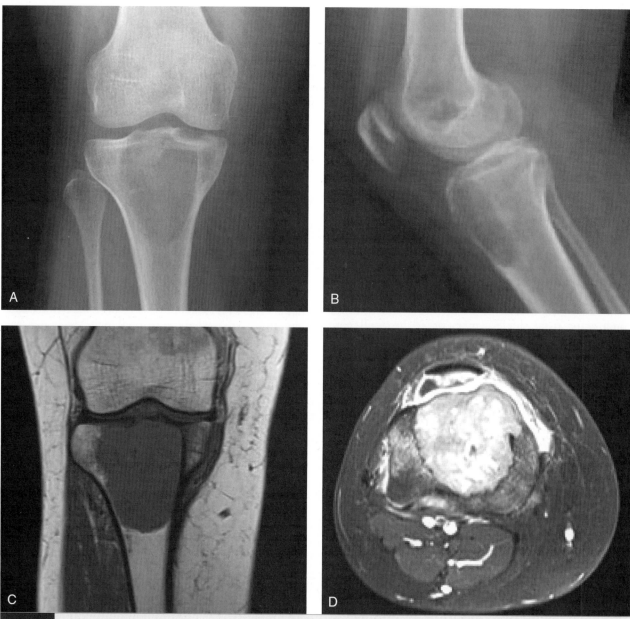

Figure 1 A 35-year-old woman delayed seeking medical attention until she felt a pop and could not bear weight on her right knee. AP (**A**) and lateral (**B**) radiographs of the knee show a lytic lesion with a narrow zone of transition, but no reactive rind of cortical bone. Such a lesion-host interface is called an active border and is given a Lodwick A2 rating. Lesions with active borders are usually in the category of benign aggressive bone lesions. **C and D,** MRI scans (T1-weighted coronal and T2-weighted axial, respectively) show a mass filling the proximal tibia, with subchondral fracture and tibial tubercle compromise. Incisional biopsy was consistent with giant cell tumor of bone. High-speed burr-enhanced intralesional excision was performed, followed by allograft reconstruction of the bone defect and reinforcement of the extensor mechanism.

time, but serial imaging remains the most definitive assessment of lesional behavior. There are few, if any, bone lesions that do not require at least a second set of imaging studies, separated in time by months, to confirm latency.

The location of the lesion in the bone also guides the differential diagnosis (**Table 3**). Most, but not all, lesions have a predilection for the metaphyses near major growth centers of the skeleton. There are few differential diagnoses for entirely epiphyseal lesions or those lo-

cated in the small bones of the wrists and ankles. Similarly, few lesions will affect the diaphysis and spare the metaphysis.

Staging is also performed by imaging, but requires distinct modalities. Local staging is achieved with MRI, which can best identify and localize any soft-tissue extension of the lesion. Although some lesions, such as giant cell tumor of bone, have characteristic appearances on MRI, this modality is primarily used for staging rather than diagnosis. For malignancies, systemic stag-

Table 3

Bone Tumor Location Within the Bone Defines the Differential Diagnosis

Epiphysis	Metaphysis	Diaphysis
Chondroblastoma Clear cell chondrosarcoma Extension of giant cell tumor of bone Osteochondromas in Trevor disease	Most common site for most bone neoplasms, primary or metastatic	Fibrous dysplasia Ewing sarcoma Langerhans cell histiocytosis Osteoid osteoma Osteoblastoma Osteofibrous dysplasia/adamantinoma Lymphoma Metastatic carcinoma Myeloma

Table 4

American Joint Committee on Cancer Staging System

Stage	Histologic Grade	Size	Location (Relative to Fascia)	Systemic/Metastatic Disease Present
IA	Low	< 5 cm	Superficial or deep	No
IB	Low	≥ 5 cm	Superficial	No
IIA	Low	≥ 5 cm	Deep	No
IIB	High	< 5 cm	Superficial or deep	No
IIC	High	≥ 5 cm	Superficial	No
III	High	≥ 5 cm	Deep	No
IV	Any	Any	Any	Yes

ing is required and usually includes a technetium Tc 99m total body bone scan and noncontrast CT of the chest to seek potential sites of metastasis. High suspicion must be maintained for false-negative bone scans in the setting of multiple myeloma or diffusely metastatic prostate carcinoma; the former for its lack of detection by bone scan, the latter because evenly increased uptake throughout whole sections of the skeleton can create a superscan effect, which can be averaged to appear negative. For myeloma, specifically, a skeletal survey is the preferred method for screening the skeleton.

Benign bone tumors are often staged according to the Campanacci[19] radiographic system, which was adapted from the Enneking clinical system. Each system includes grade 1 tumors, which are latent and surrounded by a reactive rind; grade 2 tumors, which are active but contained within at least a neocortex, if not the original cortex of the host bone; and grade 3 tumors, which include soft-tissue masses extending beyond the cortex and not contained by the neocortex.

Malignant bone neoplasms are often staged using the Enneking system, as adapted by the Musculoskeletal Tumor Society.[20] Stage I are low-grade lesions, stage II are intermediate- or high-grade lesions, and stage III are lesions with demonstrable metastatic disease. For stage I and II lesions, an intracompartmental, A, or extra-compartmental, B, designation relating to the local extent of the disease is applied. The more formal staging system of the American Joint Committee on Cancer (Table 4) is increasingly used as an alternative or adjunct to the Enneking-Musculoskeletal Tumor Society staging system and is recommended for communication with oncologists and for central registry data entry.

Iliac crest bone marrow biopsy also is included in the disease-specific staging systems for myeloma and the Ewing sarcoma family of tumors. Surgeons can facilitate the use of this evaluation tool if the biopsy is performed with the patient under general anesthesia.

Biopsy

The purpose of biopsy is to obtain diagnostic tissue as well as specimens for tissue-banking and research. Diagnostic tissue can be procured by fine-needle aspiration, core needle biopsy, incisional biopsy, or excisional biopsy and may be timed concurrent with the definitive surgery or long before it, depending on the clinical scenario. Biopsies are best performed by a team prepared to provide definitive treatment. Such interdisciplinary teams can best judge which lesions require biopsy and which biopsy method will be best suited to the patient's potential diagnoses.[21,22] Although few scenarios are safely managed with intraoperative frozen section diagnosis followed by definitive management, obtaining

2: Systemic Disorders

frozen sections to confirm the adequacy of tissue is critical to the performance of surgical incisional biopsies and thus requires a musculoskeletal pathologist. Biopsies performed without considering definitive surgical options can have severe consequences caused by poor placement of the incision, violation of otherwise non-contaminated tissue compartments, or by spreading tumor cells by hematoma formation.[21,22]

Not all lesions should be biopsied. Asymptomatic, latent-appearing bone lesions that represent no significant risk of pathologic fracture based on their size and location should be monitored with serial imaging to confirm latency, rather than exposing patients to the risks of biopsy. Cartilaginous lesions should be biopsied only with the intent of confirming their cartilaginous character if aggressive treatments are indicated because grading of such lesions has been shown to be unsatisfactory, even among skilled pathologists.[23]

Hematoxylin and eosin staining is the pathologist's primary diagnostic tool for bone neoplasms. Although immunohistochemical stains are used in specific scenarios, such as for small, round, blue cell-appearing lesions, no specific diagnostic tests are available for most bone neoplasms. This situation places increased emphasis on the experience of the interpreting pathologist. For small, round, blue cell tumors, several markers are used to identify the Ewing sarcoma family of tumors, such as immunohistochemistry against CD99 or FLI1, and molecular testing for the t(11;22) translocation or its fusion products (**Figure 2**). Other markers, such as CD45, as well as flow cytometry may be used to assess for or rule out lymphoma. For metastatic carcinomas, immunohistochemistry may guide identification of the tumor's origin; however, it is successful at identifying the primary disease type only in a minority of cases in which primary tumor tissue is not available or detectable.[24] The staging workup and serum markers help to identify the primary carcinoma in situations with less characteristic pathology.

Management Paradigms
Pathologic Fracture or Impending Fracture on Presentation
A patient presenting with a pathologic fracture or an impending pathologic fracture must be assessed with two urgent competing goals in mind. First, the diagnosis must precede any definitive surgical treatment, especially any surgery that could compromise the future possibility for margin-negative resection. Second, the fracture must be stabilized for the patient's comfort and to prevent the mechanical distribution of tumor cells into previously uncompromised compartments by hematoma or further displacement. The only situation in which a destructive bone lesion may be definitively fixed without a lesion-specific tissue diagnosis is when a tissue-confirmed skeletal metastatic carcinoma or multiple myeloma has already been diagnosed.

For pathologic fractures that raise the suspicion for sarcoma, fixation is controversial. Minimally displaced metaphyseal fractures often heal without fixation dur-

ing neoadjuvant chemotherapy. Alternatively, even with fixation, diaphyseal fractures may not heal before definitive surgical treatment. Any placed fixation devices, along with all tissues contacted during placement, must be resectable en bloc with the tumor.

Once metastatic carcinoma is diagnostically confirmed in a fractured or impending fracture lesion, decision making is refocused on restoring structural integrity. The contribution of two different types of pain must be delineated. Pain caused by tumor growth in the bone occurs primarily when the patient is at rest and is often well managed by radiotherapy. Functional pain from an impending fracture is usually not well managed by radiation alone and may require surgical stabilization. The Mirels criteria assign points for pain, location, character, and size of the lesion.[25] These criteria were developed, and are therefore only validly applied, using plain radiography. Lesions that are large and destructive on MRI or CT alone, but involve little cortical bone, may not be well characterized by the Mirels criteria. Case-by-case judgment is required.

One exception to the rule of fracture stabilization in metastatic carcinoma involves renal cell and thyroid carcinomas, which can occasionally be oligometastatic. Although controversial, some retrospective evidence suggests a survival benefit for removing metastatic renal cell foci in the presence of minimal to no visceral disease.[26] This may result from the poor radiosensitivity or the relative chemoresistance of the skeletal foci of disease. Such treatment has been applied to thyroid cancer as well, but with fewer data to support or refute the practice.

Benign Latent Lesions
With or without a diagnosis, asymptomatic lesions with proven latency and minimal risk for pathologic fracture based on size and location should receive no further treatment (Table 5). The serial observation of such lesions in growing children until skeletal maturity remains controversial.

Benign Aggressive Lesions
Lesions may be aggressive anatomically or biologically. Osteoid osteoma, for example, which usually is subcentimeter in size, is rarely anatomically aggressive. Nonetheless, it can cause severe symptoms requiring ablative treatments. Fibrous dysplasia may be biologically nearly latent, but by its size may compromise the structural integrity of the host bone, requiring stabilization to prevent fracture. The classic lesions treated by the benign-aggressive paradigm are giant cell tumors of bone, osteoblastomas, chondroblastomas, chondromyxoid fibromas, and aneurysmal bone cysts. Each of these lesions has a known predilection toward local recurrence, which should be a treatment consideration. Any small, benign, aggressive lesion may be treated with percutaneous methods such as radiofrequency ablation. Larger lesions require aggressive intralesional excision or resection. Benign aggressive lesions arising in expendable bones, such as the proximal fibula, are

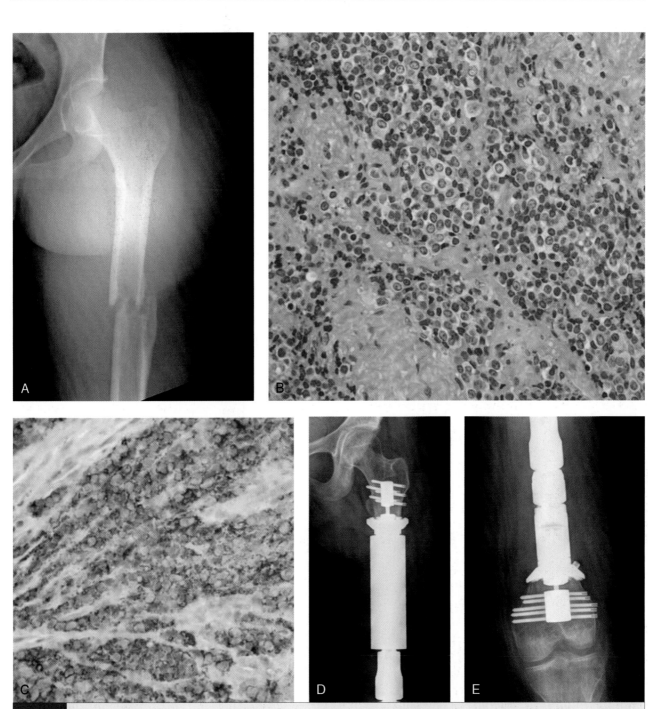

Figure 2 A 16-year-old girl had a pathologic fracture to the left femur after being kicked during a dance class. She reported experiencing antecedent proximal thigh pain for nearly 1 year, with multiple failed attempts at diagnostic imaging of the hip. **A,** AP radiograph of the fractured femur. Incisional biopsy pathology showed small, round blue cells with infiltrating bands of fibrous tissue on hematoxylin and eosin histology (**B**). Immunohistochemistry for CD99 (also called O13) showed cytoplasmic staining (**C**) and fluorescent in situ hybridization confirmed the presence of an 11;22 chromosomal translocation, consistent with a diagnosis of Ewing sarcoma. After neoadjuvant chemotherapy, the patient was treated with a limb-sparing intercalary femur resection and endoprosthetic reconstruction. AP plain radiographs of the proximal (**D**) and distal (**E**) femur show this reconstruction.

best managed with resection, whereas most arising in nonexpendable bones are removed by curettage. Curettage alone produces frequent local recurrences. Recurrence rates are greatly reduced by the use of a high-speed burr and a wide cortical window to permit full visualization of all tumor surfaces.[27,28] Additional chemical adjuvants such as phenol, ethanol, peroxide, cryotherapy, and argon beam coagulation may provide additional reductions in the rates of local recurrence, but no supporting large comparative studies have been

Table 5

Bone Neoplasms

Tissue Group	Neoplasm	Age (decades)	Location
Fibrous	Nonossifying fibroma	First through third	Metaphysis; eccentric; long bones
	Fibrous dysplasia	First through fourth	Anywhere in long bones
	Osteofibrous dysplasia	First through fourth	Anterior tibial cortex
	Adamantinoma	Second through fourth	Anterior tibia
	Malignant fibrous histiocytoma (nonosteogenic spindle cell)	Any	Metaphysis; long bones or pelvis
Cartilaginous	Enchondroma	Any	Metaphysis; central; hand; femur; humerus
	Osteochondroma	First through third	Metaphysis; long bones; pelvis; scapula
	Periosteal chondroma	Second through fourth	Metaphysis; long bones
	Chondromyxoid fibroma	Second through fourth	Metaphysis, long bones
	Chondroblastoma	Second through fourth	Epiphysis; long bones; hindfoot, wrist
	Low-grade chondrosarcoma	Third through seventh	Metaphysis; central; long bones; pelvis
	Peripheral chondrosarcoma	Third through fifth	Metaphysis; long bones; pelvis; scapula
	High-grade chondrosarcoma	Fourth through seventh	Metaphysis; central; long bones; pelvis, scapula
	Dedifferentiated chondrosarcoma	Fourth through seventh	Metaphysis; long bones; pelvis; scapula
	Chondroblastic osteosarcoma	First through fourth	Diaphyseal surface or central metaphyseal; long bones; pelvis
Osseous	Osteoid osteoma	First through third	Anywhere, spine posterior elements
	Osteoblastoma	Second through fourth	Anywhere; spine posterior elements
	Parosteal osteosarcoma	Second through fourth	Metaphysis; long bones; posterior distal femur
	Conventional osteosarcoma	Second through fourth	Metaphysis; long bones; femur; tibia; humerus
	Secondary osteosarcoma	Fifth through eighth	Anywhere
Giant cell rich	Giant cell tumor	Second through fifth	Metaphysis into epiphysis; long bones
	Aneurysmal bone cyst	First through fourth	Metaphysis; long bones; spine
Round blue cell	Langerhans cell histiocytosis	First through third	Anywhere
	Multiple myeloma	Fifth through eighth	Anywhere
	Lymphoma	Fifth through seventh	Long bones; pelvis
	Ewing sarcoma family of tumors	Second through third	Anywhere
Metastatic carcinoma	Breast carcinoma	Fifth through eighth	Spine; pelvis; femur, humerus
	Prostate carcinoma	Fifth through eighth	Spine; pelvis; femur, humerus
	Lung carcinoma	Sixth through eighth	Anywhere
	Renal cell carcinoma	Fifth through seventh	Spine; pelvis; femur/ humerus
	Thyroid carcinoma	Fourth through eighth	Spine; pelvis; femur/humerus

NSAIDs = nonsteroidal anti-inflammatory drugs, SPEP/UPEP = serum protein electrophoresis/urine protein electrophoresis
Green = surgery only necessary if bone is structurally compromised; yellow = lesion extirpation necessary, usually by curettage with adjuvant burring; orange = treated by wide resection without systemic adjuvants; red = treated by wide resection with systemic treatments; blue = surgery is aimed only at stabilization and prevention of fractures

(continued on next page)

Table 5

Bone Neoplasms (continued)

Pathology	Special Notes
Giant cells, histiocytes, hemosiderin	Misnomer, often ossifies
Disconnected trabeculae in fibrous stroma; no rimming osteoblasts	G-coupled protein receptor mutations; difficult to eradicate
Disconnected trabeculae in fibrous stroma with rimming osteoblasts	Extremely rare
Biphasic; fibrous stroma and epithelial rests	Extremely rare
Variable; fibrous stroma; histiocytes	Treated on osteosarcoma protocols
Hyaline cartilage within bone	Avoid surgery
Loosely organize physis on osseous stalk	Cortical and medullary continuity
Hyaline cartilage at bone surface	Can be painful
Stellate chondrocytes in myxoid background	Can be painful
Round, plump chondroblasts; giant cells; calcifications	Even with cortical rind, can be painful
Cellular hyaline cartilage; binucleated lacunae; bone invasion	Beware of curettage when in pelvis
Osteochondroma cap greater than 1.5 cm; hyaline cartilage	Usually secondary, usually low- to intermediate-grade
Cellular cartilage, losing hyaline features; pronounced atypia	No good treatments for high rate of metastatic disease
Tandem presence of low-grade hyaline cartilage and high-grade spindle cell neoplasm	Deadly with any treatment regimen
May be predominantly cartilage; osteoid generated by malignant cells somewhere	Periosteal osteosarcoma is intermediate grade
Variably mineralized woven bone	Treated by NSAIDs or radiofrequency ablation
Variably mineralized woven bone	Larger than 1.5 to 2 cm
Spindle cell, fibrous background, woven bone, low-grade atypia	Has long-term low metastatic potential
Malignant spindle cells making osteoid; telangiectatic areas and giant cells common	Key is systemic therapy to prevent death from metastasis, but local control is also critical
Malignant spindle cells making osteoid	Underlying Paget disease or prior radiation
Multinucleated giant cells in stromal background with matched nuclei	Many other lesions have giant cells: nonossifying fibroma, chondroblastoma, and osteosarcoma
Multinucleated giant cells, vascular spaces, peripheral woven bone	Landscape effect from minority neoplastic population
Histiocytes, multilineage inflammatory cells, prominent eosinophils	The great mimicker; always consider with Ewing sarcoma family of tumors and infection; may be self-limited
Abundant plasma cells with perinuclear hof	Can be diagnosed by SPEP/UPEP
Large round blue cells, poorly cohesive	Can cause hypercalcemia
Cohesive large round blue cells	Surgery is adjuvant to chemotherapy
Epithelial rests; strong cytokeratin staining	Long survival often possible
Epithelial rests; strong cytokeratin staining	Often blastic, less frequently surgical
Epithelial rests; strong cytokeratin staining	Often short survival
Epithelial rests; strong cytokeratin staining	Beware of hemorrhage, radiosensitive, consider excision
Epithelial rests; strong cytokeratin staining	Beware of hemorrhage

NSAIDs = nonsteroidal anti-inflammatory drugs, SPEP/UPEP = serum protein electrophoresis/urine protein electrophoresis

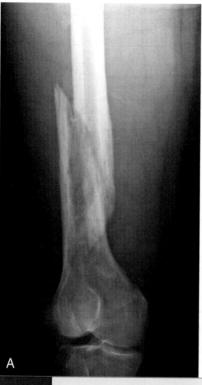 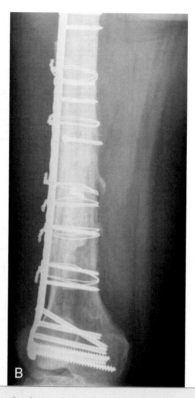 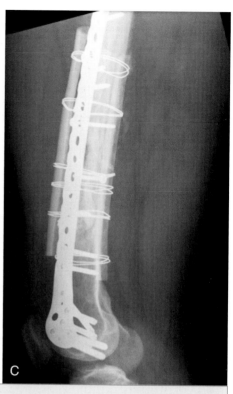

Figure 3 A, Preoperative AP radiograph of a femur fracture in a 48-year-old man who was injured while gardening in the sitting position shows an infiltrative lesion. Lymphoma of bone that was diagnosed on biopsy requires no aggressive resection. AP (**B**) and lateral (**C**) radiographs of the femur demonstrate stabilization of the fracture, preparatory to definitive chemotherapy and radiation.

published to support this hypothesis. Wide resection should be considered for some especially destructive benign aggressive neoplasms; however, intra-articular pathologic fractures through giant cell tumors of bone, although once believed to be a categoric indication for wide resection, can be managed with joint-sparing, intralesional techniques if fastidious attention is paid to complete excision.[29]

Treatment of the defect following excision also is controversial. Although filling the defect with cement with or without pin or screw augmentation is most commonly used in the United States, allograft filling and even no filling of the defect have proven safe and effective.[28]

Primary Low-Grade Malignant Neoplasms

Although primary low-grade malignant neoplasms represent a small group of tumors, separate consideration is deserved because their treatment is unique and controversial. Some low-grade malignant neoplasms of bone, such as adamantinoma and parosteal osteosarcoma, are treated with wide resections that are not surgically different from those used to treat high-grade neoplasms, other than the fact that some can be managed with hemicortical resection rather than full segmental resections. The treatment of low-grade chondrosarcoma, however, has recently trended toward less aggressive approaches.[30] Given its very low metastatic

potential, low-grade chondrosarcoma is increasingly managed more like a benign aggressive neoplasm, with adjuvant-enhanced intralesional excision. This approach has been challenged because local recurrences can be more aggressive than the primary tumor, requiring more extensive surgery; however, the spared morbidity of en bloc wide resections is advantageous for many patients. This approach may not be safely applied in the pelvis.

Primary High-Grade Malignant Neoplasms

A critical consideration in the management of malignant primary bone neoplasms derives from their sensitivity to available adjuvant treatments. Few malignant neoplasms primary to bone are radiosensitive, other than myeloma, the Ewing sarcoma family of tumors, and lymphoma of bone (**Figure 3**). From a surgical perspective, conventional osteosarcoma, the Ewing sarcoma family of tumors, and nonosteogenic spindle cell sarcomas of bone are all identically managed with biopsy, neoadjuvant chemotherapy, definitive surgical resection, and adjuvant chemotherapy (**Figure 4**). Although there are few data to support neoadjuvant chemotherapy over adjuvant chemotherapy, it permits a measurement of the effects of chemotherapy at the time of resection and remains almost universally preferred by surgeons and medical oncologists treating these disorders.

Chondrosarcoma (**Figure 5**) is not considered sensi-

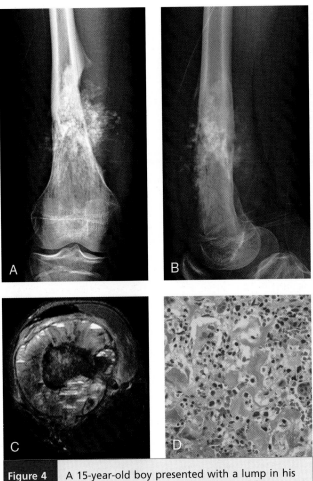

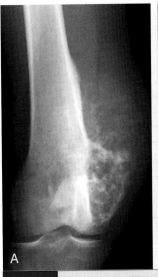

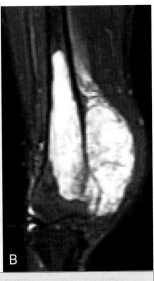

Figure 5 A 41-year-old man presented with a distal anteromedial thigh mass and reported a deep ache nightly. Classic imaging features of high-grade chondrosarcoma of bone were found. **A,** AP plain radiograph shows a destructive lesion making a cartilaginous matrix. **B,** T2-weighted MRI shows the lobular tissue structure, typical of cartilaginous neoplasms.

Figure 4 A 15-year-old boy presented with a lump in his distal thigh and reported pain waking him nightly for 3 months. The AP **(A)** and lateral **(B)** radiographs alone render a fairly confident diagnosis of osteosarcoma, with a clear Codman triangle and sunburst periosteal reaction. **C,** An axial T2-weighted MRI shows that much of the soft-tissue component was telangiectatic in character, with fluid-fluid levels marking vascular spaces. Incisional biopsy confirmed the diagnosis of conventional osteosarcoma. **D,** The photomicrograph of a hematoxylin and eosin stained section from the biopsy shows lacy osteoid formation by malignant-appearing osteoblasts with severe pleomorphic features and nuclear atypia.

tive to adjuvant treatments, but studies using radiotherapy as definitive treatment of unresectable chondrosarcomas of the spine have reported promising short-term local control.[31]

The goals of surgical resection are complete extirpation of the neoplasm with minimal functional compromise. Wide, negative margins are ideal. Even if very narrow, margins including fascia, epineurium, or vascular sheath are considered adequate; however, muscle or adipose tissue margins should be more generous in thickness. Bone marrow margins in the diaphysis should be generous in length, when possible. Margin

depth is controversial in metaphyseal and periphyseal areas.

In instances in which wide margins are not otherwise possible, neurovascular structures are sacrificed or bypassed. Limb salvage must always be measured against amputation and cannot be pursued if it significantly compromises either local control or ultimate function.

Reconstructive options for major skeletal defects present both short- and long-term challenges. In the short term, allografts and endoprostheses are prone to infections because they are implanted into massive dead spaces in immunocompromised hosts. Long-term challenges include late infections, loosening, and fractures. In the United States, trends have moved toward allograft reconstruction for intercalary resections within a bone, and endoprosthetic reconstructions of bone ends including the adjacent joints.[32]

The pelvis and shoulder girdle also present challenges to reconstruction. Most major resections of the proximal humerus and scapula require resection of too much muscle to permit useful shoulder elevation. Most shoulder reconstructions, therefore, result in a hanging arm in which the functional result is more dependent on the neuromuscular function of the elbow and hand than the shoulder itself. There has been an increase in the number of reports of satisfactory functional results of resection without reconstruction of portions of the pelvis.[33] Complication rates must be considered when deciding if reconstruction is the appropriate treatment (**Figures 6** and **7**).

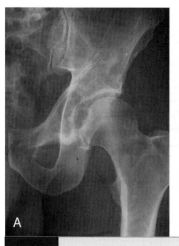
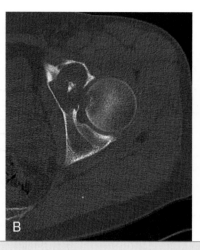
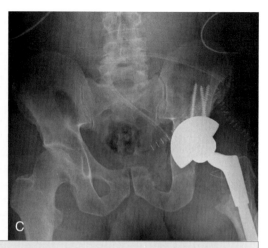

Figure 6 A 45-year-old male athlete reported worsening pain during activity that persisted through rest and woke him at night. **A,** AP radiograph shows an intermediate-grade chondrosarcoma in the periacetabular periarticular bone of the pelvis. **B,** Axial CT scan through the hip shows the lesion where it has eroded into the hip joint through the acetabulum. The CT scan also demonstrates that the posterior column is free of tumor. This anatomy was exploited by an extra-articular resection that spared the posterior column, enabling the solid acetabular component for the reconstructive total hip arthroplasty, shown in the AP pelvis postoperative radiograph (**C**).

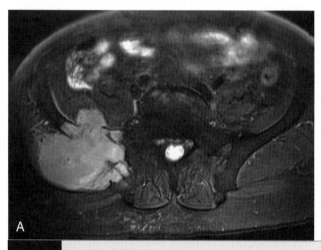
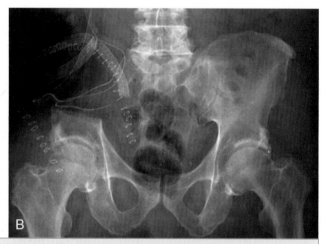

Figure 7 An 80-year-old man presented with worsening sciatica. The axial T2-weighted MRI scan (**A**) shows the large iliosacral mass causing the sciatica. A nonosteogenic spindle sarcoma of bone was noted on biopsy. Because the patient wanted to return to walking and golf, he was treated with resection of most of the ilium and sacral ala without reconstruction, shown in the postoperative AP pelvis radiograph (**B**).

Soft-Tissue Masses

Patient Presentations

The lump or bump noticed by a patient or family member may or may not be painful or changing over time. The pace of disease is critical to understanding soft-tissue masses. Occasionally, large, rapidly growing, high-grade soft-tissue sarcomas will produce mild pain, but most painful soft-tissue masses tend to be inflammatory and benign in character. Similarly, a lesion that waxes and wanes in size over time reduces the concern for malignancy. Most worrisome is a lump that inexorably and insidiously expands over time.

Physical examination of the mass should characterize the depth of the mass by assessing skin involvement, as well as mobility from fascia, muscle, and underlying bone.[34] Superficial masses are easier to remove and less likely to be malignant. Mass size also matters, with larger masses more predictive of malignancy. The palpable consistency of the mass is instructive, with fluctuant masses rarely representing true neoplasms. It is paramount to correlate the physical examination with the patient history (**Figure 8**). Some patients may fail to recall a traumatic event, but without the involvement of anticoagulation or hemophilia, there is no such entity as an atraumatic hematoma. Hemorrhagic sarcomas exist and suspicion for them should be high when eval-

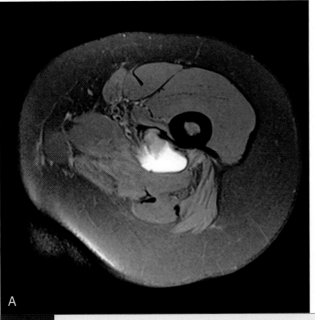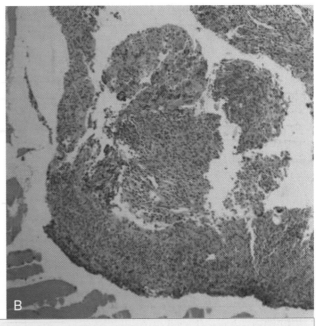

Figure 8 A 21-year-old woman presented with a fluctuant mass. The axial T2-weighted MRI of the proximal thigh (**A**) was interpreted radiologically to be a hematoma with an associated muscle tear. No history of trauma was elicited. **B**, Histologic section (hematoxylin and eosin stain) from an open biopsy showed a spindle cell neoplasm; it was also positive for the (X:18) SYT-SSX1 translocation product on fluorescent in situ hybridization.

uating any large deep hematoma for which no history of trauma can be elicited.

Careful examination of the distal neurovascular status also is critical. Direct nerve or vessel involvement is rare but has a significant impact on treatment when present. Although nodal metastasis is rare in sarcomas, regional lymph nodes should be palpated to identify mimicking lesions such as metastatic melanoma and specific subtypes of soft-tissue sarcoma that can lymphatically spread, including epithelioid sarcoma, clear cell sarcoma, rhabdomyosarcoma, angiosarcoma, and synovial sarcoma.

Imaging

MRI is the primary imaging modality used for the diagnosis and local staging of soft-tissue neoplasms. The diagnosis of some soft-tissue cysts that do not transilluminate may be confirmed by ultrasound. Plain radiographs of the mass preceding or following MRI can reveal calcification or ossification within the mass, which can suggest or confirm a diagnosis such as hemangioma (from phleboliths) or myositis ossificans (**Figure 9**). MRI alone can be nearly diagnostic for a few neoplasms such as lipomatous lesions, hemangioma, pigmented villonodular synovitis, schwannoma, and intramuscular myxoma. Gadolinium contrast can help to distinguish solid masses from cysts by measuring the depth of enhancement in the lesion. However, for most masses, MRI defines the anatomic location and surrounding involved structures rather than providing a diagnosis.

Systemic staging is achieved with technetium Tc 99m total body bone scanning and noncontrast chest

CT; however, certain mass subtypes require additional imaging. Myxoid or round cell liposarcomas can metastasize to unusual soft-tissue sites, necessitating evaluation of the retroperitoneum with contrast-enhanced CT. Alveolar soft-part sarcoma metastasizes early to the brain, usually prompting the need for a brain MRI at the time of staging.[35]

Positron emission tomography has been used in sarcoma care but usually serves as an adjunctive measure of the treatment effect of chemotherapy rather than for staging.[36] Most sarcomas are PET-avid, or detectable using positron emission tomography, but such an expensive imaging modality should be reserved for scenarios in which it serves a unique evidence-based purpose, such as in the staging of metastatic melanoma.

Biopsy

The goals, methods, and hazards of biopsy for soft-tissue neoplasms are similar to those for bone lesions. Fine-needle aspirations and core needle biopsies are more commonly performed for soft-tissue masses but require a pathologist who is experienced and comfortable with their interpretation. Excisional biopsy is also more frequently performed for soft-tissue neoplasms. If lesions are small (< 5 cm), superficial, and free from fascia, excisional biopsy is a reasonable choice but must not compromise the potential for margin-negative wide resection of the entire area of contamination. Excisional biopsy must avoid violation of the deep fascia and the development of unnecessary tissue planes.

One serious complication of biopsy is an incorrect diagnosis. As with bone lesions, there are some soft-tissue neoplasms that should not be biopsied before ex-

2: Systemic Disorders

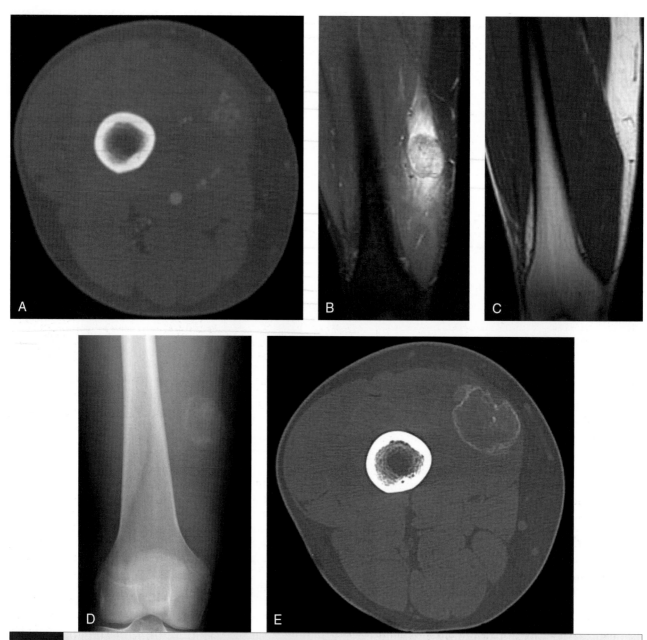

Figure 9 A 16-year-old male soccer player presented with an exquisitely painful mass of 4 weeks' duration. The patient reported receiving a hard kick to the thigh approximately 1 month prior to the onset of symptoms. Imaging studies obtained at presentation show disorganized, slight calcification on the axial CT scan **(A)**, bright T2-weighted MRI signal **(B)**, and dark T1-weighted MRI signal **(C)**, shown in these coronal images. These imaging features fit several potential diagnoses, including synovial sarcoma and soft-tissue osteosarcoma; however, the patient's history did not fit with these diagnoses. Instead of biopsy, the patient's history prompted follow-up imaging 6 weeks later. By that time, the pain was beginning to abate and both the plain AP radiograph **(D)** and axial CT scan **(E)** showed well-circumscribed peripheral ossification confirmatory of myositis ossificans circumscripta.

cision. Biopsy of lipomatous neoplasms with consistent subcutaneous fat signal characteristics throughout present a major challenge because of sampling error. The differential diagnosis for these neoplasms includes two entities, lipoma and well-differentiated lipoma-like liposarcoma, which are treated identically even though they have different propensities for local recurrence.

The pathologic interpretation of myositis ossificans can be difficult and can lead to inappropriate treat-

ments. Painful masses associated with any history of trauma, which are otherwise suspicious for myositis, are often best managed with close follow-up and serial imaging rather than biopsy so as to avoid the incorrect diagnosis of soft-tissue osteosarcoma.

The pathologic interpretation of soft-tissue neoplasms requires significant knowledge and experience. Patterns of cellular growth in bundles, fascicles, or in a storiform pattern; the production of myxoid matrix;

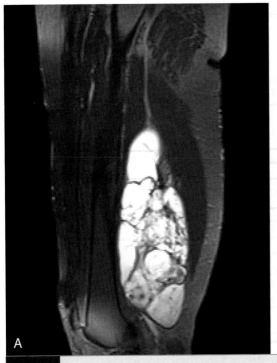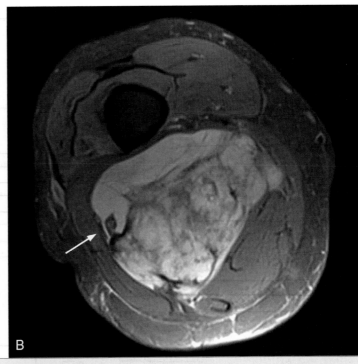

Figure 10	A 54-year-old man presented with worsening unilateral stocking foot neuropathy and a palpably enlarging mass in his posterior thigh. Core needle biopsy confirmed the diagnosis of myxoid liposarcoma, both histologically and by fluorescent in situ hybridization showing the FUS-CHOP rearrangement. Axial (**A**) and sagittal (**B**) images from a proton-density MRI scan show the sciatic nerve surrounded by the tumor (*arrow*). During preoperative radiotherapy, the tumor shrank away to a position abutting but no longer surrounding the nerve, permitting nerve-sparing resection.

the presence of necrosis; and the dominant cell type of small, round blue or spindled cells can quickly narrow the differential diagnosis based on hematoxylin and eosin staining alone; however, immunohistochemistry is the main modality for diagnosis of soft-tissue masses.

Immunohistochemical stains against cytokeratin are primarily used to rule out the presence of metastatic carcinoma, but epithelioid and synovial sarcoma will lightly stain. Endothelial markers CD31 and CD34 are used to detect vascular differentiation. S100 will stain nerve-derived tissues specifically but also stains several other sarcoma types and melanomas. TLE1 is a specific marker for synovial sarcoma because it is a target of *SYT-SSX* transcriptional amplification.[37] Markers of smooth muscle, such as smooth muscle actin, and striated muscle can be used to identify submorphologic differentiation suggestive of leiomyosarcoma or rhabdomyosarcoma.

Molecular diagnostics have revolutionized the analysis of soft-tissue neoplasms over the past decade. The dogma is increasing that the presence of subtype-specific molecular clues trump other histologic information when discrepancies arise.

Management Paradigms

Benign lesions without aggressive behavior usually can be managed conservatively (**Table 6**). Some patients elect excision for cosmetic reasons, but this choice must

be weighed against the risks involved. Elective resection of certain neoplasms should be avoided; popliteal cysts and intramuscular hemangiomas both require extensive surgeries but result in high rates of local recurrence.

Benign aggressive lesions with risk for local recurrence are challenging to treat. The prototype of this category is the extra-abdominal desmoid tumor or fibromatosis. Although lacking metastatic potential, its infiltrative growth pattern leads to high rates of local recurrence. Nonetheless, the use of adjuvant therapies remains controversial because of their adverse side effects.

Local control of soft-tissue sarcomas is primarily surgical, with adjuvant radiation used when multidisciplinary evaluation determines that achievable margins are insufficiently wide. When surgery either precedes or follows radiation, wide margins are the goal of resection. An exception is made for the salvage of critical structures such as nerves, vessels, and bones, which may be displaced or encroached on by the sarcoma (**Figure 10**). Microscopically planned positive margins along such structures do not significantly increase the rate of local recurrence when radiation is also used.[38] Such planned positive margins must be distinguished from positive margins inadvertently obtained from a poorly planned or executed resection, or by tumor infiltration beyond that apparent on imaging, which greatly increase recurrence rates. For involved vessels, resection and bypass reconstruction are used. For sar-

2: Systemic Disorders

Table 6

Soft-Tissue Masses

Tissue Group	Name	Age
Fibrous	Fibroma	Very young and adolescents
	Desmoid or fibromatosis	Young adult and middle aged
	Dermatofibroma protuberans	Middle age to older
	Myxofibrous sarcoma	Middle age to older
	Pleiomorphic undifferentiated sarcoma	Middle age to older
Lipomatous	Lipoma	Middle age
	Hibernoma	Young to middle age
	Lipoblastoma	Very young
	Well-differentiated lipoma-like liposarcoma	Middle age to older
	Myxoid liposarcoma	Young adults to middle age
	Round cell liposarcoma	Young adults to middle age
	Pleiomorphic liposarcoma	Middle age to older
Cartilaginous	Chondroma	Middle age to older
	Synovial chondromatosis	Middle age to older
	Extraskeletal myxoid chondrosarcoma	Young adults to middle age
Osseous	Myositis ossificans	Any age
	Metaplastic bone	Any age
	Soft-tissue osteosarcoma	Older adults
Vascular	Arteriovenous malformation	Adolescents through middle age
	Hemangioma	Adolescents through middle age
	Hemangiopericytoma	Middle age to older
	Epithelioid sarcoma	Young adults through older
	Angiosarcoma	Middle age to older
Neurogenic	Schwannoma	Any age
	Neurofibroma	Adolescents through middle age
	Malignant peripheral nerve sheath tumor	Young adults through middle age
Myogenic	Embryonal rhabdomyosarcoma	Very young
	Alveolar rhabdomyosarcoma	Adolescents
	Pleiomorphic rhabdomyosarcoma	Middle age to older
	Leiomyosarcoma	Middle age to older
Giant cell rich	Pigmented villonodular synovitis	Young adults to middle age
	Tenosynovial giant cell tumor	Young adults to middle age
Other	Myxoma	Any age
	Synovial sarcoma	Young adults to middle age

Green = Surgery is a last resort; yellow = Marginal excision is indicated; orange = Wide resection without adjuvants, unless recurrent; red = Wide resection with adjuvant radiation ± chemotherapy

(continued on next page)

© 2011 American Academy of Orthopaedic Surgeons

Table 6

Soft-Tissue Masses (continued)

Pathology	Special Notes
Bland fibrous tissue, low cellularity	Common on digits; recurrence common
Dense fascicles of collagen	Recurrence is a major challenge
Low-grade spindle cell neoplasm	Skin sarcoma; Moh surgery
Intermediate-grade fibrous lesion with histiocytes and myxoid features	More commonly superficial, but can have spreading growth pattern
Variable high-grade spindle cell neoplasm	Most common soft-tissue sarcoma, previously know as malignant fibrous histiocytoma
Normal adipose	Can be superficial or intramuscular
Brown adipose tissue	Rare neoplasm
Lipoblasts at variable stages of maturation	Rare and potentially self-limited
Mostly normal adipose with some lipoblasts and fibrous septae	Treated the same as intramuscular lipoma, but more recurrences
Intermediate-grade adipose/myxoid tissue, translocation	Especially radiosensitive
High-grade version of myxoid liposarcoma	Believed to be chemosensitive
High-grade spindle cell neoplasm with some lipoblasts	Second most common soft-tissue sarcoma
Hyaline cartilage	Very rare neoplasm
Hyaline cartilage undergoing endochondral ossification	Always intra-articular; behaves as low-grade malignant
Myxoid neoplasm with stellate chondrocytes, translocation	Treated on standard soft-tissue sarcoma protocols
Organized layers of ossification	Try to avoid biopsy when suspected
Woven bone area in other tumor	Can occur in synovial sarcoma, liposarcoma, and malignant peripheral nerve sheath tumors
High-grade spindle cells making osteoid matrix	Debate on whether this should get osteosarcoma chemotherapy
Large venous channels, bland	Try to avoid surgery
Variably sized bland vascular channels	Consider sclerotherapy or embolization
Round cells with fried egg appearance	Low, but not zero, metastatic potential; often treated as sarcoma
Round cells, forming nests	Often small on hands and feet
High-grade round cells forming vessel vestiges	Dreaded subtype, regionally progressive
Myxoid and spindled Schwann cells	Can be marginally excised sparing the nerve, usually
Fibrous and spindled cells	Nerve sparing is difficult
High-grade spindle cell neoplasm	Difficult to manage, radioresistant, chemoresistant
Round blue cells	Very chemosensitive
Round blue cells with stunted myogenic differentiation	Chemosensitive, surgery is adjuvant
High-grade spindle or round blue cells with striated muscle markers	Chemoresistant
High-grade spindle cells with smooth muscle markers	Extrauterine sites are treated the same as other sarcomas
Multinucleated giant cells on stromal background, hemosiderin	Complete intralesional excision is challenging, *CSF1* gene rearrangement
Multinucleated giant cells on stromal background, hemosiderin	*CSF1* gene rearrangement
Paucicellular myxoid matrix	Marginal excision usually successful
High-grade spindle cell, or biphasic with epithelial test, or round blue cell	No relationship whatsoever with synovium

2: Systemic Disorders

comas with single nerve involvements, nerve resection and limb salvage may provide adequate, although compromised, function.

The timing of radiotherapy has been studied in a randomized controlled trial. Postoperative radiotherapy requires higher doses and larger treatment volumes, which increase the adverse side effects of radiation. Preoperative radiotherapy minimizes the long-term complications of radiotherapy but increases the rate of early postoperative wound-healing complications.

The role of chemotherapy in the management of soft-tissue sarcomas remains controversial, with strong proponents and opponents among the experts. Survival benefits have not been demonstrated in large collective trials; however, some subtypes such as synovial sarcoma and round cell liposarcoma are believed to be more sensitive to chemotherapy.

Summary

Advances in population science, molecular biology, and clinical research methods have improved the understanding and accurate diagnosis of musculoskeletal neoplasia in recent years. Nonetheless, treatment protocols for this varied group of bone lesions and soft-tissue masses have remained fairly consistent over the past two decades. It is important to review the basic principles of current understanding and the clinical approach to and treatment of bone and soft-tissue neoplastic conditions, emphasizing recent modifications to long-standing accepted standards.

Annotated References

1. http://seer.cancer.gov. Accessed August 30, 2010.

    The SEER program of the National Cancer Institute provides detailed information on cancer incidence and survival data in the United States.

2. Mirabello L, Troisi RJ, Savage SA: Osteosarcoma incidence and survival rates from 1973 to 2004: data from the Surveillance, Epidemiology, and End Results Program. *Cancer* 2009;115(7):1531-1543.

    This SEER database study confirmed that osteosarcoma is bimodal in adolescents and those older than 60 years, with the latter group usually associated with underlying Paget disease or prior radiation. Treatment success has not improved in 20 years.

3. Jawad MU, Cheung MC, Min ES, Schneiderbauer MM, Koniaris LG, Scully SP: Ewing sarcoma demonstrates racial disparities in incidence-related and sex-related differences in outcome: an analysis of 1631 cases from the SEER database, 1973-2005. *Cancer* 2009;115(15):3526-3536.

    This sampling of patients with Ewing sarcoma from the SEER database showed a ninefold increased incidence but no difference in survival for Caucasians compared

with patients of African descent. Localized disease, smaller tumors, and appendicular skeletal location portend a good prognosis.

4. Giuffrida AY, Burgueno JE, Koniaris LG, Gutierrez JC, Duncan R, Scully SP: Chondrosarcoma in the United States (1973 to 2003): an analysis of 2890 cases from the SEER database. *J Bone Joint Surg Am* 2009;91(5):1063-1072.

    This analysis of 2,890 cases from the SEER database includes the largest number of patients in any single study of chondrosarcoma. The authors confirm that only the grade and stage of the tumors are predictive of survival on multivariate analysis, and that no improvement in treatment success has been observed over recent decades.

5. Gadgeel SM, Harlan LC, Zeruto CA, Osswald M, Schwartz AG: Patterns of care in a population-based sample of soft tissue sarcoma patients in the United States. *Cancer* 2009;115(12):2744-2754.

    This population evaluation study of soft-tissue sarcoma treatments confirmed the use of adjuvant radiation for survival and introduced the interesting observation that care of extremity sarcomas follows accepted guidelines more commonly than sarcomas at other anatomic sites.

6. Sultan I, Rodriguez-Galino C, Saab R, Yasir S, Casanova M, Ferrari A: Comparing children and adults with synovial sarcoma in the Surveillance, Epidemiology, and End Results program, 1983 to 2005: an analysis of 1268 patients. *Cancer* 2009;115(15):3537-3547.

    Children and adults with synovial sarcoma have similar presentations but different outcomes, which may indicate that historic treatments differed between these groups or that the underlying tumor biology changes in older patients.

7. Blazer DG III, Lazar AJ, Xing Y, et al: Clinical outcomes of molecularly confirmed clear cell sarcoma from a single institution and in comparison with data from the Surveillance, Epidemiology, and End Results registry. *Cancer* 2009;115(13):2971-2979.

    This single-institution review of patients with molecularly confirmed clear cell sarcomas was enhanced by consideration of the population-based, albeit less detailed data from the SEER database. The review confirmed that nodal metastasis is prognostically distinct from distant metastasis.

8. Jawad MU, Extein J, Min ES, Scully SP: Prognostic factors for survival in patients with epithelioid sarcoma: 441 cases from the SEER database. *Clin Orthop Relat Res* 2009;467(11):2939-2948.

    By far the largest study of epithelioid sarcoma available, this SEER database review showed an increasing incidence in diagnosis (likely resulting from improved recognition of the rare entity), but no improvement in treatment success, which was dependent entirely on surgical success and tumor stage.

9. Walkley CR, Qudsi R, Sankaran VG, et al: Conditional mouse osteosarcoma, dependent on p53 loss and poten-

tiated by loss of Rb, mimics the human disease. *Genes Dev* 2008;22(12):1662-1676.

This mouse model of osteosarcoma formation is generated from conditional ablation of the *p53* and *Rb1* tumor-suppressors, noted to be frequently disrupted in human osteosarcomas. Morphologically and molecularly (with wild chromosomal aberrations) this model matches the human disease.

10. Kirsch DG, Dinulescu DM, Miller JB, et al: A spatially and temporally restricted mouse model of soft tissue sarcoma. *Nat Med* 2007;13(8):992-997.

This mouse model of pleiomorphic undifferentiated soft-tissue sarcoma (formerly known as malignant fibrous histiocytoma) was generated from conditional ablation of *Kras* with either p53 or CDKN2a. The ablation was activated by the administration of a virus containing Cre-recombinase.

11. Riggi N, Cironi L, Provero P, et al: Expression of the FUS-CHOP fusion protein in primary mesenchymal progenitor cells gives rise to a model of myxoid liposarcoma. *Cancer Res* 2006;66(14):7016-7023.

12. Keller C, Arenkiel BR, Coffin CM, El-Bardeesy N, De-Pinho RA, Capecchi MR: Alveolar rhabdomyosarcomas in conditional Pax3:Fkhr mice: cooperativity of Ink4a/ARF and Trp53 loss of function. *Genes Dev* 2004; 18(21):2614-2626.

13. Haldar M, Hancock JD, Coffin CM, Lessnick SL, Capecchi MR: A conditional mouse model of synovial sarcoma: insights into a myogenic origin. *Cancer Cell* 2007;11(4):375-388.

The authors describe a mouse model of synovial sarcoma, generated by the expression of one of the human fusion transcripts, *SYT-SSX2*, in mouse myoblasts. This confirms that the fusion oncoprotein is sarcomagenic and specific for the synovial histologic subtype in the tumors generated.

14. Mau E, Whetstone H, Yu C, Hopyan S, Wunder JS, Alman BA: PTHrP regulates growth plate chondrocyte differentiation and proliferation in a Gli3 dependent manner utilizing hedgehog ligand dependent and independent mechanisms. *Dev Biol* 2007;305(1):28-39.

The authors follow up on a mouse model of Ollier disease using a mutated form of *PTHR1* from a patient. Additional mouse models of enchondromatosis were generated using downstream members of the same pathway.

15. Bovée JV: Multiple osteochondromas. *Orphanet J Rare Dis* 2008;3:3.

The author presents an up-to-date review of the clinical manifestations, therapeutic challenges, and remaining molecular quandaries of multiple hereditary exostoses and solitary osteochondroma formation. Level of evidence: V.

16. West RB, Rubin BP, Miller MA, et al: A landscape effect in tenosynovial giant-cell tumor from activation of CSF1 expression by a translocation in a minority of tumor cells. *Proc Natl Acad Sci U S A* 2006;103(3):690-695.

17. Oliveira AM, Perez-Atayde AR, Inwards CY, et al: USP6 and CDH11 oncogenes identify the neoplastic cell in primary aneurysmal bone cysts and are absent in so-called secondary aneurysmal bone cysts. *Am J Pathol* 2004;165(5):1773-1780.

18. Lodwick GS, Wilson AJ, Farrell C, Virtama P, Dittrich F: Determining growth rates of focal lesions of bone from radiographs. *Radiology* 1980;134(3):577-583.

19. Campanacci M: Giant-cell tumor and chondrosarcomas: grading, treatment and results (studies of 209 and 131 cases). *Recent Results Cancer Res* 1976;54:257-261.

20. Enneking WF, Spanier SS, Goodman MA: A system for the surgical staging of musculoskeletal sarcoma. *Clin Orthop Relat Res* 1980;153:106-120.

21. Mankin HJ, Lange TA, Spanier SS: The hazards of biopsy in patients with malignant primary bone and soft-tissue tumors. *J Bone Joint Surg Am* 1982;64(8):1121-1127.

22. Mankin HJ, Mankin CJ, Simon MA; Members of the Musculoskeletal Tumor Society: The hazards of the biopsy, revisited. *J Bone Joint Surg Am* 1996;78(5):656-663.

23. Skeletal Lesions Interobserver Correlation among Expert Diagnosticians (SLICED) Study Group: Reliability of histopathologic and radiologic grading of cartilaginous neoplasms in long bones. *J Bone Joint Surg Am* 2007;89(10):2113-2123.

The poor reliability of grading appendicular cartilage masses as benign, low-grade, or high-grade malignancies is confirmed even among recognized experts in bone tumor pathology and radiology. Level of evidence: II.

24. Rougraff BT: Evaluation of the patient with carcinoma of unknown origin metastatic to bone. *Clin Orthop Relat Res* 2003;(415, Suppl):S105-S109.

25. Mirels H: Metastatic disease in long bones: A proposed scoring system for diagnosing impending pathologic fractures. *Clin Orthop Relat Res* 1989;249:256-264.

26. Lin PP, Mirza AN, Lewis VO, et al: Patient survival after surgery for osseous metastases from renal cell carcinoma. *J Bone Joint Surg Am* 2007;89(8):1794-1801.

The authors provide an analysis of the largest series of patients treated for skeletal metastasis of renal cell carcinoma. They emphasize the use of tumor excision, even if intralesional, and question the use of adjuvant radiation in the same patients. Level of evidence: IV.

27. Blackley HR, Wunder JS, Davis AM, White LM, Kandel R, Bell RS: Treatment of giant-cell tumors of long bones with curettage and bone-grafting. *J Bone Joint Surg Am* 1999;81(6):811-820.

28. Prosser GH, Baloch KG, Tillman RM, Carter SR, Grimer RJ: Does curettage without adjuvant therapy provide low recurrence rates in giant-cell tumors of bone? *Clin Orthop Relat Res* 2005;435:211-218.

29. Deheshi BM, Jaffer SN, Griffin AM, Ferguson PC, Bell RS, Wunder JS: Joint salvage for pathologic fracture of giant cell tumor of the lower extremity. *Clin Orthop Relat Res* 2007;459:96-104.

   Intra-articular fractures secondary to locally advanced giant cell tumor of bone have been considered an indication for wide resection and endoprosthetic reconstruction in many centers. This study challenges that dogma with a successful series of patients treated with joint-salvage surgery. Level of evidence: III.

30. Hanna SA, Whittingham-Jones P, Sewell MD, et al: Outcome of intralesional curettage for low-grade chondrosarcoma of long bones. *Eur J Surg Oncol* 2009; 35(12):1343-1347.

   This is the largest and most recent of several studies reporting results from the technique of intralesional curettage for grade I chondrosarcoma, which is growing in popularity. Level of evidence: IV.

31. Nguyen QN, Chang EL: Emerging role of proton beam radiation therapy for chordoma and chondrosarcoma of the skull base. *Curr Oncol Rep* 2008;10(4):338-343.

   The recently burgeoning data for proton beam and other high-dose radiation technologies as isolated treatments for surgically unresectable chondrosarcomas and chordomas of the axial skeleton are discussed. Level of evidence: V.

32. Zimel MN, Cizik AM, Rapp TB, Weisstein JS, Conrad EU III: Megaprosthesis versus Condyle-sparing intercalary allograft: distal femoral sarcoma. *Clin Orthop Relat Res* 2009;467(11):2813-2824.

   This is the most recent of many studies evaluating outcomes of limb salvage with endoprosthetic or allograft reconstruction. The authors emphasize a specific technique to expand the indications for intercalary allograft reconstruction to very thin residual epiphyses. Level of evidence: IV.

33. Scwartz AJ, Kiatisevi P, Eilber FC, Eilber FR, Eckardt JJ: The Friedman-Eilber resection arthroplasty of the pelvis. *Clin Orthop Relat Res* 2009;467(11):2825-2830.

   This article reviews the very positive functional results of a large consecutive study of patients treated with pelvic resections, including resection of the hip joint without fusion, endoprosthetic reconstruction, and allograft reconstruction. Level of evidence: IV.

34. Eilber FC, Brennan MF, Eilber FR, Dry SM, Singer S, Kattan MW: Validation of the postoperative nomogram for 12-year sarcoma-specific mortality. *Cancer* 2004; 101(10):2270-2275.

35. Ogose A, Morita T, Hotta T, et al: Brain metastases in musculoskeletal sarcomas. *Jpn J Clin Oncol* 1999;29(5): 245-247.

36. Schuetze SM, Rubin BP, Vernon C, et al: Use of positron emission tomography in localized extremity soft tissue sarcoma treated with neoadjuvant chemotherapy. *Cancer* 2005;103(2):339-348.

37. Terry J, Saito T, Subramanian S, et al: TLE1 as a diagnostic immunohistochemical marker for synovial sarcoma emerging from gene expression profiling studies. *Am J Surg Pathol* 2007;31(2):240-246.

   The authors describe TLE1 as both a transcriptional target of the *SYT-SSX* fusion oncoproteins and a unique immunohistochemical marker for synovial sarcoma.

38. Clarkson PW, Griffin AM, Catton CN, et al: Epineural dissection is a safe technique that facilitates limb salvage surgery. *Clin Orthop Relat Res* 2005;438:92-96.

Chapter 18
Arthritis

SM Javad Mortazavi, MD   Javad Parvizi, MD, FRCS

Introduction

Joint disorders or arthritis affect 21% of the US population (69.9 million people) according to recent surveys by the Centers for Disease Control and Prevention.[1] Arthritis has been traditionally categorized as either inflammatory or noninflammatory, depending on the underlying pathologic processes. Inflammatory arthritis may be infectious (septic arthritis), crystal-induced (gout or pseudogout), immune-related (rheumatoid arthritis [RA]), or reactive (Reiter syndrome). Osteoarthritis (OA) is considered the prototype for noninflammatory arthritis, although in recent years the noninflammatory nature of OA has been disputed. An orthopaedic surgeon should be familiar with different types of arthritis because an accurate diagnosis is essential for planning an appropriate treatment strategy.

Osteoarthritis

OA or degenerative joint disease continues to be the leading cause of disability and impaired quality of life in developed countries.[2] It is the most common of all joint diseases that imparts substantial economic burden on health care systems and society, and it is the single greatest cause of lost work days.[3] The chronic use of analgesics and anti-inflammatory drugs and the need for surgical treatment result in additional costs. Moreover, as the baby-boomer generation ages, it is expected that the prevalence of OA will increase 66% to 100% by the year 2030.[4] Currently, approximately 800,000 total knee and total hip arthroplasties are performed in the United States annually, with the number expected to exceed 1.2 million by the year 2020.[5] Symptomatic OA of the knee (defined as the presence of knee pain on most days of a recent month plus radiographic evidence of OA in the same knee) occurs in 12% of adults age 60 years or older in the United States and in 6% of all adults age 30 years or older.[6] Symptomatic OA of the hip is approximately one third as common as OA in the knee.[7]

Pathophysiology

OA is essentially joint failure because all structures of the joint undergo pathologic changes. Traditionally, OA was considered to be a disease of articular cartilage, with loss of cartilage considered the essential pathologic process for OA. In recent years, however, it has been realized that OA affects the entire joint structure, including synovium, ligaments, and subchondral bone, along with the articular cartilage.[8] Each structure in the joint plays an important and unique role in the daily function of the joint. Articular cartilage, with its compressive stiffness and smooth surface; synovial fluid, which provides a smooth and frictionless surface for movement; the joint capsule and the ligaments, which protect the joint from excessive excursions; the periarticular muscles, which minimize focal stresses across the joint by appropriate muscle contractions; the sensory fibers, which provide feedback for muscles and tendons; and the subchondral bone, with its mechanical strength and shock-absorbing function all interact in an intricate manner to provide optimal function for the joint. Destruction of any of these structures or a disruption in the balance between them leads to the process of arthritis.

The earliest changes in OA usually appear in the hyaline articular cartilage. The cartilage matrix consists of two important macromolecules: type II collagen and aggrecan (a proteoglycan macromolecule with highly negatively charged glycosaminoglycans). Chondrocytes produce all the elements of the cartilage matrix as well as the enzymes that break down the matrix, cytokines, and growth factors. In OA, chondrocytes produce abnormally high quantities of inflammatory cytokines such as interleukin (IL)1-β and tumor necrosis factor-α (TNF-α), which in turn decrease collagen synthesis and increase degradative proteases (including matrix metalloproteinases and other inflammatory mediators, such as IL-6, IL-8, prostaglandin E_2, nitric oxide, and bone morphogenetic protein-2).[8,9] It is now clear that OA is also an inflammatory process initiated and propagated

Neither Dr. Mortazavi nor an immediate family member has received anything of value from or holds stock in a commercial company or institution related directly or indirectly to the subject of this chapter. Dr. Parvizi or an immediate family member serves as a board member, owner, officer, or committee member of the American Association of Hip and Knee Surgeons, American Board of Orthopaedic Surgery, British Orthopaedic Association, Orthopaedic Research and Education Foundation, and SmartTech; serves as a paid consultant to or an employee of Stryker; and has received research or institutional support from KCI, Medtronic, the Musculoskeletal Transplant Foundation, Smith & Nephew, and Stryker.

2: Systemic Disorders

by inflammatory mediators that lead to the demise of the articular cartilage first and damage to other structures over time.[10] The production of these mediators leads to an increase in the metabolic activity of articular cartilage, a tissue that usually has low activity. As OA progresses, the cartilage undergoes a gradual depletion of aggrecan and collagen type II; the tightly woven collagen type II then begins to unfurl. As a result, the cartilage loses its compressive stiffness and becomes more vulnerable to further injury.

The classification of OA as a noninflammatory arthritis is, in part, based on the fact that the leukocyte count in the synovial fluid of OA patients is typically less than 2,000 cells/μL. There is no question that low-grade synovial inflammation contributes to the pathogenesis of this disease. In contrast to RA, synovial inflammation in OA is mostly confined to the area adjacent to the affected cartilage and bone.

The initiation of inflammation sets up a vicious cycle whereby further inflammatory mediators, such as proteinases and cytokines, are released from the synovium and can accelerate the destruction of the nearby cartilage. In turn, cartilage breakdown products, resulting from mechanical or enzymatic destruction, can provoke the release of collagenase and other hydrolytic enzymes from synovial cells, which can lead to vascular hyperplasia in synovial membranes. This cascade sequentially results in the induction of IL-1β and TNF-α, which enhance the inflammatory process. This "cytokine storm" is more likely to occur in the earlier stages of OA.[10]

Investigations have shown that the production of reactive oxygen species plays an important role in the initiation and propagation of OA.[11] The by-products of reactive oxygen species were detected during early OA and may be used as biomarkers for detecting this condition early in the process. Future directions for treating OA will likely be based on the discovery of new biomarkers for OA, further information about the enzymatic pathways active in the disease, and the development of disease-modifying OA drugs.

Risk Factors

Several risk factors for OA have been identified. These factors either result in disruption of the protective mechanisms of the joint, rendering them dysfunctional, or cause excessive forces across the joint, which overload otherwise competent structures. The risk factors can be categorized into two groups based on the location of their effect (systemic or local).

Systemic Risk Factors
Advancing Age
Advancing age is perhaps the most important risk factor for OA because it increases the vulnerability of joints through several mechanisms.[12] With advancing age, cartilage becomes less responsive to dynamic loading and is slower to regenerate; as a result, older patients have thinner cartilage, which is more sensitive to shear stresses and is at significantly greater risk for damage. Advancing age also increases the risk of failure

in other joint protectors. Muscles become weaker, ligaments stretch and are less able to absorb stresses, and sensory input slows. It is important to note that OA is not an inevitable consequence of aging; it is not a simple wearing out of the joint. Age-related changes in the joint can be distinguished from those caused by disease. The ability of aging chondrocytes to produce and repair the extracellular matrix is compromised because of a decline in growth factor activity. This appears to be related to both a decline in the local availability of growth factors, including BMP-7 and TGF-β, as well as a decline in the response of chondrocytes to growth factors such as insulin-like growth factor-I.[13] Chondrocyte senescence, which is marked by shortened telomeres, increased levels of B-galactosidases, and decreased adenosine triphosphate production caused by mitochondrial dysfunction, has a key role in the development and progression of age-related impairments in cartilage repair. Telomere erosion and oxidative damage are the two main mechanisms for chondrocyte senescence. In the telomere erosion hypothesis, cell aging is regulated by an intrinsic genetic clock associated with the erosion of telomeres. Oxidative stress, another important cause of age-related chondrocyte senescence, is explained by the age-related degeneration of mitochondria. Mitochondria provide metabolic energy via respiration and protect cells from the toxic effects of oxygen and its free-radical derivatives; therefore, the damage to mitochondria limits energy production and exposes cells to oxidative damage.[14]

Gender
A variety of studies have reported that women are more at risk for developing OA. In addition, women have a greater number of involved joints and are more likely to have OA that affects the knees and the hands. Although the exact reason for the higher incidence of OA in women is not known, loss of estrogen over time is believed to be an important contributing factor.

Genetics
The role of genetic factors in the development of OA is well known. Many studies have confirmed the inherited element for this disease, particularly for OA of the hip and hand joints.[12,15] In one study, 50% of cases of hand and hip OA were attributed to inherited factors.[16] In addition, recent studies have identified genetic mutations that place patients at high risk for OA.[12,15] Specifically, a mutation in the *FRZB* gene is believed to put women at high risk for hip OA. This gene encodes a frizzle protein, whose role is to antagonize an extracellular Wnt ligand. Because the Wnt signaling pathway plays a critical role in matrix synthesis and joint development, it makes sense that a mutated frizzle protein would be associated with an increased incidence of OA.[17] The *ASPN* gene also is described as a susceptibility gene for OA.[18] Anatomic abnormalities of joints in patients with skeletal dysplasia are a known cause of early OA. There are known genetic bases for many of these dysplasias.[19] A recent study identified a 4-Mb re-

gion on chromosome 17q21 that was linked to developmental hip dysplasia.[20]

In addition to identifying specific genetic markers, some studies have examined the incidence of OA in different ethnic groups.[21,22] Hip OA is rare in Chinese and Chinese-American populations; however, knee OA is at least as common in the Chinese population as it is in the Caucasian population.[21] African populations (although not African Americans) appear to have much lower rates of hip OA than do Caucasians.

Local Risk Factors
Anatomy
An abnormal joint anatomy that results in an uneven distribution of load across the joint and an increase in focal stresses can be a risk factor for OA. In the hip, developmental dysplasia, Legg-Calvé-Perthes disease, and slipped capital femoral epiphysis are the most common reasons for early distortions in hip anatomy that can lead to OA later in life. The severity of the anatomic deformity determines whether OA will occur in young adulthood (seen most commonly in patients with severe abnormalities) or later in life (more common in patients with mild abnormalities). It was recently shown that subtle developmental abnormalities in the hip joint can lead to femoroacetabular impingement and secondary OA.[23] Anatomic distortion following intra-articular fractures also increases the susceptibility of a joint to early OA. Osteonecrosis secondary to a variety of etiologies, particularly if it leads to the collapse of subchondral bone, can produce joint irregularities that lead to OA. Additionally, malalignment across the joint can lead to uneven wear on the articular surfaces, also leading to OA.[24]

Trauma
Injuries such as anterior cruciate ligament tears, meniscal tears in the knee, and labral tears in the hip can increase the susceptibility of a joint to OA and can lead to premature OA. Injury to joint structures, even those that do not require surgical repair, may increase the risk of OA. This finding was shown in the Framingham study, which demonstrated that men with a history of major knee injury and no surgery had a 3.5-fold increased risk of subsequent knee OA.[25]

Body Mass Index
The relative risk of OA increases with obesity.[26] Also, obese people have more severe symptoms of OA and are more likely to have the progressive form of the disease. Obesity has been shown to be a strong risk factor for the development of knee OA and, less so, for hip OA. Interestingly, obesity has been shown to be a stronger risk factor for the disease in women than in men. In women, the relationship of weight to the risk of OA is linear; weight loss in women lowers the risk of symptomatic disease.

Repetitive Use Injury
Workers who perform repetitive occupational tasks for many years have an increased risk of the development of OA in the repeatedly used joints. For example, a high incidence of hip OA has been reported in farmers and a high incidence of knee and spine OA has been reported in miners. Certain types of exercises also may increase the risk of OA. Studies suggest that professional running increases the risk of hip and knee OA.[27,28] Patients with impaired proprioception across the joint are prone to OA and to significant progression of the disease. This trend can be observed in patients with Charcot joint.

Bone Density
The role of bone as a shock absorber for the load of impact is not well understood; however, it has been shown that people with higher bone density are at an increased risk of OA, whereas osteoporosis has a negative association with OA.[29]

Clinical Features

The initial stage of the OA disease process is silent, which explains the high prevalence of radiographic and pathologic signs of OA in clinically asymptomatic patients. Interestingly, even in the later stages of OA, there is a poor correlation between clinical symptoms and the degree of change in bone or cartilage detected directly by arthroscopy or indirectly by radiography or MRI.

The most likely sources of pain in OA are synovial inflammation, joint effusion, and bone marrow edema. The degree to which each of these three factors is present varies from patient to patient. The pain generated by OA is usually exacerbated by activity and relieved by rest. Early in the disease, the pain is episodic, triggered often by 1 or 2 days of overuse of the involved joint (for example, a person with knee OA may notice a few days of pain after a long run). More advanced OA can cause pain at rest and night pain severe enough to awaken the patient. Pain from OA is usually described as deep, aching, and poorly localized; it may radiate or be referred to surrounding structures. In diagnosing OA, it is helpful to know the location of the pain and to perform a careful physical examination to identify particular motions that aggravate the pain. Groin pain, for example, usually indicates a hip joint disorder. Some patients with hip OA, however, may report knee pain rather than hip pain. For these patients, the key to the correct diagnosis of hip OA is the finding (through physical examination) that hip rotation increases pain.

A wide range of additional symptoms tend to be present along with pain from OA. Many patients report a short-lived stiffness after inactivity (gelling). OA may be associated with joint instability or giving way. Patients may report a reduced range of motion, deformity, swelling, and crepitus. The clinician should be aware that certain clinical symptoms are not generally associated with OA. For example, even in patients with severe OA, systemic features such as fever, weight loss, anemia, and an elevated erythrocyte sedimentation rate are not normally present. In the process of taking a patient history, it is also important to ask how the pain

[Handwritten margin note at top of page:
isometric v. isotonic
- same length — same tension in muscle
- jt. angle & — concentric: muscle sho[rtens]
muscle length — eccentric: " elongates
do not change during contraction]

has affected the patient's function at home, work, and in recreational activities and how the patient is coping with the pain. The physician should look for signs of psychological distress (for example, signs of anxiety, excessive pain-avoidance posturing, or the onset of insomnia) or depression (for example, early morning wakening, weight loss, irritability, or a marked increase in memory and concentration problems).

The joints most commonly involved in primary OA are the metatarsophalangeal joint of the great toe, the proximal and distal interphalangeal joints of the fingers, the carpometacarpal joint of the thumb, and the joints of the hips, knees, and cervical and lumbar spine. Unless they are involved in a secondary form of OA, other joints are typically spared. OA is believed to be a uniformly progressive disease that invariably leads to joint arthroplasty; however, the disease appears to stabilize in many patients, with no worsening of symptoms or signs. In specific subgroups, the prognosis may be either worse or better, depending on both risk and protective factors.

Diagnosis

Classic findings of OA on plain radiographs are osteophytes, joint-space narrowing, subchondral sclerosis, and in more advanced disease, bone cysts. Because radiographs are not sensitive to the earliest pathologic features of OA, the absence of positive radiographic findings in a patient with symptoms of OA should not be interpreted as the complete absence of the disease. In clinical practice, the diagnosis of OA should be made on the basis of the patient history and physical examination. The role of radiography is to confirm clinical suspicions and rule out other conditions rather than to make an independent diagnosis.[30] This role is more distinct in patients with chronic hip and hand pain because the diagnosis can often be unclear without confirming radiographs. It has been shown in cross-sectional and longitudinal studies that there is no association, or only a weak association, between radiographic changes and functioning in patients with OA.[31] MRI can be used to diagnose other causes of joint pain (such as osteochondritis dissecans or osteonecrosis), which may otherwise be confused with OA in patients with joint pain. It should be noted that meniscal tears are nearly universally seen in patients with knee OA and are not necessarily a cause of increased symptoms.

No blood tests are routinely indicated in the workup of patients with OA unless symptoms and signs suggest inflammatory arthritis. The synovial fluid analysis in patients with noninflammatory arthritis should usually demonstrate no evidence of inflammatory reaction with few leukocytes (<1,000 per µL) and good viscosity. The presence of more than 1,000 leukocytes per µL usually is indicative of inflammatory arthritis.

Treatment
Nonsurgical
The goals in treating patients with OA are pain relief and improvement of physical function. Currently, there are no disease-modifying drugs for OA, and all available pharmacologic agents aim to provide symptomatic relief. The treatment of patients with OA should be comprehensive and should follow the stepwise formula recommended by the American College of Rheumatology.[32] Nonpharmacologic measures may include physical therapy and exercise. These treatments should be considered the base line for managing all patients with OA. Muscle weakness often accompanies OA, and increased muscle strength helps reduce the load on cartilage. Isometric (as opposed to isotonic) exercises are preferred because they put less stress on the involved joint. Perhaps some of the most important elements in therapy include activity modification, implementation of periodic rest of the affected joint, and the use of assistive walking devices to offload affected joints of the lower extremity.

For patients with intermittent and mild symptoms, reassurance and nonpharmacologic therapies usually suffice; however, patients with ongoing, disabling pain may need pharmacotherapy. The first-line medication for symptomatic pain relief is a simple analgesic such as acetaminophen. For patients with inflammatory disease (as seen in erosive OA) and for those whose symptoms cannot be well controlled with simple analgesics, nonsteroidal anti-inflammatory drugs (NSAIDs) are more effective. The new class of NSAIDS—the cyclooxygenase-2 inhibitors—are more selective and have decreased gastrointestinal toxicity; however, they also have been associated with increased cardiovascular events. Patients should be informed about risks before cyclooxygenase-2 inhibitors are prescribed.

Nutraceuticals, such as oral glucosamine and chondroitin, have been shown to reduce pain in patients with knee OA, but further research is needed to confirm the effectiveness of such treatments.

Although systemic steroids are not used in treating OA, intra-articular cortisone injections to reduce synovial inflammation are effective in relieving pain from OA. Injections should not be repeated more than a few times because they have been associated with an increased risk of cartilage breakdown. Intra-articular injection of hyaluronic acid can improve joint symptoms in a subgroup of patients with knee OA; however, the overall efficacy of this treatment over a placebo in patients with hip or knee OA remains controversial.[33]

Surgical
Joint arthroplasty is the single most effective treatment of arthritis of most joints, including the knee, hip, shoulder, elbow, ankle, and (perhaps) small joints of the hand. Joint arthroplasty is an effective treatment option for patients with advanced arthritis that compromises function and is nonresponsive to nonsurgical treatment. Currently, the failure rate for total knee and total hip arthroplasty is less than 1% per year. Better patient outcomes after joint arthroplasty have been reported in high-volume centers with surgery performed by surgeons performing more than 50 joint arthroplasties per year.[34,35] The timing of knee or hip replacement surgery

[Vertical text in left margin:] 2: Systemic Disorders

do total jt. earlier! don't wait

appears to be very important. Studies have shown that patients with more advanced disease have less improvement than those receiving the procedure earlier in the course of their disease.[36,37]

Currently, there is no efficacious treatment for cartilage regeneration in patients with OA.[38] Either chondrocyte transplantation or chondroplasty (abrasion arthroplasty), which may be useful in patients with localized cartilage damage, have no proven efficacy in OA.

Inflammatory Arthritis

Inflammatory arthritis consists of a large group of different conditions that cause inflammation in the joint. The diagnosis can be made by evaluating the patient's profile, the chronology of symptoms, the extent of joint involvement, and the precipitating factors. Systemic lupus erythematosus (SLE) and reactive arthritis occur more frequently in young patients, whereas RA is more prevalent in middle-age patients. Gout and spondyloarthropathies (such as ankylosing spondylitis) are more common in men, whereas SLE is more common in women.

The nature of the onset of the disease also can be helpful in making the diagnosis. Septic arthritis and gout tend to present abruptly, whereas RA may have an indolent presentation. Additionally, the evolution of a patient's symptoms may be intermittent (more common in crystal-induced or Lyme diseases), migratory (in rheumatic fever, gonococcal, or viral arthritis), or additive (in RA and psoriatic arthritis). Arthritides are typically classified as acute or chronic if symptoms persist for fewer than or more than 6 weeks, respectively. Reactive, infectious, or crystal-induced diseases tend to present acutely, whereas immunologic disease (such as RA) has a propensity for chronic presentation. It is also helpful in diagnosing inflammatory arthritis to note the extent and degree of articular involvement. Crystal-induced and infectious arthritis are often monoarticular, spondyloarthropathies are often oligoarticular, and RA is often polyarticular. Symmetric joint involvement is seen in RA, but spondyloarthropathies often show an asymmetric involvement. Additionally, RA often involves the joints of the upper extremities, whereas reactive arthritis and arthritis from gout tend to involve the joints of the lower extremities. Involvement of the axial skeleton (with the exception of the cervical spine) is a characteristic of spondyloarthropathies and is rare in RA.

Systemic features of inflammatory arthritis such as fever (in SLE and septic arthritis), rash (in SLE and psoriatic arthritis), and nail abnormalities (in psoriatic or reactive arthritis) should be noted. Involvement of other organ systems, including the eyes (seen in Behçet disease and spondyloarthritis), the gastrointestinal tract (seen in inflammatory bowel disease), the genitourinary tract (seen in reactive arthritis or gonococcemia), or the nervous system (seen in Lyme disease), also should be considered in diagnosing inflammatory arthritis.

Rheumatoid Arthritis

RA is a chronic multisystem disease of unknown cause. The characteristic feature of established RA is persistent inflammatory synovitis, usually involving peripheral joints in a symmetric distribution. In RA, synovial inflammation leads to cartilage damage, bony erosion, and changes in joint integrity. Despite the destructive potential of the disease, its course is quite variable. In some patients, the disease remains confined to two or three joints and may cause only minimal destruction. In most patients, however, the involvement is polyarticular, with relentless progression and marked functional impairment. RA affects 1% to 1.5% of the population worldwide.[39] Its incidence increases during adulthood and peaks at approximately age 40 to 60 years. Females are affected three times more frequently than males. The hallmarks of the disease are the symmetric involvement of multiple joints in the hands and the feet and a positive test for rheumatoid factor (immunoglobulin M antibody directed against the Fc portion of immunoglobulin G). Additional constitutional symptoms, such as weight loss, fever, and malaise, may be present. The presence of rheumatic factor does not establish the diagnosis of RA because its positive predictive value is poor; however, the presence of rheumatoid factor can have prognostic significance because patients with high titers tend to have more severe and progressive disease with extra-articular manifestation.[40]

RA usually presents initially with episodes of morning stiffness that last for more than 1 hour, joint pain and swelling, and difficulty performing the activities of daily living. RA commonly involves the wrist, elbow, knee, foot metatarsophalangeal and proximal interphalangeal joints, and the cervical spine. The distal interphalangeal joints, and the lumbosacral spine are usually spared. Cervical spine subluxation (C1-C2) secondary to RA can lead to spinal instability and cord impingement. Patients with cervical spine instability are at risk for spinal injury during intubation for general anesthesia and should be treated with fiberoptic intubation. The diagnosis of RA is made if a patient has, for more than a 6-week duration, four of the seven criteria for RA defined by the American College of Rheumatology[41] (Table 1). Extra-articular manifestations of RA are rheumatoid nodules and ocular, cardiac, or neurologic involvement. Rheumatoid nodules are pathognomonic and are seen in 30% of patients with RA, mostly on the extensor surface of the forearm. Because these nodules may be confused with gouty tophi, nodule aspiration is the best method to distinguish between the two conditions. Tophi contain monosodium urate crystals, whereas rheumatoid nodules contain cholesterol crystals.

The goal of treatment is to suppress inflammation and preserve joint structure and function. Early, aggressive use of disease-modifying antirheumatic drugs and biologic response modifiers either alone or in combination has been shown to be effective in achieving treatment goals.[42] Disease-modifying antirheumatic drugs include methotrexate, sulfasalazine, leflunomide, hy-

Table 1

The 1987 Revised Criteria for the Classification of Rheumatoid Arthritis

Guidelines for Classification

Four of seven criteria are required to classify a patient as having rheumatoid arthritis

Patients with two or more clinical diagnoses are not excluded

Criteria

Morning stiffness for at least 1 hour and present for at least 6 weeks[a]

Swelling of three or more joints[ab]

Arthritis of the hand joints: arthritis of wrist, metacarpophalangeal, or proximal interphalangeal joints for 6 weeks or more[ab]

Symmetric arthritis[ab]

Rheumatoid nodules[b]

Serum rheumatoid factor measured by a method that is positive in less than 5% of normal individuals

Radiographic changes in the hand typical of rheumatoid arthritis must include erosions or unequivocal bony decalcification

[a] Criterion must be present for at least 6 weeks
[b] Criterion must be observed by physician

droxychloroquine, and minocycline. Biologic response modifiers include etanercept, adalimumab, infliximab, and more recently, rituximab and abatacept. These medications require screening for latent tuberculosis infection before starting therapy because of the risk of reactivating the infection.[43]

For those patients with severely damaged joints, total joint arthroplasty is a viable option with better outcomes in the hip, the knee, and the shoulder joints. Several reconstructive hand surgeries can lead to functional and cosmetic improvement. Arthroscopic or open synovectomy, especially in the knee, may offer short-term relief but does not appear to retard bone destruction or alter the natural history of the disease.

Seronegative Spondyloarthropathies

The spondyloarthropathies are a group of chronic inflammatory diseases with the clinical spectrum that includes ankylosing spondylitis as a prototype, reactive arthritis (known previously as Reiter syndrome), psoriatic arthritis, enteropathic arthritis, and juvenile-onset spondyloarthropathies.[44,45] Undifferentiated spondyloarthropathy includes diseases with elements of the spondyloarthropathies that do not fulfill the accepted criteria for the diseases. The spondyloarthropathies have overlapping features and are generally characterized by peripheral arthritis and enthesitis, axial inflammation (sacroiliitis and spondylitis), and new bone formation leading to ankylosis. They often display extra-

articular manifestations such as intestinal, ocular, and skin inflammation.

These disorders are not associated with positive rheumatic factor, but show striking familial aggregation and typically are associated with HLA genes of the major histocompatibility complex. This association varies among the different forms of spondyloarthropathies and among different ethnic groups. Both men and women are affected, with an overall male predominance. Spondyloarthropathies usually begin in the late teens and early 20s, but they may also present in childhood (juvenile) or at an older age. The prevalence of spondyloarthropathies may be approximately twice as high as previously believed. Based on the validated criteria of the European Spondyloarthropathy Study Group that includes a wider disease spectrum, the overall prevalence of ankylosing spondylitis may be similar to RA.

The pathogenesis of spondyloarthropathies involves genetic susceptibility and environmental factors.[46] Genetic factors, particularly the presence of the HLA-B27 allele, heavily influence the pathogenesis of the spondyloarthropathies. Other genes probably work in concert with HLA to further augment the susceptibility and modulate the severity of the disease. Environmental factors, including infectious triggers, appear to play important roles. Reactive arthritis usually develops following infection with Chlamydia trachomatis or after dysentery caused by different enteric organisms. The microorganisms implicated in reactive arthritis share common biologic features: they can invade mucosal surfaces, replicate intracellularly, and contain lipopolysaccharide in the outer membrane. The close relationship between gut inflammation and spondyloarthropathies has been established for decades. More than 50% of patients with spondyloarthropathies have microscopic evidence of bowel inflammation; inflammatory bowel disease, particularly Crohn disease, develops in 6% to 13% of those patients.[47] These observations have raised the theory that the inciting and perpetuating event in the spondyloarthropathies may be a breakdown in the gut-blood barrier, allowing penetration of intestinal bacteria.

Ankylosing spondylitis is the most common and typical form of spondyloarthropathy. It usually presents as inflammatory back pain and stiffness in adolescence and early adulthood. It is rare for ankylosing spondylitis to present after age 45 years. The diagnosis is clinical and the presenting features are very nonspecific; for this reason, the diagnosis is often delayed for 5 to 6 years, particularly in patients with an incomplete clinical picture[48,49] (Table 2). The presence of anterior uveitis, a positive family history of spondyloarthropathy, impaired spinal mobility or chest expansion, and enthesitis further support the diagnosis. Radiologic involvement of the sacroiliac joints is still considered the hallmark of ankylosing spondylitis (Figure 1). MRI with gadolinium enhancement is a valuable imaging modality to identify sacroiliitis and enthesitis. There is no laboratory test to diagnose ankylosing spondylitis, but the HLA-B27 allele has been found in approxi-

entheses: sites where tendons or ligaments insert into bone

Table 2

Diagnostic Criteria for Ankylosing Spondylitis[a] (Modified, New York, 1984)

Criteria

1. Low back pain of at least 3 months' duration improved by exercise but not relieved by rest
2. Limitation of lumbar spine in sagittal and frontal plane
3. Chest expansion decreases relative to normal values for age and sex
4A. Unilateral sacroiliitis grade 3 to 4
4B. Bilateral sacroiliitis grade 2 to 4

[a] Definite ankylosing spondylitis if 4A or 4B and any clinical criterion (1-3)

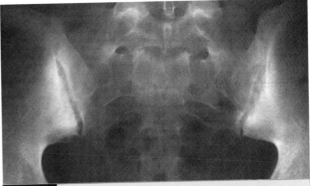

Figure 1   Radiograph of sacroiliitis in a patient with ankylosing spondylitis showing sclerosis along the iliac sides of the sacroiliac joints and loss of portions of the iliac subchondral bone, indicating erosion. (Reproduced with permission from Firestein GS: Image modalities in rheumatic disease, in Firestein G, Budd R, Harris E, eds: *Kelley's Textbook of Rheumatology*, ed 8. Philadelphia, PA, Elsevier, 2008, vol 1, pp 53-54.)

mately 90% to 95% of affected white patients. However, *HLA-B27* can be found in 8% to 10% of the white population and 2% of the black population. Moreover, ankylosing spondylitis develops in only 1% to 2% of people who are *HLA-B27* positive. The erythrocyte sedimentation rate and C-reactive protein level are elevated in 50% to 70% of patients, but the elevations are not generally associated with disease activity.

Ankylosing spondylitis is treated with both pharmacologic and nonpharmacologic modalities.[50] Pharmacologic treatment begins with NSAIDs as the first-line therapy, with sulfasalazine as the second-line therapy. Recently, data have emerged showing the efficacy of TNF-α blockers in controlling articular inflammation; however, these blockers are ineffective in preventing new bone formation and joint ankylosis, which are major features of the disease. Additionally, the expense and the adverse side-effects profile of TNF-α blockers, particularly infection, are concerns with this medication. Nonpharmacologic therapy includes patient education, outpatient physical therapy, a home exercise program (including a spinal extension program), and proper posture. In patients with end-stage joint involvement, surgical intervention, including joint arthroplasty, can be helpful. Total hip arthroplasty is the most common surgical procedure in patients with ankylosing spondylitis. Heterotopic new bone formation can be a potential complication. In patients with fixed kyphotic deformity that results in functional impairment, surgical correction of spinal deformity through osteotomy may be helpful.

Reactive arthritis is an aseptic arthritis triggered by a genitourinary or gastrointestinal tract infection. The arthritis usually begins 1 to 4 weeks after the infection as an acute and oligoarticular arthritis in the lower extremity. Enthesitis (especially in the heel), dactylitis, and inflammatory back pain are common. Constitutional symptoms, including low-grade fever and weight loss, may occur in the acute phase. Extra-articular manifestations such as conjunctivitis, urethritis, oral ulcers, and skin lesions in the palm and sole (keratoderma blennorrhagicum) are essential in supporting the

diagnosis of reactive arthritis.[51] Reactive arthritis is believed to be a self-limiting condition with a course of 3 to 12 months; symptomatic treatment with NSAIDs as first-line therapy and sulfasalazine as second-line therapy are warranted.

Psoriatic arthritis has been reported in as many as 20% of patients with psoriasis. It occurs with the same frequency in men and women. The skin manifestations precede joint involvement in 80% to 85% of patients. The severity of the arthritis usually does not correlate with the extent of the skin disease. The patterns of disease include oligoarticular arthritis, polyarticular arthritis with distal interphalangeal joint involvement, or psoriatic spondylitis. Skin lesions; nail lesions, including pitting and onycholysis; and chronic uveitis are other manifestations that are helpful in diagnosing psoriatic arthritis. The initial therapy for joint manifestations in psoriasis includes NSAIDs; other medications such as methotrexate, sulfasalazine, cyclosporine, and TNF-α blockers are used as second-line therapy.

Enteropathic arthritis occurs in up to 20% of patients with inflammatory bowel disease, particularly in patients with Crohn disease. It usually presents as peripheral arthritis involving the lower extremity; however, in one fifth of patients it manifests as spondylitis indistinguishable from ankylosing spondylitis.[52] The activity of peripheral disease correlates with the activity of intestinal disease, whereas the course of axial disease is independent of inflammatory bowel disease activity. The most common extraskeletal manifestations include uveitis and chronic skin lesions such as erythema nodosum and pyoderma gangrenosum. Treatment is different from other spondyloarthropathies in that NSAIDs should be used cautiously because of the potential exacerbation of the bowel disease. Sulfasalazine is a good medication for both inflammatory bowel disease and arthritis. Azathioprine and methotrexate have shown promising results as second-line medications.

2: Systemic Disorders

pseudogout   gout

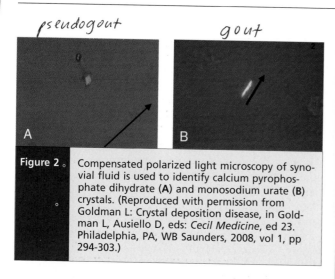

Figure 2 Compensated polarized light microscopy of synovial fluid is used to identify calcium pyrophosphate dihydrate (**A**) and monosodium urate (**B**) crystals. (Reproduced with permission from Goldman L: Crystal deposition disease, in Goldman L, Ausiello D, eds: *Cecil Medicine*, ed 23. Philadelphia, PA, WB Saunders, 2008, vol 1, pp 294-303.)

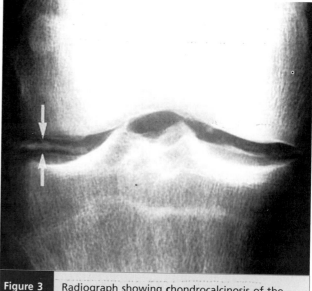

Figure 3 Radiograph showing chondrocalcinosis of the knee, which is seen particularly well in the lateral compartment (*arrows*). (Reproduced with permission from Mettler FA: Skeletal system, in Mettler FA, ed: *Essentials of Radiology*, ed 2. Philadelphia, PA, WB Saunders, 2005, vol 1, pp 253-376.)

Undifferentiated spondyloarthropathies are those that do not meet criteria for well-defined categories of spondyloarthropathy. This is not a new category or a distinct entity but it is a provisional diagnosis for differentiating patients with spondyloarthropathies from other forms of rheumatic diseases. The patients often present with nonspecific manifestations such as inflammatory back pain. Patients with undifferentiated spondyloarthropathies usually have a good prognosis and often respond well to NSAID therapy.

Crystal-Associated Arthritis

Deposition of microcrystals such as monosodium urate, calcium pyrophosphate dihydrate, calcium apatite, and calcium oxalate in the joint can result in acute or chronic arthritis. Because clinical presentations are often similar, synovial fluid analysis is needed to determine the type of arthritis. The other characteristics of synovial fluid in crystal-associated arthritis are usually nonspecific. Polarized light microscopy alone can identify most typical crystals with the exception of calcium apatite (**Figure 2**).

Acute arthritis is the most common early clinical manifestation of gout. The first metatarsophalangeal joint is the typical involved joint, but tarsal, ankle, and knee joints are also commonly affected. Trauma, surgery, excessive alcohol ingestion, and serious medical illnesses may precipitate acute gouty arthritis.[53] After several acute attacks, a proportion of patients with gouty arthritis may present with a chronic nonsymmetric synovitis, which causes potential diagnostic confusion with RA. Some patients present only with chronic gouty arthritis. Most patients (80% to 95%) are men; most women with gouty arthritis are postmenopausal and elderly. The diagnosis is usually confirmed by the presence of strongly birefringent needle-shaped monosodium urate crystals in aspirates of the involved joint. Because monosodium urate crystals often can be found in the first metatarsophalangeal joint and in knees not acutely involved with gout, arthrocentesis of these joints between attacks is a useful diagnostic tool. The serum level of uric acid has a limited role in the diagnosis of gout because it can be normal or low at the time of an acute attack. The mainstay of treatment during an acute gouty attack is the administration of anti-inflammatory medications such as colchicine or NSAIDs. For prevention of further attacks, hyperuricemic regimens and medications should be considered.

The deposition of calcium pyrophosphate dihydrate crystals in articular tissues occurs in 10% to 15% of adults 65 to 75 years of age and in 30% to 50% of those older than 85 years; therefore, this is a disease of elderly people because more than 80% of patients are older than 60 years.[54] The disease is often asymptomatic; however, when symptoms manifest, there are several patterns. Acute arthritis is very similar to acute gout and was originally termed pseudogout. Exacerbation of preexisting arthritis is another manifestation of the deposition of calcium pyrophosphate dihydrate crystals. The condition can appear with a severe destructive pattern like neuropathic arthropathy, or with symmetric proliferative synovitis, like RA. Involvement of intervertebral disk and ligaments can lead to spinal stenosis and can mimic ankylosing spondylitis. The knee joint is most frequently involved. A definitive diagnosis is verified by calcium pyrophosphate dihydrate crystals in the synovial fluid. Chondrocalcinosis involving cartilage or menisci seen on plain radiographs can be indicative of calcium pyrophosphate dihydrate crystals (Figure 3). The crystals are weakly birefringent and rhomboid in shape. The treatment of acute involvement includes NSAIDs or intra-articular glucocorticoids.[55]

Infectious Arthritis

Infectious arthritis can present as acute monoarticular, chronic monoarticular, or polyarticular arthritis. Acute bacterial infection typically precedes monoarticular or oligoarticular arthritis. Subacute or chronic monoarticular arthritis suggests mycobacterial or fungal infection, and episodic inflammation is seen in syphilis and Lyme disease.[56] Acute polyarticular inflammation occurs as an immunologic reaction during the course of endocarditis, rheumatic fever, disseminated *Neisseria* infection, and acute hepatitis B. Because acute bacterial infection can rapidly destroy the articular cartilage, it is important that all inflamed joints be promptly evaluated for the possibility of infection. The aspiration and analysis of synovial fluid is essential in the evaluation of a potentially infected joint. The definitive diagnosis of an infectious process relies on identification of the pathogen on stained smears of synovial fluid, isolation of the pathogen in the culture of the synovial fluid, or detection of the microorganism via polymerase chain reaction assays.

Staphylococcus aureus and *Neisseria gonorrhoeae* are the most common cause of infectious arthritis in adults. Although hematogenous infection can occur in healthy individuals, there is an underlying host predisposition for septic arthritis in most cases. Patients with RA, diabetes mellitus, and malignancy and those being treated with steroid therapy or hemodialysis have an increased risk of infection with *S aureus* and gram-negative bacilli. Patients with RA who are treated with TNF inhibitors are predisposed to mycobacterial and other pyogenic infections.

The treatment of nongonococcal arthritis involves prompt administration of antibiotics and drainage of the involved joint. For gonococcal arthritis, antibiotic therapy usually suffices.

There are three patterns of joint involvement in Lyme disease: intermittent episodes of monoarthritis or oligoarthritis involving knee or large joints in 50%, waxing and waning arthralgia in 20%, and chronic inflammatory arthritis with joint destruction in 10%. Lyme arthritis responds well to antibiotic therapy.

Summary

Arthritis is a common medical problem that affects about one fifth of the US population. OA is the most common joint disease and leading cause of disability and impaired quality of life. It involves pathologic changes in all structures of the joint, including cartilage, synovium, ligaments, and subchondral bone. The exact etiology of primary OA is unknown; however, several risk factors have been recognized for the disease. The diagnosis of OA is based on the classic clinical and radiologic findings; sometimes there is a need for more workup to prove the diagnosis. The main objectives in treating patients with OA are pain relief and improvement of function. The treatment should be comprehensive and includes both nonpharmacologic and pharmacologic modalities. For patients with advanced arthritis, joint arthroplasty is the most effective treatment, when timed correctly. Currently there is no effective method for cartilage regeneration in patients with OA. Inflammatory arthritis consists of a large group of diseases that lead to joint inflammation. The profile of the patient, chronology of the symptoms, pattern of joint involvement, and precipitating factors are helpful in the diagnosis of these conditions. The main objective of treatment for rheumatologic conditions is to suppress inflammation and preserve the joint. Therefore, aggressive use of disease-modifying antirheumatic drugs and biologic response modifiers early in the course of disease is promisisng. However, for those patients with severely damaged joints, total joint arthroplasty is a viable option. Crystal-associated arthritis usually manifests as acute arthritis; however, it could be present as chronic arthropathy. Infectious arthritis should always be considered in adults with acute or chronic monoarticular arthritis, especially in immunocompromised patients.

Annotated References

1. Bolen J, Schieb L, Hootman JM, et al: Differences in the prevalence and impact of arthritis among racial/ethnic groups in the United States, National Health Interview Survey, 2002, 2003, and 2006. *Prev Chronic Dis* 2010; 7(3):A64.

   The authors describe the prevalence of doctor-diagnosed OA and its impact on activities, work, and joint pain from six racial/ethnic groups. They concluded that arthritis affects 21% of the US population, but it disproportionately affects certain racial/ethnic groups.

2. Centers for Disease Control and Prevention (CDC): Prevalence of disabilities and associated health conditions among adults: United States, 1999. *MMWR Morb Mortal Wkly Rep* 2001;50(7):120-125.

3. Hootman J, Bolen J, Helmick C, Langmaid G: Prevalence of doctor-diagnosed arthritis and arthritis-attributable activity limitation—United States, 2003–2005. *MMWR Morb Mortal Wkly Rep* 2006;55(40): 1089–1092.

4. Hootman JM, Helmick CG: Projections of US prevalence of arthritis and associated activity limitations. *Arthritis Rheum* 2006;54(1):226-229.

5. Kurtz S, Ong K, Lau E, Mowat F, Halpern M: Projections of primary and revision hip and knee arthroplasty in the United States from 2005 to 2030. *J Bone Joint Surg Am* 2007;89(4):780-785.

   The authors attempt to formulate projections for the number of primary and revision total hip and knee arthroplasties that will be performed in the United States through 2030. They expect that the demand for both primary and revision joint arthroplasties will greatly increase by 2030.

6. Peat G, McCarney R, Croft P: Knee pain and osteoarthritis in older adults: A review of community burden and current use of primary health care. *Ann Rheum Dis* 2001;60(2):91-97.

7. Lawerence RC, Helmick CG, Arnett FC, et al: Estimates of the prevalence of arthritis and selected musculoskeletal disorders in the United States. *Arthritis Rheum* 1998;41(5):778-799.

8. Krasnokutsky S, Samuels J, Samuels J, Abramson SB: Osteoarthritis in 2007. *Bull NYU Hosp Jt Dis* 2007; 65(3):222-228.

   In this review article, the authors summarize the current pathophysiologic mechanism for OA and discuss relevant treatment modalities that are currently available or on the horizon.

9. Barksby HE, Milner JM, Patterson AM, et al: Matrix metalloproteinase 10 promotion of collagenolysis via procollagenase activation: Implications for cartilage degradation in arthritis. *Arthritis Rheum* 2006;54(10): 3244-3253.

10. Pelletier JP, Martel-Pelletier J, Abramson SB: Osteoarthritis, an inflammatory disease: Potential implication for the selection of new therapeutic targets. *Arthritis Rheum* 2001;44(6):1237-1247.

11. Steinbeck MJ, Nesti LJ, Sharkey PF, Parvizi J: Myeloperoxidase and chlorinated peptides in osteoarthritis: Potential biomarkers of the disease. *J Orthop Res* 2007; 25(9):1128-1135.

    The authors investigated the presence of the products of neutrophils and macrophages, specifically myeloperoxidase, in the synovial fluid of patients with OA. They found that patients with early OA showed significantly elevated levels of myeloperoxidase, whereas levels were low in control patients and patients with advanced OA.

12. Bos SD, Slagboom PE, Meulenbelt I: New insights into osteoarthritis: Early developmental features of an ageing-related disease. *Curr Opin Rheumatol* 2008; 20(5):553-559.

    The authors reviewed the possible common mechanisms by which recently identified consistent OA susceptibility genes influence the onset of OA and its progression. They proposed that these OA susceptibility genes may play a dual negative role. In early developmental processes, they may involve aberrant skeletal morphogenesis leading to malformation of joints, aberrant bone composition, or both, thereby increasing the biomechanical burden on the articular cartilage surface. Later in life, these genes may affect the propensity of articular chondrocytes in articular cartilage to become hypertrophic. As hypertrophic chondrocytes are unable to maintain cartilage homeostasis, these genes may, in part, be responsible for both the onset of OA and the progression toward clinical outcomes.

13. Loeser RF, Shanker G, Carlson CS, Gardin JF, Shelton BJ, Sonntag WE: Reduction in the chondrocyte response to insulin-like growth factor 1 in aging and osteoarthritis: Studies in a non-human primate model of naturally occurring disease. *Arthritis Rheum* 2000;43(9):2110-2120.

14. Martin JA, Buckwalter JA: The role of chondrocyte senescence in the pathogenesis of osteoarthritis and in limiting cartilage repair. *J Bone Joint Surg Am* 2003; 85(suppl 2):106-110.

15. Valdes AM, Spector TD: The contribution of genes to osteoarthritis. *Rheum Dis Clin North Am* 2008;34(3): 581-603.

    Several linkage analysis and candidate gene studies have recently revealed some of the specific genes involved in disease risks, such as *FRZB* and *GDF5*. Based on such studies, the authors discuss the impact that future genome-wide association scans can have on the understanding of the pathogenesis of OA and on identifying individuals at high risk for the development of severe OA.

16. Spector TD, MacGregor AJ: Risk factors for osteoarthritis: Genetics. *Osteoarthritis Cartilage* 2004;12(suppl A):S39-S44.

17. Velasco J, Zarrabeitia MT, Prieto JR, et al: Wnt pathway genes in osteoporosis and osteoarthritis: Differential expression and genetic association study. *Osteoporos Int* 2010;21(1):109-118.

    The authors investigated the role of Wnt activity in patients with OA. They found that genes in the Wnt pathway are upregulated in the osteoarthritic bone, suggesting their involvement not only in cartilage distortion but also in subchondral bone changes.

18. Kaliakatsos M, Tzetis M, Tzetis M, Kanavakis E, et al: Asporin and knee osteoarthritis in patients of Greek origin. *Osteoarthritis Cartilage* 2006;14(6):609-611.

19. Nakashima E, Kitoh H, Maeda K, et al: Novel COL9A3 mutation in a family with multiple epiphyseal dysplasia. *Am J Med Genet A* 2005;132A(2):181-184.

20. Feldman G, Dalsey C, Fertala K, et al: Identification of a 4 Mb region on Chromosome 17q21 linked to developmental dysplasia of the hip in one 18-member, multigeneration family. *Clin Orthop Relat Res* 2009;468(2): 327-344.

    The authors attempted to map and characterize the gene or genes responsible for developmental dysplasia of the hip by using family linkage analysis. They recruited one 18-member multigenerational affected family and observed only one chromosome region with a logarithm of the odds (LOD) score greater than 1.5 (a 4-Mb region on chromosome 17q21.32, yielding a LOD score of 1.82). Discovering the genetic basis of the disease would be an important step in understanding the etiology of this disabling condition.

21. Nevitt MC, Xu L, Zhang Y, et al: Very low prevalence of hip osteoarthritis among Chinese elderly in Beijing, China, compared with whites in the United States: The Beijing osteoarthritis study. *Arthritis Rheum* 2002; 46(7):1773-1779.

22. Dominik KL, Baker TA: Racial and ethnic differences in osteoarthritis: Prevalence, outcome, and medical care. *Ethn Dis* 2004;14(4):558-566.

2: Systemic Disorders

23. Ganz R, Leunig M, Leunig-Ganz K, Harris WH: The etiology of osteoarthritis of the hip: An integrated mechanical concept. *Clin Orthop Relat Res* 2008;466(2): 264-272.

In this article, the authors review the hypothesis that so-called primary OA is also secondary to subtle developmental abnormalities in the hip; the mechanism in these cases is femoroacetabular impingement rather than excessive contact stress. The most frequent location for femoroacetabular impingement is the anterosuperior rim area and the most critical motion is internal rotation of the hip in 90° flexion. The two major types of femoroacetabular impingement are described; however, the authors explain that most hips show a mixed pattern. Surgical attempts to restore normal anatomy to avoid femoroacetabular impingement should be performed in the early stage of the disorder before major cartilage damage is present.

24. Hunter DJ, Wilson DR: Role of alignment and biomechanics in osteoarthritis and implications for imaging. *Radiol Clin North Am* 2009;47(4):553-566.

This article details the current understanding of the etiopathogenesis of OA and examines the critical role of biomechanics in disease pathogenesis. The different ways of measuring mechanical forces across the joint are described, including those that rely on imaging methods.

25. Felson DT: The epidemiology of knee osteoarthritis: Results from the Framingham Osteoarthritis Study. *Semin Arthritis Rheum* 1990;20(3, Suppl 1):42-50.

26. Gabay O, Hall DJ, Berenbaum F, Henrotin Y, Sanchez C: Osteoarthritis and obesity: Experimental models. *Joint Bone Spine* 2008;75(6):675-679.

This study investigated the correlation between obesity and OA. The authors concluded that the link between obesity and OA may not simply result from the increased mechanical stresses on joint tissues that result from increased weight gain in individuals. Additional soluble factors such as adipokines may also play an important role in the onset of OA in obese patients.

27. Spector TD, Harris PA, Hart DJ, et al: Risk of osteoarthritis associated with long-term weight-bearing sports: A radiologic survey of the hips and knees in female ex-athletes and population controls. *Arthritis Rheum* 1996; 39:988-995.

28. Cheng Y, Macera CA, Davis DR, Ainsworth BE, Troped PJ, Blair SN: Physical activity and self-reported, physician-diagnosed osteoarthritis: Is physical activity a risk factor. *J Clin Epidemiol* 2000;53:315-322.

29. Hochberg MC, Lethbridge-Cejku M, Tobin JD: Bone mineral density and osteoarthritis: Data from the Baltimore Longitudinal Study of Aging. *Osteoarthritis Cartilage* 2004;12(suppl A):S45-S48.

30. Hunter DJ, McDougall JJ, Keefe FJ: The symptoms of osteoarthritis and the genesis of pain. *Rheum Dis Clin North Am* 2008;34(3):623-643.

The authors describe the characteristic symptoms and signs associated with OA and how they can be used to make the clinical diagnosis. The predominant symptom in most patients is pain. The causes of pain in OA and factors that contribute to its severity are discussed.

31. Cicuttini FM, Baker J, Hart DJ, Spector TD: Association of pain with radiological changes in different compartments and views of the knee joint. *Osteoarthritis Cartilage* 1996;4(2):143-147.

32. Hochberg MC, Altman RD, Brandt KD, et al: Guidelines for the medical management of osteoarthritis. *Arthritis Rheum* 1995;38(11):1535-1540.

33. Lo GH, LaValley M, McAlindon T, Felson DT: Intra-articular hyaluronic acid in treatment of knee osteoarthritis: A meta-analysis. *JAMA* 2003;290(23):3115-3121.

34. Katz JN, Barrett J, Mahomed NN, Baron JA, Wright RJ, Losina E: Association between hospital and surgeon procedure volume and the outcomes of total knee replacement. *J Bone Joint Surg Am* 2004;86:1909-1916.

35. Katz JN, Losina E, Losina E, Barrett J, et al: Association between hospital and surgeon procedure volume and outcomes of total hip replacement in the United States medicare population . *J Bone Joint Surg Am* 2001;83: 1622-1629.

36. Lingard EA, Katz JN, Wright EA, Sledge CB; Kinemax Outcomes Group: Predicting the outcome of total knee arthroplasty. *J Bone Joint Surg Am* 2004;86(10):2179-2186.

37. Nilsdotter AK, Petersson IF, Roos EM, Lohmander LS: Predictors of patient relevant outcome after total hip replacement for osteoarthritis: A prospective study. *Ann Rheum Dis* 2003;62(10):923-930.

38. Steinert AF, Nöth U, Tuan RS: Concepts in gene therapy for cartilage repair. *Injury* 2008;39(suppl 1):S97-S113.

This article reviews the current status of gene therapy as a method for regeneration of damaged cartilage. The authors describe the classes of gene products that aid cartilage repair and highlight the remaining challenges in the field.

39. Rasch EK, Hirsch R, Paulose-Ram R, Hochberg MC: Prevalence of rheumatoid arthritis in persons 60 years of age and older in the United States: Effect of different methods of case classification. *Arthritis Rheum* 2003; 48(4):917-926.

40. Bukhari M, Lunt M, Harrison BJ, Scott DG, Symmons DP, Silman AJ: Rheumatoid factor is the major predictor of increasing severity of radiographic erosions in rheumatoid arthritis: Results from the Norfolk Arthritis Register Study, a large inception cohort. *Arthritis Rheum* 2002;46(4):906-912.

2: Systemic Disorders

41. Arnett FC, Edworthy SM, Bloch DA, et al: The American Rheumatism Association 1987 revised criteria for the classification of rheumatoid arthritis. *Arthritis Rheum* 1988;31(3):315-324.

42. Finckh A, Simard JF, Duryea J, et al: The effectiveness of anti-tumor necrosis factor therapy in preventing progressive radiographic joint damage in rheumatoid arthritis: A population-based study. *Arthritis Rheum* 2006;54(1):54-59.

43. Bongartz T, Sutton AJ, Sweeting MJ, Buchan I, Matteson EL, Montori V: Anti-TNF antibody therapy in rheumatoid arthritis and the risk of serious infections and malignancies: Systematic review and meta-analysis of rare harmful effects in randomized controlled trials. *JAMA* 2006;295(19):2275-2285.

44. Khan MA: Update on spondyloarthropathies. *Ann Intern Med* 2002;136(12):896-907.

45. Olivieri I, van Tubergen A, Salvarani C, van der Linden S: Seronegative spondyloarthritides. *Best Pract Res Clin Rheumatol* 2002;16(5):723-739.

46. Reveille JD, Arnett FC: Spondyloarthritis: Update on pathogenesis and management. *Am J Med* 2005;118(6): 592-603.

47. Leirisalo-Repo M, Turunen U, Stenman S, Helenius P, Seppälä K. High frequency of silent inflammatory bowel disease in spondylarthropathy. *Arthritis Rheum* 1994; 37(1):23-31.

48. Rudwaleit M, van der Heijde D, Khan MA, Braun J, Sieper J: How to diagnose axial spondyloarthritis early. *Ann Rheum Dis* 2004;63(5):535-543.

49. van der Linden S, Valkenburg HA, Cats A: Evaluation of diagnostic criteria for ankylosing spondylitis: A proposal for modification of the New York criteria. *Arthritis Rheum* 1984;27(4):361-368.

50. Jacques P, Mielants H, De Vos M, Elewaut D: Spondyloarthropathies: Progress and challenges. *Best Pract Res Clin Rheumatol* 2008;22(2):325-337.

Unresolved issues concerning the pathogenesis of spondyloarthropathies are described. The precise sites where inflammation originates within the joints have been controversial because enthesitis, synovitis, and bone marrow inflammation can occur during the course of spondyloarthropathies. The genetic predisposition involved in the origin of the close linkage between gut and joint inflammation is described. The effects of the different TNF-blocking agents to modulate extra-articular disease manifestations are also discussed.

51. Amor B: Reiter's syndrome: Diagnosis and clinical features. *Rheum Dis Clin North Am* 1998;24(4):677-695.

52. Kataria RK, Brent LH: Spondyloarthropathies. *Am Fam Physician* 2004;69(12):2853-2860.

53. Choi HK, Curhan G: Gout: Epidemiology and lifestyle choices. *Curr Opin Rheumatol* 2005;17(3):341-345.

54. Molloy ES, McCarthy GM: Hydroxyapatite deposition disease of the joint. *Curr Rheumatol Rep* 2003;5(3): 215-221.

55. Schumacher HR Jr, Chen LX: Newer therapeutic approaches: Gout. *Rheum Dis Clin North Am* 2006;32(1): 235-244, xii.

56. Tarkowski A: Infection and musculoskeletal conditions: Infectious arthritis. *Best Pract Res Clin Rheumatol* 2006;20(6):1029-1044.

Chapter 19

Disorders of the Nervous System

Tahseen Mozaffar, MD   Ranjan Gupta, MD

Introduction

The nervous system is a complex and intricate system that enables the individual to recognize and react to the environment and to interact with the environment in a meaningful manner. Underlying this complex system is its simplicity of composition, with relatively few distinct cell types including neurons and glial cells. The nervous system is organized into the central nervous system (CNS) and the peripheral nervous system (PNS). The CNS receives, processes, and initiates signals, whereas the PNS relays signals to and from the environment and the CNS. In both systems, the neuron is the principal cell type. Neurons communicate with their targets via long cytoplasmic processes called axons. In the PNS, the peripheral nerves are primarily composed of bundles of axons and their associated Schwann cells. Schwann cells provide protection and trophic support and are found in two phenotypes—myelinating and nonmyelinating. Myelinating Schwann cells ensheathe large-caliber axons in myelin and maintain a one-to-one relationship with axons. Myelination increases the speed of action potential propagation and allows signals to reach their targets in a timely manner. In contrast, nonmyelinating Schwann cells associate with numerous axons in structures known as Remak bundles, which enclose small caliber C fibers and transmit pain and temperature sensation. The loss of myelination and changes in Remak bundles are common signs of peripheral nerve neuropathy. This chapter will describe the structure and function of the human nervous system and discuss the pathophysiology of specific neuropathies that are important in orthopaedic clinical practice.

Dr. Mozaffar or an immediate family member is a member of a speakers' bureau or has made paid presentations on behalf of Genzyme Talecris; serves as a paid consultant to or is an employee of Genzyme, Baxter, and Talcris; has received research or institutional support from Talecris Biotherapeutics; and has received nonincome support (such as equipment or services), commercially derived honoraria, or other non-research–related funding (such as paid travel) from the medical director for Crescent Healthcare. Dr. Gupta or an immediate family member has received funding from the NIH-NINDS and has received research or institutional support from Arthrex, Smith & Nephew, and Synthes.

Peripheral nerves are heterogeneous composite structures composed of neurons, Schwann cells, fibroblasts, and macrophages. The neuron is a polarized cell that forms the foundation of the nerve and consists of dendrites, the cell body, and a single axon. The cell body contains the nucleus, cytoplasmic organelles, and a cytoskeleton composed of neurofilaments and microtubules. The axon originates from a unique region of the cell body called the axon hillock, which is the site where the action potential of the neuron is produced. Axons project toward sites of innervation, where they form synapses. Synaptic transmissions from the axon to the end organ are mediated by electrochemical changes.

In the PNS, the axons are surrounded by glial cells called Schwann cells, which produce myelin. If the axonal diameter is greater than or equal to 1 μm, each Schwann cell will wrap its plasma membrane around a single region of an axon and develop myelin. This myelin, composed of 70% lipid and 30% protein, functions to provide fast and efficient conduction of the action potential propagating down an axon. Discontinuities along the length of the axon in the myelin sheath are called the nodes of Ranvier. When the action potential reaches a node, it depolarizes sodium channels. This rapid action potential propagation down the axon from node to node occurs by a process called saltatory conduction. Peripheral nerves have connective tissue layers to provide strength and protection to the nerve with its three layers: the endoneurium, perineurium, and epineurium (Figure 1). The endoneurium surrounds individual axons and their associated Schwann cells. It is composed of thin collagen strands that provide nourishment and protection. Multiple nerve fibers form a collection of axons called a fascicle. Fascicles are grouped and surrounded by the perineurium, which is composed of collagen and fibroblasts. This sheath provides the nerve with tensile strength, and the fibroblasts contribute to the formation of the blood-nerve barrier. Multiple fascicles are grouped together and surrounded by a connective tissue layer called the internal or interfascicular epineurium. This layer cushions the fascicles within the nerve and allows them to move freely against one another. The periphery of the entire nerve is covered by the external or extrafascicular epineurium, which protects the entire nerve from the surrounding environment.

The CNS consists of functions served both in the brain and in the spinal cord. The brain is structurally organized into lobes (the gray matter) named the fron-

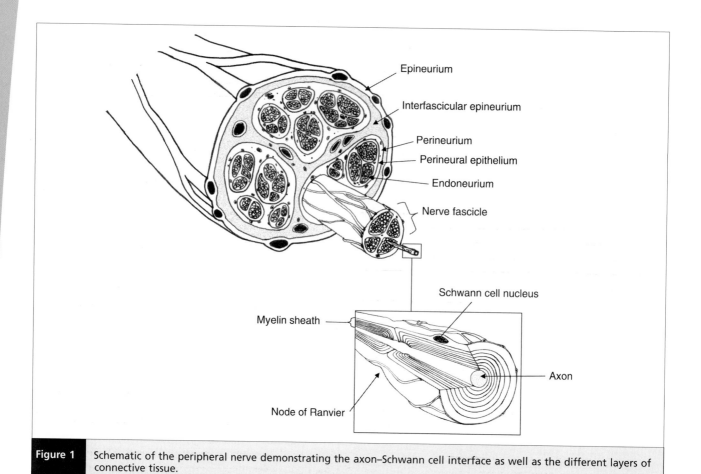

Figure 1 Schematic of the peripheral nerve demonstrating the axon–Schwann cell interface as well as the different layers of connective tissue.

tal, temporal, parietal, and occipital lobes, each with distinct functions. The frontal lobes are predominantly tasked with execution of executive and affective functions while the parietal lobes control motor and sensory functions. The temporal lobes focus on memory and cognition while the occipital lobes are concerned with vision. Language is also controlled by these structures. The various lobes connect with each other and the contralateral side through nerve fiber connections (the white matter bundle). There are also specialized nuclei deep within the brain, which are concerned with motor control, sleep, and consciousness and awareness. The caudal portion of the brain is known as the brainstem and is a densely packed region of brain with many vital structures that control autonomic functions, respiration, eye movements, swallowing, and motor and sensory functions.

The spinal cord is a vital portion of the CNS that relays sensory input from the environment to higher levels of the neuraxis, directs motor activity through somatic and visceral motor neurons, possesses intrinsic reflex properties, and influences the activity of spinal neurons through descending tracts. The spinal cord spans the distance from the foramen magnum to the second lumbar vertebrae. Axons enter and exit the spinal cord via the spinal nerves, each of which consists of a ventral or efferent root and a dorsal or afferent root.

The ventral roots carry output to the striated muscles from the myelinated nerve fibers of motor neurons in the gray matter of the ventral horn. The dorsal roots carry sensory input from myelinated and unmyelinated nerve fibers that originate from somatic sensory receptors. The cell bodies of the afferent fibers are located in the dorsal root ganglia. The spinal cord is further subdivided into white and gray matter. The descending tracts from the cortex and subcortical parts of the brain and the ascending fiber tracts are organized into well-demarcated and somatotopically arranged columns (**Figure 2**). These contain both myelinated and unmyelinated nerve axons. The gray matter is contained in the central portion of the spinal cord, which is an X-shaped structure containing longitudinally arranged neuronal cell bodies along with supporting structures such as glial cells, dendrites, and myelinated and unmyelinated axons. The gray matter is divided into the dorsal horn (predominantly sensory), the intermediate zone, and the ventral horn (purely motor). The ventral horn is populated by motor efferent neurons that project their axons out of the CNS via the ventral roots. These axons end up in various muscles in the limb and trunk and represent the pure efferent or motor fibers. The dorsal horns contain the first-order neurons that receive afferent input from the sensory dorsal root ganglion neurons (which in turn receive input from the

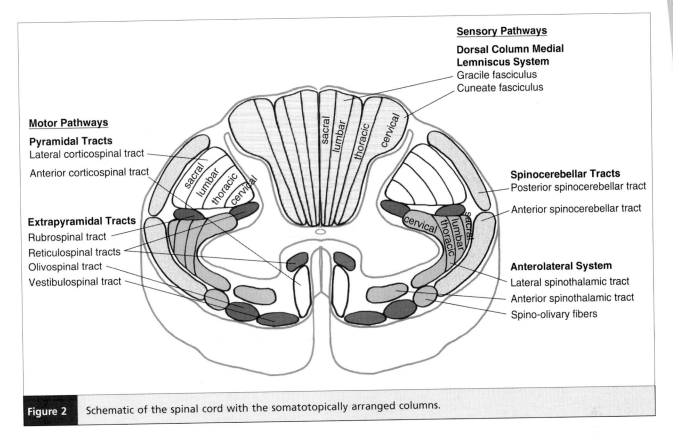

Sensory Pathways

Dorsal Column Medial Lemniscus System
- Gracile fasciculus
- Cuneate fasciculus

Motor Pathways

Pyramidal Tracts
- Lateral corticospinal tract
- Anterior corticospinal tract

Extrapyramidal Tracts
- Rubrospinal tract
- Reticulospinal tracts
- Olivospinal tract
- Vestibulospinal tract

Spinocerebellar Tracts
- Posterior spinocerebellar tract
- Anterior spinocerebellar tract

Anterolateral System
- Lateral spinothalamic tract
- Anterior spinothalamic tract
- Spino-olivary fibers

Figure 2	Schematic of the spinal cord with the somatotopically arranged columns.

skin-based and other sensory receptors). The dorsal horn is organized into columns of nerve fibers that travel in a rostral fashion, otherwise known as the "dorsal column." The dorsal columns are also organized in a lamellar structure, with sensory neurons organized in a topographical fashion. The nerve projection from the dorsal root ganglia enters the dorsal horn of the spinal cord through the dorsal column and synapse with these neurons in the dorsal column. Some of these projections either descend or ascend the dorsal column; some projections bypass the nuclei in the dorsal horns and synapse in the mid portions of the spinal cord and then ascend up in a tract of fibers, known as the spinothalamic tract. Projections within the dorsal columns as well as the spinothalamic tract eventually pass through the brainstem and end in the sensory relay nucleus, the thalamus. Descending nerve fibers from the motor cortex in the brain are organized in the lateral portions of the spinal cord and are known as the lateral corticospinal tract. These fibers, in turn, synapse on the interneurons (see below), which in turn synapse with the motor neurons in the anterior horn cells. This way the descending corticospinal tracts influence motor movements and determine the muscle tone in the extremities as well as deep tendon reflexes. Autonomic tracts and primary autonomic neurons are present in the intermediolateral column of the spinal cord in the thoracic regions; these are the primary autonomic neurons that control a number of autonomic functions, including sphincter control. The intermediate zone contains neurons whose projections remain within the

spinal cord and end on another neuron. These interneurons play an important role in generating the spinal reflexes.

Compression Neuropathies

Compression of the neural structures, either intraspinal or extraspinal, leads to neurologic dysfunction. Compression of the spinal cord within the spinal canal, either through an extrinsic lesion, such as bony outgrowth, herniated disks, bleeding (hematoma), lipoma, or metastatic lesions, or through an intrinsic lesion, such as a nerve or meningeal tumor, may create a neurologic emergency with the restoration of neurologic functions dependent on the timing of response to correct such abnormalities. Nerve compression can occur outside the spinal canal, either in the exit zone, as the nerve roots exit the spinal canal, or along the length of the nerve, often at predictable sites of entrapment. Common causes of entrapment are ligamentous or fibrous outgrowths that "pinch" a nerve. Bony outgrowth (osteophytes) in the joints or bones may also impinge a nerve. Rarely tumors (neurofibroma or lymphoma), inflammatory conditions, such as meningeal adhesions, as in arachnoiditis or amyloid deposits, or trauma may cause such entrapments.

Compression neuropathies of the upper extremity frequently occur and may require surgical treatment. Pathologic changes in peripheral nerves result from external mechanical forces of compression, with the

2: Systemic Disorders

symptoms described by patients commonly referred to as entrapment syndromes. The defining objective feature of compression neuropathies is the progressive decline in nerve conduction velocity. Chronic nerve compression injuries of the median, ulnar, and radial nerves occur in predictable locations in the wrist, forearm, and arm. Overuse and cumulative trauma in areas of restricted anatomic space can lead to compression of the nerve. The pathophysiologic changes include slowing of nerve conduction velocity, ischemia, edema, and eventually, neuropathy, which includes Schwann cell phenotypic changes, demyelination, and axonal dysfunction.

Nerve changes have classically been defined on the basis of the ensuing morphologic changes. Even with the most severe injuries to a nerve, the segment of nerve distal to the site of injury is able to maintain its integrity up to 3 to 7 days after injury. This is true even after complete injuries, where all connections to the proximal segment of the nerve, and thus the neuronal structures in the spinal cord (either the motor neurons or dorsal root ganglia), are severed. After nerve injury, the distal segment of the nerve starts to disintegrate to prepare for neural regeneration through a series of coordinated events known as wallerian degeneration. This process is initiated by granular disintegration of the axonal cytoskeleton with the ensuing recruitment of hematogenously derived macrophages. With the myelin and axonal debris cleared, the remaining Schwann cells proliferate and the distal segment is known as the bands of Bugner. Neural injuries however, are variable and may be incomplete with damage only to either the myelin sheath, with resulting segmental demyelination, or only the axon, with resulting axonal degeneration without damage to the myelin. The Seddon classification helped prognosticate these injuries. The mildest injury is when only the myelin sheath is damaged without damage to the axon. This form, known as neurapraxia, has the best prognosis. Damage to axons is termed axonotmesis, and usually is reversible, especially if only a short segment of the axon is damaged. The prognosis is fair, and recovery is possible albeit never complete and not as good as in the case of neurapraxia. However, if there is a large segment of axonal damage or if there is severe injury which not only damages the axon but the surrounding neural structures, the most severe form of nerve injury. This form was termed neurotmesis, and implies a "dying back" phenomenon where the proximal segment of the nerve (in addition to the degeneration of the distal segment – wallerian degeneration) disintegrates and the primary neurons resultantly undergo chromatolysis and eventual death.

Recent studies have shown the pathophysiology of neuropathy resulting from compression at the cellular and molecular levels.[1-5] Chronic nerve compression injuries of peripheral nerves are distinctly different from acute injuries such as those caused by crushing and transection. Initially, it was believed that axonal damage during chronic nerve compression injury triggers Schwann cells dedifferentiation and proliferation. However, research has indicated that axonal integrity is maintained and is free of pathology in chronic nerve compression injuries.[1] Compression neuropathies do not show morphometric evidence of wallerian degeneration, the hallmark of acute peripheral nerve injuries.[2] Furthermore, chronic nerve compression injuries occur in the absence of the early, dramatic inflammation and immune-mediated responses that occurs with acute injuries.[2] Chronic nerve compression injuries also lead to subsequent demyelination and remyelination of injured axons.[1] Thinner myelin is formed on remyelination, with this decrease in myelination contributing to the clinical presentation of slowing nerve conduction velocity in electrodiagnostic studies.[1] Chronic nerve compression injury also has been shown to induce a phenotypic switch in the Schwann cell phenotype.[3] An increase in the number of nonmyelinating Schwann cells and Remak bundles is observed in chronic nerve compression injuries.[1] These Remak bundles contain an increased number of C fibers, which correlate with the pain at compression sites in compressive neuropathies. Schwann cells are mechanically sensitive to shear forces and the expression of specific surface adhesion proteins are altered in response to hydrostatic pressure.[4,5] Thus, current research supports the belief that compression neuropathies are primarily a Schwann cell–mediated disease. By further understanding the mechanism of injury response by Schwann cells to mechanical stimulation, molecular therapies can be developed to prevent injury and promote regeneration.

Electrodiagnostic Studies

Nerve conduction studies and needle electromyography (EMG) are important tools in localizing areas of compression and neuropathy within the peripheral nervous system. Electrodiagnostic studies are useful in distinguishing a root lesion from compression at the spinal level from trunk, division, or cord compression at the brachial or lumbar plexus, and branch compression peripherally.[6] These studies also help determine the severity of the lesion and can be used to determine the prognosis of the lesion (neurapraxia with good prognosis versus axonotmesis/neurotmesis with a poor prognosis. Nerve conduction studies can further distinguish an axonal pathology from a demyelinating pathology and can distinguish a neurogenic lesion from a myopathic lesion. These studies complement the information obtained through imaging modalities.[7]

Nerve conduction velocity studies are routinely performed on peripheral nerves to determine their responsiveness to electrical stimuli.[8] A constant voltage electrical stimulator is used to evoke a response that is recorded either from a muscle in a motor nerve study or along the nerve in a sensory nerve study. The latency of the response (the time from the onset of the stimulus to the onset of the recorded response) is calculated and displayed in milliseconds. The distance that the stimulus had to travel (from the cathode of the stimulating electrode to the active recording electrode) is then measured with this distance then divided by the latency to obtain the nerve conduction velocity.[9] Because motor

Table 1

Findings on Nerve Conduction Velocity Studies in Various Neuromuscular Conditions

Condition	Latency	Conduction Velocity	Amplitudes	F-Wave Latency
Nerve–axonal	Normal	Normal	Reduced	Normal
Nerve–demyelinating	Prolonged	Slow	Normal or reduced	Absent or prolonged
Myopathy	Normal	Normal	Reduced	Normal
Neuromuscular junction	Normal	Normal	Reduced	Normal

nerve studies include a transit through the neuromuscular junction, where an inherent delay occurs, an additional stimulus is given along a proximal segment of the nerve, and the conduction velocity is calculated along the nerve, between the two points of stimuli (to compensate for the delay at the neuromuscular junction). The amplitude of the response also is calculated. All of the responses are compared to normative data to determine if they are normal or abnormal. A conduction block is a delay in the conduction velocity with a decrease in the amplitude of the compounded action potential from the nerve across a site of injury. A conduction block occurs because of impaired conduction across the injured segment of the nerve, with either a partial or a complete disruption of conduction. This results in a normal distal response (distal to the site of injury) but an abnormal response as the stimulator is moved proximal to the site of the injury.

An axonal injury to the nerve primarily creates a decreased amplitude on electrophysiologic examination. The latency and conduction velocity are not expected to change unless the degree of axonal injury is such that the myelin sheaths are also secondarily affected with the ensuing demyelination.[10] In that situation, a slight prolongation in latency and slowing in conduction velocity would also occur. Demyelinating lesions primarily affect the latency of the response and thus the conduction velocity. Amplitudes would only be affected with demyelinating lesions if there is a severe block in conduction or severe desynchrony of conduction created by segmental demyelination which results in a temporal dispersion of the response. Myopathic lesions tend to affect the amplitude of the motor nerve response because the motor responses are recorded from muscles; sensory nerve studies are not affected by myopathies. Table 1 details the changes seen with nerve conduction velocity studies in various nerve and muscle lesions.

Additional electrophysiologic studies can be performed to determine late responses in the motor nerve. These responses are known as F-waves (because the waves were initially recorded in the foot muscles) and are particularly useful for evaluating conduction problems in the proximal region of nerves such as in portions of nerves near the spinal cord. These studies are also very useful in evaluating disorders that affect the proximal region of nerves such as with a radiculopathy or with a demyelinating disease such as Guillain-Barré

syndrome. Another electrophysiologic study that is equally useful is the Hoffman reflex or H-reflex. The H-reflex is a true reflex with both an afferent and an efferent limb to the reflex. It is obtained by electrical stimulation of I-α afferent fibers at the knee with recording from the soleus. The resulting electrical stimulation is carried back to the spinal cord by the I-α afferents to the S1 level and then transmitted by synapses on to the anterior horn cells at that level. This results in a motor nerve discharge that can be recorded from the soleus muscle. The H-reflex is affected by sensory neuropathies, motor disorders affecting the sciatic or tibial nerves, and is asymmetrically affected by S1 root lesions.[8]

Needle EMG studies provide complementary information to nerve conduction velocity studies regarding the state of health of the skeletal muscles. These muscles can be affected by primary disease of the nerve roots, the peripheral nerves, or the skeletal muscles themselves. EMG studies help differentiate and discriminate between the various conditions. EMG studies also can determine if the nerve lesions are acute or chronic and if reinnervation has occurred. In patients with a nerve injury, this information, along with nerve conduction velocity studies, helps determine whether the nerve continuity is maintained.

To perform intramuscular EMG, a needle electrode is inserted through the skin into the muscle tissue.[9] A trained physician such as a neurologist or a physiatrist observes the electrical activity while inserting the electrode. The insertional activity provides valuable information about the state of the muscle and its innervating nerve. Normal muscles at rest produce certain normal electrical sounds when the needle is inserted into them. This baseline electrical activity is evaluated when the muscle is at rest. Abnormal spontaneous activity often indicates some nerve and/or muscle damage. Subsequently, the patient is asked to contract the muscle smoothly. The shape, size, and frequency of the resulting motor unit potentials are judged. The electrode is then retracted a few millimeters, and the activity is analyzed again until at least 10 to 20 units have been collected. Each electrode track gives only a very local picture of the activity of the whole muscle. Because the inner structures of the skeletal muscles differ, the electrode must be placed at various locations to obtain an accurate study. Table 2 describes the changes seen on EMG studies in various pathologic conditions.

2: Systemic Disorders

Table 2

Findings on Needle Electromyography Studies in Various Neuromuscular Conditions

Condition	Insertional Activity	Spontaneous Activity	Motor Unit Morphology	Recruitment	Firing Rate
Neurogenic: < 7 days	Normal	Normal	Normal	Reduced	Increased
Neurogenic: 7 days to 3 months	Increased	Fibrillations and fasciculations; complex repetitive discharges	Normal	Reduced	Increased
Neurogenic: > 3 months	Increased	Fibrillations and fasciculations; complex repetitive discharges	Increased amplitude and duration; variable polyphasia	Reduced	Increased
Myopathy: with inflammatory or necrotic elements	Increased	Fibrillations; myotonia; complex repetitive discharges	Decreased amplitude and duration; variable polyphasia	Early	Normal
Myopathy: with no inflammatory or necrotic elements	Normal	Normal	Decreased amplitude and duration; variable polyphasia	Early	Normal
Neuromuscular junction disorder	Normal	Normal	Normal; decreased amplitude and duration	Normal or early	Normal

Electrophysiologic Response to Acute Nerve Injury

Because myelin can be repaired, unless there is secondary involvement of the axonal structures, neurapraxia has a good prognosis with complete recovery over several weeks. Surgery for repair of the nerve is often not needed and patients should be carefully followed with serial electrodiagnostic studies. A more severe injury may produce axonotmesis. In addition to the disruption of myelin, the axonal tube is also damaged; however, the surrounding neural structures (the neural tube) are intact. Thus, the architectural framework for the nerve remains intact and the recovery potential is fair. With severe or large lesions, recovery may not be as robust. Surgery to perform neurolysis or bridge the defect may be required to allow maximal neural regeneration. Because axonal structures are damaged in situations with severe or large lesions, the amplitude of evoked responses on nerve conduction velocity studies decreases progressively and often may be absent. As the injury may affect both sensory and motor nerves, needle EMG examination shows evidence of denervation, such as fibrillation potentials and the reduced recruitment of motor units. In acute stages, motor units may be absent in patients with severe injuries. Follow-up studies are even more crucial in this situation, especially in patients with severe injuries, because nerve conduction changes may reverse (improve) and needle EMG examination may begin showing signs of reinnervation.

In neurotmesis, the most severe form of neural injury, all the neural structures are damaged, which results in complete disruption of the neural architecture. Nerves have inherent elastic properties, causing retraction of the cut ends and preventing any chance of spontaneous regeneration. Because of the severity of injury, and the lack of trophic support from the neural body, rapid deterioration of nerve axons occurs. Additionally, a dying-back of axons extends all the way back to the cell body (neurons) resulting in cell death. The prognosis is poor and very early surgical intervention is required in some instances to improve recovery potential. Electrophysiology shows complete absence of nerve conduction in the affected nerves. Three days after injury, EMG will show profuse denervation.[8]

Neuropathies Associated With Systemic Illnesses

A number of systemic conditions have pathologic involvement of peripheral nerves, including diabetes mellitus, uremia, thyroid disorders and nutritional deficiencies. The degree of involvement is variable as not every patient with such systemic illnesses has nerve involvement. In patients with systemic disorders, diabetes mellitus, hypothyroidism, and vitamin B_{12} deficiency routinely appear to be the most common conditions associated with neuropathies.

Diabetes

Diabetic neuropathy is a relatively common condition that is associated with multiple phenotypes and is estimated to be the cause of neuropathy in 15% to 30% of North American patients.[11] Diabetes mellitus is associated with several types of polyneuropathies: distal symmetric sensory or sensorimotor polyneuropathy, autonomic neuropathy, diabetic neuropathic cachexia, polyradiculoneuropathies, cranial neuropathies, and other mononeuropathies (**Table 3**). The exact prevalence of each subtype of neuropathy in diabetic patients is not accurately known; however, it has been estimated that neuropathy will develop in 5% to 66% of patients with diabetes.[12] Alarmingly, diabetic neuropathy can also occur in children. Long-standing, poorly controlled diabetes mellitus and the presence of retinopathy and nephropathy are risk factors for the development of peripheral neuropathy in diabetic patients. In a large community-based study, 1.3% of the population had diabetes mellitus (type 1, 27%; type 2, 73%). Of these, approximately 66% of individuals with type 1 diabetes mellitus had some form of neuropathy: generalized polyneuropathy, 54%; asymptomatic carpal tunnel syndrome, 22%; symptomatic carpal tunnel syndrome, 11%; autonomic neuropathy, 7%; and various other mononeuropathies and/or multiple mononeuropathies, 3%, which included ulnar neuropathy, peroneal neuropathy, lateral femoral cutaneous neuropathy, and diabetic amyotrophy.[13] In the group with type 2 diabetes mellitus, 45% had generalized polyneuropathy, 29% had asymptomatic carpal tunnel syndrome, 6% had symptomatic carpal tunnel syndrome, 5% had autonomic neuropathy, and 3% had other mononeuropathies and/or multiple mononeuropathies. Considering all forms of diabetes mellitus, 66% of patients had some type of objective sign of a diabetic neuropathy, but only 20% of patients with diabetes mellitus were symptomatic.

Distal symmetric sensory polyneuropathy is the most common form of diabetic neuropathy. It is a length-dependent neuropathy in which sensory loss begins in the toes and gradually progresses over time up the legs and into the fingers and arms. When severe, sensory loss may also develop in the midline of the trunk (chest and abdomen) and spread laterally toward the spine. The sensory loss is often accompanied by paresthesias, lancinating pains, burning sensations, and/or a deep aching discomfort. A severe loss of sensation can lead to increased risk from trauma to the extremities, with secondary infection, ulceration, and Charcot joints. Signs of an autonomic dysfunction may develop in patients with small fiber neuropathy because the autonomic nervous system is mediated by small myelinated and unmyelinated nerve fibers. Poor control of diabetes mellitus and the presence of nephropathy correlate with an increased risk of developing distal symmetric sensory polyneuropathy.

A neurologic examination will show loss of small fiber function, that is, pain and temperature sensation, and may also show a panmodality sensory loss. Those with large-fiber sensory loss have reduced muscle stretch reflexes, particularly at the ankles; however, reflexes can be normal in patients with only small-fiber involvement. Muscle strength and function are typically normal, although mild atrophy and weakness of intrinsic foot muscles and ankle dorsiflexors may be detected. Because patients without motor symptoms or signs on clinical examination will often have electrophysiologic evidence of subclinical motor involvement, the term distal symmetric sensorimotor peripheral neuropathy is also appropriate.

The diagnosis of diabetic neuropathy is dependent on the fulfillment of criteria outlined by the American

Table 3

Various Neuropathic Syndromes Associated With Diabetes Mellitus and Hypoglycemia

Diabetes Mellitus
Distal symmetric sensory and sensorimotor polyneuropathy
Autonomic neuropathy
Diabetic neuropathic cachexia
Radiculoplexus neuropathy
Mononeuropathy/multiple mononeuropathies

Hypoglycemia and Hyperinsulinemia
Generalized sensory or sensorimotor polyneuropathy

Diabetes Association in conjunction with one or more of the characteristic clinical diabetic neuropathy phenotypes.[14] The American Diabetes Association criteria include either an elevated fasting blood glucose level ($\geq$ 124 mg/dL) or an abnormal 2-hour glucose tolerance test ($\geq$ 200 mg/dL). Tests of glycosylated hemoglobin are usually used to assess diabetic control rather than for the initial detection of diabetes. Traditionally, neuropathy was not readily attributed to diabetes unless the diagnosis of diabetes had been established for years. More recently, a statistical association was demonstrated between impaired glucose tolerance (fasting blood sugars between 110 to 125 mg/dL; or a 2-hour serum glucose, after a 75-g glucose challenge following a 12-hour fast, 140 to 199 mg/dL) and a small-fiber neuropathy phenotype (see below).

Up to 50% of asymptomatic patients with diabetes mellitus have reduced sensory nerve action potential amplitudes along with slowed conduction velocities of the sural or plantar nerves, whereas up to 80% of symptomatic patients have abnormal sensory nerve conduction velocity studies. Quantitative sensory testing may show reduced vibratory and thermal perception. Autonomic testing may also be abnormal, particularly, quantitative sweat testing. Biopsies of nerves of patients with diabetes can show axonal degeneration, clusters of small regenerated axons, and segmental demyelination that is more pronounced distally, as expected in a length-dependent process. Although not clearly defined, the major theories about the pathogenesis of diabetic neuropathy involve a metabolic process, microangiopathic ischemia, or an immunologic disorder.[15]

The mainstay of treatment is strict control of glucose, which can reduce the risk of developing a neuropathy or can improve an existing neuropathy.[16,17] Pancreatic transplantation may stabilize or slightly improve sensory, motor, and autonomic function.[18] More than 20 trials of aldose reductase inhibitors have been performed and most have had negative results. Trials of neurotrophic growth factors also have been disappointing. A double-blind study of α-lipoic acid, an antioxidant, reported significant improvement in neuropathic sensory symptoms such as pain and several other neuropathic end points.[19]

Hypothyroidism

Although hypothyroidism is more commonly associated with a proximal myopathy, neuropathy develops in some patients, most typically carpal tunnel syndrome. Although rare, some patients may develop a generalized sensory polyneuropathy characterized by painful paresthesias and numbness in the hands and the legs. Pharmacologic correction of hypothyroidism usually halts disease progression and may improve polyneuropathy.

Inflammatory Neuropathies

Some patients develop an autoimmune response toward peripheral nerves with the immune attack directed against peripheral nerve antigens such as myelin protein zero or myelin-associated glycoprotein. In certain disorders, autoimmunity develops as an aberrant response to the normal immune response to bacterial infections. A good example of this is the autoimmunity to nerve gangliosides in patients with *Campylobacter jejuni* diarrheal infections. Two immune neuropathies – chronic inflammatory demyelinating polyradiculopathy (CIDP) and multifocal motor neuropathy (MMN) will be discussed.

CIDP is a dynamic immune-mediated neuropathy characterized by either a progressive or relapsing course. The diagnostic approach requires a detailed clinical examination, the findings of electrodiagnostic abnormalities, and occasionally, a nerve biopsy. CIDP may account for 10% to 33% of initially undiagnosed peripheral neuropathies in large tertiary referral centers. By definition, the symptoms and signs of the neuropathy must be progressive for at least 2 months, which distinguishes CIDP from Guillain-Barré syndrome or the most common form of this disorder, acute acquired inflammatory demyelinating neuropathy. Differentiating an acute acquired inflammatory demyelinating neuropathy from CIDP can be difficult in the first few weeks of disease onset because it is not always possible to determine if the disease will continue to progress for at least 2 months or will reach a plateau. Four courses of progression in patients with CIDP have been described: (1) chronic monophasic, in 15% of patients; (2) chronic relapsing with fluctuations of weakness or improvement over weeks or months, in 34%; (3) stepwise progressive, in 34%; and (4) steady progressive, in 15%.[20] In this respect, CIDP is similar to multiple sclerosis, an immune-mediated demyelinating disorder affecting the CNS.

CIDP usually presents in adults (peak incidence at approximately 40 to 60 years of age) with a slightly increased prevalence in men.[7] Most patients manifest with progressive, symmetric proximal, and distal weakness of the arms and legs. Early in the course of the illness, only distal extremity numbness and weakness may be apparent. If the weakness remains distal, other diagnoses should be considered. Although most patients (at least 80%) have both motor and sensory in-

volvement, a few patients may have pure motor (10%) or pure sensory (5% to 10%) symptoms and signs. Subjective numbness in the extremities is present in 68% to 80% of patients, whereas painful paresthesia occurs in 15% to 50%. The sensory examination is abnormal in most patients, particularly in large-fiber modalities (vibration and touch). Most patients with CIDP are areflexic or at least hyporeflexic. Most patients (80% to 95%) have an elevated cerebrospinal fluid protein level (> 45 mg/dL) with a mean of 135 mg/dL; some levels than may be greater than 1,200 mg/dL. Similar to Guillain-Barré syndrome, the cerebrospinal fluid cell count is usually normal. Elevated cerebrospinal fluid cell counts should lead to the consideration of HIV infection, sarcoidosis, Lyme disease, or lymphomatous or leukemic infiltration of nerve roots. Motor conduction studies evaluating compound muscle action potential amplitudes, distal latencies, conduction velocities, and F-wave latencies, as well as studies that look for evidence of temporal dispersion or a conduction block, are the most useful electrodiagnostic tools for CIDP. Most patients with CIDP have low-amplitude or unobtainable sensory nerve action potentials in both the upper and the lower extremities. Nerve biopsies are helpful in making the diagnosis because evidence of segmental demyelination and remyelination is often present. Although not specific for CIDP, this chronic demyelination and remyelination results in proliferation of surrounding Schwann cell processes, forming the so-called onion bulbs. Nerve biopsies are particularly useful when lymphomatous infiltration, amyloidosis, and sarcoidosis are considered in the differential diagnoses because these disorders can mimic CIDP.[21]

Although CIDP is an autoimmune disorder, the antigen(s) to which the immune attack is targeted and the specific roles of the humoral and cellular system in the pathogenesis of CIDP are not known. Corticosteroids, plasmapheresis, and infusion of intravenous immunoglobulins have been shown to be beneficial in treating patients with CIDP. Intravenous immunoglobulins have become the treatment of choice because it has fewer long-term adverse side effects than corticosteroids. Of importance, patients treated early are more likely to respond, underscoring the need for early diagnosis and treatment.[22]

In contrast, multifocal motor neuropathy (MMN) is an immune-mediated demyelinating neuropathy characterized clinically by asymmetric weakness and atrophy, typically in the distribution of individual peripheral nerves.[23] MMN is often misdiagnosed as amyotrophic lateral sclerosis (ALS).[24] Weakness in patients with MMN occurs in the distribution of individual peripheral nerves, whereas in ALS the weakness is in distribution of myotomes. MMN has a much lower incidence than ALS. MMN has a male predominance (male-to-female ratio of approximately 3:1) and an age of symptom onset usually ranging from the second to the eighth decades of life, with most occurring in the fifth decade of life. Onset in childhood is rare. Focal muscle weakness accompanied by cramps and fasciculations is usually first noted in the distal arms; however, weakness can initially develop in the legs. Most patients present with intrinsic hand weakness, wrist drop, or foot drop. The onset is usually insidious, and the weakness typically progresses over the course of several years to involve other limbs. As with CIDP, treatment of MMN can be complicated with relapses, and often patients become unresponsive to previously effective treatment.

As the name implies, MMN involves two or more motor nerves. However, MMN usually starts as a mononeuropathy. Cases of monofocal motor neuropathy may represent the early presentation of MMN and should be treated as such. The electrophysiologic hallmark of MMN is a persistent conduction block in motor nerves in segments not usually associated with compression or entrapment.[25] Sensory nerve biopsies in MMN are usually normal, although a slight reduction in myelinated fibers or axonal degeneration has been seen. Because sensory nerves are spared, the autoimmune attack is likely directed against an antigen that is relatively specific for the motor nerve. Although ganglioside antibodies are common, the pathogenic role for these antibodies is not known.

Unlike in patients with CIDP, patients with MMN generally do not respond to corticosteroids or plasmapheresis. MMN is typically responsive to intravenous immunoglobulins.[26] Rituximab also has recently been used to treat immune-mediated neuropathies, including MMN. Rituximab is a monoclonal antibody that binds to the CD20 antigen on normal and malignant B lymphocytes, destroying these cells. It is approved to treat B cell lymphoma and reduces peripheral B lymphocyte counts by 90% within 3 days.[27]

Neuropathies Associated With Infections

Nerves are commonly involved in human infectious disorders. In certain conditions, nerve involvement may occur secondary to direct invasion. For instance, both the herpes simplex virus and the HIV virus are neurotrophic and preferentially attack peripheral nerves. In other infectious conditions, nerve involvement may occur secondary to infection of the surrounding tissues or due to complications of treatment such as with leprosy.

Leprosy

Leprosy is caused by infection with the acid-fast bacteria *Mycobacterium leprae*. Leprosy is the most common cause of peripheral neuropathy in Southeast Asia, Africa, and South America. This infection has a spectrum of clinical manifestations ranging from tuberculoid leprosy to borderline leprosy to lepromatous leprosy. The clinical manifestations of the disease are determined by the immunologic response of the host to the infection. In tuberculoid leprosy, the cell-mediated immune response is intact, with focal, circumscribed inflammatory responses to the bacteria within the affected areas of the skin and nerves. The resulting skin lesions appear as well-defined, scattered, hypopig-

mented patches and plaques with raised, erythematous borders. Cutaneous nerves are often affected, resulting in a loss of sensation in the center of the skin lesions. Cooler regions of the body such as the face and limbs are more susceptible than warmer regions such as the groin or axilla.[28] The most common sites of involvement are the ulnar nerve at the medial epicondyle, the median nerve at the distal forearm, the peroneal nerve at the fibular head, the sural nerve, the greater auricular nerve, and the superficial radial nerve at the wrist. The nerves become thickened and encased with granulomas, leading to mononeuropathy or mononeuropathy multiplex.

In lepromatous leprosy, cell-mediated immunity is severely impaired, leading to extensive infiltration of the bacilli and hematogenous dissemination, which produces confluent and symmetric areas of rash, anesthesia, and anhidrosis. The clinical manifestations tend to be more severe in the lepromatous subtype.[29] As in the tuberculoid form, there is a predilection for involvement of cooler regions of the body. Infiltration of the organism in the face leads to the loss of eyebrows and eyelashes and exaggeration of the natural skin folds, leading to the so-called leonine facies. Superficial cutaneous nerves of the ears and distal limbs are also commonly affected. A slowly progressive symmetric sensorimotor polyneuropathy gradually develops because of widespread invasion of the bacilli into the epineurium, perineurium, and endoneurium. Distal extremity weakness may be seen, but large sensory fiber modalities and muscle stretch reflexes are relatively spared. Involvement of nerve trunks leads to superimposed mononeuropathies, including facial neuropathy.

Leprosy is usually diagnosed with a skin lesion biopsy and the Fite acid-fast staining method. Nerve biopsies also can be diagnostic, particularly when there are no apparent skin lesions. The immune response of the host to the bacilli determines the histopathology. The tuberculoid form is characterized by granulomas formed by macrophages and T helper 1 lymphocytes—caseation may be present, with typical lesions extending throughout the dermis. Importantly, bacilli are not seen. In contrast, in lepromatous leprosy, a large number of infiltrating bacilli, T helper 2 lymphocytes, and organism-laden foamy macrophages with minimal granulomatous infiltration are evident. Borderline leprosy can have histologic features of both tuberculoid and lepromatous leprosy. Polymerase chain reaction also may be used in making the diagnosis.

Patients are generally treated for 2 years with multiple pharmacologic agents, including dapsone, rifampin, and clofazimine. Other medications include thalidomide, perfloxacin, ofloxacin, sparfloxacin, minocycline, and clarithromycin. Treatment is sometimes complicated by the so-called reversal reaction, particularly in patients with borderline leprosy. This reversal reaction can occur at any time during treatment and develops because of a shift in the disease phenotype to the tuberculoid end of the spectrum with an increase in cellular immunity during treatment. The cellular response is upregulated, as evidenced by an increased release of

2: Systemic Disorders

tumor necrosis factor-α, gamma-interferon, and interleukin-2 with new granuloma formation. This can result in an exacerbation of the rash and the neuropathy as well as the appearance of new lesions. High-dose corticosteroids blunt this adverse reaction and may even be used prophylactically in high-risk patients at the onset of treatment. Preventing leprosy is of primary importance. It is recommended that children exposed to leprosy in the household be prophylactically treated with rifampin daily for 6 months.

Lyme Disease

Lyme disease is caused by infection with *Borrelia burgdorferi*, a spirochete, transmitted by ticks. The deer tick, *Ixodes dammini*, is usually responsible for the disease. The ticks acquire the spirochetes by feeding on an infected host (such as deer) and then transmit the spirochetes to the next hosts (such as humans) at a later feed. It takes approximately 12 to 24 hours of tick attachment to transfer the spirochetes to the next host. There are three recognized stages of Lyme disease: (1) early infection with localized erythema migrans, (2) disseminated infection, and (3) late-stage infection.

Neurologic complications may develop during the second and third stages of infection. Facial neuropathy is most common and is bilateral in approximately 50% of patients, which is rare in the differential diagnosis of Bell palsy. Involvement of nerves is frequently asymmetric. The presentation with a polyradiculoneuropathy may resemble Guillain-Barré syndrome.[30] Approximately 50% of patients have numbness, paresthesia, weakness, and cramps in the distal extremities; proprioception and vibration are reduced along with muscle stretch reflexes.

Immunofluorescent or enzyme-linked immunoabsorbent assay may detect antibodies directed against the spirochete. Because false-positive reactions are common, Western blot analysis should be performed to confirm a positive enzyme-linked immunoabsorbent assay. Examination of the cerebrospinal fluid should show lymphocytic pleocytosis and increased protein in patients with polyradiculitis, cranial neuropathies, and CNS involvement.[31]

The recommended treatment of facial nerve palsies in adults is the combination of amoxicillin plus probenecid for 2 to 4 weeks. Patients who are allergic to penicillin can be treated with doxycycline for 2 to 4 weeks. Adult patients with other types of peripheral neuropathy are treated with intravenous penicillin or ceftriaxone for 2 to 4 weeks. Those allergic to penicillin should be treated with doxycycline for 30 days.

Neuromuscular Disorders With Orthopaedic Symptomatology

Orthopaedic involvement is common in other neuromuscular conditions, including muscular dystrophy, Charcot-Marie-Tooth (CMT) disease, ALS, and Friedreich ataxia. See chapter 63 for additional information

on neuromuscular disorders. Although a detailed description of muscular dystrophies is beyond the scope of this chapter, the most common form is Duchenne muscular dystrophy, which is an X-linked muscular dystrophy, and is invariably fatal. The disease occurs secondary to a mutation in the dystrophin gene and is characterized by progressive proximal muscle weakness. Achilles tendon contractures are common early in the disease with a progressive loss of ambulation occurring by 10 years of age. Once the children are wheelchair-bound, scoliosis ensues and contributes to progressive respiratory insufficiency. If conservative management including physical therapy and orthosis fail to correct the contracture, surgical correction may be required to prevent loss of ambulation. Surgical correction of thoracic spine scoliosis is also recommended if the degree of scoliosis exceeds 40° and if there is evidence for progressive respiratory insufficiency.

Another neuromuscular disorder with prominent scoliosis is Friedreich ataxia, an autosomal recessive disorder of the spinal cord, which predominantly affects the dorsal columns, resulting in progressive sensory ataxia. Scoliosis occurs early and often is disproportionate to the amount of neurologic dysfunction. As in Duchenne muscular dystrophy, scoliosis results in progressive respiratory dysfunction, and thus eventually needs surgical correction.

Charcot-Marie-Tooth Disease

Hereditary neuropathies may account for as many as 50% of previously undiagnosed peripheral neuropathies referred for treatment to large neuromuscular centers. CMT disease is the most common type of hereditary neuropathy with the pathology focused on the Schwann cell. Rather than just one disease, CMT is a syndrome of several genetically distinct disorders.[32] The various subtypes of CMT are classified according to the nerve conduction velocities and presumed pathology (demyelinating or axonal), mode of inheritance (autosomal dominant or X-linked), age of onset (infancy, childhood, or adulthood), and the specific mutated genes. Type 1 CMT is the most common form, with individuals usually presenting with distal leg weakness in the first to third decades of life. There is an early predilection for the anterior compartment (peroneal muscle group), which results in progressive foot drop. This leads to poor clearance of the toes when walking, particularly on uneven surfaces. Patients with type 1 CMT often report frequent tripping, falling, and recurrent ankle sprains. Affected patients generally do not report numbness or tingling, which can be helpful in distinguishing CMT from acquired forms of neuropathy.

Although patients with type 1 CMT usually do not report sensory loss, reduced sensation in all modalities is apparent on examination. Muscle stretch reflexes are unobtainable or reduced throughout the body. There is often atrophy of the muscles below the knee (particularly in the anterior compartment), leading to the so-called inverted champagne bottle legs. However, in rare instances, patients have asymmetric pseudohypertrophy of the calves. Most will have pes cavus, equinovarus, or hammer toe deformities (**Figure 3**), which lead to aching in the feet. Rather than having a heel strike during ambulation, affected people land flatfooted or on their toes, and thus use a steppage gait to help prevent the toes from catching on the ground. Approximately two thirds of patients with type 1 CMT also have distal weakness and atrophy of the arms. The most severely affected patients may have clawhand deformities.

Even if there is no family history of CMT, family members of patients with possible CMT should be examined to determine if other members have features of the neuropathy. This information can be important in clarifying a diagnosis and in referral for appropriate genetic counseling. In addition to genetic testing, nerve conduction studies are the most important laboratory tests for evaluating patients with suspected CMT disease. The nerve conduction studies are invaluable in determining if the patient has an axonal or demyelinating neuropathy and in determining if a demyelinating neuropathy is uniform or multifocal, which is useful in distinguishing CMT from chronic inflammatory demyelinating polyneuropathy.[33] Although nerve biopsies on patients with suspected type 1 CMT are not routinely performed, a nerve biopsy will be strikingly abnormal. The enlarged gross appearance of the peripheral nerves led to the early designation of type 1 CMT as a hypertrophic neuropathy.

Type 1 CMT is a genetically heterogeneic disorder. Approximately 85% of patients with CMT type 1A have a 1.5-megabase duplication within chromosome 17p11.2-12 in the gene for peripheral myelin protein 22.[34] These patients carry three copies of the *PMP22* gene rather than two. In contrast, inheritance of the chromosome with the deleted segment results in affected individuals having only one copy of the *PMP-22* gene and leads to hereditary neuropathy with liability to pressure palsies.[35] Although these mutations are inherited in an autosomal dominant fashion, de novo mutations can occur. CMT type 1A is likely related to a toxic gain of function. The exact function of peripheral myelin protein 22 in the peripheral nerves is not known, but it may be important in maintaining the structural integrity of myelin, acting as an adhesion molecule, or regulating the cell cycle.

There is currently no cure for CMT disease. Orthotics play an important role in the rehabilitation of patients; however, proper attention is required to monitor patients for pressure sores. Tendon transfer and muscle transfers are often done to improve function, but there are no systemic studies showing their efficacy. Ankle fusion surgery to treat severe foot drop is not currently favored. A trial of supplementation with ascorbic acid is currently under way to determine if this vitamin will improve neural function in patients with CMT.

Amyotrophic Lateral Sclerosis

Motor neuron diseases are categorized by its pathologic affinity for the voluntary motor system including primarily the anterior horn cells of the spinal cord, certain

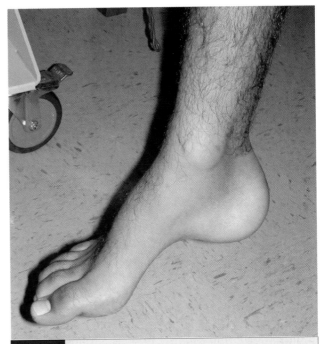

| Figure 3 | Photograph of the foot of a patient with CMT disease, showing typical features of pes cavus, hammer toes, and peroneal muscular atrophy. |

motor cranial nerve nuclei, and corticospinal/bulbar tracts. ALS, also known as Lou Gehrig's disease, is the most notorious of these disorders.[36] As in other neurodegenerative conditions, the clinical course of ALS is one of inexorable progression.[37] The cause is unknown except in the small proportion of patients who have familial forms of the disease.

The initial clinical features of ALS may be quite diverse. Typically, patients seek medical care reporting painless muscle weakness and atrophy.[7] These signs are frequently asymmetric and sometimes monomelic at the onset. The initial deficits may be restricted in distribution but involve more than a single nerve or nerve root. In instances in which patients do not seek early medical attention or if physicians do not recognize the significance of the symptoms, patients may not be seen until their disorder is fairly advanced (**Figure 4**). Less commonly, the initial symptoms may include impaired speech or swallowing, reduced head control, or disordered breathing.[38] Fasciculations are usually first recognized by the examining physician rather than by the patient, but may occasionally be the initial manifestation of the disease, particularly in those who have a preexisting awareness of their significance.[37] Fasciculations, in the presence of weakness, particularly if multifocal and continuous, strongly support the diagnosis of a motor neuron disorder.

Fasciculations in the absence of muscle weakness and EMG abnormalities, particularly if restricted in their distribution, are typically benign. Conversely, the absence of fasciculations in patients with painless weakness does not preclude the diagnosis of ALS, par-

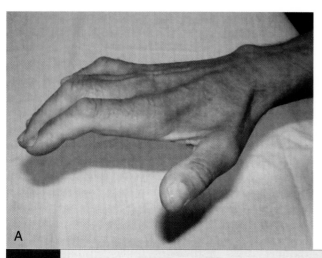
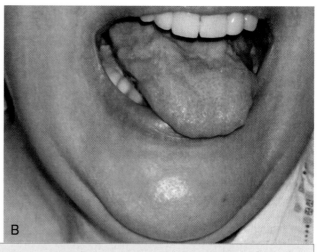

Figure 4 Photographs of the hand and tongue of a patient with ALS. **A,** Atrophy of the intrinsic muscles of the hand along with fasciculations and cramps are often the most common manifestation of ALS; these symptoms may be confused with cervical radiculopathy. **B,** Tongue atrophy and fasciculations are common in ALS and often help in making the diagnosis. (Reproduced with permission from Amato AA, Russell JA: *Neuromuscular Disorders.* New York, NY, McGraw-Hill, 2008.)

ticularly in patients with considerable subcutaneous tissue. An increased frequency of muscle cramping is common, which is often elicited during manual muscle testing.

The clinical diagnosis of ALS is dependent on the demonstration of lower motor neuron (LMN) and upper motor neuron (UMN) signs, which progress both within and between different body regions.[39] The most common ALS presentation is a patient with a combination of UMN and LMN features, limited initially in distribution, with the LMN findings typically dominating.[37] The initial involvement is typically distally located in a hand or a foot. Initial weakness may occur in proximal muscles as well. A definite diagnosis cannot be made until these combined UMN and LMN signs spread over a period of months, both within and outside the initially affected body part. A definite diagnosis of ALS is uncommon at the time of the initial examination. However, a combination of UMN and LMN signs in the same segment or a single extremity, in the absence of pain or sensory symptoms, is highly indicative of ALS. Despite the absence of a viable differential diagnosis, many patients have unnecessary surgical procedures for presumed cervical myelopathy or radiculopathy. Patients are referred for further evaluation by a neurologist only after clear progression and worsening of their symptoms. Similarly, weakness of the neck extensors and the resultant neck ptosis (neck drop) is quite common and is often mistakenly believed to be related to cervical stenosis.

With the exception of DNA mutational analysis in a patient with a mutation of the *SOD1* gene, there are no laboratory tests that currently confirm the diagnosis of sporadic ALS or most of the familial ALS genotypes.[40] There are laboratory tests, such as those that measure ventilatory function, forced vital capacity, and maximal expiratory and inspiratory pressure, that are used to monitor the course of the disease and to aid in management decisions. Although these tests may aid in the initial diagnosis, their primary purpose is to monitor progress, predict a prognosis, and aid in medical decision making. There are two primary pathologic features of ALS: (1) degeneration with the loss of myelinated fibers occurs in the corticospinal and corticobulbar pathways and (2) a loss of motor neurons within the anterior horns of the spinal cord and many motor cranial nerve nuclei.

Currently, there are no effective treatments that can reverse or arrest disease progression in patients with ALS.[41] As a result, the major goals in managing motor neuron diseases are to slow disease progression to the extent possible and maintain independent patient function, safety, and comfort. The care of patients with ALS and their families involves education, counseling, and symptom management. Two interventions that are often met with resistance by patients are percutaneous gastrostomy and noninvasive positive pressure support. In view of this, it may be prudent to introduce these concepts before the point in the patient's illness when these interventions are really needed. Both should be introduced with the idea that they will improve the quality of life rather than the duration of life, even though the latter may be achieved to a certain extent as well. Optimal management of patients with ALS and their families requires extensive effort and resources that undoubtedly surpass the capabilities of any single health care worker.[41]

Summary

It is important to have a working knowledge of neurologic conditions that are routinely encountered in orthopaedic practice. Misdiagnosis may delay treatment and result in unnecessary testing and suffering. With the assistance and early input from neurologists, treatment may begin early. Furthermore, orthopaedic interventions such as contracture and scoliosis correction may be required to improve the quality of life for these challenging patients.

Annotated References

1. Mozaffar T, Strandberg E, Abe K, Hilgenberg LG, Smith MA, Gupta R: Neuromuscular junction integrity after chronic nerve compression injury. *J Orthop Res* 2009;27(1):114-119.

   Unlike acute injuries, the neuromuscular junction is preserved with chronic nerve compression injuries even later after disease progression.

2. Gray M, Palispis W, Popovich PG, van Rooijen N, Gupta R: Macrophage depletion alters the blood-nerve barrier without affecting Schwann cell function after neural injury. *J Neurosci Res* 2007;85(4):766-777.

   Macrophage recruitment occurs with all peripheral nerve injuries. As macrophages produce Schwann cell mitogens, they are responsible in part for the increase in number of Schwann cells after acute nerve injuries. This is not true for chronic nerve injuries where hematogenously derived macrophages are responsible for the altered blood-nerve barrier but not the ensuing Schwann cell proliferation.

3. Frieboes LR, Gupta R: An in vitro traumatic model to evaluate the response of myelinated cultures to sustained hydrostatic compression injury. *J Neurotrauma* 2009;26(12):2245-2256.

   Schwann cells are mechanosensitive and have the ability to respond to mechanical stimuli such as hydrostatic compression.

4. Chao T, Pham K, Steward O, Gupta R: Chronic nerve compression injury induces a phenotypic switch of neurons within the dorsal root ganglia. *J Comp Neurol* 2008;506(2):180-193.

   Chronic nerve compression injury preferentially affects small to medium size neurons. This preferential neuronal response to injury may explain why there is not a decrease in nerve conduction velocity early in the disease process.

5. Pham K, Nassiri N, Gupta R: c-Jun, krox-20, and integrin beta4 expression following chronic nerve compression injury. *Neurosci Lett* 2009;465(2):194-198.

   Chronic nerve injury induces a demyelination and remyelination process. C-jun and Krox-20 are critical transcriptional factors in these processes. This study was one of the first to demonstrate an integrin response to compression injuries.

6. Gilchrist JM, Sachs GM: Electrodiagnostic studies in the management and prognosis of neuromuscular disorders. *Muscle Nerve* 2004;29(2):165-190.

7. Amato A, Russell J: *Neuromuscular Disorders.* New York, NY, McGraw-Hill, 2008.

   This book discusses the evaluation and management of neuromuscular disease.

8. Strandberg EJ, Mozaffar T, Gupta R: The role of neurodiagnostic studies in nerve injuries and other orthopedic disorders. *J Hand Surg Am* 2007;32(8):1280-1290.

   This review article provides a more comprehensive discussion of electrophysiology for the orthopaedic surgeon.

9. Gupta R, Mozaffar T: Neuromuscular diseases, in Buckwalter J, Einhorn T, O'Keefe R, eds: *Orthopaedic Basic Science: Biology and Biomechanics of the Musculoskeletal System*, ed 3. Rosemont, IL, American Academy of Orthopaedic Surgeons, 2007, pp 427-443.

   The authors discuss common neuromuscular conditions, the pathophysioogy of nerve injury, and factors influencing nerve regeneration.

10. Chaudhry V, Cornblath DR: Wallerian degeneration in human nerves: Serial electrophysiological studies. *Muscle Nerve* 1992;15(6):687-693.

11. Podwall D, Gooch C: Diabetic neuropathy: Clinical features, etiology, and therapy. *Curr Neurol Neurosci Rep* 2004;4(1):55-61.

12. Partanen J, Niskanen L, Lehtinen J, Mervaala E, Siitonen O, Uusitupa M: Natural history of peripheral neuropathy in patients with non-insulin-dependent diabetes mellitus. *N Engl J Med* 1995;333(2):89-94.

13. Dyck PJ, Kratz KM, Karnes JL, et al: The prevalence by staged severity of various types of diabetic neuropathy, retinopathy, and nephropathy in a population-based cohort: The Rochester Diabetic Neuropathy Study. *Neurology* 1993;43(4):817-824.

14. Dyck PJ, Karnes JL, O'Brien PC, Litchy WJ, Low PA, Melton LJ III: The Rochester Diabetic Neuropathy Study: Reassessment of tests and criteria for diagnosis and staged severity. *Neurology* 1992;42(6):1164-1170.

15. Polydefkis M, Griffin JW, McArthur J: New insights into diabetic polyneuropathy. *JAMA* 2003;290(10):1371-1376.

16. The Diabetes Control and Complications Trial Research Group: The effect of intensive treatment of diabetes on the development and progression of long-term complications in insulin-dependent diabetes mellitus. *N Engl J Med* 1993;329(14):977-986.

17. Sima AA: New insights into the metabolic and molecular basis for diabetic neuropathy. *Cell Mol Life Sci* 2003;60(11):2445-2464.

18. Kennedy WR, Navarro X, Goetz FC, Sutherland DE, Najarian JS: Effects of pancreatic transplantation on diabetic neuropathy. *N Engl J Med* 1990;322(15):1031-1037.

19. Ametov AS, Barinov A, Dyck PJ, et al; SYDNEY Trial Study Group: The sensory symptoms of diabetic polyneuropathy are improved with alpha-lipoic acid: the SYDNEY trial. *Diabetes Care* 2003;26(3):770-776.

20. Thomas PK, Lascelles RG, Hallpike JF, Hewer RL: Recurrent and chronic relapsing Guillain-Barré polyneuritis. *Brain* 1969;92(3):589-606.

21. Köller H, Kieseier BC, Jander S, Hartung H-P: Chronic inflammatory demyelinating polyneuropathy. *N Engl J Med* 2005;352(13):1343-1356.

22. Hughes RA, Bouche P, Cornblath DR, et al: European Federation of Neurological Societies/Peripheral Nerve Society guideline on management of chronic inflammatory demyelinating polyradiculoneuropathy: Report of a joint task force of the European Federation of Neurological Societies and the Peripheral Nerve Society. *Eur J Neurol* 2006;13(4):326-332.

23. Pestronk A, Cornblath DR, Ilyas AA, et al: A treatable multifocal motor neuropathy with antibodies to GM1 ganglioside. *Ann Neurol* 1988;24(1):73-78.

24. Parry GJ, Clarke S: Multifocal acquired demyelinating neuropathy masquerading as motor neuron disease. *Muscle Nerve* 1988;11(2):103-107.

25. Olney RK, Lewis RA, Putnam TD, Campellone JV Jr; American Association of Electrodiagnostic Medicine: Consensus criteria for the diagnosis of multifocal motor neuropathy. *Muscle Nerve* 2003;27(1):117-121.

26. Nobile-Orazio E, Cappellari A, Meucci N, et al: Multifocal motor neuropathy: Clinical and immunological features and response to IVIg in relation to the presence and degree of motor conduction block. *J Neurol Neurosurg Psychiatry* 2002;72(6):761-766.

27. Rüegg SJ, Fuhr P, Steck AJ: Rituximab stabilizes multifocal motor neuropathy increasingly less responsive to IVIg. *Neurology* 2004;63(11):2178-2179.

28. Ooi WW, Srinivasan J: Leprosy and the peripheral nervous system: basic and clinical aspects. *Muscle Nerve* 2004;30(4):393-409.

29. Jardim MR, Chimelli L, Faria SC, et al: Clinical, electroneuromyographic and morphological studies of pure neural leprosy in a Brazilian referral centre. *Lepr Rev* 2004;75(3):242-253.

30. Halperin J, Luft BJ, Volkman DJ, Dattwyler RJ: Lyme neuroborreliosis. Peripheral nervous system manifestations. *Brain* 1990;113(Pt 4):1207-1221.

31. Logigian EL, Steere AC: Clinical and electrophysiologic findings in chronic neuropathy of Lyme disease. *Neurology* 1992;42(2):303-311.

32. Harding AE, Thomas PK: The clinical features of hereditary motor and sensory neuropathy types I and II. *Brain* 1980;103(2):259-280.

33. Lewis RA, Sumner AJ, Shy ME: Electrophysiological features of inherited demyelinating neuropathies: A reappraisal in the era of molecular diagnosis. *Muscle Nerve* 2000;23(10):1472-1487.

34. Roa B, Garcia C, Suter U, et al: Charcot-Marie-Tooth disease type 1A: Association with point mutation in the PMP22 gene . *N Engl J Med* 1993;329(2):96-101.

35. Amato AA, Gronseth GS, Callerame KJ, Kagan-Hallet KS, Bryan WW, Barohn RJ: Tomaculous neuropathy: A clinical and electrophysiological study in patients with and without 1.5-Mb deletions in chromosome 17p11.2. *Muscle Nerve* 1996;19(1):16-22.

36. Swash M, Desai J: Motor neuron disease: Classification and nomenclature. *Amyotroph Lateral Scler Other Motor Neuron Disord* 2000;1(2):105-112.

37. Traynor BJ, Codd MB, Corr B, Forde C, Frost E, Hardiman OM: Clinical features of amyotrophic lateral sclerosis according to the El Escorial and Airlie House diagnostic criteria: A population-based study. *Arch Neurol* 2000;57(8):1171-1176.

38. Chen R, Grand'Maison F, Strong MJ, Ramsay DA, Bolton CF: Motor neuron disease presenting as acute respiratory failure: a clinical and pathological study. *J Neurol Neurosurg Psychiatry* 1996;60(4):455-458.

39. Tartaglia MC, Rowe A, Findlater K, Orange JB, Grace G, Strong MJ: Differentiation between primary lateral sclerosis and amyotrophic lateral sclerosis: Examination of symptoms and signs at disease onset and during follow-up. *Arch Neurol* 2007;64(2):232-236.

This article provides a guide for the clinician as to how to discriminate between different motor neuron disorders.

40. Siddique T, Figlewicz DA, Pericak-Vance MA, et al: Linkage of a gene causing familial amyotrophic lateral sclerosis to chromosome 21 and evidence of genetic-locus heterogeneity. *N Engl J Med* 1991;324(20):1381-1384.

41. Miller RG, Jackson CE, Kasarskis EJ, et al; Quality Standards Subcommittee of the American Academy of Neurology: Practice parameter update: The care of the patient with amyotrophic lateral sclerosis: drug, nutritional, and respiratory therapies (an evidence-based review). Report of the Quality Standards Subcommittee of the American Academy of Neurology. *Neurology* 2009;73(15):1218-1226.

Evidence on the management of patients with ALS was systematically reviewed. Topics studied included slowing disease progression, nutrition, and respiratory management. Several recommendations were made.

Chapter 20
Musculoskeletal Infection

Edward J. McPherson, MD, FACS   Christopher L. Peters, MD

Introduction

Infections involving the musculoskeletal system can ravage soft tissue and bone, resulting in significant destruction of an extremity. The lingering effects of an orthopaedic infection can cause significant residual pain and deformity. Despite the expanding growth of antibiotics and antibiotic classes, musculoskeletal infections remain problematic. Treatment of musculoskeletal infections imposes a significant economic strain to the health care system. In addition, the fear factor highlighted by multidrug-resistant bacterial infections has increased the anxiety level of the general population. This fear has created a perception that hospitalization increases the risk of serious health consequences, including death.

Infection Pathomechanics in the Hospital Setting

Most postoperative musculoskeletal infections occur via bacterial inoculation at the time of surgery. Some postoperative infections can occur as a result of bacterial contamination of the wound via open pathways to the deep tissue layers. Understanding the pathomechanics of bacterial contamination of a surgical wound is paramount in training operating room staff in appropriate "best care" standards to minimize bacterial inoculation risk. The Venn diagram (**Figure 1**) depicts the general parameters involved in eliciting a musculoskeletal infection. In the Venn diagram, a surgical infection occurs when bacteria of sufficient quantity are able to enter the human host, sustain their presence, replicate, and liberate toxin to cause damage to the host. The exposure risk is the open surgical wound itself. Bacteria are delivered to the open wound, and the open wound provides the surface area for bacterial adherence. The host can thwart the bacterial inoculation via its innate immune system. The human skin serves as the outer barrier to bacterial penetration. An intact and healthy

skin layer prevents further bacterial introduction into the deep host tissue layers. For bacteria, virulence in the orthopaedic realm relates to a bacteria's ability to attach, reproduce, and subsequently damage the host (for example, human host) tissue. The factors of bacterial adherence, reproduction rates, and toxin production are genetically determined.

The operating room personnel are the primary culprits in providing the "bacterial load" in the operating room. Traditionally, wound contamination has been thought to be the result of direct seeding from nasopharyngeal fallout. The ecologic niche for *Staphylococcus aureus* in humans is the anterior nares, where *S aureus* can be indentified most consistently in humans. However, the mechanism of operating room wound contamination is more complex than just nasopharyngeal fallout. Current theory of operating room wound contamination will be discussed in subsequent paragraphs. The function of the host immunity plays a sig-

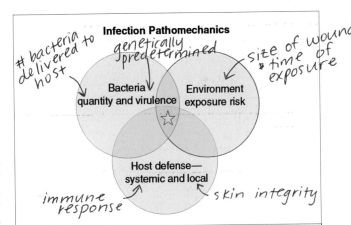

Figure 1	Venn diagram depicting the three major factors that interact to cause a musculoskeletal infection. The bacterial quantity is dependent upon delivery of bacteria to the host. Virulence is genetically predetermined. The environmental exposure includes the size of the surgical wound and the time the wound is exposed. The role of human host defense against microorganisms is the final key factor in infection pathogenesis. Local defense (that is, skin integrity) combined with human systemic immune response both determine whether contamination proceeds to colonization and overt infection. The relative contribution from each circle can grow or shrink according to each individual clinical scenario.

Dr. McPherson or an immediate family member has received royalties from Biomet and serves as an unpaid consultant to Biomet. Dr. Peters or an immediate family member has received royalties from Biomet; serves as an unpaid consultant to Biomet; and has received research or institutional support from Biomet.

2: Systemic Disorders

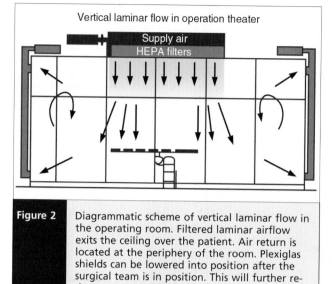

Vertical laminar flow in operation theater

Supply air
HEPA filters

Figure 2 Diagrammatic scheme of vertical laminar flow in the operating room. Filtered laminar airflow exits the ceiling over the patient. Air return is located at the periphery of the room. Plexiglas shields can be lowered into position after the surgical team is in position. This will further reduce any potential vortex flow into the wound area.

nificant role by determining whether wound contamination proceeds to colonization and subsequent infection. By recognizing weak immune hosts, the surgeon can use measures to help mitigate the risk of wound infection.

Operating Room

People inside the hospital are the source of the bacterial load delivered to a wound in the operating room and hospital setting. Bacteria are shed from the external body skin of each person at various rates.[1] The rate of shedding is genetically predetermined. Shedding from the human body typically is in the range of 10^2 to 10^4 bacteria per minute. High-rate shedders can release greater than 10^4 bacteria per minute. Bacteria that are shed from human skin attach to fomites, any inanimate object or substance capable of carrying infectious organisms. In the hospital setting, typical fomites include stethoscopes, ties, shirt sleeves, bed handrails, and doorknobs.[2] However, the more significant fomites are microscopic. Small pieces of skin detritus also serve as fomites. These microscopic particles have a large surface area and can float within the air. When bacteria are shed from the human body, they are attached to microscopic skin-derived fomites.

In the operating room, the sum total bacterial load available for delivery is conceptually represented by the following formula:

$$TE = P(SR_P) + A(SR_A) + B(SR_B) + C(SR_C)... + X(SR_X)$$

TE = total bacterial load exposure to patient in operating room (OR);

SR= shedding rate   P = patient

A = OR person A   B = OR person B

C = OR person C   X = OR person X

The number of personnel in the operating room suite has a significant effect on bacterial delivery into a surgical wound. The more health care personnel in the room, the greater number of bacteria available to potentially inoculate the wound area.

Operating room dynamics also play an important role in bacterial delivery into the surgical wound and onto operating room equipment. Movement of a person through a room generates turbulent airflow. Pressure waves of air and vortices (whirlwind circulation) are generated in front of and behind the moving person, respectively. In addition, the mere opening and closing of doors and movement of equipment creates wind vortices.[3] All of these movements create currents whereby bacteria (attached to microscopic fomites) are circulated throughout the room. With continued movement, bacteria can eventually be deposited within the wound and onto operating room equipment. Minimization of movement of operating room personnel will curtail vortex airflow. It is important that health care personnel understand the importance of making all movements within the operating room succinct and efficient. The surgeon and all health care personnel should envision themselves as working in a bacterial nebula. The denser the human interaction, the higher the bacterial concentration within the nebula. This increases the chance of bacterial delivery to an open portal on the human body. By limiting the bacterial cloud concentration, rates of bacterial colonization can be significantly decreased.

Elimination of bacteria is a key factor in thwarting bacterial wound contamination in the operating room. Two techniques to neutralize bacteria are mechanical filtration and ultraviolet light deactivation. Modern operating room suites have positive pressure flow filtration systems. The next level of filtration is laminar airflow systems, whereby concentrated positive pressure flow is directed across the room (horizontal laminar flow) or from a ceiling surface (vertical laminar flow). The return air within these systems is filtered with high-efficiency particulate air (HEPA) filters. HEPA filters significantly reduce the airborne particulate quantity within the room. Because health care personnel can stand in front of a horizontal laminar flow system, turbulent airflow around that person can create significant wind vortices that can deposit microscopic fomites into a surgical wound. It is preferable for vertical laminar airflow systems to be directly situated over the wound site. The minimization of wind vortices is enhanced in vertical laminar flow systems when Plexiglas shields are lowered into position around the table (**Figure 2**).

The use of personal isolator suits (also called operating room space suits) to reduce the risk of musculoskeletal infection is controversial, although their use has resulted in a significant reduction in total hip infection rates. However, current personal isolator suits are different from what was used in the past. The early suits had an inflow and outflow tube that was connected to the surgeon. The exhaust side had a negative flow pressure, which removed a significant load of bacterial shedding from the person wearing the suit. The more

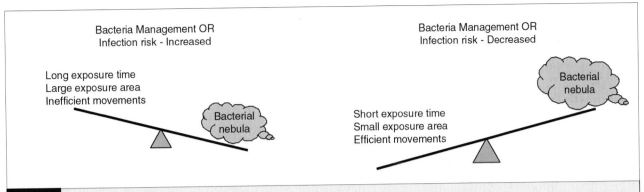

Figure 3	Schematic diagram illustrating strategic goals to reduce infection risk in the operating room (OR) when using medically implanted devices. **A,** When bacterial quantity is high, surgical time is long, and incision exposure is large, this risk for bacteria deposition into the wound area is increased. **B,** When bacterial quantity is low, surgical time is short, and incision exposure is small, the risk for bacteria deposition into the wound area is decreased.

personnel who used the personal isolator suits, the greater the reduction in bacterial load. The personal isolator suits in current use are not closed systems. Fans attached to the isolator system circulate operating room air into the isolator suit. Exhaled air is exhausted through a paper filter (not HEPA) around the head, or flows under the surgical gown to the floor. Therefore, turbulent flow around the bottom of the surgical gown or head is created. Furthermore, the total bacterial burden is unchanged. The lack of bacterial load reduction with the current personal isolator suits likely explains the variable reduction in infection rates when these current systems are studied as a method for infection control.

The methods to reduce bacterial wound contamination in the operating room depend on many factors, including the physical limitations of the physical plant, the financial resources available for filtration equipment (and maintenance), and the skill level of operating room health care personnel. **Figure 3** depicts strategic goals of the operating room team to reduce bacterial wound inoculation. Surgery involving implant insertion should be done by highly skilled health care personnel, and should be given priority to operating rooms that allow personnel to work efficiently and minimize bacterial loads. Best-care practices by operating room personnel to reduce bacterial load concentrations are listed in **Table 1**.

Hospital Floor

Postoperative bacterial wound contamination can occur via direct contamination of an incision that has not yet been completely sealed off from the outer environment, or by hematogenous seeding of bacteria. Although wound inoculation on the hospital floor involves many variables, the same basic tenets similar to the operating room setting apply. First, patients are exposed to a bacterial load introduced by health care personnel and visitors inside the hospital; patients located nearby, either in the same room or adjacent rooms, also can contribute to the bacterial shedding load. Hospitalized patients often are immunologically challenged, and

their intrinsic skin bacterial reservoir becomes populated with resistant bacteria. These patients can shed resistant bacteria. On the hospital floor, the sum total bacterial load available for delivery to a patient is conceptually represented by the following **formula:**

$$TE = P_i(SR_i) + P_A(SR_A) + P_B(SR_B)... + P_X(SR_X) + H_A(SR_A) + H_B(SR_B)... + H_X(SR_X) + V_1(SR_1) + V_2(SR_2)... + V_X(SR_X)$$

TE = total bacterial load exposure to patient in hospital bed

P_i = index patient 　　　　　　SR = shedding rate

P_A = adjacent patient A 　　　　H_A = health care person A
　(same room)

P_B = adjacent patient B 　　　　H_B = health care person B

P_X = adjacent patient X 　　　　H_X = health care person X

V_A = patient visitor 1 　　　　　V_B = patient visitor 2

V_X = patient visitor X

In general, the higher the density of the resident population (health care personnel+patients+visitors), the greater the overall bacterial load available within the physical plant. On the hospital floor, bacterial wound contamination occurs mainly via direct contact of the wound from health care personnel, the patient, or visitors who assist in patient care. The delivery of fomites to the wound site allows transmission of bacteria to the surgical area. All personnel involved with direct patient care should follow universal precautions (hand washing before patient contact and the wearing of gloves) to minimize wound contamination. In addition, measures to reduce overall bacterial load to the patient (such as single-patient rooms) can also help reduce the risk of fomite transfer to the wound. This is especially important in those patients receiving medically implanted devices.

The dynamics of bacterial flow within the air on the hospital floor is far less controlled than that of the operating room environment. Turbulent vortices can al-

Table 1

Best-Care Practices in the Operating Room When Patients Are Receiving Implanted Medical Devices

Technique	Reason
Least amount of OR personnel needed to efficiently complete surgical procedure in timely fashion • Highly skilled OR personnel required	Fewer personnel lowers number of bacterial shedders
Restriction of OR personnel rotations during surgical procedure • No mandatory breaks	Limits turbulent airflow Lowers number of bacterial shedders Prevents disruption of surgical procedure and increases efficiency and reduces surgical time Limits opening/closing of doors
Minimal traffic flow in OR theater	Limits turbulent airflow
Restriction of door openings	Limits turbulent airflow Keeps nonessential OR personnel from entering room
All necessary equipment and implant supplies are positioned in OR before start of procedure	Reduces door openings Reduces turbulent airflow Increases OR efficiency and reduces surgical time
Strict adherence to sterile technique Accepting environment of recognized contamination	Reduced risk of wound contamination
Complete change of surgical attire anytime personnel leave confines of OR suite	Reduced fomite contamination from outside sources
Restriction of unsterilized equipment applied to patient; for example, reusable tourniquets and Velcro safety straps	Reduced fomite contamination from other patients who may have resistant bacteria
Fresh surgical attire daily (including cloth surgical caps)	Reduced fomite load from dirty attire Reduced fomite contamination from outside sources
Unscrubbed personnel wash hands before entering OR room	Reduced fomite contamination from outside sources and other patients
Vigorous terminal cleaning of OR at end of day and after any potentially infected case Includes top side of OR lights and fixed equipment	Reduced fomite contamination from other patients who may have resistant bacteria
Culture surveillance of OR on regular basis	Assesses quality of decontamination procedures Assesses for presence of resistant bacteria
All OR personnel shower every morning before work	Reduced fomite load brought to OR theater

OR = operating room

low microcurrents to flow into a patient's room when the doors are open. The movement of equipment and the disruption of the local physical plant structures (when structural repairs are needed) create additional turbulent airflow. Furthermore, the increased fomite reservoirs on the hospital ward allow bacteria additional chances for patient inoculation.

On the hospital floor, the bacterial elimination process is less robust than that of the operating room environment. Filtration systems are more dependent on the age of the physical plant and the ventilation schemes for each floor. The particulate quantity allowed in the air on the hospital floor is generally no better than any other office building. Best-care practices to reduce bacterial load concentrations and wound colonization on the hospital ward are listed in Table 2.

Bacteria Characteristics and Defense Mechanisms

Biofilm

Bacteria involved in musculoskeletal infections exist primarily in the human host as a biofilm, a phenotypic expression of a bacterial species representing a unique form of existence. The first evidence of a biofilm on a medically implanted device was presented in 1980, and biofilm (glycocalyx) associated with musculoskeletal infection was first described in 1984.[4] It is estimated that 500,000 people in the United States die as a result of biofilm-associated infections. The anticipated occurrence of biofilm infections on medically implanted devices is expected to rise in the next decade.

All bacterial species, including many fungi, are capable of producing a biofilm. Bacteria can exist either in a planktonized state (similar to individual plankton that

Table 2

Postoperative Wound Care Measures to Reduce Wound Contamination

Multilayered wound closure
  Especially avoid sutures that run from skin through to deep tissue layers; bacterial biofilm will track along sutures

Single hospital rooms for patients receiving implanted medical devices
  Eliminates exposure to bacterial shedding from patients who may harbor resistant bacteria

Modify anticoagulation technique when needed to minimize deep wound drainage
  Any conduit out is an open conduit for bacteria to enter

Keep wounds dry with frequent dressing changes
  Bacteria on moist skin can exist deeper than on dry skin

Clean surrounding incision edges at time of dressing change with bactericidal/static agent (that is, alcohol, betadine, soap and water)

Positive airflow from patient room outward to floor

Rigorous postdischarge decontamination of hospital rooms. Aggressive environmental ward cleaning when MRSA or other highly resistant bacteria are isolated

Hospital screening of HCP and patients for highly resistant organisms when hospital related outbreaks are documented.

HCP = health care personnel, MRSA = methicillin-resistant *Staphylococcus aureus*.

exist in the sea) or in a biofilm state.[5] A bacterial biofilm comprises bacterial cells and a hydrated extracellular matrix (ECM). The extracellular matrix is a polysaccharide coating made by bacteria that contains host proteins acquired by the bacterial network. The ECM holds the bacterial cells together, forming a "collective" colony, which in its mature form has a well-defined sophisticated architecture (Figure 4). Most of the biofilm is filled by the ECM. Depending on species, less than 30% of the volume is filled by bacterial cells.[6] The biofilm forms a base layer that allows adherence to the target interface. The outer layers form discrete structures such as columns and mushrooms. Streamers can form in the outer layers that may break off to infect contiguous areas or enter the bloodstream to seed distant sites hematogenously. Within the biofilm exists channels that provide access to environmental nutrients and also allow communication between each other via signaling molecules.[7] In addition, bacteria communicate with each other in the biofilm with nanowires, which are small cellular connections between bacteria that allow direct cell-to-cell communication[8] (Figure 5). Biofilms also form on human body tissues that are compromised. Examples of human tissue biofilm infections include chronic infections involving bone, inner ear, bladder, prostate, and lung.[9]

A biofilm forms when the quantity of bacteria reaches a quorum, a genetically determined level. Lactone-derived molecules known as quorum-sensing molecules are produced by bacteria and are released into the extracellular environment. As bacteria adhere and complete their rate of exponential growth, quorum-sensing molecules are released. Once bacteria reach a quorum, the concentration of quorum-sensing molecules is high enough to trigger the phenotype expression of the biofilm state.[10] The biofilm state represents a metamorphosis whereby all bacteria that exist within the biofilm state work as a "collective."

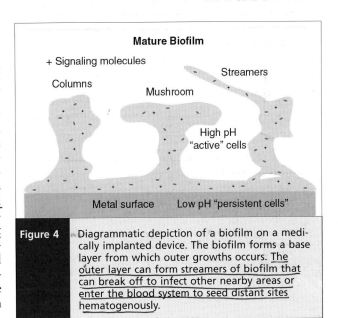

Figure 4 Diagrammatic depiction of a biofilm on a medically implanted device. The biofilm forms a base layer from which outer growths occurs. The outer layer can form streamers of biofilm that can break off to infect other nearby areas or enter the blood system to seed distant sites hematogenously.

The biofilm state confers significant resistance to host immunologic attack using multiple defenses.[5] These immunologic defense mechanism are outlined in Table 3. To date, biofilms cannot be completely removed once they form. Mechanical scrubbing can remove a biofilm from an implant, but small areas always remain.

Host Defense

Host defense mechanisms consist of two major categories: systemic defense and local defense.[11] The human host has developed a complex and adaptive immune system that monitors all areas of the body for microorganism invasion. Through a combination of antibodies, signaling molecules, and specialized cells, the human

2: Systemic Disorders

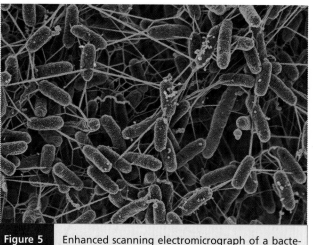

Figure 5 Enhanced scanning electromicrograph of a bacterial biofilm that shows intricate connections between bacteria that allow cell-to-cell communication within the biofilm network. The other form of communication is via signaling molecules liberated by bacteria within the biofilm. (Copyright Yuri Gorby, PhD, San Diego, CA.)

immune system is able to maintain a vigilant defense. Maintenance of optimum immune system surveillance requires multiorgan support. There are many associated medical conditions and disease states that affect proper function of the immune system. In addition, congenital defects in immune systemic development and function also predispose the host to infection. Furthermore, viral infections can attack specific immune cell lines, resulting in immune system compromise.[12] The major conditions associated with altered immune system function are listed in **Table 4**. Of the factors listed, some conditions can be treated to improve immune system function. For example, improving patient nutrition and cessation of immune suppressive drugs (when possible) can improve immune function. Optimizing diabetic care, smoking cessation, and alcohol cessation will also improve system function. Other conditions cannot be changed. In this situation, hypervigilance in surgical technique and during postoperative care are required to optimize infection prevention.

Local defense consists of the skin and endothelial linings of the alimentary canal and respiratory tract,

---

Table 3

General Biofilm Properties That Promote Infection in Humans

- Biofilm acts as a mechanical barrier that presents inward diffusion of several antimicrobial agents. This can increase minimal bactericidal contractions by 100-fold

- Within the biofilm there are pH differences that allow some bacteria to become dormat while others remain active. Those dormant cells are able to resist antibiotic attack and subsequently develop resistance to antibiotics

- Biofilms display antiphagocytic properties allowing bacteria to evade clearance by the host immune system

- Biofilm protects the organism from direct antibody and complement-mediated bactericidal mechanisms and opsonophagocytosis

- There are currently no methods or chemicals to completely dissolve a biofilm. Current research is focusing on developing signaling molecules that signal the biofilm collective to dissolve and disperse

---

Table 4

Factors That Impair Systemic Immune Function

Advanced age (older than 80 years)	Immune deficiency states
Allogeneic blood transfusion (during and shortly after transfusion)	Aquired immune deficiency (for example, HIV-1)
Alcoholism	Congenital immune deficiency (for example, chronic granulomatous disease, Di George syndrome)
Asplenia	Dysplasia/neoplasia immune system (leukemia, lymphoma, myelodysplasia)
Autoimmune disease states (for example, rheumatoid arthritis, SLE)	Immunosuppressive drugs (for example, corticosteroids, methotrexate, anti TNF-α agents)
Chronic hypoxia (for example, COPD)	Intravenous drug abuse
Hemaglobinopathy (for example, sickle cell disease, β thalasemia)	Malignancy
	Malnutrition
Hepatic insufficiency – cirrhosis	Renal insufficiency – chronic uremia
	Tobacco abuse

SLE = systemic lupus crythematosus, COPD = chronic obstructive pulmonary disease, HIV-1 = human immunodeficiency virus type 1, TNF-α = tumor necrosis factor α

---

and also includes the limb vasculature and neural innervations that support normal limb function. Damage to any of these systems raises the risk of local bacterial entry and subsequent infection to the musculoskeletal system. In the skin, small portals of entry are created by conditions that damage the protective skin layer. Patients having chronic venous insufficiency develop lower leg swelling from valvular incompetence and chronic hydrostatic loads to the lower legs. Areas of taut, shiny skin are easily traumatized on a microscopic level, causing the creation of entry points for bacteria. In addition, local hypoxia occurs in the areas of increased hydrostatic tension, which limits systemic immune response. Chronic lymphedema in an extremity results in infection susceptibility by a similar mechanism of persistent limb swelling and increased skin tension. Intrinsic skin conditions also provide areas for bacterial entry. Chronic dermatitis, psoriasis, traumatic burns, and rashes from medicines all can create portals for microorganism entry.[11]

Neuropathic conditions also predispose to localized skin trauma. The lack of feeling in weight-bearing regions allows excess mechanical stress to be applied to the skin, resulting in blisters, skin cracks, and tears. Mechanical alterations in gait as a result of neurologic disorders apply abnormal mechanical loads to the skin in weight bearing regions. Furthermore, the disruption of autonomic regulatory control to the peripheral extremity alters the functions of sweating and oil production. Disruption of these functions predisposes the skin to localized trauma, again creating portals of entry for bacteria. Better patient education and surveillance are needed to enhance long-term preventive care. Furthermore, regular inspections and early intervention by health care professionals can mitigate the effects of crippling musculoskeletal infections.

Vascular insufficiency at all levels of delivery plays an important role in the initiation and persistence of musculoskeletal infection. Localized hypoxia at an infection site inhibits immune system function. The inability to deliver immune-functional cells, combined with chronic local hypoxia, limits the immune cellular response to microorganism attack. Many methods are used to assess the vascular status of a limb. Generally, measurement of cutaneous oxygen tension at the local site, along with pulse pressure measurements to the limb, are accepted screening techniques. Local scarring as a result of multiple surgeries and trauma is a risk factor for infection. The local tissue area lacks an adequate vascular supply, which inhibits immune system function. An area of significant scarring (multiple incisions or loss of the normal soft tissue layer) lacks pliability and is more prone to superficial tearing. This creates small portals of entry for bacteria. In addition, if an incision is made through an area of nonpliable scar tissue, wound healing is delayed and the local area is at risk for bacterial inoculation. Similarly, radiation fibrosis significantly alters soft-tissue pliability and local host defense is compromised.

In the mouth, dental disrepair is frequently overlooked by health care personnel when evaluating for musculoskeletal infection. A multitude of bacterial species exist on teeth as a biofilm state. Chronic tooth decay allows the biofilm to penetrate deeper within the mucosal layer and closely appose bone. Furthermore, chronic gingival inflammation allows entry of bacteria and biofilm plaques into the body any time the mouth is mechanically disturbed, such as during mastication and tooth brushing. Recurrent bacteremia at increased levels is a major risk factor for hematogenous seeding, especially of the hosts who are immunocompromised. When elective major reconstructive surgery with medically implanted devices is planned, specific questioning and examination should be conducted to determine the need for dental care and restoration before surgery.

Chronic conditions within the respiratory tract and digestive system can also predispose to bacteremia. Conditions in the digestive tract such as Crohn disease and diverticulosis, if not carefully controlled, can lead to repetitive episodes of bacteremia. Similarly, within the respiratory tract chronic bronchitis or other parenchymal diseases also predispose to bacterial invasion. Close monitoring and treatment is needed to maintain the health of these systems. For example, in patients with diverticular disease or colonic polyps, maintenance endoscopic examinations will help to assess and treat the disease process.

Musculoskeletal Infection Conditions

Adult Osteomyelitis

The three major routes of bacterial bone inoculation in adult osteomyelitis are hematogenous, direct inoculation (penetrating wounds, open fractures, surgery), and contiguous spread from an adjacent infection. The other less frequent source of infection is reactivation of a bone infection that has occurred in infancy or childhood. Unlike pediatric osteomyelitis where hematogenous seeding is the most common source, the more common mechanisms of bacterial delivery in adults are from direct inoculation and contiguous spread. These mechanisms are more common in adults for several reasons. First, high-energy injuries are more frequent. Second, there is a trend toward more frequent use of medically implanted devices to stabilize fractures. Third, the rich vascular supply present in the metadiaphyseal region of growing long bones in pediatric patients is reduced in the adult. Fourth, as medical technology increases life expectancy, more patients with vascular compromise of the extremities are being treated. These patients develop localized extremity infections that can spread to bone.

S aureus is the most common organism involved. Staphylococcus species have numerous mechanisms for adherence to bony surfaces, making this species the most commonly involved in bone infection. However, any opportunistic organism can be involved if a patient's systemic immunity and local wound protection are compromised. Pseudomonas aeruginosa and gram-negative organisms must be suspected in intravenous

Table 5

Cierny-Mader Staging System for Osteomyelitis

Anatomic type

Stage 1 Medullary osteomyelitis

Stage 2 Superficial osteomyelitis

Stage 3 Localized osteomyelitis

Stage 4 Diffuse osteomyelitis

Physiologic class

A Host: normal host

B Host: systemic compromise (Bs)

Local compromise (Bl)

Systemic and local compromise (Bls)

C Host: treatment worse than disease

Systemic (Bs)-systemic	Local (Bl)-local
Malnutrition	Chronic lymphedema
Renal, hepatic failure	Venous stasis
Diabetes mellitus	Major vessel compromise
Chronic hypoxia	Arteritis
Immune disease	Extensive scarring
Malignancy	Radiation fibrosis
Extremes of age	Small vessel disease
Immunosuppression or immune deficiency	Neuropathy
Asplenic patients	
HIV/AIDS	
Alcohol and/or tobacco abuse	

drug users. Host deficiencies in immunity that lead to bacteremia predispose a patient to hematogenous seeding of bone.

In acute osteomyelitis, suppurative infection can compromise the vascular supply to bone. When the medullary and periosteal blood supplies are both disrupted, bone necrosis occurs. The dead bone, a sequestra, serves as a platform for biofilm formation. Once a biofilm forms, the disease process becomes chronic.[13] At this point, the only method to eradicate the infection is removal of the dead bone (sequestrectomy) along with radical débridement of nonviable soft tissue. Therefore, prompt diagnosis and treatment of acute osteomyelitis is needed to prevent the dreaded protracted course of chronic osteomyelitis. In chronic osteomyelitis, viable new bone will form around the infection region to support the weakened bone. The new periosteal bone that is seen encasing an area of dead infected bone is called an involucrum. In addition, endosteal new bone can form, which can obliterate the medullary canal. This appears radiographically as bony sclerosis.

In acute osteomyelitis the clinical presentation is variable. This is a function of host immunity response (full function versus suppression). The surgeon must be vigilant when the patient has a blunted response to infection (with conditions such as diabetic peripheral neuropathy or anergy due to advanced age). Acute symptoms include fever, chills, local pain, swelling, and erythema over the infected bone. An infection can also present as vague, nonspecific pain along with generalized malaise. In the situation of direct inoculation or contiguous spread, localized bone pain, swelling, and erythema are present. Wound drainage is frequently noted in the area of the previous trauma, surgical wound, or infected wound. In a chronic infection, a local draining sinus is frequently noted. Localized pain is noted at the infection site. If a sinus tract closes, a localized abscess can develop. The patient will usually note increasing redness, swelling, and pain at the infection site. Systemic bacteremia may ensue if not treated. In addition, a chronic draining sinus can undergo malignant transformation into squamous cell carcinoma in approximately 1% of patients.[14]

The diagnosis of osteomyelitis requires a high index of suspicion. Patient groups that should be suspected of osteomyelitis include those with systemic immune suppression, open fractures, chronic open wounds, and medically implanted devices into bone. Laboratory examination should include complete blood count (CBC), erythrocyte sedimentation rate (ESR), and assessment of C-reactive protein (CRP) level. The white blood cell (WBC) count may be elevated in patients with acute osteomyelitis, but is often normal in those with chronic osteomyelitis. The ESR and CRP are most often elevated in both acute and chronic osteomyelitis. However, if the patient is immunosuppressed (because of medications or malnutrition) these markers can remain low. In this scenario, the surgeon must be diligent in the diagnostic evaluation. The CRP level is used to monitor effective treatment. With effective treatment, the CRP level will start to decline after several weeks. With curative treatment, it should return to normal. Imaging studies include radiographs, MRI, and bone scintigraphy. MRI will show changes in cortical bone, the medullary canal, and surrounding soft tissues 2 to 3 weeks before any changes are seen radiographically.[15] Definitive diagnosis of osteomyelitis is provided by obtaining bone specimens for culture. All bone specimens should be sent for Gram stain and cultures (aerobic, anaerobic, fungal, and mycobacterial). Cultures of draining sinus tracts are not reliable for predicting which organism is growing in the infected bone site. If the clinical situation allows, all bone cultures should be obtained before antibiotics are initiated.

Treatment of adult osteomyelitis is best assessed in the context of the host's capacity to respond to an infection. A commonly used staging system for treatment in adult osteomyelitis that takes into account the location and type of infection[11] is the Cierny-Mader classification system (Table 5). More importantly, the classification rates the quality of the host to respond to an infection. A weak host will require more aggressive treatment to eradicate the infection.

In acute osteomyelitis, surgical débridement is almost always required. In primary hematogenous seeding, any abscess in bone and surrounding tissue requires prompt surgical débridement and decompression before sequestration occurs. In cases of direct inoculation (open fracture or open surgical stabilization with implanted hardware) the wound is fully opened, débrided, and vigorously lavaged. Soft-tissue deficiencies over bone require coverage with a muscle flap transfer (rotational or free flap depending on location). In cases of contiguous spread from chronic open wounds, definitive treatment also requires careful assessment of the vascular supply to the local area. Local perfusion to a wound area is evaluated with cutaneous oxygen tension measurements. If perfusion is inadequate, vascular bypass surgery is needed to reestablish local tissue perfusion. If bypass surgery is not possible, limb ablation may be required for definitive treatment. Bone takes 3 to 4 weeks to revascularize after débridement. During this time period, it is important to protect this "at risk" area with antibiotics until healing and revascularization occur. Patients should be treated with antibiotics for 4 to 6 weeks, starting when the last débridement procedure ended.

The goal of treatment of chronic osteomyelitis is to eradicate all tissue surfaces that allow biofilm to persist. Surgical débridement requires removal of all medically implanted devices, dead bone, and devascularized scar tissue (the avascular fibroinflammatory rind surrounding a chronic bone infection). Bone is removed to a region where visible bleeding is noted. Punctate bleeding from the surface of cortical bone is termed the paprika sign. The infected bone is stabilized either with splinting/casting or with application of an external fixator. Fixation pins are placed remotely away from the infection site. Dead spaces within bone are filled with polymethylmethacrylate antibiotic-loaded beads. Once the bone dead space is treated, the antibiotic beads are removed, usually after 4 to 6 weeks. Definitive stabilization is performed along with a bone grafting procedure, or bone transport (distraction osteogenesis) as indicated. Overlying soft-tissue deficiencies must be covered at the time of the débridement surgery. A muscle flap transfer is used to cover deficient areas. A muscle flap provides soft-tissue coverage, but also brings to the local area a rich vascular supply that promotes healing and neogenesis. Furthermore, a muscle flap also allows systemic antibiotic delivery to the infected area.

Adult Septic Arthritis

Acute septic arthritis by pyogenic bacteria can cause significant long-term joint debility if not properly recognized and treated. Almost every organism has been reported to cause septic arthritis. The three mechanisms of bacterial joint inoculation are hematogenous seeding, direct inoculation (surgery, needle injection, traumatic puncture), and contiguous spread from an adjacent infection. The most frequently involved joints in adults, in descending order, are the knee, hip, elbow, and ankle.[16]

Acute septic arthritis in adults can be separated into two major patient groups: young (age 15 to 40 years), healthy, sexually active patients with gonococcal pyogenic arthritis and elderly or immunocompromised patients with nongonococcal septic arthritis.[17] In gonococcal septic arthritis, the infecting organism is *Neisseria gonorrhoeae*. It is the most common cause of acute joint infection in persons 15 to 40 years of age in the United States. The clinical presentation is variable but typically includes migratory polyarthralgias, fever, rash, urethral or vaginal discharge, and tenosynovitis. A patient with disseminated gonnococcal infection may report few genital symptoms. More than 50% of these infections are polyarticular. The infected joint shows irritability to active and passive range, and a joint effusion is present. Blood cultures most often are negative (less than 10%). Joint aspiration cultures are also frequently negative (less than 25%). Because patients with gonococcal septic arthritis are healthy, prompt treatment results in a generally good prognosis.

In elderly or immunocompromised patients, the infection is most often monoarticular.[18] Blood and joint aspiration cultures are frequently positive. *S aureus* is the most common organism involved followed by *Streptococcus* species. In patients with sickle cell disease, *Salmonella* species is frequently isolated. In HIV-infected patients, *S aureus* is still the most frequently isolated organism. However, there is a much wider array of opportunistic organisms isolated from this group of patients. In patients with direct inoculation via a dog or cat bite, *Pasteurella multocida* is commonly noted. In human bites, *Eikenella corrodens* is an organism frequently associated with septic joint infection. In patients with a history of intravenous drug abuse, both *P aeruginosa* and *S aureus* are frequently found.

Elderly patients and patients with immune system compromise are more likely to develop bacteremia and hematogenous seeding of a joint. Elderly patients are more prone to septic arthritis because the immune system response displays a reduced vigor with age. Furthermore, concomitant medial comorbidities also impair immune system response. Common medical conditions that impair host immunity include diabetes, cancer, smoking abuse, alcoholism, inflammatory autoimmune conditions, renal failure, cirrhosis, malnutrition, HIV, and intravenous drug abuse. In addition, medications that are used to treat life-threatening conditions, such as corticosteroids, antineoplastic agents, and anti–tumor necrosis factor-α agents, also impair host immunity.[19]

The clinical presentation of a patient with a septic joint may be blunted because of coexisting medical conditions and significant immunosuppression. Therefore, a high index of suspicion is the first requirement for successful diagnosis. The patient with a suspected joint infection typically notes a rapid onset of pain in the affected join. Limping and an inability to bear weight on the affected limb occur. Irritability and withdrawal to attempted passive range are noted. The infected joint is warm and an effusion is present. The overlying skin will often have a pink-colored erythema.

Radiographs are required to assess for adjacent bone involvement and to detect intra-articular hardware (plates, screws, anchors). When indicated, MRI is obtained to assess for adjacent infections in the periarticular soft tissues and bone. Any case of suspected joint infection requires a blood culture. Serum blood tests include CBC, CRP, and ESR. Serum leukocyte count is often elevated, but can be normal. The CRP level is almost always elevated. The ESR is usually elevated, but can be normal.

Aspiration of the suspected joint is mandatory to establish the diagnosis and to identify an organism. Joint fluid is analyzed for cell count with differential, cultures (aerobic, anaerobic, fungal, and mycobacterial cultures), glucose level, Gram stain (including acid-fast stain), and crystal analysis (urate and calcium pyrophosphate). In septic arthritis, the joint fluid glucose level is less than 60% of the simultaneous serum glucose level. The fluid lacks a positive string sign (mucin clot). The joint fluid appears cloudy or purulent. Typically, joint fluid with greater than 50,000 WBC per mL and greater than 75% polymorphonuclear leukocytes (PMNs) is indicative of infection, whereas lower cell counts suggest noninfectious causes. However, there can be substantial overlap. In patients in whom immune suppression medications have been aggressively used, the cutoff value of 50,000 cells/mm³ may be too high. When the clinical presentation is equivocal but suggests infection (acute-onset joint pain, clinical immune suppression, and joint fluid WBC 30,000 to 50,000 cells/mm²), the joint should be considered infected.[20] Waiting for culture results can cause untoward joint destruction and debility. In addition, bacteria may fail to grow from infected joint fluid, particularly if the patient was pretreated with antibiotics, the organism is fastidious, or the fluid was not optimally processed.

The decompression of a septic joint is controversial. Treatment modalities include serial needle aspiration, arthroscopic lavage, and arthrotomy with or without synovectomy. The main goal of treatment is to prevent the rapid destruction of articular cartilage. The suppurative process in septic arthritis releases proteolytic enzymes from PMNs, which irreversibly break down articular cartilage. Therefore, the more thorough clearing of PMNs from the joint, the less chance for long-term joint damage. The choice of treatment should take into consideration the following factors: lifespan of the joint (young patients need a healthy joint for a long period of time), associated medical comorbidities, and the ability of the patient to sustain a surgical procedure. As a general rule, immunocompromised patients require more help in infection eradication, and more often require aggressive lavage and débridement. Open procedures have a greater chance to clear out bacteria and PMNs. If serial aspiration is initially chosen to treat septic arthritis, the joint fluid PMN count must be carefully monitored. If the PMN count remains high despite appropriate antibiotic treatment, open surgical débridement is mandatory. Serial aspiration should not be performed on deep joints such as the hip and small joints.

Intravenous antibiotic therapy is initiated immediately after joint and blood cultures have been obtained. In young, healthy adults, coverage should encompass treatment of S aureus and N gonorrhoeae. In the immunocompromised patient, treatment should cover S aureus and P aeruginosa. Peak antibacterial serum concentrations should exceed the minimal inhibitory concentration of the infecting organisms by fivefold to tenfold, and will generally provide optimal antibiotic treatment. For gonococcal septic arthritis, the duration of antibiotic treatment is 1 week. For all other cases, treatment duration is 4 weeks with a minimum of 2 weeks of parenteral antibiotics. An oral antibiotic may be used only if it is sensitive to the infecting organism. In addition, the patient must be able to tolerate the antibiotic, and must be compliant with the dosing regimen.

In chronic septic arthritis or recurring disease, the goal is to eradicate the infection in preparation for later salvage reconstruction (arthroplasty or fusion). In chronic or recurrent disease, a radical synovectomy is required. In addition, all abscesses and bony lesions surrounding the joint are aggressively débrided. Parenteral antibiotics are administered for 4 to 6 weeks. Effectiveness of treatment is determined by aspirations of the joint after completion of a full course of antibiotic therapy. In addition, treatment is monitored by following the serum CBC, CRP, and ESR levels during and after the treatment period.

Pediatric Osteomyelitis

Children have a propensity to develop musculoskeletal infection from hematogenous seeding. Other routes of bacteria delivery include direct seeding (from trauma, foreign body inoculation, or surgery). In addition, infection can result from contiguous spread from an adjacent infection site. Children have more frequent episodes of bacteremia; thus, bacterial delivery to bone can develop.[21] Osteomyelitis generally affects children younger than 13 years; males are more commonly affected. Children younger than 13 years are generally more susceptible for infection because the immune system has yet to fully develop. Fifty percent of cases occur in patients younger than 5 years.

In primary hematogenous osteomyelitis, the metaphysis of long bones is most frequently affected by bacterial inoculation. At this site in long bones, nonanastomosing capillary vessels make sharp loops under the growth plate and enter a system of large venous sinusoids. Blood flow slows and becomes turbulent, and bacteria can lodge in this region. In addition, the area adjacent to the growth plate has a lower oxygen tension and lower pH level, which gives bacteria a tactical advantage. Furthermore, the end capillary region and sinusoids lack phagocytic lining cells. These factors combined make the area more susceptible as a nidus for bone infection.[22]

The most common organism causing pediatric osteomyelitis is S aureus.[23] The next most common organism is group A β-hemolytic streptococci (GABHS). GABHS

© 2011 American Academy of Orthopaedic Surgeons

is more commonly seen in neonates. *Haemophilius influenzae* is a much less common pathogen due to vaccination against this species.[24]

The acute infection, once developed, can spread to adjacent bony areas through the haversian and Volkmann canal systems. The infection can perforate through the cortical bone and can further spread along the bone under the periosteum, which is elevated by the inflammatory process. In the neonate, the infection can spread to the epiphysis and joint surfaces through capillaries that cross the growth plate. In the infant older than 1 year, the capillaries that extend into the epiphysis atrophy, confining the infection to the metaphysis and diaphysis. Adjacent joint infection can occur when the metaphyseal portion of the bone is intracapsular (proximal radius, humerus, and femur). Cortical perforation of a metaphyseal region that is intracapsular will deliver bacteria directly into the joint.[24] → *septic arthritis*

The clinical presentation of pediatric osteomyelitis varies according to age groups. In neonates, findings include local edema and decreased motion of the limb (pseudoparalysis). Joint swelling of the adjacent joint is common (60%). Joint swelling requires an arthrocentesis to evaluate for septic arthritis. Not infrequently, fever is absent. In children, the immune system response is more developed. Findings typically include acute onset of fever, irritability, and lethargy. Local findings include localized swelling, inflammation, and erythema. The child will either limp or may not be able to bear weight on the affected limb. Older children and adolescents will describe pain that is nearly constant. Pain is localized to the infection site.

The evaluation for pediatric osteomyelitis includes a CBC, CRP, and ESR. The CRP is almost always elevated (98% of cases with acute hematogenous osteomyelitis). The ESR is less reliable in neonates and in patients with sickle cell disease.[25] Measurement of plasma procalcitonin (PCT) is a newer serologic test. PCT levels rise rapidly with bacterial infections but remain low in viral infections and other inflammatory processes. In pediatric osteomyelitis, plasma PCT levels were elevated in 58% of cases.[26] Because most cases of pediatric osteomyelitis originate from hematogenous seeding, blood cultures are mandatory. The imaging modality of choice is MRI.[27] Hematogenous osteomyelitis in older children usually involves a single site. In neonates, polyostotic involvement occurs in 30% of patients and can be detected by bone scintigraphy.[28] In addition, in young children who refuse to walk and are unable to localize the source of pain, a bone scan is useful to help identify a site of infection.

Definitive diagnosis of the pathogen is obtained via bone aspiration. The technique involves insertion of an 18-gauge spinal needle at the site of maximal tenderness. Aspiration should start as the needle reaches the cortex. If pus is obtained, which is indicative of subperiosteal abscess formation, the fluid is sent for culture and analysis. If no pus is obtained, the needle is advanced gently through the cortex and into the cancellous bone of the metaphysis. If pus is obtained, the diagnosis of medullary osteomyelitis is confirmed. If only

blood is obtained, the fluid is still sent for culture and analysis. Fifty percent to 85% of patients have a positive bone aspiration.

Treatment of acute pediatric osteomyelitis consists of prompt evaluation and subsequent administration of intravenous antibiotics. The antibiotics should cover *S aureus* and GABHS. In communities where methicillin-resistant *S aureus* (MRSA) is prevalent, antibiotics for treatment of MRSA should be used until definitive culture results are available.[29] Patients with sickle cell disease should have coverage for *S aureus* and *Salmonella* species.[30] Intravenous antibiotics should be administered for 4 to 6 weeks. Treatment can be transitioned to oral antibiotics provided that the patient is compliant, the organism is adequately sensitive to the antibiotic, the antibiotic has good bioavailability to achieve adequate serum levels, and the clinical picture continues to improve. A minimum of 2 weeks of intravenous antibiotics is recommended before changing to an oral regimen. Serial monitoring with CBC, ESR, and CRP is required for effective treatment. Surgical intervention is required when an abscess is present. Abscess is detected by bone biopsy (pus upon aspiration) or MRI. Surgery is also required if sepsis of the adjacent joint is present.

In some cases, a low-grade (subacute) osteomyelitis slowly develops over a period of months.[31] The patient is initially asymptomatic and later presents with pain or a limp. The radiographic findings show bone loss that can often resemble a tumor. A Brodie abscess describes a localized, well-circumscribed bone abscess that is not associated with systemic illness. The most common site is the distal tibial metaphysis. In the case of subacute osteomyelitis, a bone biopsy will help determine the diagnosis. It is important to remember the general rule: always "culture what you biopsy and biopsy what you culture." Treatment of subacute osteomyelitis is surgical débridement followed by a course of parenteral antibiotics for 4 to 6 weeks.

Pediatric Septic Arthritis

As in pediatric osteomyelitis, the source of infection in pediatric septic arthritis is dependent on developmental age. The bacterial spectrum in septic arthritis is similar to that seen in pediatric osteomyelitis. In addition, *Kingella kingae* is detected in pediatric arthritis based on PCR studies, but is difficult to grow in culture.[32] The knee and hip are the most commonly affected joints. In neonates in whom small capillaries still cross the epiphyseal growth plate, the most common source of infection is adjacent osteomyelitis. However, neonates still can develop septic arthritis from hematogenous seeding. In infants and children, the most common source of infection is hematogenous seeding. Septic arthritis can occur in cases where the metaphyseal portion of a joint is intracapsular (proximal radius, humerus, or femur). Pediatric osteomyelitis primarily involves the metaphyseal region of the long bone. If the infection breaks through the relatively thin metaphyseal cortex in the neonate and infant, the infection will be contiguously delivered into the joint. Septic arthritis

2: Systemic Disorders

can develop from direct inoculation (traumatic puncture and surgery).[33]

A septic joint presents with localized joint swelling, warmth, and irritability with active and passive motion. Refusal by the neonate to use the extremity (pseudoparalysis) is noted. In the older child, significant limp or refusal to bear weight on the extremity is noted. Fever and malaise are frequent. Laboratory tests include CBC with differential, CRP, and ESR. In almost all cases, the CRP and ESR will be elevated in septic arthritis. In contrast, the serum leukocyte count may be normal in up to 50% of cases. In a deep joint (such as the hip) in which clinical examination is difficult, ultrasonography or MRI can be used to determine joint inflammation and distention. MRI is also needed to rule out osteomyelitis in the adjacent bone. Aspiration of a swollen, irritable joint is mandatory to provide a definitive diagnosis and determine the need for surgical drainage and lavage. Joint fluid studies should include cell count with differential, cultures with sensitivities, Gram stain, glucose level, and protein levels. The differential diagnosis of a reactive joint effusion includes contiguous osteomyelitis, toxic synovitis, trauma, and autoimmune inflammatory arthritis (such as juvenile rheumatoid arthritis, acute rheumatic fever, Kawasaki disease, and serum sickness). Sometimes the clinical presentations and laboratory examination overlap, making early definitive diagnosis difficult. The destructive process of proteolytic enzymes upon articular cartilage can have long-term disabling consequences. Thus, if clinical doubt is present, surgical drainage should be considered and the diagnosis of infection made in retrospect. A joint fluid PMN count greater than 50,000 cells/mm³ warrants immediate surgical drainage. In inflammatory disease, the joint fluid leukocyte count ranges from 20,000 to 50,000 cells/mm³, the overlap region with septic arthritis. In this scenario, careful review of patient history, family history, Gram stain, and joint fluid differential must all be considered to determine the need for surgical drainage.

Surgical decompression of an acute septic joint can be accomplished by open arthrotomy or arthroscopy.[34] A vigorous lavage is used to flush out proteolytic enzymes and bacteria. Prompt surgical decompression of the hip is required to prevent collateral damage. Specifically, protracted joint distention of the hip with pus can cause osteonecrosis from vessel compression. Also, capsular destruction can cause joint subluxation/dislocation.[35] In any joint, prolonged joint infection can lead to adjacent bone infection. Serial joint aspiration has been used to treat septic arthritis in joints readily accessible to needle aspiration. However, careful monitoring is required. If the clinical picture fails to improve within 24 to 36 hours, surgical decompression is required. Serial joint aspiration is not recommended for small joints or the hip.

Antibiotics should be started immediately after cultures have been obtained. Antibiotic therapy should target those pathogens based on age and medical comorbidities. In a septic joint in a patient older than 12 years, antibiotics should include coverage for gonococcal septic arthritis. Intravenous antibiotics are initially administered. Conversion to oral antibiotics is allowed once the clinical situation improves and definitive sensitivities are obtained.[36] Total duration of antibiotics in septic arthritis is 3 weeks. Monitoring of the joint by clinical examination and serial testing of serum CBC, CRP, and ESR is used to assess effectiveness of treatment. If clinical relapse occurs, the evaluation should focus on the presence of adjacent osteomyelitis.

Foot Puncture Wounds

The musculoskeletal structures of the foot are vulnerable to puncture injuries due to the significant mechanical stress placed on the sole of the foot during gait. Puncture wounds sometimes cause infection. The penetrating object, when it travels through a shoe, collects bacteria from the inner sole, which itself serves as a bacterial culture medium.[37] As a result, *Pseudomonas* species and *S aureus* are the most frequently encountered organisms involved with puncture infections.

Treatment of foot puncture wounds depends on the time of presentation. In an early presentation (within hours of injury), the focus is on preventing a deep infection. The shoe is inspected to see if any fragments are missing that may have been pushed into the wound. The offending puncture object is inspected (if brought in) to see if it is intact or broken. Radiographs are required to examine for a retained foreign body and to look for any bony violations. Any puncture near the metatarsal head should be carefully assessed for intra-articular puncture. If a retained foreign body is suspected, or an intra-articular puncture is strongly suspected, formal surgical irrigation and débridement are required. If a foreign body is not suspected, the irrigation and débridement can be performed with local anesthesia in the clinic. Close follow-up is mandatory to reassess for developing infection. Prophylactic oral antibiotic administration after acute puncture injury is controversial. If indicated, antibiotic selection should include coverage for *Pseudomonas* species and *S aureus*.[38]

When a patient presents several days after a foot puncture and reports increasing pain and a swollen foot, the focus is on assessing the extent of infection. Radiographs are used to look for retained foreign bodies and any bony violations. A careful examination of foot joints is required to assess for intra-articular infection (most typically the metatarsophalangeal joint). Pain during passive motion of a suspected joint is a worrisome sign of septic arthritis that warrants arthrotomy, lavage, and débridement. When the joint is not involved, débridement is required when a retained foreign object is suspected, or the clinical presentation suggests a deep soft-tissue infection.[39] Prompt intervention is required to prevent infection from spreading along fascial planes. Surgical débridement includes débridement of the puncture tract, curettement of bone, culturing of soft tissues and bone, copious irrigation, and open packing of the wound. Intravenous antibiotics should be administered for 2 weeks, and should in-

[handwritten margin note: consequences of hip septic arthritis]

clude coverage for *Pseudomonas* species and *S aureus*.[40] For any patient who presents with a penetrating foot wound, tetanus immunization status must be verified; if status is unclear, tetanus vaccination is required.

Periprosthetic Joint Infection

Infection of a joint with a medically implanted device is termed a periprosthetic joint infection. The term periprosthetic is used because the surrounding soft tissues and bone are frequently affected by the infection process. It also emphasizes the principle that all structures of the joint (soft tissues, bone, and implant) need to be addressed during surgical débridement procedures. The most common reason for reinfection of a two-stage exchange arthroplasty procedure is inadequate débridement of the periprosthetic soft tissue and bone. With current surgical technique, the incidence of periprosthetic infection in major joint replacement centers in the United States is less than 1% (0.39% to 0.97%).[39,41,42] Most periprosthetic infections manifest with overt clinical symptoms within the first year of the joint replacement.

The mechanisms of joint inoculation in periprosthetic joint infection are direct inoculation of the joint, hematogenous seeding, and contiguous spread from an adjacent infection focus. The knee is the most commonly affected joint, followed by the hip. The most common organisms involved in periprosthetic joint infection are *Staphylococcus epidermidis* (or coagulase-negative *Staphylococcus* species) and *S aureus*. The high incidence of *S epidermidis* infections reflects the mechanism of fomite delivery into the surgical wound at the time of surgery. *S epidermidis* is shed by operating room personnel. With dynamic turbulent flow in the operating room theater, bacteria are delivered to the surgical site and to operating room equipment. *S aureus* is a frequent organism due to its multiple mechanisms of bacterial adherence, which provide a tactical advantage for this organism.[43] Hematogenous seeding of a prosthetic joint more often occurs in immunocompromised patients. In this situation, a wide variety of organisms can infect the joint, including *Enterococcus*, gram-negative rods, anaerobic organisms, and fungi.

Many staging systems are used to categorize periprosthetic joint infection.[44,45] The more recent staging system introduced by the Musculoskeletal Infection Society incorporates three major categories to objectively describe the infection and the patient in a progressive system to reflect worsening disease severity[46] (Tables 6 and 7). The first category describes the temporal presentation and infection state of the periprosthetic joint infection. An early postoperative infection is defined as an infection that presents less than 3 weeks from the index joint arthroplasty procedure. An early postoperative infection is an acute infection defined as a nonbiofilm state. A late infection occurs in a medically implanted joint device of any age and also is defined as a nonbiofilm state. The infection is clinically determined to be less than 3 weeks in duration. Bacteria are delivered to the joint via hematogenous transport or from direct seeding from adjacent soft tissues that are infected (such as abscess, cellulitis, or traumatic wound). A chronic infection is currently defined as an infection in any joint arthroplasty that is judged to be of 3 weeks' duration or longer. In a chronic periprosthetic infection, a biofilm coating has enveloped the prosthetic implant, ensuring perpetual survival of the infection.

The second category of the staging system rates the ability of the patient or host to combat the infection with a systemic immune response. The objective factors defining this category focus on the competency of the host immune system and related medical conditions that affect proper functioning of the immune system. A patient is considered either uncompromised, compromised, or significantly compromised. The third category grades the extent of osseous and soft-tissue compromise surrounding the affected joint. This category includes local soft-tissue factors that can potentially impair local wound healing, and also allow subsequent reinfection at the index site. The staging system incorporates all three categories in the following fashion: stage equals infection type plus systemic host grade plus local extremity grade. Examples of the nomenclature include I-A-1, II-B-2, III-C-1.

A chronic periprosthetic infection is defined by the Musculoskeletal Infection Society as an infection where the infecting organism has transformed into a biofilm state. At present, the sobering reality is that once a biofilm has formed, it cannot be completely eradicated unless prosthetic implants are surgically removed and the surrounding wound is radically débrided. Thus, in this staging system, an acute infection of a joint implant is considered salvageable. In a chronic infection, the infected implant is considered nonsalvageable and should be removed. At present, any prosthetic arthroplasty where the infection is clinically judged to be of 3 weeks' duration or longer is considered chronic. However, it has been shown that in an optimum environment, a biofilm can form on an implant in as few as 72 hours. Therefore, the definition of chronic infection may change to an even shorter time interval. It is hoped that a simple testing method to detect the presence of a biofilm on a medically implanted device will be developed soon. When this test is available, the definition of a chronic periprosthetic infection will no longer be arbitrary.

Similar to adult osteomyelitis, the health of the host is an important aspect of periprosthetic infection care. The inability of a weak host to vigorously fight an infection with systemic immune support may result in persistent infection at a low-grade level, or even at life-threatening levels. In a patient who is medically compromised, one of two options must be chosen. The first option (when possible) is to improve medical host grading with therapy designed to positively affect the patient's immune system. Treatment of the host would hopefully improve the systemic immune response and positively affect infection eradiation. In the future, medical therapy may allow modification of treatment of periprosthetic joint infection. If the host immune sys-

2: Systemic Disorders

Table 6

Musculoskeletal Infection Society Staging for Periprosthetic Infection

Category	Grading	Description
Infection type	I	Early postoperative infection (< 3 weeks postoperative) Nonbiofilm state
	II	Late occurring infection (< 3 weeks' duration) Nonbiofilm state
	III	Late chronic infection (≥ 3 weeks' duration) Biofilm state Either from early postoperative infection or late-occurring infection
Systemic host grade (medical/immune status)	A	Uncompromised (no compromising factors)
	B	Compromised (1 to 2 compromising factors)
	C	Significant compromise (Fewer than two compromising factors) or one of the following: Absolute neutrophil count < 1,000 CD4 T-cell count < 100 Intravenous drug abuse Chronic active infection at other site Dysplasia/neoplasm of immune system (For example, myelodysplasia, chronic lymphocytic leukemia)
Local extremity grade	1	Uncompromised (no compromising factors)
	2	Compromised (one to two compromising factors)
	3	Significant compromise (fewer than two compromising factors) or one of the following: Soft-tissue loss requiring muscle transposition or free flap transfer Bone loss requiring structural allograft or substituting megaprosthesis Local wound irradiation ≥ 4,000 rad

Stage = infection type + systemic host grade + local extremity grade; eg, I-A-1, III-B-2

tem cannot assist in the eradication of the bacterial infection, then treatment must be modified to extirpate the infection surgically (with wide radical resection or amputation). This method is described as a "tumoresque" removal of the infection.

The third factor is the grading of the local wound. An intact soft-tissue envelope with normal tissue perfusion is critical to eradicating the infection at the local site. An intact vasculature, at all levels of tissue support, is necessary to deliver oxygen, immune cells, and signaling mediators to the area of infection. If the local wound is damaged significantly, then undamaged fresh tissue can be used to help fill deficits and reestablish a sound local environment. Local muscle rotational flaps are helpful in this regard. If there is poor extremity perfusion, then a vascular bypass procedure may be needed to improve blood flow to the local wound. Sometimes the local wound is so pervasively damaged by the infection that satisfactory salvage is impossible, and an amputation is recommended.

The presentation of a periprosthetic joint infection is variable due to host factors and the inherent virulence of the infecting organism. Most frequently, joint pain, effusion, and loss of joint range of motion are noted. In an acute presentation, a significant limp and inability to bear weight are evident. Often the affected joint is warm and overlying erythema is present. In chronic infections, a draining sinus or boil is seen around the joint. In low-grade infections, there is a paucity of systemic symptoms.

Evaluation of periprosthetic infection first includes a high index of suspicion. All joint arthroplasty procedures cause pain, warmth, and swelling for up to 3 to 4 weeks after the index procedure. However, the surgeon should be suspicious of infection when pain and narcotic use escalates rather than recedes; range of motion decreases; swelling of the joint increases; skin erythema is noted; and wound drainage develops. For a suspected periprosthetic joint infection, recommended studies include a serum CRP, ESR, and CBC with differential. An elevated CRP level is the most frequently elevated serum test. An elevated CRP level can also be present in other conditions such as autoimmune inflammatory disease states. Therefore, review of the cell count and clinical picture are also needed. The combination of normal CRP and ESR levels reliably predicts the absence of infection. A joint aspiration is required to confirm the presence of infection. Joint fluid studies should include Gram stain, culture (aerobic, anaerobic, fungal, and mycobacterial), cell count with differential, crystal analysis, and mucin clot quality. With a periprosthetic joint infection, joint fluid analysis will show an elevated WBC count with a preponderance of PMNs. Because host immunity can be blunted, the threshold WBC level in joint fluid in a periprosthetic joint infection can be low. As a general guide, when the joint fluid WBC is greater than 10,000 cells/mm^3 and there is a preponderance of PMNs, joint infection should be strongly suspected.[47] Radiographs of the affected joint are needed to rule out other sources of joint irritability (such as bone fracture, mechanical breakage, or dislocation). Bone scintigraphy is useful when evaluating for a chronic periprosthetic infection where the diagnosis of the painful joint arthroplasty is unclear. An indium-labeled WBC scan is a useful technique to detect a chronic periprosthetic infection.

The treatment of periprosthetic joint infection is outlined in Table 8. In an acute infection (nonbiofilm state) the goal is prompt surgical lavage and débridement of the infected joint arthroplasty to prevent biofilm formation. If an acute periprosthetic joint infection is suspected and laboratory data corroborate, immediate surgical intervention is recommended. One should not wait for culture results because biofilm formation on an implant can occur quickly. Open surgical débridement with component retention is recommended. During the débridement procedure, modular parts should be removed. The thin, light, yellow fibrin layer that is seen between metal and polyethylene modular parts serves as a site for bacterial adherence and persistence. The débridement procedure should include debulking of inflammatory synovium and copious lavage. Arthroscopic lavage of an acute periprosthetic joint infection does not accomplish all technical goals of periprosthetic joint infection débridement and is not routinely recommended. The best prospect for arthroscopic lavage is a patient who is very ill and cannot tolerate the stress of an open débridement procedure. Intravenous antibiotics are administered for 6 weeks af-

ter the débridement procedure. The prognosis for infection for recovery is good (generally 90% success). Recurrence is more likely seen in medical C hosts. In chronic periprosthetic infection bacteria have formed a biofilm and have had time to invade the prosthetic bone interface. Curative treatment requires removal of prosthetic implants, infected bone, and devascularized soft tissues. The two-stage exchange protocol is considered the most prudent course and is recommended for a chronic periprosthetic joint infection.[48] A single-stage exchange protocol can provide a good rate of success in experienced centers. A single-stage exchange is best suited for patients who are medically uncompromised (type A host) and have normal soft tissues (type 1 wound). A single-stage exchange protocol requires meticulous, coordinated care by the entire operating room team. This technique is best reserved for those centers logistically able to handle an arduous single-stage exchange protocol.

Table 7

Musculoskeletal Infection Society Staging for Periprosthetic Infection - Compromising Factors

Systemic Host Compromising Factors

Age ≥ 80 years

Alcoholism

Chronic active dermatitis/cellulitis

Chronic indwelling catheter (out through skin)

Chronic malnutrition (albumin ≤ 3.0 g/dL)

Current nicotine use (inhalational or oral)

Diabetes (requiring oral agents and/or insulin)

Hepatic insufficiency (cirrhosis)

Immunosuppressive drugs (eg, methotrexate, prednisone, cyclosporine, anti-TNF agents)

Malignancy (history of, or active)

Renal insufficiency with uremia (dialysis)

Systemic autoimmune inflammatory disease (for example, rheumatoid arthritis, systemic lupus erythematosus)

Systemic immune compromise from infection or disease (eg, HIV, sickle cell disease, splenectomy)

Local Extremity Grade (Wound) Compromising Factors

Infection of a revision arthroplasty

Recurrent infection after joint débridement with prosthesis retention

Recurrent infection after prosthetic exchange protocol

Recurrent open foot sores (neuropathic or structural)

Multiple incisions (creating skin bridges)

Sinus tract

Vascular insufficiency to extremity: absent extremity pulses, calcific arterial disease, venous insufficiency with skin plaques or intermittent sores

Table 8

Management of Periprosthetic Joint Infection

Infection Type	Duration	Treatment

Early postoperative infection	Less than 3 weeks from initial joint arthroplasty
	Nonbiofilm state
		1. I and D with retention of components
		    Exchange of modular polyethylene parts
		    Postoperative IV antibiotics (6 weeks)
		2. Arthroscopic lavage if patient is too medically ill to undergo an open débridement procedure
		3. Treat as chronic infection if I and D fails

Late-occurring infection	Less than 3 weeks from joint seeding event
	    Hematogenous seeding or
	    Local spread to joint from adjacent infection
	Nonbiofilm state
		1. I and D with retention of components
		    Exchange of modular polyethylene parts
		    Postoperative IV antibiotics (6 weeks)
		2. Arthroscopic lavage if patient is too medically ill to undergo an open débridement procedure
		3. Treat as chronic infection if I and D fails

Chronic Infection	More than 3 weeks from initial joint replacement
	Seeding event
	Biofilm state
		1. Two-stage exchange with interval period IV antibiotics
		    Interpositional high-dose antibiotic-loaded polymethylmethacrylate spacer
		    IV antibiotics 4 to 6 weeks after resection
		    Reimplantation in 9 to 12 weeks if free of infection
		    Indicated when anticipated joint function is good
		2. Single-stage exchange
		    IV antibiotics 4 to 6 weeks after exchange
		    Best reserved to centers specialized in periprosthetic joint infection management
		    Best indication: Medial A host, type 1 wound
		3. Two-stage arthrodesis with an interval period of IV antibiotics
		    Indicated when surrounding musculoskeletal tissues are severely damaged and anticipated joint function is poor
		    Interpositional high-dose antibiotic-loaded polymethylmethacrylate spacer when needed for joint stabilization
		4. Permanent resection arthroplasty with IV antibiotics
		    IV antibiotics 4 to 6 weeks
		    Indicated when risk of reinfection is high (medial C host) and patient unable to tolerate major reconstructive procedure
		    Joint provides functional mobility with bracing
		5. Amputation/disarticulation
		    IV antibiotics 4 to 6 weeks
		    Indications
		        Painful neuropathic arthropathy
		        Uncontrolled recurrent infection (usually medial C host)
		        Severe soft-tissue destruction and patient unable to tolerate multiple reconstructive procedures to salvage limb
		        Permanent resection will not provide functional mobility with bracing

IV = intravenous, I and D = irrigation and débridement.

In a two-stage protocol, the resected joint is stabilized with an acrylic antibiotic-loaded polymethylmethacrylate spacer to provide sustained, high-dose antibiotic delivery to the infected joint tissue and exposed bone.[49] If supporting ligaments and bone are intact, an articulating spacer construct can be used; one that allows limited motion helps to maintain soft-tissue pliability.[50] Joint motion exercises are to be limited because excess motion and weight bearing can cause an acrylic synovitis to develop. If supporting ligamentous and/or bony structures are deficient, then a static spacer must be used. Intravenous antibiotics are administered for 4 to 6 weeks. Reevaluation for infection is performed after antibiotic administration has been completed (usually 10 to 14 days after completion). Reconstruction of the infected joint is predicated on a benign clinical examination, a normal serum laboratory analysis (normal CBC, CRP, and ESR val-

Table 9

Dental Prophylaxis for Prosthetic Joint Arthroplasty Patients

Patient Status	Recommended Antibiotic	Regimen
Patients not allergic to penicillin	Cephalexin, cephradine, or amoxicillin	2 g orally 1 h before dental procedure
Patients not allergic to penicillin and unable to take oral medications	Cefazolin or ampicillin	Cefazolin 1 g or ampicillin 2 g Intramuscularly or intravenously 1 h before dental procedure
Patients allergic to penicillin	Clindamycin	600 mg orally 1 h before dental procedure
Patients allergic to penicillin and unable to take oral medications	Clindamycin	600 mg intravenously 1 h before dental procedure

ues), and aspiration cultures showing no growth. In the second stage, the type of reconstructive process depends on the patient's medical status and local wound condition.

For most patients, the medical status after the initial resection procedure is stable, and the reconstructive procedure can proceed. The quality of the local wound determines the type of reconstructive process. In most cases, joint arthroplasty can be performed. A requirement for total joint reconstruction includes an intact neuromuscular status to support the joint. Medullary stem support and adjacent screw fixation are needed to support the prosthesis. Joint constraint built into the prosthetic system is often required to support attenuated ligamentous structures. Endoprosthetic implants or bulk support allografts may be required to replace segmental deficiencies in bone. The disadvantage of using a bulk support allograft for reconstruction is that the surrounding tissues (damaged by infection) may have an attenuated blood supply, limiting host-graft healing. Furthermore, if an allograft is placed in a superficial position (such as the proximal tibia) it can become easily infected from minor wound dehiscence or prolonged drainage. Once the allograft is colonized with bacteria, eradication of the infection is nearly impossible. The allograft is a dead porous structure in which bacteria can easily hide. In contrast, deficits filled by solid metal have only an outer surface to which bacteria can adhere. If colonization does occur, successful treatment with irrigation and débridement before a biofilm is allowed to form is possible. In the second-stage procedure, soft tissues are covered with a rotational muscle flap if a secure water-tight and tension-free closure cannot be attained. The vascular status of the limb requires careful assessment when considering a rotational muscle flap procedure. Inadequate arterial supply to the extremity can result in flap necrosis.

When severe soft-tissue and bone damage has occurred, alternative techniques for joint salvage are required. In cases where the medical status is compromised and the risk of recurrent infection is high, a permanent resection arthroplasty is an alternative treatment. The infected implant is removed and the infec-

tion is treated with intravenous antibiotics. The joint is supported with external bracing. The patient is allowed ambulation with assistive devices (cane, crutch, or walker). Permanent resection arthroplasty is chosen over amputation when the resected joint can provide acceptable support for ambulation and pain levels are acceptable. An amputation is chosen when the infection process is life or limb threatening or anticipated pain and suffering will be great. Chronic neuropathic pain in an extremity in the face of a severe periprosthetic joint infection is an indication for amputation. When severe soft-tissue damage and bone loss has occurred, an amputation is chosen when the reconstructive process is too arduous for the patient to handle (such as multiple procedures in a compromised host). When the infection becomes life threatening, an urgent amputation/disarticulation is the recommended procedure. Limb ablation removes the infection mass, thus allowing the immune system to focus on primary wound healing.

Dental prophylaxis is recommended for all patients who have undergone a joint arthroplasty. Prophylactic antibiotic coverage for dental procedures should be given for the first 2 years after surgery. Patients who are immunocompromised or immunosuppressed should receive lifetime prophylactic antibiotics. Examples of immunocompromised conditions include inflammatory arthropathies (rheumatoid arthritis, systemic lupus erythematosus) and medication-induced immunosuppression. Patients with comorbidities that alter immune system function should also receive lifetime dental prophylaxis. Examples include previous prosthetic joint infection, diabetes, and malignancy. **Table 9** outlines the recommended prophylactic antibiotic coverage for dental procedures.

In communities where MRSA is endemic, preoperative office screening for MRSA is advocated for those patients considered at risk for MRSA colonization.[51,52] At-risk groups include patients who have recently been or reside in a hospital or extended-stay care facility, patients with a history of MRSA colonization, and patients who are immune compromised. Screening can be performed in the office with a nares and/or axillary swab culture. Eradication of the MRSA carrier state is recommended before any elective joint arthroplasty or

2: Systemic Disorders

Table 10

Treatment Protocol for MRSA-Colonized Patient

14-day protocol

Bactroban intranasal ointment 2%. Apply to nares twice daily

Rifampin 300 mg by mouth twice daily

Bactrim DS by mouth twice daily

Hibiclens (chlorhexidine gluconate) bath daily for 5 minutes. Immerse entire body (including scalp) to face. Wash face with wash cloth. Use 1 oz of Hibiclens solution (chlorhexidine gluconate 4%) in warm bath water.

Repeat MRSA screen

orthopaedic procedure. This reduces MRSA bioburden to patients within the health care facility. A treatment protocol for MRSA carriers is listed in **Table 10**.

Summary

The competition between human host defense and environmental microorganisms is a battle that will continue in perpetuity. Infection prevention remains the best method to thwart microorganism destruction seen in musculoskeletal infections. An understanding of the concept of bacterial shedding and microorganism inoculation allows the orthopaedic surgeon and health care team to maximize efforts to ameliorate the risk of orthopaedic infections. An understanding of the concept of bacterial biofilm is key to providing appropriate care once a musculoskeletal infection is established. Compromise in human host defense requires a more aggressive surgical treatment regimen to eradicate an established musculoskeletal infection. By using staging systems for osteomyelitis and periprosthetic joint infection, treatment regimens can be evaluated and tailored to address various levels of host weakness. Future research is directed toward developing methods to eradicate a biofilm that do not require surgical extirpation of host tissue and implanted medical devices. Research also is focused on biofilm dissolution with detergents or signaling molecules that will instruct a biofilm to dissipate. It is hoped that methods to boost host immunity to combat musculoskeletal infections will be developed. The goal is to rely less on antibiotic therapy and surgical débridement to help maintain limb function and quality of life.

Annotated References

1. Bethune DW, Blowers R, Parker M, Pask EA: Dispersal of *Staphylococcus aureus* by patients and surgical staff. *Lancet* 1965;1(7383):480-483.

2. Miller LG, Diep BA: Clinical practice: colonization, fomites, and virulence: rethinking the pathogenesis of community-associated methicillin-resistant *Staphylococcus aureus* infection. *Clin Infect Dis* 2008;46(5):752-760.

   The authors discuss community-associated MRSA infection and strategies for prevention.

3. Ritter MA: Surgical wound environment. *Clin Orthop Relat Res* 1984;190(190):11-13.

4. Gristina AG, Costerton JW: Bacterial adherence and the glycocalyx and their role in musculoskeletal infection. *Orthop Clin North Am* 1984;15(3):517-535.

5. Donlan RM, Costerton JW: Biofilms: survival mechanisms of clinically relevant microorganisms. *Clin Microbiol Rev* 2002;15(2):167-193.

6. Shirtliff ME, Leid JG, Costerton JW: The basic science of musculoskeletal infection, in *Musculoskeletal Infections*. Calhoun JH, Mader JT, eds: Marcel Dekker Inc. New York, NY, 2003, pp 1-61.

7. Balaban N, Novick RP: Autocrine regulation of toxin synthesis by *Staphylococcus aureus*. *Proc Natl Acad Sci U S A* 1995;92(5):1619-1623.

8. Reguera G, McCarthy KD, Mehta T, Nicoll JS, Tuominen MT, Lovley DR: Extracellular electron transfer via microbial nanowires. *Nature* 2005;435(7045):1098-1101.

9. Hall-Stoodley L, Costerton JW, Stoodley P: Bacterial biofilms: from the natural environment to infectious diseases. *Nat Rev Microbiol* 2004;2(2):95-108.

10. Cirioni O, Giacometti A, Ghiselli R, et al: RNAIII-inhibiting peptide significantly reduces bacterial load and enhances the effect of antibiotics in the treatment of central venous catheter-associated *Staphylococcus aureus* infections. *J Infect Dis* 2006;193(2):180-186.

11. Mader JT, Calhoun JH: Staging and staging application in osteomyelitis, in Calhoun JH, Mader JT, eds: *Musculoskeletal Infections* New York, NY, Marcel Dekker Inc. 2003, pp 149-182.

12. Globerson A, Effros RB: Ageing of lymphocytes and lymphocytes in the aged. *Immunol Today* 2000;21(10):515-521.

13. Brady RA, Leid JG, Calhoun JH, Costerton JW, Shirtliff ME: Osteomyelitis and the role of biofilms in chronic infection. *FEMS Immunol Med Microbiol* 2008;52(1):13-22.

    The authors discuss current understanding of biofilms and molecular interactions of bacteria.

14. Bauer T, David T, Rimareix F, Lortat-Jacob A: [Marjolin's ulcer in chronic osteomyelitis: Seven cases and a review of the literature]. *Rev Chir Orthop Reparatrice Appar Mot* 2007;93(1):63-71.

The authors report on seven patients with squamous cell skin carcinoma in whom wounds related to deep bone infections had developed. Nonsurgical treatment was unsuccessful in four patients, and three required amputation.

15. Pineda C, Vargas A, Rodríguez AV: Imaging of osteomyelitis: Current concepts. *Infect Dis Clin North Am* 2006;20(4):789-825.

16. Favero M, Schiavon F, Riato L, Carraro V, Punzi L: [Septic arthritis: A 12 years retrospective study in a rheumatological university clinic]. *Reumatismo* 2008; 60(4):260-267.

    The authors reevaluated septic arthritis cases discharged over a 12-year period to study risk factors, clinical and laboratory characteristics, causative microorganisms, and possible increase in frequency.

17. Frazee BW, Fee C, Lambert L: How common is MRSA in adult septic arthritis? *Ann Emerg Med* 2009;54(5): 695-700.

    The authors studied the proportion of MRSA in emergency department patients with adult septic arthritis.

18. Geirsson AJ, Statkevicius S, Víkingsson A: Septic arthritis in Iceland 1990-2002: Increasing incidence due to iatrogenic infections. *Ann Rheum Dis* 2008;67(5):638-643.

    The authors studied the effect of the increase in diagnostic and therapeutic joint procedures on the incidence and type of septic arthritis. The importance of sterile technique and firm indications for joint procedures is emphasized.

19. Mathews CJ, Coakley G: Septic arthritis: Current diagnostic and therapeutic algorithm. *Curr Opin Rheumatol* 2008;20(4):457-462.

    An evidence-based algorithm for diagnosis and treatment of bacterial septic arthritis is discussed.

20. McGillicuddy DC, Shah KH, Friedberg RP, Nathanson LA, Edlow JA: How sensitive is the synovial fluid white blood cell count in diagnosing septic arthritis? *Am J Emerg Med* 2007;25(7):749-752.

    The authors studied the sensitivity of the current standard for synovial fluid leukocytosis analysis in the diagnosis of infectious arthritis or a septic joint.

21. De Boeck H: Osteomyelitis and septic arthritis in children. *Acta Orthop Belg* 2005;71(5):505-515.

22. Jansson A, Jansson V, von Liebe A: [Pediatric osteomyelitis]. *Orthopade* 2009;38(3):283-294.

    The authors discuss diagnostic and therapeutic approaches for childhood osteomyelitis.

23. Gafur OA, Copley LA, Hollmig ST, Browne RH, Thornton LA, Crawford SE: The impact of the current epidemiology of pediatric musculoskeletal infection on evaluation and treatment guidelines. *J Pediatr Orthop* 2008;28(7):777-785.

The authors compared the current epidemiology of musculoskeletal infection with historical data and evaluated the degree of disease severity within the current epidemiology.

24. McCarthy JJ, Dormans JP, Kozin SH, Pizzutillo PD: Musculoskeletal infections in children: Basic treatment principles and recent advancements. *Instr Course Lect* 2005;54:515-528.

25. Khachatourians AG, Patzakis MJ, Roidis N, Holtom PD: Laboratory monitoring in pediatric acute osteomyelitis and septic arthritis. *Clin Orthop Relat Res* 2003; 409:186-194.

26. Hügle T, Schuetz P, Mueller B, et al: Serum procalcitonin for discrimination between septic and non-septic arthritis. *Clin Exp Rheumatol* 2008;26(3):453-456.

    The authors studied the diagnostic value of serum procalcitonin and determined that it is highly sensitive and specific for septic arthritis, depending on the clinical setting.

27. Blickman JG, van Die CE, de Rooy JW: Current imaging concepts in pediatric osteomyelitis. *Eur Radiol* 2004;14(suppl 4):L55-L64.

28. Schmit P, Glorion C: Osteomyelitis in infants and children. *Eur Radiol* 2004;14(suppl 4):L44-L54.

29. Hawkshead JJ III, Patel NB, Steele RW, Heinrich SD: Comparative severity of pediatric osteomyelitis attributable to methicillin-resistant versus methicillin-sensitive *Staphylococcus aureus*. *J Pediatr Orthop* 2009;29(1): 85-90.

    The authors attempted to determine whether there were significant differences in predetermined measures of disease severity among 97 patients with hematogenous osteomyelitis of varying etiologies.

30. Al-Ola K, Mahdi N, Al-Subaie AM, Ali ME, Al-Absi IK, Almawi WY: Evidence for HLA class II susceptible and protective haplotypes for osteomyelitis in pediatric patients with sickle cell anemia. *Tissue Antigens* 2008; 71(5):453-457.

    The authors determined that specific HLA haplotypes influence sickle cell anemia osteomyelitis risk, and specific HLA types may be markers for identifying sickle cell anemia patients at high risk for osteomyelitis.

31. Hughes LO, Mader JT: Pediatric osteomyelitis, in Calhoun JH, Mader JT, eds: *Musculoskeletal Infections.* New York, NY, Marcel Dekker Inc. 2003, pp 473-493.

32. Yagupsky P: Kingella kingae: From medical rarity to an emerging paediatric pathogen. *Lancet Infect Dis* 2004; 4(6):358-367.

33. Yuan HC, Wu KG, Chen CJ, Tang RB, Hwang BT: Characteristics and outcome of septic arthritis in children. *J Microbiol Immunol Infect* 2006;39(4):342-347.

2: Systemic Disorders

34. El-Sayed AM: Treatment of early septic arthritis of the hip in children: Comparison of results of open arthrotomy versus arthroscopic drainage. *J Child Orthop* 2008;2(3):229-237.

In a prospective controlled study, the authors compared results of open arthrotomy compared with those of arthroscopic drainage in the treatment of septic arthritis of the hip in children.

35. Rutz E, Brunner R: Septic arthritis of the hip: Current concepts. *Hip Int* 2009;19(suppl 6):S9-S12.

The authors discuss etiology and therapeutic options for septic arthritis of the hip.

36. Ballock RT, Newton PO, Evans SJ, Estabrook M, Farnsworth CL, Bradley JS: A comparison of early versus late conversion from intravenous to oral therapy in the treatment of septic arthritis. *J Pediatr Orthop* 2009;29(6):636-642.

The authors studied records of 186 patients from two children's hospitals and concluded that clinical outcome in patients with septic arthritis converted to oral antibiotic therapy early in treatment based on defined criteria was similar to those patients converted later.

37. Chang HC, Verhoeven W, Chay WM: Rubber foreign bodies in puncture wounds of the foot in patients wearing rubber-soled shoes. *Foot Ankle Int* 2001;22(5):409-414.

38. Raz R, Miron D: Oral ciprofloxacin for treatment of infection following nail puncture wounds of the foot. *Clin Infect Dis* 1995;21(1):194-195.

39. Lavery LA, Peters EJ, Armstrong DG, Wendel CS, Murdoch DP, Lipsky BA: Risk factors for developing osteomyelitis in patients with diabetic foot wounds. *Diabetes Res Clin Pract* 2009;83(3):347-352.

The results of this prospective study suggest that independent risk factors for developing osteomyelitis are deep, recurrent, multiple wounds; these findings may help in the diagnosis of foot osteomyelitis in high-risk patients.

40. Jacobs RF, McCarthy RE, Elser JM: Pseudomonas osteochondritis complicating puncture wounds of the foot in children: A 10-year evaluation. *J Infect Dis* 1989;160(4):657-661.

41. Peersman G, Laskin R, Davis J, Peterson M: Infection in total knee replacement: A retrospective review of 6489 total knee replacements. *Clin Orthop Relat Res* 2001;392:15-23.

42. Pulido L, Ghanem E, Joshi A, Purtill JJ, Parvizi J: Periprosthetic joint infection: The incidence, timing, and predisposing factors. *Clin Orthop Relat Res* 2008;466(7):1710-1715.

The authors identified current risk factors of periprosthetic joint infection after modern joint arthroplasty. The incidence and timing of periprosthetic joint infection were also determined. Level of evidence: II.

43. Herrmann M, Vaudaux PE, Vaudaux PE, Pittet D, et al: Fibronectin, fibrinogen, and laminin act as mediators of adherence of clinical staphylococcal isolates to foreign material. *J Infect Dis* 1988;158(4):693-701.

44. Jämsen E, Huhtala H, Huhtala H, Puolakka T, Moilanen T: Risk factors for infection after knee arthroplasty: A register-based analysis of 43,149 cases. *J Bone Joint Surg Am* 2009;91(1):38-47.

The authors used a large register-based series to study risk factors for infection after primary and revision knee replacement.

45. McPherson EJ, Woodson C, Holtom P, Roidis N, Shufelt C, Patzakis M: Periprosthetic total hip infection: Outcomes using a staging system. *Clin Orthop Relat Res* 2002;403(403):8-15.

46. McPherson EJ: Periprosthetic total knee infection, in Calhoun JH, Mader JT, eds: *Musculoskeletal Infections*. New York, NY, Marcel Dekker Inc, 2003, pp 293-324.

47. Ghanem E, Parvizi J, Burnett RS, et al: Cell count and differential of aspirated fluid in the diagnosis of infection at the site of total knee arthroplasty. *J Bone Joint Surg Am* 2008;90(8):1637-1643.

The authors used receiver operating characteristic curves to determine cutoff values for fluid leukocyte count and neutrophil differential to help diagnose infection at the site of a prosthetic joint.

48. Burnett RS, Kelly MA, Hanssen AD, Barrack RL: Technique and timing of two-stage exchange for infection in TKA. *Clin Orthop Relat Res* 2007;464:164-178.

The authors present classification and alternatives to a two-stage exchange procedure for infection in total knee arthroplasty and discuss current diagnosis and monitoring of infection. Level of evidence: V.

49. Greene N, Holtom PD, Warren CA, et al: In vitro elution of tobramycin and vancomycin polymethylmethacrylate beads and spacers from Simplex and Palacos. *Am J Orthop (Belle Mead NJ)* 1998;27(3):201-205.

50. Yamamoto K, Miyagawa N, Masaoka T, Katori Y, Shishido T, Imakiire A: Cement spacer loaded with antibiotics for infected implants of the hip joint. *J Arthroplasty* 2009;24(1):83-89.

The authors used antibiotic-impregnated cement spacers in 17 cases of infection after total hip arthroplasty and bipolar arthroplasty. Results were good, with no recurring infection after a 3-year, 2-month follow-up period.

51. Mohanty SS, Kay PR: Infection in total joint replacements: Why we screen MRSA when MRSE is the problem? *J Bone Joint Surg Br* 2004;86(2):266-268.

52. Sankar B, Hopgood P, Bell KM: The role of MRSA screening in joint-replacement surgery. *Int Orthop* 2005;29(3):160-163.

Chapter 21

Pain Management

Sharon M. Weinstein, MD, FAAHPM

2: Systemic Disorders

Introduction

Orthopaedic surgeons should be familiar with the basic assessment, diagnosis, and treatment of pain in various clinical settings (Table 1). Injury and surgery can cause acute pain. Some orthopaedic conditions may be associated with persistent or chronic pain that can significantly limit the patient's functional status if not adequately managed. Collaboration between orthopaedic surgeons and other caregivers is required to provide state-of-the-art pain management in patients requiring both acute and chronic care.

Pain remains medically undertreated for several reasons, including deficient professional education, societal concerns regarding the use of opioid analgesics (narcotics), and professional fear of regulatory agency influence. The lack of availability of analgesic drugs is also a significant problem in many areas of the world.

The direct costs of unrelieved pain can be measured in dollars, in lost productivity, and in lives lost to suicide. Pain costs $60 to $100 billion each year in the United States alone.[1] The loss of functional status and poor quality of life are frequent, intangible costs of unrelieved pain.

Pain associated with noncancerous chronic conditions is highly prevalent. An estimated 75 million Americans suffer from chronic pain. Headache and low back pain are the most common types of noncancer-related pain in developed countries. More than 26 million Americans between the ages of 20 and 64 years experience frequent back pain, and two thirds of American adults will have back pain during their lifetime.[2] Other common conditions include inflammatory and degenerative musculoskeletal conditions, headache, jaw and lower facial pain (temporomandibular dysfunction, temporomandibular joint syndrome), neuropathic pain syndromes, and fibromyalgia (a complex condition involving generalized body pain and other symptoms). Chronic painful conditions in underdeveloped countries are more likely to be related to malnutrition; infectious diseases; and trauma, including limb amputation. Millions of the world's inhabitants are affected by these conditions.

Dr. Weinstein or an immediate family member serves as a paid consultant to or is an employee of Wyeth Optum.

General Considerations

Basic Physiology of Pain

Pain is defined as a complex psychophysiologic phenomenon. It is the perceptual product of a complex integration of multiple brain circuits. Pain is a necessary and physiologic function of the nervous system. Pathologic pain results from abnormal nervous system functioning (neuropathic pain). A great deal of information has been learned in recent decades about the peripheral and central neurophysiologic mechanisms of human pain, including how acute pain states can become chronic conditions. A discrete human brain locus for the conscious perception of pain probably does not exist.

Within the human nervous system there are mechanisms to transmit nociceptive signals, to inhibit nociception and produce analgesia, and to release analgesic mechanisms (antianalgesia) that facilitate healing and recovery. Human pain has both sensory (discriminative) and affective dimensions. The process of nociception begins when a noxious stimulus is transduced in the peripheral tissues. Nociceptive signals are transmitted over peripheral nerves to the central nervous system. Ascending transmission and modulation occur at

Table 1

Basic Assessment and Treatment of Pain

Preoperative Assessment

Orthopaedic surgeon
Anesthesiologist
Primary care provider
Pain specialist

Intraoperative Care

Orthopaedic surgeon
Anesthesiologist

Immediate Postoperative Care

Orthopaedic surgeon
Anesthesiologist
Pain specialist

Follow-up Care

Orthopaedic surgeon
Primary care provider
Pain specialist

Table 2

Pathophysiologic Classification of Pain

Nociceptive

Somatic
Visceral

Nonnociceptive

Neuropathic
Psychogenic (rare)

Unclassified Soft-Tissue Pain Syndromes

Myofascial pain syndrome
Fibromyalgia pain syndrome

(Adapted with permission from Weinstein SM: Non-malignant pain, in Walsh D: *Palliative Medicine.* Philadelphia, PA, WB Saunders, 2009, pp 931-937.)

spinal and supraspinal levels. Neuroanatomic pathways of nociceptive processing involve a human thalamic nucleus specific for pain and widely distributed cerebral cannabinoid receptors. Another receptor also widely distributed in the brain is termed the orphan opioid receptor; its natural ligand (nociceptin or orphanin FQ) appears to facilitate pain perception in animals and may be involved in learning and memory. Many chemical mediators and neurotransmitters involved in pain transduction, transmission, modulation, and perception have been identified. It is known that opioid receptors are widely distributed in nonneural tissues throughout the nervous system, leading to specific targets for pain relief, such as opioid joint injections. The contribution of other neurotransmitters, such as serotonin and norepinephrine, to the inhibition of pain signaling also is known.

Pathophysiology and Pain Diagnosis

Advances in neuroscience research in learning, memory, and neural plasticity have helped to elucidate the pathophysiology of chronic pain states. It has been observed that both membrane excitability and synaptic transmission are enhanced in sensory neurons with damaged axons. Signal proteins that are synthesized in response to such sensitization are probably distributed throughout the neuronal arbor and thus affect structural remodeling. Perceptions are encoded in both anatomic structures and temporal patterns of neural activity in the brain.

Pain is a dynamic perceptual product of higher cortical processing. It is important to note that the central nervous system responds to nociceptive signals acutely with activity at the spinal cord, the brainstem, and the thalamus, and with immediate alterations in cortical somatosensory synaptic patterns. Structural as well as functional changes occur with repeated noxious stimuli, persistent damaging stimuli, or as a result of direct injury to the nervous system itself. Chronic noncancerous pain in humans may be attributable to pathologic functioning of a damaged nervous system at any level. A working classification of pain states, based on the

two broad categories of pain (nociceptive and nonnociceptive), is summarized in **Table 2.** Simple mechanisms for myofascial and fibromyalgia pain have not been identified.

Acute Pain

In the setting of injury, adequate control of acute pain is a necessary part of stabilizing the injured patient for further diagnostic evaluation and treatment. When surgery is planned, pain should be anticipated and a pain management plan should be developed before surgery whenever possible. Patients may be most cooperative when they are advised in advance of what can be expected and how pain will be managed. Medical evidence has accumulated indicating that applying nonpharmacologic and pharmacologic interventions in both preoperative (preemptive or preventive) and postoperative phases produces the best outcomes.[3-6] These outcomes include pain prevention, faster recovery, shorter hospitalization time, and improved patient satisfaction.

Current standards of pain management include the formal assessment of pain, the diagnosis of different physiologic mechanisms of pain, and the development of individualized treatment with nonpharmacologic and pharmacologic strategies. The synthesis of knowledge of how to minimize acute pain and improve postoperative recovery continues to advance, permitting some major orthopaedic procedures to be done in the outpatient or day-surgery setting.[7,8] Specific pain management protocols are suggested for particular clinical situations such as geriatric hip fracture repair[9] and for more refined perioperative analgesic techniques.[10-12] The optimal combination of analgesic medications and the use of vitamin C for postoperative pain prevention have been reported.[13,14] The orthopaedic surgeon is in a pivotal position to prevent chronic pain by identifying unrelieved pain in the acute setting and by collaborating with other clinicians providing pain management. Consultation with pain specialists is suggested when patients with acute pain are not progressing as expected and for the collaborative management of persistent pain.

Persistent Pain in Orthopaedic Patients

Steps in the management of persistent (chronic) pain are (1) evaluating the patient and establishing the pain diagnoses, (2) identifying any curative treatments, (3) maximizing nonpharmacologic analgesic interventions, (4) tailoring analgesic medications to the individual, and (5) monitoring the patient for response to treatment and modifying the treatment plan accordingly.

Patient Evaluation

A thorough evaluation of the patient with persistent pain includes a comprehensive history, a physical exam-

Table 3

PQRST Mnemonic for Eliciting a Complete History of Pain

P = palliative, provocative factors (what factors make pain better or worse)

Q = quality, word descriptors (such as burning or stabbing)

R = region, radiation, referral (where does it hurt? does pain move or travel? radicular or nonradicular pattern?)

S = severity (pain intensity rating scales or word descriptors)

T = temporal factors (such as onset, duration, daily fluctuations, when did it start, constant and/or intermittent, how long does it last, better or worse at certain times of the day)

(Adapted with permission from Weinstein SM: Non-malignant pain, in Walsh D: *Palliative Medicine*. Philadelphia, PA, WB Saunders, 2009, pp 931-937.)

Table 4

Physical Examination of the Patient With Pain

General

Patient's appearance and vital signs
Evidence of abnormalities such as weight loss, muscle atrophy, deformities, trophic changes

Pain Site Assessment

Inspect the pain site(s) for abnormal appearance or color of overlying skin, change of contour, visible muscle spasm
Palpate the site(s) for tenderness and texture
Use percussion to elicit, reproduce, or evaluate the pain and any tenderness on palpation
Determine the effects of physical factors such as position, pressure, and motion

Neurologic Examination

Mental status: level of alertness, higher cognitive functions, affect
Cranial nerves
Motor system: muscle bulk and tone, abnormal movements, manual motor testing, reflexes
Sensory system: light touch and pin prick test to assess for allodynia, evoked dysesthesia, hypoesthesia, hyperesthesia, hypoalgesia, hyperalgesia, hyperpathia
Coordination, station, and gait

Musculoskeletal Examination

Body type, posture, and overall symmetry
Abnormal spine curvature, limb alignment, and other deformities
Range of motion (spine, extremities)
For muscles in neck, upper extremities, trunk, and lower extremities: observe for any abnormalities such as atrophy, hypertrophy, irritability, tenderness, trigger points

(Adapted with permission from Weinstein SM: Non-malignant pain, in Walsh D: *Palliative Medicine*. Philadelphia, PA, WB Saunders, 2009, pp 931-937.)

ination, and a review of diagnostic information. The gold standard of pain assessment remains the patient's self-report. Clinicians can use the PQRST mnemonic to elicit a complete pain history (Table 3). Certain characteristics suggestive of neuropathic pain should be elicited. Typically, patients describe burning or lancinating pain. Some patients report unusual symptoms such as painful numbness, itching, or crawling sensations. Neuropathic pain may also manifest as new, bizarre sensations that may frighten the patient and confuse clinicians. The detailed history is crucial to the diagnosis of specific pathophysiologic mechanisms of persistent pain.

Pain intensity rating scales are used in clinical practice to establish a baseline against which the efficacy of analgesic interventions can be assessed. Many patients must be encouraged to verbalize their pain, and most need to learn how to report pain intensity. In circumstances in which patients are unable to communicate, behavioral observations may substitute for the patient's report of pain intensity. Standardized tools are available to assess preverbal children and impaired adults. The Behavioral Pain Scale (BPS) and the FLACC Behavioral Pain Assessment Scale (acronym FLACC: face, legs, activity, cry, and consolability) have been validated in adult and pediatric populations.[15,16]

There are different temporal patterns of persistent pain: constant pain, daily pain, intermittent/recurring pain that is predictable or regular, and intermittent/recurring pain that is unpredictable or irregular. Analgesic treatment approaches vary considerably according to the temporal pattern of the painful condition.

Standardized pain assessment tools capture the impact of pain on mood, sleep, appetite, physical activities and social functioning. A psychosocial assessment should be performed and the meaning of pain to the individual and family should be explored. The expression of pain is influenced by a patient's prior experience and social and cultural milieu. Psychosocial stressors should be elicited. A patient's usual coping strategies and social

support system should be understood. When formulating a medical treatment plan that includes the prescription of controlled substances, it is especially important to identify prior or current psychological dependency on licit or illicit drugs, including alcohol. Prior pain treatments, including prescription and nonprescription medications, and their relative efficacies should be recorded.

It is important to assess the patient's general physical condition and to identify physical findings that help to elucidate the pathophysiology of the reported pain (Table 4). The physiologic signs of acute pain—elevated blood pressure, respiratory rates, and pulse rates—are not reliable in patients with subacute and chronic pain.

The pain specialist will perform a complete physical examination including a detailed neurologic examination, especially if neuropathic pain is suspected. Pain in an area of reduced sensation, allodynia (pain elicited by normally nonpainful stimuli), and hyperpathia (summation of painful stimuli) indicate neural dysfunction. The diagnosis of a complex regional pain syndrome,

2: Systemic Disorders

Table 5

Diagnostic Testing for Persistent Pain Associated With a Noncancerous Condition

Types of Tests	Uses for the Tests
Screening laboratory test: complete blood cell count, chemistry profile (for example, electrolytes, liver, enzymes, blood urea nitrogen, creatinine), urinalysis, erythrocyte sedimentation rate	Screen for medical illnesses, organ dysfunction
Disease-specific laboratory tests: includes autoantibodies and sickle cell test	Autoimmune disorders, sickle cell disease
Imaging studies: radiographs, CT, MRI, ultrasound, myelography	Detection of tumors, other structural abnormalities
Diagnostic procedures: lumbar puncture for cerebrospinal fluid analysis	Detection of various central nervous system illnesses
Electrophysiologic tests: electromyography (direct examination of skeletal muscle), nerve conduction velocity (examination of conduction along peripheral nerves)	Detection of myopathy, neuropathy, radiculopathy
Diagnostic nerve block: injection of a local anesthetic to determine the source and/or mechanism of the pain	Identification of structures responsible for the pain (such as sacroiliac or facet joint blocks), differentiation of pain pathophysiology

(Adapted with permission from Weinstein SM: Non-malignant pain, in Walsh D: *Palliative Medicine*. Philadelphia, PA, WB Saunders, 2009, pp 931-937.)

previously termed sympathetically maintained pain (causalgia or reflex sympathetic dystrophy), is suggested when there are signs of marked sympathetic nervous dysfunction and other physical abnormalities.

A careful mechanical and soft-tissue evaluation is part of the comprehensive pain evaluation. Soft-tissue conditions may contribute to ongoing pain. Muscle spasms, tender musculotendinous points of fibromyalgia, or discrete muscle trigger points may be palpated; when stimulated, pain may be referred to another site in a predictable pattern (criteria for myofascial pain syndrome).

Pain Diagnosis

Correlation should be made between clinical symptoms; physical signs; and diagnostic, laboratory, and radiographic information to establish the pain diagnosis (Table 5). There is no definitive test to confirm pain, and the pain diagnosis depends not only on clinical assessment, but also on the clinician's complete understanding of normal and abnormal nervous system physiology as previously described. In patients with chronic orthopaedic conditions, there are likely to be multiple pathophysiologic mechanisms underlying the patient's reported pain; each should be clearly identified to form the basis of a multimodal treatment plan.

Low back pain, arthritides, neuropathic pain (such as painful diabetic neuropathy, postherpetic neuralgia, and pain from nerve injury),[17,18] and other conditions require daily management on the part of the patient that includes lifestyle modifications. Published guidelines for the management of chronic painful conditions outline the proper diagnosis, nonpharmacologic approaches, and pharmacologic treatment.[19]

Pain Treatment

Nonpharmacologic Interventions
Anesthetic and Neurosurgical Procedures
Many anesthetic procedures can be done in the outpatient setting.[20]

Patients with pain may also be evaluated by the neurosurgeon to determine the indication for implanted intrathecal systems for opioid delivery, neuroaugmentation (nervous system stimulation), or neuroablative (destructive) surgical procedures. Nonpharmacologic strategies using neurostimulation or neuroaugmentation techniques are being refined and may produce pain relief that lessens the requirement for systemic medications.[21]

Physical Treatment and Psychological and Behavioral Interventions
Specific treatments (such as soft-tissue manipulation) for myofascial pain and musculoskeletal disorders may be performed in the clinic. Patients with pain should be referred to physical medicine and rehabilitation physicians to determine the need for rehabilitation and occupational and physical therapy programs.

Pain specialists work closely with psychiatrists and mental health practitioners to evaluate and treat pain along with concurrent psychiatric or psychological conditions. Cognitive and behavioral therapy, relaxation training, hypnosis, individual therapy, family psychotherapy, and psychoeducational support groups are useful as adjunctive outpatient pain treatments.[20] Spiritual support is a part of maintaining overall wellness especially in the setting of life-threatening illness and end-of-life care. Many patients with chronic noncancerous pain use a variety of complementary and alternative medicine techniques for pain relief.[22] Clinicians should inquire about their patients' use of these methods.

Pharmacologic Treatment

Analgesic medications are considered to have broad effects, including reducing transduction of painful peripheral stimuli, altering pain transmission within the central nervous system, or altering pain perception at the higher cortical level. Nonsteroidal anti-inflammatory drugs (NSAIDs) and acetaminophen, the opioids, and an assorted group of medications referred to as adjuvant analgesics or coanalgesics are the three main classes of drugs used to treat pain.

Complex pharmacotherapy is the rational combination of analgesic medications that work through different mechanisms within the human nervous system to produce pain relief. Many patients with chronic noncancerous pain are prescribed medications from more than one drug class. The best results are obtained by individualized medication management in the context of a well-established therapeutic relationship. NSAIDs and acetaminophen are used for mild nociceptive pain. Patients requiring long-term treatment should be monitored for cumulative renal and hepatic toxicity.

Opioid Analgesics

Oral administration of opioid analgesics is preferred because of convenience and costs. Modified release or long-acting preparations are recommended to produce more uniform serum drug levels and to enhance patient compliance with dosing. Alternative methods of administration are considered when the oral method is unavailable, if oral dosing is impractical, or if systemic adverse side effects are unmanageable. Patients may remain ambulatory with external pumps for subcutaneous, intravenous, or intraspinal (epidural, intrathecal) drug delivery. Implantable systems for the administration of intrathecal opioid and nonopioid medications are available.

Adjuvant Analgesics

Adjuvant analgesics are a heterogeneous class of medications, which are administered to provide additive analgesic effects, to counteract the adverse side effects of more traditional analgesics such as NSAIDs and opioids, and/or to treat a concurrent symptom. Adjuvant analgesics include antidepressants, anticonvulsants, antihistamines, psychostimulants, muscle relaxants, antispasmodics, and oral local anesthetics. Topical agents are useful to spare systemic drug burden.[23]

Evidence-Based Guidelines

Numerous professional societies and government agencies have developed guidelines and policies for the treatment of chronic noncancerous pain.[19,24-27] General policies emphasize the obligation of clinicians to properly assess and treat pain. Clinical guidelines detail the management approaches and outline specific considerations for special populations, such as children, elderly

people, and marginalized people. It is recognized that societal concerns related to drug abuse and diversion should not outweigh a patient's rights to compassionate, effective pain treatment.

Outcomes of Pain Management

The successful management of chronic noncancerous pain is dependent on individualized care. Clinicians working with patients on a long-term basis to manage pain follow several outcome variables to judge the efficacy of the pain management plan. These include the patient's self-report of pain intensity, pain relief, side effects of treatment, adverse events, quality of life, and functional status. Patients with severe persistent pain related to orthopaedic conditions that are not expected to resolve will likely benefit from pain specialty care in conjunction with primary orthopaedic care. Ongoing communication between care providers is important, especially when patients are treated with complex pharmacotherapy, including controlled substances.

Special Considerations

The Pediatric Population

Although much progress has been made in identifying pain in children, pain management in the pediatric population remains challenging.[28,29] Medications for pain are generally tested in only adults, leaving questions regarding appropriate pediatric dosing, efficacy, and safety. In 2001, the American Academy of Pediatrics developed guidelines for managing acute pain in infants, children, and adolescents.[30] More recently, organizational changes needed for improved pain management in hospitalized children have been identified.[31] Regional anesthesia and spinal techniques for postoperative pain control in children have been tested.[32-34] A specific approach to acute postoperative pain control in children with chronic disabilities has been described. A conceptual model and practice framework for managing chronic pain in children and adolescents also has been proposed.[35] Parental beliefs and worries regarding adolescent chronic pain have been explored, relating to the meaning of pain itself and concerns with effects of medications.[36]

The Elderly Population

Pain management in elderly patients also has been a focus for guideline development. In 2009, the American Geriatric Society updated its guideline for the pharmacologic management of chronic pain in older persons, specifying risks and benefits of different analgesics and outlining the role of opioid analgesics in the treatment of pain.[37] A higher prevalence of chronic painful orthopaedic conditions requiring clinical management can be expected in the aging US population. Interdisciplinary programs to reduce pain and improve function in older adults after orthopaedic surgery have been tested.[9] Given the prevalence of hip fractures, coordinated orthogeriatric care is suggested for this subpopulation;[38] the perception of pain as an important clinical variable in this setting is recognized.[39]

2: Systemic Disorders

Opioid Therapy

The management of chronic pain with long-term opioid therapy remains controversial, although some patients clearly benefit from this treatment approach.[40] Federal standards indicate that prescribers have dual responsibilities to treat patients adequately while taking steps to minimize prescription drug diversion and abuse. Current guidelines emphasize the comprehensive evaluation and multidisciplinary treatment of patients with severe chronic pain. The use of written treatment agreements and regular monitoring, including drug screening, are suggested when controlled substances are prescribed.[19] Long-term opioid therapy should be prescribed only by clinicians with adequate knowledge, skill, and the necessary clinical infrastructure with interdisciplinary support. There are no established patient selection criteria for opioid therapy; clinicians are advised to follow relevant literature as it emerges.

Methadone Therapy

Methadone is an effective, inexpensive analgesic that is generally available. It is a potent, synthetic diphenylheptane-derivative opioid agonist. Its pharmacokinetics and pharmacodynamics vary considerably from those of morphine. Methadone has high oral bioavailability, three times that of morphine. Methadone is metabolized extensively by the cytochrome P450 system. Unlike modified or time-released opioid formulations, methadone has a rapid and extensive initial distribution phase, which occurs within 2 to 3 hours, and a prolonged elimination phase, which may last from 15 to 60 hours. Methadone can accumulate to high levels with repeated dosing. Rates of elimination from the body vary widely. The broad interindividual variability in methadone metabolism also confers special risks when patients are undergoing dose conversion from other opioids to methadone.[41-43]

There is emerging concern that patients prescribed methadone by inexperienced practitioners may be at increased risk of death from inadvertent drug accumulation and its resultant respiratory depression.[44] As a result of this evidence, in November 2006 the United States Food and Drug Administration issued a specific warning to prescribers regarding methadone.[45]

There also has been increasing attention to the potential cardiac toxicity associated with methadone. Daily doses of more than 100 mg may be associated with cardiac arrhythmias, including the potentially fatal torsades de pointes. Caution in prescribing methadone is advised in the opioid-naïve patient (a patient who has not taken opioids). Equianalgesic conversion ratios should be used conservatively when converting opioid prescriptions, especially in conversions from other opioids to methadone. Clinicians prescribing methadone for the first time are strongly encouraged to consult with a qualified pain specialist regarding doses and titration schedules.[46-49]

The Role of the Orthopaedic Surgeon in Palliative and End-of-Life Care

The World Health Organization defines palliative care as "an approach to care that improves quality of life of patients facing life-threatening illness and their families, through the prevention and relief of suffering by means of early identification and impeccable assessment and treatment of pain and other problems, physical, psychosocial, and spiritual."[50] Although palliative care specialists have become more widely available for consultation, the care of patients at the end of life is central to the practice of medicine and surgery.

There are three elements which define palliative care: (1) medical symptom management, (2) psychosocial and spiritual support of the patient and family, and (3) advanced care planning.[51] An integrated palliative care model implies treatment of patients starting at the time of diagnosis and continuing throughout the course of the illness—from treatment to cure, in disease relapse, or through disease progression to death.

Regardless of the prognosis, soon after receiving a diagnosis of a life-limiting condition, most patients will receive disease-modifying therapy, medical supportive care, and palliative care aimed at relief of symptoms (the integrated model). However, as the disease progresses to death, the goals of care for the terminally ill patient shift away from cure-oriented medical treatment to providing comfort and dignity at the end of life. Specifically, goals shift to relief of pain and other distressing symptoms, maintenance of function, support of family and personal relationships, avoidance of impoverishment, and attentiveness to meaningful activities and spiritual issues.

Orthopaedic surgeons play varied clinical roles in the setting of life-limiting illness. They may act as the primary treating physician for patients with conditions that are curable by surgical intervention (for example, certain sarcomas). They may provide intensive care of critically ill surgical patients, some of whom have a poor prognosis. The orthopaedic surgeon may also act as a partner in the management of patients with various life-limiting illnesses such as cancer. They may be called on to evaluate the use of possible palliative surgical care in patients with advanced illness. For example, procedures such as hip joint replacement may significantly improve functional status and overall quality of life even in patients with incurable widely metastatic bone disease. The fundamental principles of palliative care should be understood by the orthopaedic surgeon and applied in the settings in which they practice, regardless of if they are acting in a primary or collaborative role.

During the past decade, numerous policy statements and guidelines have been developed for palliative and end-of-life care in the United States. It has been noted that historically there is little discussion of palliative and end-of-life care in surgical textbooks, despite the important contributions surgeons can make.[52]

Multispecialty, interdisciplinary care of seriously ill and dying patients is now standard practice. This re-

Table 6

Palliative Orthopaedic Surgical Interventions

General Goals

Reconstruction
Restoration of function
Symptom control
Disease control
    Tumor resection
Control of hemorrhage, discharge, odor
Wound management

Specific Procedures

Bone
    Fracture stabilization
Spine
    Laminectomy
    Decompression of spinal cord or cauda equina
    Stabilization
    Vertebroplasty
    Kyphoplasty

quires teamwork in both the inpatient and outpatient settings. Orthopaedic surgeons will relate to other physicians, nurses, mental health professionals, spiritual advisors and clinical support staff of various disciplines. Extensive discussions with patients, families, and other health care professionals in this setting require time and patience.[53,54] Surgeons should have palliative care competencies in five areas: patient care, medical knowledge, communication, professionalism, and systems-based practice.[55]

It is important for the orthopaedic surgeon to characterize planned surgeries as either curative or palliative. When terminally ill patients present with advanced disease that requires palliative surgery, the patient must be assessed with the intent of resolving symptoms; controlling pain, the morbidity of disease, and therapy regimens; and improving the patient's quality of life. After assessing the patient, the orthopaedic surgeon will recommend the intervention that will best maximize symptom relief and minimize complications. When a procedure is selected and performed with palliative intent, treatment goals must be clearly defined and communicated to the patient and family. Because treatment choices can greatly affect a patient's final days, effective palliation of terminally ill patients demands the highest level of surgical judgment.[56] Preoperative assessment and discussions are important because the goals of the patient, family, and orthopaedic surgeon should be complementary[57,58] (**Table 6**).

Ethical Considerations

Ethical considerations may arise in relation to declining to intervene and withdrawing specific medical interventions. Advance care planning is essential for the prevention of unwanted interventions and, more importantly, for supporting families when they act as surrogate decision makers in choosing to accept, decline, or stop specific interventions.

Health care professionals have an obligation to provide treatments that carry a favorable balance of benefits to burdens or risks. Treatments with a favorable balance should be offered with the appropriate recommendation. In many circumstances the balance of benefits to burdens or risks are not clearly overwhelming and are regarded as optional; these decisions may be more difficult for patients and families. Treatments that have only a minimal chance of benefit but which have overwhelming burdens or risks for the patient should not be offered.

The moral dilemmas that arise in palliative care and end-of-life care regarding treatments intended primarily to prolong or sustain life relate to the balance between the benefits and the burdens of treatment. Medical professions do not have a duty to extend life at all costs. In certain circumstances, such as when treatment is considered futile, when burdens and risks greatly outweigh the benefits of treatment, when treatment will not further the total good of the patient, and when treatments are not available because of resource constraints, it is ethical for providers not to offer life-prolonging treatment. This last aspect may pose the most difficult dilemma for physicians. A more extensive discussion of these ethical issues is beyond the scope of this chapter.

Health care professionals practicing palliative and end-of-life care are encouraged to read, reflect, and discuss difficult issues as they arise. Orthopaedic surgeons are strongly encouraged to be familiar with principles of medical ethics and to participate in family conferences, interdisciplinary treatment planning meetings, and ethics committees.

Summary

With continued basic and clinical research, improvements are anticipated in diagnostic imaging, which will better define clinical pain states; new pharmacologic and nonpharmacologic treatments of pain; and in the development of standardized measures of clinical outcomes in pain management. To best serve their patients in all clinical settings, orthopaedic surgeons should have a basic understanding of pain physiology and familiarity with state-of-the-art pain management techniques.

Annotated References

1. *The NIH Guide: New Directions in Pain Research I.* Washington, DC: Government Printing Office, 1998.

2. American Pain Society: Pain Facts. 2005. http://www.ampainsoc.org

3. Hebl JR, Dilger JA, Byer DE, et al: A pre-emptive multimodal pathway featuring peripheral nerve block improves perioperative outcomes after major orthopedic surgery. *Reg Anesth Pain Med* 2008;33(6):510-517.

The authors report that a comprehensive, preemptive, multimodal analgesic regimen improved perioperative outcomes and resulted in fewer adverse events, shorter hospitalization times, and a significant reduction in urinary retention and ileus formation in patients treated with total hip or total knee arthroplasty. Level of evidence: III.

4. Reuben SS, Buvanendran A: Preventing the development of chronic pain after orthopaedic surgery with preventive multimodal analgesic techniques. *J Bone Joint Surg Am* 2007;89(6):1343-1358.

Effective multimodal analgesic techniques are reviewed in this article.

5. Grape S, Tramer MR: Do we need preemptive analgesia for the treatment of postoperative pain? *Best Pract Res Clin Anaesthesiol* 2007;21:51-63.

The authors suggest that routine multimodal analgesic treatment is better supported than preemptive approaches at this time.

6. Duellman TJ, Gaffigan C, Milbrandt JC, Allan DG: Multi-modal, pre-emptive analgesia decreases the length of hospital stay following total joint arthroplasty. *Orthopedics* 2009;32(3):167.

The authors of this retrospective study reported that, compared to standard patient-controlled analgesia, multimodal preemptive analgesia resulted in better outcomes for patients, including a decrease in the likelihood of discharge to a skilled nursing facility. Level of evidence: III.

7. Berger RA, Sanders SA, Thill ES, Sporer SM, Della Valle C: Newer anesthesia and rehabilitation protocols enable outpatient hip replacement in selected patients. *Clin Orthop Relat Res* 2009;467(6):1424-1430.

The authors report that newer anesthesia and outpatient rehabilitation protocols may result in better outcomes at a higher cost. Level of evidence: IV.

8. Parvizi J, Porat M, Gandhi K, Viscusi ER, Rothman RH: Postoperative pain management techniques in hip and knee arthroplasty. *Instr Course Lect* 2009;58:769-779.

The authors present a review of current multimodal and preemptive analgesia techniques.

9. Morrison RS, Flanagan S, Fischberg D, Cintron A, Siu AL: A novel interdisciplinary analgesic program reduces pain and improves function in older adults after orthopedic surgery. *J Am Geriatr Soc* 2009;57(1):1-10.

The authors report the results of a study to evaluate the effect of a multicomponent intervention on pain and function after orthopaedic (hip and knee) surgery in a large metropolitan hospital. Level of evidence: I.

10. Hudcova J, McNicol E, Quah C, Lau J, Carr DB: Patient controlled opioid analgesia versus conventional opioid analgesia for postoperative pain. *Cochrane Database Syst Rev* 2006;4:CD003348.

11. Parker RD, Streem K, Schmitz L, Martineau PA; Marguerite Group: Efficacy of continuous intra-articular bupivacaine infusion for postoperative analgesia after anterior cruciate ligament reconstruction: A double-blinded, placebo-controlled, prospective, and randomized study. *Am J Sports Med* 2007;35(4):531-536.

The authors report the results of this study to evaluate outcomes of continuous intra-articular bupivacaine infusion for postoperative analgesia after anterior cruciate ligament reconstruction. This technique produced no distinct advantage in terms of reported pain and analgesic consumption in the postoperative period. Level of evidence: I.

12. Choi PT, Bhandari M, Scott J, Douketis J: Epidural analgesia for pain relief following hip or knee replacement. *Cochrane Database Syst Rev* 2003;3:CD003071.

13. Montane E, Vallano A, Vallano A, Aguilera C, Vidal X, Laporte JR: Analgesics for pain after traumatic or orthopaedic surgery: What is the evidence. A systematic review. *Eur J Clin Pharmacol* 2006;62(11):971-988.

14. Besse JL, Gadeyne S, Galand-Desmé S, Lerat JL, Moyen B: Effect of vitamin C on prevention of complex regional pain syndrome type I in foot and ankle surgery. *Foot Ankle Surg* 2009;15(4):179-182.

This quasi-experimental study demonstrates the effect of vitamin C in preventing complex regional pain syndrome type I after foot and ankle surgery. Level of evidence: II.

15. Nilsson S, Finnström B, Kokinsky E: The FLACC behavioral scale for procedural pain assessment in children aged 5-16 years. *Paediatr Anaesth* 2008;18(8):767-774.

The FLACC tool is appropriate for use in pediatric settings.

16. Cade CH: Clinical tools for the assessment of pain in sedated critically ill adults. *Nurs Crit Care* 2008;13(6):288-297.

The Behavioral Pain Scale has been validated for use in pediatric and adult populations.

17. Morley-Foster P: Prevalence of neuropathic pain and need for treatment. *Pain Res Manag* 2006;11(suppl A):5A-10A.

18. DworkinRH, Backonja M, Rowbotham MC, et al: Advances in neuropathic pain: Diagnosis, mechanisms, and treatment recommendations. *Arch Neurol* 2003;60(11):1524-1534.

19. *Model Policy for the Use of Controlled Substances for the Treatment of Pain.* Dallas, TX, Federation of State Medical Boards of the United States, Inc., 2004.

20. Weinstein SM: Non-malignant pain, in Walsh D, Caraceni AT, Fainsinger R, eds: *Palliative Medicine.* Miamisburg, OH, Elsevier, 2008.

A review of the assessment and interdisciplinary management of chronic noncancerous pain is presented.

21. Nicolaidis S: Neurosurgical treatments of intractable pain. *Metabolism* 2010;59(suppl 1):S27-S31.

    A thorough review of state-of-the art neurosurgical pain interventions is presented.

22. Nation Center for Complementary and Alternative Medicine Web site. http://Nccam.nih.gov. Accessed January 22, 2010.

    This site provides information on the safety and effectiveness of alternative therapies not considered part of conventional allopathic medicine.

23. *Principles of Analgesic Use in the Treatment of Acute Pain and Cancer Pain*, ed 6. Skokie, IL, American Pain Society, 2008.

    This text is an updated guide to medication management of pain.

24. *Guidelines for the Management of Pain in Osteoarthritis, Rheumatoid Arthritis, and Juvenile Chronic Arthritis*, ed 2. Skokie, IL, American Pain Society, 2002.

25. *Guidelines for the Management of Acute and Chronic Pain in Sickle Cell Disease*. Skokie, IL, American Pain Society, 1999.

26. *Guidelines for the Management of Fibromyalgia Syndrome Pain in Adults and Children*. Skokie, IL, American Pain Society, 2005.

27. *Pain Control in the Primary Care Setting*. Skokie, IL, American Pain Society, 2006.

28. Greco C, Berde C: Pain management for the hospitalized pediatric patient. *Pediatr Clin North Am* 2005;52(4):995-1027.

29. Walker SM: Pain in children: Recent advances and ongoing challenges. *Br J Anaesth* 2008;101(1):101-110.

    The author reviews current practice challenges and research initiatives in pediatric pain management.

30. American Academy of Pediatrics, Committee on Psychosocial Aspects of Child and Family Health; Task Force on Pain in Infants, Children, and Adolescents: The assessment and management of acute pain in infants, children, and adolescents. *Pediatrics* 2001;108(3):793-797.

31. Dowden S, McCarthy M, Chalkiadis G: Achieving organizational change in pediatric pain management. *Pain Res Manag* 2008;13(4):321-326.

    Deficiencies in pediatric pain management and barriers to achieving effective pain management are discussed. Institutional improvement strategies are presented.

32. Dadure C, Bringuier S, Raux O, et al: Continuous peripheral nerve blocks for postoperative analgesia in children: Feasibility and side effects in a cohort study of 339 catheters. *Can J Anaesth* 2009;56(11):843-850.

    A study to evaluate the indications, efficacy, and adverse events of the use of continuous peripheral nerve blocks in a large pediatric cohort demonstrated feasibility and safety. Level IV.

33. Khoury CE, Dagher C, Ghanem I, Naccache N, Jawish D, Yazbeck P: Combined regional and general anesthesia for ambulatory peripheral orthopedic surgery in children. *J Pediatr Orthop B* 2009;18(1):37-45.

    The authors report on pain control and parental satisfaction in this prospective study of combined regional anesthesia and general anesthesia to support ambulatory surgery in children. Combined techniques resulted in improved patient pain control and better parental satisfaction. Level of evidence: IV.

34. Tobias JD: A review of intrathecal and epidural analgesia after spinal surgery in children. *Anesth Analg* 2004;98(4):956-965.

35. Kozlowska K, Rose D, Khan R, Kram S, Lane L, Collins J: A conceptual model and practice framework for managing chronic pain in children and adolescents. *Harv Rev Psychiatry* 2008;16(2):136-150.

    The integrated, family-based assessment and treatment approach to pain is aimed at restoration of normal functioning and improved symptom control. Level of evidence: IV.

36. Guite JW, Logan DE, McCue R, Sherry DD, Rose JB: Parental beliefs and worries regarding adolescent chronic pain. *Clin J Pain* 2009;25(3):223-232.

    This retrospective review indicates that parental beliefs about pain may have implications for treatment in adolescents. Level of evidence: III.

37. American Geriatrics Society Panel on Pharmacological Management of Persistent Pain in Older Persons: Pharmacological management of persistent pain in older persons. *J Am Geriatr Soc* 2009;57(8):1331-1346.

    An updated review of guidelines for best practices in the medical management of persistent pain in elderly patients is presented.

38. Pioli G, Giusti A, Barone A: Orthogeriatric care for the elderly with hip fractures: Where are we? *Aging Clin Exp Res* 2008;20(2):113-122.

    The coordinated, multidisciplinary care for elderly patients with hip fractures provided by an orthogeriatric center is described.

39. Arinzon Z, Gepstein R, Shabat S, Berner Y: Pain perception during the rehabilitation phase following traumatic hip fracture in the elderly is an important prognostic factor and treatment tool. *Disabil Rehabil* 2007;29(8):651-658.

    Pain intensity is a prognostic factor that predicts outcomes of rehabilitation following hip fractures in elderly patients. Level of evidence: II.

40. Trescot AM, Helm S, Hansen H, et al: Opioids in the management of chronic non-cancer pain: An update of American Society of the Interventional Pain Physicians' (ASIPP) Guidelines. *Pain Physician* 2008;11(2, suppl) S5-S62.

2: Systemic Disorders

The authors present a review of the current guidelines for opioid therapy of noncancerous pain.

41. Corkery JM, Schifano F, Ghodse AH, Oyefeso A: The effects of methadone and its role in fatalities. *Hum Psychopharmacol* 2004;19(8):565-576.

42. Karch SB, Stephens BG: Toxicology and pathology of deaths related to methadone: Retrospective review. *West J Med* 2000;172(1):11-14.

43. Wolff K: Characterization of methadone overdose: Clinical considerations and the scientific evidence. *Ther Drug Monit* 2002;24(4):457-470.

44. Centers for Disease Control and Prevention (CDC): Increase in poisoning deaths caused by non-illicit drugs – Utah, 1991-2003. *MMWR Morb Mortal Wkly Rep* 2005;54(2):33-36.

45. US Food and Drug Administration Web site. Public Health Advisory: Methadone Use for Pain Control May Result in Death and Life-Threatening Changes in Breathing and Heart Beat. http://www.fda.gov/Drugs/DrugSafety/PublicHealthAdvisories/ucm124346.htm. Accessed January 25, 2010.

46. Martell BA, Arnsten JH, Krantz MJ, Gourevitch MN: Impact of methadone treatment on cardiac repolarization and conduction in opioid users. *Am J Cardiol* 2005;95(7):915-918.

47. Pearson EC, Woosley RL: QT prolongation and torsades de pointes among methadone users: Reports to the FDA spontaneous reporting system. *Pharmacoepidemiol Drug Saf* 2005;14(11):747-753.

48. Peles E, Bodner G, Kreek MJ, Rados V, Adelson M: Corrected-QT intervals as related to methadone dose and serum level in methadone maintenance treatment (MMT) patients: A cross-sectional study. *Addiction* 2007;102(2):289-300.

A clinical review of methadone dose-related cardiac conduction changes is presented, showing that in some patients dangerous prolongation of QT interval can be dose related.

49. Fanoe S, Hvidt C, Hvidt C, Ege P, Jensen GB. Syncope and QT prolongation among patients treated with methadone for heroin dependence in the city of Copenhagen. *Heart* 2007;93(9):1051-1055.

The authors present the findings of a clinical review of methadone-related cardiac conduction changes and adverse effects.

50. WHO Expert Committee: *Cancer Pain Relief and Palliative Care*. Geneva, Switzerland, World Health Organization, 1998.

51. Weinstein SM: Integrating palliative care in oncology. *Cancer Control* 2001;8(1):32-35.

52. Easson AM, Crosby JA, Librach SL: Discussion of death and dying in surgical textbooks. *Am J Surg* 2001;182(1):34-39.

53. Lee KF, Purcell GP, Hinshaw DB, Krouse RS, Baluss M: Clinical palliative care for surgeons: Part 1. *J Am Coll Surg* 2004;198(2):303-319.

54. Lee KF, Johnson DL, Purcell GP, Hinshaw DB, Krouse RS, Baluss M: Clinical palliative care for surgeons: Part 2. *J Am Coll Surg* 2004;198(3):477-491.

55. Surgeons Palliative Care Workshop: Robert Wood Johnson Foundation Office of Promoting Excellence in End-of-Life Care: Executive summary of the report from the field. *J Am Coll Surg* 2003;196(5):807-815.

56. Cullinane CA, Borneman T, Smith DD, Chu DZ, Ferrell BR, Wagman LD: The surgical treatment of cancer: A comparison of resource utilization following procedures performed with a curative and palliative intent. *Cancer* 2003;98(10):2266-2273.

57. Miner TJ, Jaques DP, Shriver CD: A prospective evaluation of patients undergoing surgery for the palliation of an advanced malignancy. *Ann Surg Oncol* 2002;9(7):696-703.

58. Frasscia FJ, Frasscia DA, Jacofsky DJ, Sim FH: Palliative orthopaedic surgery, in Berger AM, Portenoy RK, Weissman DE, eds: *Principles and Practice of Palliative Care and Supportive Oncology*, ed 2. Philadelphia, PA, Lippincott Williams and Wilkins, 2002, pp 722-730.

Section 3

Upper Extremity

SECTION EDITOR:

PEDRO BEREDJIKLIAN, MD

Chapter 22

Shoulder Trauma: Bone

Joseph A. Abboud, MD   N. Douglas Boardman III, MD

Clavicle Fractures

The clavicle, one of the <u>most commonly fractured bones</u>, accounts for 2.6% to 4% of all adult fractures and approximately 35% of injuries to the shoulder girdle.[1] Clavicle fractures can involve the midshaft (69% to 83%), lateral end (28%), and/or medial end (2% to 3%) and are typically caused by either a <u>fall on an outstretched arm</u> or a <u>direct blow</u>. Shaft fractures occur most commonly in young adults, whereas lateral and medial fractures are more common in elderly patients.[2]

Presentation

In displaced <u>midshaft</u> fractures, the <u>sternocleidomastoid</u> and <u>trapezius</u> muscles pull the medial fragment superiorly and posteriorly, respectively, whereas the <u>weight of the arm</u> and <u>pectoralis major</u> pull the lateral fragment inferomedially, producing ptosis of the involved shoulder. With severely angulated or comminuted fractures, <u>fragments may buttonhole subcutaneously through the platysma muscle</u> (**Figure 1**). Because the clavicle is in close proximity to the <u>brachial plexus</u> and <u>subclavian vessels</u>, associated neurovascular injury may occur (3%).[2]

Radiographic Evaluation

A clavicle fracture is typically initially visualized on AP radiographs of the shoulder or the chest. A <u>true AP view of the clavicle</u> and a <u>30° cephalic tilt</u> view should be obtained to allow biplanar assessment of the bony deformity. <u>CT</u> with three-dimensional reconstructions may be helpful in special situations, such as the evaluation of medial clavicular physeal fractures or sternoclavicular fracture-dislocations.

[handwritten: cephalic tilt: sup-inf. displacement]
[handwritten: caudal tilt: A/P displacement]

Dr. Abboud or an immediate family member serves as a board member, owner, officer, or committee member of the American Academy of Orthopaedic Surgeons Multimedia subcommittee; is a member of a speakers' bureau or has made paid presentations on behalf of DePuy, and serves as a paid consultant to or is an employee of DePuy. Dr. Boardman or an immediate family member is a member of a speakers' bureau or has made paid presentations on behalf of GlaxoSmithKline, DePuy, and Merck and serves as a paid consultant to or is an employee of DePuy.

Classification

A classification system for clavicle fractures based solely on the anatomic location of the fracture (lateral, medial, or midshaft) has been proposed, and lateral end fractures have been classified as nondisplaced (type I) or displaced (type II). Displaced lateral fractures can be further subclassified according to the integrity of the conoid and trapezoid ligaments (**Figure 2**). The Edinburgh classification has been used to subclassify shaft fractures according to displacement and degree of comminution.[1] This classification scheme has acceptable levels of interobserver and intraobserver variation. Medial and lateral end fractures are subclassified with the Edinburgh system according to their displacement and articular involvement.

Midshaft Fractures

Fractures of the middle third of the clavicle usually proceed to bony union uneventfully without the need for surgery. Studies have reported that significant risk factors for nonunion include age, female sex, fracture displacement, and comminution; shortening of the fracture (> 20 mm) is also a risk factor for the development of nonunion.[3]

Previous studies have reported a nonunion rate of only 0.13% to 0.8%. Shortcomings of these studies are inclusion of the pediatric population and absence of

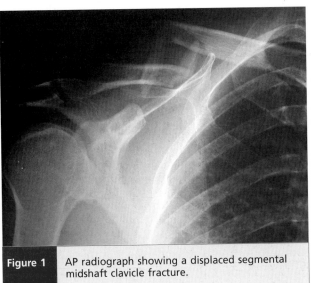

Figure 1 AP radiograph showing a displaced segmental midshaft clavicle fracture.

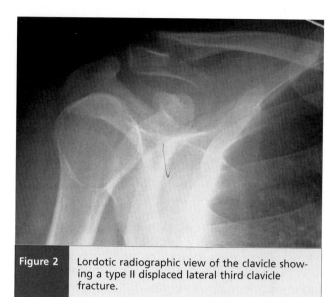

Figure 2 Lordotic radiographic view of the clavicle showing a type II displaced lateral third clavicle fracture.

modern methods for assessing functional outcomes. It is generally accepted that midshaft clavicle fractures will heal in most adults. The standard of care is initial immobilization in either a sling or figure-of-8 bandage, with immobilization discontinued when the level of pain allows.

Until recently, there was little evidence available to suggest that early surgical treatment of displaced clavicle fractures conferred a functional benefit when compared with the results of initial nonsurgical treatment. A recent multicenter trial comparing nonsurgical treatment with primary plate fixation for displaced fractures in 132 patients reported better functional outcomes, lower rates of malunion and nonunion, and a shorter time to union in the latter group.[4] However, the group treated with primary plate fixation had a complication rate of 34% and a reoperation rate of 18%, although most reoperations were for hardware removal. In a retrospective review of 30 patients who had been treated nonsurgically for displaced midshaft clavicle fractures, a higher prevalence of patient dissatisfaction was reported when shortening was greater than 2 cm, which corroborates previous reports.[5]

Plate Fixation

Plate fixation provides immediate rigid stabilization and pain relief and facilitates early mobilization. Most commonly, the plate is implanted on the superior aspect of the clavicle; biomechanical studies have shown this to be advantageous, especially in the presence of inferior cortical comminution.[6] Superior plating techniques have greater load to failure and bending failure stiffness than anterior inferior plating.[7] Despite the biomechanical advantages, the superior approach is associated with a greater risk of injury to the underlying neurovascular structures during fracture manipulation and drilling. In addition, plate prominence with the superior approach may require hardware removal in symptomatic patients. Currently, the implants most commonly used

are either dynamic compression or locking plates. Site-specific precontoured locking plates have become increasingly popular and may be less prominent after healing, leading to lower rates of hardware removal after union.[6]

If nonsurgical treatment of the fracture leads to symptomatic malunion or nonunion, surgical management, including plate fixation with autologous bone grafting, can be considered. In 47 patients treated with superior plating for clavicular nonunions, 93% of the fracture nonunions united after one surgery.[8] The authors reported that treating patients with a superiorly applied plate without a distant autogenous bone graft was efficacious in obtaining fracture union.

Intramedullary Nailing

Intramedullary nailing is another option in the surgical treatment of clavicle fractures. Intramedullary repair of midshaft clavicle fractures with a titanium elastic nail can be safe and minimally invasive;[9] however, implant-related complications can include medial perforations, lateral penetrations, nail breakage, and hardware irritations.[10] More studies are needed to fully define the role of intramedullary nail fixation in clavicular fractures.

Distal Third Fractures

Lateral third clavicle fractures can be classified based on the location relative to the coracoclavicular ligaments. Type I fractures are interligamentous and only minimally displaced, as both the proximal and distal fragments continue to be stabilized by the coracoclavicular ligaments. For these injuries, nonsurgical management is the treatment of choice, and the protocol is similar to that of shaft fractures. Type II fractures occur medial to the coracoclavicular ligaments. Deforming forces, such as the weight of the arm and muscular attachments, lead to inferior and medial displacement of the distal fragment via its ligamentous attachments. These fracture patterns are associated with delayed union and nonunion. Type III fractures extend into the articular surface of the acromioclavicular joint with no ligamentous injury and are generally stable.

Although several retrospective studies have reported high rates of nonunion after nonsurgical treatment of displaced lateral end fractures, a recent study showed a low incidence of nonunion after nonsurgical treatment.[3] In addition, high complication rates have been reported with surgical fixation.[11] Because most of these injuries occur in middle-aged and elderly patients, nonunion is often tolerated, with few patients requiring delayed surgical intervention.[3,11] In the small number of patients in whom substantial arthritis develops, resection of the lateral segment may result in a functional shoulder.[2]

Many primary surgical techniques have been described for the treatment of type II fractures and many surgical techniques used to treat displaced lateral end fractures have been adapted from those used to treat acromioclavicular separations. Treatment options include coracoclavicular screws, hook-plate fixation, locking plates, Kirschner wire fixation, and suture techniques.

Intra-articular fractures (type III) carry an increased risk of late acromioclavicular osteoarthritis, which may require further treatment. Type III fractures are generally adequately managed nonsurgically, although open reduction and internal fixation (ORIF) may be indicated if a large fragment resulting in significant articular step-off is present. Delayed distal clavicle resection is the procedure of choice if symptomatic degenerative disease occurs.[2]

Medial Third Clavicle Fractures

Medial third clavicle fractures are rare, and most are extra-articular and minimally displaced.[1] Often, these fractures are physeal fracture-dislocations, usually in a posterior direction. Stability depends on the integrity of the costoclavicular ligaments. If the ligaments are ruptured, the lateral fragment displaces anteriorly and may overlap the medial fragment. These fractures are usually managed nonsurgically, unless fracture displacement produces mediastinal compromise. In such circumstances, an emergent attempt at closed reduction should be made, with open reduction performed next if that is unsuccessful. If surgical stabilization of this fracture is required, a thoracic surgeon should be available. A variety of internal fixation techniques, including use of the modified Balser plate and use of polyester fiber suture or other strong braided interosseous sutures, have been described.[12] However, supporting evidence is limited for each technique, and there is a lack of consensus regarding the optimal treatment of fractures that require surgical treatment.

General Complications of Clavicular Fracture Fixation

The main intraoperative complication in clavicular fracture fixation is injury to the subclavian artery or vein at the time of fracture mobilization or from drill penetration. As with any ORIF, postoperative wound complications, scar dysesthesia, infection, fixation failure, and nonunion can occur and may require revision surgery.

Proximal Humerus Fractures

Fractures of the proximal humerus are common injuries, representing 4% to 6% of all fractures. There is a 2:1 female to male distribution, and increasing age has been shown to correlate with an increasing fracture risk in women, suggesting an association with osteoporosis. Fractures of the proximal humerus represent the third most common fracture in elderly patients, with hip fractures and distal radius fractures being more common. Approximately 85% of proximal humerus fractures are minimally displaced; however, there is a fairly significant amount of controversy over the diagnosis and treatment of the remaining 15% of patients (**Figure 3**). Although proximal humerus fractures frequently re-

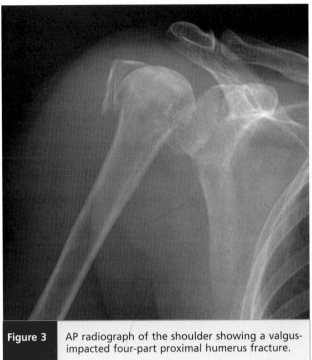

Figure 3 AP radiograph of the shoulder showing a valgus-impacted four-part proximal humerus fracture.

sult from falls and involve osteoporotic bone, these fractures can occur secondary to high-energy mechanisms in younger patients, who often sustain more severe trauma with concomitant soft-tissue and neurovascular injuries.

Presentation

In a patient with a proximal humerus fracture, the shoulder is often swollen and tender to palpation. There is abundant ecchymosis that progresses down the arm and into the forearm and chest. Because most patients are elderly, the etiology of the fall should be discerned and associated injuries evaluated. The presence of associated peripheral nerve injury has typically been underappreciated. It has been shown that 67% of all patients with proximal humerus fractures have acute neurologic injury most commonly affecting the axillary nerve and/or the suprascapular nerve.[13]

Vascularity

Blood supply to the proximal humerus is important in determining survival of the humeral head. The anterior humeral circumflex artery contributes the major blood supply to the humeral head through the ascending anterolateral branch, which enters the proximal aspect of the bicipital groove. Other vascular contributors include vessels entering the tuberosities through the rotator cuff insertions and direct branches of the circumflex vessels.

An emphasis on the importance of the vascularity of the proximal humerus has led surgeons to try to ascertain a deeper understanding of fracture configuration because it relates to perfusion of the articular segment. Recently, patients treated with hemiarthroplasty received tetracycline labeling to measure humeral head viability after three- or four-part proximal humerus fractures. It was found that the vascular supply was preserved in both three- and four-part fractures of the proximal humerus and that patient age was inversely proportional to the amount of vascularity in the area.[14]

In a recent report, intraoperative assessment of humeral head perfusion was performed by means of bore hole drillings, laser Doppler flowmetry, or both.[15] Osteonecrosis did not develop in 8 of 10 humeral heads that were initially ischemic at the time of surgery; this finding led the authors to believe that revascularization can occur and that the rate of osteonecrosis may not be as high as traditionally believed. As a result of these findings, osteosynthesis with preservation of the humeral head may be considered when adequate reduction and stable fixation, which are optimal conditions for revascularization, can be obtained. A recent study analyzed a proximal humerus fracture classification scheme and outlined factors that predicted the likelihood of humeral head ischemia.[16] Such factors included disruption of the medial periosteal hinge, medial metadiaphyseal extension less than 8 mm, increasing fracture complexity, and displacement greater than 10 mm or angulation greater than 45°.

Radiographic Evaluation and Classification

The trauma series of radiographs, consisting of AP, scapular Y, and axillary views, is the standard for evaluating proximal humerus fractures. CT with three-dimensional reconstruction is useful for evaluating the size and displacement of fracture fragments. The classification of proximal humerus fractures is commonly based on the four-part system of Neer. This scheme is based on the identification of the four anatomic fragments (humeral head, greater tuberosity, lesser tuberosity, and humeral shaft) and the determination of displacement and angulation between these parts greater than 1 cm or 45°, respectively. Another classification scheme assesses predictors of ischemia, including medial hinge disruption greater than 2 mm and metaphyseal head extension less than 8 mm.[17] A third scheme, the AO/Orthopaedic Trauma Association (OTA) system, classifies fractures into types A, B, and C. Type A is a two-part extracapsular fracture with an intact vascular supply, type B is a three-part partially intracapsular fracture with possible vascular compromise, and type C is a four-part intracapsular fracture with a likelihood of vascular compromise.[16]

A recent study evaluated the impact of stereovisualization of three-dimensional volume-rendering CT datasets on the interobserver and intraobserver reliability of the AO/OTA and Neer classification systems in the assessment of proximal humerus fractures.[18] Both classification systems showed moderate interobserver reliability with plain radiographs and two-dimensional CT. Three-dimensional volume-rendered CT improved interobserver reliability to good for both classification systems, and the intraobserver reliability for the three-dimensional scans improved to good for the AO/OTA

classification and to excellent for the Neer classification.

Nonsurgical Treatment

The treatment of proximal humerus fractures is based on many factors, including patient age, bone quality, medical comorbidities, concurrent injuries, and fracture type. Nonsurgical treatment with early passive motion remains the treatment of choice for minimally displaced or nondisplaced fractures. Open treatment is reserved for displaced fractures that cannot be reduced with closed means. A recent study found that immediate physiotherapy after a minimally displaced proximal humerus fracture resulted in a faster recovery with maximum functional benefits being achieved at 1 year.[19] The authors of a recent study reported that nonsurgical treatment of proximal humerus fractures is safe and effective, specifically in AO/OTA fracture types A and B, but can also be extended to three-part fractures.[20] Of the fractures regarded suitable for conservative treatment, few required later surgical stabilization. When complex proximal humerus fractures are managed nonsurgically, there is usually some degree of malunion, and osteonecrosis leading to collapse of the humeral head may occur. As mentioned previously, this osteonecrosis appears to occur at lower rates than have been described previously.[21]

Surgical Treatment

When the humeral head is amenable to fixation, many methods are available. Fractures considered for ORIF include displaced greater tuberosity fractures with more than 5 mm of displacement, lesser tuberosity fractures with involvement of the articular surface, displaced or unstable surgical neck fractures, displaced anatomic fractures in young patients, and displaced reconstructible three- and four-part fractures.

Fractures amenable to closed reduction and percutaneous pinning include two-part fractures of the surgical neck, greater tuberosity, and lesser tuberosity; three-part surgical neck fractures with involvement of the greater or lesser tuberosity; and valgus-impacted four-part fractures. Closed reduction and percutaneous pinning is a demanding surgical technique (**Figure 4**). For this technique to be used successfully, several conditions are required: (1) a stable closed reduction; (2) good bone stock; (3) minimal comminution, particularly involving the tuberosity; (4) an intact medial calcar; and (5) a cooperative patient. It has been shown that the posteromedial hinge is a mechanical structure that provides support for percutaneous reduction and stabilization of a proximal humerus fracture by ligamentotaxis.[22] If acceptable alignment cannot be obtained, the technique should be abandoned in favor of more traditional open reduction.

Greater Tuberosity Fractures

Two-part fractures of the greater tuberosity commonly occur in the setting of a glenohumeral dislocation. After closed reduction of the glenohumeral dislocation, the tu-

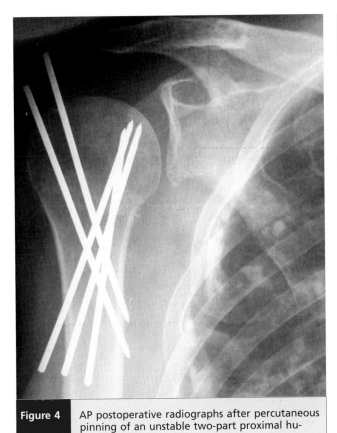

Figure 4 AP postoperative radiographs after percutaneous pinning of an unstable two-part proximal humerus fracture.

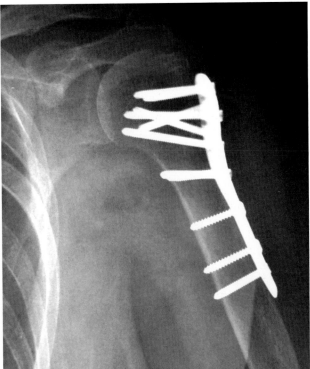

Figure 5 AP radiograph of a left shoulder showing precontoured plate fixation used in the treatment of a displaced three-part proximal humerus fracture. Note the inferior placement of the plate relative to the top of the greater tuberosity as well as the purposeful placement of the screws in the humeral head well short of the subchondral surface.

berosity should be assessed for displacement. If superior and posterior displacement greater than 5 mm to 10 mm persists, ORIF of the tuberosity fragment is considered. Untreated residual displacement greater than 5 mm may cause impingement of the superiorly displaced greater tuberosity against the acromion. Fixation of the tuberosity is often achieved with intraosseous sutures incorporating the cuff insertion. If the tuberosity is a single large piece, screw fixation can be used.

ORIF With Precontoured Locking Plates

Short-term outcomes of precontoured locking plates for fixation of displaced proximal humerus fractures have recently been described. In a study of 187 patients with acute proximal humerus fractures who were treated with ORIF with a locking proximal humeral plate, 62 complications occurred in 52 patients at 1-year follow-up.[23] Twenty-five complications (40%) were related to incorrect surgical technique and were present at the end of the surgical procedure. The most common complication, reported in 21 of 155 patients, was intraoperative screw perforation of the humeral head.

In a study using a proximal humerus internal locking system plate (Philos, Synthes, Oberdorf, Switzerland) in the treatment of displaced proximal humerus fractures in 157 patients (158 fractures), the complication rate was relatively high (35%), particularly because of primary and secondary screw perforation into the gleno-

humeral joint.[24] The authors reported that the surgical treatment of displaced proximal humerus fractures with use of a proximal humeral plate can lead to good functional outcomes provided that the correct surgical technique is used. Accurate length measurements and the selection of shorter screws were recommended to prevent primary screw perforation. Awareness of the need to obtain anatomic reduction of the tubercles and restoration of medial support should reduce the incidence of secondary screw penetrations even in osteoporotic bone (Figure 5).

New Techniques in Fixation

Several new techniques being introduced for fixation of proximal humerus fractures include the humeral block system, the block-bridge, and the use of helix wire.[25,26] Because there is a paucity of information regarding the outcomes of treatment with these modalities, they should be considered with care.

Hemiarthroplasty

Hemiarthroplasty is an option for fractures involving young or middle-aged patients with a nonreconstructible articular surface, severe head splits, or extruded anatomic neck fractures, and elderly patients

3: Upper Extremity

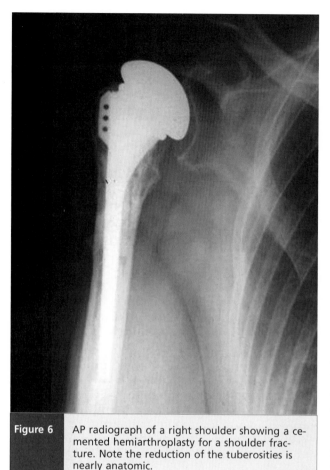

Figure 6 AP radiograph of a right shoulder showing a cemented hemiarthroplasty for a shoulder fracture. Note the reduction of the tuberosities is nearly anatomic.

with markedly comminuted severely osteoporotic three- and four-part fractures as well as three- and four-part fracture-dislocations. Primary hemiarthroplasty for fracture of the proximal humerus can result in good patient satisfaction and pain relief. Intraoperative restoration of the anatomic humeral height, version, and tuberosity reconstruction have been identified as important factors in the improvement of outcomes after arthroplasty for shoulder fractures (**Figure 6**). Humeral length reconstruction and centering of the prosthetic head in hemiarthroplasty for proximal humerus fractures using the pectoralis major as a reference point were evaluated in a 2008 study.[27] In 21 of 30 patients, the humeral length reconstruction was performed using the pectoralis major tendon as a reference; in 9 patients this reference was not used. Patients appeared to have improved outcomes when the pectoralis major tendon was used as a reference point.

In a recent study, 82 patients treated with primary hemiarthroplasty for a severely displaced proximal humerus fracture were evaluated at an average follow-up of 4.4 years.[28] Primary hemiarthroplasty generally prevented shoulder pain, but most patients had only moderate function and poor strength. The reduced function appeared to be related to lack of rotator cuff integrity. In a 2008 review of 50 patients treated with hemiar-

throplasty for proximal humerus fractures with a minimum 5-year follow-up, satisfactory results were reported in 27 patients and unsatisfactory results in 30 patients.[29] The study data suggest that patients treated with arthroplasty for an acute fracture of the proximal humerus may achieve satisfactory long-term pain relief. However, the result for overall shoulder motion is less predictable. Based on these results, it has been suggested that the current indications, surgical technique, and postoperative treatment of these fractures be reevaluated.

Reverse Arthroplasty
With the increasing use of reverse shoulder arthroplasty, indications for this procedure have been extended to the treatment of comminuted fractures in elderly patients. Forty-three consecutive patients with a mean age of 78 years who sustained three- and four-part proximal humerus fractures were evaluated after reverse shoulder arthroplasty.[30] This group had a postoperative mean active forward elevation of 97° and mean active external rotation of 30°. The study authors concluded that compared with conventional hemiarthroplasty, satisfactory mobility was obtained despite frequent migration of the tuberosities at short-term follow-up.

Twenty-nine patients were treated with reverse arthroplasty after failure of primary hemiarthroplasty for fracture treatment.[31] In patients treated with revision from a hemiarthroplasty for fracture to a reverse shoulder prosthesis, the average forward flexion improved from 38° to 73° and abduction improved from 34° to 70°. In these instances, the reverse shoulder prosthesis offered a salvage-type solution to the complication of failed hemiarthroplasty because of glenoid arthrosis and rotator cuff deficiency following tuberosity failure. The study authors caution that long-term results are required before reverse shoulder arthroplasty can be recommended as a routine procedure in treating complex fractures of the proximal humerus in elderly patients.

Proximal Humeral Nonunion and Malunion
Although rare, proximal humeral nonunion tends to involve the surgical neck or the greater tuberosity. Malunion tends to occur as a result of failure of the primary surgical procedure or as a sequelae of nonsurgical treatment. Shoulder arthroplasty in the setting of a malunited proximal humerus fracture has been performed with caution because of the higher rate of complications and unpredictable functional results.[32] Patients with surgical neck nonunions may be candidates for revision ORIF with bone grafting.[33] Greater tuberosity nonunions are often not amenable to revision ORIF or anatomic shoulder arthroplasty. For severe nonunions, particularly those affecting the tuberosities, there are increasing data to support the use of reverse shoulder arthroplasty, although this approach should be carefully considered on an individual basis.

Scapular Fractures

Scapular fractures account for approximately 4% of all shoulder girdle fractures. Because of the extensive soft-tissue coverage from the rotator cuff musculature and the thoracic cavity, significant forces are required to fracture the scapula. As such, most scapular fractures (11% to 25%) occur secondary to high-energy injuries.[34]

Presentation

In the setting of high-energy trauma, the context in which scapular fractures typically occur, the patient should be assessed using the Advanced Trauma Life Support protocol. Scapular fractures also can occur secondary to low-energy mechanisms, such as a fall onto outstretched hands. In the awake patient, palpation of the scapula as well as abduction of the arm causes pain. The arm is typically held in the adducted position and the forearm is held against the chest wall. Pseudorupture of the rotator cuff may be seen with intramuscular hemorrhage and consequent muscular dysfunction.[35]

Associated Injuries

The high incidence (35% to 98%) of associated injuries mandates a thorough evaluation of the patient with a scapular fracture. In a retrospective review, the incidence of associated injuries was reported as follows: rib fractures, 52%; pulmonary contusion, 41%; spinal fractures, 29%; clavicular fractures, 25%; and pneumothorax, 32%.[36] Patients with a brachial plexus injury and a scapular fracture have a 57% chance of arterial injury.[37]

Radiographic Evaluation

Scapular fractures are seen only 57% of the time on initial chest radiographs.[38] A true AP radiograph of the scapula, a scapular Y view, and an axillary view should be obtained. A Stryker notch view (AP radiography with the beam centered over the coracoid process directed 10° cephalad) can also be obtained to visualize coracoid fractures. CT is helpful in evaluating the glenoid and the coracoid, and may show body fractures not initially seen with plain imaging.

Classification

Scapular fractures are divided into the following types: body, acromion, coracoid, glenoid neck, and intra-articular glenoid fractures (glenoid fossa). Acromial fractures are further subdivided into minimally displaced, displaced without subacromial impingement, and displaced with subacromial impingement. Coracoid fractures are classified by the location of the fracture, either proximal (type 1) or distal (type 2) to the coracoclavicular ligaments. Extra-articular glenoid neck fractures are differentiated by the presence or absence of a clavicle fracture or acromioclavicular separation (such as the presence or absence of the so-called floating shoulder). The Ideberg fracture classification for intra-articular glenoid fractures was modified into six types.[39] Type I is a fracture of the glenoid rim, type II a transverse fracture through the fossa with a subluxated humeral head, types III-V include scapular body fractures, and type VI has severe glenoid fossa comminution.

Treatment

Scapular Body Fractures

Nonsurgical treatment of scapular body fractures, the most common scapular fractures, generally yields good outcomes in most patients. Early pendulum, passive, and active-assisted exercises should preferably begin soon after the injury. In a study of 123 scapular body fractures, 106 (86%) had either good or excellent results.[40] Patient dissatisfaction with treatment was caused by weakness, crepitus, or pain. Patients with isolated scapular body fractures usually regain good function; however, multiple trauma patients tend to have poorer outcomes.

Acromial Fractures

Fractures of the acromion process usually result either from a direct blow to the shoulder or from an indirect blow through the humerus. Stress fractures also have been reported in advanced-stage rotator cuff tear arthropathy, and recently have been seen following reverse total shoulder arthroplasty. It may be difficult to differentiate between an acromial fracture and os acromiale, the latter occurring bilaterally in up to 60% of patients.[41,42] MRI of the shoulder should be obtained to rule out a rotator cuff tear if superior displacement of the humeral head is present. Acromial fractures that do not cause subacromial impingement are amenable to nonsurgical treatment. An abduction orthosis may help decrease the pull of the deltoid on the acromion to prevent an increase in fracture displacement. If subacromial impingement occurs, the acromion process fracture can be repaired with figure-of-8 wiring, cannulated screws, plating, or if the fragment is small, surgical excision.[43-45]

Coracoid Fractures

Direct blows, avulsion injury, anterior shoulder dislocation, acromioclavicular dislocation, superior escape of the humerus, and coracoclavicular taping have all been implicated as causes of coracoid fractures. These fractures most commonly occur at the coracoid base and are usually minimally displaced because of multiple soft-tissue attachments. Surgical fixation has been advocated for avulsion injuries in athletes as well as those who perform heavy labor. However, even with marked displacement, nonsurgical management has produced excellent results and is the mainstay of treatment.[46,47] Fracture healing generally occurs in 6 weeks with nonsurgical treatment.

Glenoid Neck Fractures

A glenoid neck fracture is the second most common pattern of scapular fracture. True glenoid neck fractures exit along the lateral scapular border as well as

3: Upper Extremity

superiorly, either medial or lateral to the coracoid base. The major deforming force is the long head of the triceps. More than 90% of all glenoid neck fractures are minimally displaced and can be treated nonsurgically with good to excellent functional results. An intact clavicle and acromioclavicular joint enhance fracture stability, and healing usually occurs in the position documented at the primary examination.

Surgical treatment has been recommended for patients with greater than 40° of angulation or greater than 1 cm of medial translation.[48] Study results of 113 patients showed that nonsurgical treatment of these fractures resulted in continued pain in 50% of the patients, weakness with exertion in 40%, persistent mechanical symptoms in 25%, and decreased range of shoulder motion in 20%.[48] Greater loss of shoulder abduction was associated with increased medialization of the glenoid. The surgical approach to the glenoid neck is typically posterior, with preservation of the deltoid origin.

Glenoid Fossa Fractures

Most (90%) of all glenoid fossa fractures are minimally displaced and can be treated nonsurgically. In addition to standard scapular imaging, a Stryker notch view and CT are often helpful in assessing the fracture for displacement and joint congruity.

Type I

Glenoid rim fractures occur when the humeral head eccentrically loads the glenoid cavity. Surgical management should be considered in patients with persistent subluxation, with fracture displacement of more than 10 mm, or with 25% anterior or 33% posterior fracture involvement.[49] The approach to these fractures is dictated by fracture location—anterior via a deltopectoral approach or posterior.

Types II-V

Surgery is indicated in patients with more than 5 mm of step-off of the articular surface, continued humeral head subluxation, or severe separation of the glenoid fragments.[50] The approach may require a combination of multiple surgical approaches (anterior, posterior, and/or superior).

Type VI

Severely comminuted glenoid cavity fractures are best treated with early motion. Surgery may disrupt soft-tissue support, potentially hastening chondral damage.

The Floating Shoulder

The superior shoulder suspensory complex is an osseous and soft-tissue structure that maintains a stable relationship between the axial skeleton and upper extremity. The components of the superior shoulder suspensory complex form a ring composed of the acromion, glenoid, coracoid, coracoclavicular ligaments, distal clavicle, and acromioclavicular joint with its respective ligaments. Injuries involving the disruption of a single component of the superior shoulder suspensory complex are stable, whereas a disruption of two or more components leads to instability.[51]

The classic floating shoulder has a fracture to both the glenoid neck and the clavicle. Management of these injuries continues to be controversial. Nonsurgical care consists of a period of immobilization followed by physical therapy. Nonsurgical outcomes are good to excellent for fractures with minimal displacement; however, there is debate on the degree of acceptable displacement. In nonsurgically treated patients with more than 10 mm of clavicular displacement and more than 5 mm of scapular displacement, outcomes were comparable to those of patients with nondisplaced fractures.[52] Patients with glenoid medialization of more than 30 mm fared better with surgery.

Fixation of the clavicle and/or glenoid neck also has been debated. In the absence of coracoclavicular disruption, fixation of the clavicle lengthens the soft tissues, neutralizes deforming forces, prevents displacement and malrotation of the glenoid, allows earlier physical therapy, and is a relatively uncomplicated procedure. Good to excellent results have been consistently achieved.[53,54] Proponents for surgical fixation of the glenoid argue that it facilitates postoperative rehabilitation and provides greater stability to the humerus. Although several approaches have been used, surgical fixation of the clavicle is generally addressed first. An intraoperative evaluation of the glenoid should occur; fixation should be done if necessary.

Humeral Shaft Fractures

Humeral shaft fractures account for approximately 4% of all fractures and occur in a bimodal distribution, with the first peak occurring in males in the third decade of life (largely secondary to high-energy trauma). The second peak occurs in the seventh decade of life, with an increased incidence in females, typically resulting from falls. Appropriate recognition of the mechanism of injury and patient characteristics are important for treatment.

Presentation

Patients with fractures of the humeral shaft will typically present with pain and deformity of the affected extremity. A thorough examination of the skin and neurovascular status must be performed as an integral component of the evaluation. Radial nerve palsy is the most common nerve injury seen with humeral shaft fractures, with a reported incidence of 3% to 34%.[55,56] This rate increases with open fractures, multiple trauma, vascular injury, and multiple ipsilateral fractures.

Radiographic Evaluation

The initial radiographic evaluation of humerus fractures should include orthogonal plain radiographs. In addition, dedicated views of both the ipsilateral shoul-

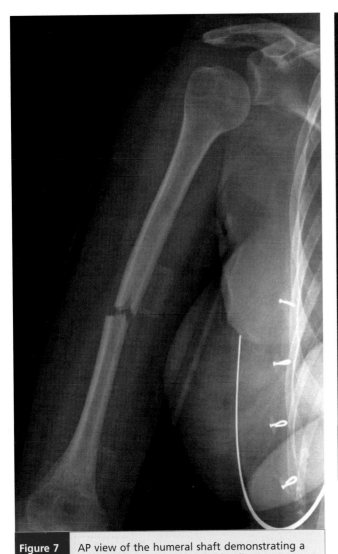

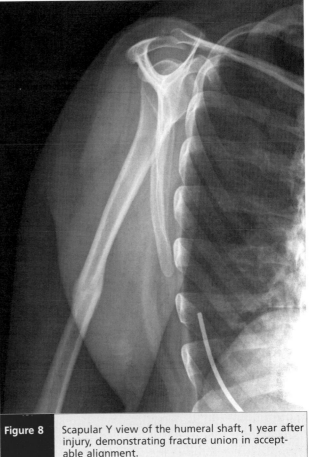

Figure 8 | Scapular Y view of the humeral shaft, 1 year after injury, demonstrating fracture union in acceptable alignment.

Figure 7 | AP view of the humeral shaft demonstrating a midshaft fracture in acceptable alignment treated with a Sarmiento brace.

der and elbow should be obtained (**Figure 7**). Angiography should be considered for fractures with apparent associated vascular injury. CT may provide benefit acutely in the evaluation of fracture extension into joint surfaces, and later in the evaluation of humeral rotational malunions.

Management

Nonsurgical treatment with functional bracing is an important mainstay in the treatment of midshaft humerus fractures, permitting early range of motion, patient comfort, and cost containment (**Figure 8**). Time to union varies from 3 to 40 weeks, with closed fractures averaging 10.7 weeks. The nonunion rate has been reported at 5.5% (79 of 1,428 fractures).[57] Malunion represents one of the potential disadvantages of functional bracing, with varus angulation the most common deformity. However, varus angulation in excess of 10° has been reported to occur in less than 15% of patients treated with functional bracing. In a recent study of

452 fractures, an average sagittal angulation of 3.7° was reported, and only 2% of patients had more than 20° of angulation in the sagittal plane.[57] No studies reported shortening exceeding 2 cm. Alignment is considered acceptable for fractures that heal with up to 20° of anterior angulation, 30° of varus angulation, and/or 3 cm of shortening.

Although excellent clinical results have been reported with nonsurgical management, there are several indications for the surgical treatment of humeral shaft fractures. These indications include open fractures, fractures with vascular injury, associated ipsilateral upper extremity fractures, multiple trauma, and fractures with intra-articular extension.

Surgical options include plate osteosynthesis, intramedullary nailing, and external fixation. Whereas functional bracing is the mainstay for nonsurgical treatment, plate osteosynthesis remains the gold standard for surgical treatment. Union rates in the 93% to 96% range have been consistently reported. Low complication rates also have been reported, including radial nerve palsy (2%), infection (2%), and refracture (1%).[58] The surgical approach (anterolateral, lateral, or posterior) is largely dictated by the surgeon's preference as well as the fracture site. As a rule, middle to proximal shaft fractures are amenable to an anterolateral approach, whereas more distal fractures may benefit from

3: Upper Extremity

a posterior approach. A 3.5- or 4.5-mm dynamic compression plate with three screws proximal and distal to the fracture site is preferred, with lag screw placement when possible. Fractures with comminution, poor screw purchase, or poor bone quality may require more robust fixation and the use of a fixed-angle locking plate.

Intramedullary nailing has not shown the same success rates in the upper extremity as seen in the lower extremity. Antegrade, retrograde, and lateral antegrade insertion entry points have been devised to permit nail placement. In a meta-analysis of more than 155 patients, humeral nailing had higher rates of reoperation, radial nerve injury, chronic subacromial pain, and iatrogenic fracture compared with compression plating.[59] However, intramedullary nailing of the humerus plays a role in the treatment of pathologic fractures, morbidly obese patients, and fractures with soft-tissue compromise that preclude a safe surgical approach for plate fixation.

External fixation traditionally has been used as a temporizing measure in the context of contaminated wounds, infected nonunions, or the need for quick stabilization in unstable patients or those with vascular injury. Constant motion from the shoulder and elbow in the presence of a large soft-tissue envelope has led to complications, including delayed union, pin tract irritation, and infection.

Radial Nerve Palsy

Radial nerve palsy in the setting of humerus fractures requires special mention. As previously noted, the incidence of radial nerve palsy associated with humeral shaft fractures is 3% to 34%.[60] In a recent meta-analysis, the most frequently reported fracture location with a radial nerve injury was the distal third of the humerus (23.6%), followed by the middle third (15.2%), and the proximal third (1.8%).[61] Most of these radial nerve injuries are neurapraxias with a good chance for recovery of nerve function. In a study of 1,045 patients with humerus fractures and radial nerve palsy, 921 recovered nerve function.[56,62-65] However, patients with open fractures recovered nerve function less frequently (85.7%) than those with closed fractures (97.1%). The mean time to onset of recovery was 7.3 weeks. If no recovery is apparent, a baseline nerve conduction velocity study and electromyography should be obtained at approximately 3 to 4 weeks after injury. If there is no return of nerve function, repeat electrodiagnostic studies should be obtained at approximately 4 to 6 months after injury and before surgery is considered. If a transected nerve is involved, surgical repair or tagging of the nerve for a delayed repair should be performed.

Nonunion

Nonunion occurs in 2% to 10% of nonsurgically treated fractures and in up to 15% of fractures treated with internal fixation, more often occurring with intramedullary nailing than with plating.[66] An increased incidence of nonunion is associated with open fractures, high-energy injuries, impaired blood supply, infection, unstable fracture patterns, obesity, osteoporosis, patient noncompliance, smoking, and malnutrition. Humeral shaft fracture nonunion should be treated with excision of the nonunion site, opening of the humeral canal, bone graft application, and dynamic compression plating. Union is achievable in 83% to 100% of nonunion cases.[67-69] If an intramedullary nail has been placed, the nail must be removed. In a retrospective study, nine of nine intramedullary nailed nonunions healed after plating.[70] Union rates of 88% to 95% have been reported with irrigation, débridement, intravenous antibiotics, and an external fixator for infected nonunions.[71] Free fibular grafting offers a viable treatment option for recalcitrant, atrophic nonunions.[72-74]

Annotated References

1. Robinson CM: Fractures of the clavicle in the adult: Epidemiology and classification. *J Bone Joint Surg Br* 1998;80(3):476-484.

2. Khan LA, Bradnock TJ, Scott C, Robinson CM: Fractures of the clavicle. *J Bone Joint Surg Am* 2009;91(2):447-460.

   Nonsurgical treatment of displaced shaft fractures may be associated with a higher rate of nonunion and functional deficits than previously reported. However, it remains difficult to predict which patients will have these complications.

3. Robinson CM, Court-Brown CM, McQueen MM, Wakefield AE: Estimating the risk of nonunion following nonoperative treatment of a clavicular fracture. *J Bone Joint Surg Am* 2004;86(7):1359-1365.

4. Canadian Orthopaedic Trauma Society: Nonoperative treatment compared with plate fixation of displaced midshaft clavicular fractures: A multicenter, randomized clinical trial. *J Bone Joint Surg Am* 2007;89(1):1-10.

   The authors concluded that primary plate fixation of completely displaced midshaft clavicular fractures in active adults is an acceptable treatment method.

5. McKee MD, Pedersen EM, Jones C, et al: Deficits following nonoperative treatment of displaced midshaft clavicular fractures. *J Bone Joint Surg Am* 2006;88(1):35-40.

6. Iannotti MR, Crosby LA, Stafford P, Grayson G, Goulet R: Effects of plate location and selection on the stability of midshaft clavicle osteotomies: A biomechanical study. *J Shoulder Elbow Surg* 2002;11(5):457-462.

7. Robertson C, Celestre P, Mahar A, Schwartz A: Reconstruction plates for stabilization of mid-shaft clavicle fractures: Differences between nonlocked and locked plates in two different positions. *J Shoulder Elbow Surg* 2009;18(2):204-209.

The authors present an evaluation of the biomechanical stability of locking and nonlocking clavicle reconstruction plates for treating midshaft transverse fractures, comparing anterior-inferior to superior plate position. Level of evidence: I.

8. Endrizzi DP, White RR, Babikian GM, Old AB: Nonunion of the clavicle treated with plate fixation: A review of forty-seven consecutive cases. *J Shoulder Elbow Surg* 2008;17(6):951-953.

    Forty-seven patients were treated with superior plating for clavicular nonunions. Distant autogenous bone graft is usually not necessary to obtain union. Level of evidence: III.

9. Mueller M, Rangger C, Striepens N, Burger C: Minimally invasive intramedullary nailing of midshaft clavicular fractures using titanium elastic nails. *J Trauma* 2008;64(6):1528-1534.

    Thirty-one midshaft clavicular fractures were treated with intramedullary nailing with a titanium elastic nail. Nonunion was not observed. No patient sustained a refracture after nail removal. Medial migration of the titanium elastic nail in seven patients and iatrogenic perforation of the lateral cortex in one patient required secondary shortening on five occasions. Nail breakage after fracture healing was observed twice. Level of evidence: III.

10. Frigg A, Rillmann P, Perren T, Gerber M, Ryf C: Intramedullary nailing of clavicular midshaft fractures with the titanium elastic nail: Problems and complications. *Am J Sports Med* 2009;37(2):352-359.

    Thirty-four patients were treated with intramedullary nailing. A standard titanium elastic nail was used in 19 patients and a titanium elastic nail with an end cap in 15 patients. A short incision at the fracture site was made for open reduction if needed. In 62% of patients, open reduction was necessary independent of fracture type, flattening of the titanium elastic nail, or transverse fragments. In 70% of patients, complications occurred. Level of evidence: IV.

11. Robinson CM, Cairns DA: Primary nonoperative treatment of displaced lateral fractures of the clavicle. *J Bone Joint Surg Am* 2004;86(4):778-782.

12. Franck WM, Siassi RM, Hennig FF: Treatment of posterior epiphyseal disruption of the medial clavicle with a modified Balser plate. *J Trauma* 2003;55(5):966-968.

13. Visser CP, Coene LN, Brand R, Tavy DL: Nerve lesions in proximal humeral fractures. *J Shoulder Elbow Surg* 2001;10(5):421-427.

14. Crosby LA, Finnan RP, Anderson CG, Gozdanovic J, Miller MW: Tetracycline labeling as a measure of humeral head viability after 3- or 4-part proximal humerus fracture. *J Shoulder Elbow Surg* 2009;18(6):851-858.

    Nineteen patients were treated with hemiarthroplasty as definitive treatment of 20 displaced three- and four-part proximal humerus fractures after receiving 500 mg of tetracycline hydrochloride. Humeral head biopsies were taken from four predetermined locations intraoperatively. The authors concluded that the vascular supply is preserved in displaced three- and four-part proximal humerus fractures, especially in younger patients in the anterosuperior aspect of the humeral head.

15. Bastian JD, Hertel R: Initial post-fracture humeral head ischemia does not predict development of necrosis. *J Shoulder Elbow Surg* 2008;17(1):2-8.

    The authors evaluated the functional outcome and the occurrence of osteonecrosis in 51 consecutive patients (26 women) with intracapsular fractures of the proximal humerus treated with ORIF. Osteosynthesis with preservation of the humeral head warrants consideration when adequate reduction and stable conditions for revascularization can be obtained. Level of evidence: II.

16. Robinson BC, Athwal GS, Sanchez-Sotelo J, Rispoli DM: Classification and imaging of proximal humerus fractures. *Orthop Clin North Am* 2008;39(4):393-403.

    Understanding the particular proximal humeral fracture pattern in each case is complicated. Three-dimensional reconstructions based on CT currently available in most institutions allow a better understanding of complex fractures. Level of evidence: IV.

17. Hertel R, Hempfing A, Stiehler M, Leunig M: Predictors of humeral head ischemia after intracapsular fracture of the proximal humerus. *J Shoulder Elbow Surg* 2004; 13(4):427-433.

18. Brunner A, Honigmann P, Treumann T, Babst R: The impact of stereo-visualisation of three-dimensional CT datasets on the inter- and intraobserver reliability of the AO/OTA and Neer classifications in the assessment of fractures of the proximal humerus. *J Bone Joint Surg Br* 2009;91(6):766-771.

    The authors evaluated the impact of stereovisualization of three-dimensional volume-rendering CT datasets on the interobserver and intraobserver reliability assessed by kappa values on the AO/OTA and Neer classifications in the assessment of proximal humeral fractures. Level of evidence: I.

19. Hodgson SA, Mawson SJ, Saxton JM, Stanley D: Rehabilitation of two-part fractures of the neck of the humerus (two-year follow-up). *J Shoulder Elbow Surg* 2007;16(2):143-145.

    The 2-year results of a randomized, prospective, controlled trial of minimally displaced proximal humeral fractures treated either by immediate physiotherapy or after 3 weeks of immobilization are reported. Delayed rehabilitation by 3 weeks of shoulder immobilization produces a slower recovery, which continues for at least 2 years after the time of injury. Level of evidence: I.

20. Hanson B, Neidenbach P, de Boer P, Stengel D: Functional outcomes after nonoperative management of fractures of the proximal humerus. *J Shoulder Elbow Surg* 2009;18(4):612-621.

    Patients older than 18 years presenting with a closed proximal humeral fracture who were considered suitable for functional treatment by the surgeon in charge were enrolled in a prospective, externally monitored, observational study. This study may provide reference values for future investigations; it stresses ceiling effects that will make it difficult to demonstrate a significant advantage of surgical over nonsurgical treatment in patients with proximal humeral fractures. Level of evidence: IV.

21. Edelson G, Safuri H, Salami J, Vigder F, Militianu D: Natural history of complex fractures of the proximal humerus using a three-dimensional classification system. *J Shoulder Elbow Surg* 2008;17(3):399-409.

The natural history of 63 patients with complex fractures of the proximal humerus was followed prospectively for 2 to 9 years with a nonrandomized protocol. Status comparable to a successful surgical shoulder fusion was achieved in most cases (termed nature's fusion). Osteonecrosis, even in severely displaced injuries, is rare. Level of evidence: II.

22. Kralinger F, Unger S, Wambacher M, Smekal V, Schmoelz W: The medial periosteal hinge, a key structure in fractures of the proximal humerus: A biomechanical cadaver study of its mechanical properties. *J Bone Joint Surg Br* 2009;91(7):973-976.

The authors investigated the biomechanical properties of the medial periosteum in fractures of the proximal humerus using a standard model in 20 fresh-frozen cadaver specimens comparable in age, sex, and bone mineral density. Periosteal rupture started at a mean displacement of 2.96 mm with a mean load of 100.9 N. A statistically significant but low correlation between bone mineral density and the maximum load uptake was observed. Level of evidence: I.

23. Konrad GG, Mehlhorn A, Kühle J, Strohm PC, Südkamp NP: Proximal humerus fractures: Current treatment options. *Acta Chir Orthop Traumatol Cech* 2008; 75(6):413-421.

Nondisplaced fractures and fractures with minimal displacement and adequate stability are usually successfully treated nonsurgically. Recently invented implants with angular stability provide better biomechanical properties and enhanced anchorage, especially in the osteoporotic bone. These implants have the potential for achieving better results in the treatment of these complex injuries.

24. Brunner F, Sommer C, Bahrs C, et al: Open reduction and internal fixation of proximal humerus fractures using a proximal humeral locked plate: A prospective multicenter analysis. *J Orthop Trauma* 2009;23(3):163-172.

One hundred fifty-seven patients with 158 fractures were treated with ORIF with a Philos plate. The authors concluded that a good functional outcome can be expected. However, complication incidence proportions are high. Level of evidence: II.

25. Bogner R, Hübner C, Matis N, Auffarth A, Lederer S, Resch H: Minimally-invasive treatment of three- and four-part fractures of the proximal humerus in elderly patients. *J Bone Joint Surg Br* 2008;90(12):1602-1607.

Seventy-six patients older than 70 years with three- or four-part fractures were treated with percutaneous reduction and internal fixation using the Humerusblock (Synthes, Salzburg, Austria) This technique can provide a comfortable and mobile shoulder in elderly patients and is a satisfactory alternative to replacement and traditional techniques of internal fixation. Level of evidence: IV.

26. Russo R, Visconti V, Lombardi LV, Ciccarelli M, Giudice G: The block-bridge system: A new concept and surgical technique to reconstruct articular surfaces and tuberosities in complex proximal humeral fractures. *J Shoulder Elbow Surg* 2008;17(1):29-36.

The block-bridge system is a new technique for the reconstruction of the proximal humerus around a triangular-shaped bone block positioned inside the head and the metaphysis. The results were excellent or good in 23 patients. The mean active anterior elevation was 160° and all patients were pain free and returned to their preoperative activities, including sports. One patient had a symptomatic osteonecrosis that was treated with a hemiarthroplasty. Level of evidence: IV.

27. Greiner SH, Kääb MJ, Kröning I, Scheibel M, Perka C: Reconstruction of humeral length and centering of the prosthetic head in hemiarthroplasty for proximal humeral fractures. *J Shoulder Elbow Surg* 2008;17(5):709-714.

This study analyzed clinical outcome, reconstruction of humeral length, centering of the prosthetic head in the glenoid, and tuberosity positioning and healing, using the pectoralis major tendon as a reference intraoperatively. Clinical outcome depended significantly on greater tuberosity healing and centering of the prosthetic head in the glenoid. Level of evidence: III.

28. Grönhagen CM, Abbaszadegan H, Révay SA, Adolphson PY: Medium-term results after primary hemiarthroplasty for comminute proximal humerus fractures: A study of 46 patients followed up for an average of 4.4 years. *J Shoulder Elbow Surg* 2007;16(6): 766-773.

This study evaluated 82 patients treated with primary hemiarthroplasty for a severely displaced proximal humerus fracture. The mean Constant score for all patients was 42 of 100 points. Radiologic evaluation showed that 24 prostheses had migrated superiorly, ectopic bone developed in 25 patients, 16 had glenoid erosion, and 5 had displaced tuberosities. Level of evidence: IV.

29. Antuña SA, Sperling JW, Cofield RH: Shoulder hemiarthroplasty for acute fractures of the proximal humerus: A minimum five-year follow-up. *J Shoulder Elbow Surg* 2008;17(2):202-209.

The study data suggest that patients undergoing arthroplasty as treatment of an acute fracture of the proximal humerus may achieve satisfactory long-term pain relief; however, the result for overall shoulder motion is less predictable. All efforts should be aimed at reconstructing the tuberosities anatomically and delaying aggressive physical therapy until there is radiographic evidence of tuberosity healing.

30. Bufquin T, Hersan A, Hubert L, Massin P: Reverse shoulder arthroplasty for the treatment of three- and four-part fractures of the proximal humerus in the elderly: A prospective review of 43 cases with a short-term follow-up. *J Bone Joint Surg Br* 2007;89(4):516-520.

Reverse shoulder arthroplasty was used in 43 patients with a three- or four-part fracture of the proximal humerus. Complications included three patients with reflex sympathetic dystrophy and five with neurologic complications; most of these complications resolved. One patient had an anterior dislocation. Level of evidence: II.

31. Levy JC, Virani N, Pupello D, Frankle M: Use of the reverse shoulder prosthesis for the treatment of failed hemiarthroplasty in patients with glenohumeral arthritis and rotator cuff deficiency. *J Bone Joint Surg Br* 2007;89(2):189-195.

The authors report on the reverse shoulder prosthesis in the revision of a failed shoulder hemiarthroplasty in 19 shoulders in 18 patients with severe pain and loss of function. Statistically significant improvements were seen in pain and functional outcome. There were six prosthesis-related complications in six shoulders (32%), five of which had severe bone loss of the glenoid, proximal humerus, or both. Level of evidence: IV.

32. Boileau P, Trojani C, Walch G, Krishnan SG, Romeo A, Sinnerton R: Shoulder arthroplasty for the treatment of the sequelae of fractures of the proximal humerus. *J Shoulder Elbow Surg* 2001;10(4):299-308.

33. Walch G, Badet R, Nové-Josserand L, Levigne C: Nonunions of the surgical neck of the humerus: Surgical treatment with an intramedullary bone peg, internal fixation, and cancellous bone grafting. *J Shoulder Elbow Surg* 1996;5(3):161-168.

34. McGahan JP, Rab GT: Fracture of the acromion associated with an axillary nerve deficit: A case report and review of the literature. *Clin Orthop Relat Res* 1980;147: 216-218.

35. Neviaser JS: Traumatic lesions: Injuries in and about the shoulder joint. *Instr Course Lect* 1956;13:187-216.

36. Baldwin KD, Ohman-Strickland P, Mehta S, Hume E: Scapula fractures: A marker for concomitant injury? A retrospective review of data in the National Trauma Database. *J Trauma* 2008;65(2):430-435.

The authors studied whether there was a relationship between scapula fractures and concomitant injury and determined that injuries to the upper extremity and pelvic ring and thoracic injuries were associated with greater frequency in patients with scapular fracture.

37. Folman Y, el-Masri W, Gepstein R, Messias R: Fractures of the scapula associated with traumatic paralysis: A pathomechanical indicator. *Injury* 1993;24(5):306-308.

38. Harris RD, Harris JH Jr: The prevalence and significance of missed scapular fractures in blunt chest trauma. *AJR Am J Roentgenol* 1988;151(4):747-750.

39. Goss TP: Fractures of the glenoid cavity. *J Bone Joint Surg Am* 1992;74(2):299-305.

40. Gosens T, Speigner B, Minekus J: Fracture of the scapular body: Functional outcome after conservative treatment. *J Shoulder Elbow Surg* 2009;18(3):443-448.

Isolated scapular body fractures healed after nonsurgical treatment, leading to a functional shoulder score level equal to that of the general population and a range of motion equal to the uninjured shoulder. Multitrauma patients had a less favorable outcome.

41. Liberson F: Os acromiale: A contested anomaly. *J Bone Joint Surg Am* 1937;19:683-689.

42. Sammarco VJ: Os acromiale: Frequency, anatomy, and clinical implications. *J Bone Joint Surg Am* 2000;82(3): 394-400.

43. Wong-Pack WK, Bobechko PE, Becker EJ: Fractured coracoid with anterior shoulder dislocation. *J Can Assoc Radiol* 1980;31(4):278-279.

44. Mick CA, Weiland AJ: Pseudoarthrosis of a fracture of the acromion. *J Trauma* 1983;23(3):248-249.

45. Gorczyca JT, Davis RT, Hartford JM, Brindle TJ: Open reduction internal fixation after displacement of a previously nondisplaced acromial fracture in a multiply injured patient: Case report and review of literature. *J Orthop Trauma* 2001;15(5):369-373.

46. Asbury S, Tennent TD: Avulsion fracture of the coracoid process: A case report. *Injury* 2005;36(4):567-568.

47. Zlowodzki M, Bhandari M, Zelle BA, Kregor PJ, Cole PA: Treatment of scapula fractures: Systematic review of 520 fractures in 22 case series. *J Orthop Trauma* 2006; 20(3):230-233.

48. Ada JR, Miller ME: Scapular fractures: Analysis of 113 cases. *Clin Orthop Relat Res* 1991;269:174-180.

49. DePalma A, ed: *Surgery of the Shoulder*, ed 3. Philadelphia, PA, JB Lippincott; 1983.

50. Soslowsky LJ, Flatow EL, Bigliani LU, Mow VC: Articular geometry of the glenohumeral joint. *Clin Orthop Relat Res* 1992;285:181-190.

51. Goss TP: Double disruptions of the superior shoulder suspensory complex. *J Orthop Trauma* 1993;7(2):99-106.

52. Egol KA, Connor PM, Karunakar MA, Sims SH, Bosse MJ, Kellam JF: The floating shoulder: Clinical and functional results. *J Bone Joint Surg Am* 2001;83(8):1188-1194.

53. DeFranco MJ, Patterson BM: The floating shoulder. *J Am Acad Orthop Surg* 2006;14(8):499-509.

54. Owens BD, Goss TP: The floating shoulder. *J Bone Joint Surg Br* 2006;88(11):1419-1424.

55. Tingstad EM, Wolinsky PR, Shyr Y, Johnson KD: Effect of immediate weightbearing on plated fractures of the humeral shaft. *J Trauma* 2000;49(2):278-280.

56. Ring D, Chin K, Jupiter JB: Radial nerve palsy associated with high-energy humeral shaft fractures. *J Hand Surg Am* 2004;29(1):144-147.

57. Papasoulis E, Drosos GI, Ververidis AN, Verettas DA: Functional bracing of humeral shaft fractures: A review of clinical studies. *Injury* 2010;41(7):e1-e7.

   The authors conducted a literature review to determine the efficacy of functional bracing and found that humeral shaft fractures heal in an average of 10.7 weeks after treatment and proximal third and AO type A fractures have a higher nonunion rate. Residual deformity and joint stiffness are the main disadvantages of this treatment.

58. McKee MD: Fractures of the shaft of the humerus, in Bucholz RW, Heckman JD, Brown CC, eds: *Rockwood and Green's Fractures in Adults*, ed 6. Philadelphia, PA, Lippincott Williams & Wilkins, 2006, vol 1, pp 1117-1159.

59. Bhandari M, Devereaux PJ, McKee MD, Schemitsch EH: Compression plating versus intramedullary nailing of humeral shaft fractures: A meta-analysis. *Acta Orthop* 2006;77(2):279-284.

60. Hak DJ: Radial nerve palsy associated with humeral shaft fractures. *Orthopedics* 2009;32(2):111.

   The authors discussed the need for surgical exploration in patients with radial nerve palsy associated with humeral shaft fractures.

61. Shao YC, Harwood P, Grotz MR, Limb D, Giannoudis PV: Radial nerve palsy associated with fractures of the shaft of the humerus: A systematic review. *J Bone Joint Surg Br* 2005;87(12):1647-1652.

62. Larsen LB, Barfred T: Radial nerve palsy after simple fracture of the humerus. *Scand J Plast Reconstr Surg Hand Surg* 2000;34(4):363-366.

63. Pollock FH, Drake D, Bovill EG, Day L, Trafton PG: Treatment of radial neuropathy associated with fractures of the humerus. *J Bone Joint Surg Am* 1981;63(2):239-243.

64. Shaw JL, Sakellarides H: Radial-nerve paralysis associated with fractures of the humerus: A review of forty-five cases. *J Bone Joint Surg Am* 1967;49(5):899-902.

65. Postacchini F, Morace GB: Fractures of the humerus associated with paralysis of the radial nerve. *Ital J Orthop Traumatol* 1988;14(4):455-464.

66. Pugh DM, McKee MD: Advances in the management of humeral nonunion. *J Am Acad Orthop Surg* 2003;11(1):48-59.

67. Otsuka NY, McKee MD, Liew A, et al: The effect of comorbidity and duration of nonunion on outcome after surgical treatment for nonunion of the humerus. *J Shoulder Elbow Surg* 1998;7(2):127-133.

68. Ring D, McKee MD, Perey BH, Jupiter JB: The use of a blade plate and autogenous cancellous bone graft in the treatment of ununited fractures of the proximal humerus. *J Shoulder Elbow Surg* 2001;10(6):501-507.

69. Healy WL, White GM, Mick CA, Brooker AF Jr, Weiland AJ: Nonunion of the humeral shaft. *Clin Orthop Relat Res* 1987;219:206-213.

70. McKee MD, Miranda MA, Riemer BL, et al: Management of humeral nonunion after the failure of locking intramedullary nails. *J Orthop Trauma* 1996;10(7):492-499.

71. Patel VR, Menon DK, Pool RD, Simonis RB: Nonunion of the humerus after failure of surgical treatment: Management using the Ilizarov circular fixator. *J Bone Joint Surg Br* 2000;82(7):977-983.

72. Healy WL, Jupiter JB, Kristiansen TK, White RR: Nonunion of the proximal humerus: A review of 25 cases. *J Orthop Trauma* 1990;4(4):424-431.

73. Chhabra AB, Golish SR, Pannunzio ME, Butler TE Jr, Bolano LE, Pederson WC: Treatment of chronic nonunions of the humerus with free vascularized fibula transfer: A report of thirteen cases. *J Reconstr Microsurg* 2009;25(2):117-124.

   The authors reviewed 13 cases of chronic nonunion of the humerus treated with vascularized fibula transfer and found that healing occurred in 12 of the 13 patients after an average of 18 weeks.

74. Jupiter JB: Complex non-union of the humeral diaphysis: Treatment with a medial approach, an anterior plate, and a vascularized fibular graft. *J Bone Joint Surg Am* 1990;72(5):701-707.

Chapter 23

Shoulder Reconstruction

Anand M. Murthi, MD   Jesse A. McCarron, MD

Glenohumeral Degenerative Joint Disease

Glenohumeral degenerative joint disorders are caused by numerous disease processes and injury patterns. Common disease processes include osteoarthritis (OA), rheumatoid (inflammatory) arthritis, osteonecrosis, posttraumatic arthritis, rotator cuff arthropathy, and postoperative or iatrogenic arthropathy. Each of these entities has associated symptomatology, examination findings, radiographic changes, and therapeutic interventions.

Primary OA is a disease of cartilage and, as such, is the most common degenerative process in the shoulder. Classic physical findings include painful loss of motion, early morning stiffness, and loss of strength. Radiographic findings include osteophyte formation, loss of joint space, and subchondral sclerosis (Figure 1). A late finding is posterior glenoid wear, which is important in planning surgical reconstruction and potential glenoid resurfacing.

Rheumatoid arthritis is a synovial fluid–based disease that more commonly occurs in older women. Physical findings are similar to those of OA, although range of motion may not be as limited. Classic radiographic findings include central glenoid wear, osteopenia, subchondral cysts, and bony erosions. When considering surgical reconstruction and arthroplasty, pathologic abnormality of the rotator cuff is very common and must be evaluated.

Osteonecrosis is a less frequently occurring disease process that can manifest as significant deep-seated shoulder pain, although the patient is often able to maintain motion and strength. Stiffness occurs during late stages, with complete loss of the humeral head architecture. Osteonecrosis is caused by disruption of the vascular supply to the humeral head, which can lead to cartilage death and collapse. Osteonecrosis is character-ized by early radiographic sclerosis, then humeral head collapse, and later glenoid changes. Common causes include steroid intake, alcoholism, and trauma. A careful diagnosis with radiography or MRI to determine the presence of humeral head collapse will guide the choice of surgical treatment from core decompression to total shoulder replacement.

Posttraumatic arthritis presents in many forms, from proximal humerus malunions and subsequent irregular glenoid contact stresses to intra-articular glenoid fractures leading to glenohumeral arthroses. Previous trauma or fracture may predispose a patient to this disorder. Numerous case reports and small series have shown that rapid chondrolysis may be an issue in young patients presenting with painful, stiff shoulders after arthroscopic surgery.[1-3] Chondrolysis may result from pain pump insertion, infection, and/or thermal procedures. Although there has been no definitive correlation, rapid chondrolysis along with infection should be considered in the differential diagnosis of the rapid loss of joint space.

Dr. Murthi or an immediate family member serves as a paid consultant to or is an employee of Zimmer and Ascension Orthopaedics and has received research or institutional support from Arthrex, DePuy, and Synthes. Dr. McCarron or an immediate family member is a member of a speakers' bureau or has made paid presentations on behalf of Mitek, serves as a paid consultant to or is an employee of Wyeth, and has received research or institutional support from Wyeth.

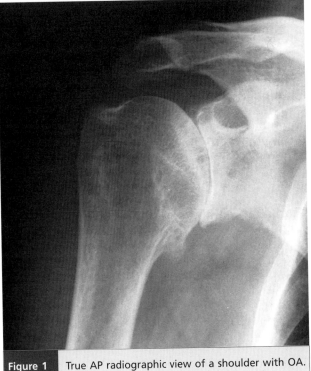

Figure 1   True AP radiographic view of a shoulder with OA.

Postoperative arthropathy is difficult to diagnose accurately and develop a treatment strategy for, especially in a shoulder treated with stabilization or capsulorrhaphy. For example, in a common scenario, a 50-year-old man presents with a stiff, painful, arthritic shoulder many years after undergoing open subscapularis shortening and/or a disruptive procedure (such as Putti-Platt, Magnuson-Stack, or Bristow-Latarjet). The eccentric forces placed on the glenoid lead to severe arthritis (posterior glenoid wear) and extreme loss of external rotation. These shoulders require complex treatments, especially when performing arthroplasty procedures, because regaining motion can be difficult when soft-tissue balancing is needed to provide stability and motion.

Understanding the many origins of degenerative shoulder disease permits proper surgical planning and the best chance for a successful outcome because each disease process lends itself to various treatment modalities.

Nonsurgical Treatment

Nonsurgical treatment in the form of activity modification, pharmacotherapy, and physical therapy remains the first-line treatment option for patients with glenohumeral arthritis, although the effectiveness of these modalities is inconclusive. Nonsurgical, multimodality therapies should be tried in all patients (especially younger patients) before surgical treatment is considered.

Physical therapy is often prescribed for mild or moderate glenohumeral arthritis to preserve motion and optimize function, but its efficacy has not been established.[4-6] Determining the efficacy of physical therapy for glenohumeral arthritis has been complicated by the failure of most studies and systematic reviews to distinguish between different etiologies of shoulder pain and by the lack of consistency in the type of therapy prescribed. Similarly, acupuncture and transcutaneous electrical nerve stimulation are reasonable treatment options for the arthritic shoulder; however, no studies have evaluated the specific efficacy of these modalities in the management of glenohumeral arthritis. Symptomatic improvement with these modalities likely results in large part from the alleviation of neck and upper back pain often associated with shoulder dysfunction; these treatments have shown great efficacy in relieving such pain.[7-10]

Acetaminophen, nonsteroidal anti-inflammatory drugs (NSAIDs), and narcotic medications are frequently prescribed for arthritis-related shoulder pain and have demonstrated efficacy in reducing symptoms. However, all of these medications can have deleterious side effects that must be taken into consideration. A meta-analysis of randomized controlled trials suggests that NSAIDs are more effective than acetaminophen for treating pain related to OA, but are also associated with a higher risk of complications.[11] Patients with an increased risk of gastrointestinal complications are best treated with either a cyclooxygenase-2 selective NSAID or a nonselective NSAID with coprescription of a proton pump inhibitor.[4] Although the risk of gastrointestinal and renal complications is considered lower with acetaminophen than with NSAIDs, a new focus on the potential for liver toxicity with acetaminophen or medications that contain acetaminophen (including many narcotics) emphasizes the need to consider these risk factors when prescribing these medications.

Glenohumeral steroid injections are commonly used for shoulder arthritis to reduce pain, but there are no studies showing the efficacy of these injections in the shoulder and their effectiveness is inconclusive. Generally, the administration of glenohumeral steroid injections is likely to be more effective when treating an inflammatory synovitis component of the pain, which may accompany many forms of arthritis. Pain that is related to the strenuous use of the arm or caused by mechanical problems, such as pain at the extremes of motion caused by capsular tightness or osteophytes, is less likely to be successfully treated by steroid injections. Guidelines at this time are based on level V evidence.

Viscosupplementation for joints affected by OA has a delayed onset but improved duration in relieving pain when compared with steroid injections or placebo.[4,12] The only multicenter randomized controlled trial to evaluate viscosupplementation for shoulder arthritis showed modest but statistically significant improvements in pain (2 to 8 points better than placebo on a 100-point visual analog scale) over a 26-week period.[12]

Nonprosthetic Joint-Sparing Techniques

Surgical options for the treatment of shoulder OA that avoid hemiarthroplasty or total shoulder arthroplasty include glenohumeral débridement, lavage and microfracture, autologous chondrocyte implantation, osteochondral autologous transplantation, and capsular release. The effectiveness of treating OA by these means remains inconclusive.

Arthroscopic glenohumeral débridement, with removal of loose debris and resection of unstable cartilage flaps back to a stable edge, is considered a reasonable treatment option for a patient who does not have end-stage arthritis or diffuse full-thickness cartilage defects and has been unsuccessfully managed with nonsurgical treatment. In two case reports and in one limited retrospective review, it was shown that in a young patient with focal, full-thickness, cartilage lesions, débridement and lavage with microfracture of the full-thickness cartilage defects can yield good short-term and midterm outcomes compared with the patient's preoperative condition.[13-15] These outcomes are equivalent to those of patients with lesser (Outerbridge grade 2 or 3) chondral lesions at 12- to 33-month follow-ups.[15] Patients with bipolar lesions (involving both the glenoid and humeral sides of the joint) did significantly worse than patients with unipolar lesions.

More involved treatment strategies involving autologous chondrocyte implantation, osteochondral autograft transplantation, or osteochondral allografting procedures for focal, full-thickness articular cartilage defects are intended to regenerate or replace lost cartilage as opposed to creating a fibrocartilage scar, which is associated with the microfracture technique. There is only one case report in the literature involving the use of autologous chondrocyte implantation in the shoulder. The procedure resulted in a good patient outcome at 3 months postoperatively, but no long-term follow-up was available.[16] Osteochondral autografting for the treatment of full-thickness cartilage defects of the shoulder has been reported in a group of seven patients.[17] All patients showed improved function, decreased pain, and good range of motion at a mean follow-up of 9-years; however, the procedure did not prevent the radiographic progression of glenohumeral OA.

Débridement with capsular release of full-thickness cartilage defects has achieved mixed results.[18-20] Although good pain relief and improved function has been reported in some patient groups at a mean 34-month follow-up,[18] other reports have suggested more modest results with the return of pain within 1 year of surgery (after an initial pain-free period),[19] and a 30% failure rate requiring conversion to hemiarthroplasty.[20] The initial success and durability of the results for these types of procedures are likely highly dependent on appropriate patient selection and management of expectations, with less favorable outcomes in younger patients with higher demands and those with larger, more diffuse chondral lesions.

Shoulder Resurfacing Arthroplasty

Recent information has shown that select patients with pathologic conditions of the shoulder may benefit from shoulder resurfacing arthroplasty.[20-23] Degenerative conditions such as inflammatory arthritis, OA, osteonecrosis, posttraumatic conditions, and focal articular defects have benefited from shoulder resurfacing arthroplasty. Short- and long-term improvements in pain and function have been reported after treatment with this bone-preserving technique.[20,24]

Prerequisites for shoulder resurfacing arthroplasty include adequate proximal humeral bone stock to contain the short peg and support the implant. Bone loss up to 25% has not precluded shoulder resurfacing arthroplasty according to one study.[25] Technically, the starting position of the centrally placed guidewire remains the reference point in all designs to recreate the anatomic position and function of the shoulder. Obtaining the proper amount of lateral offset will position the rotator cuff to function properly. In patients with significant anatomic distortion (for example, surgical neck malunion) or long-stem total elbow replacements, humeral stem placement may not be possible, thus providing an indication for shoulder resurfacing arthroplasty.

Advantages of the shoulder resurfacing arthroplasty design include the ability to replicate native anatomic humeral version, inclination, offset, and head size while preserving bone stock. In physiologically younger, active patients who may require future revision surgery, preservation of bone stock is beneficial. Although hemiarthroplasty may provide similar functional outcomes, revising stemmed implants results in potentially significant proximal bone loss and soft-tissue disruption. Complications with humeral stems, such as periprosthetic fracture, loosening, bone resorption, and deep infection, do not occur with shoulder resurfacing arthroplasty. When properly implanted, a shoulder resurfacing arthroplasty device provides a stable shoulder replacement option that can mirror native offset; allows proper soft-tissue balancing; and preserves the glenoid, thus preventing the risk of polyethylene glenoid failure (**Figure 2**). The caveat remains that an overstuffed, lateralized, improperly positioned shoulder resurfacing arthroplasty can lead to rapid progression of pain and stiffness and potential cuff rupture. Selecting patients with relatively preserved motion and minimal and centralized glenoid wear (without static posterior subluxation or biconcavity) can lead to good results. Several studies have shown shoulder resurfacing arthroplasty to be an appropriate choice for the younger patient who meets these criteria.[20,21,23] Shoulder resurfacing arthroplasty, however, may not be appropriate for patients with end-stage degenerative stiff shoulder with posterior static subluxation because stability and tissue balancing will be a consideration.

Hemiarthroplasty

Historically, hemiarthroplasty or humeral head replacement has been indicated for most degenerative shoulder conditions, including OA, inflammatory arthritis, posttraumatic sequelae (osteochondral defects, malunions, and chondrolysis), osteonecrosis, and certain cuff tear arthropathies.[24,26-28] Although the recent trend has been to use total shoulder arthroplasty to treat the arthritic shoulder with an intact rotator cuff, glenoid loosening must still be regarded as a source of potential failure in shoulder arthroplasty. Humeral head replacement continues to be an option in select, physiologically younger, active patients.[28] Proper patient selection is paramount for success, and is considerably dependent on understanding glenoid morphology and wear patterns. Selecting patients with a centralized glenoid wear pattern without posterior wear or static subluxation should lead to improved outcomes. Soft-tissue balancing and appropriate capsular releases with subscapularis mobilization are required, just as with a total shoulder arthroplasty, to optimize results. A recent study indicated that concentric reaming with humeral head replacement, as performed during the "ream and run" procedure, may also benefit younger, active patients with degenerative arthritis.[28]

The current literature has described a spectrum of results achieved in using humeral head replacement for degenerative joint disease.[24,26-30] Guidelines indicate that obtaining proper height, version, and offset to balance the shoulder is essential to improve function. This theory of anatomic replacement allows proper tensioning in both the rotator cuff and deltoid to allow an in-

3: Upper Extremity

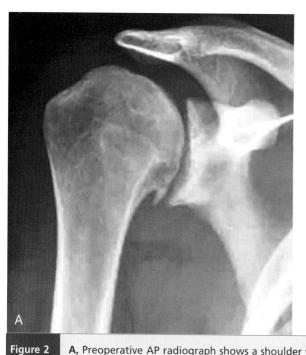
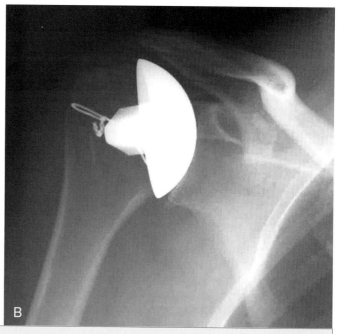

Figure 2 **A,** Preoperative AP radiograph shows a shoulder with degenerative arthritis. **B,** Postoperative AP radiograph of the shoulder after successful surface replacement arthroplasty.

crease in motion and decrease in pain. Anatomic sizing and the proper level of humeral head osteotomy (resection) are often misunderstood, leading to either over-stuffing or instability. Resection is based on the level of the rotator cuff insertion, which results in anatomic version (approximately 20°), with retroversion usually ranging from 20° to 40°. Technical complications include malpositioning and overstuffing the joint (using too large a head size) to compensate for instability. Complications may include stiffness, progressive glenoid wear, periprosthetic fracture, infection, and instability (subscapularis dysfunction). Revision or conversion to total shoulder arthroplasty is complex, difficult, and rarely provides results similar to those achieved with primary total shoulder arthroplasty.[29]

Biologic Total Shoulder Arthroplasty

Humeral head hemiarthroplasty with soft-tissue resurfacing of the glenoid (biologic total shoulder arthroplasty) is an option for treating patients with glenohumeral arthritis if younger age or a higher activity level makes implantation of a polyethylene glenoid component less desirable. The objective of this procedure is to reduce the rate of progressive glenoid erosions, arthrosis, and glenoid-side pain that is often reported following hemiarthroplasty at midterm and longer-term follow-up, while avoiding the increased risk of polyethylene wear and traditional glenoid component failure associated with younger, active patients. The biomechanical justification for soft-tissue resurfacing of the glenoid was demonstrated in a cadaver model that showed that lateral meniscal interposition reduced mean glenoid contact pressures by 10% and transferred more load to the periphery of the glenoid and away

from the glenoid center.[31] It is unclear if similar benefits would be derived from using other interposition materials. The role for glenoid recontouring (or glenoid reaming) in distributing forces across the glenoid also is unclear.

Lateral meniscus or Achilles tendon allograft, fascia lata or anterior joint capsule autograft, and dermal extracellular matrix patches have been used for glenoid resurfacing. Only small series and case reports are available on the short-term and midterm outcomes with this procedure, and results have been highly variable. Studies have described the use of anterior joint capsule, autologous fascia lata, Achilles tendon allograft or GraftJacket (Wright Medical, Arlington, VA) as the interposition material, reporting 50% excellent, 36% satisfactory, and 14% unsatisfactory results at a mean of 7 years (range, 2 to 15 years) after surgery.[32,33] Early techniques using anterior joint capsule and fascia lata resulted in persistent pain and glenoid erosions, which led to the more recent use of Achilles tendon, lateral meniscus, or dermal extracellular matrix devices.[34]

A 92% failure rate (defined as persistent pain, glenoid erosions, and loss of the joint space on radiographs) was reported in 13 shoulders treated with humeral hemiarthroplasty and Achilles tendon allograft glenoid resurfacing.[35] Other investigators have reported short-term (12- to 18-month) outcomes with mixed results using lateral meniscus allografts. Complication rates as high as 17% have been reported, with loss of graft fixation, mechanical symptoms, graft failure, recurrent pain, or progressive glenoid bone erosions sighted as the most common causes of failure.[36,37] Several reports, at 2- to 5-year follow-up, showed good functional outcomes and patient satisfaction with the

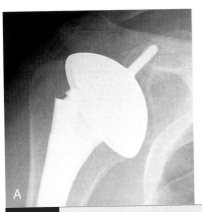
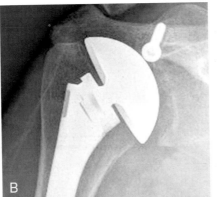
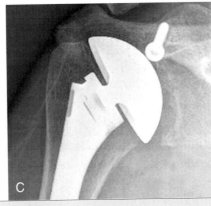

Figure 3 **A,** AP radiograph showing good joint space 2 weeks after hemiarthroplasty and glenoid resurfacing with anterior joint capsule. An opening wedge coracoid osteotomy also was done. **B,** AP radiograph 6 months postoperatively. **C,** AP radiograph 18 months postoperatively showing areas of glenoid erosion and loss of joint space despite a good clinical outcome.

procedure; however, progressive joint-space narrowing and glenoid erosion were reported, which raises concerns about the ability of this procedure to serve as a durable treatment option for the glenoid and to prevent progressive glenoid bone loss.[38,39] (Figure 3).

Despite these unresolved questions, hemiarthroplasty with glenoid soft-tissue resurfacing is still considered a reasonable treatment option for a young patient with end-stage arthritis. Current recommendations to minimize the risk of complications are to avoid the use of anterior joint capsule or fascia lata, appropriately prepare the glenoid surface to create a healing environment for the graft, delay range-of-motion exercises, and select fewer high-demand patients for the procedure.

Total Shoulder Arthroplasty

Total shoulder arthroplasty has consistently achieved good pain relief and improved function in patients with glenohumeral posttraumatic arthritis, inflammatory arthritis, and OA with short-term, midterm, and long-term follow-up; however, functional outcomes are usually more modest in patients with posttraumatic and inflammatory arthritis than in those with OA. Both cemented and press-fit humeral components have shown good longevity and a low incidence of loosening.[40,41] Glenoid component wear and glenoid loosening continue to present a clinical challenge and are the main source of failures, recurrent pain, and the need for revision surgery after total shoulder arthroplasty.

Several clinical studies have recently reported the presence of progressive radiolucent lines around the glenoid component and/or glenoid component settling in 50% of patients as early as 3 to 4 years after total shoulder arthroplasty.[40,42] The presence of radiographic glenoid lucencies or glenoid seating did not correlate with poor patient functional outcomes or pain at 3- to 7-year follow-up.

Recent data suggest that pegged glenoid designs instead of keeled designs, and cross-linked ultra-high–molecular-weight polyethylene may reduce the rate of glenoid failure and improve the survivorship of total shoulder arthroplasties. In cyclic mechanical testing, cross-linked ultra-high–molecular-weight polyethylene demonstrated an 85% reduction in the glenoid polyethylene wear rate compared with a conventional, non–cross-linked glenoid component.[43] With similar particulate size and morphology of the wear debris from both the cross-linked and non–cross-linked components, the osteolytic potential should be similar on a per volume basis, resulting in a theoretic 85% reduction in clinically observed glenoid lucency secondary to polyethylene wear.

A recent study evaluating the 5- to 15-year clinical and radiographic outcomes of total shoulder arthroplasty with different glenoid component designs showed the lowest failure rates at 5 years when using cemented peg glenoid designs (99% survival) compared with cemented keeled or metal-backed designs.[44] Uncemented, metal-backed keeled glenoid designs have shown the highest rates of glenoid lucencies,[45,46] which likely result from the combination of backside wear between the metal and the polyethylene, and the inferior mechanical stability of the keeled component design and the bone-component interface.[47] Because pegged glenoid designs and cross-linked ultra-high–molecular-weight polyethylene have only been used in shoulder arthroplasty in recent years, long-term follow-up is not yet available to determine if these advances will lead to reduced failure and revision rates.

Rotator Cuff Tear Arthropathy

Rotator cuff tear arthropathy (RCTA) is a pathoanatomic condition described during the 1800s.[48] In 1983, Neer et al[49] provided a thorough description of this entity, which included both mechanical and nutritional responses in the shoulder, leading to the subsequent development of arthritis in the setting of massive attritional rotator cuff tearing (Figure 4). The pathogenesis of this disorder is unknown despite previous theories. However, evidence suggests that RCTA is a

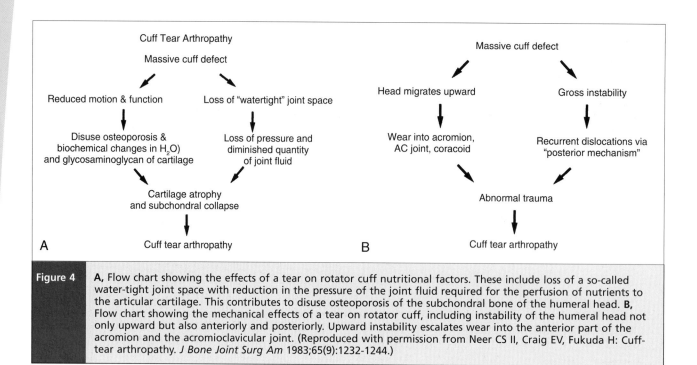

Figure 4 **A,** Flow chart showing the effects of a tear on rotator cuff nutritional factors. These include loss of a so-called water-tight joint space with reduction in the pressure of the joint fluid required for the perfusion of nutrients to the articular cartilage. This contributes to disuse osteoporosis of the subchondral bone of the humeral head. **B,** Flow chart showing the mechanical effects of a tear on rotator cuff, including instability of the humeral head not only upward but also anteriorly and posteriorly. Upward instability escalates wear into the anterior part of the acromion and the acromioclavicular joint. (Reproduced with permission from Neer CS II, Craig EV, Fukuda H: Cuff-tear arthropathy. *J Bone Joint Surg Am* 1983;65(9):1232-1244.)

crystalline-induced arthropathy in which synovial fluid–based matrix degradation proteins act to degrade tendons and cartilage. Calcium phosphate crystal deposition has been reported in end-stage disease. Characteristics of RCTA include massive chronic rotator cuff tears, glenohumeral cartilage destruction, subchondral bone osteoporosis, and humeral head collapse. This disease process usually occurs in the dominant shoulder, with a mean patient age of 69 years and a 3:1 female predominance. Classic physical findings include shoulder effusions, painful arcs of motion, spinati atrophy, and weakness in rotation; late-stage findings include pseudoparalysis with the inability to raise the arm. Radiographic findings include acromial acetabularization, femoralization of the humeral head, eccentric superior glenoid wear, lack of typical peripheral osteophytes of OA, osteopenia, subarticular sclerosis (snowcap sign), and loss of the coracoacromial arch (anterosuperior escape). MRI is not routinely necessary for the diagnosis.

A classification scheme has been developed[50] to categorize the various radiographic stages of RCTA, which are described in Table 1. This classification scheme may guide the surgeon in the proper selection of arthroplasty reconstruction. A type II shoulder may not improve with humeral head replacement because it has lost coracoacromial arch support and is unstable and uncompensated.

Treatment of RCTA includes nonsurgical modalities such as rest, anti-inflammatory drugs, corticosteroid injections, and therapy to strengthen the deltoid. Arthroscopic treatments include extensive débridement (greater tuberosity tuberoplasty) with concomitant biceps tenotomy and/or tenodesis. Although useful, these options achieve unpredictable results.

When nonsurgical treatments fail, shoulder arthroplasty may be necessary. The objectives of reconstruction are to decrease discomfort and improve shoulder motion. The two arthroplasty options are hemiarthroplasty and reverse shoulder replacement. Traditional unconstrained total shoulder arthroplasty is contraindicated because of evidence of early glenoid loosening. Hemiarthroplasty is recommended for younger patients with RCTA who have relatively active lifestyles. Better results are achieved with maintained elevation (greater than 90°) and intact force couples.[51] An intact subscapularis appears to be key in maintaining postoperative elevation and rotation. Anatomic sizing is important to prevent joint-line lateralization and subsequent deltoid stretching. Soft-tissue balancing and repair of any residual posterior superior rotator cuff may lead to improved results. Surgical techniques include maintaining the anterior cuff and working through the superior cuff defect. The deltoid insertion and coracoacromial arch and/or ligament must be maintained to prevent anterior-superior escape. Results may deteriorate over time, with loss of motion and pain from superior glenoid erosion.[52] Specially designed hooded and/or extended coverage prostheses built to articulate with the acromion with less friction may provide improved pain relief and function; however, few well-controlled studies are available for comparison. Rehabilitation is slow, with the focus on deltoid strengthening and limited-goals outcomes.

Reverse shoulder arthroplasty is reserved for the physiologically older patient with a painful pseudoparalytic shoulder from RCTA.[53-55] Relative indications include glenohumeral arthritis with cuff tearing, failed previous cuff surgery, a massive rotator cuff tear without arthritis, proximal humerus malunions and/or nonunions, and acute four-part fractures in an elderly pa-

Table 1

Radiographic Classification of Cuff Tear Arthropathy

Type IA Centered Stable	Type IB Centered Medialized	Type IIA Decentered Limited Stable	Type IIB Decentered Unstable
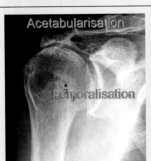	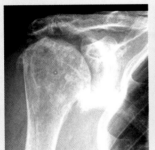	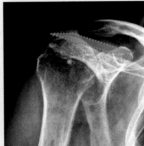	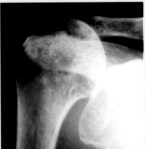
Intact anterior restraints	Intact anterior restraints	Compromised anterior restraints	Incompetent anterior structures
Minimal superior migration	Force couple intact/ compensated	Compromised force couple	Anterior superior escape
Dynamic joint stabilization	Minimal superior migration	Superior translation	Absent dynamic joint stabilization
Acetabularization of coracoacromial arch and femoralization of humeral head	Compromised dynamic joint stabilization	Insufficient dynamic joint stabilization	No stabilization by coracoacromial arch
	Medial erosion of the glenoid	Minimum stabilization by coracoacromial arch	Deficient anterior structures
	Acetabularization of coracoacromial arch	Superior-medial erosion	
	Femoralization of humeral head	Extensive acetabularization of coracoacromial arch	
		Femoralization of humeral head	

(Adapted with permission from Visotsky JL, Basamania C, Seebauer L, et al: Cuff tear arthropathy. *J Bone Joint Surg Am* 2004;86:35-40.)

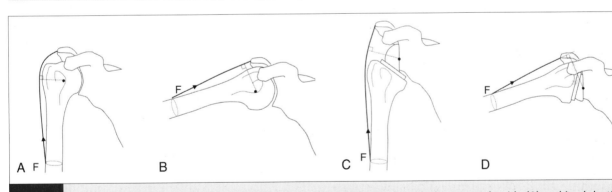

Figure 5 Center of rotation and position of the humerus and deltoid muscles with the arm at the side (**A**) and in abduction (**B**) in normal shoulder anatomy. **C** and **D**, Reverse total shoulder arthroplasty medializes the center of rotation, distalizes the humerus, and elongates the deltoid. The lever arm of the deltoid muscle (*dotted line*) is lengthened so that for any given angular displacement of the humerus, shortening of the deltoid is greater than with total shoulder arthroplasty. F = deltoid line of action. (Reproduced from Gerber C, Pennington SD, Nyffeler RW: Reverse total shoulder arthroplasty. *J Am Acad Orthop Surg* 2009;17:284-295.)

tient with osteoporosis. Reverse shoulder arthroplasty is another treatment option for the patient with failed shoulder arthroplasty, especially those with dysfunctional rotator cuffs and humeral and/or glenoid bone loss. Prerequisites for surgery include a functional deltoid, adequate glenoid bone stock for base plate implantation, and specific patient expectations. Contraindica-tions include deltoid dysfunction, chronic infection, and poor glenohumeral bone stock. With the semicon-strained reverse shoulder prosthesis, the center of rota-tion is moved inferior and medial onto the scapula to assist the deltoid fulcrum in raising the arm (Figure 5). Early results in European and American studies are very promising for improved elevation and pain relief.[53-55]

Table 2

AAOS Clinical Practice Guideline on the Treatment of Glenohumeral Arthritis

Recommendation	Strength of Recommendation
Recommend for or against physical therapy for the initial treatment of patients with osteoarthritis of the glenohumeral joint.	Inconclusive
Recommend for or against the use of pharmacotherapy in the initial treatment of patients with glenohumeral joint osteoarthritis.	Inconclusive
Recommend for or against the use of injectable corticosteroids when treating patients with glenohumeral joint osteoarthritis.	Inconclusive
The use of injectable viscosupplementation as an option when treating patients with glenohumeral joint osteoarthritis.	Weak
Recommend for or against the use of arthroscopic treatments for patients with glenohumeral joint osteoarthritis. These treatments include débridement, capsular release, chondroplasty, microfracture, removal of loose bodies, and biologic and interpositional grafts, subacromial decompression, distal clavicle resection, acromioclavicular joint resection, biceps tenotomy or tenodesis, and labral repair or advancement.	Inconclusive
Recommend for or against open débridement and/or nonprosthetic or biologic interposition arthroplasty in patients with glenohumeral joint osteoarthritis. These treatments include allograft, biologic and interpositional grafts, and autograft.	Inconclusive
Recommend for total shoulder arthroplasty and hemiarthroplasty as options when treating patients with glenohumeral joint osteoarthritis.	Weak
Recommend for total shoulder arthroplasty over hemiarthroplasty when treating patients with glenohumeral joint osteoarthritis.	Moderate
An option for reducing immediate postoperative complication rates is for patients to avoid shoulder arthroplasty by surgeons who perform fewer than two shoulder arthroplasties per year.	Weak
In the absence of reliable evidence, it is the opinion of this work group that physicians use perioperative mechanical and/or chemical venous thromboembolism prophylaxis for shoulder arthroplasty patients.	Consensus
The use of either keeled or pegged all-polyethylene cemented glenoid components are options when performing total shoulder arthroplasty.	Weak
In the absence of reliable evidence, it is the opinion of this work group that total shoulder arthroplasty not be performed in patients with glenohumeral osteoarthritis who have an irreparable rotator cuff tear.	Consensus
Recommend for or against biceps tenotomy or tenodesis when performing shoulder arthroplasty in patients who have glenohumeral joint osteoarthritis.	Inconclusive
Recommend for or against a subscapularis trans-tendonous approach or a lesser tuberosity osteotomy when performing shoulder arthroplasty in patients who have glenohumeral joint osteoarthritis.	Inconclusive
Recommend for or against a specific type of humeral prosthetic design or method of fixation when performing shoulder arthroplasty in patients with glenohumeral joint osteoarthritis.	Inconclusive
Recommend for or against physical therapy following shoulder arthroplasty	Inconclusive

(AAOS Evidence-Based Clinical Practice Guidelines: American Academy of Orthopaedic Surgeons web site. http://www.aaos.org/research/guidelines/guide.asp. Accessed August 4, 2010.)

Complications include instability, component failure, infection, and scapular notching (which may predispose the patient to base plate failure). With improved component design and postoperative rehabilitation, recent evidence suggests decreased complication rates and the maintenance of good functional outcomes (Figure 6).

Clinical Practice Guidelines

The American Academy of Orthopaedic Surgeons (AAOS) work group on the treatment of glenohumeral OA has provided a summary of clinical practice guidelines based on available evidence. A summary of these recommendations is provided in Table 2.

Future Directions

Advances in medical therapies, such as immune modulatory drugs for the treatment of inflammatory arthritis, selective cyclooxygenase-2 inhibitors, viscosupplementation, and other nonsurgical treatment options, are preventing or delaying the need for surgery. At the same time, less invasive and minimally invasive treatment strategies, including arthroscopic débridement

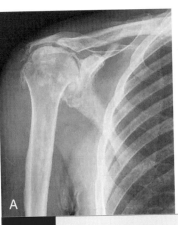
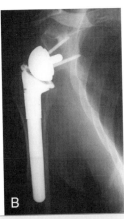

Figure 6 A, Preoperative AP radiograph of classic RCTA.
B, Postoperative AP radiograph of a reverse shoulder arthroplasty.

and osteochondral autografts, are allowing intervention at an earlier stage in the disease process to preserve the native tissues before nonrecoverable damage is done. When end-stage glenohumeral arthritis requires reconstructive procedures, many prosthetic designs and treatment strategies are available depending on the nature of the disorder. Current trends suggest that future approaches will use more extensive preoperative planning through the use of surgical simulators and advanced imaging techniques,[56,57] and intraoperative procedures will use computer-assisted navigation to optimize implant placement.[58-60] Although still in its nascent stages, the field of bioengineering will likely shift the focus of treatment strategies for end-stage shoulder pathology away from reconstructive procedures, which replace damaged tissue with inert composite materials, and toward regenerative strategies intended to restore lost or degenerated tissues through biologics.

Annotated References

1. Levy JC, Virani NA, Frankle MA, Cuff D, Pupello DR, Hamelin J: Young patients with shoulder chondrolysis following arthroscopic shoulder surgery treated with total shoulder arthroplasty. *J Shoulder Elbow Surg* 2008; 17(3):380-388.

   Total shoulder arthroplasty has been shown to improve pain and function in patients with shoulder chondrolysis after arthroscopic surgery.

2. Levy JC, Frankle M: Bilateral shoulder chondrolysis following arthroscopy: A report of two cases. *J Bone Joint Surg Am* 2008;90(11):2546-2547.

   The authors discuss two patients with bilateral shoulder chondrolysis after arthroscopy.

3. Greis PE, Legrand A, Burks RT: Bilateral shoulder chondrolysis following arthroscopy. A report of two cases. *J Bone Joint Surg Am* 2008;90(6):1338-1344.

   The authors discuss two patients with bilateral shoulder chondrolysis after arthroscopy.

4. Zhang W, Moskowitz RW, Nuki G, et al: OARSI recommendations for the management of hip and knee osteoarthritis: Part II. OARSI evidence-based, expert consensus guidelines. *Osteoarthritis Cartilage* 2008;16(2): 137-162.

   This study presents the systematic review of current guidelines and literature related to the management of lower extremity arthritis performed by 16 experts from four disciplines (rheumatology, orthopaedics, primary care, and evidence-based medicine).

5. Burbank KM, Stevenson JH, Czarnecki GR, Dorfman J: Chronic shoulder pain: Part II. Treatment. *Am Fam Physician* 2008;77(4):493-497.

   Review of general practice guidelines for initial nonsurgical treatment of common causes of shoulder pain.

6. Smidt N, de Vet HC, Bouter LM, et al; Exercise Therapy Group: Effectiveness of exercise therapy: A best-evidence summary of systematic reviews. *Aust J Physiother* 2005;51(2):71-85.

7. Kelly RB: Acupuncture for pain. *Am Fam Physician* 2009;80(5):481-484.

   A syystematic literature review on the use of acupuncture for treatment of musculoskeletal pain and pain syndromes is presented. The author's analysis of available literature suggests some potential benefits may be seen with the use of acupuncture to treat shoulder pain, although definitive data are lacking.

8. Wang ZL, Chen LF, Zhu WM: Observation on the transient analgesic effect of abdominal acupuncture TENS on pain of neck, shoulder, loin and legs. *Zhongguo Zhen Jiu* 2007;27(9):657-659.

   One hundred twenty patients with neck, shoulder, or leg pain were randomized into four groups to receive different modalities of combined acupuncture and transcutaneous electrical nerve stimulation (TENS) treatment for musculoskeletal pain. Visual analog scores were measured before and after treatment. Patients receiving abdominal acupuncture and TENS treatment saw significantly better transient reductions in pain as compared to other acupuncture/TENS treatment modalities.

9. Vas J, Ortega C, Olmo V, et al: Single-point acupuncture and physiotherapy for the treatment of painful shoulder: A multicentre randomized controlled trial. *Rheumatology (Oxford)* 2008;47(6):887-893.

   A randomized controlled trial evaluating the efficacy of acupuncture in the treatment of shoulder pain arising from the subacromial space is described. The authors found that acupuncture was effective in reducing pain and the consumption of analgesic medication.

10. Vance CG, Radhakrishnan R, Skyba DA, Sluka KA: Transcutaneous electrical nerve stimulation at both high and low frequencies reduces primary hyperalgesia in rats with joint inflammation in a time-dependent manner. *Phys Ther* 2007;87(1):44-51.

The authors studied Sprague-Dawley rats with intra-articular injection and chemically induced knee inflammation as a model for joint pain. Sham TENS application, low-frequency (4-Hz) TENS, and high-frequency (100-Hz) TENS were applied to the affected knee at 4 hours, 24 hours, and 2 weeks after injection. Low- and high-frequency TENS application both reduced the withdrawl from pain response at 24 hours and 2 weeks as compared to placebo (sham) treatment.

11. Zhang W, Jones A, Doherty M: Does paracetamol (acetaminophen) reduce the pain of osteoarthritis? A meta-analysis of randomised controlled trials. *Ann Rheum Dis* 2004;63(8):901-907.

12. Blaine T, Moskowitz R, Udell J, et al: Treatment of persistent shoulder pain with sodium hyaluronate: A randomized, controlled trial. A multicenter study. *J Bone Joint Surg Am* 2008;90(5):970-979.

The authors present the results of a randomized controlled trial of three or five hyaluronate injections versus placebo to treat arthritic pain, adhesive capsulitis, or rotator cuff pathology. Hyaluronate injections were effective in reducing pain for patients with arthritis but not for those with adhesive capsulitis or rotator cuff pathology.

13. Gogus A, Ozturk C: Osteochondritis dissecans of the glenoid cavity: A case report. *Arch Orthop Trauma Surg* 2008;128(5):457-460.

A case report of a 60-year-old woman with shoulder pain and an articular cartilage flap overlying a cystic glenoid lesion who was treated with arthroscopic debridement of the loose flap and microfracture of the glenoid is presented. At 4 years after surgery, the patient reported full motion and no pain. Level of evidence: IV.

14. Koike Y, Komatsuda T, Sato K: Osteochondritis dissecans of the glenoid associated with the nontraumatic, painful throwing shoulder in a professional baseball player: A case report. *J Shoulder Elbow Surg* 2008; 17(5):e9-e12.

The authors discuss a case report of a 22-year-old male baseball pitcher who underwent joint débridement and microfracture of a full-thickness glenoid cartilage defect. The patient returned to training 4 months after surgery. Japan Shoulder Society and Constant scores improved from 43 to 88 and from 86 to 98, respectively. Further follow-up and ability to return to competitive pitching was not reported. Level of evidence: IV. ain. Level of evidence: IV.

15. Kerr BJ, McCarty EC: Outcome of arthroscopic débridement is worse for patients with glenohumeral arthritis of both sides of the joint. *Clin Orthop Relat Res* 2008;466(3):634-638.

The authors describe their retrospective review of 19 patients (20 shoulders) with shoulder arthritis who were treated arthroscopically. The patients were age 55 years or younger. Focal, full-thickness defects are effectively managed with débridement and microfracture; however, patients with involvement of both sides of the joint have worse outcomes. Level of evidence: IV.

16. Romeo AA, Cole BJ, Mazzocca AD, Fox JA, Freeman KB, Joy E: Autologous chondrocyte repair of an articular defect in the humeral head. *Arthroscopy* 2002;18(8): 925-929.

17. Kircher J, Patzer T, Magosch P, Lichtenberg S, Habermeyer P: Osteochondral autologous transplantation for the treatment of full-thickness cartilage defects of the shoulder: Results at nine years. *J Bone Joint Surg Br* 2009;91(4):499-503.

Reported outcomes at 8 years postoperatively of seven patients treated with osteochondral autologous transplantation for full-thickness cartilage defects of the shoulder are presented. Assessments were made using the Constant score, radiographs, and MRI.

18. Cameron BD, Galatz LM, Ramsey ML, Williams GR, Iannotti JP: Non-prosthetic management of grade IV osteochondral lesions of the glenohumeral joint. *J Shoulder Elbow Surg* 2002;11(1):25-32.

19. Richards DP, Burkhart SS: Arthroscopic debridement and capsular release for glenohumeral osteoarthritis. *Arthroscopy* 2007;23(9):1019-1022.

The authors present a case-series of eight patients with a diagnosis of glenohumeral arthritis treated with arthroscopic capsular release and joint débridement. The mean postoperative range of motion improved by 22° of forward flexion, 16° of external rotation, and 31° of internal rotation. Patients also reported decreased pain. The surgical technique is described. Level of evidence: IV.

20. Bailie DS, Llinas PJ, Ellenbecker TS: Cementless humeral resurfacing arthroplasty in active patients less than fifty-five years of age. *J Bone Joint Surg Am* 2008; 90(1):110-117.

A review of young patients with arthritis treated with hemiarthroplasty and multiple other ancillary procedures is presented. Good outcomes with regard to function and pain were reported at 3-year follow-up.

21. Uribe JW, Botto-van Bemden A: Partial humeral head resurfacing for osteonecrosis. *J Shoulder Elbow Surg* 2009;18(5):711-716.

Partial humeral head resurfacing had successful results in advanced focal osteonecrosis in patients with a mean age of 56 years and average follow-up of 30 months.

22. Levy O, Copeland SA: Cementless surface replacement arthroplasty (Copeland CSRA) for osteoarthritis of the shoulder. *J Shoulder Elbow Surg* 2004;13(3):266-271.

23. Raiss P, Kasten P, Baumann F, Moser M, Rickert M, Loew M: Treatment of osteonecrosis of the humeral head with cementless surface replacement arthroplasty. *J Bone Joint Surg Am* 2009;91(2):340-349.

Cementless surface replacement arthroplasty provides good functional results as a bone-preserving procedure in humeral heads with osteonecrosis and up to 31% bone loss.

24. Lo IK, Litchfield RB, Griffin S, Faber K, Patterson SD, Kirkley A: Quality-of-life outcome following hemiar-

throplasty or total shoulder arthroplasty in patients with osteoarthritis: A prospective, randomized trial. *J Bone Joint Surg Am* 2005;87(10):2178-2185.

25. Raiss P, Aldinger PR, Kasten P, Rickert M, Loew M: Total shoulder replacement in young and middle-aged patients with glenohumeral osteoarthritis. *J Bone Joint Surg Br* 2008;90(6):764-769.

    The authors evaluated the outcome of total shoulder replacement in young and middle-aged patients with glenohumeral arthritis and found a low rate of complications and excellent results.

26. Pfahler M, Jena F, Neyton L, Sirveaux F, Molé D: Hemiarthroplasty versus total shoulder prosthesis: Results of cemented glenoid components. *J Shoulder Elbow Surg* 2006;15(2):154-163.

27. Wirth MA, Tapscott RS, Southworth C, Rockwood CA Jr: Treatment of glenohumeral arthritis with a hemiarthroplasty: A minimum five-year follow-up outcome study. *J Bone Joint Surg Am* 2006;88(5):964-973.

28. Lynch JR, Franta AK, Montgomery WH Jr, Lenters TR, Mounce D, Matsen FA III: Self-assessed outcome at two to four years after shoulder hemiarthroplasty with concentric glenoid reaming. *J Bone Joint Surg Am* 2007; 89(6):1284-1292.

    Patients with a mean age of 57 years treated with hemiarthroplasty with concentric glenoid reaming showed improved self-assessment shoulder scores for comfort and function at a minimum 2-year follow-up. Twenty-two of 37 patients maintained radiographic joint space.

29. Carroll RM, Izquierdo R, Vazquez M, Blaine TA, Levine WN, Bigliani LU: Conversion of painful hemiarthroplasty to total shoulder arthroplasty: Long-term results. *J Shoulder Elbow Surg* 2004;13(6):599-603.

30. Radnay CS, Setter KJ, Chambers L, Levine WN, Bigliani LU, Ahmad CS: Total shoulder replacement compared with humeral head replacement for the treatment of primary glenohumeral osteoarthritis: A systematic review. *J Shoulder Elbow Surg* 2007;16(4):396-402.

    This systematic review provides evidence that total shoulder replacement significantly improves pain relief, range of motion, and patient satisfaction and has a lower rate of revision surgery when compared with hemiarthroplasty.

31. Creighton RA, Cole BJ, Nicholson GP, Romeo AA, Lorenz EP: Effect of lateral meniscus allograft on shoulder articular contact areas and pressures. *J Shoulder Elbow Surg* 2007;16(3):367-372.

    The authors present a cadaver biomechanical study of the influence of lateral meniscus transplant on glenoid contact area and contact pressures under compressive loads of 220N and 440N. A statistically significant decrease in total force was seen at 220N and 440N of loading, and decreased contact area was seen at 220N loading when comparing glenoid loading with meniscal allograft to glenoid loading without glenoid allograft.

32. Burkhead WZ Jr, Krishnan SG, Lin KC: Biologic resurfacing of the arthritic glenohumeral joint: Historical review and current applications. *J Shoulder Elbow Surg* 2007;16(5, suppl)S248-S253.

    A historical review of the use of interposition resurfacing arthroplasties in orthopaedics is presented, as well as current surgical techniques for soft-tissue resurfacing of the glenoid. Clinical outcomes from 5- to 13-year follow-up from a select case series are reported. Level of evidence: IV.

33. Krishnan SG, Nowinski RJ, Harrison D, Burkhead WZ: Humeral hemiarthroplasty with biologic resurfacing of the glenoid for glenohumeral arthritis: Two to fifteen-year outcomes. *J Bone Joint Surg Am* 2007;89(4):727-734.

    A case series is discussed describing the surgical technique and outcomes of 36 patients treated with humeral hemiarthroplasty and biologic glenoid resurfacing for a diagnosis of glenohumeral arthritis. Three different glenoid resurfacing materials were investigated: anterior joint capsule (19%), fascia lata (31%), and Achilles tendon allograft (50%). Pain relief was excellent or good in 86% of patients, and increased activity levels and range of motion were reported at most recent follow-up (minimum 2 years). Poor outcomes were associated with use of anterior joint capsule as an interposition material.

34. Krishnan SG, Reineck JR, Nowinski RJ, Harrison D, Burkhead WZ: Humeral hemiarthroplasty with biologic resurfacing of the glenoid for glenohumeral arthritis: Surgical technique. *J Bone Joint Surg Am* 2008;90(suppl 2, pt 1):9-19.

    The surgical technique and concepts used when performing hemiarthroplasty and biologic glenoid resurfacing are described.

35. Elhassan B, Ozbaydar M, Diller D, Higgins LD, Warner JJ: Soft-tissue resurfacing of the glenoid in the treatment of glenohumeral arthritis in active patients less than fifty years old. *J Bone Joint Surg Am* 2009;91(2):419-424.

    The authors retrospectively reviewed 13 shoulders in patients with a mean age of 34 years treated with hemiarthroplasty and biologic resurfacing of the glenoid. A 92% failure rate was reported.

36. Nicholson GP, Goldstein JL, Romeo AA, et al: Lateral meniscus allograft biologic glenoid arthroplasty in total shoulder arthroplasty for young shoulders with degenerative joint disease. *J Shoulder Elbow Surg* 2007;16(5, suppl)S261-S266.

    In a case series, 30 patients (ages 18 to 52 years) underwent humeral hemiarthroplasty and glenoid resurfacing with lateral meniscus allograft for treatment of multiple etiologies of glenohumeral arthrosis. Ninety-four percent of patients said they would have the procedure again. Average American Shoulder and Elbow Surgeons score increased from 38 to 69 points. A 17% complication rate was reported during the first year, all of which required re-operation. Duration of postoperative follow-up was not given. Level of evidence: IV.

3: Upper Extremity

37. Ellenbecker TS, Bailie DS, Lamprecht D: Humeral resurfacing hemiarthroplasty with meniscal allograft in a young patient with glenohumeral osteoarthritis. *J Orthop Sports Phys Ther* 2008;38(5):277-286.

In this case report, a 36-year-old male manual laborer underwent humeral hemiarthroplasty and meniscal allograft glenoid resurfacing for postinstability glenohumeral arthritis. A detailed description of the postoperative rehabilitation program is presented. American Shoulder and Elbow Surgeons scores improved from 17 preoperation to 85 at 1 year postoperation but decreased to 68 at 2-year follow-up. Level of evidence: IV.

38. Lee KT, Bell S, Salmon J: Cementless surface replacement arthroplasty of the shoulder with biologic resurfacing of the glenoid. *J Shoulder Elbow Surg* 2009;18(6):915-919.

In this retrospective case series, 18 patients (mean age, 55 years) were treated with humeral head surface replacement and biologic glenoid resurfacing. At a mean follow-up of 4.8 years, 83% of patients were satisfied with their results. Radiographic examination demonstrated moderate to severe glenoid erosions in 55% of shoulders. Level of evidence: IV.

39. Wirth MA: Humeral head arthroplasty and meniscal allograft resurfacing of the glenoid. *J Bone Joint Surg Am* 2009;91(5):1109-1119.

In this case series, 27 patients were followed for a minimum of 2 years (mean, 3 years) following humeral hemiarthroplasty and meniscal allograft glenoid resurfacing for treatment of glenohumeral arthritis. Function and pain were significantly improved from their preoperative status at last follow-up. Progressive glenoid joint space narrowing but no glenoid erosions were observed radiographically. Level of evidence: IV.

40. Raiss P, Aldinger PR, Kasten P, Rickert M, Loew M: Total shoulder replacement in young and middle-aged patients with glenohumeral osteoarthritis. *J Bone Joint Surg Br* 2008;90(6):764-769.

A review of 21 patients treated with total shoulder arthroplasty at a mean age of 55 years old is presented. The authors report good functional outcomes and pain relief; however, there was a 48% rate of glenoid lucent lines at 51-month follow-up.

41. Cil A, Veillette CJ, Sanchez-Sotelo J, Sperling JW, Schleck C, Cofield RH: Revision of the humeral component for aseptic loosening in arthroplasty of the shoulder. *J Bone Joint Surg Br* 2009;91(1):75-81.

Thirty-eight humeral components were revised for loosening over a 28-year period at a high-volume shoulder reconstruction service. Revision humeral stems were cemented in 29 and press-fit in 9. Humeral component survivorship was 89% at 10 years after revision, with one humeral component demonstrating recurrent loosening. Level of evidence: III.

42. Levy JC, Virani NA, Frankle MA, Cuff D, Pupello DR, Hamelin JA: Young patients with shoulder chondrolysis following arthroscopic shoulder surgery treated with total shoulder arthroplasty. *J Shoulder Elbow Surg* 2008; 17(3):380-388.

Eleven shoulders with chondrolysis were reviewed to evaluate the etiology and assess functional and radiographic outcomes after total shoulder arthroplasty. Functional outcomes were good at 3 years, but high rates of glenoid lucency and seating were observed.

43. Wirth MA, Klotz C, Deffenbaugh DL, McNulty D, Richards L, Tipper JL: Cross-linked glenoid prosthesis: A wear comparison to conventional glenoid prosthesis with wear particulate analysis. *J Shoulder Elbow Surg* 2009;18(1):130-137.

Biomechanical testing of cross-linked and conventional glenoid polyethylene was performed. Cross-linked glenoid polyethylene showed an 85% reduction in volume of particulate debris generated, with similar particulate size and morphology compared with conventional glenoid components.

44. Fox TJ, Cil A, Sperling JW, Sanchez-Sotelo J, Schleck CD, Cofield RH: Survival of the glenoid component in shoulder arthroplasty. *J Shoulder Elbow Surg* 2009; 18(6):859-863.

The authors present the results of a retrospective review of 1,542 total shoulder arthroplasties performed with several different glenoid component designs between 1984 and 2004. Cemented, all-polyethylene, and pegged glenoid components had the lowest rate of revision surgery for glenoid failure.

45. Taunton MJ, McIntosh AL, Sperling JW, Cofield RH: Total shoulder arthroplasty with a metal-backed, bone-ingrowth glenoid component: Medium to long-term results. *J Bone Joint Surg Am* 2008;90(10):2180-2188.

Retrospective review of 83 total shoulder arthroplasties performed with metal-back, press-fit ingrowth glenoid components. Mean clinical follow-up was 9.5 years. Five-year glenoid survival rate was 71.6%, and 10-year survival rate was 51.9%. Excessive polyethylene and metal wear with glenoid loosening was the common cause of failure. Level of evidence: III.

46. Tammachote N, Sperling JW, Vathana T, Cofield RH, Harmsen WS, Schleck CD: Long-term results of cemented metal-backed glenoid components for osteoarthritis of the shoulder. *J Bone Joint Surg Am* 2009; 91(1):160-166.

Retrospective review of 95 total shoulder arthroplasties performed with cemented metal-backed glenoid components. At minimum follow-up of 2 years, two glenoids were revised for loosening, and one was revised for periprosthetic lucency. Eighty-three percent of shoulders demonstrated radiographic evidence of periprosthetic glenoid lucency. Level of evidence: III.

47. Pelletier MH, Langdown A, Gillies RM, Sonnabend DH, Walsh WR: Photoelastic comparison of strains in the underlying glenoid with metal-backed and all-polyethylene implants. *J Shoulder Elbow Surg* 2008; 17(5):779-783.

A biomechanical study comparing cortical glenoid shear strain measurements with uncemented, keeled metal-backed glenoid components and cemented, all-polyethylene pegged glenoid components was performed. Loading was performed in 0°, 30°, 60°, and 90° of abduction. Uncemented, keeled metal-backed components demonstrated higher cortical strains than cemented all-polyethylene pegged components.

48. Frankle MA, ed: *Rotator Cuff Deficiency of the Shoulder.* New York, NY, Thieme, 2008.

    This comprehensive text covers the pathomechanics and pathophysiology, and diagnostic and treatment options for rotator cuff pathology. Level of evidence: V.

49. Neer CS II, Craig EV, Fukuda H: Cuff-tear arthropathy. *J Bone Joint Surg Am* 1983;65(9):1232-1244.

50. Visotsky JL, Basamania C, Seebauer L, Rockwood CA, Jensen KL: Cuff tear arthropathy: Pathogenesis, classification, and algorithm for treatment. *J Bone Joint Surg Am* 2004;86(suppl 2):35-40.

51. Goldberg SS, Bell JE, Kim HJ, Bak SF, Levine WN, Bigliani LU: Hemiarthroplasty for the rotator cuff-deficient shoulder. *J Bone Joint Surg Am* 2008;90(3):554-559.

    Hemiarthroplasty for arthritic, cuff-deficient shoulders can provide good long-term results, especially in those with maintained elevation of more than 90°. A low complication rate was noted in the 34 shoulders reviewed.

52. Sanchez-Sotelo J, Cofield RH, Rowland CM: Shoulder hemiarthroplasty for glenohumeral arthritis associated with severe rotator cuff deficiency. *J Bone Joint Surg Am* 2001;83(12):1814-1822.

53. Wall B, Nové-Josserand L, O'Connor DP, Edwards TB, Walch G: Reverse total shoulder arthroplasty: A review of results according to etiology. *J Bone Joint Surg Am* 2007;89(7):1476-1485.

    The authors showed, in a large cohort of 191 patients, that reverse shoulder arthroplasty can produce good functional results for multiple complex shoulder disorders in addition to RCTA. Higher complication rates were reported in the revision arthroplasty group and in patients with posttraumatic arthritis. The mean follow-up was 39.9 months.

54. Boileau P, Gonzalez JF, Chuinard C, Bicknell R, Walch G: Reverse total shoulder arthroplasty after failed rotator cuff surgery. *J Shoulder Elbow Surg* 2009;18(4):600-606.

    Reverse shoulder arthroplasty provided improved functional results in 40 patients after failed rotator cuff surgery. The mean follow-up was 50 months, with a 12% complication rate.

55. Werner CM, Steinmann PA, Gilbart M, Gerber C: Treatment of painful pseudoparesis due to irreparable rotator cuff dysfunction with the Delta III reverse-ball-and-socket total shoulder prosthesis. *J Bone Joint Surg Am* 2005;87(7):1476-1486.

56. Hoenecke HR Jr, Hermida JC, Dembitsky N, Patil S, D'Lima DD: Optimizing glenoid component position using three-dimensional computed tomography reconstruction. *J Shoulder Elbow Surg* 2008;17(4):637-641.

    Computer-based virtual implantation of 3 glenoid implant designs (keel, standard pegs, and modified pegs) was performed into 40 glenoid vault CT scans. The ability to implant the glenoid component without perforation of the glenoid vault and still correct for glenoid retroversion was greatest with a modified peg design. Retroverted glenoid components were well tolerated.

57. Scalise JJ, Codsi MJ, Bryan J, Iannotti JP: The three-dimensional glenoid vault model can estimate normal glenoid version in osteoarthritis. *J Shoulder Elbow Surg* 2008;17(3):487-491.

    Preoperative templating using CT scan–based three-dimensional reconstruction in a surgical simulator allows accurate assessment of glenoid version and bone loss.

58. Kircher J, Wiedemann M, Magosch P, Lichtenberg S, Habermeyer P: Improved accuracy of glenoid positioning in total shoulder arthroplasty with intraoperative navigation: A prospective-randomized clinical study. *J Shoulder Elbow Surg* 2009;18(4):515-520.

    In a small, prospective randomized clinical study, two groups (10 patients in each group) were assessed. Intraoperative navigation resulted in greater correction of glenoid retroversion at the time of total shoulder arthroplasty based on preoperative and postoperative CT. Level of evidence: II.

59. Nguyen D, Ferreira LM, Brownhill JR, et al: Improved accuracy of computer assisted glenoid implantation in total shoulder arthroplasty: An in-vitro randomized controlled trial. *J Shoulder Elbow Surg* 2009;18(6):907-914.

    Sixteen paired cadaver shoulders were randomized to two groups and underwent glenoid component implantation either with or without computer-assisted navigation. Computer-navigated glenoid implantation was more accurate at reproducing the planned glenoid position determined during preoperative templating. Non-navigated glenoid implantation trended toward increased glenoid retroversion.

60. Edwards TB, Gartsman GM, O'Connor DP, Sarin VK: Safety and utility of computer-aided shoulder arthroplasty. *J Shoulder Elbow Surg* 2008;17(3):503-508.

    The authors discuss a case series of 27 patients who underwent implantation of total shoulder arthroplasty using an image-free navigation system. No navigation-related complications were reported. The navigation system was safe and provided real-time information on the patient-specific anatomy and angles of resection and reaming. Level of evidence: IV.

3: Upper Extremity

Chapter 24

Shoulder Instability and Rotator Cuff Tears

Charles L. Getz, MD   Jonathan E. Buzzell, MD   Sumant G. Krishnan, MD

[handwritten annotation: glenoid — labrum — capsule + thickening in capsule = GH ligament]

Shoulder Instability

The pathologic increase in glenohumeral motion is a common disorder in physically active patients. Diagnosis and treatment of patients with shoulder instability continues to evolve with a better understanding of pathology and treatment outcomes.

Anatomy

Shoulder stability is the end result of the shoulder stabilizing structures working properly together. The constraints on shoulder motion can be divided into static stabilizers and dynamic stabilizers (Table 1).

Static stability is chiefly maintained by joint congruency, the labrum, and the shoulder ligaments. The glenohumeral joint is a ball and shallow socket joint with a constant mismatch between the radii of curvatures. The unconstrained bony relationship allows the shoulder to obtain a large excursion and range of motion. The glenoid socket is deepened by the glenoid labrum,

Dr. Getz or an immediate family member has received research or institutional support from Zimmer, Smith & Nephew, Johnson & Johnson, and Biomet. Dr. Krishnan or an immediate family member serves as a board member, owner, officer, or committee member of the American Shoulder and Elbow Surgeons and the Arthroscopy Association of North America; has received royalties from Innovation Sports, Tornier, and TAG Medical; is a member of a speakers' bureau or has made paid presentations on behalf of Mitek and Tornier; serves as a paid consultant to or is an employee of Tornier and TAG Medical; has received research or institutional support from Wolters Kluwer Health—Lippincott Williams & Wilkins, Mitek, Tornier, and TAG Medical; has stock or stock options held in Johnson & Johnson, Pfizer, and Merck; and has received nonincome support (such as equipment or services), commercially derived honoraria, or other non–research-related funding (such as paid travel) from Mitek and Tornier. Neither Dr. Buzzell nor any immediate family member has received anything of value from or owns stock in a commercial company or institution related directly or indirectly to the subject of this chapter.

which is made of fibrocartilage. The labrum serves as the attachment site for the glenohumeral capsule and biceps tendon, and decreases the glenoid radius of curvature to more closely match the humeral curvature. Discrete thickening of the capsule in consistent locations form the glenohumeral ligaments (Figure 1). The glenohumeral capsule connects to the humerus at the rotator cuff insertion and inferiorly onto the humeral neck.[1]

The main dynamic stabilizers are the rotator cuff, scapulothoracic rhythm, and the long head of the biceps. The neurologic feedback that connects the dynamic stabilizers to each other and to the static stabilizers is called proprioception. A dysfunction of any of the stabilizers can lead to instability, dysfunction, and pain in the shoulder. The rotator cuff consists of four muscles (subscapularis, supraspinatus, infraspinatus, and teres minor) whose tendons coalesce to dynamically stabilize the humeral head in the center of the glenoid cavity throughout the full range of shoulder motion by generating force couples in the coronal and transverse planes of the glenohumeral joint.[2,3] Loss of the coronal plane force couple results in superior head migration, but not necessarily loss of function. Disruption of the transverse force couple can result in pain and loss of function.

Biomechanics

The ligaments of the shoulder limit the extremes of motion. The labrum acts as a wedge to limit sliding and increases the wall height to prevent dislocation.[4] When the arm is abducted and externally rotated, the anteroinferior glenohumeral ligament is stretched. An anterior dislocation can occur with a failure of the anterior stabilizing structures, from the anterior glenoid rim, labrum, capsule (ligaments), or humeral insertion.

With the arm in the adducted, forward flexed position, a force applied to the arm stresses the posterior glenoid, posterior labrum, and posterior capsule. Posterior dislocation or subluxation of the joint results in an injury to one or more of these structures. Repetitive submaximal stress to the ligaments can produce a pathologic increase in joint range of motion. The subsequent atraumatic instability pattern often is associated with generalized laxity, instability in multiple planes, abnormal proprioception, and scapulohumeral rhythm dysfunction.

3: Upper Extremity

Table 1

Static and Dynamic Constraints to Joint Instability

Type	Subtypes
Static	
Osteochondral	Proximal humerus: articular surface (Hill-Sachs lesion, posttraumatic defect, osteonecrosis), abnormal humeral version Glenoid: articular surface; bony defect, fracture, or erosion; abnormal morphology (dysplasia); abnormal glenoid version
Capsulolabral complex	Glenoid labrum Glenohumeral ligaments Coracohumeral ligament
Coracoacromial ligament	
Negative intra-articular pressure	
Synovial fluid adhesion-cohesion	
Rotator cuff	
Dynamic	
Rotator cuff	
Long head of biceps	
Scapulothoracic rhythm	
Concavity-compression	
Proprioception	

(Reproduced from Costouros JG, Warner JP: Classification, clinical assessment, and imaging of glenohumeral instability, in Galatz, LM, ed: *Orthopaedic Knowledge Update: Shoulder and Elbow 3*. Rosemont, IL, American Academy of Orthopaedic Surgeons, 2008, pp 67-81.)

[handwritten margin notes: "RTC in both categories]"

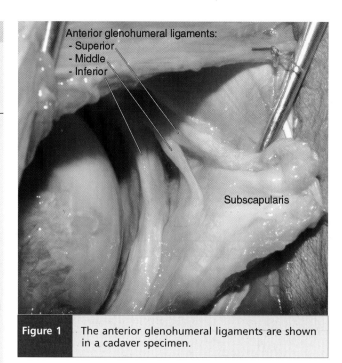

Figure 1 The anterior glenohumeral ligaments are shown in a cadaver specimen.

[image labels: Anterior glenohumeral ligaments: - Superior, - Middle, - Inferior; Subscapularis]

The role of glenoid bone loss in patients with recurrent anterior instability has received considerable recent attention. Anterior glenoid bone loss of up to 25% was classically treated with open soft-tissue repair.[5] Reports of higher rates of recurrent instability after arthroscopic repairs in patients with substantial bone loss has heightened interest in this problem.[6] A biomechanical study has shown a significant decrease in anterior shoulder stability with bone loss of at least 21% of the glenoid.[7]

The type of anterior glenoid bone loss may also play a role in treatment. Patients with recent onset of recurrent dislocations will likely have identifiable bone at the time of repair. Patients with long-standing instability will likely have resorption of the bone and blunting of the glenoid margin.[8] Humeral bone loss from a Hill-Sachs lesion or reverse Hill-Sachs lesion can contribute to instability because the glenoid can fall into the humeral head defect. The location and size of these engaging lesions and the importance of the lesions in regard

[handwritten margin notes: "aka, humeral Hill-Sachs lesion can engage in glenoid Bony ant defect"]

to anterior bone loss continues to be explored.

As previously stated, the rotator cuff provides dynamic shoulder stability by generating force couples in the coronal and transverse planes of the glenohumeral joint (**Figure 2**). A force couple is composed of two equal but oppositely directed forces that act simultaneously on opposite sides of an axis of rotation. Translational forces are cancelled out, linear motion is eliminated, and torque is produced. Loss of the coronal plane force couple results in superior head migration, but not necessarily loss of function. The transverse force couple is composed of the subscapularis anteriorly and the infraspinatus/teres minor posteriorly, and provides anterior-posterior glenohumeral stability throughout active elevation. Disruption of the transverse force couple results in loss of concavity compression, a pathologic increase in translation or subluxation of the humeral head toward the cuff deficiency, and decreased active abduction.

The functions of the long head of the biceps tendon, described as the fifth tendon of the rotator cuff,[9] are proposed to involve shoulder flexion, abduction, and glenohumeral joint stabilization during rotation. One study provided radiographic evidence of the superior stabilizing effect of the biceps tendon,[10] and another study evaluated biceps activity electromyographically during 10 basic shoulder motions and reported very little biceps activity.[11] Although its functional contributions are debated, painful lesions of the biceps tendon can coexist with rotator cuff tears.[12]

Classification

Instability can be classified into categories based on timing, etiology, and the direction of instability. Instability can be acute or insidious in onset, can occur after

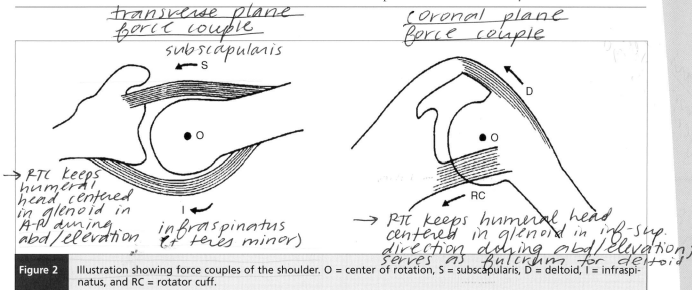

transverse plane force couple (handwritten)
coronal plane force couple (handwritten)

subscapularis (handwritten)

→ RTC keeps humeral head centered in glenoid in A-P during abd/elevation (handwritten)

infraspinatus (+ teres minor) (handwritten)

→ RTC keeps humeral head centered in glenoid in inf-sup. direction during abd/elevation; serves as fulcrum for deltoid (handwritten)

Figure 2 Illustration showing force couples of the shoulder. O = center of rotation, S = subscapularis, D = deltoid, I = infraspinatus, and RC = rotator cuff.

a single traumatic event, or can be the result of repetitive microtraumas. Instability can occur in a single plane or in multiple directions. An understanding of the spectrum of disorders that result from shoulder instability can help in diagnosing and treating patients.

Anterior Instability

The most common direction of dislocation is anterior, that is, the humeral head comes to lie anterior to the glenoid. A subluxation event can occur that may not produce a dislocation but can result in continued instability.[13]

When an anterior dislocation occurs, a lesion to the anterior stabilizing structures has occurred. The injury can take the form of a labral detachment from the glenoid (Bankart lesion), bone and labral detachment (bony Bankart lesion), ligament stretching or tearing, or detachment of the capsule/ligament from the humerus. When the Bankart lesion heals along the medial glenoid neck, it is often referred to as an anterior periosteal sleeve avulsion.[14] The anterior periosteal sleeve avulsion lesion highlights the fact that healing of a Bankart lesion does not stabilize the shoulder; the labrum must be in the proper location on the glenoid edge to stabilize the shoulder.

MRI may be helpful in determining the presence of anterior glenoid rim fractures, labral tears, the size of humeral defects, and rotator cuff tears. CT provides better detail of the bony defects compared with MRI, but does not allow visualization of the soft tissues.

Treatment

When a shoulder dislocation is diagnosed, closed reduction of the joint is attempted. The patient typically is given pain medication and muscle relaxants for closed reduction in the emergency department. The patient should be evaluated for rotator cuff tears and neurologic injury after the shoulder is reduced. Inability to reduce the shoulder dislocation can result from chronic dislocation, interposed soft tissue, and buttonholing of the humerus under the conjoined tendon. If the shoulder remains dislocated, the patient should be treated with closed reduction while under general anesthesia. Open reduction is also a possibility. Consideration should be given to advanced imaging before surgical reduction (if it can be obtained expeditiously) because the studies may show an interposed rotator cuff, large losses of humeral bone, or associated fractures; these findings may alter surgical treatment.

Natural History

The role of nonsurgical treatment in young, active patients with anterior instability continues to be defined. Physical therapy does not decrease dislocation recurrence rates except in a very tightly controlled population. Immobilization in external rotation can reduce the labrum back to a more anatomic position compared with traditional immobilization in internal rotation.[15] There appears to be a clinically significant reduction in recurrent dislocation if the shoulder is immobilized for 3 weeks in external rotation. In contrast, one study reported no difference in instability when comparing traditional to external rotation immobilization after an anterior dislocation in a young active population.[16]

but debatable (handwritten)

Several large cohorts of first-time dislocators were evaluated with variable incidences of recurrent instability ranging from 8% to 75%.[17-19] These studies reported lower rates of recurrent instability compared with smaller studies with patient-based outcomes.[17,20,21]

A 2007 study reported on a cohort of patients with dislocations and associated large (> 5 mm) and displaced (> 2 mm) fractures of the anteroinferior glenoid rim. Patients were followed for an average of 5.6 years.[22] Nonsurgical treatment was used only in patients with a concentrically reduced joint. No patient in the cohort had a dislocation, and the average outcome score was excellent.

Fifty percent to 80% of patients younger than 20 years at the time of the initial dislocation have a recurrent dislocation. The rate of recurrent instability declines with age.[18,23] Patients older than 40 years appear to be at increased risk for rotator cuff tears and neuro-

Bankart lesion v. ALPSA (ant. periosteal sleeve avulsion) ↳ higher rate recurrent dislocation after labral repair (handwritten)

Latarjet if bony glenoid defect > 25-30% [handwritten margin note]

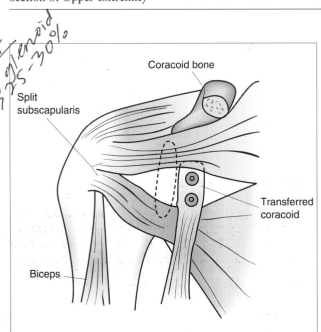

Figure 3 The Latarjet procedure involves a transfer of the coracoid process to the medial glenoid via a split of the subscapularis. The coracoid provides for glenohumeral stability by augmenting the anterior glenoid rim, whereas the conjoined tendon acts as a stabilizer with the arm abducted and externally rotated. (Reproduced from Burns JP, Snyder SJ: Shoulder instability, in Fischgrund JS, ed: *Orthopaedic Knowledge Update 9.* Rosemont, IL, American Academy of Orthopaedic Surgeons, 2008, pp 301-311.)

Labels in figure: Coracoid bone; Split subscapularis; Transferred coracoid; Biceps

logic injury.[24]

For young and active patients, the recurrence of instability is an indication for either open or arthroscopic stabilization. With the high recurrence rates reported after nonsurgical treatment in young, active patients, some authors recommend surgical repair for these patients at the time of the first shoulder dislocation. A randomized controlled trial compared arthroscopic stabilization with joint lavage alone after a primary dislocation. In the group of patients with arthroscopically stabilized shoulders, there was an 82% risk reduction for recurrent instability and a 76% risk reduction for dislocation 2 years after the initial injury.[25]

Arthroscopic Versus Open Repair

Patients with recurrent anterior shoulder instability can be treated using open or arthroscopic repair. Multiple studies have reported excellent results for open repair, with an approximate 5% rate of recurrent instability after surgery. With older arthroscopic repair techniques, results are less reliable, with recurrent instability rates of 15% to 33%.[9,23,26] With improvement in arthroscopic repair techniques, results have approached those of open repair, with successful outcomes in 90% to 96% of patients.[27-29]

In a randomized controlled trial comparing open and arthroscopic repair for recurrent anterior shoulder instability, the two groups had similar outcome scores

and rates of recurrence.[30] In two studies that systematically reviewed the literature,[31,32] the authors reported that when modern suture anchor techniques were used, outcome scores were similar or appeared to favor arthroscopic repair over open repair.

Recurrent Instability After Repair

When instability occurs after shoulder repair, multiple potential sources can be considered, including excessive bone loss from the anterior glenoid or humerus, capsular laxity, failure of labrum healing, medialization of the labrum, and unrepaired humeral avulsion of the inferior glenohumeral ligament. An 89% instability recurrence rate was reported for contact athletes when the anterior bony deficiency of 20% to 30% of the joint surface was treated with soft-tissue repair only.[9] Significant bone lesions can be treated arthroscopically by incorporating the lesions into the repair. A 93% success rate was reported in patients with an average defect measuring 24% of the joint surface.[33] However, the quality of the bony fragments may be an important consideration because a significantly higher instability recurrence rate was identified in patients with attritional fragments.[11] An association of recurrent instability with attritional bone loss on the glenoid has been reported.[26]

For defects of the anterior glenoid covering more than 25% to 30% of the joint surface, an open or arthroscopic coracoid transfer procedure (Figure 3) or structural iliac crest graft can be used. This technique can also be considered in the primary setting. A 4.4% instability recurrence rate was reported in patients with significant anterior glenoid bone loss who were treated with the Latarjet procedure.[34] The use of structural iliac crest has been supported by reports of high rates of patient satisfaction;[35,36] however, concerns regarding humeral head articulation on the graft, which leads to degenerative changes, have been raised.[37]

Large Hill-Sachs lesions (> 25% of the joint surface) can be considered for osteochondral allograft,[38] remplissage,[39] or infraspinatus transfer into the defect. There appears to be a biomechanical correlation between the size and location of a Hill-Sachs lesion and the ability of the humeral head to track on the glenoid.[40] Bone grafting of defects larger than 37.5% of the joint surface has been recommended based on biomechanical testing.[41]

Posterior Instability

Although posterior shoulder dislocations are less common than anterior dislocations, posterior dislocations are commonly missed. Mechanisms involved in posterior dislocations include trauma to the anterior aspect of the shoulder, an indirect force applied through an adducted or flexed arm, seizure, and electrocution.

Acute Posterior Dislocation

Unlike anterior instability, posterior instability does not lead to frequent recurrent dislocations. Once the dislocation is reduced, a short period of immobilization in external rotation is recommended, followed by physical therapy and range-of-motion exercises. The diagnosis of a posterior dislocation can be difficult. Diagnostic modalities such as CT can be a valuable adjunct in establishing the diagnosis.

Surgical Treatment

Patients with recurrent posterior shoulder instability or those with continued pain with loading of the arm in the forward flexed position (bench press or football pass blocking) are candidates for surgical posterior shoulder stabilization. Stabilization can be performed through an open posterior approach or arthroscopically. The goal of any repair is to address the posterior labral detachment, repair any capsular tears, and/or reduce the volume of the posterior capsule. Success has been reported with both open and arthroscopic approaches. Results for open surgery have been successful in 80% to 85% of patients at 5- to 7-year follow-ups.[42,43] With shorter follow-ups, arthroscopic repairs have been reported to have similar results.[44,45]

Chronic Posterior Dislocation

After several weeks of posterior dislocation, the bone of the humeral head and the glenoid begins to erode. If left untreated, destruction of the humerus and glenoid can occur. After 2 to 3 weeks, a closed reduction is unlikely to achieve a reduction of a posterior dislocation; an open repair will be required.

Prior to proceeding with open reduction, CT can help determine the extent and location of bone loss. After reduction, the shoulder can be assessed for stability. Options to improve stability include subscapularis or lesser tuberosity transfer into the reverse Hill-Sachs lesion, osteochondral bone grafting, segmental humeral head replacement, and humeral head replacement. For glenoid bone loss, iliac crest bone graft can be used to restore bone stock.

As the dislocation becomes more chronic, the bone of the humeral head becomes osteoporotic and arthritic. If humeral head arthritis is extensive, if the head collapses during reduction, or if bone loss is more than 50% of the articular surface, humeral head replacement is needed to restore stability and treat the arthritis. Total shoulder replacement can be considered when significant glenoid arthritis is present.

Multidirectional Instability

When instability occurs in more then one plane, the term multidirectional instability (MDI) is used. Patients with MDI often have generalized shoulder laxity, have had no acute trauma, and do not have a true dislocation of the joint. MDI can result from poor technique during athletic activities, genetics (Ehlers-Danlos syndrome), poor scapulohumeral mechanics, and rotator cuff dysfunction.

Comparison with the unaffected side will help to identify instability and increased motion in multiple planes. Provocative testing for anterior or posterior instability as described previously can be positive, and in-

ferior instability may be present. Inferior instability is characterized by a positive sulcus test and a sulcus that does not reduce with external rotation; both are signs of rotator interval injury. MRI with intra-articular administration of gadolinium can be helpful to determine the presence of labral tears. In most patients with MDI, no labral pathology is present and the capsular volume is increased.

Nonsurgical Treatment

Treatment for MDI is nonsurgical and includes prolonged abstinence from the sporting activity that provoked the symptoms. Results of nonsurgical treatment have been variable, with success rates reported as high as 80%.[46] One report outlined significant dysfunction after nonsurgical treatment, with one third of patients with poor outcomes at 8-year follow-up.[47]

Surgical Treatment

Moderate success in treating MDI has been achieved with open capsular shift, with the goal of reducing the capsular volume of the shoulder. Open techniques can be performed from an anterior or posterior approach, with some surgeons choosing the approach based on the direction of primary instability. An 88% success rate was reported following inferior capsular shift surgery.[48] Similarly, techniques have been developed to accomplish volume reduction during arthroscopy. Early results for arthroscopic plication have been promising, with success rate reported from 85% to 88%.[49,50]

Rotator Cuff Disorders

The understanding, evaluation, and treatment of rotator cuff tears have evolved since the 1934 publication of Codman's landmark text, *The Shoulder*.[51] Codman proposed that cuff tears have a traumatic origin, described the fundamental pathology and pathophysiology of the rotator cuff, and detailed the associated clinical findings and treatment options. In 1937, the theory of outlet impingement was introduced and it was proposed that rotator cuff tears occur secondary to chronic, repetitive contact between the greater tuberosity and the acromion.[52] A later study introduced the three stages of outlet impingement (Table 2), which represent the spectrum of disease severity, and described the technique of anterior acromioplasty designed to remove the offending structures that contribute to symptomatic outlet impingement of the rotator cuff tendon.[53] It is likely that all of these theories of rotator cuff tear etiology are correct, and that one simplified mechanism does not apply to all situations.

An age-dependent increase in the incidence of full-thickness rotator cuff tears has been reported in patients older than 50 years.[54,55] A 22% to 23% rate of asymptomatic tears was reported in two studies with a combined total of 999 patients; the incidence of asymptomatic full-thickness tears increased dramatically for each decade after 50 years of age.[54,55]

Table 2

Neer Stages of Impingement[a]

Stage	Patient Age (years)	Findings	Treatment
I	Younger than 25	Reversible edema, hemorrhage	Conservative
II	25-40	Irreversible tendon fibrosis, tendinosis	Conservative, surgical
III	Older than 40	Rotator cuff tear	Subacromial decompression/acromioplasty and rotator cuff repair

[a]The Neer stages of impingement progress from reversible changes to irreversible tendonosis, and finally to full-thickness rotator cuff tears. As the severity of staging increases, the likelihood of successful conservative therapy decreases.
(Reproduced with permission from Neer CS: Impingement lesions. *Clin Orthop Relat Res* 1983;173:70-77.

Table 3

Patient Factors Associated With Poor Healing After Rotator Cuff Repair[a]

Age older than 65 years

Female sex

Smoking

Duration of symptoms

Medical comorbidities

Inability to elevate > 100°

Weak elevation and external rotation

[a]Patient factors that have been associated with diminished tendon healing after cuff repair must be considered in conjunction with tear characteristics (fatty infiltration, retraction, atrophy) when determining treatment options.

The spectrum of rotator cuff disease occurs in a wide range of patients, from the young, elite, overhead athlete who presents with a partial-thickness rotator cuff tear to the elderly patient with a massive, irreparable tear.

History and Physical Examination

A thorough history and physical examination is the first step in evaluating a patient with shoulder pain. Patient factors associated with poor healing after rotator cuff repair, when considered individually, may not preclude an attempt at repair (Table 3). The examination of a patient with a suspected rotator cuff tear begins with the cervical spine, which must be ruled out as the source of the patient's symptoms. The shoulder girdle is then inspected in both shoulders. The deltoid is evaluated for atrophy, detachment, swelling, and/or evidence of anterosuperior escape. The supraspinatus and infraspinatus fossae are inspected for evidence of muscular atrophy. Tenderness to palpation over the acromioclavicular (AC) joint and the insertion of the supraspinatus on the greater tuberosity (the Codman point) should also be evaluated. Active and passive ranges of motion are compared, and rotator cuff strength is measured and compared with the normal contralateral side, if asymptomatic.

The supraspinatus is tested at 30° abduction and internal rotation, and the infraspinatus is tested in adduction with the elbows flexed to 90° and in maximal external rotation. Subscapularis strength is tested with the belly press test (upper subscapularis) and the lift-off test (lower subscapularis).[56] The teres minor muscle is an external rotator that is tested with the shoulders in 90° of abduction. At this point, a diagnostic subacromial injection of local anesthetic is used to determine if existing motion and/or strength deficits are caused by a rotator cuff tear or pain. Any differences in strength and/or motion are retested and the patient is evaluated for the presence of lag signs, which are indicative of full-thickness tears of the respective rotator cuff muscles shown in Table 4.

Associated Lesions

The biceps tendon, glenohumeral and AC joints, os acromiale, and the suprascapular nerve may be involved in the symptom complex of rotator cuff disease; each lesion should be identified during the workup phase and treated appropriately for the best outcome.

AC joint arthritis is fairly common in patients with rotator cuff disease. Specific findings include radiographic degenerative changes, tenderness to palpation directly over the AC joint, and pain in the AC joint with cross-arm adduction and/or the active compression test. An os acromiale is found in approximately 8% of the population[57] and should be recognized preoperatively. The potential for poorer outcomes after rotator cuff repair in patients with stable or unstable meso-os acromiale has been reported.[58] Suprascapular nerve compression can cause shoulder pain and weakness that can mimic full-thickness supraspinatus and/or infraspinatus tears, or may be seen in conjunction with tears that include supraspinatus retraction of 2 cm or more.[59]

It is important to evaluate the patient for associated symptomatic lesions so that the lesions may be appropriately treated. The use of diagnostic injections with 1% plain lidocaine requires a small investment of time in the clinic, but provides a wealth of information for treatment planning.

Table 4

Lag Signs for Rotator Cuff Tear[a]

Muscle	Test	Positive Finding
Supraspinatus	Drop arm test	Examiner places patient's arm in 90° elevation; patient unable to maintain
Infraspinatus	External rotation lag test	Examiner places patient's arm in maximum external rotation with arm in adduction; patient unable to maintain
Teres minor	Hornblower sign	Examiner places patient's arm in 90° abduction, 90° external rotation; patient unable to maintain external rotation
Upper subscapularis	Belly press test	Patient places hands on abdomen and must maintain elbows anterior to midsagittal plane of body
Lower subscapularis	Lift-off test	Examiner lifts patient's hand off lumbosacral spine; patient unable to maintain hand position

[a]The various lag signs are useful in determining the integrity of each muscle of the rotator cuff. Diagnostic injections help determine if weakness is caused by pain, full-thickness tearing, or both.

Diagnostic Imaging

Plain radiographs are obtained in the plane of the scapula and include AP views in internal and external rotation, a scapular Y view (10° to 15° of caudal tilt in the lateral scapular plane), and an axillary lateral view. Greater tuberosity sclerosis and excrescences, subacromial spurs and/or sclerosis (sourcil sign), and narrowing of the acromiohumeral distance are indications of rotator cuff tears. Radiographs should also be evaluated for glenohumeral arthritis, which may preclude cuff repair.

CT is useful in evaluating rotator cuff tears and is ideal for grading the severity of bone loss in severe cuff tear arthropathy. The Goutallier grading system (Table 5) of rotator cuff muscle fatty infiltration is based on CT imaging and remains an important method for determining whether a tear is reparable.[60] A higher degree of preoperative fatty infiltration on CT (≥ grade 3) is associated with recurrent tears and lower Constant scores.

MRI is an excellent method to confirm the diagnosis of a rotator cuff tear because it shows the number of tendons involved, the degree of retraction, fatty infiltration, and muscle atrophy.[61] This information is crucial for determining the potential for healing after repair. The addition of intra-articular contrast is particularly beneficial for detecting small, full-thickness tears and for improved prediction of the extent of partial articular-sided tears.

Ultrasound is an accurate, noninvasive method of detecting rotator cuff tears, is less expensive than MRI or CT arthrography, but requires an experienced technician and may not provide the same degree of information for evaluating concomitant pathology. Some evidence indicates that ultrasound is comparable to MRI for assessing rotator cuff tears.[62]

Tear Classification

Rotator cuff tears have been classified according to the depth (full- versus partial-thickness), etiology, age of

Table 5

Goutallier Classification of Fatty Infiltration[a]

Grade	Finding
0	No fat within the muscle
1	Some fatty streaks
2	Fat < muscle
3	Fat = muscle
4	Fat > muscle

[a]Fatty infiltration of the rotator cuff muscles was first based on CT, but is now more commonly evaluated on MRI studies. Fatty infiltration greater than grade 2 is associated with a higher rate of failure.
(Reproduced with permission from Goutallier D, Postel JM, Bernageau J, Lavau L, Voisin MC. Fatty muscle infiltration in cuff ruptures: Pre- and postoperative evaluation by CT scan. *Clin Orthop Relat Res* 1994;304:78-83.)

the tear, size, shape, number of tendons involved, and topography/trophicity of the tear. As such, there is no standard classification for rotator cuff tears. The Patte classification[61] is the most elaborate system and includes anatomic and pathologic considerations that are important for defining an individual treatment plan for each patient (Table 6 and Figure 4).

Treatment

There are three arms of treatment for disorders of the rotator cuff: (1) preventive, (2) conservative, and (3) surgical. Prevention focuses on body mechanics, proper use and strengthening of core body and shoulder girdle musculature, and avoiding aggravating activities. When cuff symptoms develop in the absence of a full-thickness tear, conservative therapy, including rest, activity modification, gentle passive and active motion exercises, anti-inflammatory medication, and periodic subacromial corticosteroid injections, can provide relief.[63] Therapeutic corticosteroid injections should be used with knowledge of the potential detrimental effects on the tendon and bone and decreased potential

Table 6

Patte Classification of Rotator Cuff Tears

Extent of Tear

Group I: Partial tears or full-substance tears < 1 cm in sagittal diameter at bony detachment

    a. Deep, partial tears

    b. Superficial tears

    c. Small, full-substance tears

Group II: Full-substance tears of entire supraspinatus

Group III: Full-substance tears involving more than one tendon

Group IV: Massive tears with secondary osteoarthritis

Topography of Tear in Sagittal Plane

Segment 1: Subscapularis tear

Segment 2: Coracohumeral ligament tear

Segment 3: Isolated supraspinatus tear

Segment 4: Tear of entire supraspinatus and one half of infraspinatus

Segment 5: Tear of supraspinatus and infraspinatus

Segment 6: Tear of subscapularis, supraspinatus, and infraspinatus

Topography of Tear in Frontal Plane

Stage 1: Proximal stump close to bony insertion

Stage 2: Proximal stump at level of humeral head

Stage 3: Proximal stump at level of glenoid

Quality of Muscle

1. Minimal fatty streaking

2. Less fat than muscle

3. Equal fat and muscle

4. More fat than muscle

State of the Biceps Tendon

1. Intact

2. Subluxated

3. Dislocated

---

for healing after repair.[64,65] For patients whose symptoms are not relieved by conservative measures, or for those who have a full-thickness rotator cuff tear,[66] surgical treatment is recommended.

Surgical Treatment

Surgical treatment of rotator cuff tears can be performed through open, arthroscopically assisted mini-open, or all-arthroscopic techniques.[67-69] Acromioplasty and subacromial decompression have therapeutic and technical roles in rotator cuff surgery; the goal is to smooth the undersurface of the arch to relieve pressure on the cuff without disrupting the deltoid origin or destabilizing the coracoacromial arch.

Open Rotator Cuff Repair: Basic Principles

Diagnostic arthroscopy results enable the surgeon to visualize and address concomitant pathology before proceeding with a rotator cuff repair. In large and massive tears, the degree of glenohumeral arthritis may be more severe than suggested by preoperative imaging; therefore, the treatment plan may be altered to exclude repair and proceed with arthroscopic débridement, subacromial decompression, and biceps tenotomy or tenodesis as dictated by the pathology (Table 7).

With open repair, portals should be closed and the shoulder reprepped and draped to prevent infection.[70] Skin incisions should be made with consideration for the current surgery and any potential revision surgery, particularly with open repair of large and massive tears. An oblique incision from the posterior edge of the AC joint to the anterolateral corner of the acromion that extends 2 to 3 cm distally over the raphe between the anterior and middle deltoid provides excellent visualization for cuff repair and allows anterosuperior access for revision surgery (reverse shoulder arthroplasty) through the same incision.

Distal clavicle excision and two-step acromioplasty[71] improve access to the subacromial space without the need to extend the deltoid split (Figure 5). Subacromial bursectomy improves visualization and is facilitated by rotating the arm. The coracohumeral ligament is palpated in external rotation, adduction, and released if it is tight. This exposes the rotator cuff for evaluation, mobilization, and repair. Advances in arthroscopic surgery have made repair techniques (single-row, double-row, transosseous, and transosseous equivalent) similar in arthroscopic and open surgery. Following repair, the deltoid is meticulously repaired.

Arthroscopic Repair

Arthroscopic rotator cuff surgery, which requires a methodic, stepwise approach for successful and timely completion of a sturdy repair, is becoming increasingly popular. Patient positioning depends on the surgeon's preference. The beach chair position with an articulated arm holder can be used. This positioning allows for easy conversion to an open procedure if necessary, and the arm holder allows flexibility of arm positioning throughout the surgery. Two-step acromioplasty, as previously described, is performed. The coracoacromial ligament may be preserved in large and massive repairs.

Partial-Thickness Tears

Surgical treatment of partial-thickness tears includes débridement, transtendinous in situ repair, or tear completion and repair.[72] Tears that are at least 50% (6 mm) of the tendon thickness should be considered for repair because, over time, these tears may progress to full-thickness tears.[73] Patient factors must be considered when evaluating treatment options. No prospective study compares in situ repair with tear completion and repair despite reported good and excellent results with both techniques.[74,75] Tear completion allows for débridement of the degenerative tendon, thorough tuber-

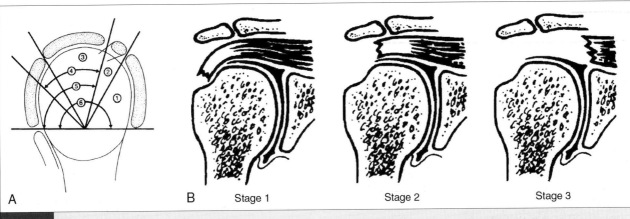

| Figure 4 | Patte classification of rotator cuff tears. **A,** Rotator cuff tear topography in the sagittal plane is divided into six segments: Anterosuperior tears (segments 1, 2, and 3), superior tears (segments 2, and 3), posterosuperior tears (segments 4 and 5), and total cuff tears (segment 6). **B,** The topography of tears in the frontal plane is divided into three stages. Stage 1: the proximal stump shows little retraction; stage 2: retracted to the level of the humeral head; stage 3: retracted to the level of the glenoid. (Reproduced with permission from Patte D: Classification of rotator cuff lesions. *Clin Orthop Relat Res* 1990;254:81-86.) |

osity preparation, and repair of healthy tendon to bone. The proposed benefit of transtendinous repair is avoiding the creation of a full-thickness tear.

Single-Row Versus Double-Row Repair

There is no clear consensus on whether single- or double-row repair of rotator cuff tears is better.[33,76] Double-row fixation is more costly, time-consuming, and technically more difficult when performed arthroscopically. Biomechanical studies comparing the two techniques have reported higher initial fixation strength and stiffness, improved footprint restoration, and decreased gap formation and strain with double-row fixation.[77-79] Recent prospective randomized studies have failed to demonstrate a convincing difference in effectiveness between the two techniques, but tear size may prove to be a determining factor.[80-82] At 2-year follow-up, higher American Shoulder and Elbow Surgeon and Constant scores were reported with double-row fixation in tears larger than 3 cm; however, cuff integrity was not evaluated with MRI at follow-up.[83] In a nonrandomized retrospective comparison, a clinical difference was not found between repair techniques at 2 years, but improved healing for double-row compared with single-row fixation was shown with CT arthrography.[84] These data suggest that double-row fixation may prove better for larger tears, whereas single-row fixation is probably adequate for smaller (< 3 cm) tears.

Transosseous and Transosseous Equivalent Repairs

Transosseous and transosseous equivalent rotator cuff repair techniques produce low bone-tendon interface motion, excellent footprint restoration, a high number of cycles to failure, and favorable distribution of stress over the repair in biomechanical and clinical evaluations.[85-88]

Table 7

Biceps Pathology Indicating the Need for Tenodesis or Tenotomy[a]

Subluxation

Fraying

Tenosynovitis

Insertional detachment

Hypertrophy

[a]The functional contributions of the long head of the biceps tendon are debated, but biceps pathology is well-recognized as a pain generator. Sometimes, only subtle changes are found at diagnostic arthroscopy and, if left untreated (with tenotomy or tenodesis), the biceps can be a source of postoperative pain.

Repair Augmentation: Grafts and Patches

Recurrent tears of the repaired rotator cuff occur more frequently with large and massive tears,[89] with up to 94% of these repairs failing by 1-year follow-up.[90] Augmentation of large and massive rotator cuff repairs with allograft or xenograft tissues is proposed to improve repair strength and provide a bioreplaceable collagen network in an effort to decrease failure rates. Commonly used materials for grafts include human dermal allograft, porcine dermis, and porcine smooth intestine submucosa. Based on a randomized trial of large and massive cuff repairs, the authors recommended against porcine smooth intestine submucosa augmentation for cuff repair because of adverse graft reactions and failure to demonstrate improved outcomes.[91] There are no similar randomized trials evaluating if augmented repair with human dermal allograft is beneficial, but there are no reports of adverse graft reactions, and the potential benefit of mechanical and biologic augmentation are worthy of consideration in young patients with large or massive cuff tears.

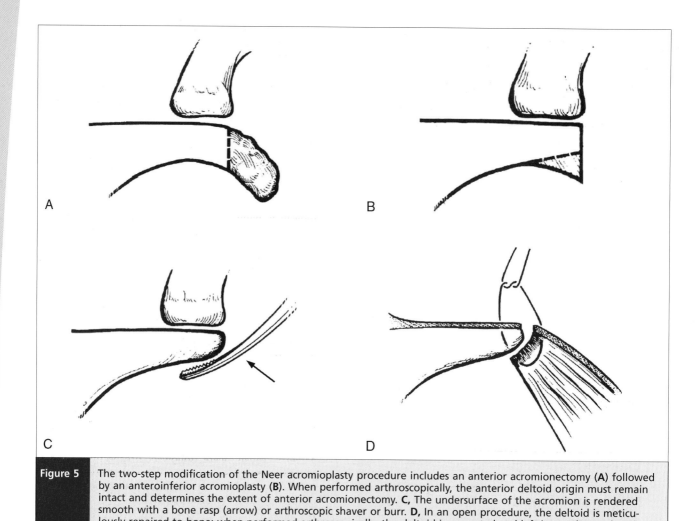

Figure 5 The two-step modification of the Neer acromioplasty procedure includes an anterior acromionectomy (**A**) followed by an anteroinferior acromioplasty (**B**). When performed arthroscopically, the anterior deltoid origin must remain intact and determines the extent of anterior acromionectomy. **C,** The undersurface of the acromion is rendered smooth with a bone rasp (arrow) or arthroscopic shaver or burr. **D,** In an open procedure, the deltoid is meticulously repaired to bone; when performed arthroscopically, the deltoid is respected and left intact. (Reproduced with permission from Rockwood CA Jr, Lyons FR: Shoulder impingement syndrome: Diagnosis, radiographic evaluation, and treatment with a modified Neer acromioplasty. *J Bone Joint Surg Am* 1993;75:409-424.)

Tendon Transfers

Irreparable large and massive tears are challenging to treat, especially in younger patients (60 years or younger) with higher functional demands. Tendon transfers are a viable option to reduce pain and restore function when the rotator cuff cannot be mobilized for repair. Latissimus dorsi tendon transfer is suited for irreparable posterosuperior cuff tears,[92-94] and pectoralis major tendon transfer is designed for treating anterosuperior tears with an irreparable subscapularis tendon.[95]

Study results support the recommendation of latissimus dorsi tendon transfer for patients with an intact subscapularis, an irreparable posterosuperior rotator cuff tear with external rotation deficit, and grade 2 or less fatty infiltration of the teres minor on preoperative imaging.[92,94] In contrast, other authors have reported improved results in patients with posterosuperior tears associated with preoperative teres minor dysfunction.[93] Each of these studies report improvements in external rotation and forward elevation, as well as subjective improvements that support latissimus dorsi tendon transfer as a viable option for patients who have pain-

ful, irreparable posterosuperior cuff tears and an external rotation deficit.

The results of pectoralis major tendon transfer in 30 shoulders were reviewed. The authors reported Constant scores improved from 47 to 70 points at an average follow-up of 32 months.[95] The pectoralis major was transferred superficial to the conjoined tendon. Worse outcomes were observed in patients with concomitant irreparable supraspinatus tears, whereas a reparable supraspinatus tear did not affect the postoperative outcome. Pectoralis major tendon transfer underneath the conjoined tendon has been described in a group of 12 older patients (average age 65 years); the Constant score improved from 26.9 points preoperatively to 67.1 points at a mean of 28 months postoperatively.[96] Dramatic improvement in pain scores was noted in addition to the reported functional gains.

Postoperative Rehabilitation

Postoperatively, patients are maintained in a shoulder sling and pillow that positions the arm in approximately 20° to 30° of abduction to take tension off the repair. Traditionally, passive-assisted forward elevation and external rotation are started immediately. Internal rotation of the arm up the back is delayed 3 weeks (for small or medium tears) to 6 weeks (for large or massive tears). Active motion combined with terminal stretching commences at approximately 6 weeks, depending on the extent of the tear.[97] Resistive motion is added according to each patient's individual progress, usually at 10 weeks. Despite advances in repair techniques, recurrent cuff defects remain a treatment challenge for the orthopaedic surgeon. As such, there is a trend toward decelerated postoperative rehabilitation that delays passive elevation and external rotation in an effort to improve tendon healing.

Annotated References

1. Turkel SJ, Panio MW, Marshall JL, Girgis FG: Stabilizing mechanisms preventing anterior dislocation of the glenohumeral joint. *J Bone Joint Surg Am* 1981;63(8): 1208-1217.

2. Inman VT, Saunder CM, Abbott LC: Observations on the function of the shoulder joint. *J Bone Joint Surg Am* 1944;26:1-30.

3. Saha AK: Dynamic stability of the glenohumeral joint. *Acta Orthop Scand* 1971;42(6):491-505.

4. Howell SM, Galinat BJ: The glenoid-labral socket: A constrained articular surface. *Clin Orthop Relat Res* 1989;243(243):122-125.

5. Rowe CR, Patel D, Southmayd WW: The Bankart procedure: A long-term end-result study. *J Bone Joint Surg Am* 1978;60(1):1-16.

6. Burkhart SS, De Beer JF: Traumatic glenohumeral bone defects and their relationship to failure of arthroscopic Bankart repairs: Significance of the inverted-pear glenoid and the humeral engaging Hill-Sachs lesion. *Arthroscopy* 2000;16(7):677-694.

7. Itoi E, Lee SB, Berglund LJ, Berge LL, An KN: The effect of a glenoid defect on anteroinferior stability of the shoulder after Bankart repair: A cadaveric study. *J Bone Joint Surg Am* 2000;82(1):35-46.

8. Mologne TS, Provencher MT, Menzel KA, Vachon TA, Dewing CB: Arthroscopic stabilization in patients with an inverted pear glenoid: Results in patients with bone loss of the anterior glenoid. *Am J Sports Med* 2007; 35(8):1276-1283.

   In patients with postoperative instability with moderate anterior bone loss treated with arthroscopic repair, a 14.2% rate of recurrent instability was found in those patients with attritional bone loss. No instability was reported when significant bone was incorporated into the repair.

9. Habermeyer P, Walch G: The biceps tendon and rotator cuff disease, in Burkhead WZ Jr, ed: *Rotator Cuff Disorders*. Baltimore, MD, Williams and Wilkins, 1996, pp 142-159.

10. Warner JJ, McMahon PJ: The role of the long head of the biceps brachii in superior stability of the glenohumeral joint. *J Bone Joint Surg Am* 1995;77(3):366-372.

11. Yamaguchi K, Riew KD, Galatz LM, Syme JA, Neviaser RJ: Biceps activity during shoulder motion: An electromyographic analysis. *Clin Orthop Relat Res* 1997; 336(336):122-129.

12. Bioleau P, Baqué F, Valerio L, Ahrens P, Chuinard C, Trojani C: Isolated arthroscopic biceps tenotomy or tenodesis improves symptoms in patients with massive irreparable rotator cuff tears. *J Bone Joint Surg Am* 2007; 89(4):747-757.

    Arthroscopic biceps tenotomy or tenodesis is an effective method to relieve pain and improve function in patients with massive irreparable cuff tears with no pseudoparalysis or glenohumeral arthritis. Patients with an intact teres minor have a better outcome. Level of evidence: IV.

13. Owens BD, Duffey ML, Nelson BJ, DeBerardino TM, Taylor DC, Mountcastle SB: The incidence and characteristics of shoulder instability at the United States Military Academy. *Am J Sports Med* 2007;35(7):1168-1173.

    Military cadets were followed prospectively for 9 months and all instability episodes were recorded. Most instability events (85%) were subluxations without true dislocation. Level of evidence: I.

14. Neviaser TJ: The anterior labroligamentous periosteal sleeve avulsion lesion: A cause of anterior instability of the shoulder. *Arthroscopy* 1993;9(1):17-21.

15. Itoi E, Hatakeyama Y, Sato T, et al: Immobilization in external rotation after shoulder dislocation reduces the risk of recurrence: A randomized controlled trial. *J Bone Joint Surg Am* 2007;89(10):2124-2131.

    A total of 198 patients with anterior dislocation of the shoulder were randomized to treatment with immobilization in internal rotation or external rotation for 3 weeks. Immobilization in external rotation reduced the risk of recurrence and was beneficial in patients age 30 years or younger.

16. Finestone A, Milgrom C, Radeva-Petrova DR, et al: Bracing in external rotation for traumatic anterior dislocation of the shoulder. *J Bone Joint Surg Br* 2009;91(7): 918-921.

    The authors found that bracing in external rotation may not be as effective as previously believed in the prevention of anterior dislocation of the shoulder because further dislocation occurred a mean 33.4 months after treatment.

17. Jakobsen BW, Johannsen HV, Suder P, Søjbjerg JO: Primary repair versus conservative treatment of first-time traumatic anterior dislocation of the shoulder: A ran-

3: Upper Extremity

domized study with 10-year follow-up. *Arthroscopy* 2007;23(2):118-123.

Patients were randomized to open Bankart repair versus nonsurgical treatment. At a minimum 2-year follow-up, the stabilization group had 3% recurrent instability compared with 56% in the cohort treated nonsurgically. Level of evidence: I.

18. Hovelius L, Olofsson A, Sandström B, et al: Nonoperative treatment of primary anterior shoulder dislocation in patients forty years of age and younger: A prospective twenty-five-year follow-up. *J Bone Joint Surg Am* 2008;90(5):945-952.

The authors studied the results of nonsurgical treatment of primary anterior shoulder dislocation and found that half of the dislocations had not recurred or had stabilized over time.

19. Sachs RA, Lin D, Stone ML, Paxton E, Kuney M: Can the need for future surgery for acute traumatic anterior shoulder dislocation be predicted? *J Bone Joint Surg Am* 2007;89(8):1665-1674.

One hundred thirty-one patients were followed prospectively after an initial dislocation. Approximately one third of the patients experienced recurrent instability of the shoulder. Level of evidence: I.

20. Kirkley A, Werstine R, Ratjek A, Griffin S: Prospective randomized clinical trial comparing the effectiveness of immediate arthroscopic stabilization versus immobilization and rehabilitation in first traumatic anterior dislocations of the shoulder: Long-term evaluation. *Arthroscopy* 2005;21(1):55-63.

21. Kirkley S: Primary anterior dislocation of the shoulder in young patients. A ten-year prospective study. *J Bone Joint Surg Am* 1998;80(2):300-301.

22. Maquieira GJ, Espinosa N, Gerber C, Eid K: Nonoperative treatment of large anterior glenoid rim fractures after traumatic anterior dislocation of the shoulder. *J Bone Joint Surg Br* 2007;89(10):1347-1351.

Patients with large displaced Bankart lesions, a single dislocation, and a postreduction concentric humeral head were followed after nonsurgical treatment. No patients experienced recurrent instability.

23. Arciero Ra, Wheeler JH, Ryan JB, McBride JT: Arthroscopic Bankart repair versus nonoperative treatment for acute, initial anterior shoulder dislocations. *Am J Sports Med* 1994;22(5):589-594.

24. Neviaser RJ, Neviaser TJ, Neviaser JS: Concurrent rupture of the rotator cuff and anterior dislocation of the shoulder in the older patient. *J Bone Joint Surg Am* 1988;70(9):1308-1311.

25. Robinson CM, Jenkins PJ, White TO, Ker A, Will E: Primary arthroscopic stabilization for a first-time anterior dislocation of the shoulder: A randomized, double-blind trial. *J Bone Joint Surg Am* 2008;90(4):708-721.

Patients with first-time anterior shoulder dislocations were randomized to arthroscopic stabilization versus joint lavage alone. Patients treated with stabilization had a risk reduction for instability of 82% and dislocation rate of 76%. Level of evidence: I.

26. Bioleau P, Villalba M, Héry JY, Balg F, Ahrens P, Neyton L: Risk factors for recurrence of shoulder instability after arthroscopic Bankart repair. *J Bone Joint Surg Am* 2006;88(8):1755-1763.

27. Kim SH, Ha KI, Cho YB, Ryu BD, Oh I: Arthroscopic anterior stabilization of the shoulder: Two to six-year follow-up. *J Bone Joint Surg Am* 2003;85(8):1511-1518.

28. Carreira DS, Mazzocca AD, Oryhon J, Brown FM, Hayden JK, Romeo AA: A prospective outcome evaluation of arthroscopic Bankart repairs: Minimum 2-year follow-up. *Am J Sports Med* 2006;34(5):771-777.

29. Marquardt B, Witt KA, Liem D, Steinbeck J, Pötzl W: Arthroscopic Bankart repair in traumatic anterior shoulder instability using a suture anchor technique. *Arthroscopy* 2006;22(9):931-936.

30. Bottoni CR, Smith EL, Berkowitz MJ, Towle RB, Moore JH: Arthroscopic versus open shoulder stabilization for recurrent anterior instability: A prospective randomized clinical trial. *Am J Sports Med* 2006;34(11):1730-1737.

31. Hobby J, Griffin D, Dunbar M, Boileau P: Is arthroscopic surgery for stabilisation of chronic shoulder instability as effective as open surgery? A systematic review and meta-analysis of 62 studies including 3044 arthroscopic operations. *J Bone Joint Surg Br* 2007;89(9):1188-1196.

The authors report on a systematic review with meta-analysis of articles from 1985 to 2006 dealing with open compared with arthroscopic Bankart repair. When older techniques were eliminated, no significant difference in outcomes was found.

32. Lenters TR, Franta AK, Wolf FM, Leopold SS, Matsen FA III: Arthroscopic compared with open repairs for recurrent anterior shoulder instability: A systematic review and meta-analysis of the literature. *J Bone Joint Surg Am* 2007;89(2):244-254.

A systematic literature review and meta-analysis found higher outcomes score for patients treated with modern arthroscopic technique compared with open repair. Higher instability scores were reported in patients treated with arthroscopic repairs. Level of evidence: II.

33. Sugaya H, Moriishi J, Kanisawa I, Tsuchiya A: Arthroscopic osseous Bankart repair for chronic recurrent traumatic anterior glenohumeral instability. *J Bone Joint Surg Am* 2005;87(8):1752-1760.

34. Burkhart SS, De Beer JF, Barth JR, et al: Results of modified Latarjet reconstruction in patients with anteroinferior instability and significant bone loss. *Arthroscopy* 2007;23(10):1033-1041.

In a therapeutic case series, the authors demonstrate the

effectiveness of the modified Latarjet procedure in the treatment of patients with dramatic bone loss in whom open or arthroscopic soft-tissue reconstruction is not an option. Level of evidence: IV.

35. Warner JJ, Gill TJ, O'hollerhan JD, Pathare N, Millett PJ: Anatomical glenoid reconstruction for recurrent anterior glenohumeral instability with glenoid deficiency using an autogenous tricortical iliac crest bone graft. *Am J Sports Med* 2006;34(2):205-212.

36. Haaker RG, Eickhoff U, Klammer HL: Intraarticular autogenous bone grafting in recurrent shoulder dislocations. *Mil Med* 1993;158(3):164-169.

37. Hindmarsh J, Lindberg A: Eden-Hybbinette's operation for recurrent dislocation of the humero-scapular joint. *Acta Orthop Scand* 1967;38(4):459-478.

38. Gerber C, Lambert SM: Allograft reconstruction of segmental defects of the humeral head for the treatment of chronic locked posterior dislocation of the shoulder. *J Bone Joint Surg Am* 1996;78(3):376-382.

39. Purchase RJ, Wolf EM, Hobgood ER, Pollock ME, Smalley CC: Hill-Sachs "remplissage": An arthroscopic solution for the engaging Hill-Sachs lesion. *Arthroscopy* 2008;24(6):723-726.

    The authors used arthroscopic capsulotenodesis of the posterior capsule and infraspinatus tendon to treat traumatic shoulder instability in patients with glenoid bone loss and a large Hill-Sachs lesion.

40. Yamamoto N, Itoi E, Abe H, et al: Contact between the glenoid and the humeral head in abduction, external rotation, and horizontal extension: A new concept of glenoid track. *J Shoulder Elbow Surg* 2007;16(5):649-656.

    The authors used a custom device to test nine fresh-frozen cadaver shoulders in an assessment of contact between the glenoid and humeral head.

41. Sekiya JK, Wickwire AC, Stehle JH, Debski RE: Hill-Sachs defects and repair using osteoarticular allograft transplantation: Biomechanical analysis using a joint compression model. *Am J Sports Med* 2009;37(12):2459-2466.

    The authors concluded that the size and orientation of humeral head defects greatly contributes to glenohumeral joint function. An increase in the size of the defect required less anterior translation before dislocation and decreased the stability ration. As a result, the risk of recurrent instability was increased.

42. Hawkins RJ, Koppert G, Johnston G: Recurrent posterior instability (subluxation) of the shoulder. *J Bone Joint Surg Am* 1984;66(2):169-174.

43. Pollock RG, Bigliani LU: Recurrent posterior shoulder instability: Diagnosis and treatment. *Clin Orthop Relat Res* 1993;291(291):85-96.

44. Bradley JP, Baker CL III, Kline AJ, Armfield DR, Chhabra A: Arthroscopic capsulolabral reconstruction for posterior instability of the shoulder: A prospective study of 100 shoulders. *Am J Sports Med* 2006;34(7):1061-1071.

45. Provencher MT, Bell SJ, Menzel KA, Mologne TS: Arthroscopic treatment of posterior shoulder instability: Results in 33 patients. *Am J Sports Med* 2005;33(10):1463-1471.

46. Burkhead WZ Jr, Rockwood CA Jr: Treatment of instability of the shoulder with an exercise program. *J Bone Joint Surg Am* 1992;74(6):890-896.

47. Misamore GW, Sallay PI, Didelot W: A longitudinal study of patients with multidirectional instability of the shoulder with seven- to ten-year follow-up. *J Shoulder Elbow Surg* 2005;14(5):466-470.

48. Hamada K, Fukuda H, Nakajima T, Yamada N: The inferior capsular shift operation for instability of the shoulder: Long-term results in 34 shoulders. *J Bone Joint Surg Br* 1999;81(2):218-225.

49. Gartsman GM, Roddey TS, Hammerman SM: Arthroscopic treatment of multidirectional glenohumeral instability: 2- to 5-year follow-up. *Arthroscopy* 2001;17(3):236-243.

50. Treacy SH, Savoie FH III, Field LD: Arthroscopic treatment of multidirectional instability. *J Shoulder Elbow Surg* 1999;8(4):345-350.

51. Codman EA: *The Shoulder*. Brooklyn, NY, G Miller & Company, 1934.

52. Meyer AW: Chronic functional lesions of the shoulder. *Arch Surg* 1937;35:646-674.

53. Neer CS: Impingement lesions. *Clin Orthop Relat Res* 1983;173:70-77.

54. Tempelhof S, Rupp S, Seil R: Age-related prevalence of rotator cuff tears in asymptomatic shoulders. *J Shoulder Elbow Surg* 1999;8(4):296-299.

55. Yamaguchi K, Ditsios K, Middleton WD, Hildebolt CF, Galatz LM, Teefey SA: The demographic and morphological features of rotator cuff disease: A comparison of asymptomatic and symptomatic shoulders. *J Bone Joint Surg Am* 2006;88(8):1699-1704.

56. Tokish JM, Decker MJ, Ellis HB, Torry MR, Hawkins RJ: The belly-press test for the physical examination of the subscapularis muscle: Electromyographic validation and comparison to the lift-off test. *J Shoulder Elbow Surg* 2003;12(5):427-430.

57. Sammarco VJ: Os acromiale: Frequency, anatomy, and clinical implications. *J Bone Joint Surg Am* 2000;82(3):394-400.

58. Abboud JA, Silverberg D, Pepe M, et al: Surgical treatment of os acromiale with and without associated rota-

3: Upper Extremity

tor cuff tears. *J Shoulder Elbow Surg* 2006;15(3):265-270.

59. Albritton MJ, Graham RD, Richards RS II, Basamania CJ: An anatomic study of the effects on the suprascapular nerve due to retraction of the supraspinatus muscle after a rotator cuff tear. *J Shoulder Elbow Surg* 2003; 12(5):497-500.

60. Goutallier D, Postel JM, Gleyze P, Leguilloux P, Van Driessche S: Influence of cuff muscle fatty degeneration on anatomic and functional outcomes after simple suture of full-thickness tears. *J Shoulder Elbow Surg* 2003;12(6):550-554.

61. Patte D: Classification of rotator cuff lesions. *Clin Orthop Relat Res* 1990;254(254):81-86.

62. Teefey SA, Rubin DA, Middleton WD, Hildebolt CF, Leibold RA, Yamaguchi K: Detection and quantification of rotator cuff tears: Comparison of ultrasonographic, magnetic resonance imaging, and arthroscopic findings in seventy-one consecutive cases. *J Bone Joint Surg Am* 2004;86(4):708-716.

63. Kuhn JE: Exercise in the treatment of rotator cuff impingement: A systematic review and a synthesized evidence-based rehabilitation protocol. *J Shoulder Elbow Surg* 2009;18(1):138-160.

This review synthesizes a new "gold standard" rehabilitation program for rotator cuff impingement syndrome based on level I and II studies evaluating nonsurgical treatment of this disorder in an effort to standardize therapy for improved outcome comparisons. Level of evidence: I.

64. Watson M: Major ruptures of the rotator cuff: The results of surgical repair in 89 patients. *J Bone Joint Surg Br* 1985;67(4):618-624.

65. Mikolyzk DK, Wei AS, Tonino P, et al: Effect of corticosteroids on the biomechanical strength of rat rotator cuff tendon. *J Bone Joint Surg Am* 2009;91(5):1172-1180.

A single dose of corticosteroids significantly weakened intact and injured rat rotator cuff tendons at 1 week. Decreased maximum load, stress, and stiffness returned to baseline after 3 weeks.

66. Nho SJ, Brown BS, Lyman S, Adler RS, Altchek DW, MacGillivray JD: Prospective analysis of arthroscopic rotator cuff repair: Prognostic factors affecting clinical and ultrasound outcome. *J Shoulder Elbow Surg* 2009; 18(1):13-20.

Single-tendon tears were nine times more likely to heal after arthroscopic repair than tears involving more than one tendon. Early repair of full-thickness rotator cuff tears will prevent tear progression and will likely improve patient outcomes. Level of evidence: IV.

67. Mohtadi NG, Hollinshead RM, Sasyniuk TM, Fletcher JA, Chan DS, Li FX: A randomized clinical trial comparing open to arthroscopic acromioplasty with mini-open rotator cuff repair for full-thickness rotator cuff tears: Disease-specific quality of life outcome at an average 2-year follow-up. *Am J Sports Med* 2008;36(6):1043-1051.

A randomized controlled trial comparing open acromioplasty and rotator cuff repair to arthroscopic acromioplasty and mini-open rotator cuff repair demonstrated significantly better quality of life and shoulder-specific outcome scores at 3 months in the mini-open group. However, at 1 and 2 years postoperatively there was no difference in outcome between the groups. Level of evidence: I.

68. Zumstein MA, Jost B, Hempel J, Hodler J, Gerber C: The clinical and structural long-term results of open repair of massive tears of the rotator cuff. *J Bone Joint Surg Am* 2008;90(11):2423-2431.

Long-term follow-up of open cuff repairs showed durable clinical results, despite a retear rate of 57%. A wide lateral extension of the acromion was identified as a previously unknown risk factor for retearing. Level of evidence: IV.

69. More K, Davis AD, Afra R, Kaye EK, Schepsis A, Voloshin I: Arthroscopic versus mini-open rotator cuff repair: A comprehensive review and meta-analysis. *Am J Sports Med* 2008;36(9):1824-1828.

A meta-analysis of case series comparing arthroscopic to mini-open repair reported no difference in functional outcomes or complication rates. A variety of repair methods were reviewed in the selected series. Level of evidence: III.

70. Herrera MF, Bauer G, Reynolds F, Wilk RM, Bigliani LU, Levine WN: Infection after mini-open rotator cuff repair. *J Shoulder Elbow Surg* 2002;11(6):605-608.

71. Rockwood CA Jr, Lyons FR: Shoulder impingement syndrome: Diagnosis, radiographic evaluation, and treatment with a modified Neer acromioplasty. *J Bone Joint Surg Am* 1993;75(3):409-424.

72. Liem D, Alci S, Dedy N, Steinbeck J, Marquardt B, Möllenhoff G: Clinical and structural results of partial supraspinatus tears treated by subacromial decompression without repair. *Knee Surg Sports Traumatol Arthrosc* 2008;16(10):967-972.

Forty-six patients with grade I or II (Ellman) partial-thickness, articular-sided, cuff tears were treated with arthroscopic subacromial decompression and débridement (grade II only). At 50.6 months, only three patients progressed to a full-thickness tear. Good or excellent results were reported in 87% of patients. Level of evidence: IV.

73. Kartus J, Kartus C, Rostgård-Christensen L, Sernert N, Read J, Perko M: Long-term clinical and ultrasound evaluation after arthroscopic acromioplasty in patients with partial rotator cuff tears. *Arthroscopy* 2006;22(1):44-49.

74. Kamath G, Galatz LM, Keener JD, Teefey S, Middleton W, Yamaguchi K: Tendon integrity and functional out-

come after arthroscopic repair of high-grade partial-thickness supraspinatus tears. *J Bone Joint Surg Am* 2009;91(5):1055-1062.

Arthroscopic completion and repair of partial-thickness cuff tears resulted in 88% healing rate. Advanced age was associated with repair failure. Level of evidence: IV.

75. Castagna A, Delle Rose G, Conti M, Snyder SJ, Borroni M, Garofalo R: Predictive factors of subtle residual shoulder symptoms after transtendinous arthroscopic cuff repair: A clinical study. *Am J Sports Med* 2009; 37(1):103-108.

Transtendinous repair techniques resulted in residual shoulder discomfort at the extremes of motion in 41% of patients. Large tendon retraction and/or a relatively small exposure footprint area in an older patient without a traumatic etiology were predictive of residual symptoms. Level of evidence: IV.

76. Grasso A, Milano G, Salvatore M, Falcone G, Deriu L, Fabbriciani C: Single-row versus double-row arthroscopic rotator cuff repair: A prospective randomized clinical study. *Arthroscopy* 2009;25(1):4-12.

In a prospective study comparing single- versus double-row arthroscopic cuff repair, the authors found no difference in clinical or functional outcome at 2 years. Age, sex, and baseline strength significantly and independently influenced outcome. Level of evidence: I.

77. Kim DH, Elattrache NS, Tibone JE, et al: Biomechanical comparison of a single-row versus double-row suture anchor technique for rotator cuff repair. *Am J Sports Med* 2006;34(3):407-414.

78. Ma CB, Comerford L, Wilson J, Puttlitz CM: Biomechanical evaluation of arthroscopic rotator cuff repairs: Double-row compared with single-row fixation. *J Bone Joint Surg Am* 2006;88(2):403-410.

79. Lo IK, Burkhart SS: Double-row arthroscopic rotator cuff repair: Re-establishing the footprint of the rotator cuff. *Arthroscopy* 2003;19(9):1035-1042.

80. Burks RT, Crim J, Brown N, Fink B, Greis PE: A prospective randomized clinical trial comparing arthroscopic single- and double-row rotator cuff repair: Magnetic resonance imaging and early clinical evaluation. *Am J Sports Med* 2009;37(4):674-682.

The authors compared arthroscopic single- and double-row rotator cuff repairs. No substantial difference was found between repair types at a minimum of 12 months. The average tear size was 1.8 cm, and most tears (82.5%) were small or medium size (1 to 3 cm).

81. Franceschi F, Ruzzini L, Longo UG, et al: Equivalent clinical results of arthroscopic single-row and double-row suture anchor repair for rotator cuff tears: A randomized controlled trial. *Am J Sports Med* 2007;35(8): 1254-1260.

Sixty patients prospectively randomized to single- or double-row arthroscopic rotator cuff repair showed no difference in outcome clinically or on MRI arthrography at 2 years. Level of evidence: I.

82. Sugaya H, Maeda K, Matsuki K, Moriishi J: Repair integrity and functional outcome after arthroscopic double-row rotator cuff repair: A prospective outcome study. *J Bone Joint Surg Am* 2007;89(5):953-960.

On postoperative MRI, the retear rate was 5% for small to medium size tears and 40% for large and massive tears. The average clinical outcome improved significantly, but large postoperative defects were associated with lower functional scores. Level of evidence: IV.

83. Park JY, Lhee SH, Choi JH, Park HK, Yu JW, Seo JB: Comparison of the clinical outcomes of single- and double-row repairs in rotator cuff tears. *Am J Sports Med* 2008;36(7):1310-1316.

A cohort study of 78 patients retrospectively compared arthroscopic single- and double-row cuff repairs. There was no difference in clinical or functional outcome for tears smaller than 3 cm. Patients with tears larger than 3 cm had better clinical results with double-row repairs. No postoperative imaging was used. Level of evidence: II.

84. Charousset C, Grimberg J, Duranthon LD, Bellaiche L, Petrover D: Can a double-row anchorage technique improve tendon healing in arthroscopic rotator cuff repair? A prospective, nonrandomized, comparative study of double-row and single-row anchorage techniques with computed tomographic arthrography tendon healing assessment. *Am J Sports Med* 2007;35(8):1247-1253.

The authors compared arthroscopic single- and double-row cuff repairs and found no significant clinical difference between the repair types. Postoperative CT arthrography showed significantly better healing with double-row repairs at 6-month follow-up. Level of evidence: II.

85. Park MC, Cadet ER, Levine WN, Bigliani LU, Ahmad CS: Tendon-to-bone pressure distributions at a repaired rotator cuff footprint using transosseous suture and suture anchor fixation techniques. *Am J Sports Med* 2005; 33(8):1154-1159.

86. Park MC, ElAttrache NS, Tibone JE, Ahmad CS, Jun BJ, Lee TQ: Part I: Footprint contact characteristics for a transosseous-equivalent rotator cuff repair technique compared with a double-row repair technique. *J Shoulder Elbow Surg* 2007;16(4):461-468.

An arthroscopic transosseous equivalent rotator cuff repair technique showed improved pressurized contact area and overall pressure between tendon and footprint when compared with a double-row technique.

87. Zheng N, Harris HW, Andrews JR: Failure analysis of rotator cuff repair: A comparison of three double-row techniques. *J Bone Joint Surg Am* 2008;90(5):1034-1042.

A biomechanical study comparing double-row fixation with corkscrew anchors, knotless anchors, and transosseous tunnels showed a higher individual failure rate with corkscrew anchors compared to knotless anchor and transosseous techniques. Level of evidence: controlled laboratory study.

3: Upper Extremity

88. Frank JB, ElAttrache NS, Dines JS, Blackburn A, Crues J, Tibone JE: Repair site integrity after arthroscopic transosseous-equivalent suture-bridge rotator cuff repair. *Am J Sports Med* 2008;36(8):1496-1503.

Retrospective analysis of arthroscopic transosseous equivalent cuff repair showed that 88% of small and medium, and 86% of large and massive tears were healed on 12-month postoperative MRIs. Persistent tears were not correlated with patient age or the initial tear size. Level of evidence: IV.

89. Klepps S, Bishop J, Lin J, et al: Prospective evaluation of the effect of rotator cuff integrity on the outcome of open rotator cuff repairs. *Am J Sports Med* 2004;32(7):1716-1722.

90. Galatz LM, Ball CM, Teefey SA, Middleton WD, Yamaguchi K: The outcome and repair integrity of completely arthroscopically repaired large and massive rotator cuff tears. *J Bone Joint Surg Am* 2004;86(2):219-224.

91. Iannotti JP, Codsi MJ, Kwon YW, Derwin K, Ciccone J, Brems JJ: Porcine small intestine submucosa augmentation of surgical repair of chronic two-tendon rotator cuff tears: A randomized, controlled trial. *J Bone Joint Surg Am* 2006;88(6):1238-1244.

92. Gerber C, Maquieira G, Espinosa N: Latissimus dorsi transfer for the treatment of irreparable rotator cuff tears. *J Bone Joint Surg Am* 2006;88(1):113-120.

93. Nové-Josserand L, Costa P, Liotard JP, Safar JF, Walch G, Zilber S: Results of latissimus dorsi tendon transfer for irreparable cuff tears. *Orthop Traumatol Surg Res* 2009;95(2):108-113.

The authors recommend latissimus dorsi tendon transfer for irreparable posterosuperior rotator cuff tears with loss of active external rotation associated with a deficient teres minor muscle. They caution against latissimus dorsi tendon transfer in the absence of active motion deficiency. Level of evidence: IV.

94. Costouros JG, Espinosa N, Schmid MR, Gerber C: Teres minor integrity predicts outcome of latissimus dorsi tendon transfer for irreparable rotator cuff tears. *J Shoulder Elbow Surg* 2007;16(6):727-734.

A retrospective review of 22 patients who underwent latissimus dorsi tendon transfer for massive irreparable posterior-superior rotator cuff tears demonstrated significant improvement in mean absolute Constant scores, age-adjusted Constant scores, and subjective shoulder values. Patients with preoperative teres minor fatty infiltration less than or equal to grade 2 demonstrated significantly better postoperative Constant scores, active elevation, and external rotation. Level of evidence: IV.

95. Jost B, Puskas GJ, Lustenberger A, Gerber C: Outcome of pectoralis major transfer for the treatment of irreparable subscapularis tears. *J Bone Joint Surg Am* 2003;85(10):1944-1951.

96. Resch H, Povacz P, Ritter E, Matschi W: Transfer of the pectoralis major muscle for the treatment of irreparable rupture of the subscapularis tendon. *J Bone Joint Surg Am* 2000;82(3):372-382.

97. Hawkins RJ, Misamore GW, Hobeika PE: Surgery for full-thickness rotator-cuff tears. *J Bone Joint Surg Am* 1985;67(9):1349-1355.

Chapter 25

Shoulder and Elbow Disorders in the Athlete

Joseph Bernstein, MD   Matthew Pepe, MD   Lee Kaplan, MD

Shoulder Disorders

The throwing athlete is at increased risk for injury to the shoulder because of the large and repetitive forces generated during the throwing motion. Injuries may occur from a single supraphysiologic load or from repeated subthreshold loads that cumulatively damage the tissue.

The act of throwing has been classified, with some variation, into five stages: windup, early cocking, late cocking, acceleration, and deceleration with follow-through. This classification centers on the essential physical challenge of each phase (Figure 1). In the late cocking phase, the throwing arm is externally rotated with the arm abducted; the greater this external rotation, the greater the velocity that can be obtained from the internal rotator muscles in the acceleration phase. At the completion of the throwing motion, the arm has been internally rotated through an arc of approximately 180°. This arc is traversed at speeds approaching 7,000° per second, with great forces applied to both accelerate and decelerate the arm.[1] As such, the arm is structurally challenged to move within a wide arc while maintaining the location of the humeral head within the glenoid fossa.

The needed range of motion is attained by allowing just enough soft-tissue laxity, and the humeral location is maintained by the action of both static and dynamic stabilizers. Static stability is provided by the capsule and ligaments, and dynamic stability is conferred by the eccentric contraction of the rotator cuff muscles. If the capsule and ligaments are insufficiently lax, the forces of throwing applied to these tight tissues may damage them. Likewise, if the capsule and ligaments

are too loose or if the rotator cuff does not hold the humeral head in contact against the glenoid, forceful abutment between the articular surfaces may lead to injury. The cuff itself is subject to repetitive microtrauma with every throw as it eccentrically contracts to stabilize the humeral head in the glenoid.

Clinical Evaluation

The clinical evaluation of a throwing athlete begins with careful consideration of the shoulder symptoms. Although some throwers may report nonspecific symptoms, such as constant pain or a "dead arm," others may describe focal complaints that localize the pathology, either in terms of the anatomic structure or the phase of throwing that induces the symptoms. A general history, to exclude a cause not associated with throwing, must also be obtained.

The physical examination includes palpation of all of the bony and soft-tissue landmarks. Range of motion should be assessed, with particular attention to the total arc of motion. It should be remembered that the shoulders of throwing athletes may undergo adaptive changes that begin during early adolescence. As such, throwers may have decreased internal rotation and increased external rotation in the abducted arm. Likewise, the coracohumeral ligament and the anterior band of the inferior glenohumeral ligament, which restrain external rotation in the abducted arm, can become lax in the throwing shoulder.[2,3] The main osseous change is increased retroversion of the proximal humerus, which enables the throwing shoulder to achieve additional external rotation while keeping the glenohumeral joint located.[4] The examiner must also remember that laxity of the medial collateral ligament of the elbow (either symptomatic or asymptomatic) may increase apparent external rotation of the shoulder by valgus gapping of the elbow.[5] Close attention to scapular dynamic is also important. Although the scapula and surrounding muscles may not be painful, poor scapular dynamics may predispose the arm to a compensatory injury in the glenohumeral joint.

Special and eponymous physical examination maneuvers for specific lesions have been developed, but the hallmark of preoperative anatomic diagnosis is MRI, typically enhanced with an injection of contrast material. The limitations of MRI are its inability to

Dr. Bernstein or an immediate family member has received royalties from Clinical Orthopaedics and Related Research. Neither Dr. Kaplan nor any immediate family member has received anything of value from or owns stock in a commercial company or institution related directly or indirectly to the subject of this chapter. Dr. Pepe or an immediate family member is a member of a Speakers' bureau or has made paid presentations on behalf of Tornier.

3: Upper Extremity

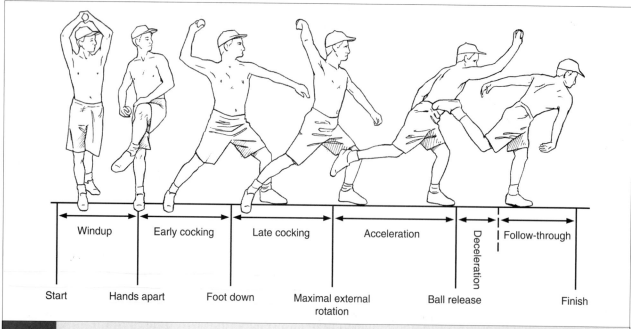

Figure 1 Illustration showing the five main stages of overhead throwing motion. (Adapted with permission from DiGiovine NM, Jobe FW, Pink M, Perry J: An electromyographic analysis of the upper extremity in pitching. *J Shoulder Elbow Surg* 1992;1:15–25.)

portray the dynamic relationship between structures and its inability to identify specifically the source of symptoms (as opposed to simply identifying structures that are incidentally abnormal in appearance). An over-reliance on MRI and excessive focus on every anatomic perturbation may lead to diagnostic excess, overtreatment, and an increase in iatrogenic complications.

Instability and Laxity

The term shoulder instability typically refers to subluxation or dislocation, with the patient often describing a sensation indicating excessive humeral head translation on the glenoid.[6] This sensation is rarely reported by the throwing athlete. Rather, the throwing athlete will present with what has been termed subtle or microinstability—a form of pathologic laxity that predisposes the shoulder to secondary injury; that is, the athlete will report pain with throwing or loss of mechanical effectiveness whose occult cause is instability.[7] The thrower may also report paresthesias in the arm because of possible traction on the nerves about the shoulder girdle caused by the glenohumeral instability. A sense of subluxation or frank dislocation is atypical.

The proposed causes of the pathologic laxity include repetitive microtrauma to the anterior capsule (as the arm is maximally externally rotated) or contracture of the posterior capsule, causing secondary damage to the anterior structures. Repeated forceful loading of the humeral head may create primary laxity of the anterior stabilizing soft tissues; conversely, a tight posterior capsule that shifts the humeral head forward may result in excessive stresses on the anterior structures. A combination of factors may be involved.

If instability is considered, the shoulder examination should attempt to measure anterior translation and the presence of apprehension when the arm is abducted and externally rotated. A positive relocation test, defined as relief of the pain or apprehension when a posterior force is applied, can be helpful. Tightness of the posterior capsule should be ascertained by measuring the arc of rotation with the patient supine (or by other means that hold the scapula fixed) and the arm abducted.

Treatment of pathologic laxity depends on the severity of the laxity and the presence of concomitant abnormalities. Most throwers with evidence of pathologic laxity without labral detachment can be treated by a program of rehabilitation. Particular emphasis should be placed on stretching (to minimize any capsular contractures) and on strengthening the rotator cuff (to increase dynamic stability of the glenohumeral joint). Surgery is reserved for patients who have not been successfully treated with nonsurgical care. The precise surgical plan is defined by the physical findings. Any frank tissue damage, such as a Bankart lesion, should be repaired. Labral repairs, capsular repair shifts and plication, and rotator interval closures have been recommended, but excellent results are not uniformly obtained. If a tight posterior capsule contributes to the instability, a release may be indicated.

Superior Labrum Anterior Posterior Tears

Superior labrum anterior posterior (SLAP) tears are common injuries in the throwing athlete, causing pain with throwing and loss of velocity. SLAP tears have been categorized into various types,[8] but the main dis-

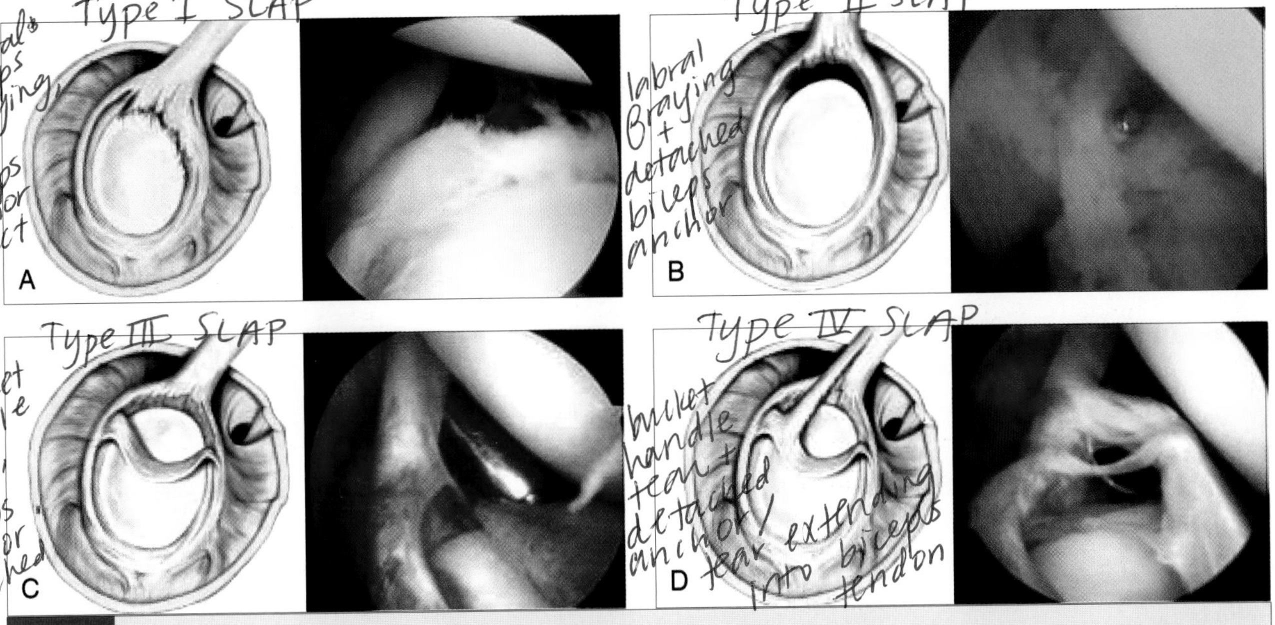

[Handwritten note: ⊛ remember labral variants!! (see back page)]

[Handwritten annotations on figures:]
- *Type I SLAP — labral biceps fraying but biceps anchor intact*
- *Type II SLAP — labral fraying + detached biceps anchor*
- *Type III SLAP — bucket handle tear but biceps anchor attached*
- *Type IV SLAP — bucket handle tear + detached anchor, tear extending into biceps tendon*

Figure 2 Illustrations and arthroscopic images of SLAP lesions. **A,** Type I lesion characterized by superior labral fraying with degeneration. **B,** Type II lesion characterized by detachment of the superior labrum/biceps anchor from the glenoid. **C,** Type III lesion with a bucket-handle tear of the superior labrum with an intact biceps anchor. **D,** Type IV lesion with a bucket-handle tear of the superior labrum with extension of the labral tear into the biceps tendon. (Illustrations © Stephen J. Snyder, MD, Van Nuys, CA.)

[Handwritten note: type II SLAP most common]

tinction is whether the biceps anchor and capsule are intact (**Figure 2**). The most common variant is a tear with the biceps anchor detached. These injuries are believed to result from a peelback mechanism, namely, when the shoulder is abducted and maximally externally rotated and the distal part of the biceps anchor becomes avulsed from the posterior-superior glenoid rim.[1]

The throwing athlete with a SLAP tear often reports decreased throwing velocity and pain in the late cocking phase of the throwing motion. Mechanical symptoms, such as catching or locking, may be reported. Many physical examination maneuvers have been proposed for detecting SLAP tears, but these maneuvers might be too unreliable for clinical use.[9] A SLAP tear is best diagnosed visually on imaging studies or arthroscopically. Correlating the patient's symptoms with radiographic and intraoperative findings is often challenging.

The initial treatment for a patient with a suspected SLAP tear is strengthening and stretching of the shoulder with physical therapy; surgery is indicated if non-surgical treatments fail. Surgical treatment consists of débriding frayed tissue and stabilizing the biceps anchor and labrum back to the glenoid. Range-of-motion exercises for the elbow, wrist, and fingers should be started just after surgery; however, the shoulder should be immobilized for 2 weeks and external rotation should be avoided for 4 weeks. A recent study showed that arthroscopic repair of SLAP tears in throwing athletes allowed 70% to 80% of patients to return to a preinjury level of performance.[10] The most common complication seen after a type II SLAP repair is over-

tightening of the repair causing postoperative stiffness and loss of motion.[11] Although controversial, biceps tenotomy or tenodesis can be considered in nonthrowing athletes.

Internal Impingement

Partial, articular-sided, rotator cuff tears are common in the throwing athlete. In throwing athletes, these tears are believed to be caused by either a tensile or compressive failure of the tendon. Tensile failure results from repetitive eccentric contractions.[12] Compressive failure is believed to occur when the cuff is compressed in a position of arm abduction and external rotation between the greater tuberosity of the humeral head and the posterior glenoid. This produces internal impingement of the articular side of the rotator cuff.[13] The term internal impingement is used to contrast this condition with subacromial (external) impingement on the bursal surface of the cuff (**Figure 3**).

The first-line treatment for patients with a suspected cuff lesion from internal impingement is a physical therapy program dedicated to restoring normal kinematics to the shoulder and stretching to relieve capsular contractures.[14] Specific stretches, such as the "sleeper" stretch and the cross-body adduction stretch, can be helpful in eliminating posterior capsule tightness. Subacromial injections and nonsteroidal anti-inflammatory drugs (NSAIDs) can be used judiciously during the initial treatment period. As shoulder motion improves and pain decreases, therapy should focus on strengthening the rotator cuff and periscapular musculature. An interval throwing program can be initiated. If improvement does not occur, surgery may be warranted; however, ar-

[Sidebar: 3: Upper Extremity]

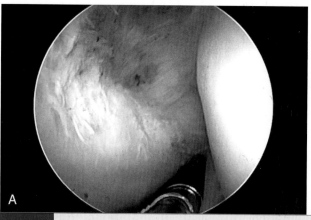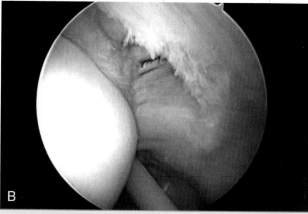

Figure 3	Arthroscopic view through the posterior portal of a small partial-thickness tear of the articular side of the rotator cuff. (Reproduced from Wolff AB, Sethi P, Sutton KM, Covey AS, Magit DP, Medvecky M: Partial-thickness rotator cuff tears. *J Am Acad Orthop Surg* 2006;14:715-725.)

throscopic débridement of partial tears has achieved inconsistent results, with some athletes having difficulty in returning to sports participation.[15] Compression between the greater tuberosity and the posterior glenoid in the position of arm abduction and external rotation is also seen in asymptomatic throwers.[16]

Scapular Dyskinesis

Scapular dysfunction during throwing disrupts normal throwing biomechanics and places the athlete at risk for injury to the labrum, rotator cuff, and capsule. Overuse and accompanying fatigue of the shoulder complex causes an imbalance of the periscapular musculature. Such power imbalances lead to protraction of the scapula and alterations of the geometric relationship of the glenoid and humeral head. If the scapula fails to retract normally, excessive angulation of the humerus occurs relative to the glenoid and excessive stress is placed on the anterior capsule of the shoulder and posterosuperior labrum.

Throwers with scapular dyskinesis present with a range of symptoms, including anterior shoulder pain, posterosuperior scapular pain, and proximolateral (subacromial) discomfort; a loss of velocity and pain with throwing may also be reported. The affected scapula is usually lower and more protracted than the scapula on the uninjured side, and the inferomedial border of the scapula is prominent. Tenderness in the coracoid region is a common finding. Treatment of scapular dyskinesis begins with strengthening the core musculature. After core stability is corrected and scapular motion is normalized, emphasis is placed on strengthening the periscapular muscles, especially the serratus anterior and lower trapezius. These muscles help hold the scapula in the correct retracted position and can be strengthened with low row, inferior glide, and lawn mower pull exercises.[17] The last phase of rehabilitation, after scapular motion has normalized and periscapular strength has returned, focuses on rotator cuff strengthening, with exercises that emphasize closed kinetic chain strengthening. Successful treatment of scapular dyskinesis requires a 2- to 3-month course of therapy.

Acromioclavicular Joint Injuries

Although acromioclavicular (AC) joint injuries are common in contact sports, the AC joint infrequently causes acute pain in the throwing athlete. Over a long career, repetitive throwing can produce inflammation and microtrauma in the AC joint. Some athletes have a hyperemic response in the distal clavicle that results in bone resorption and secondary arthritic changes. Reports of pain with overhead motion and reaching across the body are common. When taking the patient's history, information on previous trauma should be elicited because low-grade AC joint separations can induce arthritic changes.

Classic physical examination findings include tenderness to palpation over the AC joint and discomfort during the cross-body test. Radiographic analysis of AC joint pathology should include AP, axillary, and Zanca views. The Zanca view is taken with 10° to 15° of cephalic tilt, with the patient in an upright position and without any support to the injured arm. These views may show distal clavicle osteolysis and arthritic changes not seen otherwise. An injection with a combination of steroid and local anesthetic may be helpful for diagnosis as well as initial treatment.

As with many conditions in the throwing athlete, the treatment of AC joint arthrosis begins with NSAIDs and physical therapy, with a program emphasizing strengthening and stretching of the shoulder girdle. A distal clavicle resection may be performed if improvement does not occur with nonsurgical management. If there is any doubt regarding the source of the symptoms, a diagnostic shoulder arthroscopy should be part of the surgical procedure. The most common cause of failed surgery is inadequate posterior-superior resection of bone; however, care should be taken not to resect more than 1 cm of clavicle because this can injure the coracoclavicular ligaments and produce instability.[18] The athlete can usually return to sports 3 months after surgery if motion and strength have been restored.

Neurovascular Injuries

Although neurovascular injuries are rare in throwers, such injuries have been described in overhead athletes and should be considered in the differential diagnosis of the painful shoulder. The theme common to these conditions is extrinsic pressure on nerves or adjacent blood vessels. For example, the suprascapular nerve can be compressed at the suprascapular and spinoglenoid notches and can mimic intrinsic rotator cuff disease. Entrapment at the suprascapular notch will affect the supraspinatus and infraspinatus, whereas compression at the spinoglenoid notch will weaken the infraspinatus. Injuries to the suprascapular nerve are well described in volleyball players, but the exact incidence of these injuries in baseball players is unknown. The extremes of arm positioning and the forces generated by the throwing motion have been postulated to cause stretching and compression of the suprascapular nerve, causing a type II SLAP tear and the development of paralabral cysts. Overhead athletes with suprascapular nerve injuries present with poorly localized pain in the posterolateral shoulder, weakness, and pain that may radiate down the arm. In the later stages of the injury, examination of the shoulder may show atrophy of the supraspinatus and/or infraspinatus. On examination, significant weakness is usually revealed when testing external rotation, with a presentation that may be very similar to rotator cuff tendinitis. Magnetic resonance arthrography is useful in identifying labral cysts or a hypertrophied scapular ligament, in quantifying the degree of atrophy of the muscles, and in assessing the integrity of the rotator cuff tendons. Electromyography can be helpful in making the diagnosis and in providing information regarding the severity and location of the compression.

Treatment for a suprascapular nerve injury depends on the underlying etiology. For patients without an anatomic cause for the compression, activity modification is the best initial treatment, along with NSAIDs and strengthening exercises for the rotator cuff, deltoid, and scapula. Most patients respond positively to this treatment protocol. Athletes with evidence of early muscle atrophy, anatomic compression, or those in whom nonsurgical management fails are candidates for surgery. If the nerve compression is located at the suprascapular notch, open or arthroscopic release of the transverse scapular ligament using a superior approach may be needed. Paralabral cysts can be treated with arthroscopic repair of the labrum, with anchors and indirect decompression of the cyst. Spinoglenoid cysts usually respond to arthroscopic treatment, although successful open treatment has been reported.[19]

Quadrilateral space syndrome is a compression neuropathy of the axillary nerve within the four-sided area bounded by the teres minor superiorly, the teres major inferiorly, the long head of the triceps medially, and the proximal humerus laterally. As is the case with many other conditions affecting the throwing athlete, the compression of the structures within the quadrilateral space appears to be greatest in the late cocking phase of throwing. Symptoms of quadrilateral space syndrome are initially vague. Athletes may report mild discomfort and weakness with throwing activities. There may be associated night pain and lateral arm paresthesias. Physical findings may include weakness with abduction, loss of sensation in the axillary nerve distribution, and atrophy of the deltoid muscle. Tenderness over the quadrilateral space has been suggested as a reliable physical examination finding in the throwing athlete.[20]

Arteriography is the study of choice for diagnosing quadrilateral space syndrome; however, for maximal accuracy the dye must be injected with the arm at the side and in the late cocking phase position of abduction and external rotation. The diagnosis is made when the artery is occluded in the abduction-external rotation position and relieved when the arm is brought down to the side. Nonsurgical management, consisting of rest, NSAIDs, and physical therapy focused on stretching and strengthening the posterior shoulder, is the preferred initial treatment option. If success is not achieved after 6 months of nonsurgical treatment, decompression has been shown to be a beneficial option.

Thoracic outlet syndrome is a rare (and controversial) cause of neurovascular disorders in throwing athletes. In thoracic outlet syndrome, anomalous bands of the pectoralis minor,[21] an anomalous first rib, or extremes of arm positioning (for example, the late cocking phase of throwing) are believed to compress the neurovascular structures as they exit the thoracic cavity. Symptoms caused by the ischemia include arm heaviness, fatigue, cold intolerance, paresthesias, and coolness and numbness in the fingers. During the physical examination, the radial pulse should be checked with the arm at the side and then with the shoulder in the abducted, externally rotated position (the Wright test). Surgical options for thoracic outlet syndrome that is recalcitrant to rest and therapy include first rib resection, release of anomalous bands of fascia, scalenectomy, and pectoralis minor tenotomy.

Elbow Disorders

Elbow Instability

During the late cocking and acceleration phases of throwing, the elbow is rapidly extended more than 90° and is exposed to high valgus stresses. These forces can lead to attenuation, partial tears, or even complete rupture of the medial ligament complex. Because throwing creates tension on the medial side specifically, the lateral ligament complex is not typically injured in the throwing athlete.

Valgus instability usually manifests as pain occurring in the medial epicondyle region during the late cocking/early acceleration phase of throwing. Ulnar nerve symptoms can be induced by traction (secondary to instability) or from direct mechanical irritation of the nerve by the ligament. Arthrosis of the elbow joint occurs as a secondary adaptation to the stress, with osteophyte formation along the posteromedial olecranon and calcification in the ligament. Posteromedial impingement will typically cause pain in a more posterior location at or near the terminal extension.

A thorough history and physical examination is the key to diagnosing ulnar collateral ligament injuries in a throwing athlete. It is important to elicit information about previous symptoms or injuries. Throwers may report having experienced an acute "pop" or sharp medial elbow pain. Some throwers have an insidious onset of pain without a specific inciting event; throwing velocity, command, and control are affected. Mechanical symptoms may signal the presence of loose bodies. In younger pitchers, it is important to obtain information on pitch counts and the types of pitches thrown because elevated pitch counts and curveballs and sliders have been associated with pain.[22] More recent studies have shown that the type of pitch has substantially less effect on shoulder and elbow loads than the absolute number of pitches thrown and that throwing a fastball causes higher elbow loads than throwing a curveball.[23] Discussions with coaches and athletic trainers also can be beneficial because correct pitching mechanics lower valgus elbow loads and increase pitching efficiency.[24]

The physical examination of the thrower with medial elbow pain involves evaluating the entire extremity. It is important to exclude pathology in the shoulder and scapula because problems there can produce referred elbow pain or induce a secondary injury at the elbow (by abnormal mechanics). Particular attention should be paid to examining the shoulder for a posterior capsular contracture as a cause of medial elbow pain. A substantial percentage of throwers with an ulnar collateral ligament insufficiency have a glenohumeral internal rotation deficit when compared with asymptomatic pitchers.[25] The cervical spine also should be examined in any thrower with neurologic symptoms because cervical nerve root pathology can mimic ulnar neuropathy at the elbow. The range of motion of the affected elbow in flexion and extension and in pronation and supination should be measured with a goniometer and compared with the contralateral side. It is common for even asymptomatic pitchers to have a flexion contracture of the elbow. Measurements taken before and after pitching show a significant decrease in elbow extension both immediately and 24 hours after throwing.[26]

Valgus stress testing is performed at both 0° and 30° to evaluate the medial collateral ligament. Asymptomatic throwers typically have a degree of developmental laxity of the medial restraints of the injured elbow when compared with the contralateral side.[27] A dynamic valgus stress test is believed to be sensitive and specific for ulnar collateral ligament tears. In this test, a constant valgus load is applied to the maximally flexed elbow as it is brought rapidly into extension. A positive finding occurs when medial pain is reproduced between

the arcs of 120° and 70°.[28] Tenderness in valgus extension overload occurs along the posteromedial olecranon. Pain is reproduced with valgus and forced extension of the elbow. Flexor pronator tendinitis may also manifest as medial-sided elbow pain. Tenderness is noted at or just distal to the medial epicondyle, and pain is reproduced with resisted wrist flexion and forearm pronation. The ulnar nerve is palpated for tenderness and instability. Tinel and cubital tunnel compression tests can be used to check for ulnar nerve irritability, which can occur in isolation or concomitant with ulnar collateral insufficiency.

Standard AP, lateral, and oblique radiographs are routinely obtained and may show calcification within the ligament as well as posterior compartment osteophytes. MRI is a useful tool in evaluating the soft tissues of the elbow, including the collateral ligaments, articular surface, and ulnar nerve. Noncontrast MRI can identify full-thickness tears of the ulnar collateral ligament, hypertrophy, or tears of the flexor pronator origin. Consideration must be given, however, to the very high rate of abnormal findings in the asymptomatic high-level thrower.[29,30] In a study that evaluated the elbows of professional pitchers with plain radiographs, a significant number of radiographic abnormalities were reported; however, the pathologic findings did not correlate with impairment.[30] The pathologic findings did correlate with activity (the number of innings pitched professionally). Using contrast material adds to the sensitivity of the MRI study, particularly for partial-thickness tears; however, the instillation of this fluid may cause discomfort that may interfere with athletic performance for several days. Dynamic ultrasound has been used to evaluate the medial collateral ligament but produces a high rate of abnormal findings in the asymptomatic major league pitcher.[31,32] Ultrasound also has been shown to have high accuracy in diagnosing medial epicondylitis.[33] The accuracy of ultrasound may be dependent on the skill of the examiner.

Nonsurgical treatment is the preferred first step in treating medial-sided elbow pain. Rest, coupled with stretching and strengthening exercises, should be prescribed. Corticosteroid injections may offer short-term relief in the patient with refractory medial elbow pain but have not been shown to be better than placebo. Platelet-rich plasma injections may avoid the possible adverse side effects of corticosteroid injections, but they too may rely on a placebo effect.[34] The authors of one study reported that nonsurgical treatment of an ulnar collateral ligament injury in a pitcher has a success rate of 42%,[35] with success defined as a return to the same or a higher level of competition. No factors from either the patient's history or physical examination could predict a successful outcome.

Direct repair of the ulnar collateral ligament is possible if rupture occurs at the proximal or distal end and if the remaining ligament tissue is adequate. This scenario is more typical in younger, adolescent athletes who have not experienced much wear and tear. A preoperative MRI or ultrasound will define the location of the tear and the quality of the remaining tissue and

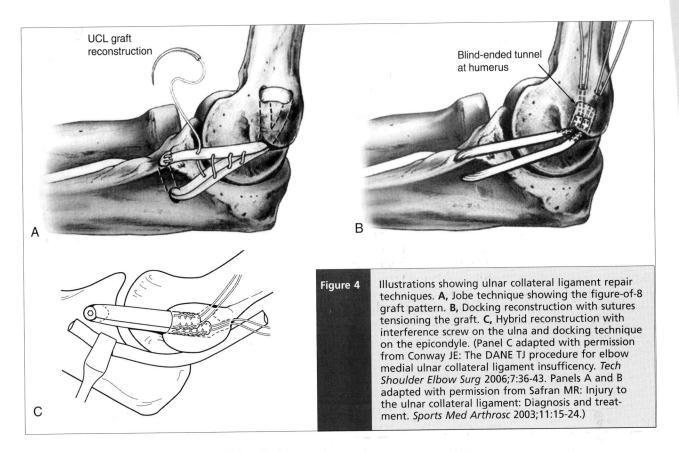

Figure 4 | Illustrations showing ulnar collateral ligament repair techniques. **A,** Jobe technique showing the figure-of-8 graft pattern. **B,** Docking reconstruction with sutures tensioning the graft. **C,** Hybrid reconstruction with interference screw on the ulna and docking technique on the epicondyle. (Panel C adapted with permission from Conway JE: The DANE TJ procedure for elbow medial ulnar collateral ligament insufficiency. *Tech Shoulder Elbow Surg* 2006;7:36-43. Panels A and B adapted with permission from Safran MR: Injury to the ulnar collateral ligament: Diagnosis and treatment. *Sports Med Arthrosc* 2003;11:15-24.)

plan the treatment, though final treatment decisions are made intraoperatively, based on visualization of the ligament. The repair is best performed using suture anchors with braided nonabsorbable suture. In one study, nearly all the athletes achieved a good to excellent result and returned to the same level of competition.[36] Various techniques have been described for reconstruction, including the traditional Jobe technique, the docking procedure, and interference screw fixation[37-39] (Figure 4). When performed by an experienced surgeon, ligament reconstruction of the anterior band of the ulnar collateral ligament (without ulnar nerve transposition) offers athletes a good chance for successful return to their preinjury level of competition.[37]

Medial Epicondylitis

Medial epicondylitis is a syndrome characterized by medial elbow pain and is associated with degeneration of the flexor pronator origin. It may also be associated with ulnar collateral ligament insufficiency or ulnar nerve symptoms. Physical examination findings include tenderness over the anterior aspect of the medial epicondyle and pain that is reproduced with resisted pronation and wrist flexion. It is important to rule out concomitant medial instability in the throwing athlete. Although nonsurgical management has a very high success rate,[40] the condition may take several months for overall resolution. Surgical treatment involves excising the area of tendinopathy. The ulnar nerve may be transposed if there is also cubital tunnel compression.

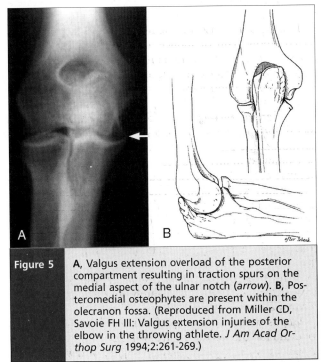

Figure 5 | A, Valgus extension overload of the posterior compartment resulting in traction spurs on the medial aspect of the ulnar notch (*arrow*). B, Posteromedial osteophytes are present within the olecranon fossa. (Reproduced from Miller CD, Savoie FH III: Valgus extension injuries of the elbow in the throwing athlete. *J Am Acad Orthop Surg* 1994;2:261-269.)

Valgus Extension Overload

Posteromedial impingement of the olecranon against the medial wall of the olecranon fossa is believed to result from valgus loads placed on the elbow in the early acceleration phase of throwing (**Figure 5**). This stress causes reactive osteophyte formation along the postero-medial wall of the olecranon, a spur that causes impingement in extension. Pain is typically located posteromedially and is reported in the deceleration phase of throwing. The pain may be mild at first, but progression over the course of the game is common.[41] An axial view of the olecranon with the elbow flexed to 110°, MRI, or CT will define the osteophyte and identify any loose bodies if present. Nonsurgical treatment, which is always attempted first, typically has a poor prognosis if a posteromedial osteophyte is present.

Surgical treatment of isolated posteromedial impingement involves excision of the posterior and medial olecranon osteophytes, either arthroscopically or through a miniopen approach. Care must be taken not to remove more than 3 mm of the normal olecranon because greater resection will cause a substantial increase in the strain in the anterior band of the medial collateral ligament.[42] In patients with signs and symptoms of valgus instability in addition to impingement, resection of the posteromedial osteophyte alone is not indicated. Because the olecranon osteophytes were likely caused by elbow instability,[43] the athlete will continue to have instability pain postoperatively if the primary cause of the instability is not treated. In such cases, the ulnar collateral ligament should be reconstructed and the osteophytes should be removed.

Annotated References

1. Burkhart SS, Morgan CD, Kibler WB: The disabled throwing shoulder: Spectrum of pathology. Part I: Pathoanatomy and biomechanics. *Arthroscopy* 2003; 19(4):404-420.

2. Kuhn JE, Bey MJ, Huston LJ, Blasier RB, Soslowsky LJ: Ligamentous restraints to external rotation of the humerus in the late-cocking phase of throwing: A cadaveric biomechanical investigation. *Am J Sports Med* 2000;28(2):200-205.

3. Fitzpatrick MJ, Tibone JE, Grossman M, McGarry MH, Lee TQ: Development of cadaveric models of a thrower's shoulder. *J Shoulder Elbow Surg* 2005;14(1, suppl S)49S-57S.

4. Crockett HC, Gross LB, Wilk KE, et al: Osseous adaptation and range of motion at the glenohumeral joint in professional baseball pitchers. *Am J Sports Med* 2002; 30(1):20-26.

5. Mihata T, Safran MR, McGarry MH, Abe M, Lee TQ: Elbow valgus laxity may result in an overestimation of apparent shoulder external rotation during physical examination. *Am J Sports Med* 2008;36(5):978-982.

    The authors perform a controlled laboratory study to determine if an increase in elbow valgus laxity affects assessment of shoulder external rotation measured during physical examination at 90° of elbow flexion.

6. Braun S, Kokmeyer D, Millett PJ: Shoulder injuries in the throwing athlete. *J Bone Joint Surg Am* 2009;91(4): 966-978.

    A current concepts review of pathologic conditions affecting the shoulder of the throwing athlete is presented along with associated treatment options. The authors emphasize the importance of physical therapy and rehabilitation as the initial treatment for most throwing-related conditions. Level of evidence: V.

7. Ryu RK, Dunbar WH, Kuhn JE, McFarland EG, Chronopoulos E, Kim TK: Comprehensive evaluation and treatment of the shoulder in the throwing athlete. *Arthroscopy* 2002;18(9, suppl 2):70-89.

8. Snyder SJ, Karzel RP, Del Pizzo W, Ferkel RD, Friedman MJ: SLAP lesions of the shoulder. *Arthroscopy* 1990;6(4):274-279.

9. Calvert E, Chambers GK, Regan W, Hawkins RH, Leith JM: Special physical examination tests for superior labrum anterior posterior shoulder tears are clinically limited and invalid: A diagnostic systematic review. *J Clin Epidemiol* 2009;62(5):558-563.

    A review of the current literature with epidemiologic methodology was performed. The authors concluded that physical examination maneuvers to detect SLAP lesions are not valid or reliable. Level of evidence: I.

10. Ide J, Maeda S, Takagi K: Sports activity after arthroscopic superior labral repair using suture anchors in overhead-throwing athletes. *Am J Sports Med* 2005; 33(4):507-514.

11. Brockmeier SF, Voos JE, Williams RJ III, Altchek DW, Cordasco FA, Allen AA; Hospital for Special Surgery Sports Medicine and Shoulder Service: Outcomes after arthroscopic repair of type-II SLAP lesions. *J Bone Joint Surg Am* 2009;91(7):1595-1603.

    The authors discuss the results of type II SLAP lesions treated with arthroscopic suture anchor fixation. Thirty-four of 47 patients were throwing athletes. With a minimum 2-year follow-up, 25 of the athletes (74%) returned to sports. The major complication with this procedure was postoperative stiffness, which occurred in four patients. Level of evidence: IV.

12. Nakagawa S, Yoneda M, Hayashida K, Wakitani S, Okamura K: Greater tuberosity notch: An important indicator of articular-side partial rotator cuff tears in the shoulders of throwing athletes. *Am J Sports Med* 2001; 29(6):762-770.

13. Heyworth BE, Williams RJ III: Internal impingement of the shoulder. *Am J Sports Med* 2009;37(5):1024-1037.

    A comprehensive review on internal impingement is presented. The authors discuss the clinical presentation and physical examination and imaging findings seen with this condition and review treatment options. A treatment algorithm for internal impingement is included. Level of evidence: V.

14. Matava MJ, Purcell DB, Rudzki JR: Partial-thickness

rotator cuff tears. *Am J Sports Med* 2005;33(9):1405-1417.

15. Payne LZ, Altchek DW, Craig EV, Warren RF: Arthroscopic treatment of partial rotator cuff tears in young athletes: A preliminary report. *Am J Sports Med* 1997;25(3):299-305.

16. Halbrecht JL, Tirman P, Atkin D: Internal impingement of the shoulder: Comparison of findings between the throwing and nonthrowing shoulders of college baseball players. *Arthroscopy* 1999;15(3):253-258.

17. Kibler WB, McMullen J: Scapular dyskinesis and its relation to shoulder pain. *J Am Acad Orthop Surg* 2003; 11(2):142-151.

18. Zvijac JE, Popkin CA, Botto-van Bemden A: Salvage procedure for chronic acromioclavicular dislocation subsequent to overzealous distal clavicle resection. *Orthopedics* 2008;31(12):pii.

    The authors describe a technique to treat AC instability after excessive distal clavicle resection. Level of evidence: IV.

19. Ringel SP, Treihaft M, Carry M, Fisher R, Jacobs P: Suprascapular neuropathy in pitchers. *Am J Sports Med* 1990;18(1):80-86.

20. McAdams TR, Dillingham MF: Surgical decompression of the quadrilateral space in overhead athletes. *Am J Sports Med* 2008;36(3):528-532.

    This study reports on quadrilateral space syndrome in four overhead throwing athletes who required surgical decompression. The cause was fibrous bands in three patients and venous dilatation in one. All athletes returned to full activity by 3 months. Level of evidence: IV.

21. Simovitch RW, Bal GK, Basamania CJ: Thoracic outlet syndrome in a competitive baseball player secondary to the anomalous insertion of an atrophic pectoralis minor muscle: A case report. *Am J Sports Med* 2006;34(6): 1016-1019.

22. Lyman S, Fleisig GS, Andrews JR, Osinski ED: Effect of pitch type, pitch count, and pitching mechanics on risk of elbow and shoulder pain in youth baseball pitchers. *Am J Sports Med* 2002;30(4):463-468.

23. Dun S, Loftice J, Fleisig GS, Kingsley D, Andrews JR: A biomechanical comparison of youth baseball pitches: Is the curveball potentially harmful? *Am J Sports Med* 2008;36(4):686-692.

    The authors studied the kinetics of the fastball, curveball, and change-up baseball pitches in youth pitchers and determined that the curveball may not be more harmful than the fastball. Recent epidemiologic research indicates that amount of pitching is a stronger risk factor for injury than type of pitches thrown.

24. Davis JT, Limpisvasti O, Fluhme D, et al: The effect of pitching biomechanics on the upper extremity in youth and adolescent baseball pitchers. *Am J Sports Med* 2009;37(8):1484-1491.

    The authors performed a descriptive laboratory study and determined that proper pitching mechanics may help prevent pain and injuries to the shoulder and elbow in youth pitchers.

25. Dines JS, Frank JB, Akerman M, Yocum LA: Glenohumeral internal rotation deficits in baseball players with ulnar collateral ligament insufficiency. *Am J Sports Med* 2009;37(3):566-570.

    The authors studied throwers with ulnar collateral ligament insufficiency and determined that pathologic glenohumeral internal rotation deficit may be associated with elbow valgus instability. Level of evidence: III.

26. Reinold MM, Wilk KE, Macrina LC, et al: Changes in shoulder and elbow passive range of motion after pitching in professional baseball players. *Am J Sports Med* 2008;36(3):523-527.

    In a controlled laboratory study, the authors noted a substantial decrease in passive range of motion immediately after baseball pitching that is present 24 hours after throwing. These results may suggest a newly defined mechanism to adaptations in range of motion resulting from acute musculoskeletal and potential osseous and capsular adaptations.

27. Ellenbecker TS, Mattalino AJ, Elam EA, Caplinger RA: Medial elbow joint laxity in professional baseball pitchers: A bilateral comparison using stress radiography. *Am J Sports Med* 1998;26(3):420-424.

28. O'Driscoll SW, Lawton RL, Lawton RL, Smith AM: The "moving valgus stress test" for medial collateral ligament tears of the elbow. *Am J Sports Med* 2005;33(2): 231-239.

29. Kooima CL, Anderson K, Craig JV, Teeter DM, van Holsbeeck M: Evidence of subclinical medial collateral ligament injury and posteromedial impingement in professional baseball players. *Am J Sports Med* 2004;32(7): 1602-1606.

30. Wright RW, Steger-May K, Klein SE: Radiographic findings in the shoulder and elbow of Major League Baseball pitchers. *Am J Sports Med* 2007;35(11):1839-1843.

    The authors found that degenerative changes in the dominant shoulder and elbow of professional pitchers develop over time because of chronic repetitive stresses across joints. Level of evidence: IV.

31. De Smet AA, Winter TC, Best TM, Bernhardt DT: Dynamic sonography with valgus stress to assess elbow ulnar collateral ligament injury in baseball pitchers. *Skeletal Radiol* 2002;31(11):671-676.

32. Nazarian LN, McShane JM, Ciccotti MG, O'Kane PL, Harwood MI: Dynamic US of the anterior band of the ulnar collateral ligament of the elbow in asymptomatic major league baseball pitchers. *Radiology* 2003;227(1): 149-154.

3: Upper Extremity

33. Park GY, Lee MY: Diagnostic value of ultrasonography for clinical medial epicondylitis. *Arch Phys Med Rehabil* 2008;89(4):738-742.

In a prospective, single-blind study, the authors attempted to determine the value of ultrasonography as a diagnostic tool for detecting clinical medial epicondylitis.

34. Mishra A, Pavelko T: Treatment of chronic elbow tendinosis with buffered platelet-rich plasma. *Am J Sports Med* 2006;34(11):1774-1778.

35. Rettig AC, Sherrill C, Snead DS, Mendler JC, Mieling P: Nonoperative treatment of ulnar collateral ligament injuries in throwing athletes. *Am J Sports Med* 2001; 29(1):15-17.

36. Savoie FH III, Trenhaile SW, Roberts J, Field LD, Ramsey JR: Primary repair of ulnar collateral ligament injuries of the elbow in young athletes: A case series of injuries to the proximal and distal ends of the ligament. *Am J Sports Med* 2008;36(6):1066-1072.

The authors concluded that primary repair of proximal and distal injuries of the medial ulnar collateral ligament is an acceptable treatment option in young athletes. Level of evidence: IV.

37. Thompson WH, Jobe FW, Yocum LA, Pink MM: Ulnar collateral ligament reconstruction in athletes: Muscle-splitting approach without transposition of the ulnar nerve. *J Shoulder Elbow Surg* 2001;10(2):152-157.

38. Dodson CC, Thomas A, Dines JS, Nho SJ, Williams RJ III, Altchek DW: Medial ulnar collateral ligament reconstruction of the elbow in throwing athletes. *Am J Sports Med* 2006;34(12):1926-1932.

39. Dines JS, ElAttrache NS, Conway JE, Smith W, Ahmad CS: Clinical outcomes of the DANE TJ technique to treat ulnar collateral ligament insufficiency of the elbow. *Am J Sports Med* 2007;35(12):2039-2044.

The authors studied 22 athletes over a 3-year period and determined that the use of the DANE TJ technique for ulnar collateral ligament reconstruction led to favorable results. Level of evidence: IV.

40. Gabel GT, Morrey BF: Operative treatment of medical epicondylitis: Influence of concomitant ulnar neuropathy at the elbow. *J Bone Joint Surg Am* 1995;77(7): 1065-1069.

41. Wilson FD, Andrews JR, Blackburn TA, McCluskey G: Valgus extension overload in the pitching elbow. *Am J Sports Med* 1983;11(2):83-88.

42. Kamineni S, ElAttrache NS, O'driscoll SW, et al: Medial collateral ligament strain with partial posteromedial olecranon resection: A biomechanical study. *J Bone Joint Surg Am* 2004;86(11):2424-2430.

43. Ahmad CS, Park MC, Elattrache NS: Elbow medial ulnar collateral ligament insufficiency alters posteromedial olecranon contact. *Am J Sports Med* 2004;32(7): 1607-1612.

Labral Variants

1st: most common position of long head of biceps on labrum (supra-glenoid tubercle) is just post. to 12 o'clock

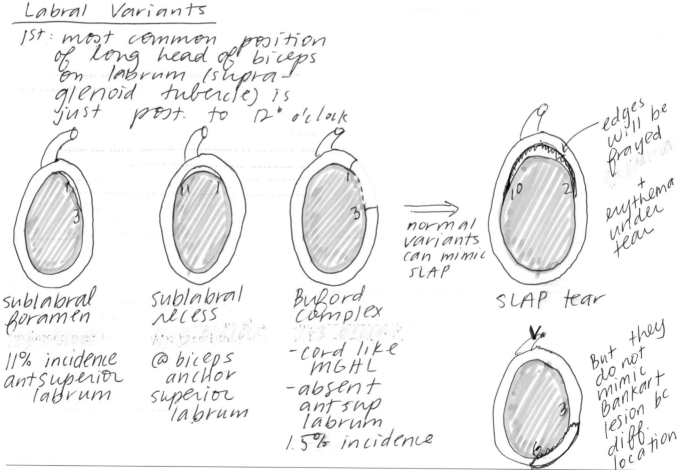

sublabral foramen

11% incidence ant superior labrum

sublabral recess

@ biceps anchor superior labrum

Buford complex

- cord like MGHL
- absent ant sup labrum
1.5% incidence

normal variants can mimic SLAP

edges will be frayed + erythema under tear

SLAP tear

But they do not mimic bankart lesion bc diff location

Bankart

Chapter 26

Elbow and Forearm Trauma

David L. Glaser, MD   April D. Armstrong, MD

Radial Head Fractures

Fractures of the radial head are among the most common elbow fractures, occurring in approximately 20% of all elbow fractures. The typical mechanism of injury is a fall on an outstretched hand with the forearm in pronation.

Classification

Several classification systems have been used to describe radial head fractures but the observer reliability of these systems has been questioned.[1] There have been several variations of the original Mason system, which classified radial head fractures into three categories: type I, a nondisplaced fracture; type II, a displaced partial articular fracture with or without comminution; and type III, a comminuted radial head fracture involving the whole head (**Figure 1**). This system was modified to quantify the extent of the radial head involvement and to include radial neck fractures.[2] Type I was defined as a fracture of the radial head or neck with less than 2 mm of displacement, type II as a fracture of the radial head or neck displaced 2 mm or more and involving 30% or more of the articular surface, type III as a comminuted fracture of the radial head or neck, and type IV as an elbow dislocation with any fracture of the radial head. The Mason classification was later modified to include clinical examination and intraoperative findings so that it could help guide treatment decisions.[3]

Patient Examination and Imaging

Lateral elbow pain and tenderness or limitation in elbow or forearm motion should alert the examiner to the possibility of a radial head fracture. Although tenderness over the radial head is expected, tenderness at other sites suggests the presence of an associated injury.[4] Point tenderness over the lateral epicondyle may indicate a lateral collateral ligament (LCL) injury. Tenderness over the sublime tubercle or medial epicondyle or ecchymosis on the medial aspect of the elbow may indicate a medial collateral ligament (MCL) injury. Pain and tenderness at the distal radioulnar joint or in the forearm should raise suspicion of an interosseous ligament disruption leading to axial forearm instability, termed an Essex-Lopresti lesion.[3]

AP and lateral radiographs of the elbow are typically sufficient to diagnose a radial head injury. The radiocapitellar view is obtained by positioning the patient for a lateral view but angling the tube 45° toward the shoulder. CT is commonly used to better define details of the fracture. Joint aspiration with an injection of a local anesthetic helps assess mechanical blocks to motion.

Treatment

Nondisplaced fractures of the radial head may cause elevation of the anterior and posterior fat pads (the sail sign) by an intra-articular hemarthrosis. These fractures can be treated nonsurgically with a brief period of immobilization in a sling, followed by early motion. Good results have been reported in 85% to 95% of patients with these injuries.[5,6]

For displaced fractures, the decision for surgical fixation and the type of surgical treatment remains controversial. Surgical approaches vary based on the specific pathology of the fracture. For isolated radial head fractures in which a single lateral approach is planned, the patient is positioned supine with an arm board or the affected arm is placed over the body. An extensile posterior skin incision, which will allow access to the medial elbow if needed, is also possible from the supine position. The Kocher approach is preferred if the LCL is known to be disrupted, whereas the more anterior extensor digitorum communis-splitting approach is used if the LCL is intact; this approach avoids injury to the lateral ulnar collateral ligament.

Excision of capitellum or radial head fragments should be avoided if the fragments comprise more than approximately 25% to 33% of the capitellar surface area or 25% of the surface area of the radial head.[6,7] Historically, radial head resection has been considered in patients with isolated, displaced, and comminuted radial head fractures without associated ligamentous injury. Excision alone should generally be considered an option only in low-demand, sedentary patients. Radial head replacement in the absence of demonstrable instability or associated injuries is controversial. Biome-

3: Upper Extremity

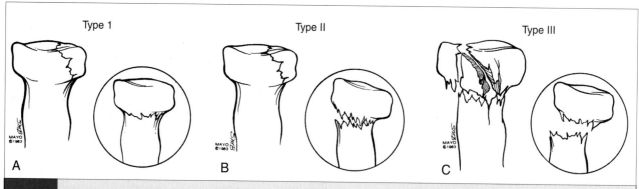

Figure 1 Mason classification of radial head fractures. **A,** Type I are minimally or nondisplaced fractures. **B,** Type II fractures have more than 2 mm of displacement. **C,** Type III fractures are severely comminuted. (Reproduced with permission from the Mayo Foundation for Medical Education and Research, Rochester, MN, 1983.)

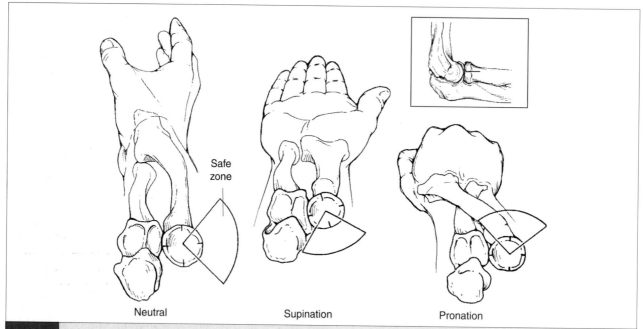

Figure 2 Safe zone for the application of hardware on the radial head. (Reproduced from Hotchkiss RN: Displaced fractures of the radial head: Internal fixation or excision? *J Am Acad Orthop Surg* 1997;5:8.)

chanical studies following radial head resection have shown altered kinematics and stability, which may contribute to the increased rate of radiographic degeneration.[8] The biomechanical implications of radial head resection suggest that restoration of radiocapitellar contact with a radial head replacement is advisable.

In those fractures amenable to repair, stable fixation of the articular surface and restoration of the head-neck relationship can be achieved using a variety of devices. In fractures in which a portion of the head is still connected to the neck, the intact head can be used as a scaffold for securing the fractured fragments using either small standard screws (1.5 to 3.0 mm), fully threaded Kirschner wires, or headless screws. For more complex fracture patterns or those involving the radial neck, mini-implant plates are useful.[9]

The safe zone has been identified as the posterolateral aspect of the radial head that does not articulate with the sigmoid notch of the ulna during forearm rotation[3] (Figure 2). With the forearm in neutral rotation, the safe zone is the portion of the radial head that presents laterally in the wound. Alternatively, this zone can be found within the 90° angle bound by the radial styloid and the Lister tubercle distally.

For displaced radial head fractures with more than three fracture fragments, radial head replacement may be the preferred technique.[6] Appropriately sized radial head replacement implants will restore the length of the radius and radiocapitellar contact. Good clinical results have been reported with metallic radial head implants for comminuted radial head fractures.[10-13] Long-term effects on the capitellar articular cartilage and complications such as implant loosening and failure require further study.

Various implants are available for radial head replacement. However, clinical evidence supporting a particular design, such as bipolar versus monopolar, cemented versus uncemented, and anatomic versus asymmetric head shape, is not yet available.

Attention to the technical aspects of radial head replacement will ensure the best possible outcomes. The resected radial head serves as the optimal template for sizing the prosthetic implant. After the implant has been inserted, the elbow should be moved through a range of motion while the surgeon observes the radiocapitellar contact for congruency and tracking and scrutinizes the height and diameter of the implant. Elbow alignment and implant sizing also can be assessed for parallelism by using fluoroscopy to examine the medial ulnotrochlear joint space.

Distal Humerus Fractures

Classification

Fractures of the distal humerus can be classified according to the Orthopaedic Trauma Association/AO comprehensive classification of fractures of long bones: type A (nonarticular), type B (partial articular), and type C (complete articular).[14] These categories are further subdivided based on the position of the fracture line and the degree of comminution.

Treatment

Nonsurgical management of distal humerus fractures is rarely recommended. Although nonsurgical treatment may be appropriate for nondisplaced fractures, surgical fixation allows immediate motion and is generally preferred. In low-demand patients with preexisting neurologic impairment or if surgery is contraindicated because of medical comorbidities, nonsurgical management may be the only treatment option.

The elbow joint can be exposed through several different surgical approaches. A longitudinal posterior approach can permit the elevation of broad skin flaps and provide extensile exposure of both the medial and lateral sides of the elbow. For isolated condylar fractures, a medial or a lateral approach can be considered. An ulnar nerve transposition should be considered in all cases. Several options exist for approaching the fracture itself, including an olecranon osteotomy, a triceps-sparing approach, and a triceps-splitting approach. The Bryan-Morrey approach involves subperiosteal reflection of the triceps insertion from medial to lateral in continuity with the forearm fascia and anconeus muscle.[15] The triceps-reflecting anconeus pedicle approach described by O'Driscoll[16] may also be used. When treating complex articular fractures, a chevron-shaped osteotomy with the apex pointing distally facilitates anatomic repositioning, enhances stability, and provides a broader interface of cancellous bone. The osteotomy should be located at the depth of the semilunar notch,

where there is the least amount of articular cartilage. Osteotomy should be avoided if total elbow arthroplasty is being considered.

An anatomic study showed that the percentage of articular surface visible after triceps-splitting, triceps-sparing, and olecranon osteotomy were 35%, 46%, and 57%, respectively.[17] If an osteotomy is performed it can be fixed by either compression plating, tension band wiring, or with an intramedullary compression screw. Predrilling helps achieve an anatomic reduction when an intramedullary screw will be used. Variations of the olecranon osteotomy have been reported. Recently, the anconeus flap transolecranon approach, which combines a proximally based anconeus flap with an apex distal chevron osteotomy of the olecranon, has been described.[18] This procedure involves incising the Kocher interval (between the extensor carpi ulnaris and anconeus muscles) and elevating the anconeus muscle in a proximal direction off the ulna. The anconeus remains attached to the proximal olecranon and triceps, which preserves its neurovascular supply. This process maintains the dynamic stabilizing effect of the anconeus muscle and also provides a vascularized bed over the osteotomy, which is hypothesized to reduce the incidence of nonunion. A recent study of olecranon osteotomies in 67 patients reported no nonunions and an 8% rate of hardware removal.[19]

Surgical treatment of intra-articular distal humerus fractures that follows the principles of stable internal fixation with two-column plating, anatomic restoration of the articular surface, and early mobilization yields satisfactory functional and radiographic outcomes.[20,21] Methods of internal fixation include parallel, orthogonal, triple, and fixed-angle plating.[22-26] The findings of a 2009 study support the literature regarding the high success rate of parallel plating, although many techniques lead to successful healing if properly applied.[27]

Although there is controversy regarding optimal plate positioning, it is generally agreed that, if applied appropriately with adequate plates, both parallel and orthogonal placement can provide necessary stability. In addition to screws that are placed through the plate, interfragmentary screws of various sizes and threaded Kirschner wires (if needed) cut at the edge of the fracture fragments can be used to achieve stable fixation. A compression plate, 3.5-mm pelvic reconstruction plates, and precontoured plates are sufficiently rigid to provide stable fixation. In contrast, one third semitubular plates have insufficient strength and are susceptible to breakage in this location; therefore, they are not adequate for fixation of distal humerus fractures.

Primary total elbow arthroplasty for treating comminuted distal humerus fractures has become a viable option for elderly, low-demand patients.[28-32] In a series of 43 fractures treated with primary total elbow arthroplasty, patients achieved a mean range of motion from 24° to 131° at 7-year follow-up.[28] Thirty-two of 49 patients had no further surgery and had no complications. Five revision arthroplasties were required. In an extensive review of 92 elbows treated with total elbow arthroplasty as a salvage procedure for distal humeral

3: Upper Extremity

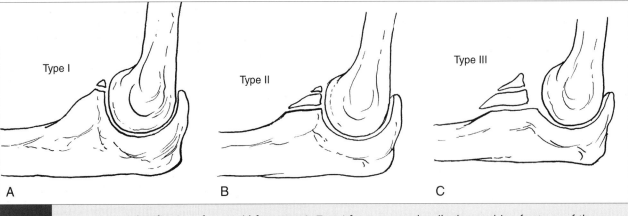

Figure 3   Regan-Morrey classification of coronoid fractures. **A,** Type I fractures are described as avulsion fractures of the tip of the coronoid, and usually do not require surgical treatment. **B,** Type II fractures involve 50% or less of the height of the coronoid, and frequently do not require treatment. **C,** Type III fractures involve more than 50% of the height of the coronoid. (Reproduced with permission from Regan WD, Morrey BF: Coronoid process and Monteggia fractures, in Morrey BF, ed: *The Elbow and Its Disorders*, ed 3. Philadelphia, PA, WB Saunders, 2000, pp 396-408.)

nonunion, improvements were reported in most patients.[30] No pain or mild pain was reported in 74% of patients and 85% had satisfactory subjective results. However, the reoperation rate was 35%. Implant survival was 96% at 2 years, 82% at 5 years, and 65% at 10 and 15 years. Another study of total elbow arthroplasty reported good results with a 29% single complication rate.[31]

In a retrospective review of 24 patients older than 65 years treated with total elbow arthroplasty or open reduction and internal fixation for type C2 or C3 distal humerus fractures, the authors concluded that total elbow arthroplasty was supported in this patient population, particularly in those with osteoporosis and rheumatoid arthritis.[32] However, the study size was small and follow-up was only 2 years. In a prospective study evaluating fracture fixation versus total elbow arthroplasty in elderly patients, the authors reported no difference in functional outcomes at 2-year follow-up using the Disabilities of the Arm, Shoulder and Hand scoring system.[33] The authors stated that arthroplasty is the preferred method of treatment if stable fixation cannot be achieved.

Complications

Complications following fixation of distal humerus fractures are surprisingly common, ranging from 25% to 48%.[25,28-32] Complications include heterotopic ossification, olecranon nonunion, infection, ulnar neuropathy, nonunion, and fixation failure.

Coronoid Fractures

Classification

The classic method for classifying coronoid fractures is based on the height of the coronoid fragment (**Figure 3**). Type I represents a fracture of the coronoid tip that is

believed to be related to a shearing mechanism. This injury was originally described as a brachialis avulsion fracture, but the insertion of the brachialis is more distal to the coronoid tip. Typically, the fragment remains attached to the anterior capsule.[34] Type II fractures involve 50% or less of the coronoid height, and type III involve more than 50% of the coronoid height and can include the attachment of the MCL. Based on biomechanical studies, it has been proposed that, in an otherwise stable elbow, coronoid fractures of 50% or more of the coronoid height should be fixed.[35-37] In a retrospective review of 103 coronoid fractures, patients with associated injuries, particularly radial head fractures, scored lower on the Mayo elbow performance score, had less elbow extension, more pain, and less pronation/supination than those without associated injuries.[38]

Biomechanics and Treatment

In an elbow that is unstable because of a fracture-dislocation, the coronoid process plays an important role in elbow stability. CT scans of elbows with a terrible triad injury showed that the average height for the coronoid fragment was 35% of the total height of the coronoid.[39] Coronoid fractures related to terrible triad injuries tend to have a transverse fracture pattern.[40] It is typically recommended that all coronoid fractures be fixed when the elbow is unstable, especially type II and III injuries. Results of testing in biomechanical cadaver models have suggested that the terrible triad injury patterns could be rendered stable with fixation or replacement of the radial head and LCL repair, without fixation of the small (type I) coronoid fragments.[37,41] It also has been suggested that MCL repair may be more important than type I coronoid fracture fixation.[41] However, there are no randomized clinical studies addressing these issues. Therefore, it is more routinely advocated that type I fractures be fixed because they represent an anterior capsular injury, which can have an impact on elbow stability. A recent biomechanical study highlighted the fact that open reduction and internal fixation of type II coronoid fractures is particularly important in a tenuous collateral ligament repair.[42] Isolated repair and overtightening of a collateral ligament can "off balance" the elbow if the opposing collateral ligament is torn, particularly with a type II coronoid fracture.

The coronoid fracture may be fixed with suture through drill holes in the ulna, or larger fragments may be treated with screw fixation. Biomechanically, it has been shown that a screw inserted from posterior to anterior yielded greater strength and fixation stiffness compared with anterior to posterior placement.[43] Precontoured plates are also commercially available for coronoid fixation. Small series of arthroscopically assisted open reduction and internal fixation of coronoid fractures have reported good results.[44,45]

Capitellum and Trochlea Fractures

Classification

Coronal fractures of the distal humerus are rare, accounting for fewer than 1% of distal humeral fractures. Early classification systems for capitellar and trochlear fractures have not been useful for guiding treatment.[46] More recently, a new classification system has been proposed that also helps to direct treatment.[47] Capitellar and trochlear fractures are divided into three types. Type I fractures primarily involve the capitellum, with or without the lateral trochlear ridge. Type II fractures involve both the capitellum and trochlea as one piece, and type III fractures involve both the capitellum and trochlea as separate pieces. These groups are further subdivided into class A (without) and B (with) posterior condylar comminution (Figure 4). Patients with isolated noncomminuted fractures have better results and fewer complications than those with more complex fractures.[47,48] However, on average, most patients will achieve functional range of motion; functional results appear durable over time.[47,48]

Surgical Treatment

Capitellar and trochlear fractures may be approached through a posterior midline skin incision, a bicolumn approach with separate medial and lateral incisions, or even an olecranon osteotomy.[47] For type I fractures, a lateral interval approach (Kaplan and/or Kocher approach) with screw fixation may be used (Figure 5). Type II fractures also require visualization of the medial aspect of the trochlea, which can be achieved through a flexor pronator-splitting approach, olecranon osteotomy, or sectioning of the LCL. The optimal approach for visualizing the trochlea requires further study. Typically, screws are used for fixation. Type III fractures will often require an olecranon osteotomy for adequate exposure. It may be possible to visualize the fracture from the lateral approach if the LCL is disrupted. A variety of fixation methods have been described, including lag screws, headless compression screws, bioab-

sorbable screws, threaded Kirschner wires, and plate fixation (particularly if there is posterior comminution). For the subtype B fractures with posterior comminution, plate fixation with or without bone graft is advocated. There has been some mention of using a distal humerus hemiarthroplasty with an anatomically shaped component for these more comminuted articular fractures.[29]

Results and Complications

Although surgical treatment results are generally favorable with capitellar and trochlear fractures, there are notable complication and reoperation rates associated with these fractures. Reported reoperation rates are 43% to 48%.[46,47] Reasons for reoperation include prominent hardware, nonunion, and contracture release. Osteonecrosis is not commonly reported.

Olecranon Fractures

Fractures of the olecranon occur in approximately 10% of all elbow fractures as either an isolated injury or part of a more complex fracture pattern.[49] These fractures result from either a direct blow to the bone or indirectly as an avulsion from forces generated by the triceps muscle.

Classification

The Mayo classification of olecranon fractures is based on three variables: displacement, stability, and comminution.[50] Type I fractures are nondisplaced; type II fractures are displaced, but the ulnohumeral joint is stable; and type III fractures are displaced and unstable. Each fracture type is subdivided into noncomminuted (A) and comminuted (B) fractures.

Treatment

Several treatment options for internal fixation of olecranon fractures have been described, including tension-band wiring, plate fixation, intramedullary screw fixation, and triceps advancement after fragment excision. The method of internal fixation is based primarily on the fracture type.

Nondisplaced fractures of the olecranon (Mayo type IA and IB), although exceedingly rare, can be treated nonsurgically. These fractures are defined by displacement less than 2 mm, and no change in position with gentle flexion to 90° or extension of the elbow against gravity. Type IA and IB fractures are immobilized in a long arm cast for 3 to 4 weeks followed by protected range-of-motion exercises. Flexion past 90° should be avoided until radiographic bone healing is complete at approximately 6 to 8 weeks. In elderly patients, range of motion may be initiated earlier than 3 weeks if tolerated by the patient, with the goal of preventing stiffness. A follow-up radiograph should be obtained within 5 to 7 days after cast application to ensure that fracture displacement has not occurred. Immobilization in full extension is not recommended because stiffness

3: Upper Extremity

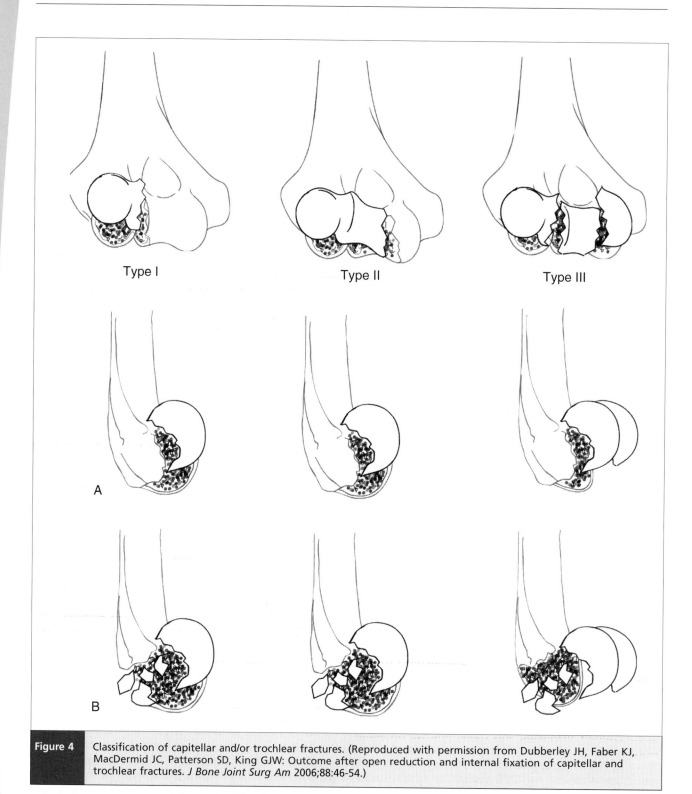

Type I   Type II   Type III

A

B

Figure 4 Classification of capitellar and/or trochlear fractures. (Reproduced with permission from Dubberley JH, Faber KJ, MacDermid JC, Patterson SD, King GJW: Outcome after open reduction and internal fixation of capitellar and trochlear fractures. *J Bone Joint Surg Am* 2006;88:46-54.)

is more likely. Fractures that require full extension for reduction should be surgically treated.

Displaced olecranon fractures (Mayo types IIA, IIB, IIIA, and IIIB) require surgical treatment. Several types of internal fixation are available, including tension-band wiring, plate fixation, intramedullary screw fixation, and triceps advancement after fragment excision. The goal of internal fixation is to restore the joint surfaces without changing the shape of the greater sigmoid notch using fixation that is sufficiently stable to permit early motion. Transverse fractures without comminution (Mayo type IIA) are amenable to tension-band wiring or plating, depending on the relationship to the midpoint of the greater sigmoid notch. The tension band construct can be fashioned using either Kirschner wires or an intramedullary screw.

In fractures with comminution (Mayo type IIB and IIIB) or following a fracture-dislocation (Mayo type IIIA or IIIB), optimal fixation can be achieved with plate fixation. Treatment with the tension-band technique may not provide a sufficiently stable construct, which can lead to displacement.

Complications

Hardware irritation requiring removal is one of the most common complications after internal fixation of olecranon fractures. Complaints related to prominent hardware are common. Although a mild loss of motion (of approximately 10° to 15° primarily in extension) is common, it is rarely a significant problem. Nonunion of olecranon fractures has been reported in up to 1% of patients.

Diaphyseal Forearm Fractures

Plate osteosynthesis is considered the standard treatment for diaphyseal radius and ulna forearm fractures. Patient-based functional outcomes show that plate fixation restores the normal anatomy of the bones and normal motion; however, a moderate reduction (30%) in forearm, wrist, and grip strength has been reported.[51] Recently, an interlocking intramedullary nail system has been described for treating radial and ulnar fractures, and has achieved a high rate of osseous consolidation for simple (noncomminuted) diaphyseal fractures.[52] Patients with poor soft-tissue integrity have been suggested as candidates for treatment with this technique. Reported disadvantages of this approach are the need for a brace and longer periods of immobilization.

Elbow Dislocation

The elbow is the second most commonly dislocated large joint, following the shoulder.[53] The management of the unstable elbow has evolved considerably over recent years as knowledge of the anatomic stabilizers of the elbow and the pathoanatomy of instability has increased. The goals of treating an unstable elbow are to restore functional stability and motion. Achieving these goals requires managing soft-tissue injuries (in simple dislocations) or addressing these injuries in conjunction with fracture management (in complex instability). Simple dislocations, which account for approximately 50% to 60% of elbow dislocations, often can be managed with closed reduction and treatment, whereas complex injury patterns often require surgical treatment.[54]

Elbow stability is provided by both static and dynamic constraints. The three primary static constraints are the ulnohumeral bony articulation, the anterior bundle of the MCL, and the LCL complex. The secondary static constraints include the capsule and the radial head. The dynamic constraints refer to any muscle

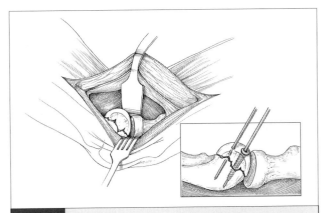

Figure 5 Lateral approaches for capitellar fracture fixation. (Reproduced from Ruchelsman DE, Tejwani NC, Kwon YW, Egol KE: Coronal plane partial articular fractures of the distal humerus: Current concepts in management. *J Am Acad Orthop Surg* 2008;16:716-728.)

crossing the elbow joint that provides a compressive force to the joint (the common flexor and extensor muscle groups).

Simple Dislocations

Most dislocations occur in a posterior or posterolateral direction, although anterior, medial, lateral, and divergent patterns have been reported. Biomechanical testing has demonstrated that a combination of valgus force, axial load, supination, and external rotation can result in a posterolateral dislocation.[55] Other biomechanical models have shown posterior dislocation following varus rather than valgus loading.[56]

Although a variety of mechanisms may result in elbow dislocation, the primary lesion appears to be injury to the LCL, with a spectrum of injury to other ligamentous and osseous structures following a circular path laterally to medially (Figure 6). The LCL ligament is composed of the lateral ulnar collateral ligament, radial collateral ligament, accessory collateral ligament, and annular ligament. Although it is generally agreed that the lateral ulnar collateral ligament appears to be the primary restraint to posterolateral rotatory instability,[57] some investigators believe that the radial collateral ligament and accessory collateral ligament also contribute significantly to lateral elbow stability.[58,59]

Controversy exists regarding the involvement of the MCL in elbow dislocations. The MCL is composed of an anterior oblique, posterior oblique, and transverse ligament. The anterior oblique band resists valgus stress throughout the elbow range of motion. Although some biomechanical models have demonstrated that posterior dislocation is possible with an intact anterior band,[55] other studies have suggested that the anterior oblique band is disrupted following posterior dislocation.[60,61] The variability of pathoanatomy associated with elbow instability highlights the importance of carefully assessing and recognizing all potential sources of instability.

3: Upper Extremity

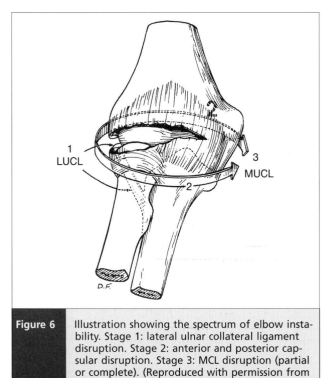

Figure 6 Illustration showing the spectrum of elbow instability. Stage 1: lateral ulnar collateral ligament disruption. Stage 2: anterior and posterior capsular disruption. Stage 3: MCL disruption (partial or complete). (Reproduced with permission from O'Driscoll SW, Morrey BF, Korinek S, An KH: Elbow subluxation and dislocation: A spectrum of instability. *Clin Orthop Relat Res* 1992;280: 186-197.)

The treatment algorithm for simple elbow dislocations has shifted toward early mobilization to prevent flexion contracture of the elbow[62] (**Figure 7**). The bony constraint of the elbow is already highly congruous and the compressive forces of the dynamic stabilizers protect the soft-tissue injury. Following reduction of an elbow dislocation, it is typically immobilized for 5 to 7 days at 90°, with the forearm positioned to allow for concentric reduction of the ulnohumeral articulation. At follow-up, the splint is removed and active range of motion is commenced through the stable flexion and extension arc (stable forearm position);[63] an extension block brace is commonly used for 3 to 4 weeks. The extension block is progressively decreased so that by 6 to 8 weeks the patient achieves full stable extension. Forearm active pronation and supination at 90° of elbow flexion is started early to prevent rotational contracture. A drop sign refers to a static widening of the ulnohumeral joint on the lateral radiograph.[64] Ulnohumeral incongruence must be corrected by changing the forearm position, splinting, or surgery to repair soft-tissue injury or remove entrapped osteochondral or soft-tissue structures. If the LCL complex is disrupted and the MCL is intact, the elbow may be more stable with the forearm in pronation.[65] If the LCL is intact and the MCL is ruptured, the elbow may be more stable with the forearm in supination.[66] If both ligaments are disrupted, the elbow may be placed in neutral rotation to protect both the medial and lateral ligamentous structures. A posterior impaction fracture

on the capitellum is common, and is analogous to a Hill-Sachs lesion in the shoulder. The stability of the joint is not affected by this impaction fracture.

Complex Dislocation

The "terrible triad" injury to the elbow refers to an elbow dislocation with an associated fracture, typically a fracture of the radial head and coronoid process (**Figure 8**). Disruption of the LCL is a critical component of the terrible triad lesion, and is almost uniformly observed in a fracture-dislocation of the elbow.[67] The ligament often avulses from its isometric origin on the lateral aspect of the capitellum (**Figure 9**), along with a component of the extensor origin lesion from the lateral epicondyle. Cadaver testing has shown that fracture repair of the radial head and coronoid alone does not restore stability, and that optimal stability and kinematics require isometric and appropriately tensioned repair of the LCL.[68]

The MCL, especially the anterior band, is well established as a primary restraint to valgus instability of the elbow. Complex instability often can result in MCL injury, either as an intrasubstance lesion or as an avulsion of the origin along with a sleeve of the common flexor origin. Although the MCL is critical to normal valgus stability, routine repair or reconstruction following complex instability may not be necessary because of the role of the radial head as a secondary stabilizer, especially in the setting of an intact or repaired coronoid process.[69]

The potential for elbow instability increases with the increasing height of the fragment.[70] In a cadaver model, a 30% loss of coronoid height in association with removal of the radial head in a ligamentously intact elbow resulted in elbow instability.[71] Because isolated loss of 50% or more of the coronoid height also results in elbow instability, it is critical to repair coronoid fractures, especially type II and III fractures. Although small fragments (type I) may not directly impart significant instability, they are often a hallmark of an anterior capsular injury, which can have an impact on stability and repair.[34]

Historically, treatment results of terrible triad injuries have been suboptimal and have been associated with a high complication rate, recurrent instability, arthrosis, and stiffness.[72] The use of a systematic algorithmic approach to this injury pattern, which appreciates both the bony and soft-tissue injuries, has improved clinical results.[69,73-75]

A standard approach to treating terrible triad injuries is to sequentially repair injured structures from deep to superficial (**Figure 10**). A midline posterior incision is advocated to allow access to both the medial and lateral joint spaces; or a bicolumn approach can be used with separate medial and lateral approaches. The coronoid is initially fixed through a space created by the fractured radial head or through a medial approach. There is often a rent in the flexor pronator mass that allows access to the coronoid. The coronoid is fixed with sutures or screws depending on the size of

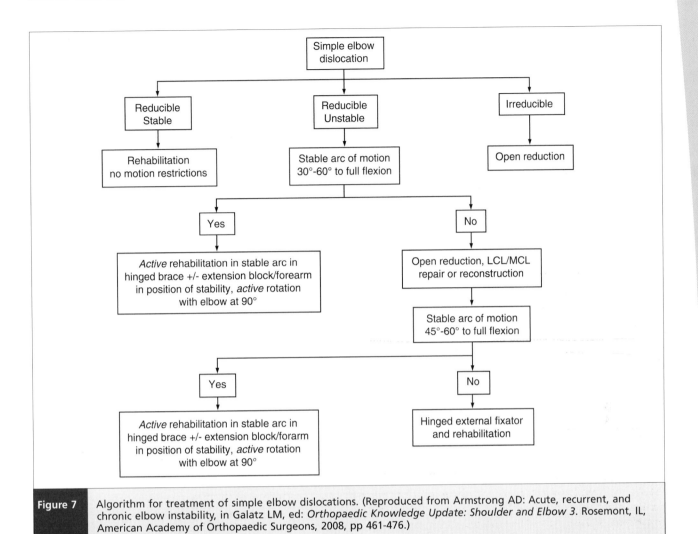

```
                        ┌─────────────────┐
                        │  Simple elbow   │
                        │  dislocation    │
                        └────────┬────────┘
        ┌────────────────────────┼────────────────────────┐
┌───────────────┐       ┌─────────────────┐       ┌───────────────┐
│   Reducible   │       │    Reducible    │       │  Irreducible  │
│    Stable     │       │    Unstable     │       │               │
└───────┬───────┘       └────────┬────────┘       └───────┬───────┘
        │                        │                        │
┌───────────────┐      ┌───────────────────┐     ┌───────────────┐
│ Rehabilitation │     │ Stable arc of motion│    │ Open reduction │
│ no motion      │     │ 30°-60° to full     │    └───────────────┘
│ restrictions   │     │ flexion             │
└───────────────┘      └──────────┬──────────┘
              ┌───────────────────┴───────────────────┐
          ┌───────┐                               ┌───────┐
          │  Yes  │                               │  No   │
          └───┬───┘                               └───┬───┘
```

Active rehabilitation in stable arc in hinged brace +/- extension block/forearm in position of stability, active rotation with elbow at 90°

Open reduction, LCL/MCL repair or reconstruction

Stable arc of motion 45°-60° to full flexion

Yes — Active rehabilitation in stable arc in hinged brace +/- extension block/forearm in position of stability, active rotation with elbow at 90°

No — Hinged external fixator and rehabilitation

Figure 7   Algorithm for treatment of simple elbow dislocations. (Reproduced from Armstrong AD: Acute, recurrent, and chronic elbow instability, in Galatz LM, ed: *Orthopaedic Knowledge Update: Shoulder and Elbow 3*. Rosemont, IL, American Academy of Orthopaedic Surgeons, 2008, pp 461-476.)

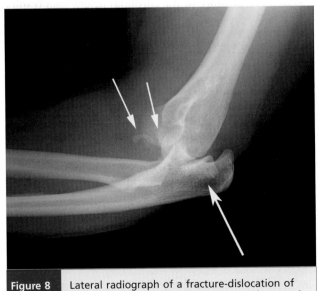

Figure 8   Lateral radiograph of a fracture-dislocation of the elbow. The small arrows point to the anteriorly displaced coronoid fractures, which may be confused for radial head fragments (*large arrow*). (Courtesy of Bradford Parsons, MD, New York, NY.)

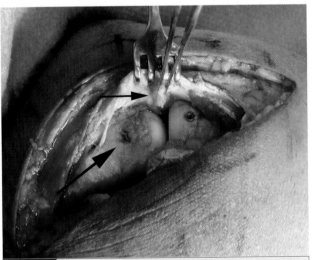

Figure 9   The LCL (*small arrow*) typically avulses from its isometric origin (*large arrow* pointing to cautery mark on lateral capitellum) and often can be repaired isometrically in the acute injury. (Courtesy of Bradford Parsons, MD, New York, NY.)

3: Upper Extremity

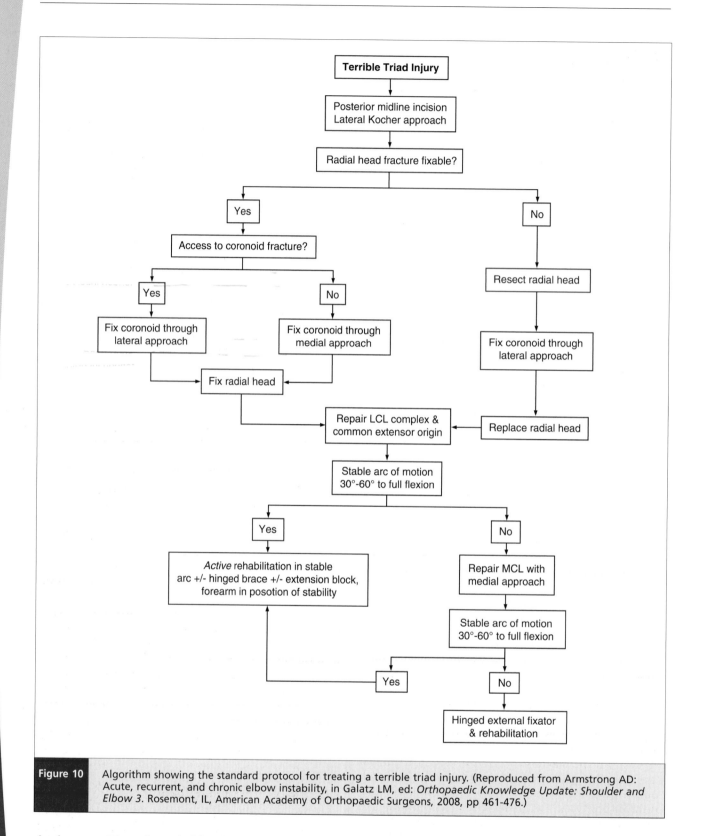

Terrible Triad Injury

Posterior midline incision
Lateral Kocher approach

Radial head fracture fixable?

Yes → Access to coronoid fracture?

No → Resect radial head

Access to coronoid fracture?
- Yes → Fix coronoid through lateral approach
- No → Fix coronoid through medial approach

Fix radial head

Resect radial head → Fix coronoid through lateral approach → Replace radial head

Repair LCL complex & common extensor origin

Stable arc of motion 30°-60° to full flexion
- Yes → *Active* rehabilitation in stable arc +/- hinged brace +/- extension block, forearm in posotion of stability
- No → Repair MCL with medial approach

Repair MCL with medial approach → Stable arc of motion 30°-60° to full flexion
- Yes → (to Active rehabilitation)
- No → Hinged external fixator & rehabilitation

Figure 10 Algorithm showing the standard protocol for treating a terrible triad injury. (Reproduced from Armstrong AD: Acute, recurrent, and chronic elbow instability, in Galatz LM, ed: *Orthopaedic Knowledge Update: Shoulder and Elbow 3*. Rosemont, IL, American Academy of Orthopaedic Surgeons, 2008, pp 461-476.)

the fracture. Next, the radial head is either fixed or replaced. Internal fixation of the radial head will improve joint stability, but only if it can be fixed with a construct that is as stable as the native radial head. Radial head replacement should be anatomic, restoring normal length and size.

Recent biomechanical studies have shown the importance of the radial head as a secondary valgus stabilizer; however, full valgus stability of the elbow will not be achieved unless the MCL is repaired or reconstructed.[76] The radial head is also an important constraint to varus and external rotatory forces about the elbow, but less important than the LCL. Biomechanically, varus and external rotator instability of the elbow is worsened with radial head excision with a deficient LCL complex.[68] Radial head replacement improves the varus and external rotator stability of the elbow, but stability is not fully restored until the LCL is repaired. Biomechanical studies also have shown the combined importance of the radial head and the coronoid fracture in a terrible triad injury. The radial head alone could not stabilize the elbow joint when 50% to 70% of the coronoid was resected, despite an intact MCL and LCL.[41,70,71]

Following repair of the bony injuries, the soft-tissue injuries are treated. LCL rupture is universal to these injuries and must be repaired to the anatomic axis of rotation of the elbow at the center of the capitellar curvature. Avulsion of the common extensor origin from the lateral epicondyle, leaving it devoid of any soft tissue, is a common occurrence. Lateral soft-tissue repair also should include the common extensor muscles. In most instances, the joint is rendered stable by this point; however, if the elbow is still unstable, consideration should be given to repair of the medial structure and ultimately to the use of an external fixator if the elbow cannot be stabilized. Early consideration of hinged external fixation has been advocated.[77] Postoperative rehabilitation should follow the same protocol as previously described for simple elbow dislocations. The primary goal of surgery is to achieve a stable elbow, which will allow early range of motion.

Distal Biceps Tendon Injuries

Recent studies focusing on the treatment of distal biceps rupture have described the normal anatomy of the tendon along with different fixation techniques and surgical approaches. The biceps tendon inserts on the ulnar aspect of the bicipital tuberosity,[78,79] which has surgical implications for anatomic repair of the tendon. A patient with limited supination may not be a good candidate for a single-incision approach because anatomic repair would be difficult.[79] There are two distinct insertion points of the tendon—the anteromedial fibers (short head) insert more inferiorly, whereas the posterolateral fibers (long head) insert more proximally[80] (Figure 11). This gives the tendon a twisted appearance at its insertion. The short head of the biceps tendon is the origin of the lacertus fibrosus, which is key to proper anatomic alignment at surgery.[81]

Although the diagnosis of distal biceps tendon rupture is largely clinical, MRI can be helpful in establishing the diagnosis. Because of the anatomic positioning of the biceps tendon, visualizing a rupture and the tendon itself with standard positioning can be difficult. Recently, a modified positioning technique involving a flexed elbow, abducted shoulder, and supinated forearm (termed FABS) has been popularized. This technique significantly enhances the visualization of the biceps tendon with MRI.[82]

The two current surgical approaches for distal biceps repair are the two-incision and anterior single-incision techniques. Surgical treatment is typically advocated for patients who are more active or those who often perform twisting motions of the forearm. Nonsurgical treatment of distal biceps tendon injuries results in a modest reduction in supination strength and minimal reduction in elbow flexion strength.[83] Classically, the two-incision Boyd-Anderson approach was used for distal biceps reconstruction. The single-incision anterior approach evolved in an attempt to decrease the incidence of radioulnar synostosis; however, heterotopic ossification also has been reported with the single-incision anterior approach.[84] Excellent clinical results have been reported with both approaches.

A variety of fixation methods have been reported in the literature, including bone tunnels, suture anchors, interference screws, or button.[85-87] Biomechanically the Endobutton (Smith & Nephew, Memphis, TN) may have a higher initial load-to-failure strength;[87,88] however, in contrast, it has also been shown to have comparable strength to suture anchor fixation.[89] Overall, surgical fixation techniques have shown similar clinical results.[84,90-92] Small case series for late reconstruction of chronic distal biceps injuries with either Achilles tendon allograft or autologous hamstring graft have shown promising results for improving supination strength.[93,94]

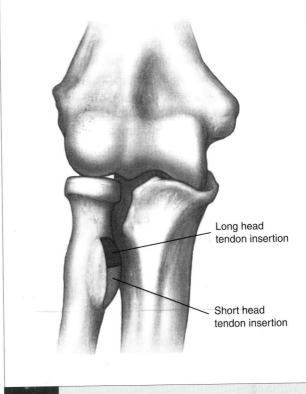

Long head tendon insertion

Short head tendon insertion

Figure 11 Illustration of the biceps tendon insertions. (Reproduced with permission from Athwal GS, Steinmann SP, Rispoli DM: The distal biceps tendon: Footprint and relevant clinical anatomy. *J Hand Surg Am* 2007;32:1225-1229.)

3: Upper Extremity

Annotated References

1. Sheps DM, Kiefer KR, Boorman RS, et al: The interobserver reliability of classification systems for radial head fractures: The Hotchkiss modification of the Mason classification and the AO classification systems. *Can J Surg* 2009;52(4):277-282.

   The interobserver reliability of two commonly used classification systems, the Hotchkiss modification of the Mason classification and the AO classification system, were evaluated. The authors concluded that, according to the criteria of Landis and Koch, there was moderate interobserver reliability for the Hotchkiss modification of the Mason classification, and fair interobserver reliability for the AO classification. Collapsing the Hotchkiss classification improved the reliability to substantial, and collapsing the AO system improved reliability to the lower end of moderate.

2. Broberg MA, Morrey BF: Results of treatment of fracture-dislocations of the elbow. *Clin Orthop Relat Res* 1987;216:109-119.

3. Hotchkiss RN: Displaced fractures of the radial head: Internal fixation or excision? *J Am Acad Orthop Surg* 1997;5(1):1-10.

4. van Riet RP, Morrey BF: Documentation of associated injuries occurring with radial head fracture. *Clin Orthop Relat Res* 2008;466(1):130-134.

   This article reviews the authors' experience with 333 radial head fractures with the purpose of describing the spectrum of associated injuries that commonly occur in conjunction with a radial head fracture. A system based on the Mason fracture classification was proposed to document the presence of additional articular and ligamentous injuries.

5. Caputo AE, Burton KJ, Cohen MS, King GJ: Articular cartilage injuries of the capitellum interposed in radial head fractures: A report of ten cases. *J Shoulder Elbow Surg* 2006;15(6):716-720.

6. Ring D, Quintero J, Jupiter JB: Open reduction and internal fixation of fractures of the radial head. *J Bone Joint Surg Am* 2002;84(10):1811-1815.

7. Bain GI, Ashwood N, Baird R, Unni R, Oka Y: Management of Mason type-III radial head fractures with a titanium prosthesis, ligament repair, and early mobilization: Surgical technique. *J Bone Joint Surg Am* 2005;87(pt 1, suppl 1)136-147.

8. Beingessner DM, Dunning CE, Gordon KD, Johnson JA, King GJ: The effect of radial head fracture size on elbow kinematics and stability. *J Orthop Res* 2005;23:210-217.

9. Lindenhovius AL, Felsch Q, Ring D, Kloen P: The long-term outcome of open reduction and internal fixation of stable displaced isolated partial articular fractures of the radial head. *J Trauma* 2009;67(1):143-146.

   The authors report on the long-term outcome of surgically treated Mason type II radial head fractures. They concluded that surgical treatment of stable, isolated, displaced partial articular (Mason type II) fractures of the radial head show no appreciable advantage over the long-term results of nonsurgical treatment of these fractures as described in prior reports. The appeal of surgical treatment is diminished by potential complications.

10. Smets S, Govaers K, Jansen N, Van Riet R, Schaap M, Van Glabbeek F: The floating radial head prosthesis for comminuted radial head fractures: A multicentric study. *Acta Orthop Belg* 2000;66(4):353-358.

11. Doornberg JN, Linzel DS, Zurakowski D, Ring D: Reference points for radial head prosthesis size. *J Hand Surg Am* 2006;31(1):53-57.

12. van Riet RP, van Glabbeek F, de Weerdt W, Oemar J, Bortier H: Validation of the lesser sigmoid notch of the ulna as a reference point for accurate placement of a prosthesis for the head of the radius: A cadaver study. *J Bone Joint Surg Br* 2007;89(3):413-416.

    A review of the Antwerp University Hospital's experience with radial head fractures from 1997 to 2002 showed that 88 of 333 radial head fractures (26%) had associated injuries. Based on this clinical experience, an accurate and comprehensive description of associated injuries was developed. The proposed system offered a reproducible (98%) extension of the current Mason fracture classification system to document the presence of additional articular and ligamentous injuries.

13. Pike JM, Athwal GS, Faber KJ, King GJ: Radial head fractures: An update. *J Hand Surg Am* 2009;34(3):557-565.

    The authors summarize diagnosis and treatment options for treatment of radial head fractures.

14. Muller M, Nazanan S, Koch P, et al: Fracture and dislocation compendium: Orthopaedic trauma association committee for coding and classification. *J Orthop Trauma* 2001;10(suppl 1):311-324.

15. Bryan RS, Morrey BF: Extensive posterior exposure of the elbow: A triceps-sparing approach. *Clin Orthop Relat Res* 1982;166(166):188-192.

16. O'Driscoll SW: The triceps-reflecting anconeus pedicle (TRAP) approach for distal humeral fractures and nonunions. *Orthop Clin North Am* 2000;31(1):91-101.

17. Wilkinson JM, Stanley D: Posterior surgical approaches to the elbow: A comparative anatomic study. *J Shoulder Elbow Surg* 2001;10(4):380-382.

18. Athwal GS, Rispoli DM, Steinmann SP: The anconeus flap transolecranon approach to the distal humerus. *J Orthop Trauma* 2006;20(4):282-285.

19. Coles CP, Barei DP, Nork SE, Taitsman LA, Hanel DP, Bradford Henley M: The olecranon osteotomy: A six-year experience in the treatment of intraarticular frac-

tures of the distal humerus. *J Orthop Trauma* 2006; 20(3):164-171.

20. Doornberg JN, van Duijn PJ, Linzel D, et al: Surgical treatment of intra-articular fractures of the distal part of the humerus: Functional outcome after twelve to thirty years. *J Bone Joint Surg Am* 2007;89(7):1524-1532.

    This investigation addressed the long-term clinical and radiographic results of surgical treatment of intra-articular distal humeral fractures (AO type C) as assessed with use of standardized outcome measures. The authors concluded that long-term results of open reduction and internal fixation of AO type C fractures of the distal part of the humerus are similar to those reported in the short term, suggesting that the results are durable. Functional ratings and perceived disability were predicated more on pain than on functional impairment and did not correlate with radiographic signs of arthrosis.

21. Pollock JW, Faber KJ, Athwal GS: Distal humerus fractures. *Orthop Clin North Am* 2008;39(2):187-200, vi.

    This review article focused on the management of intra-articular fractures of the distal humerus. The surgical management of these cases using careful preoperative planning, adequate exposure, and stable fixation was emphasized.

22. Sanchez-Sotelo J, Torchia ME, O'Driscoll SW: Complex distal humeral fractures: Internal fixation with a principle-based parallel-plate technique. *J Bone Joint Surg Am* 2007;89(5):961-969.

    The goal of this study was to determine the outcome of treating complex distal humerus fractures with a principle-based technique that maximizes fixation in the articular fragments and stability at the supracondylar level. The study demonstrated that stable fixation and a high rate of union of complex distal humeral fractures can be achieved when a principle-based surgical technique that maximizes fixation in the distal segments and stability at the supracondylar level is used. The early stability achieved with this technique permits intensive rehabilitation to restore elbow motion.

23. Ek ET, Goldwasser M, Bonomo AL: Functional outcome of complex intercondylar fractures of the distal humerus treated through a triceps-sparing approach. *J Shoulder Elbow Surg* 2008;17(3):441-446.

    This study aimed to review the functional outcome of complex intra-articular fractures of the distal humerus (AO/ASIF type C) managed with open reduction and internal fixation through a posterior triceps-sparing approach. All patients achieved good clinical scores as determined by the Mayo Clinic Performance Index. Quality of life assessment (SF-36) revealed no significant difference compared to the general population. The authors concluded that the posterior triceps-sparing approach provides adequate exposure to the fracture site and allows early rehabilitation.

24. Huang TL, Chiu FY, Chuang TY, Chen TH: The results of open reduction and internal fixation in elderly patients with severe fractures of the distal humerus: A critical analysis of the results. *J Trauma* 2005;58(1):62-69.

25. Gofton WT, Macdermid JC, Patterson SD, Faber KJ, King GJ: Functional outcome of AO type C distal humeral fractures. *J Hand Surg Am* 2003;28(2):294-308.

26. Greiner S, Haas NP, Bail HJ: Outcome after open reduction and angular stable internal fixation for supra-intercondylar fractures of the distal humerus: Preliminary results with the LCP distal humerus system. *Arch Orthop Trauma Surg* 2008;128(7):723-729.

    This study evaluated the surgical reposition, fracture healing, pain, function, and patient satisfaction after open reduction with an angular stable fixation. Anatomically preshaped, angular stable implants facilitate surgical reduction and stabilization of the fracture and may allow early postoperative rehabilitation. Clinical and radiological results are promising, with good range of motion and flexion and extension force.

27. Athwal GS, Hoxie SC, Rispoli DM, Steinmann SP: Precontoured parallel plate fixation of AO/OTA type C distal humerus fractures. *J Orthop Trauma* 2009;23(8): 575-580.

    This study reports on the clinical effectiveness of precontoured parallel plating for the management of Orthopaedic Trauma Association type C distal humerus fractures and provides support for prior reports of the successful use of parallel plating techniques. The complication rate of 53% in procedures performed by experienced surgeons highlights the complexity of these fractures. Preoperative patient counseling is paramount.

28. Müller LP, Kamineni S, Rommens PM, Morrey BF: Primary total elbow replacement for fractures of the distal humerus. *Oper Orthop Traumatol* 2005;17(2):119-142.

29. Athwal GS, Goetz TJ, Pollock JW, Faber KJ: Prosthetic replacement for distal humerus fractures. *Orthop Clin North Am* 2008;39(2):201-212, vi.

    This article focuses on the evaluation and management of distal humerus fractures with prosthetic replacements.

30. Cil A, Veillette CJ, Sanchez-Sotelo J, Morrey BF: Linked elbow replacement: A salvage procedure for distal humeral nonunion. *J Bone Joint Surg Am* 2008;90(9): 1939-1950.

    This article reports the long-term experience with linked semiconstrained total elbow arthroplasty as a salvage procedure for patients with distal humeral nonunion not amenable to internal fixation. The authors concluded that linked semiconstrained total elbow arthroplasty is a salvage procedure that can provide pain relief and restore motion and function in patients with a distal humeral nonunion that is not amenable to internal fixation.

31. Kamineni S, Morrey BF: Distal humeral fractures treated with noncustom total elbow replacement. *J Bone Joint Surg Am* 2004;86(5):940-947.

32. Frankle MA, Herscovici D Jr, DiPasquale TG, Vasey MB, Sanders RW: A comparison of open reduction and internal fixation and primary total elbow arthroplasty

in the treatment of intraarticular distal humerus fractures in women older than age 65. *J Orthop Trauma* 2003;17(7):473-480.

33. McKee MD, Veillette CJ, Hall JA, et al: A multicenter, prospective, randomized, controlled trial of open reduction-internal fixation versus total elbow arthroplasty for displaced intra-articular distal humeral fractures in elderly patients. *J Shoulder Elbow Surg* 2009; 18(1):3-12.

This paper reports the results of a prospective randomized controlled trial to compare functional outcomes, complications, and reoperation rates in elderly patients with displaced intra-articular, distal humeral fractures treated with open reduction and internal fixation (ORIF) or primary semiconstrained total elbow arthroplasty (TEA). Patients who underwent TEA had substantially better Mayo Elbow Performance Scores at 3 months (83 versus 65, *P* = .01), 6 months (86 versus 68, *P* = .003), 12 months (88 versus 72, *P* = .007), and 2 years (86 versus 73, *P* = .015) compared with the ORIF group. Patients who underwent TEA had significantly better Disabilities of the Arm, Shoulder and Hand (DASH) scores at 6 weeks (43 versus 77, *P* = .02) and 6 months (31 versus 50, *P* = .01) but not at 12 months (32 versus 47, *P* = .1) or 2 years (34 versus 38, *P* = .6). The mean flexion-extension arc was 107° (range, 42°-145°) in the TEA group and 95° (range, 30°-140°) in the ORIF group (*P* = .19). Reoperation rates for TEA (3 of 25, 12%) and ORIF (4 of 15, 27%) were not statistically different (*P* = .2). They concluded that TEA is a preferred alternative for ORIF in elderly patients with complex distal humeral fractures that are not amenable to stable fixation. Elderly patients have an increased baseline DASH score and appear to accommodate objective limitations in function with time.

34. Ablove RH, Moy OJ, Howard C, Peimer CA, S'Doia S: Ulnar coronoid process anatomy: Possible implications for elbow instability. *Clin Orthop Relat Res* 2006;449: 259-261.

35. Closkey RF, Goode JR, Kirschenbaum D, Cody RP: The role of the coronoid process in elbow stability: A biomechanical analysis of axial loading. *J Bone Joint Surg Am* 2000;82(12):1749-1753.

36. Hull JR, Owen JR, Fern SE, Wayne JS, Boardman ND III: Role of the coronoid process in varus osteoarticular stability of the elbow. *J Shoulder Elbow Surg* 2005; 14(4):441-446.

37. Beingessner DM, Dunning CE, Stacpoole RA, Johnson JA, King GJ: The effect of coronoid fractures on elbow kinematics and stability. *Clin Biomech (Bristol, Avon)* 2007;22(2):183-190.

The authors report on a biomechanical study determining the effect of coronoid fractures on elbow kinematics and stability. Elbow kinematics are altered with increasing fracture size. Repair of type II and III coronoid fractures and LCL repair is recommended.

38. Adams JE, Hoskin TL, Morrey BF, Steinmann SP: Management and outcome of 103 acute fractures of the cor-

onoid process of the ulna. *J Bone Joint Surg Br* 2009; 91(5):632-635.

A retrospective review 103 coronoid fractures is presented. Coronoid fracture with associated injuries have a higher rate of complications and poorer results.

39. Doornberg JN, van Duijn J, Ring D: Coronoid fracture height in terrible-triad injuries. *J Hand Surg Am* 2006; 31(5):794-797.

40. Doornberg JN, Ring D: Coronoid fracture patterns. *J Hand Surg Am* 2006;31(1):45-52.

41. Beingessner DM, Stacpoole RA, Dunning CE, Johnson JA, King GJ: The effect of suture fixation of type I coronoid fractures on the kinematics and stability of the elbow with and without medial collateral ligament repair. *J Shoulder Elbow Surg* 2007;16(2):213-217.

The authors of this biomechanical study examined the effect of type I coronoid fracture and ligament repair on elbow kinematics. MCL repair may be more important than fixation of type I coronoid fractures.

42. Pollock JW, Pichora J, Brownhill J, et al: The influence of type II coronoid fractures, collateral ligament injuries, and surgical repair on the kinematics and stability of the elbow: An in vitro biomechanical study. *J Shoulder Elbow Surg* 2009;18(3):408-417.

This biomechanical study examined elbow kinematics with type II coronoid fractures and ligament repair. Repair of type II coronoid fractures and ligament repair should be performed when possible to restore normal kinematics and care should be taken to prevent overtensioning of the ligament repair.

43. Moon JG, Zobitz ME, An KN, O'Driscoll SW: Optimal screw orientation for fixation of coronoid fractures. *J Orthop Trauma* 2009;23(4):277-280.

Posteroanterior screw placement was biomechanically superior to anteroposterior screw placement in fixing coronoid fractures.

44. Hausman MR, Klug RA, Qureshi S, Goldstein R, Parsons BO: Arthroscopically assisted coronoid fracture fixation: A preliminary report. *Clin Orthop Relat Res* 2008;466(12):3147-3152.

Four patients were treated with arthroscopically assisted reduction of a coronoid fracture. The patients had no recurrent instability and all had a functional arc of motion.

45. Adams JE, Merten SM, Steinmann SP: Arthroscopic-assisted treatment of coronoid fractures. *Arthroscopy* 2007;23(10):1060-1065.

In seven coronoid fractures treated arthroscopically, all achieved functional, pain-free motion.

46. Ring D, Jupiter JB, Gulotta L: Articular fractures of the distal part of the humerus. *J Bone Joint Surg Am* 2003; 85(2):232-238.

47. Dubberley JH, Faber KJ, Macdermid JC, Patterson SD,

King GJ: Outcome after open reduction and internal fixation of capitellar and trochlear fractures. *J Bone Joint Surg Am* 2006;88(1):46-54.

48. Guitton TG, Doornberg JN, Raaymakers EL, Ring D, Kloen P: Fractures of the capitellum and trochlea. *J Bone Joint Surg Am* 2009;91(2):390-397.

In 27 patients treated for capitellar/trochlea fractures who were followed for 1 year or longer, those with more complex fractures had worse results and a higher complication rate; however, results were durable over time.

49. Veillette CJ, Steinmann SP: Olecranon fractures. *Orthop Clin North Am* 2008;39(2):229-236, vii.

The treatment of olecranon fractures is summarized, with an emphasis on anatomic reduction and stable fixation using one of the many techniques available to surgeons.

50. Morrey BF: Current concepts in the treatment of fractures of the radial head, the olecranon, and the coronoid. *Instr Course Lect* 1995;44:175-185.

51. Droll KP, Perna P, Potter J, Harniman E, Schemitsch EH, McKee MD: Outcomes following plate fixation of fractures of both bones of the forearm in adults. *J Bone Joint Surg Am* 2007;89(12):2619-2624.

In 30 patients treated with open reduction and internal fixation of a both-bone forearm fracture, anatomy and motion were restored; however, a moderate reduction in upper extremity strength was reported.

52. Lee YH, Lee SK, Chung MS, Baek GH, Gong HS, Kim KH: Interlocking contoured intramedullary nail fixation for selected diaphyseal fractures of the forearm in adults. *J Bone Joint Surg Am* 2008;90(9):1891-1898.

Interlocking contoured intramedullary nail fixation of the radius and ulna was used to treat 27 patients with forearm fractures. A high rate of osseous consolidation was reported but a longer period of immobilization was required. The authors reported 81% excellent and 11% good results. This fixation technique should be considered in patients with soft-tissue defects.

53. Safran MR, Baillargeon D: Soft-tissue stabilizers of the elbow. *J Shoulder Elbow Surg* 2005;14(1, suppl S):179S-185S.

54. de Haan J, Schep NW, Tuinebreijer WE, Patka P, den Hartog D: Simple elbow dislocations: A systematic review of the literature. *Arch Orthop Trauma Surg* 2010;130(2):241-249.

The authors present a systematic review of the literature, with an overview of the management and outcome of simple elbow dislocations.

55. O'Driscoll SW, Morrey BF, Korinek S, An KN: Elbow subluxation and dislocation: A spectrum of instability. *Clin Orthop Relat Res* 1992;280:186-197.

56. Deutch SR, Jensen SL, Olsen BS, Sneppen O: Elbow joint stability in relation to forced external rotation: An experimental study of the osseous constraint. *J Shoulder Elbow Surg* 2003;12(3):287-292.

57. O'Driscoll SW, Bell DF, Morrey BF: Posterolateral rotatory instability of the elbow. *J Bone Joint Surg Am* 1991;73(3):440-446.

58. McAdams TR, Masters GW, Srivastava S: The effect of arthroscopic sectioning of the lateral ligament complex of the elbow on posterolateral rotatory stability. *J Shoulder Elbow Surg* 2005;14(3):298-301.

59. Dunning CE, Zarzour ZD, Patterson SD, Johnson JA, King GJ: Ligamentous stabilizers against posterolateral rotatory instability of the elbow. *J Bone Joint Surg Am* 2001;83(12):1823-1828.

60. Deutch SR, Jensen SL, Tyrdal S, Olsen BS, Sneppen O: Elbow joint stability following experimental osteoligamentous injury and reconstruction. *J Shoulder Elbow Surg* 2003;12(5):466-471.

61. Josefsson PO, Gentz CF, Johnell O, Wendeberg B: Surgical versus non-surgical treatment of ligamentous injuries following dislocation of the elbow joint: A prospective randomized study. *J Bone Joint Surg Am* 1987;69(4):605-608.

62. Maripuri SN, Debnath UK, Rao P, Mohanty K: Simple elbow dislocation among adults: A comparative study of two different methods of treatment. *Injury* 2007;38(11):1254-1258.

Simple elbow dislocations treated with cast versus sling immobilization are compared. The authors advocate early mobilization of the elbow following a simple elbow dislocation.

63. Duckworth AD, Kulijdian A, McKee MD, Ring D: Residual subluxation of the elbow after dislocation or fracture-dislocation: Treatment with active elbow exercises and avoidance of varus stress. *J Shoulder Elbow Surg* 2008;17(2):276-280.

The authors describe their clinical experience with the drop sign and support that slight residual subluxation can reduce with active mobilization.

64. Coonrad RW, Roush TF, Major NM, Basamania CJ: The drop sign, a radiographic warning sign of elbow instability. *J Shoulder Elbow Surg* 2005;14(3):312-317.

65. Armstrong AD, Dunning CE, Faber KJ, Duck TR, Johnson JA, King GJ: Rehabilitation of the medial collateral ligament-deficient elbow: An in vitro biomechanical study. *J Hand Surg Am* 2000;25(6):1051-1057.

66. Dunning CE, Zarzour ZD, Patterson SD, Johnson JA, King GJ: Muscle forces and pronation stabilize the lateral ligament deficient elbow. *Clin Orthop Relat Res* 2001;388(388):118-124.

67. McKee MD, Schemitsch EH, Sala MJ, O'driscoll SW: The pathoanatomy of lateral ligamentous disruption in

3: Upper Extremity

complex elbow instability. *J Shoulder Elbow Surg* 2003; 12(4):391-396.

68. Jensen SL, Olsen BS, Tyrdal S, Søjbjerg JO, Sneppen O: Elbow joint laxity after experimental radial head excision and lateral collateral ligament rupture: Efficacy of prosthetic replacement and ligament repair. *J Shoulder Elbow Surg* 2005;14(1):78-84.

69. Forthman C, Henket M, Ring DC: Elbow dislocation with intra-articular fracture: The results of operative treatment without repair of the medial collateral ligament. *J Hand Surg Am* 2007;32(8):1200-1209.

  In 34 complex elbow dislocations with coronoid and radial head fractures, the patients were treated with lateral ligament repair, without MCL repair. Thirty-two of 34 elbows remained stable and averaged 120° of ulnohumeral motion. The authors concluded that MCL repair is not required. Level of evidence: IV.

70. Fern SE, Owen JR, Ordyna NJ, Wayne JS, Boardman ND III: Complex varus elbow instability: A terrible triad model. *J Shoulder Elbow Surg* 2009;18(2):269-274.

  Using a cadaver terrible triad model, the authors demonstrated that repair of a radial head and LCL injury, when associated with at least 50% coronoid bone loss, fails to restore varus stability of the elbow.

71. Schneeberger AG, Sadowski MM, Jacob HA: Coronoid process and radial head as posterolateral rotatory stabilizers of the elbow. *J Bone Joint Surg Am* 2004;86(5):975-982.

72. Ring D, Jupiter JB, Zilberfarb J: Posterior dislocation of the elbow with fractures of the radial head and coronoid . *J Bone Joint Surg Am* 2002;84:547-551.

73. Pugh DM, Wild LM, Schemitsch EH, King GJ, McKee MD: Standard surgical protocol to treat elbow dislocations with radial head and coronoid fractures. *J Bone Joint Surg Am* 2004;86:1122-1130.

74. McKee MD, Pugh DM, Wild LM, Schemitsch EH, King GJ: Standard surgical protocol to treat elbow dislocations with radial head and coronoid fractures: Surgical technique. *J Bone Joint Surg Am* 2005;87(pt 1, suppl 1):22-32.

75. Winter M, Chuinard C, Cikes A, Pelegri C, Bronsard N, de Peretti F: Surgical management of elbow dislocation associated with non-reparable fractures of the radial head. *Chir Main* 2009;28(3):158-167.

  Thirteen patients treated with a standard surgical approach for a terrible triad injury had reliable and reproducible results.

76. Beingessner DM, Dunning CE, Gordon KD, Johnson JA, King GJ: The effect of radial head excision and arthroplasty on elbow kinematics and stability. *J Bone Joint Surg Am* 2004;86:1730-1739.

77. Zeiders GJ, Patel MK: Management of unstable elbows following complex fracture-dislocations: The "terrible triad" injury. *J Bone Joint Surg Am* 2008;90(suppl 4):75-84.

  The authors describe an approach to terrible triad injuries involving the earlier consideration of external fixation.

78. Mazzocca AD, Cohen M, Berkson E, et al: The anatomy of the bicipital tuberosity and distal biceps tendon. *J Shoulder Elbow Surg* 2007;16(1):122-127.

  This anatomic study provides dimensions and describes the angular relationship of the radial head and styloid.

79. Hutchinson HL, Gloystein D, Gillespie M: Distal biceps tendon insertion: An anatomic study. *J Shoulder Elbow Surg* 2008;17:342-346.

  This anatomic study quantifies the angular relationships of the distal biceps tendon.

80. Kulshreshtha R, Singh R, Sinha J, Hall S: Anatomy of the distal biceps brachii tendon and its clinical relevance. *Clin Orthop Relat Res* 2007;456:117-120.

  The authors offer descriptive analysis of the distal biceps tendon anatomic insertion.

81. Athwal GS, Steinmann SP, Rispoli DM: The distal biceps tendon: Footprint and relevant clinical anatomy. *J Hand Surg Am* 2007;32(8):1225-1229.

  This anatomic study showed that the short head of the distal biceps tendon has a consistent relationship to the lacertus fibrosus, which has implications for orienting the tendon during surgical repair.

82. Chew ML, Giuffrè BM: Disorders of the distal biceps brachii tendon. *Radiographics* 2005;25(5):1227-1237.

83. Freeman CR, McCormick KR, Mahoney D, Baratz M, Lubahn JD: Nonoperative treatment of distal biceps tendon ruptures compared with a historical control group. *J Bone Joint Surg Am* 2009;91(10):2329-2334.

  Eighteen patients with 20 unrepaired distal biceps tendon ruptures were retrospectively assessed. The medial supination and elbow flexion strengths for the injured arm and contralateral arm were 63% and 93%, respectively. Nonsurgical treatment yielded modest reduction in supination strength.

84. El-Hawary R, Macdermid JC, Faber KJ, Patterson SD, King GJ: Distal biceps tendon repair: Comparison of surgical techniques. *J Hand Surg Am* 2003;28(3):496-502.

85. Lemos SE, Ebramzedeh E, Kvitne RS: A new technique: In vitro suture anchor fixation has superior yield strength to bone tunnel fixation for distal biceps tendon repair. *Am J Sports Med* 2004;32(2):406-410.

86. Krushinski EM, Brown JA, Murthi AM: Distal biceps tendon rupture: Biomechanical analysis of repair strength of the Bio-Tenodesis screw versus suture anchors. *J Shoulder Elbow Surg* 2007;16(2):218-223.

  The authors compared the strength and stiffness of distal biceps repairs using biotenodesis screw or suture anchor techniques in cadavers. The biotenodesis screw technique showed more initial pullout strength compared with suture anchors.

87. Mazzocca AD, Burton KJ, Romeo AA, Santangelo S, Adams DA, Arciero RA: Biomechanical evaluation of 4 techniques of distal biceps brachii tendon repair. *Am J Sports Med* 2007;35(2):252-258.

In a biomechanical comparison of four techniques of distal biceps tendon repair, the Endobutton technique had the highest load to failure.

88. Kettler M, Tingart MJ, Lunger J, Kuhn V: Reattachment of the distal tendon of biceps: Factors affecting the failure strength of the repair. *J Bone Joint Surg Br* 2008; 90(1):103-106.

The Endobutton-based method had the highest load-to-failure in a biomechanical comparison of distal biceps tendon repair techniques.

89. Spang JT, Weinhold PS, Karas SG: A biomechanical comparison of EndoButton versus suture anchor repair of distal biceps tendon injuries. *J Shoulder Elbow Surg* 2006;15(4):509-514.

90. Peeters T, Ching-Soon NG, Jansen N, Sneyers C, Declercq G, Verstreken F: Functional outcome after repair of distal biceps tendon ruptures using the endobutton technique. *J Shoulder Elbow Surg* 2009;18(2):283-287.

The authors reported that distal biceps repair using the Endobutton technique yielded good results in 26 patients.

91. John CK, Field LD, Weiss KS, Savoie FH III: Single-incision repair of acute distal biceps ruptures by use of suture anchors. *J Shoulder Elbow Surg* 2007;16(1): 78-83.

The authors of this study showed that the one-incision approach and fixation with suture anchors is a safe and effective method for distal biceps repair.

92. Hartman MW, Merten SM, Steinmann SP: Mini-open 2-incision technique for repair of distal biceps tendon ruptures. *J Shoulder Elbow Surg* 2007;16(5):616-620.

Distal biceps tendon repair using the two-incision technique achieved good results in 33 patients.

93. Patterson RW, Sharma J, Lawton JN, Evans PJ: Distal biceps tendon reconstruction with tendoachilles allograft: A modification of the endobutton technique utilizing an ACL reconstruction system. *J Hand Surg Am* 2009;34(3):545-552.

This article describes reconstruction of distal biceps injuries with tendo Achilles allograft, with the Endobutton technique for fixation.

94. Wiley WB, Noble JS, Dulaney TD, Bell RH, Noble DD: Late reconstruction of chronic distal biceps tendon ruptures with a semitendinosus autograft technique. *J Shoulder Elbow Surg* 2006;15(4):440-444.

3: Upper Extremity

Chapter 27

Elbow Instability and Reconstruction

Bradford O. Parsons, MD   Matthew L. Ramsey, MD

Arthritis

Osteoarthritis

Osteoarthritis of the elbow joint can occur primarily or secondary to trauma. Primary osteoarthritis usually occurs in middle-aged men who often have performed manual labor. In the early stages, nonsurgical management with nonsteroidal anti-inflammatory drugs, activity modification, and corticosteroid injections can be helpful. Arthroscopic débridement and synovectomy, and débridement or interpositional arthroplasty are generally recommended for younger, active patients who do not respond to nonsurgical management. For older and more sedentary patients, total elbow arthroplasty is considered the procedure of choice.

A 2008 study reported on arthroscopic osteophyte resection and capsulectomy in 41 patients with primary osteoarthritis.[1] At follow-up of more than 2 years, the authors identified significant improvements in flexion and extension, supination, and functional scores. Many patients (81%) reported good to excellent results with a significant decrease in pain; complications were rare.

In a study with seven patients, the outcomes of treating osteochondral lesions in the elbow with autologous osteochondral transplantation were reported.[2] The grafts were harvested from the lateral femoral condyle. Significant improvements occurred in pain and functional scores. Graft viability was confirmed in all patients with postoperative MRI.

A recent study reported on 11 patients younger than 50 years who were treated with arthroscopic ulnohumeral arthroplasty for degenerative arthritis of the elbow after failed nonsurgical treatment.[3] An all-arthroscopic technique was used. It was concluded that the procedure resulted in significant short-term pain relief, restoration of motion, and improved function.

In a recent radiographic study of arthritic elbows using CT scanning, a higher incidence of ulnohumeral osteophytes (95%) was identified compared with radiocapitellar joint osteophytes (59%).[4] The study authors challenged the notion that osteoarthritis originates in the radiohumeral joint.

Inflammatory Arthritis

The Larsen classification is generally used for the stratification of elbow joint involvement in rheumatoid arthritis (Figure 1). Surgical arthroscopy remains an important modality for treatment, especially when the inflammatory component is significant and the bony structures are relatively well preserved.

In a study reviewing the use of either open or arthroscopic synovectomy in 58 rheumatoid elbows, no significant differences between the techniques were identified in elbows with a preoperative arc of flexion of less than 90°.[5] In patients with an elbow arc of motion greater than 90°, arthroscopic synovectomy provided better function than the open approach.

In patients with inflammatory changes with symptoms and dysfunction refractory to nonsurgical measures, semiconstrained total elbow arthroplasty remains a reliable method of treatment. A 2009 study compared complication rates between patients with and without rheumatoid arthritis who were treated with total elbow arthroplasty.[6] Data from 3,617 patients were analyzed; 888 patients were identified as having rheumatoid arthritis and the remainder were classified as nonrheumatic patients. Complication rates were low in both groups; however, there were more medical complications and longer hospital stays in the nonrheumatic group. The authors concluded that complications after total elbow arthroplasty were rare and nearly equivalent in rheumatoid and nonrheumatoid patients.

In 49 patients age 40 years or younger treated with total elbow arthroplasty (6 bilateral procedures), 30 patients had inflammatory arthritis and 19 had post-

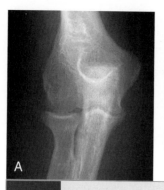
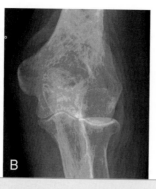
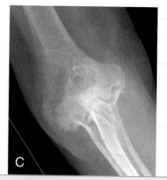
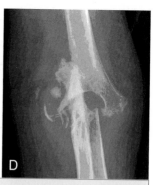

Figure 1 Larsen classification system for the rheumatoid elbow. **A,** Stage I: normal architecture and osteoporosis. Synovitis is present. **B,** Stage II: joint-space narrowing and intact joint architecture. Synovitis is present. **C,** Stage III: alteration of joint architecture. **D,** Stage IV, gross joint destruction and minimal synovitis. (Reproduced from Athwal GS, Faber KJ, King GJW: Elbow reconstruction, in Fischgrund JS, ed: *Orthopaedic Knowledge Update 9*. Rosemont, IL, American Academy of Orthopaedic Surgeons, 2008, pp 333-342.)

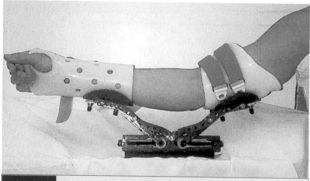

Figure 2 A progressive static splint is used to manage elbow stiffness. (Reproduced from Bruno RJ, Lee ML, Strauch RJ, Rosenwasser MP: Posttraumatic elbow stiffness: Evaluation and management. *J Am Acad Orthop Surg* 2002;10(2):106-116.)

traumatic arthritis.[7] During the recorded follow-up (minimum of 5 years), 12 of the elbows required a second surgical procedure. The rate of revision was higher for patients with posttraumatic arthritis.

Stiffness

Loss of motion after injury or elbow surgery can lead to significant functional disability. Although the exact cause of the development of elbow contracture remains unclear, several factors have been theorized to contribute to this disorder, including the high degree of congruity of the elbow joint, its propensity for developing heterotopic bone, cocontraction of the periarticular muscle groups, and irritability of the ulnar nerve.

Treatment of posttraumatic or postoperative elbow stiffness can be unreliable. As a result, prevention with range-of-motion exercises and other modalities, including static progressive splinting, is critical in managing these patients (Figure 2). Any injury that does not require surgical treatment (for example, nondisplaced radial head fractures) should be treated with an early range-of-motion program. Injuries that require surgical treatment should be fixed in a stable manner so that the

rehabilitation process can begin a few days following the surgical procedure.

If nonsurgical management fails to restore mobility, arthroscopic or open contracture release can restore motion in patients with dysfunction. Arthroscopic release is generally reserved for patients with mild contractures, whereas open releases are performed in patients with severe stiffness, a significant amount of heterotopic bone, or those with ankylosis. Manipulation under anesthesia is commonly performed in the knee for treating stiffness following total knee arthroplasty. In 51 patients treated with manipulation under anesthesia for contracture release of a stiff elbow an average of 40 days after surgery, the mean postmanipulation arc of motion increased to 78° from 40° preoperatively.[8] The authors concluded that manipulation under anesthesia is a safe and valuable adjunct in the treatment of elbow stiffness.

Continuous passive motion (CPM) after elbow contracture release has been used to maintain motion in the early postoperative period. CPM after open contracture release in two matched cohorts of 16 patients was evaluated in a 2009 study. The preoperative arc of motion (flexion and extension) averaged 38° in the CPM group and 42° in the group with no CPM.[9] The improvement and the final arc of motion between both groups were comparable, differing by 5°. The authors concluded that there was no demonstrable benefit of postoperative CPM after open contracture release.

Elbow Instability

The elbow joint is stabilized by a combination of static and dynamic constraints. The static stabilizers are divided between a set of primary and secondary stabilizers. The primary stabilizers of the elbow include the ulnohumeral articulation (coronoid process), the medial collateral ligament (MCL), and the lateral collateral ligament (LCL) complex. The secondary stabilizers include the radiocapitellar articulation and the common flexor and extensor origins. The anterior capsule also

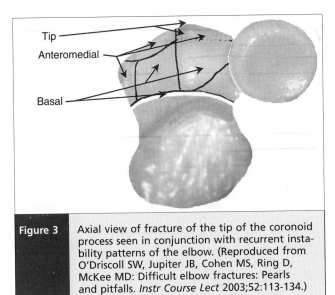

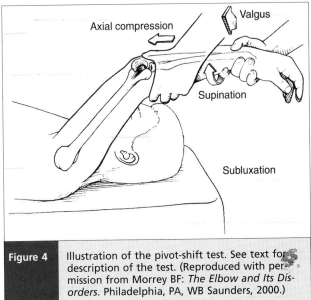

| Figure 3 | Axial view of fracture of the tip of the coronoid process seen in conjunction with recurrent instability patterns of the elbow. (Reproduced from O'Driscoll SW, Jupiter JB, Cohen MS, Ring D, McKee MD: Difficult elbow fractures: Pearls and pitfalls. *Instr Course Lect* 2003;52:113-134.) |

| Figure 4 | Illustration of the pivot-shift test. See text for description of the test. (Reproduced with permission from Morrey BF: *The Elbow and Its Disorders*. Philadelphia, PA, WB Saunders, 2000.) |

contributes to the stability of the elbow as an anterior restraint, especially in terminal extension. Further stability is conferred by the action of the muscles spanning the elbow, including the brachialis, triceps, and anconeus, which impart compressive forces across the joint. Traumatic injury to any single primary stabilizer may lead to elbow instability, with most injuries involving a spectrum of pathology.

In addition to acute instability, a variety of recurrent instability patterns of the elbow have been described, including posterolateral rotatory instability, varus posteromedial rotatory instability, and valgus instability. Chronic dislocation or failed management of complex instability may also occur, although more rarely.

Recurrent Instability
Recurrent instability of the elbow is rare and often subtle, with most patients describing pain as the primary symptom. A history of recurrent dislocation is extremely rare. As such, a high index of suspicion is required to diagnose this condition because static imaging studies may appear normal and physical examination findings may be limited by pain and guarding. Three pathologic entities of recurrent instability have been described: posterolateral rotatory instability, varus posteromedial rotatory instability, and valgus instability. A new classification of fractures of the coronoid process has furthered the understanding of the role of this structure in these instability patterns (Figure 3).

Posterolateral Rotatory Instability
The most common etiology of symptomatic recurrent instability occurs following injury to the LCL, specifically the lateral ulnar collateral ligament (LUCL) complex, resulting in posterolateral rotatory instability.[10] This condition describes a sequence of instability that occurs with supination, axial loading, valgus stress, and extension of the elbow, resulting in subluxation of the

radial head posterior to the capitellum, and rotation of the semilunar notch away from the trochlea. Most commonly, posterolateral rotatory instability occurs following traumatic injury (elbow dislocation), which can result in an attenuated LUCL complex. Other etiologies also have been described, including iatrogenic injury during lateral elbow procedures, such as lateral epicondylitis release, or from progressive ligament attenuation secondary to chronic cubitus varus malunion.

Most patients with posterolateral rotatory instability report pain and occasional "catching" or "clunking" sensations, often when pushing off from the arm of a chair. The lateral pivot-shift test has been shown to be a provocative test that can identify posterolateral rotatory instability, although it can be difficult to perform in an awake patient because of apprehension and guarding (Figure 4). This test is often more reliable in an anesthetized patient. The test is performed with the arm flexed over the head of a supine patient. The forearm is supinated, elbow extended, and a valgus load is placed across the elbow. In this position the elbow is subluxated. As the elbow is slowly flexed, maintaining a supinated forearm and valgus load, the radial head will reduce, often with a clunk (in an anesthetized patient), confirming LCL insufficiency. When performed under fluoroscopy, the radial head can be visualized posterior to the capitellum on lateral imaging when the elbow is extended. Additionally, the ulnohumeral joint can appear widened; both the radiocapitellar and ulnohumeral joint congruencies are restored to normal with elbow flexion.

More recently, other diagnostic tests have been described, including the tabletop relocation test,[11] chair push-up test, and floor push-up test.[12] All of these tests mimic the subluxating force associated with posterolateral rotatory instability, involving active extension of the elbow with the forearm supinated and the hand on a platform (either the floor, table, or armchair). In all

3: Upper Extremity

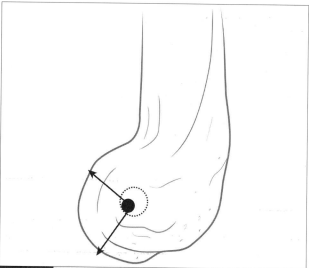

Figure 5 Illustration of the location of the isometric point of the origin of the LUCL on the lateral aspect of the capitellum. Docking hole placement requires the hole to be centered slightly posterior and proximal to the isometric point to keep the ligament graft tensioned in extension. (Reproduced from Armstrong AD: Acute, recurrent, and chronic elbow instability, in Galatz LM, ed: *Orthopaedic Knowledge Update: Shoulder and Elbow 3*. Rosemont, IL, American Academy of Orthopaedic Surgeons, 2008, pp 461-476.)

tests, a positive finding is indicated by patient apprehension or a report of pain with elbow extension. Similar to a relocation test for anterior shoulder instability, in the tabletop relocation test the examiner places their thumb over the radial head and posterolateral gutter of the elbow to prevent instability; this minimizes the patient's symptoms. These tests are reliable and reproducible in an awake patient.

Standard imaging studies are often of little value in evaluating posterolateral rotatory instability. Static radiographs are often normal. Although MRI can identify acute avulsion of the origin of the LUCL from the lateral humerus, as seen in acute instability, in recurrent instability the LUCL is often attenuated, and MRI may not be helpful. Fluoroscopic evaluation during a pivot shift test or other provocative test may demonstrate subluxation of the radial head posterior to the capitellum.

The management of symptomatic, recurrent posterolateral rotatory instability most often involves reconstruction of the LUCL complex, using either autograft or allograft. Repair of the LUCL in patients with recurrent elbow instability yields inferior results to reconstruction with tendon graft, often because of attenuation of the native ligament tissue.[13] However, repair has been successfully performed for acute instability, both with open, or more recently, arthroscopic techniques.[14] A variety of reconstruction techniques have been described, with the original technique using tendon graft placed through a tunnel in the supinator crest of the

ulna and then weaved in a figure-of-8 fashion through a "Y" tunnel configuration in the humerus, with the graft tied to itself over the lateral column.[10] Conversely, the graft may be "docked" on the humeral side with sutures exiting the "Y" tunnels and tied over the column, or a single-strand graft can be docked on both the ulnar and humeral side with interference screws or sutures through bone tunnels.[15] Reconstruction techniques using lateral triceps tissue also have been described.[16,17]

Regardless of the technique, the critical aspect of repair and reconstruction remains the reestablishment of the isometric origin of the LUCL on the lateral aspect of the capitellum. The isometric point is the exact center of rotation of the joint, which is located in the center of the lateral face of the hemisphere of the capitellum (**Figure 5**). An important technical aspect of tunnel placement is to establish the humeral tunnel so that the distal corner of the tunnel is at the isometric point, not the center of the tunnel, ensuring appropriate tension. The graft is secured with the arm in neutral rotation and 45° of flexion. Postoperatively, patients are protected from varus stress across the elbow and shoulder abduction is avoided; early range-of-motion therapy is started.

Intermediate results of the surgical management of posterolateral rotatory instability have recently been described in 45 patients, with 12 repairs and 33 reconstructions with tendon graft.[13] Eighty-six percent of patients were subjectively satisfied, with better results observed in patients with a posttraumatic etiology and those treated with elbow reconstruction. Patients with primary reports of instability had better outcomes than those who reported pain.

Varus Posteromedial Rotatory Instability

More recent attention has focused on fractures involving the anteromedial facet of the coronoid, resulting in a complex pattern of instability termed varus posteromedial rotatory instability. This type of instability develops as a result of injury to the anteromedial facet of the coronoid and rupture of the LCL complex. In this setting, a varus force fractures the anteromedial facet of the coronoid with rupture of the LCL, leading to subluxation of the ulnohumeral joint into the defect created by the anteromedial coronoid fracture.[18-21] As a result, fracture to the anteromedial facet can be subtle but can lead to significant ulnohumeral instability. An important aspect of anteromedial facet injuries in relationship to elbow stability is the involvement of the sublime tubercle, which is the insertion point of the anterior bundle of the MCL.

The mechanism of injury is different from the valgus stress to an axially loaded and supinated forearm that is involved in posterolateral rotatory instability. In posteromedial rotatory instability, the radial head does not impact the capitellum, as occurs in most fracture-dislocations of the elbow; therefore, the radial head is often spared. Repair of posteromedial rotatory instability requires both a medial and lateral approach that fixes the coronoid fragment and repairs the LCL com-

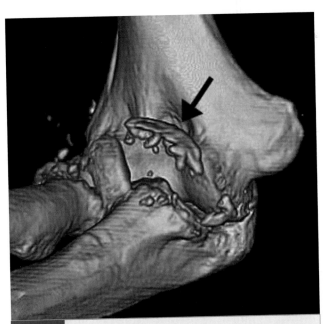

Figure 6 Three-dimensional CT scan of an anteromedial coronoid fracture. The arrow indicates the fracture fragment. (Reproduced from Steinmann SP: Coronoid process fracture. *J Am Acad Orthop Surg* 2008;16(9):519-529.)

plex. In a biomechanical study, it has been shown that it may be possible for small subtype I anteromedial coronoid fractures to be managed with isolated repair of the LCL if the MCL is intact.[22]

To identify posteromedial rotatory instability, a high index of suspicion is required because elbow radiographs may appear relatively normal on AP and lateral views. Some radiographic clues may include a double density of the coronoid subchondral plate on lateral images, or a narrowing of the anteromedial ulnohumeral joint space on AP images. Varus stress radiographs may highlight LCL insufficiency and show trochlear-coronoid contact. CT scans can help identify the anteromedial coronoid fracture and confirm the diagnosis (Figure 6).

Although the diagnosis may be difficult, it is critical because nonsurgical treatment often results in persistent incongruity of the elbow, altered kinematics, and early arthrosis of the ulnohumeral joint.[20,22] Surgical treatment is necessary to restore the coronoid architecture, often using an anteromedial buttress plate via a medial approach, followed by LCL isometric repair. At an average follow-up of 26 months, 18 patients with anteromedial facet fractures of the coronoid were evaluated.[21] Six patients had varus subluxation of the elbow; four had not had fixation of the anteromedial facet and two had loss of fixation. Arthrosis developed in all six of these patients; results were fair to poor. The 12 patients with secure fixation of the anteromedial facet fracture had good to excellent elbow function.

Early range of motion is started after surgical repair.[21] Anatomic repair and healing of the coronoid and LCL has yielded favorable results.[20]

Valgus Instability

Disruption of the MCL, specifically the anterior band of the MCL, can result in recurrent valgus instability of the elbow. MCL injuries may occur secondary to trauma (such as a dislocation) or as the result of repetitive stress (most commonly observed in throwing athletes). As opposed to lateral-sided instability, medial instability was historically believed to be well tolerated in most patients because little valgus load is placed across the elbow during the activities of daily living. Secondary stabilizers such as the radial head often minimize the severity of instability so that frank recurrent dislocation is rare. As such, findings of valgus instability may be subtle, and often can be confused with medial epicondylitis or an inflamed cubital tunnel.

Most patients who report symptomatic valgus instability are overhead athletes, predominantly baseball players. The elbow is subjected to a high valgus load during the acceleration phase of throwing, placing tremendous stress on the anterior band of the MCL. Throwers may report experiencing a "pop" associated with a sudden drop in velocity following acute rupture of the anterior band of the MCL. However, some patients cannot identify any cardinal event and primarily report pain during throwing motion, or a loss of velocity or accuracy. Adding to the diagnostic difficulty, many throwers with anterior band MCL insufficiency also report posteromedial elbow pain resulting from posteromedial impingement of the olecranon during the deceleration phase of throwing, termed valgus extension overload.

The physical examination centers on provocative testing of the MCL. Tenderness is often elicited over the MCL origin. Integrity of the flexor pronator mass is assessed, as is the ulnar nerve and cubital tunnel. Posteromedial tenderness over the olecranon may indicate valgus extension overload. A variety of provocative maneuvers have been described to identify MCL injury, including the valgus stress test, milking maneuver, and moving valgus stress test. Valgus stress testing is performed with the elbow in 30° flexion, unlocking the olecranon from the fossa. The milking maneuver is performed with the elbow in 90° flexion. With the examiner holding the patient's ipsilateral thumb, a valgus stress is placed on the elbow with the forearm supinated. Pain at the MCL origin is considered a positive finding. More recently, a variant of the milking maneuver, the moving valgus stress test, was reported to be 100% sensitive and 75% specific for MCL injury when compared with arthroscopic or open visualization of the ligament.[23] In this maneuver, the arm is positioned in the same manner used in the milking maneuver, but the elbow is taken through a range of motion while a maximal valgus stress is applied across the joint. Reproducible pain in the medial elbow between 70° and 120° is considered a positive test.

Similar to posterolateral and posteromedial rotatory instability, static radiographs of patients with valgus instability are often normal. A posteromedial osteophyte of the olecranon in patients with valgus extension overload may be apparent on radiographs but is often sub-

3: Upper Extremity

tle. Valgus stress radiographs may show medial ulnohumeral joint widening, especially in posttraumatic valgus instability. MRI can be helpful in identifying acute ruptures of the anterior band of the MCL, chronic thickening associated with repetitive injury, and injury to the flexor-pronator origin.

Patients with symptomatic valgus instability are initially managed nonsurgically, with therapy aimed at strengthening the flexor-pronator muscles, along with rest from throwing for a minimum of 6 weeks. Patients can resume throwing if symptoms abate, with careful attention placed on throwing mechanics. Nonsurgical treatment has been used with success in some throwing athletes, with 13 of 31 athletes (42%) returning to their preinjury level of sports activity at an average of 24 weeks following rehabilitation and rest.[24]

If nonsurgical treatment is unsuccessful, patients can be candidates for MCL reconstruction with tendon graft. Primary repair, as is the case in posterolateral rotatory instability, is often inferior to reconstruction in recurrent valgus instability, except in rare cases of early identification of acute avulsion injuries.[25] Similar to LUCL reconstruction, a variety of reconstruction techniques for the anterior band of the MCL have been described, including figure-of-8 graft passage through the ulnar and humeral tunnels, docking techniques, and the use of fixation devices such as Endobuttons (Smith & Nephew, Memphis, TN) or interference screws with single- or double-strand tendon grafts.

Recently, a biomechanical study evaluated four conventional reconstruction methods: figure-of-8 fixation, humeral docking, interference screw fixation, and single-strand Endobutton reconstruction. The humeral docking and Endobutton techniques were stronger than the figure-of-8 and interference screw fixation methods, although none were as strong as the native ligament.[26] Conversely, another biomechanical analysis found that interference screw fixation of the ulnar side, associated with humeral docking, yields graft fixation strength equal to 95% of that provided by the native MCL under valgus loading.[27]

Conventional approaches use a flexor-pronator split rather than the original technique with reflection of the flexor mass off the epicondyle in an effort to preserve the role of the flexor group as a dynamic stabilizer of the medial elbow. Management of the ulnar nerve is dictated by the presence of preoperative ulnar nerve symptoms; routine transposition has been abandoned because of the potential for ulnar nerve irritation. Although not truly isometric, the anterior band of the MCL is nearly isometric, with the origin at the center of rotation of the medial aspect of the trochlea; humeral fixation should be placed at this site.[26]

Results following reconstruction have been excellent, with most series reporting more than 90% of patients returning to preinjury levels of throwing and sports participation.[28-30] Few clinical data are available to demonstrate the superiority of one technique over another.

Chronic Instability

Chronic instability of the elbow is rare. Management of a chronic simple dislocation or the more common complex dislocation is challenging, with results inferior to those obtained following appropriate closed treatment or surgical management of an acute dislocation. Failed prior surgical stabilization, especially following complex instability, is the most common etiology of chronic instability and requires careful assessment of the osseous and ligamentous structures critical for elbow stability. In addition to the inherent ligamentous and osseous pathophysiology, articular derangement is often present, as are fibrous adhesions of the joint that fill the widened joint space of a chronically dislocated elbow. Heterotopic ossification, which may encase the neurovascular structures around the elbow, adds complexity to treating the disorder. The periarticular muscles, especially the triceps, are often contracted, potentially requiring lengthening or release. Most studies show that closed reduction of a chronically dislocated elbow is unlikely to achieve successful restoration of stability or function, especially after 3 to 4 weeks of being dislocated.[31]

Surgical management is aimed at concentric reduction of the joint, with removal of any fibrous tissue or adhesions preventing reduction, ligament reconstruction, and triceps lengthening (when necessary). Chronic complex dislocations require restoration of the osseous constraints, especially the coronoid process. Unfortunately, coronoid insufficiency is frequently present after neglected or failed prior surgical stabilization of terrible triad injuries, and carries a guarded prognosis, especially when bone loss exceeds 50%. Reconstruction of coronoid bone loss is very challenging.[32]

Hinged external fixation is often required when managing the chronically dislocated elbow, and has been used with success in limited series.[33,34] When greater then 50% of the articular surface is damaged, interposition arthroplasty or prosthetic replacement is considered, depending on the patient's physiologic age and activity level. Regardless of the reconstructive technique, patients should be aware of the potential goals of treatment, which are restoration of concentric reduction and a functional range of motion. Persistent pain and limitation of motion, especially in extension, often occur following successful management of this complex disorder.

Annotated References

1. Adams JE, Wolff LH III, Merten SM, Steinmann SP: Osteoarthritis of the elbow: Results of arthroscopic osteophyte resection and capsulectomy. *J Shoulder Elbow Surg* 2008;17(1):126-131.

   In this series the authors present the retrospective results of 41 patients who underwent arthroscopic osteophyte removal and capsulectomy. At minimum 2-year follow-up, total flexion improved from 117.3° to 131.6° and extension improved from 21.4° to 8.4°. Overall the authors cited 81% good to excellent results according to Mayo Elbow Performance Scores.

2. Ansah P, Vogt S, Ueblacker P, Martinek V, Woertler K, Imhoff AB: Osteochondral transplantation to treat osteochondral lesions in the elbow. *J Bone Joint Surg Am* 2007;89(10):2188-2194.

This series reviews the results of seven patients with osteochondral lesions of the elbow (five capitellar, one trochlea, and one radial head) who were managed with autologous lateral femoral condyle cylindrical osteochondral plugs. At an average follow-up of 59 months, Broberg-Morrey and pain scores were significantly improved and all grafts were viable and congruent on MRI scans.

3. Krishnan SG, Harkins DC, Pennington SD, Harrison DK, Burkhead WZ: Arthroscopic ulnohumeral arthroplasty for degenerative arthritis of the elbow in patients under fifty years of age. *J Shoulder Elbow Surg* 2007; 16(4):443-448.

In their series of 11 patients younger than 50 years with symptomatic elbow osteoarthritis managed by arthroscopic ulnohumeral arthroplasty, the authors demonstrated an average improvement in arc of motion of 73° and improved pain scores at minimum follow-up of 2 years.

4. Lim YW, van Riet RP, Mittal R, Bain GI: Pattern of osteophyte distribution in primary osteoarthritis of the elbow. *J Shoulder Elbow Surg* 2008;17(6):963-966.

In a consecutive series of 22 patients with osteoarthritis of the elbow, 95% of patients demonstrated ulnohumeral osteophytes on three-dimensional CT scans. Conversely, radiohumeral osteophytes were observed in only 59% of patients.

5. Tanaka N, Sakahashi H, Hirose K, Ishima T, Ishii S: Arthroscopic and open synovectomy of the elbow in rheumatoid arthritis. *J Bone Joint Surg Am* 2006;88(3):521-525.

6. Cook C, Hawkins R, Aldridge JM III, Tolan S, Krupp R, Bolognesi M: Comparison of perioperative complications in patients with and without rheumatoid arthritis who receive total elbow replacement. *J Shoulder Elbow Surg* 2009;18(1):21-26.

Using data analyzed from the Nationwide Inpatient Sample database, the authors found that in 3,617 total elbow arthroplasties, overall complication rates were low and nearly equivalent between patients with rheumatoid arthritis (888 patients) compared to other diagnoses. Length of stay was longer in patients without rheumatoid arthritis.

7. Celli A, Morrey BF: Total elbow arthroplasty in patients forty years of age or less. *J Bone Joint Surg Am* 2009; 91(6):1414-1418.

The authors retrospectively reviewed the results of 49 patients (55 elbows) younger than 40 years with elbow arthritis managed with total elbow arthroplasty. Thirty patients had a diagnosis of inflammatory arthritis, and the remaining 19 patients, posttraumatic arthritis. At an average follow-up of 91 months, 22% of elbows had undergone additional surgery, and 93% (51) were graded as good-excellent according to Mayo Elbow Performance Scores. The revision rate is higher in patients with a posttraumatic etiology.

8. Araghi A, Celli A, Adams R, Morrey B: The outcome of examination (manipulation) under anesthesia on the stiff elbow after surgical contracture release. *J Shoulder Elbow Surg* 2010;19(2):202-208.

In a series of 44 patients with stiff postsurgical elbows, an examination (with manipulation) of the elbow under anesthesia at a mean postoperative date of 40 days yielded an improvement in arc of motion from 33° to 73°. Three patients had worsening of ulnar paresthesias, with one requiring ulnar nerve transposition.

9. Lindenhovius AL, van de Luijtgaarden K, Ring D, Jupiter J: Open elbow contracture release: Postoperative management with and without continuous passive motion. *J Hand Surg Am* 2009;34(5):858-865.

In a retrospective matched series of patients undergoing open contracture release of stiff elbows, outcomes were compared between 16 patients who underwent postoperative CPM compared with 16 control subjects. At final follow-up of 6 months, no difference was observed in flexion or extension motion between groups.

10. O'Driscoll SW, Bell DF, Morrey BF: Posterolateral rotatory instability of the elbow. *J Bone Joint Surg Am* 1991;73(3):440-446.

11. Arvind CH, Hargreaves DG: Tabletop relocation test: A new clinical test for posterolateral rotatory instability of the elbow. *J Shoulder Elbow Surg* 2006;15(6):707-708.

12. Regan W, Lapner PC: Prospective evaluation of two diagnostic apprehension signs for posterolateral instability of the elbow. *J Shoulder Elbow Surg* 2006;15(3):344-346.

13. Sanchez-Sotelo J, Morrey BF, O'Driscoll SW: Ligamentous repair and reconstruction for posterolateral rotatory instability of the elbow. *J Bone Joint Surg Br* 2005; 87(1):54-61.

14. Savoie FH III, Field LD, Gurley DJ: Arthroscopic and open radial ulnohumeral ligament reconstruction for posterolateral rotatory instability of the elbow. *Hand Clin* 2009;25(3):323-329.

The authors report on a series of 54 patients with posterolateral rotatory instability of the elbow managed with open repair or reconstruction (30 patients) or arthroscopic repair (24 patients). The authors report improvement in Andrews-Carson scores of 145 to 180 at an average follow-up of 41 months. Acute repairs (10) demonstrated the best outcome, and no difference was observed between open and arthroscopic repairs. Level of evidence: IV.

15. King GJ, Dunning CE, Zarzour ZD, Patterson SD, Johnson JA: Single-strand reconstruction of the lateral ulnar collateral ligament restores varus and posterolat-

3: Upper Extremity

eral rotatory stability of the elbow. *J Shoulder Elbow Surg* 2002;11(1):60-64.

16. DeLaMora SN, Hausman M: Lateral ulnar collateral ligament reconstruction using the lateral triceps fascia. *Orthopedics* 2002;25(9):909-912.

17. Olsen BS, Søjbjerg JO: The treatment of recurrent posterolateral instability of the elbow. *J Bone Joint Surg Br* 2003;85(3):342-346.

18. O'Driscoll SW, Jupiter JB, Cohen MS, Ring D, McKee MD: Difficult elbow fractures: Pearls and pitfalls. *Instr Course Lect* 2003;52:113-134.

19. Sanchez-Sotelo J, O'Driscoll SW, Morrey BF: Medial oblique compression fracture of the coronoid process of the ulna. *J Shoulder Elbow Surg* 2005;14(1):60-64.

20. Ring D, Doornberg JN: Fracture of the anteromedial facet of the coronoid process: Surgical technique. *J Bone Joint Surg Am* 2007;89(suppl 2, pt 2):267-283.

    The authors evaluated 18 patients with anteromedial facet coronoid fracture and varus posteromedial rotatory instability. Early ulnohumeral arthrosis developed and a fair or poor outcome was reported in six patients with coronoid fracture malalignment. The remaining 12 patients with anatomic coronoid healing had good or excellent elbow function. Level of evidence: III.

21. Doornberg JN, Ring DC: Fracture of the anteromedial facet of the coronoid process. *J Bone Joint Surg Am* 2006;88(10):2216-2224.

22. Pollock JW, Brownhill J, Ferreira L, McDonald CP, Johnson J, King G: The effect of anteromedial facet fractures of the coronoid and lateral collateral ligament injury on elbow stability and kinematics. *J Bone Joint Surg Am* 2009;91(6):1448-1458.

    Using an in vitro cadaver model, the authors assessed the impact of the size of an anteromedial facet coronoid fracture on elbow stability and kinematics. Elbows with subtype I and repaired LCL demonstrated kinematics similar to an intact elbow. Subtype II and III fractures were unstable with varus and valgus stress.

23. O'Driscoll SW, Lawton RL, Smith AM: The "moving valgus stress test" for medial collateral ligament tears of the elbow. *Am J Sports Med* 2005;33(2):231-239.

24. Rettig AC, Sherrill C, Snead DS, Mendler JC, Mieling P: Nonoperative treatment of ulnar collateral ligament injuries in throwing athletes. *Am J Sports Med* 2001; 29(1):15-17.

25. Richard MJ, Aldridge JM III, Wiesler ER, Ruch DS: Traumatic valgus instability of the elbow: Pathoanatomy and results of direct repair. *J Bone Joint Surg Am* 2008;90(11):2416-2422.

    The authors report on a study of 11 collegiate athletes with acute rupture of the anterior band of the MCL. After MCL repair, 9 of 11 patients returned to college athletics. Level of evidence: IV.

26. Armstrong AD, Ferreira LM, Dunning CE, Johnson JA, King GJ: The medial collateral ligament of the elbow is not isometric: An in vitro biomechanical study. *Am J Sports Med* 2004;32(1):85-90.

27. Ahmad CS, Lee TQ, ElAttrache NS: Biomechanical evaluation of a new ulnar collateral ligament reconstruction technique with interference screw fixation. *Am J Sports Med* 2003;31(3):332-337.

28. Thompson WH, Jobe FW, Yocum LA, Pink MM: Ulnar collateral ligament reconstruction in athletes: Muscle-splitting approach without transposition of the ulnar nerve. *J Shoulder Elbow Surg* 2001;10(2):152-157.

29. Dodson CC, Thomas A, Dines JS, Nho SJ, Williams RJ III, Altchek DW: Medial ulnar collateral ligament reconstruction of the elbow in throwing athletes. *Am J Sports Med* 2006;34(12):1926-1932.

30. Dines JS, ElAttrache NS, Conway JE, Smith W, Ahmad CS: Clinical outcomes of the DANE TJ technique to treat ulnar collateral ligament insufficiency of the elbow. *Am J Sports Med* 2007;35(12):2039-2044.

    Following DANE TJ reconstruction of the ulnar collateral ligament of the elbow, 19 of 22 patients had excellent Conway scores at a mean follow-up of 36 months. Level of evidence: IV.

31. Lyons RP, Armstrong A: Chronically unreduced elbow dislocations. *Hand Clin* 2008;24(1):91-103.

    The authors present a review of current options for treating a chronically dislocated elbow.

32. Papandrea RF, Morrey BF, O'Driscoll SW: Reconstruction for persistent instability of the elbow after coronoid fracture-dislocation. *J Shoulder Elbow Surg* 2007;16(1): 68-77.

    At a minimum 2-year follow-up, 13 of 21 patients (62%) treated for chronic instability with associated coronoid fracture had successful objective outcomes. Eight patients had persistent elbow instability; 16 patients required hinged external fixation as part of their treatment. Level of evidence: IV.

33. Jupiter JB, Ring D: Treatment of unreduced elbow dislocations with hinged external fixation. *J Bone Joint Surg Am* 2002;84(9):1630-1635.

34. Ring D, Hannouche D, Jupiter JB: Surgical treatment of persistent dislocation or subluxation of the ulnohumeral joint after fracture-dislocation of the elbow. *J Hand Surg Am* 2004;29(3):470-480.

3: Upper Extremity

Chapter 28

Hand and Wrist Trauma

Virak Tan, MD   Leonid I. Katolik, MD

Fractures and Dislocations of the Hand

Fractures and dislocations of the hand are common injuries occurring across the age spectrum. These injuries may be classified as irreducible, reducible-stable, and reducible-unstable. Reducible-stable injuries are typically best managed with immobilization. Irreducible or unstable injuries are best treated surgically. When possible, treatment should allow for early functional rehabilitation and should avoid periods of lengthy immobilization.

Phalangeal Fractures

Distal phalanx fractures are common, are frequently associated with a nail bed injury, and can remain painful or sensitive long after fracture healing has occurred. Most of these fractures can be treated with splinting or compressive wrapping. Unstable transverse fractures or those associated with displaced injuries to the sterile matrix can be treated with supplemental longitudinal Kirschner wire (K-wire) fixation. If the nail bed is injured, consideration should be given to using fine absorbable sutures for the repair, with splinting of the fold with either the native nail plate or foil.

The treatment of extra-articular fractures of the proximal and middle phalanges is predicated on restoring the bony anatomy, maintaining reduction until bony union, and achieving functional rehabilitation. Fracture stability depends more on the injury mechanism than on the fracture pattern. Injuries that are easily reducible and stable following reduction may be treated with immobilization and rehabilitation beginning 3 to 4 weeks after injury. Traction splinting is an effective means of maintaining fracture reduction while allowing for early motion.[1] High-energy injuries with marked angulation (> 10°), malrotation (≥ 50% overlap of adjacent digit), shortening, comminution, and associated

Dr. Tan or an immediate family member has received royalties from Wright Medical Technology; serves as a paid consultant to or is an employee of Wright Medical Technology; and has stock or stock options held in Wright Medical Technology. Neither Dr. Katolik nor any immediate family member has received anything of value from or owns stock in a commercial company or institution related directly or indirectly to the subject or this chapter.

soft-tissue injuries are typically managed surgically. Multiple ipsilateral injuries are also typically treated surgically.

The surgical treatment of extra-articular fractures of the proximal and middle phalanges must take into account the overlying soft tissues. Failure to do so may result in injury to the flexor or extensor apparatus and a stiff, dysfunctional finger. With open surgical approaches, meticulous soft-tissue handling and the use of soft-tissue "sleeve" approaches[2] may minimize surgical trauma and the formation of postoperative adhesions. Further advancements in microplate design, plate materials, surface anodization, and the advent of microlocking technology may extend the safe application for open treatment of fractures while minimizing complications. The choice of fixation is largely dependent on the surgeon's preference. A recent prospective randomized study found no difference in outcomes for surgically treated phalangeal fractures when K-wire and lag screw fixation were compared.[3]

Distal Interphalangeal Joint Injuries

← *more non-op tx*

There is no consensus on the treatment of intra-articular injuries of the distal interphalangeal joint. Comminuted fractures can be treated with a short period of immobilization, followed by early active motion, which often reestablishes secondary congruity. Surgical reduction and stabilization, while yielding an aesthetically pleasing radiograph, often results in significant stiffness. Bony mallet injuries should almost universally be treated with immobilization. For large fragments, simple pin fixation or dorsal blocking pin fixation can be considered;[4] however, splinting alone will also yield a satisfactory clinical outcome.

Proximal Interphalangeal Joint Injuries

The proximal interphalangeal (PIP) joint is central to functional digital motion; injury to this joint can be challenging to treat and rehabilitate. Closed, simple dislocations are reduced under digital block anesthesia and tested for stability following reduction. If the joint requires less than 40° of flexion to maintain stability, a dorsal block splint is applied, and early active flexion is started. Long-term thickening of the PIP joint and residual stiffness are common sequelae.

Hyperextension and axial loading injuries of the PIP joint often result in dorsal dislocation with varying degrees of fracture to the volar surface of the middle pha-

[handwritten margin note: thumb UCL injury / acute: skiier's thumb / chronic: gamekeeper's thumb / hyper AB or ext @ MCP / UCL resists valgus F]

langeal base. Fractures comprising less than 30% of the joint surface can typically be stablized with dorsal block splinting alone. Fractures occupying 30% to 50% of the joint have tenuous stability. If closed treatment is selected for these injuries, careful follow-up is essential to recognize recurrent instability. Fractures requiring more than 40° of PIP joint flexion to maintain stability or those involving more than 50% of the joint surface should be treated surgically.

The ideal surgical procedure for unstable PIP joint fracture-dislocations has not been determined.[5] Static dorsal block pinning is favored in some instances because it is simple and avoids a larger surgical exposure. It can be effective in acute settings when joint involvement is less than 40% and a dorsal block splint provides a poor fit. The joint must be concentrically reduced before pin application.

Open reduction and internal fixation of the volar lip is effective if the fragment is large. Unfortunately, most PIP joint dislocations result in comminution of the volar lip. Dynamic external fixation is another option. When properly applied, it allows concentric joint motion and distraction throughout range of motion. Although fracture reduction may not be perfect, the applied traction stabilizes articular and metaphyseal comminution, allowing sufficient joint remodeling so that stable proximal phalangeal condylar containment is maintained.

Volar plate arthroplasty advances the fibrocartilaginous volar plate into the defect left after resecting the comminuted and irreparable volar lip. Some surgeons have found this procedure to be durable, with high patient satisfaction in long-term follow-up.[6] Success appears to be more favorable in acute (present ≤ 6 weeks) versus chronic injuries (present > 6 weeks).

Hemihamate arthroplasty is an alternative to volar plate arthroplasty. It is based on reestablishing the anatomic concavity of the volar lip and is indicated for comminuted fractures involving 50% or more of the volar lip; these fractures are not amenable to fixation. Although technically difficult, hemihamate arthroplasty is useful in restoring a functional range of motion and long-term stability for severely injured joints. Acute injuries have a better rate of success than chronic cases.[7]

Metacarpophalangeal Joint Injuries

Although many metacarpophalangeal (MCP) joint injuries are irreducible, dorsal dislocations of the MCP joint warrant an attempt at closed reduction. Irreducible dislocations generally result from the interposition of the volar plate in the joint and buttonholing of the metacarpal head between the flexor tendons and the radial lumbrical.

Open reduction can be safely performed through a dorsal or volar approach. With the volar approach, great care must be taken to protect the digital nerves, which may be severely tented over the metacarpal head. The A1 pulley may be released to allow retraction of the flexor tendons. The volar plate is then incised longitudinally, allowing for reduction.

Injuries to the radial or ulnar collateral ligaments of the MCP joint are common, particularly involving the thumb. Immobilization is adequate to treat partial tears or nondisplaced avulsion fractures. Distinguishing partial from complete tears can be clinically difficult. Asymmetric laxity is an unreliable diagnostic finding given inherent side-to-side differences. The absence of a firm end point with stress testing or the presence of static subluxation should be used to predict the presence of a complete tear. Surgical repair may be performed using a variety of surgical techniques, including suture anchors, with no significant differences in outcomes reported between techniques.[8]

Traditionally, acute injuries have been treated with primary repair and chronic injuries with tendon graft reconstruction. However, with the advent of microbone anchors, it appears that primary repair of some ligament injuries in a chronic setting may be satisfactorily performed.

Metacarpal Fractures

Metacarpal neck fractures may be treated nonsurgically with excellent functional outcomes for angulations of 40° to 50° in the small finger, 30° in the ring finger, 20° in the middle finger, and 10° in the index finger. Deformities exceeding these limits should be reduced. If open reduction is necessary, pinning across the fracture should be considered.

Metacarpal shaft fractures may be grouped into three general categories: transverse, oblique, or comminuted. Transverse fractures are unstable but easily reducible. Some dorsal angulation is acceptable, but generally, dorsal angulation exceeding 30° for the small finger, 20° for the ring finger, and any dorsal angulation for the index and middle fingers should be treated surgically.

Oblique fractures introduce the potential for shortening and rotational malalignment, which is poorly tolerated. Five degrees of malrotation can produce 1.5 cm of digital overlap. The presence of malrotation is a key indicator for surgical management. Comminuted fractures lack inherent stability and should be treated surgically.

Surgical treatment is indicated in the presence of multiple fractures because of the loss of supporting architecture in the adjacent digits. It is also indicated for oblique fractures (especially those with multiple comminuted fractures) and in open fractures (especially those associated with significant soft-tissue injuries). Fractures should be surgically treated in polytrauma patients who cannot tolerate cast immobilization.

A variety of percutaneous, interosseous, internal, and external fixation devices and techniques are available for metacarpal fracture fixation. Each option offers the surgeon relative advantages with respect to construct strength, ease of application, and cost. These factors should be evaluated by the surgeon when selecting the appropriate treatment. All options can afford excellent outcomes when properly applied.

Carpometacarpal Joint Injuries

Injuries to the carpometacarpal (CMC) joints are relatively uncommon. The metacarpals are very congruously seated onto the distal carpal row with stout volar, dorsal, and intermetacarpal ligament attachments. The CMC joints of the small and ring fingers act as a mobile hinge allowing flexion, extension, and rotation toward the thumb; this mobility predisposes those joints to injury more so than any of the other CMC joints. Although pure dislocation is possible, these injuries more commonly occur as fracture-dislocations with variable degrees of fracture through the hamate, metacarpal bases, or both. Closed reduction and percutaneous pinning of the metacarpal base to its neighbor or to the carpus is frequently sufficient. If a large portion of the hamate has been avulsed, open reduction and screw or plate fixation may be performed.

A Bennett fracture is an intra-articular fracture of the thumb metacarpal base involving avulsion of the thumb from the volar oblique ligament of the thumb CMC joint. Nonsurgical treatment is possible for the small number of these injuries that present with a congruent joint and minimal fracture step-off. In most instances, the adductor pollicis and the abductor pollicis longus act together to pull the metacarpal radially, proximally, and into supination, thereby causing subluxation of the joint. These injuries should be reduced with traction, extension, and pronation toward the small finger. Once reduced, the position can be held with K-wires to the index metacarpal or into the carpus. The volar oblique fragment does not necessarily need to be captured by the wires. If the fracture cannot be reduced by closed means, an open approach may afford better visualization. Although congruous reduction without articular step-off is the goal, no absolute agreement exists among surgeons regarding the acceptable limits of reduction and long-term functional implications.[9]

A Rolando fracture is a pilon-type injury to the thumb CMC joint following axial loading. This splits the thumb into diaphyseal, radial, and ulnar articular fragments. Occasionally, the joint surface is fragmented. Rolando fractures should generally be treated closed with joint unloading by means of a mini-external fixator and supplemental K-wire stabilization of larger fragments. As with Bennett fractures, joint congruity does not necessarily correlate with functional outcome.[10]

Fractures and Dislocations of the Wrist

Carpal Fractures and Nonunion

Acute Fractures

Fractures of a carpal bone are usually caused by a fall onto an outstretched hand or by a motor vehicle crash. Other causes include injuries caused by contact sports or a sudden impact to the palm, as can occur in baseball players or golfers. Carpal bone fractures account for 18% of hand fractures, with the bones of the proximal carpal row being the most frequently fractured. These injuries may be difficult to see on plain radiographs and may require advanced imaging techniques (CT or MRI) to confirm the diagnosis.

The location of the carpal bone fracture depends on the hand and wrist position at impact and the forces applied. The scaphoid is the most frequently fractured carpal bone, followed by the triquetrum and lunate. Scaphoid fractures account for up to 80% of all carpal fractures. Approximately 345,000 scaphoid fractures occur annually in the United States and most occur in younger individuals (15 to 60 years of age).[11] Because the scaphoid is largely covered by cartilage and receives most of its blood supply in a retrograde manner, fractures of this bone are more prone to complications than fractures of the other carpal bones.

In general, scaphoid fractures that are nondisplaced or minimally displaced (< 1 mm) can be treated by immobilization and have a union rate of approximately 90%. There is no clear consensus on the type of immobilization needed, such as long arm versus short arm or thumb-spica versus nonspica immobilization. Over the past decade, there has been a trend toward surgical fixation of nondisplaced or minimally displaced waist fractures; however, a systematic literature review did not demonstrate better union rates, grip strength, wrist motion, patient satisfaction, or shorter return-to-work times after surgical fixation.[12] One recent study showed that an evaluation of long-term outcomes indicated that surgical treatment seems to cause more complications and is associated with a higher risk of scaphotrapezial osteoarthritis based on radiographic findings.[13]

Surgery is indicated for scaphoid fractures that are displaced, comminuted, located at the proximal pole, have an intrascaphoid angle greater than 35°, or those associated with an ipsilateral distal fracture or perilunate dislocation. A cannulated, headless screw placed in the central axis appears to provide the most stability and avoids prominence. Open reduction can either be done through the volar or dorsal approach. The volar approach is preferred for distal pole and waist fractures, whereas the proximal pole is best accessed from the dorsal side. The blood supply is at risk with the dorsal approach. Indirect or arthroscopically assisted reduction has facilitated percutaneous screw fixation of displaced fractures.

Most triquetral and lunate fractures are avulsion injuries of the dorsal capsule and are the bony equivalent of a wrist sprain. These fractures can be treated with immobilization for 4 to 6 weeks. Kienböck disease should be ruled out if a fracture line is seen in the coronal plane through the body of the lunate. Fractures of the hamate generally occur through the hook from a direct blow to the palm. Nondisplaced fractures can be treated with immobilization. Internal fixation or fragment excision can be considered for displaced hamate hook fractures. Symptomatic partial union or nonunion of the hook of the hamate is treated by excision. Grip strength has not been shown to be adversely affected by excision of the hook of the hamate in most clinical series; however, decreased strength with wrist extension and ulnar deviation has been suggested in a biomechanical study.[14]

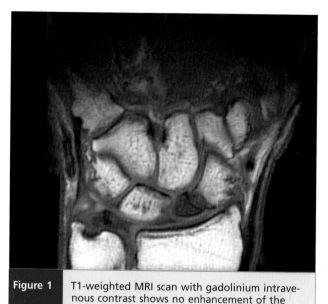

Figure 1 T1-weighted MRI scan with gadolinium intravenous contrast shows no enhancement of the proximal pole of the scaphoid, indicating osteonecrosis in a patient with a scaphoid nonunion. (Courtesy of Virak Tan, MD, Newark, NJ.)

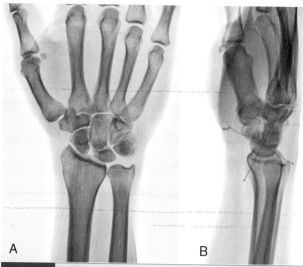

Figure 2 Radiographs of a scapholunate dissociation injury. **A,** PA view shows widening of the scapholunate interval and a signet ring of the scaphoid. **B,** Lateral view shows dorsal intercalated segment instability with a scapholunate angle of 90°. (Courtesy of Virak Tan, MD, Newark, NJ.)

Nonunion

Risk factors for scaphoid nonunion include proximal pole fractures, delayed diagnosis and treatment, patient noncompliance, and comminution or displacement at the fracture site. MRI with intravenous contrast is used to assess the vascularity of the proximal pole (such as in cases of osteonecrosis) and the extent of arthritis (**Figure 1**). CT is helpful in determining scaphoid morphology, including any humpback deformity. The treatment of scaphoid nonunion is based on the location of the fracture, the presence of osteonecrosis, the amount of deformity/collapse, and the extent of arthrosis. Percutaneous screw fixation has been successful in treating selected nonunions without displacement, collapse, or osteonecrosis. In the presence of humpback deformity, structural autologous bone graft from the volar side and rigid fixation is necessary for healing. If there is osteonecrosis of the proximal pole, vascularized bone grafting should be considered. In long-standing, symptomatic nonunions with significant secondary wrist arthrosis (such as a scaphoid nonunion advanced collapse wrist), motion-sparing salvage procedures, such as proximal row carpectomy or four-corner fusion, are most appropriate.

Carpal Instability

In an uninjured wrist, the bones of the proximal carpal row act together as an intercalated segment to coordinate movements between the distal radius and ulna and the distal carpal row. It is believed that the scaphoid functions as a stabilizer of the midcarpal joint, acting as a bridge between the proximal and distal carpal rows. In the proximal row, the lunate is attached to the scaphoid through the U-shaped scapholunate interosseous ligament and to the triquetrum through the

C-shaped lunotriquetral interosseous ligament. The opposing forces acting through these interosseous ligaments hold the lunate in a balanced position. As the hand is radially deviated, the scaphoid flexes, causing the lunate and triquetrum to follow into flexion. With ulnar deviation, the reverse occurs and the proximal row goes into extension.

Scapholunate Dissociation

Injury to the scapholunate interosseous ligament is the most common form of wrist instability and can be dynamic or static. Disruption of the scapholunate interosseous ligament removes the scaphoid flexion moment from the lunate, allowing it to assume an extended position under the influence of the triquetrum. The scaphoid, in turn, falls into further flexion and supination, creating incongruity at the radioscaphoid facet. This condition is termed dorsal intercalated segment instability. It is generally believed that if the condition is left untreated, it will progress to carpal collapse and an arthritic (scapholunate advanced collapse) wrist.

Most patients with scapholunate dissociation will report wrist pain or weakness with loading. Some patients will report a painful click or snapping sensation with motion. Examination will often reveal mild swelling in the scapholunate interval, which may be confused with a ganglion. The scaphoid shift test will often increase pain and may produce a clunk.

Radiographs of a suspected scapholunate interosseous ligament injury should include PA views in neutral, along with clenched fist, ulnar deviation, and lateral views (**Figure 2**). Comparing radiographs of the injured and uninjured side may be helpful. Bone scintigraphy and plain film arthrography have largely been replaced

Table 1

Treatment of Scapholunate Dissociation Based on the Garcia-Elias Classification of Stages

Stage	Description	Treatment
1	Partial scapholunate (or stretch) injury	Arthroscopic débridement K-wire stabilization
2	Complete scapholunate ligament tear with repairable dorsal ligament	Direct dorsal ligament repair (± dorsal capsulodesis) Dorsal capsulodesis
3	Complete scapholunate tear with nonrepairable dorsal ligament but a normally aligned scaphoid	Ligament reconstruction with tendon graft (± dorsal capsulodesis) Dorsal capsulodesis
4	Complete scapholunate tear with nonrepairable tissue and a reducible rotary subluxation of the scaphoid	Ligament reconstruction with tendon graft (± dorsal capsulodesis) Dorsal capsulodesis
5	Complete scapholunate tear with irreducible malalignment but no evidence of cartilage degeneration	Partial carpal fusion
6	Complete scapholunate tear with irreducible malalignment and cartilage degeneration	Motion-preserving procedure (proximal row carpectomy [or four-corner fusion]) Total wrist fusion

because of their low specificity for ligamentous injuries. MRI and magnetic resonance and CT arthrography are the principal imaging techniques for diagnosing tears of the wrist ligaments. Recent studies reported CT arthrography to be more accurate than 1.5-tesla (T) MRI and magnetic resonance arthrography for detecting tears of the scapholunate and lunotriquetral ligaments. In general, there is improvement in the diagnostic capability and quality of 3.0-T MRI compared with 1.5-T MRI;[15] however, arthroscopy remains the gold standard for diagnosis.

The treatment of scapholunate instability continues to be an ongoing challenge for hand surgeons because outcomes have been inconsistent. Partial tears can be managed with immobilization or arthroscopic débridement. Complete ligament disruption requires reduction and pinning, and primary dorsal ligament repair or ligament reconstruction. The authors of a 2006 study proposed six stages of scapholunate dissociation and described a treatment algorithm based on these stages[16] (Table 1).

Lunotriquetral Dissociation

Lunotriquetral interosseous ligament tears usually occur in combination with other intercarpal or radiocarpal ligament injuries, such as lunate or perilunate dislocations. Isolated injuries have been reported from a fall on a pronated, extended, and radially deviated hand or with the wrist in flexion. Provocative maneuvers, such as the ballottement maneuver, and shuck and shear tests may be positive. Radiographs may show evidence of carpal instability with flexion of the lunate (such as the volar intercalated segmental instability pattern). Magnetic resonance arthrography may show a dye leak at the lunotriquetral joint; however, similar to other soft-tissue injuries about the wrist, arthroscopy remains

the best method for assessing the tear. Immobilization is used to treat stable lunotriquetral ligament tears. Midcarpal corticosteroid injection or arthroscopic débridement of the lunotriquetral interosseous ligament may be considered for patients with persistent symptoms and normal carpal alignment. The treatment of an unstable lunotriquetral ligament can range from pinning the joint to direct repair or reconstruction of the ligament to limited fusions with the goal of correcting rotational malalignment of the proximal carpal row.

Lunate and Perilunate Dislocations

Lunate and perilunate instability patterns are uncommon and represent injuries from high-energy trauma. The common defining feature is capitate dislocation from the distal articulation of the lunate. In lunate dislocation, the lunate is completely displaced from its fossa (and capitate) and comes to rest volar to the distal radius (Figure 3, A). In a perilunate dislocation, the relationship between the distal radius and lunate is maintained, but the capitate assumes a position dorsal to the lunate (Figure 3, B). Variations in this injury spectrum can involve a pure ligamentous disruption around the lunate (lesser arc injury) or a combination of bony and ligamentous structures (greater arc injury).

Young men are most prone to these injuries and often have associated injuries that may require more urgent attention. Closed reduction should be attempted for acute dislocations to prevent median nerve compression. Patients with progressive median nerve symptoms should be treated with a carpal tunnel release; direct digital pressure on the lunate (through an extended carpal tunnel incision) should readily reduce the dislocation. Definitive treatment requires open repair of the scapholunate interosseous ligament (some surgeons also repair the lunotriquetral interosseous ligament)

3: Upper Extremity

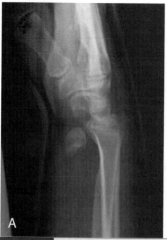
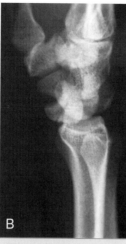

Figure 3 **A,** Lateral radiograph of a wrist with lunate dislocation. The lunate is completely displaced from the fossa and is volar to the remainder of the carpus and distal radius. **B,** Lateral radiograph of a wrist with perilunate dislocation. The lunate remains in contact with the lunate fossa of the distal radius but the capitate is dislocated from the lunate and is sitting dorsal to the lunate. (Courtesy of Virak Tan, MD, Newark, NJ.)

with intercarpal K-wire fixation. Surgical exposure for this injury can be through a single dorsal incision or a combined volar-dorsal approach. Great arc injuries are treated with fracture fixation and suture augmentation of the ligaments if they are ruptured or attenuated. Poor results can be expected after open injury or delayed treatment, and a primary proximal row carpectomy should be considered.

Distal Radius Fractures

Distal radius fractures are the most common fractures of the upper limb and account for approximately 20% of all fractures. A large percentage of these injuries occur in older women with osteoporosis. Despite the myriad of treatment options, restoration of painless function of the injured wrist remains the ultimate goal. Plain radiographs (PA, true, fossa lateral, and oblique views) are usually sufficient to assess the initial displacement, angulation, and articular involvement. A CT scan, if needed, may be helpful in delineating the extent of articular disruption.

The management of distal radius fractures should be individualized on the basis of the fracture pattern, degree of displacement, other associated injuries, the patient's activity level, and the surgeon's experience and preference. Despite the enthusiasm for internal fixation, closed reduction and immobilization should be attempted for most distal radius fractures that have minimal metaphyseal comminution and articular incongruity. Surgery is generally indicated for fractures that are open, unstable, have 2 mm or more of articular displacement, or those that are a part of a multitraumatic injury. The advantage of closed reduction and casting of distal radius fractures is its nonsurgical nature; how-

ever, there is a known risk of secondary displacement (up to 89% in patients older than 65 years) as seen on radiographs.[17] Predictors for redisplacement include increasing age, metaphyseal comminution, and shortening at presentation.[17,18] In older patients, some degree of malalignment of the distal radius is well tolerated. Several studies found no relationship between anatomic position at healing and functional outcomes.[19,20]

The surgical treatment of distal radius fractures has become commonplace, although conclusive scientific evidence of improved patient outcomes is lacking. Surgical fixation is typically recommended for fractures with postreduction radial shortening of more than 3 mm, dorsal tilt greater than 10°, or intra-articular displacement of more than 2 mm.[21] The following conclusions can be reached from the literature on distal radius fractures.[22] (1) Closed management or percutaneous pinning alone has worse radiographic outcomes than external fixation augmented with percutaneous pins. (2) Internal fixation yields radiographic and clinical results that are at least comparable with augmented external fixation. (3) Because internal fixation produces radiographic results comparable to external fixation, internal fixation can be expected to provide radiographic results that are better than those of casting or percutaneous pinning.

The trend in surgical fixation is away from percutaneous pinning and external fixation, and toward internal fixation. Advocates of internal fixation suggest that fractures of the distal radius, like other periarticular fractures, are best treated by internal fixation that is sufficiently stable to allow immediate active motion of the wrist while maintaining alignment. Internal fixation, especially with volar fixed-angle locking plates, is seemingly the preferred treatment for most displaced or unstable distal radius fractures. Currently, there are more than 30 implant designs available worldwide. Although the use of volar plates and low-profile dorsal plates may decrease complications related to hardware prominence, these implants do not entirely eliminate complications. Additionally, there also has been an increased focus on contracture of the pronator quadratus as a cause of limited forearm rotation after fixation with a volar plate. Although locked plating is an acceptable form of treatment of distal radial fractures, it should be realized that data are lacking indicating clear superiority of one treatment modality over another.

The American Academy of Orthopaedic Surgeon's work group on the treatment of distal radius fractures has summarized the clinical practice guidelines for treating distal radius fractures[21] (Table 2).

Distal Radioulnar Joint

The ulnar side of the wrist contains important anatomic structures that contribute to stability yet allow for motion of the distal radioulnar joint (DRUJ). The prime stabilizers of the DRUJ are the dorsal and volar radioulnar ligaments and the triangular fibrocartilage. The diagnosis of instability can be made with plain radiographs, although dynamic CT with contralateral

Table 2

AAOS Clinical Practice Guideline on the Treatment of Distal Radius Fractures

Recommendation	Strength of Recommendation
We are unable to recommend for or against performing nerve decompression when nerve dysfunction persists after reduction.	Inconclusive
We are unable to recommend for or against casting as definitive treatment for unstable fractures that are initially adequately reduced.	Inconclusive
We suggest surgical fixation for fractures with postreduction radial shortening > 3 mm, dorsal tilt > 10°, or intra-articular displacement or step-off > 2 mm as opposed to cast fixation.	Moderate
We are unable to recommend for or against any one specific surgical method for fixation of distal radius fractures.	Inconclusive
We are unable to recommend for or against surgical treatment for patients older than 55 years with distal radius fractures.	Inconclusive
We are unable to recommend for or against locking plates in patients older than 55 years who are treated surgically.	Inconclusive
We suggest rigid immobilization in preference to removable splints when using nonsurgical treatment for the management of displaced distal radius fractures.	Moderate
The use of removable splints is an option when treating minimally displaced distal radius fractures.	Weak
We are unable to recommend for or against immobilization of the elbow in patients treated with cast immobilization.	Inconclusive
Arthroscopic evaluation of the articular surface is an option during surgical treatment of intra-articular distal radius fractures.	Weak
Surgical treatment of associated ligament injuries (SLIL injuries, LT, or TFCC tears) at the time of radius fixation is an option.	Weak
Arthroscopy is an option in patients with distal radius intra-articular fractures to improve diagnostic accuracy for wrist ligament injuries, and CT is an option to improve diagnostic accuracy for patterns of intra-articular fractures.	Weak
We are unable to recommend for or against the use of supplement bone grafts or substitutes when using locking plates.	Inconclusive
We are unable to recommend for or against the use of bone graft (autograft or allograft) or bone graft substitutes for the filling of a bone void as an adjunct to other surgical treatments.	Inconclusive
In the absence of reliable evidence, it is the opinion of the work group that distal radius fractures that are treated nonsurgically be followed by ongoing radiographic evaluation for 3 weeks and at cessation of immobilization.	Consensus
We are unable to recommend whether two or three K-wires should be used for distal radius fracture fixation.	Inconclusive
We are unable to recommend for or against using the occurrence of distal radius fractures to predict future fragility fractures.	Inconclusive
We are unable to recommend for or against concurrent surgical treatment of DRUJ instability in patients with surgically treated distal radius fractures.	Inconclusive
We suggest that all patients with distal radius fractures receive a postreduction true lateral radiograph of the carpus to assess DRUJ alignment.	Moderate
In the absence of reliable evidence, it is the opinion of the work group that all patients with distal radius fractures and unremitting pain during follow-up be reevaluated.	Consensus
A home exercise program is an option for patients prescribed therapy after distal radius fracture.	Weak
In the absence of reliable evidence, it is the opinion of the work group that patients perform active finger motion exercises following diagnosis of distal radius fractures.	Consensus
We suggest that patients do not need to begin early wrist motion routinely following stable fracture fixation.	Moderate

(continued on next page)

3: Upper Extremity

Table 2

AAOS Clinical Practice Guideline on the Treatment of Distal Radius Fractures (continued)

Recommendation	Strength of Recommendation
In order to limit complications when using external fixation, it is an option to limit the duration of fixation.	Weak
We are unable to recommend against overdistraction of the wrist when using an external fixator.	Inconclusive
We suggest adjuvant treatment of distal radius fractures with vitamin C for the prevention of disproportionate pain.	Moderate
Ultrasound and/or ice are options for adjuvant treatment of distal radius fractures.	Weak
We are unable to recommend for or against fixation of ulnar styloid fractures associated with distal radius fractures.	Inconclusive
We are unable to recommend for or against using external fixation alone for the management of distal radius fractures where there is depressed lunate fossa or four-part fracture (sagittal split).	Inconclusive

SLIL = scapholunate interosseous ligament, LT = lunotriquetral, TFCC = triangular fibrocartilage complex, DRUJ = distal radioulnar joint
(Reproduced from the American Academy of Orthopaedic Surgeons: *Clinical Practice Guideline on the Treatment of Distal Radius Fractures.* Rosemont, IL, American Academy of Orthopaedic Surgeons, Dec 2009. http://www.aaos.org/research/guidelines/DRFguideline.asp.)

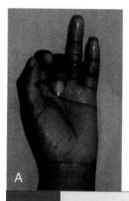
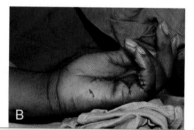

Figure 4 **A,** Preoperative clinical photograph shows loss of the normal cascade of the ring and small fingers caused by disruption of the flexor tendons from a flexor tendon laceration. **B,** The cascade is restored after primary repair of the flexor tendons. (Courtesy of Virak Tan, MD, Newark, NJ.)

wrist comparison is more accurate. DRUJ instability most commonly results from a fracture of the distal radius. When the instability is purely ligamentous, it usually can be reduced by closed manipulation; the forearm can be immobilized in the position of stability for 4 weeks. Dorsal instability (the distal ulna is dorsal to the distal radius) is usually stable when the forearm is in supination, and vice versa for instability in the volar direction. If the DRUJ is highly unstable, pinning across the joint with 0.062-inch K-wires or repair of the radioulnar ligaments should be considered.

In the setting of a distal radius fracture, anatomic reduction to re-create a concentric sigmoid notch is an important factor in determining DRUJ stability. The conventional practice has been to fix associated ulnar styloid base fractures because of the potential DRUJ in-

stability caused by disruption of the radioulnar ligaments. However, a recent study concluded that an unrepaired ulnar styloid base fracture does not appear to influence function or outcome after plate fixation of a distal radial fracture.[23]

Soft-Tissue and Vascular Injuries

Trauma to the hand and wrist can result in injury to multiple structures depending on the injury mechanism. Tendons, joints, and bone are at risk with blunt trauma, whereas skin, blood vessels, and nerves may be injured by sharp lacerations. Partial tendon disruption from a closed injury may be difficult to diagnose with physical examination; therefore, MRI or ultrasound may be needed.

Extensor Tendon Injuries
The treatment of extensor tendon injuries is largely dependent on the location and type of injury. Closed injury to the central slip (PIP boutonnière deformity) or terminal extensor tendon (distal interphalangeal mallet finger) should be managed with splinting; in rare instances, surgery will be needed. Injury to the radial sagittal band can cause subluxation of the extensor digitorum communis ulnarly, which can be managed with splinting or surgery to centralize the tendon over the MCP joint. More proximal extensor tendon lacerations require direct repair with either figure-of-8 or core sutures.[24]

Flexor Tendon Injuries
Suspected flexor tendon injury warrants a careful examination to identify loss of active flexion strength or motion, and any associated digital nerve injury (Figure 4). Injuries are classified by the anatomic zones. Zone I

injury is distal to the flexor digitorum sublimis insertion, and the flexor digitorum profundus is either avulsed from the distal phalanx or transected distal to the A4 pulley. Tendon avulsion (such as a jersey finger) should be reattached to its insertion site. Although suture anchors in the distal phalanx are increasing in popularity, the traditional pull-out suture tied over a button is acceptable.

Zone II flexor tendon injuries occur between the A1 and A4 pulleys. Both the flexor digitorum sublimis and flexor digitorum profundus (along with the digital neurovascular structures) can be involved. Tendon repair in this zone frequently requires working around the A2 and A4 pulleys to avoid bowstringing. If the laceration occurs at either of these pulleys, repair with a small-caliber monofilament suture is recommended at the end of the procedure. Both the flexor digitorum profundus and flexor digitorum sublimis should be repaired with core and epitendinous sutures. Studies have shown improved gliding when only one slip of the flexor digitorum sublimis is repaired.[25] Numerous articles have been dedicated to the study of intrasynovial flexor tendon repair. Different suture techniques are described and many suture materials are available; however, it is believed that it is desirable to increase the number of core strands with stronger suture material, which leaves minimal suture bulk (from the knots). Great interest has been shown in reducing adhesions with various agents, but these agents generally remain experimental. Meticulous atraumatic handling of the tendon ends, precise suturing techniques, repair of the flexor tendon sheath, and early motion rehabilitation protocols reduce peritendinous adhesions. Although early controlled motion is widely accepted, a Cochrane review found insufficient evidence from published controlled trials to determine the best mobilization protocol.[26]

Flexor tendon injuries that occur more proximally (zones III to V) are less common. Acute lacerations should be repaired, but tendon transfers may be required for attritional ruptures.

Nerve Injuries

Traumatic peripheral nerve injuries are a heterogeneous group of disorders that commonly occur in conjunction with other soft-tissues trauma. When possible, primary repair of the nerve should be done within the first 2 days after injury to achieve the best possible functional result. Urgent repair is not needed. The nerve ends should be trimmed back to healthy axons and reapproximated with epineural or group fascicular sutures. There should be minimal tension on the repair to allow for motion within 2 to 3 weeks.

When primary end-to-end coaptation is not possible because of tension or gapping, autografting is the gold standard for treatment. However, because autografts result in donor-site deficits and are a limited resource, nerve graft substitutes have been developed. Biologic and synthetic axonal guidance channels (nerve conduits) are effective substitutes for short gaps (approximately up to 2 cm). For longer gaps, enhancement of

the conduits with nerve growth factor, brain-derived neurotrophic factor, glial growth factor, Schwann cells, and segments of normal nerve tissue are being actively investigated. Future improvements may include engineered conduits that closely mimic the internal organization of an uninjured nerve.[27]

Tendon transfer can supplement a motor nerve repair. If done early, the transfer can act as an internal splint to support function and prevent deformity during nerve recovery.

High-Pressure Injection Injuries

Despite a relatively benign appearing entry wound, high-pressure injection injuries may result in extensive soft-tissue damage. The nondominant index finger is most commonly involved. The force of the injection, the volume injected, the composition of the injected substance, and the latency from injury to treatment affect the degree of mechanical and chemical injury. Local tissue necrosis and vascular occlusion can lead to digit loss. Grease, chlorofluorocarbon, and water-based paints are relatively less destructive. Less severe injuries may be successfully treated nonsurgically with parenteral antibiotics, elevation, and early mobilization.[28,29] Industrial solvents and oil-based paints produce a high degree of tissue necrosis. An amputation rate of 50% was reported in one large study of oil-based paint injection injuries.[30]

Emergent surgical débridement and decompression is typically required following high-pressure injection injuries. A surgical delay of more than 10 hours from the time of injury was found to result in higher rates of amputation.[31] Despite wide and aggressive initial surgical débridement, it is generally not possible to remove all the injected material. Broad-spectrum antibiotic coverage is important because the necrotic tissue resulting from these injuries is a good culture medium for bacterial growth.

Compartment Syndrome

The hand can be divided into dorsal and volar interosseous compartments, thenar and hypothenar compartments, and a separate digital compartment. Compartment syndrome has many causes, including decreased compartment volume resulting from tight closure of fascial defects, the application of excessive traction to fractured limbs, and the use of tourniquets, tight dressings, or splints. Alternatively, increased content within the compartment caused by bleeding, postrevascularization changes, trauma, metabolic derangement, or fluid extravasation also can lead to compartment syndrome.

It has been shown that no distinct fascia completely surrounds any of the intrinsic muscles of the hand. The unyielding nature of the surrounding skin, however, can contribute to the development of compartment syndrome. As in all limbs, compartment syndrome of the

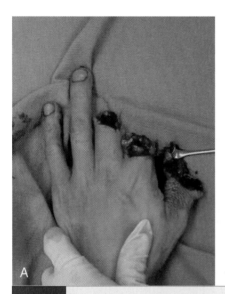
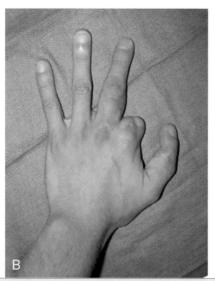
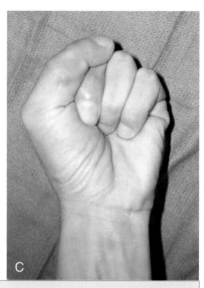

Figure 5   **A,** Clinical photograph of multiple finger amputations caused by a table saw injury. The amputated part of the thumb was not salvageable, therefore orthotopic replantation of the amputated middle finger to the thumb and amputated index finger to the middle finger stump were performed. **B** and **C,** Clinical photographs taken 9 months postoperatively. (Courtesy of Virak Tan, MD, Newark, NJ.)

hand is a surgical emergency. If not treated within 24 hours, contracture becomes established in a matter of days with muscle necrosis ultimately leading to fibrosis. Late changes in missed diagnoses of compartment syndrome vary with the compartment, but generally lead to a stiff hand and prolonged pain.

Digital Replantation

Digital replantation is among the most technically challenging procedures for the hand surgeon. Educational, economic, and practical factors discourage many surgeons from attempting microsurgery.[32] The procedures themselves are typically performed in large tertiary referral centers and academic institutions only.

The criteria for digital replantation varies based on the experience of the surgeon, but the goals are return of function of the replanted part and low morbidity to the remainder of the limb and the patient as a whole. Survivability of the digit alone should not be the main indication. Typical indications include multiple digit traumatic amputations (**Figure 5**), thumb amputations, through-the-palm amputations, major limb replantation, and almost any level of digital amputation in a child. Single digit amputation distal to the flexor digitorum sublimis insertion is suitable for replantation after a careful discussion with the patient regarding potential morbidity and long-term functional expectations.

Typical contraindications to replantation include severe mangling of the amputated part, segmental injury, serious comorbidities, and severely arteriosclerotic vessels. Digital replantation in patients with psychiatric comorbidities is typically contraindicated. Single digits, particularly border digits and digits proximal to the

flexor digitorum sublimis insertion, are relative contraindications for replantation.

Patient selection may also be influenced by other risk factors. A large meta-analysis[33] reported a worse prognosis in patients with a history of diabetes or smoking, those younger than 9 years, and patients with injuries caused by a crush or avulsion mechanism. Amputations of the distal phalanx and thumb, male sex, and ischemia time greater than 12 hours are associated with a somewhat worse prognosis. A history of alcohol use did not affect the prognosis. Regardless of the zone of injury, repair of as many vessels as possible is correlated with better implant survivability.[34] Postoperative anemia, hemodilution, and the use of dextrans negatively affected digital implant survival rates.[35]

Annotated References

1. Collins AL, Timlin M, Thornes B, O'Sullivan T: Old principles revisited: Traction splinting for closed proximal phalangeal fractures. *Injury* 2002;33(3):235-237.

2. Henry M: Soft tissue sleeve approach to open reduction and internal fixation of proximal phalangeal fractures. *Tech Hand Up Extrem Surg* 2008;12(3):161-165.

   The author describes specific technical aspects of optimizing soft-tissue management for open fixation of proximal phalanx fractures.

3. Horton TC, Hatton M, Davis TR: A prospective randomized controlled study of fixation of long oblique and spiral shaft fractures of the proximal phalanx: Closed reduction and percutaneous Kirschner wiring versus open reduction and lag screw fixation. *J Hand Surg Br* 2003;28(1):5-9.

4. Badia A, Riano F: A simple fixation method for unstable bony mallet finger. *J Hand Surg Am* 2004;29(6): 1051-1055.

5. McAuliffe JA: Dorsal fracture dislocation of the proximal interphalangeal joint. *J Hand Surg Am* 2008; 33(10):1885-1888.

   This evidence-based medicine article discusses the best treatment of an unstable dorsal fracture-dislocation of the PIP joint.

6. Dionysian E, Eaton RG: The long-term outcome of volar plate arthroplasty of the proximal interphalangeal joint. *J Hand Surg Am* 2000;25(3):429-437.

7. Calfee RP, Kiefhaber TR, Sommerkamp TG, Stern PJ: Hemi-hamate arthroplasty provides functional reconstruction of acute and chronic proximal interphalangeal fracture-dislocations. *J Hand Surg Am* 2009;34(7): 1232-1241.

   The authors report on 33 patients treated with autologous hemihamate bone graft for reconstructing a PIP fracture-dislocation. They conclude that the procedure is valuable for treating severe injuries.

8. Katolik LI, Friedrich J, Trumble TE: Repair of acute ulnar collateral ligament injuries of the thumb metacarpophalangeal joint: A retrospective comparison of pull-out sutures and bone anchor techniques. *Plast Reconstr Surg* 2008;122(5):1451-1456.

   Two cohorts (30 patients each) were treated with repair of the thumb MCP ulnar collateral ligament with either an intraosseous suture anchor or a pull-out suture tied over a button. Both methods were effective, but the cohort treated with the suture anchor had improved range of motion and pinch strength at follow-up.

9. Carlsen BT, Moran SL: Thumb trauma: Bennett fractures, Rolando fractures, and ulnar collateral ligament injuries. *J Hand Surg Am* 2009;34(5):945-952.

   The authors of this review article summarize recent advancements in the realm of thumb trauma.

10. Langhoff O, Andersen K, Kjaer-Petersen K: Rolando's fracture. *J Hand Surg Br* 1991;16(4):454-459.

11. Boles CA: Wrist, scaphoid fractures and complications. eMedicine: Medscape. http://emedicine.com/radio/topic747.htm. Accessed September 30, 2010.

    Scaphoid fractures are discussed in this review article.

12. Yin ZG, Zhang JB, Kan SL, Wang P: Treatment of acute scaphoid fractures: Systematic review and meta-analysis. *Clin Orthop Relat Res* 2007;460:142-151.

    The results of a meta-analysis showed that the surgical treatment of acute nondisplaced or minimally displaced scaphoid waist fractures does not provide greater benefits regarding nonunion rate, return to work, grip strength, range of wrist motion, or patient satisfaction than nonsurgical treatment.

13. Vinnars B, Pietreanu M, Bodestedt A, Ekenstam F, Gerdin B: Nonoperative compared with operative treatment of acute scaphoid fractures: A randomized clinical trial. *J Bone Joint Surg Am* 2008;90(6):1176-1185.

    This randomized study did not show improved benefits of internal fixation compared with nonsurgical treatment for acute nondisplaced or minimally displaced scaphoid fractures at 10-year follow-up. Level of evidence: I.

14. Demirkan F, Calandruccio JH, DiAngelo D: Biomechanical evaluation of flexor tendon function after hamate hook excision. *J Hand Surg [Br]* 2003;28(1): 138-143.

15. Magee T: Comparison of 3-T MRI and arthroscopy of intrinsic wrist ligament and TFCC tears. *AJR Am J Roentgenol* 2009;192(1):80-85.

    This study showed that 3-T MRI is sensitive and specific for detecting wrist ligament tears.

16. Garcia-Elias M, Lluch AL, Stanley JK: Three-ligament tenodesis for the treatment of scapholunate dissociation: Indications and surgical technique. *J Hand Surg Am* 2006;31(1):125-134.

17. Makhni EC, Ewald TJ, Kelly S, Day CS: Effect of patient age on the radiographic outcomes of distal radius fractures subject to nonoperative treatment. *J Hand Surg Am* 2008;33(8):1301-1308.

    The authors evaluated 124 nonsurgically treated distal radius fractures at union. The displacement rate was associated with increasing patient age.

18. Mackenney PJ, McQueen MM, Elton R: Prediction of instability in distal radial fractures. *J Bone Joint Surg Am* 2006;88(9):1944-1951.

19. Jaremko JL, Lambert RG, Rowe BH, Johnson JA, Majumdar SR, Lambert RG: Do radiographic indices of distal radius fracture reduction predict outcomes in older adults receiving conservative treatment? *Clin Radiol* 2007;62(1):65-72.

    Seventy-four patients (older than 50 years) with nonsurgically managed distal radius fractures were enrolled in a prospective cohort study. Self-reported outcomes were not related to the "acceptability" of radiographic fracture reduction.

20. Synn AJ, Makhni EC, Makhni MC, Rozental TD, Day CS: Distal radius fractures in older patients: Is anatomic reduction necessary? *Clin Orthop Relat Res* 2009; 467(6):1612-1620.

    In a study of 53 patients (older than 55 years) with distal radius fractures, the authors reported no relationship between anatomic reduction, as evidenced by radiographic outcomes, and subjective or objective functional outcomes. Level of evidence: II.

21. Guideline on the Treatment of Distal Radius Fractures. American Academy of Orthopaedic Surgeons Web site. http://www.aaos.org/Research/guidelines/DRFguideline.asp. Accessed September 30, 2010.

    The AAOS workgroup presents their guideline on the treatment of distal radius fractures.

3: Upper Extremity

22. Chen NC, Jupiter JB: Management of distal radial fractures. *J Bone Joint Surg Am* 2007;89(9):2051-2062.

    The authors discuss the management of distal radial fractures in this review article.

23. Souer JS, Ring D, Matschke S, Audige L, Marent-Huber M, Jupiter JB; AOCID Prospective ORIF Distal Radius Study Group: Effect of an unrepaired fracture of the ulnar styloid base on outcome after plate-and-screw fixation of a distal radial fracture. *J Bone Joint Surg Am* 2009;91(4):830-838.

    Two cohorts of 76 matched patients (fracture of the ulnar styloid base versus no ulnar fracture) were retrospectively analyzed. The authors found that not fixing the ulnar styloid base fracture did not appear to influence function or outcome after plate fixation of a distal radial fracture.

24. Soni P, Stern CA, Foreman KB, Rockwell WB: Advances in extensor tendon diagnosis and therapy. *Plast Reconstr Surg* 2009;123(2):52e-57e.

    The authors present a summary of a literature review of extensor tendon injury articles published since 1989.

25. Tang JB, Xie RG, Cao Y, Ke ZS, Xu Y: A2 pulley incision or one slip of the superficialis improves flexor tendon repairs. *Clin Orthop Relat Res* 2007;456:121-127.

    In a chicken model, incision of the pulley or partial flexor digitorum superficialis resection improved outcomes of tendon repairs.

26. Thien TB, Becker JH, Theis J-C: Rehabilitation after surgery for flexor tendon injuries in the hand. *Cochrane Database Syst Rev* 2004;4:CD00397910.1002/14651858.CD003979.pub2.

27. de Ruiter GC, Malessy MJ, Yaszemski MJ, Windebank AJ, Spinner RJ: Designing ideal conduits for peripheral nerve repair. *Neurosurg Focus* 2009;26(2):E5.

    The authors present a review article that discusses the ideal nerve conduit for peripheral nerve repair.

28. Goetting AT, Carson J, Burton BT: Freon injection injury to the hand: A report of four cases. *J Occup Med* 1992;34(8):775-778.

29. Snarski JT, Birkhahn RH: Non-operative management of a high-pressure water injection injury to the hand. *CJEM* 2005;7(2):124-126.

30. Mirzayan R, Schnall SB, Chon JH, Holtom PD, Patzakis MJ, Stevanovic MV: Culture results and amputation rates in high-pressure paint gun injuries of the hand. *Orthopedics* 2001;24(6):587-589.

31. Stark HH, Ashworth CR, Boyes JH: Paint-gun injuries of the hand. *J Bone Joint Surg Am* 1967;49(4):637-647.

32. Payatakes AH, Zagoreos NP, Fedorcik GG, Ruch DS, Levin LS: Current practice of microsurgery by members of the American Society for Surgery of the Hand. *J Hand Surg Am* 2007;32(4):541-547.

    A survey of members of the American Society for Surgery of the Hand showed that 44% of surgeons do not perform replantation surgery. Reasons for not performing replantations included busy elective schedules (51%), inadequate confidence in performing replantations (39%), and disappointment in results (23%).

33. Chung KC, Watt AJ, Kotsis SV, Margaliot Z, Haase SC, Kim HM: Treatment of unstable distal radial fractures with the volar locking plating system. *J Bone Joint Surg Am* 2006;88(12):2687-2694.

34. Lee BI, Chung HY, Kim WK, Kim SW, Dhong ES: The effects of the number and ratio of repaired arteries and veins on the survival rate in digital replantation. *Ann Plast Surg* 2000;44(3):288-294.

35. Ridha H, Jallali N, Butler PE: The use of dextran post free tissue transfer. *J Plast Reconstr Aesthet Surg* 2006;59(9):951-954.

Chapter 29

Hand and Wrist Reconstruction

Tamara D. Rozental, MD   Dawn M. LaPorte, MD

Posttraumatic Arthritis of the Wrist

Scapholunate Advanced Collapse Wrist

Scapholunate advanced collapse (SLAC) wrist is the most common form of posttraumatic arthritis of the wrist and typically stems from disruption of the scapholunate interosseous ligament. This condition results in palmar rotatory subluxation of the scaphoid and abnormal wrist mechanics, leading to the development of degenerative changes in the radioscaphoid and capitolunate joints (Figure 1). Arthrosis progresses in a predictable fashion and is reflected in the radiographic staging of SLAC wrist (Table 1). The radiolunate articulation is typically spared.

Once a SLAC wrist develops, reconstruction of the scapholunate ligament alone is no longer adequate to correct rotatory subluxation of the scaphoid and eliminate pain from underlying arthrosis. At this stage, a radial styloidectomy and/or scapholunate reconstruction is typically the procedure of choice. For stage II and III SLAC wrists, elimination of the radioscaphoid joint is necessary. This is usually accomplished through a proximal row carpectomy, scaphoid excision with four-corner fusion, or partial or total radiocarpal fusions.[1,2] Stage IV SLAC wrists, with pancarpal involvement, are treated with a total wrist arthrodesis.

Proximal row carpectomies can be performed in patients whose proximal capitate is intact (no evidence of degenerative changes). The procedure preserves motion and strength and results in good long-term outcomes. In some instances, conversion to a total wrist arthrodesis may be required. A scaphoid excision with four-corner fusion (SLAC procedure) is a better alternative in patients with midcarpal joint involvement. Overall, both procedures lead to similar functional outcomes.[2] Traditionally, four-corner arthrodesis is believed to provide better short-term grip strength.[3]

Scaphoid Nonunion Advanced Collapse Wrist

Untreated scaphoid nonunions also can lead to posttraumatic wrist arthritis. Staging for scaphoid nonunion advanced collapse (SNAC) wrist is similar to staging for SLAC wrist except that the joint surface between the proximal scaphoid fragment and scaphoid fossa of the distal radius is preserved (Table 2).

Treatment methods for SNAC wrist are similar to those for SLAC wrist. In the early stages, fixation of the nonunion and radial styloidectomy are attempted. Fixation with vascularized bone grafts is also an option and has met with varying success.[4] Excision of the distal pole of the scaphoid can be performed in patients with distal nonunions and an intact midcarpal joint. In later stages of SNAC wrist, salvage procedures such as a proximal row carpectomy or four-corner fusion are preferred. Once the capitolunate joint is involved, a four-corner fusion or wrist arthrodesis achieves more predictable results.

Arthritis at the Distal Radioulnar Joint

Patients with arthritis at the distal radioulnar joint (DRUJ) typically present with pain over the dorsum of

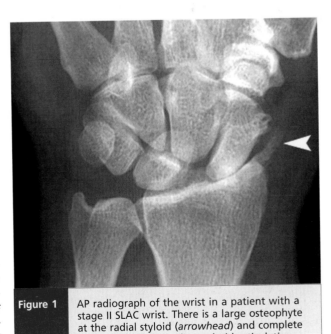

Figure 1   AP radiograph of the wrist in a patient with a stage II SLAC wrist. There is a large osteophyte at the radial styloid (*arrowhead*) and complete destruction of the radioscaphoid articulation.

3: Upper Extremity

Table 1

Progression of SLAC Wrist Deformity

Radiographic Stage	Description	Treatment Options
I	Arthrosis between radial styloid and distal scaphoid	Radial styloidectomy and scapholunate reconstruction
II	Arthrosis of entire radioscaphoid joint	Proximal row carpectomy Four-corner fusion Radioscapholunate fusion
III	Arthrosis involving capitolunate joint with proximal migration of the capitate	Proximal row carpectomy Four-corner fusion Total wrist arthrodesis
IV	Pancarpal arthrosis	Total wrist arthrodesis Wrist arthroplasty (sedentary patients)

Table 2

Progression of SNAC Wrist Deformity

Radiographic Stage	Description	Treatment Options
I	Arthrosis between radial styloid and distal scaphoid	Radial styloidectomy and fixation of scaphoid nonunion
II	Arthrosis of scaphocapitate joint	Proximal row carpectomy Four-corner fusion
III	Capitolunate arthrosis	Four-corner fusion Total wrist arthrodesis
IV	Pancarpal arthrosis (except radiolunate joint)	Total wrist arthrodesis Wrist arthroplasty (sedentary patients)

the wrist and limitation of forearm rotation. No classification or radiographic staging is used for DRUJ arthrosis and treatment is typically aimed toward restoration of motion and pain relief. If conservative management is unsuccessful in patients with mild involvement, the patient may be treated with débridement of the DRUJ and/or an ulnar shortening osteotomy to alter the contact surface of the joint. In patients with more advanced disease, options include resection of the entire ulnar head (Darrach resection), partial ulnar head resection (hemisection with soft-tissue interposition), or arthrodesis of the DRUJ with resection of the proximal ulnar segment (Sauve-Kapandji procedure). More recently, prosthetic replacement of the ulnar head has been attempted with promising early results.[5]

Osteoarthritis

Thumb Carpometacarpal Joint

The carpometacarpal (CMC) joint of the thumb is commonly affected by osteoarthritis (second only to the distal interphalangeal [DIP] joint). The anterior oblique ligament (beak ligament) is believed to be the primary stabilizing force of the CMC joint; deficiency leads to the typical pattern of arthrosis. Patients present with pain at the base of the thumb and have difficulty with pinching and gripping activities. Most patients are initially treated conservatively, independent of the degree of involvement. Treatment consists of anti-inflammatory drugs, splinting, activity modification, and corticosteroid injections.

The Eaton classification system is used for radiographic staging of CMC joint arthritis (Table 3). For early stages, surgical treatment may consist of joint débridement (open or arthroscopic) or metacarpal extension osteotomy.[6] For later stages, there are a variety of described procedures, but all involve either partial or complete excision of the trapezium. Most commonly, patients are treated with trapezium excision (partial or complete), tendon interposition, and reconstruction of the anterior oblique ligament (with the flexor carpi radialis or abductor pollicis longus). Some surgeons prefer trapezium excision alone or excision and the insertion of an allograft spacer. Most described forms of CMC joint arthroplasty provide good results in terms of pain relief although pinch strength is never fully restored.[7] Compensatory metacarpophalangeal hyperextension should be treated with metacarpophalangeal capsulodesis or arthrodesis. The scaphotrapezoid joint also should be evaluated. If degenerative changes are present, a partial trapeziectomy should be performed.

Table 3

Eaton Staging and Treatment Classification System for CMC Joint Arthritis

Radiographic Stage	Description	Treatment Options
1	Widened CMC joint	CMC débridement Ligament reconstruction Metacarpal osteotomy
2	Joint space narrowing Mild subchondral sclerosis Osteophytes < 2 mm	CMC débridement Trapeziectomy ± tendon interposition Arthrodesis
3	Joint space narrowing Sclerosis or cystic changes Osteophytes > 2 mm	Trapeziectomy ± tendon interposition Arthrodesis
4	Pantrapezial arthrosis	Trapeziectomy ± tendon interposition Arthroplasty

As a treatment alternative to procedures involving excision of the trapezium, trapeziometacarpal arthrodesis can result in reliable long-term results, helping to preserve pinch strength at the expense of some loss of thumb mobility.[8] Arthrodesis has been recommended in young, active patients who have trapeziometacarpal arthritis and require strong pinch and grip strength.[9]

Scaphotrapezial Trapezoid Joint

Scaphotrapezial trapezoid joint arthritis may be present with or without concomitant CMC joint changes. Symptoms are similar to CMC joint arthritis and radiographs are often necessary to make the diagnosis. If conservative care is unsuccessful, patients can be treated with scaphotrapezial fusion if the CMC joint is intact. Distal pole scaphoid or scaphotrapezial trapezoid excision also can be considered for symptomatic scaphotrapezial arthritis. If the CMC joint is also involved, a trapezium excision with tendon interposition and partial trapezoid excision is the procedure of choice.

Metacarpophalangeal Joint

Metacarpophalangeal joint arthritis is most common in the thumb. If the CMC joint and interphalangeal joints are not involved, arthrodesis is typically the procedure of choice, although implants for joint arthroplasty are available. In the digits, metacarpophalangeal joint fusions are functionally limiting and arthroplasty is preferred. Options include silicone implants or newer pyrolytic carbon implants. In rheumatoid arthritis patients with ulnar drift, metacarpophalangeal joint arthroplasty should be accompanied by soft-tissue reconstruction and realignment of the extensor mechanism.

Proximal and Distal Interphalangeal Joints

Osteoarthritis of the proximal interphalangeal (PIP) joint and DIP joint is common and often associated with enlargement of the joints (Heberden nodes at the DIP joint and Bouchard nodes at the PIP joint). At the DIP joint, bone spurs often result in the formation of mucous cysts, which can drain and lead to infection.

Treatment involves resection of the cyst as well as removal of the underlying bone spur. For patients with more advanced disease, arthrodesis in 10° to 20° of flexion is the procedure of choice.[10] At the PIP joint, mild osteoarthritis with contractures and nodular involvement can be treated with joint débridement and collateral ligament excision. Options for more advanced osteoarthritis include arthroplasty or arthrodesis. Arthroplasty with silicone implants leads to good pain relief but is often complicated by implant fractures in the long term. Newer two-piece prostheses have been designed to address this problem but significant complications have been reported, including dislocations, extensor lag, and stiffness.[11,12] Arthrodesis is the traditional option for the management of degenerative changes in the PIP joint. The optimal position for PIP joint fusion is 30° to 45° of flexion, in 5° increments from the index to the small finger. In general, arthroplasty is a better option for the long and ring fingers, whereas border digits (index and small finger) are best treated with arthrodesis.

Osteonecrosis

Kienböck Disease

A patient with Kienböck disease or osteonecrosis of the lunate often presents with pain, limited range of motion, and weakness. The etiology is not well understood but is associated with mechanical factors (ulnar negative variance leading to increased loads) as well as vascular factors (single nutrient vessel and poor collateral circulation, elevated intraosseous pressure).[13] Plain radiographs may show increased sclerosis but MRI may be required to make a definitive diagnosis (Figure 2). Kienböck disease is classified according to the Lichtman classification system (Table 4). Early stages of the disease are treated with joint-leveling procedures designed to decrease the mechanical load on the lunate,[14] with or without vascularized bone grafts from the distal radius. Once fixed scaphoid rotation occurs, the

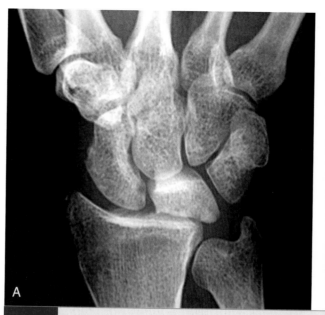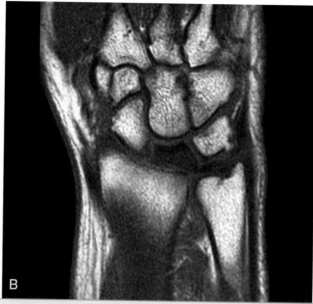

Figures 2 **A,** AP radiograph of the wrist of a patient with stage IIIA Kienböck disease showing lunate sclerosis and collapse without rotation of the scaphoid. **B,** The corresponding T1-weighted MRI shows signal change in the entire lunate.

Table 4

Staging and Treatment of Kienböck Disease

Radiographic Stage	Description	Treatment Options
Stage I	Normal radiographs Low signal on MRI	Observation Activity modification/immobilization
Stage II	Lunate sclerosis without collapse	Radial shortening for ulnar negative Capitate shortening for ulnar neutral/positive Vascularized grafts
Stage IIIA	Sclerosis with lunate collapse	Radial shortening for ulnar negative Capitate shortening for ulnar neutral/positive Vascularized grafts
Stage IIIB	Lunate collapse with rotatory scaphoid deformity	Scaphotrapezial arthrodesis Scaphocapitate arthrodesis Proximal row carpectomy
Stage IV	Radiocarpal and/or midcarpal arthrosis	Proximal row carpectomy Wrist arthrodesis

scaphoid must be stabilized with a limited arthrodesis or treated with a proximal row carpectomy.[15] If radiocarpal or midcarpal arthrosis is present, wrist fusion is the procedure of choice. Early in the disease process, MRI should be used to differentiate Kienböck disease from ulnar impaction. Kienböck disease involves the entire lunate, whereas ulnar impaction typically only affects the ulnar facet.

Preiser Disease

Preiser disease, or idiopathic osteonecrosis of the scaphoid, is much less common than Kienböck disease.[16] Radiographs or MRI may show sclerosis of the proxi-

mal pole of the scaphoid without any evidence of fracture. Observation and immobilization may be effective in up to 20% of patients. Surgery includes vascularized grafting,[17] scaphoid excision, and four-corner fusion or proximal row carpectomy.

Osteonecrosis of the Capitate

Patients with idiopathic osteonecrosis of the capitate, a rare condition, present with pain and limitation of motion. This condition can be posttraumatic or can be associated with steroid use or chemotherapy. Radiographs show sclerosis and fragmentation of the proximal pole of the capitate. Idiopathic osteonecrosis of the capitate is initially treated with observation and/or immobilization. Excision of the avascular head of the capitate with tendon interposition can be used for recalcitrant cases. Other options are vascularized grafting or limited arthrodesis.

Nerve Compression Syndromes

Although the term "compression neuropathy" suggests that the affected nerve is compressed by an anatomic structure, the cause of the compression is often multifactorial. There are several sites between the cervical spine and the hand where nerve compression is common (Table 5). Compression at one point on a peripheral nerve will lower the threshold for the occurrence of a compression neuropathy at a more proximal or distal level on the same nerve. This is referred to as a double crush phenomenon. Cervical radiculopathy in a patient with carpal tunnel syndrome is the most common manifestation of the double crush phenomenon; both sites of compression should be treated to achieve an optimal result.

Median Nerve

Carpal Tunnel Syndrome

Compression neuropathy of the median nerve at the wrist is the most common compression neuropathy of the upper extremity and affects up to 10% of the general population. Carpal tunnel syndrome is primarily a clinical diagnosis. In addition to an accurate patient history, sensory examination with Semmes-Weinstein monofilaments (a threshold test) is considered to be the most sensitive test for detecting early disease. Manual motor testing of the upper extremity should be performed with attention to ascertaining the presence of thenar atrophy, which has a high predictive value in carpal tunnel syndrome. Provocative maneuvers, including the carpal compression test, the Phalen maneuver, and the Tinel sign can be helpful in establishing the diagnosis. The American Academy of Orthopaedic Surgeons (AAOS) Clinical Practice Guideline on the Diagnosis of Carpal Tunnel Syndrome recommends obtaining electrodiagnostic studies if clinical and/or provocative tests are positive and surgery is being considered[18] (Table 6). However, many surgeons believe that the diagnosis can satisfactorily be made based on the clinical examination alone (Table 7). Good surgical outcome is correlated with a combination of positive clinical and electrodiagnostic tests. Although electrodiagnostic testing is generally considered the gold standard for assessing peripheral compression neuropathies, a negative nerve study does not universally rule out carpal tunnel syndrome, which may improve following carpal tunnel release.

The initial treatment of mild or moderate carpal tunnel syndrome includes nighttime splinting to avoid flexion/extension and the use of nonsteroidal anti-inflammatory drugs. Corticosteroid injection into the carpal canal also can be very effective for symptom re-

Table 5

Sites of Nerve Compression

Nerve	Sites of Compression	Syndrome
Median	Ligament of Struthers	
	Lacertus fibrosus	
	Pronator teres	Pronator
	Flexor digitorum superficialis origin	Anterior interosseous
	Flexor carpi radialis	
	Gantzer muscle	
	Transverse carpal ligament	Carpal tunnel
Ulnar	Arcade of Struthers	Cubital tunnel
	Intermuscular septum	
	Medial epicondyle	
	Cubital tunnel	
	Anconeus epitrochlearis	
	Flexor carpi ulnaris aponeurosis	
	Guyon canal	Ulnar tunnel
Radial	Fibrous band at radial head	Posterior interosseous nerve
	Recurrent leash of Henry	Radial tunnel
	Extensor carpi radialis brevis fibrous edge	
	Arcade of Frohse (most common) proximal supinator	
	Distal supinator	
	Between extensor carpi radialis longus and extensor carpi radialis brevis	Wartenberg

lief. Patients who have temporary relief after injection are likely to have a good response to surgical carpal tunnel release. Surgical carpal tunnel release is recommended if symptoms persist. Improvement in symptoms can be anticipated in up to 98% of patients following surgery. Although treatment in elderly and diabetic patients has been controversial, studies support carpal tunnel release in both of these populations.[19-21] Carpal tunnel release can be performed via open or endoscopic techniques; there does not appear to be an appreciable difference in outcomes at 1 year postoperatively.[22] No proven benefit to neurolysis of the median nerve or tenosynovectomy of the flexor tendons has been shown.[23] Pillar pain, associated with a painful palmar scar at the site of transverse carpal ligament release, is the most common complication after carpal tunnel release. Persistent or recurrent carpal tunnel symptoms are likely caused by an incomplete release. The initial recommended treatment for recurrent or persistent carpal tunnel syndrome is revision surgery.[24]

3: Upper Extremity

Table 6

AAOS Clinical Practice Guideline on the Diagnosis of Carpal Tunnel Syndrome: Summary of Recommendations

Recommendation 1.1	The physician should obtain an accurate patient history (level V, grade C).
Recommendation 2.1	The physician should perform a physical examination of the patient that may include: Personal characteristics (level V, grade C) Performing a sensory examination (level V, grade C) Performing a manual muscle testing of the upper extremity (level V, grade C) Performing provocative tests (level V, grade C), and/or Performing discriminatory tests for alternative diagnoses (level V, grade C)
Recommendation 3.1a	The physician may obtain electrodiagnostic tests to differentiate among diagnoses (level V, grade C)
Recommendation 3.1b	The physician may obtain electrodiagnostic tests in the presence of thenar atrophy and/or persistent numbness (Level V, grade C)
Recommendation 3.1c	The physician should obtain electrodiagnostic tests if clinical and/or preventive tests are positive and surgical management is being considered (level II and III, grade B)
Recommendation 3.2	If the physician orders electrodiagnostic tests, the testing protocol should follow the AAN/AANEM/AAPMR guidelines for diagnosis of carpal tunnel syndrome (level IV and V, grade C)
Recommendation 3.3[a]	The physician should not routinely evaluate patients suspected of having carpal tunnel syndrome with new technology, such as MRI, CT, and pressure-specified sensorimotor devices in the wrist and hand. (level V, grade C)

[a]Please note that recommendation 3.3 is not based on a systematic literature review. An additional abbreviated review was completed following the face-to-face meeting of the Work Group on February 24, 2007.
AAN = American Academy of Neurology, AANEM = American Association of Neuromuscular and Electrodiagnostic Medicine, AAPMR = American Academy of Physical Medicine and Rehabilitation
(Reproduced from the American Academy of Orthopaedic Surgeons: Clinical Practice Guideline on the Diagnosis of Carpal Tunnel Syndrome. Rosemont, IL, American Academy of Orthopaedic Surgeons, May 2007. Http://www.aaos.org/Research/guidelines/CTStreatmentguide.asp.)

Table 7

Diagnostic Tests for Carpal Tunnel Syndrome

Name of Test	How Performed	Condition Measured	Positive Result	Interpretation of Positive Result
Phalen test	Patient places elbows on table, forearms vertical, wrists flexed	Paresthesia in response to position	Numbness or tingling on radial side digits within 60 seconds	Probable carpal tunnel syndrome (sensitivity 0.75, specificity 0.47)
Percussion test (Tinel sign)	Examiner lightly taps along median nerve at the wrist, proximal to distal	Site of nerve lesion	Tingling response in fingers at site of compression	Probable carpal tunnel syndrome if response is at the wrist (sensitivity 0.60, specificity 0.67)
Carpal tunnel compression test	Direct compression of median nerve by examiner	Paresthesias in response to pressure	Paresthesias within 30 seconds	Probable carpal tunnel syndrome (sensitivity 0.87, specificity 0.90)
Hand diagram	Patient marks sites of pain or altered sensation on the outline diagram of the hand	Patient's perception of site of nerve deficit	Signs on palmar side of radial digits without signs in the palm	Probable carpal tunnel syndrome (sensitivity 0.96, specificity 0.73, negative predictive value of a negative test 0.91)

(Data from Szabo RM: Nerve compression syndromes, in Hand Surgery Update 1. Rosemont, IL, American Academy of Orthopaedic Surgeons, 1996, pp 221-231.)

An AAOS work group has provided a summary of recommendations for the treatment of carpal tunnel syndrome in a clinical practice guideline based on available evidence[25] (Table 8).

Anterior Interosseous Nerve Syndrome

A patient with anterior interosseous nerve syndrome presents with anterior forearm pain and weakness or motor loss of one or more of the flexor pollicis longus,

Table 8

AAOS Clinical Practice Guideline on the Treatment of Carpal Tunnel Syndrome: Summary of Recommendations

Recommendation 1	A course of nonsurgical treatment is an option in patients diagnosed with carpal tunnel syndrome. Early surgery is an option when there is clinical evidence of median nerve denervation or the patient elects to proceed directly to surgical treatment.	(Grade C, level V)
Recommendation 2	We suggest another nonsurgical treatment or surgery when the current treatment fails to resolve the symptoms within 2 to 7 weeks.	(Grade B, level I and II)
Recommendation 3	We do not have sufficient evidence to provide a specific treatment recommendations for carpal tunnel syndrome when found in association with the following conditions: diabetes mellitus, coexistent cervical radiculopathy, hypothyroidism, polyneuropathy, pregnancy, rheumatoid arthritis, and carpal tunnel syndrome in the workplace.	(Inconclusive, No evidence found)
Recommendation 4a	Local steroid injection or splinting is suggested when treating patients with carpal tunnel syndrome, before considering surgery.	(Grade B, level I and II)
Recommendation 4b	Oral steroids or ultrasound are options when treating patients with carpal tunnel syndrome.	(Grade C, level II)
Recommendation 4c	We recommend carpal tunnel release as treatment of carpal tunnel syndrome.	(Grade A, level I)
Recommendation 4d	Heat therapy is not among the options that should be used to treat patients with carpal tunnel syndrome.	(Grade C, level II)
Recommendation 4e	The following treatments carry no recommendation for or against their use: activity modifications, acupuncture, cognitive behavioral therapy, cold laser, diuretics, exercise, electric stimulation, fitness, graston instrument, iontophoresis, laser, stretching, massage therapy, magnet therapy, manipulation, medications (including anticonvulsants, antidepressants, and nonsteroidal anti-inflammatory drugs), nutritional supplements, phonophoresis, smoking cessation, systemic steroid injection, therapeutic touch, vitamin B_6 (pyridoxine), weight reduction, yoga.	(Inconclusive, level II and V)
Recommendation 5	We recommend surgical treatment of carpal tunnel syndrome by complete division of the flexor retinaculum regardless of the specific surgical technique.	(Grade A, level I and II)
Recommendation 6	We suggest that surgeons do not routinely use the following procedures when performing carpal tunnel release: Skin nerve preservation Epineurotomy The following procedures carry no recommendation for or against use: Flexor retinaculum lengthening Internal neurolysis Tenosynovectomy Ulnar bursa preservation	(Grade B, level I) (Grade C, level II) (Inconclusive, level II and V)
Recommendation 7	The physician has the option of prescribing preoperative antibiotics for carpal tunnel surgery.	(Grade C, level III)
Recommendation 8	We suggest that the wrist not be immobilized postoperatively after routine carpal tunnel surgery. We make no recommendation for or against the use of postoperative rehabilitation.	(Grade B, level II) (Inconclusive, level II)
Recommendation 9	We suggest physicians use one or more of the following instruments when assessing patients' responses to carpal tunnel syndrome treatment of research: Boston Carpal Tunnel Questionnaire (disease-specific) DASH: Disabilities of the Arm, Shoulder and Hand (region-specific; upper limb) MHQ: Michigan Hand Outcomes Questionnaire (region-specific; hand/wrist) PEM: Patient Evaluation Measure (region-specific; hand) SF-12 or SF-36 Medical Outcomes Short Form Health Survey (generic; physical health component for global health impact)	(Grade B, level I, II, and III)

(Reproduced from the American Academy of Orthopaedic Surgeons: Clinical Practice Guideline on the Treatment of Carpal Tunnel Syndrome. Rosemont, IL, Sept 2008. Http://www.aaos.org/Research/guidelines/CTstreatmentguide.asp.)

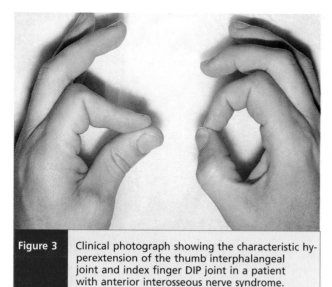

Figure 3 Clinical photograph showing the characteristic hyperextension of the thumb interphalangeal joint and index finger DIP joint in a patient with anterior interosseous nerve syndrome.

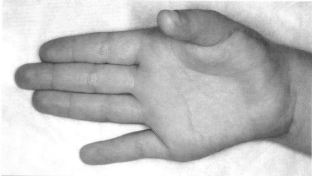

Figure 4 Clinical photograph of a hand showing the Wartenberg sign. Ulnar deviation of the small finger occurs secondary to the unopposed force of the extensor digiti minimi in patients with advanced ulnar nerve compression.

index finger and/or long flexor digitorum profundus, and the pronator quadratus muscle. There is no clinically observable or measurable sensory loss, and if present, sensory involvement suggests other diagnoses. A partial palsy with isolated involvement of the flexor digitorum profundus to the index finger or the flexor pollicis longus can be seen. When attempting a tip to tip pinch, the distal joints hyperextend with the pinch creating pulp-to-pulp contact (Figure 3). The differential diagnosis of anterior interior nerve syndrome includes tendon rupture; proximal compression; or brachial neuritis/Parsonage-Turner syndrome, which often follows a viral illness. More than one third of cases are idiopathic. In many patients, anterior interior nerve syndrome resolves spontaneously; therefore, observation is recommended for a minimum of 3 to 6 months. If there is no improvement, surgical treatment may be indicated with a longitudinal/extensile exposure and neurolysis of the entire anterior interior nerve. If there is no electrodiagnostic evidence of reinnervation, a nerve transfer (radial to median) may be considered at 7 to 10 months after surgery.[26] Tendon transfers (brachioradialis to flexor pollicis longus and flexor digitorum profundus small/ring to index/long or extensor carpi radialis longus to index profundus) can be helpful in reestablishing pinch strength.

Pronator Syndrome

Pronator syndrome is a proximal entrapment of the median nerve that results in primarily sensory changes in the median nerve distribution in the hand and the palmar cutaneous distribution of the palm and thenar eminence. It is less common than carpal tunnel syndrome, is more common in women, and often occurs in the fifth decade of life. It has been associated with repetitive activities and in patients with well-developed forearm muscles, such as weight lifters. Provocative tests, which should reproduce symptoms in the median nerve distribution, include resisted forearm pronation,

resisted elbow flexion with the forearm supinated, and resisted flexion of the long finger flexor digitorum superficialis. Electrodiagnostic studies are not reliable in diagnosing proximal median nerve compression. Nonsurgical management includes activity modification, nonsteroidal anti-inflammatory drugs, and splinting. If nonsurgical treatment fails (in approximately 50% of patients) and the clinical diagnosis is clear, surgical exploration and release of the nerve at all potential sites of compression is indicated.

Ulnar Nerve
Cubital Tunnel

Compression of the ulnar nerve at the cubital tunnel is the second most common compression neuropathy after carpal tunnel syndrome. The diagnosis can often be made clinically. Physical examination findings include numbness and paresthesias in the small and ring finger and occasional pain at the medial elbow. The Tinel sign over the ulnar nerve at the cubital tunnel is often positive, but this test may be overly sensitive. More severe compression may result in motor changes, including atrophy of ulnar-innervated muscles, claw deformity of the small and ring fingers, and positive Froment and Wartenberg signs (Figure 4). Electrodiagnostic studies may be used to confirm the diagnosis and to evaluate other sites of nerve compression or other disease processes that may be present. Electromyographic changes in ulnar-innervated muscles are more sensitive than nerve conduction velocity studies in the early stages of the disorder.

As in all other compression neuropathies, treatment outcomes are generally better before muscle atrophy develops. Nonsurgical management includes nighttime elbow extension splinting and education to avoid positioning that places the elbow in flexion or creates pressure on the ulnar nerve. If symptoms persist or progress, surgery may be indicated. Surgery may involve in situ decompression, medial epicondylectomy, or anterior transposition (subcutaneous, submuscular, or intramuscular). No significant difference has been reported in outcomes between these procedures, although fewer complications have been observed in patients treated with in situ decompression.[27] Endoscopically assisted cubital tunnel release with or without transposition also has been described with favorable early results.[28] The most common reasons for reoperation are inadequate decompression, perineural scarring, or tethering at the intermuscular septum or flexor carpi ulnaris fascia. Submuscular transposition has traditionally been preferred to revise a failed ulnar nerve procedure.[29]

Ulnar Tunnel Syndrome

The ulnar nerve divides in the Guyon canal at the hypothenar region of the wrist and can be compressed in this area. Compression at this level is uncommon and can be secondary to trauma (acute or repetitive); anomalous muscles; or space-occupying lesions such as ganglia (most commonly), thrombosis, or pseudoaneurysms. The anatomy is divided into three zones: zone 1 is proximal to the bifurcation of the nerve and includes both sensory and motor fibers, zone 2 surrounds the motor branch distal to the bifurcation, and zone 3 encompasses the superficial sensory branches distal to the bifurcation. The site of compression impacts the presenting symptoms, which can include strictly motor, strictly sensory, or a mix of both motor and sensory loss. If a space-occupying lesion is suspected, MRI can identify the mass. The Allen test along with vascular testing, and in some cases ultrasound, can identify thrombosis of the ulnar artery. CT is the most cost-efficient method for evaluating the hook of the hamate fracture or fracture nonunion of the hook. When surgery is indicated, all three zones must be explored and released. Care should be taken to identify and release the deep motor branch of the ulnar nerve.

Radial Nerve

Compression of the radial nerve in the proximal forearm can result in motor weakness without pain (posterior interosseous nerve syndrome) or in pain without weakness (radial tunnel syndrome). Compression of the radial sensory nerve in the distal forearm (Wartenberg syndrome or cheiralgia paresthetica) can cause pain and, occasionally, sensory loss on the dorsal radial aspect of the distal forearm and hand.

Posterior Interosseous Nerve Syndrome

Posterior interosseous nerve syndrome results in weakness of the muscles without clinically measurable loss of sensory function. This syndrome may occur spontaneously, after trauma, or may present secondary to a mass at the elbow. The diagnosis is based on clinical examination findings and electrodiagnostic testing. MRI is indicated to evaluate the possible presence of a space-occupying lesion. A baseline electromyogram should be obtained at 3 to 4 weeks after onset of symptoms and a repeat electromyogram should be obtained after 4 to 5 months if there is no return of function. Although posterior interosseous nerve syndrome resolves spontaneously in many instances, surgery may be indicated if there is no clinical improvement and no recovery from baseline measurements on repeat electrodiagnostic testing. In patients who have no return of function, nerve decompression or tendon transfer surgery should be considered.

Radial Tunnel Syndrome

Radial tunnel syndrome is characterized by pain without motor deficit. The pain is typically localized to the lateral aspect of the proximal forearm, and has been associated with lateral epicondylitis. Electrodiagnostic studies are usually negative. Nonsurgical management is appropriate in most patients. If nonsurgical treatment fails, surgical radial tunnel release may yield good outcomes.[30] A recent study has reported good treatment results for radial tunnel syndrome with surgical decompression of the superficial branch of the radial nerve.[31]

Wartenberg Syndrome (Cheiralgia Paresthetica)

Radial sensory nerve entrapment at the distal forearm is characterized by pain. It may be related to closed trauma, laceration, or wearing a tight wristwatch or handcuffs. The nerve is compressed in pronation by the scissoring effect of the tendons of the brachioradialis and extensor carpi radialis longus. The physical examination will show a positive Tinel sign. Provocative testing includes wrist flexion and ulnar deviation and pronation. The Finkelstein maneuver places traction on the nerve and may increase symptoms. Electrodiagnostic testing is rarely useful in the diagnosis. Nonsurgical management includes splinting, activity modification, and local corticosteroid injections. Surgical release is occasionally needed if symptoms persist.

Tendon Transfers

Tendon transfers can provide an alternative to functional deficits secondary to nerve palsy. Adherence to certain principles is critical for successful tendon transfer surgery (Table 9). Planning for tendon transfer surgery requires identifying the key lost functions and the motor resources available to treat the deficit(s).

Radial Nerve Palsy

Radial nerve palsy is the most common indication for tendon transfer in the upper extremity. It can be classified as a high (radial nerve proper) or a low (posterior interosseous nerve syndrome) palsy. It is important to maintain full passive range of motion in the hand and wrist before proceeding with tendon transfer. Nonsurgical treatment includes wrist splint immobilization (including the metacarpophalangeal joints in extension) or a dynamic splint. Early tendon transfers can be considered as an "internal splint" as opposed to definitive treatment. Although there are several tendon transfer options to treat radial nerve palsy deficits, all generally include using the pronator teres to the extensor carpi radialis brevis for wrist extension in high radial nerve

Table 9

Principles of Tendon Transfer Surgery

One tendon, one function	A split transfer will only function to the shortest excursion of the recipient tendons.
Straight line of pull	A straight line between motor and recipient maximizes function of the transfer.
Similar excursion	Donor excursion should approximate recipient excursion.
Similar strength	Donor strength should approximate recipient strength.
Expendable donor	Transferred tendons should not sacrifice existing function.
Tissue equilibrium	Tendon transfer surgery should be done at a time when surrounding soft tissue and bone is healed and mature.
Joint mobility	Soft-tissue maturity includes the correction of contracture. Range of motion of affected joints must be maximized prior to transfer.
Synergy	Tendon transfers that take advantage of the stabilization effect of antagonistic muscles result in improved recipient function.
Tenodesis	The normal tenodesis effect of the hand enhances the function of tendon transfers. Wrist fusion should be a measure of last resort as this compromises the results of tendon transfers.
Power versus positional motors	The use of weaker transfers for position and stronger transfers for power uses available motor resources more efficiently.

From Dorf ER, Chhabra AB: Tendon transfer surgery, in Trumble TE, Budoff JE, eds: *Hand Surgery Update IV*. Rosemont, IL, American Society for Surgery of the Hand, 2007, pp 439-453.

palsy, the palmaris longus to extensor pollicis longus for thumb extension, and either the flexor carpi ulnaris or flexor carpi radialis to the extensor digitorum communis for finger extension.

One area of controversy is when to explore radial nerve palsy associated with a humeral fracture. Because many patients with closed injuries will achieve full recovery of the radial nerve without surgical treatment, nonsurgical management is recommended. A baseline electrodiagnostic study may be obtained at 3 to 4 weeks after injury. If there is no evidence of return of function of the brachioradialis or radial wrist extensor by 4 to 5 months, a repeat electrodiagnostic study can be obtained for comparison with the baseline study. If there is no evidence of recovery, surgical treatment may be indicated. In patients with open fractures or fractures with vascular injury, the radial nerve should be explored acutely. Indications for nerve exploration for radial nerve palsy occurring after fracture manipulation remain controversial.

Median Nerve Palsy

Median nerve injuries are classified as high or low based on whether the lesion is proximal or distal to the origin of the anterior interosseous nerve in the proximal forearm. The benefits and prognosis of tendon transfer surgery are largely influenced by the quality of hand sensation, function in the uninvolved hand, and patient motivation.

Low Median Nerve Palsy

Low median nerve palsy is the second most common reason for tendon transfer in the upper extremity after radial nerve palsy. Thumb opposition, largely motored by the abductor pollicis brevis, is the primary functional loss in low median nerve palsy. Surgery is indicated when loss of thumb opposition causes a functional deficit for the patient. There are four reliable tendon transfers for opposition (opponensplasties): the flexor digitorum superficialis of the ring finger opponensplasty (Boyes transfer), the extensor indicis proprius opponensplasty, abductor digiti minimi or Huber transfer, and the palmaris longus or Camitz procedure. The extensor indicis proprius and flexor digitorum superficialis-ring finger are most commonly selected. The Huber transfer is most beneficial in pediatric patients with congenital hypoplastic thumb because it also improves the hand's appearance by increasing the bulk of the thenar musculature. The Camitz procedure is most commonly performed for loss of opposition secondary to severe carpal tunnel syndrome.

High Median Nerve Palsy

In high median nerve palsy, along with loss of thumb opposition, flexion is also lost in the thumb, index finger, and long finger. Patients may also have loss of active pronation. In high median nerve palsy, thumb opposition is typically provided by transfer of the extensor indicis proprius as previously described. Alternatively, the extensor digiti minimi or extensor carpi ulnaris can be used for opponensplasty. As useful sensory recovery is often unlikely in these cases, opponensplasty may not benefit the patient. The preferred method to restore index and long finger flexion is a side-to-side transfer of the small and ring finger flexor digitorum profundus to the index and long flexor digitorum profundus. Flexor pollicis longus function is typically restored through transfer of the brachioradialis.

Ulnar Nerve Palsy

Ulnar nerve palsy is characterized by loss of function of ulnar-innervated musculature as well as deformity and contractures. A high ulnar nerve palsy is distinguished from a low ulnar nerve palsy by ring and small finger flexor digitorum profundus involvement. The primary deformity seen with ulnar nerve deficit is clawing, which results from an imbalance between the intrinsic and extrinsic muscles.

Low Ulnar Nerve Palsy

An injury to the ulnar nerve below the elbow results in loss of power pinch, abduction of the small finger, and clawing. Although tendon transfers typically improve function, they can also correct deformity in ulnar nerve palsy. The deficit in power pinch is a result of paralysis of the adductor pollicis and the first dorsal interosseous muscles. With this functional loss, patients compensate by using the extensor pollicis longus to adduct the thumb and the flexor pollicis longus to flex the thumb interphalangeal joint against the index finger (the compensation is known as the Froment sign). The unopposed extension force of the extensor digiti minimi results in ulnar deviation of the small finger. Clawing results because the intrinsic muscles are not functioning to flex the metacarpophalangeal joints and extend the interphalangeal joints. Tendon transfers for correcting clawing must pass volar to the transverse metacarpal ligament to flex the proximal phalanx. Many different motors have been used to correct clawing, including the extensor carpi radialis longus, extensor carpi radialis brevis, and palmaris longus. The grafts are attached by either a two- or four-tailed graft to the A2 pulleys or the radial lateral bands of the small and ring digits or all four digits. Power pinch can be restored with a Smith transfer (using extensor carpi radialis brevis) or with flexor digitorum superficialis of the ring finger. Abduction of the small finger (Wartenberg sign) can be corrected with transfer of the ulnar insertion of extensor digiti minimi to the radial collateral ligament or A1 pulley of the small finger.

High Ulnar Nerve Palsy

Loss of function of the ring and small finger flexor digitorum profundus is the primary distinguishing deficit between low and high ulnar nerve palsy. Clawing will not be as pronounced in high ulnar nerve palsy as in low ulnar nerve palsy because the extrinsic flexors are not functioning. Restoring DIP flexion in the small and ring fingers is achieved via side-to-side transfer between the long, ring, and small finger flexor digitorum profundus muscles as is the case in a high median nerve palsy. Extensor carpi radialis brevis transfer should be used to treat the deficit in power pinch because flexor digitorum superficialis transfer will further weaken grip strength.

Combined Nerve Palsies

Combined nerve palsies lead to significant disability. A combination of low median and low ulnar nerve injury is the most common of these combined palsies. Function in this combined nerve palsy is most impacted by the loss of thumb adduction and opposition, thumb to index finger pinch, intrinsics, and sensibility. Sensibility may be restored through transfer of a dorsal metacarpal artery flap with superficial radial nerve innervated skin from the index finger proximal phalanx to the palmar surface of the thumb. Combined high median and high ulnar nerve palsy is the second most common combined nerve injury and results in even greater loss of function. Clawing of all four fingers occurs because of the imbalance between the extrinsic flexors and extensors. The goals of surgery are to help restore simple grasp and key pinch. A volar neurovascular cutaneous island flap from the ring finger may be used to achieve sensation for pinch. A recent study has reported promising results with nerve transfers in the hand and upper extremity and has indicated that there may be an increasing role for nerve transfer in treating motor and sensory deficits.[26]

Ulnar Wrist Pain

The differential diagnosis of ulnar-sided wrist pain includes arthritis, fracture, and instability, along with nerve, tendon, and vascular injuries.

Triangular Fibrocartilage Complex

The triangular fibrocartilage complex (TFCC) is a major stabilizer of the DRUJ and of the ulnar carpus. It is composed of a central articular disk, dorsal and volar radioulnar ligaments, a meniscus homolog, the ulnar collateral ligament, and the sheath of the extensor carpi ulnaris.[32] The central disk extends from the sigmoid notch of the radius to its insertion at the base of the ulnar styloid. The vascular supply extends to the peripheral 10% to 40% of the TFCC with the central component being avascular.[33]

Palmer[34] divided TFCC injuries into traumatic (type I) and degenerative (type II) categories. Injuries are further classified by the location of the tear and the articular pathology (Table 10). Plain radiographs should be obtained and the ulnar variance evaluated (a zero rotation PA view is best). A dynamic PA grip view with the forearm in pronation also is helpful. MRI may show tears and signal changes at the ulnar part of the lunate, which are consistent with ulnocarpal impaction. The sensitivity of MRI arthrography for detecting TFCC tears ranges from 74% to 100%. Dedicated wrist coils, high-resolution pulsed sequences, and high-strength magnets can increase diagnostic sensitivity.

Arthroscopy is the most accurate modality in diagnosing lesions of the TFCC and can help to directly evaluate the size and stability of a tear and detect coincident ligament or chondral injuries. Arthroscopy is indicated for patients with symptomatic TFCC injuries after failed conservative treatment (typically wrist splinting and activity modification for several months). Wrist arthroscopy should include midcarpal portals be-

Table 10

Classification and Treatment of TFCC Injuries

Type	Description	Treatment
I	**Traumatic Tears**	
IA	Isolated central TFCC tear; no instability	Nonsurgical or arthroscopic débridement of unstable portion: leave at least 2 mm peripherally to avoid instability
IB	Peripheral tear at base of ulnar styloid; mild DRUJ instability; may have extensor carpi ulnaris instability	Arthroscopic repair of TFCC tear; if ulnar styloid ununited with tear, need open procedure: pathognomonic finding is loss of triangular fibrocartilage normal tension as determined with a probe
IC	TFCC disruption from the ulnar extrinsic ligaments	Arthroscopic reefing or tenodesis procedure; open repair for large defect—can augment with a strip of flexor carpi ulnaris
ID	Radial detachment of the TFCC from the sigmoid notch of the distal radius	Open radial-sided TFCC repair; Munster cast for 4 weeks if TFCC repair
II	**Degenerative Tears Associated With Ulnar Impaction**	
IIA	TFCC wear without perforation or chondromalacia	Arthroscopic evaluation and synovectomy; open ulnar shortening
IIB	TFCC wear with chondromalacia of the lunate or ulna	Same as IIA
IIC	Perforation of TFCC with lunate chondromalacia	Débridement of central tear and arthroscopic wafer versus open ulnar shortening osteotomy
IID	TFCC perforation with ulna and/or lunate chondromalacia and lunotriquetral ligament injury but without carpal instability (no volar intercalated segmental instability)	TFCC débridement and arthroscopic wafer (open ulnar shortening if lunotriquetral unstable)
IIE	TFCC perforation with arthritic changes involving ulna and lunate; lunotriquetral ligament injury	Ulnar shortening osteotomy with lunotriquetral débridement; lunotriquetral pinning if unstable after ulnar shortening

cause these are more sensitive than radiocarpal arthroscopy for evaluating scapholunate and lunotriquetral ligament instability.[35]

Degenerative Ulnocarpal Impaction

Chronic overloading of the ulnocarpal joint can lead to ulnocarpal impaction, which may include wear of the ulnar head, lunate, triquetrum, and/or TFCC. Patients will present with reports of ulnar-sided wrist pain and possibly swelling or decreased range of motion. Pain is increased with ulnar deviation, especially when combined with pronation and supination. Positive ulnar variance is a known risk factor for ulnar impaction syndrome because of the resultant increase in ulnocarpal loading. Degenerative ulnocarpal impaction can be developmental or acquired, static or dynamic. Several months of nonsurgical treatment should be attempted before surgery is considered. Surgical treatment involves an ulnar shortening osteotomy or partial distal ulna resection (arthroscopic wafer or hemiresection arthroplasty) to decrease force transmission through the ulnar side of the wrist. Newer techniques for ulnar shortening use subcondylar osteotomies, require less surgical exposure, and may achieve more rapid healing in metaphyseal rather than diaphyseal bone.[36]

Annotated References

1. Chung KC, Watt AJ, Kotsis SV: A prospective outcomes study of four-corner wrist arthrodesis using a circular limited wrist fusion plate for stage II scapholunate advanced collapse wrist deformity. *Plast Reconstr Surg* 2006;118(2):433-442.

2. Mulford JS, Ceulemans LJ, Nam D, Axelrod TS: Proximal row carpectomy vs four corner fusion for scapholunate (Slac) or scaphoid nonunion advanced collapse (Snac) wrists: A systematic review of outcomes. *J Hand Surg Eur Vol* 2009;34(2):256-263.

   The authors present a meta-analysis comparing proximal row carpectomy and four-corner fusion. Outcomes were similar in both groups.

3. Cohen MS, Kozin SH: Degenerative arthritis of the wrist: Proximal row carpectomy versus scaphoid excision and four-corner arthrodesis. *J Hand Surg Am* 2001;26(1):94-104.

4. Jones DB Jr, Bürger H, Bishop AT, Shin AY: Treatment of scaphoid waist nonunions with an avascular proximal pole and carpal collapse: A comparison of two vascularized bone grafts. *J Bone Joint Surg Am* 2008; 90(12):2616-2625.

This retrospective review compares distal radial pedicle grafts to medial femoral condyle grafts for scaphoid nonunions with an avascular proximal pole. Union rates and time to healing were better for medial femoral condyle grafts. Level of evidence: III.

5. Greenberg JA: Reconstruction of the distal ulna: Instability, impaction, impingement, and arthrosis. *J Hand Surg Am* 2009;34(2):351-356.

   The authors present a review of the etiology and treatment options for distal radioulnar joint pathology.

6. Parker WL, Linscheid RL, Amadio PC: Long-term outcomes of first metacarpal extension osteotomy in the treatment of carpal-metacarpal osteoarthritis. *J Hand Surg Am* 2008;33(10):1737-1743.

   A small retrospective review of metacarpal osteotomies for early and moderate CMC arthritis showed good outcomes at an average 9-year follow-up.

7. Shuler MS, Luria S, Trumble TE: Basal joint arthritis of the thumb. *J Am Acad Orthop Surg* 2008;16(7):418-423.

   The authors present a comprehensive review of treatment modalities for CMC joint arthritis.

8. Rizzo M, Moran SL, Shin AY: Long-term outcomes of trapeziometacarpal arthrodesis in the management of trapeziometacarpal arthritis. *J Hand Surg Am* 2009;34(1):20-26.

   The authors report on a large retrospective review of patients treated with CMC arthrodesis. Improvements in pinch and grip strength as well as average pain scores were reported. Despite the development of arthritis in adjacent joints, patient satisfaction scores were excellent several years postoperatively. Level of evidence: IV.

9. Klimo GF, Verma RB, Baratz ME: The treatment of trapeziometacarpal arthritis with arthrodesis. *Hand Clin* 2001;17(2):261-270.

10. Tomaino MM: Distal interphalangeal joint arthrodesis with screw fixation: Why and how. *Hand Clin* 2006;22(2):207-210.

11. Chung KC, Ram AN, Shauver MJ: Outcomes of pyrolytic carbon arthroplasty for the proximal interphalangeal joint. *Plast Reconstr Surg* 2009;123(5):1521-1532.

    A prospective evaluation of pyrolytic carbon implants for PIP arthritis revealed improvements in grip and pinch strength as well as functional outcome scores. Implant squeaking and dislocation were the most common complications.

12. Jennings CD, Livingstone DP: Surface replacement arthroplasty of the proximal interphalangeal joint using the PIP-SRA implant: Results, complications, and revisions. *J Hand Surg Am* 2008;33(9):1565, e1-e11.

    The authors present a retrospective review of PIP joint arthroplasties performed with surface replacement arthroplasty implants. Although range of motion did not improve, pain scores were significantly better. The complication rate was 26%. Loosening in noncemented

prostheses was the most common reason for revision surgery. Level of evidence: IV.

13. Bonzar M, Firrell JC, Hainer M, Mah ET, McCabe SJ: Kienböck disease and negative ulnar variance. *J Bone Joint Surg Am* 1998;80(8):1154-1157.

14. Watanabe T, Takahara M, Tsuchida H, Yamahara S, Kikuchi N, Ogino T: Long-term follow-up of radial shortening osteotomy for Kienbock disease. *J Bone Joint Surg Am* 2008;90(8):1705-1711.

    The authors present results of a follow-up questionnaire administered to patients treated with radial shortening osteotomy for Kienbock disease. Most patients reported mild pain and little functional loss. Level of evidence: IV.

15. Croog AS, Stern PJ: Proximal row carpectomy for advanced Kienböck's disease: Average 10-year follow-up. *J Hand Surg Am* 2008;33(7):1122-1130.

    A long-term follow-up of proximal row carpectomies for Kienböck disease showed reliable results and minimal functional limitations. Patients with more advanced disease were more likely to require conversion to arthrodesis. Level of evidence: IV.

16. Kalainov DM, Cohen MS, Hendrix RW, Sweet S, Culp RW, Osterman AL: Preiser's disease: Identification of two patterns. *J Hand Surg Am* 2003;28(5):767-778.

17. Moran SL, Cooney WP, Shin AY: The use of vascularized grafts from the distal radius for the treatment of Preiser's disease. *J Hand Surg Am* 2006;31(5):705-710.

18. Keith MW, Masear V, Chung K, et al: Diagnosis of carpal tunnel syndrome. *J Am Acad Orthop Surg* 2009;17(6):389-396.

    The authors discuss the clinical practice guideline for diagnosis of carpal tunnel syndrome developed by AAOS.

19. Weber RA, Rude MJ: Clinical outcomes of carpal tunnel release in patients 65 and older. *J Hand Surg Am* 2005;30(1):75-80.

20. Hobby JL, Venkatesh R, Motkur P: The effect of age and gender upon symptoms and surgical outcomes in carpal tunnel syndrome. *J Hand Surg Br* 2005;30(6):599-604.

21. Thomsen NO, Cederlund R, Rosén I, Björk J, Dahlin LB: Clinical outcomes of surgical release among diabetic patients with carpal tunnel syndrome: Prospective follow-up with matched controls. *J Hand Surg Am* 2009;34(7):1177-1187.

    The authors report on a prospective, consecutive matched series of diabetic and nondiabetic patients treated with carpal tunnel release. Diabetic patients had the same beneficial outcome as nondiabetic patients. Level of evidence: I.

22. Keith MW, Masear V, Amadio PC, et al: Treatment of carpal tunnel syndrome. *J Am Acad Orthop Surg* 2009;17(6):397-405.

3: Upper Extremity

Clinical practice guidelines for the treatment of carpal tunnel syndrome are discussed. Nine specific recommendations are made.

23. Scholten RJ, Gerritsen AA, Uitdehaag BM, van Geldere D, de Vet HC, Bouter LM: Surgical treatment options for carpal tunnel syndrome. *Cochrane Database Syst Rev* 2004;4(4):CD003905.

24. Amadio PC: Interventions for recurrent/persistent carpal tunnel syndrome after carpal tunnel release. *J Hand Surg Am* 2009;34(7):1320-1322.

   This case report-based article presents an algorithm for evaluation and treatment recommendations for recurrent or persistent carpal tunnel syndrome.

25. Guideline on the Treatment of Carpal Tunnel Syndrome. American Academy of Orthopaedic Surgeons Web site. http://www.aaos.org/research/guidelines/CTStreatmentguide.asp. Accessed October 5, 2010.

   The AAOS work group recommendations on the guideline for treating carpal tunnel syndrome are summarized. A list of the work group members also is provided.

26. Brown JM, Mackinnon SE: Nerve transfers in the forearm and hand. *Hand Clin* 2008;24(4):319-340, v.

   This review article presents nerve transfer options for restoring motor and sensory deficits in each nerve in the hand and forearm.

27. Zlowodzki M, Chan S, Bhandari M, Kalliainen L, Schubert W: Anterior transposition compared with simple decompression for treatment of cubital tunnel syndrome: A meta-analysis of randomized, controlled trials. *J Bone Joint Surg Am* 2007;89(12):2591-2598.

   The authors present a meta-analysis of randomized controlled studies evaluating the efficacy of simple decompression of the ulnar nerve compared with anterior transposition. Results showed no significant difference in motor nerve conduction velocities or clinical outcome scores between the two procedures.

28. Ahcan U, Zorman P: Endoscopic decompression of the ulnar nerve at the elbow. *J Hand Surg Am* 2007;32(8):1171-1176.

   In a retrospective review of endoscopically assisted ulnar nerve decompression at the elbow, the authors reported only one complication (hematoma). All patients had electrophysiologic improvement after surgery, were satisfied with the procedure, and returned to full activities within 3 weeks.

29. Vogel RB, Nossaman BC, Rayan GM: Revision anterior submuscular transposition of the ulnar nerve for failed subcutaneous transposition. *Br J Plast Surg* 2004;57(4):311-316.

30. Lee JT, Azari K, Jones NF: Long term results of radial tunnel release: The effect of co-existing tennis elbow, multiple compression syndromes and workers' compensation. *J Plast Reconstr Aesthet Surg* 2008;61(9):1095-1099.

   The authors of this retrospective analysis of outcomes of radial tunnel release at an average of 57 months after surgery reported better outcomes in patients with radial tunnel pathology alone compared with patients with additional pathologies.

31. Bolster MA, Bakker XR: Radial tunnel syndrome: Emphasis on the superficial branch of the radial nerve. *J Hand Surg Eur Vol* 2009;34(3):343-347.

   In a study reporting results on 12 patients with radial tunnel syndrome treated with surgical decompression of the superficial branch of the radial nerve, 11 patients were satisfied with the results.

32. Palmer AK, Werner FW: The triangular fibrocartilage complex of the wrist: Anatomy and function. *J Hand Surg Am* 1981;6(2):153-162.

33. Bednar MS, Arnoczky SP, Weiland AJ: The microvasculature of the triangular fibrocartilage complex: Its clinical significance. *J Hand Surg Am* 1991;16(6):1101-1105.

34. Palmer AK: Triangular fibrocartilage complex lesions: A classification. *J Hand Surg Am* 1989;14(4):594-606.

35. Hofmeister EP, Dao KD, Dao KD, Glowacki KA, Shin AY: The role of midcarpal arthroscopy in the diagnosis of disorders of the wrist. *J Hand Surg Am* 2001;26(3):407-414.

36. Slade JF III, Gillon TJ: Osteochondral shortening osteotomy for the treatment of ulnar impaction syndrome: A new technique. *Tech Hand Up Extrem Surg* 2007;11(1):74-82.

   A new technique for ulnar shortening osteotomy is described that preserves the articular surface of the distal ulna. The osteotomy is secured with headless compression screws and, therefore, complications associated with plating are avoided.

3: Upper Extremity

Lower Extremity

SECTION EDITOR:

LISA K. CANNADA, MD

Chapter 30

Fractures of the Pelvis and Acetabulum

Henry Claude Sagi, MD   Frank A. Liporace, MD

Introduction

Traumatic pelvic and acetabular fractures result from high-energy accidents such as motor vehicle crashes, auto-pedestrian collisions, falls, and crush injuries. Because of the great forces that are required to disrupt the pelvic ring, traumatic pelvic fractures and the accompanying visceral and soft-tissue injuries are associated with diverse outcomes. Prior to the 1980s, there was a substantial lack of both clinical and scientific information regarding the biomechanics and techniques for stabilization of pelvic ring disruptions. Modern strategies and philosophies regarding surgical and nonsurgical treatment of injuries to the pelvic ring continue to evolve to include early open reduction and internal fixation to restore normal anatomic relationships in hopes of improving functional outcomes.

Current Issues and Controversies in the Treatment of Pelvic Ring Injuries

Four controversies concerning the treatment of pelvic ring injuries currently exist. (1) Malunion of one hemipelvis may result in leg length inequality, mechan-

Dr. Sagi or an immediate family member serves as a board member, owner, officer, or committee member of the Orthopaedic Trauma Association of the American Academy of Orthopaedic Surgeons; is a member of a speakers' bureau or has made paid presentations on behalf of Stryker, Smith & Nephew, and AO; serves as a paid consultant to or is an employee of Smith & Nephew, Synthes, and Stryker; and has received research or institutional support from Smith & Nephew, Synthes, and Stryker. Dr. Liporace or an immediate family member is a member of a speakers' bureau or has made paid presentations on behalf of DePuy, A Johnson & Johnson Company, Osteotech, Synthes, and Smith & Nephew; serves as a paid consultant to or is an employee of DePuy, A Johnson & Johnson Company, Osteotech, Synthes, and Smith & Nephew; serves as an unpaid consultant to AO; and has received research or institutional support from Synthes and Smith & Nephew.

ical low back pain, sitting imbalance, dyspareunia, and bowel and/or bladder dysfunction. However, the exact relationship of pelvic malunion to functional outcome remains unclear.

(2) Ligamentous injuries (symphyseal disruptions and sacroiliac (SI) joint dislocations) heal less predictably than fractures and may result in chronic pain secondary to pelvic instability. Accurately identifying those injuries that exhibit sufficient ligamentous instability to warrant surgical stabilization remains difficult.

(3) Completely unstable injuries of the posterior ring managed with posterior fixation should be supplemented with some form of anterior fixation to improve stability and restore the normal loading response of the unstable hemipelvis.[1] However, this may depend on whether the anterior injury is ligamentous (symphysis) or bony (ramus).

(4) Anatomic reduction and stable fixation is more critical for the unstable posterior pelvic ring than anterior. However, considerable debate exists regarding the order of fixation and reduction maneuvers as it pertains to the nature and extent of posterior injury.

Initial Evaluation and Management of Patients With Pelvic Fractures

Established standard prehospital transport protocols and emergency department management algorithms have documented benefit and should be followed to decrease patient morbidity and mortality. The multiply injured patient is at risk for thoracic, intra-abdominal, soft-tissue, pelvic, and extremity hemorrhage, and requires a coordinated multidisciplinary team approach. The most common injuries associated with pelvic fractures are chest injury in up to 63% of patients, long bone fractures in 50%, brain and abdominal injury (spleen, liver, bladder, and urethra) in 40%, and spine fractures in 25%.[2]

Injuries to the bladder and urethra have a reported incidence of 15% to 20% (21% in males and 8% in females). Bladder and urethral trauma occur with relatively equal frequency (approximately 7%). When pelvic fractures are accompanied by bladder rupture, associated mortality can be as high as 22% to 34% because of the significant force required to rupture a hollow viscus within the pelvis. The clinical finding most

Table 1

Clinical Findings That May Be Present in Patients With a Pelvic Fracture

External rotation of one or both extremities

Limb-length discrepancy

Scrotal, labial, and/or perineal ecchymosis

Urethral, vaginal, and/or rectal bleeding

Neurologic deficit

consistently observed after bladder or urethral injury is gross hematuria, which is present in approximately 95% of patients; most bladder ruptures are extraperitoneal.[3]

Gastrointestinal injuries and open pelvic fractures are seen in 4% to 5% of patients with pelvic fracture, and significantly increase the incidence of deep pelvic and soft-tissue infection, osteomyelitis, mortality, and long-term disability. Diverting colostomy and distal washout are performed to reduce the chance of pelvic wound infection when damage to the anal sphincter with a perineal laceration exists or fecal soiling of an open perineal wound that communicates with the fracture is possible. Diverting colostomy should be performed within the first 6 to 8 hours following injury to reduce the incidence of sepsis and death.[4]

Modern evaluation of a patient with blunt abdominal and pelvic trauma routinely involves the use of plain radiographs; CT of the chest, abdomen, and pelvis; diagnostic peritoneal lavage (DPL); and focused abdominal sonography for trauma (FAST) examination for free fluid and bleeding within the peritoneal and preperitoneal cavities. The sequence of assessments outlined in the Advanced Trauma Life Support course and handbook is helpful for organizing an approach to managing potentially unstable trauma patients.[5] **Table 1** lists the clinical findings that may be present in patients with a pelvic fracture.

Persistent pelvic hemorrhage and hemodynamic instability despite appropriate fluid resuscitation is usually the result of coagulopathy and/or pelvic arterial bleeding and requires urgent intervention to prevent ongoing blood loss, shock, and death. In a recent review of the German Trauma Registry, the rate of mortality directly attributable to pelvic injury and hemorrhage was 7%.[6]

External compression devices such as inflatable garments, pelvic binders/sheets applied over the greater trochanters, and external fixators are generally the first line of intervention for persistent hypotension after appropriate fluid resuscitation in a patient with pelvic fracture and no other potential source of hemorrhage. Internal rotation and adduction of the lower extremities (if possible) can be helpful in reducing external rotation deformities of the pelvic ring. Anterior pelvic external fixation frames function by internally rotating an externally rotated (open book) hemipelvis around a sufficiently intact posterior ring that functions as a

hinge. With skillful placement of the pins and lateral to medial translation of the hemipelvis, some control of the posterior ring is also possible.

For patients who present in shock and/or have persistent hemodynamic instability despite pelvic compression, appropriate resuscitation and exclusion of thoracic, abdominal, and extremity hemorrhage, laparotomy with pelvic packing or angiography should be considered. The basic tenets are well outlined in the practice management guidelines promulgated by the Eastern Association for the Surgery of Trauma.[7]

The use of transfemoral angiography with selective embolization of injured arteries should be based on initial response to resuscitation and the presence of a contrast blush on CT. Necrosis of pelvic viscera, sexual dysfunction, and soft-tissue necrosis (particularly gluteal) are potential complications seen with aggressive angiography, particularly with bilateral internal iliac arterial occlusion in patients who have had large extensile exposures.[8] For those patients in extremis, pelvic packing may be preferable to taking a desperately ill, unstable patient to the angiography suite.[9]

Radiologic Evaluation

Apart from the standard AP pelvic radiograph taken as part of the traditional "trauma series," radiologic evaluation of the pelvic ring should include the inlet and outlet projections. The pelvic inlet view is obtained with the x-ray beam directed caudally approximately 40° to 60° to the radiographic film. The inlet view is helpful in imaging external or internal rotation of the hemipelvis, diastasis of the SI joint, and impaction fractures of the sacral ala. The pelvic outlet is obtained by directing the x-ray beam approximately 30° to 60° cephalad to the radiographic film. The outlet view is helpful in imaging cephalad "vertical" shift of the hemipelvis and the location of sacral fractures relative to the foramina. CT is performed routinely using 2- to 3-mm axial sections (or 3 mm of vertical travel per 360° rotation of the gantry in a spiral CT). Images with this resolution should disclose most injuries and allow for good-qualtiy three-dimensional and multiplanar reconstructions.

Classification of Pelvic Fractures

The Young and Burgess classification scheme,[10] currently the most widely used, focuses on the mechanism of injury and represents further refinement and modification of the work performed by Pennal and Tile.[11] These two classification schemes are summarized in **Tables 2** and **3**.

Nonsurgical Treatment of Pelvic Ring Injuries

The following injury patterns can be considered sufficiently stable to warrant a trial of nonsurgical care: nondisplaced or minimally displaced ramus fractures; symphyseal disruptions with less than 2.5 cm of widening (anteroposterior compression injury); and impacted sacral fractures without cephalad displacement or "excessive" internal rotation of the hemipelvis (lateral compression injury).

Table 2

Young and Burgess Classification Scheme

Lateral Compression (LC type): rami fractures plus:

LC I: sacral fracture on side of impact (usually impacted fracture).

LC II: crescent fracture on side of impact.

LC III: type I or II injury on side of impact with contra-lateral open book injury.

Anteroposterior Compression (APC type): symphysis diastasis or rami fractures plus:

APC I: minor opening of symphysis and SI joint anteriorly (SI, STL, and SSL intact)

APC II: opening of anterior SI (sacrospinous and sacrotuberous ligaments), intact posterior SI ligaments

APC III: complete disruption of SI joint and all supporting ligaments

Vertical Shear (VS type)

Vertical displacement of hemipelvis with symphysis diastasis or rami fractures anteriorly

Iliac wing fracture, sacral facture or SI dislocation posteriorly

Combination (CM type): any combination of above injuries

Table 3

Pennal and Tile Classification Scheme

Type A: Pelvic Ring Stable

A1: fractures not involving the ring (ie, avulsions, iliac wing or crest fractures).

A2: stable minimally displaced fractures of the pelvic ring

Type B: Pelvic Ring Rotationally Unstable, Vertically Stable

B1: open book

B2: lateral compression, ipsilateral

B3: lateral compression, contralateral or bucket-handle type injury

Type C: Pelvic Ring Rotationally and Vertically Unstable

C1: unilateral

C2: bilateral

C3: associated with acetabular fracture

Although some authors have used single-leg stance views to diagnose occult instability in the subacute or chronic setting, these tests have limited utility in the acute phase of the injury.[12,13] Examination under anesthesia with dynamic intraoperative stress fluoroscopic views can be used to diagnose occult instability of the pelvic ring; however, the tolerable ranges of motion of the pelvic ring under stress examination are not well defined (**Figure 1**). Some lateral compression injuries of the sacrum in patients with good bone quality may be treated successfully in some circumstances with immediate weight bearing as tolerated without the risk of further displacement. Because the consequences of malunion can significantly affect function and quality of life for patients, a course of nonsurgical care requires a compliant patient and frequent serial physical and radiographic examinations to detect early displacement.

Indications for Surgical Reduction and Fixation of Anterior Pelvic Ring Injuries

The indications for surgical reduction and fixation of anterior pelvic ring injuries include symphyseal dislocations demonstrating greater than 2.5 cm of diastasis (implying disruption of the sacrospinous and sacrotuberous ligaments) with static or dynamic (examination under anesthesia) imaging; augmentation of posterior fixation in vertically displaced unstable pelvic ring injuries; a locked symphysis; pain and immobility; or the presence of tilt fractures.

External Anterior Fixation

Some of the more frequent complications that have limited the use of external fixation devices for definitive treatment of unstable pelvic injuries include pin site complications, interference with abdominal access, their cumbersome nature, inability to maintain accurate reductions, and bladder entrapment.[14] However, when formal open reduction and internal fixation is contraindicated by open pelvic fractures, contaminated abdominal incisions, or complex bladder and urethral injuries, external fixation may be a good treatment option. Recent biomechanical studies have demonstrated that supra-acetabular frames[15] (**Figure 2**) are similar to traditional iliac crest frames in resisting flexion and extension but superior in resisting internal and external rotation.[16] Five-millimeter Schanz pins for both constructs have been shown to be significantly stronger than 4-mm pins.[17]

Open Reduction and Internal Fixation of Symphyseal Disruptions

One recent study has shown a higher rate of fixation failure and pelvic malunion with two-hole symphyseal plating, recommending a plating configuration that has at least two points of fixation on either side of the symphysis.[18] Dual plating and multiplanar symphyseal plates have not been shown to offer improved stability in biomechanical studies and are currently used only in revision or failed fixation cases.[19] The role of locking plates for symphyseal fixation remains undefined. Four- and six-hole precontoured symphyseal plates with 3.5- or 4.5-mm cortical screws are the constructs most commonly used by most pelvic reconstruction surgeons (**Figure 3**).

Open Reduction and Internal Fixation of Ramus Fractures

Many ramus fractures can be treated nonsurgically because of the surrounding periosteal sleeve that enhances stability and provides rapid, predictable bony healing. Surgical fixation of widely displaced ramus fractures should be considered for augmenting posterior fixation

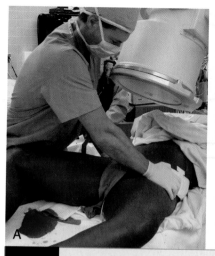
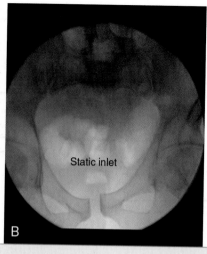
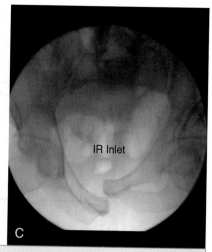

Static inlet

IR Inlet

Figure 1   **A,** Technique for examination under anesthesia of pelvic ring. **B,** Preoperative static film of pelvic ring injury. **C,** Intraoperative dynamic stress view of the pelvis showing an unstable pelvic ring.

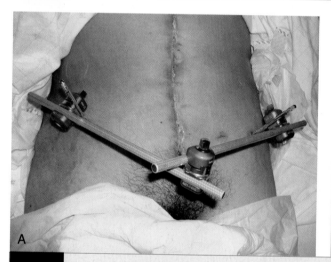
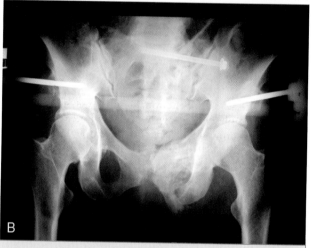

Figure 2   **A,** Clinical photograph of a supra-acetabular pelvic external fixator. **B,** Radiograph demonstrating pin placement for the supra-acetabular frame.

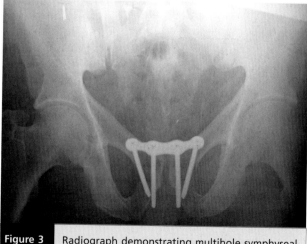

Figure 3   Radiograph demonstrating multihole symphyseal plating.

constructs to increase the stability of the pelvic ring. Where indicated, the use of percutaneously placed intramedullary ramus screws can be considered for stabilization of the anterior pelvic ring. Medially located fractures can be stabilized with a retrograde ramus screw, whereas those fractures located laterally near the pubic root may be better treated with an anterior column screw[20] (**Figure 4**).

Indications for Surgical Reduction and Fixation of Posterior Pelvic Ring Injuries

The indications for surgical reduction and fixation of posterior pelvic ring injuries are: displaced iliac wing fractures that enter and exit both the crest and greater sciatic notch or sacroiliac (SI) joint (crescent fractures); disruption of the posterior SI ligaments, resulting in multiplanar instability of the SI joint; nonimpacted, comminuted sacral fractures; any posterior ring injury that has demonstrated or has the propensity for cepha-

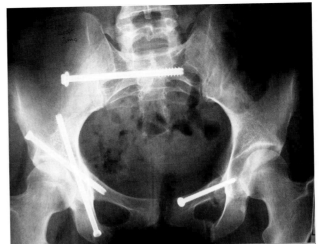

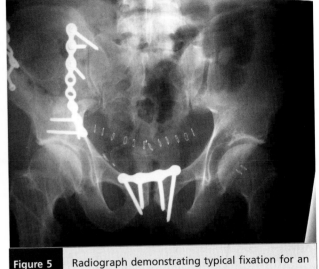

| Figure 4 | Radiograph demonstrating the use of both anterior column (right) and retrograde rami screws (left) for anterior pelvic fixation. | Figure 5 | Radiograph demonstrating typical fixation for an iliac wing fracture. |

lad (vertical) displacement; and U-shaped sacral fractures with spinal-pelvic dissociation.

Iliac Wing Fractures and Fracture-Dislocations (Crescent Fractures)

A single pelvic reconstruction plate or lag screw along the crest supplemented with a second reconstruction plate or lag screw at the level of the pelvic brim (anterior approach) or sciatic buttress (posterior approach) will usually suffice in neutralizing deforming forces until healing has occurred[21] (**Figure 5**).

Iliac wing fractures are more often associated with open wounds than other pelvic ring injuries and may be associated with entrapped bowel.[22] Careful examination of the wound and evaluation of the CT scan for subcutaneous air or entrapped bowel is imperative. Early reconstruction of the ilium and serial débridements with open packing and delayed closure, along with appropriate prophylactic antibiotic therapy, is recommended.

Iliac wing fractures that enter the SI joint (crescent fractures) result in disruption of some or all of the SI ligaments.[23] Reduction of crescent fractures involving only a small portion of the SI joint are treated similar to extra-articular iliac wing fractures, and no iliosacral screws are needed. Standard fixation involves a superiorly placed pelvic reconstruction plate along the iliac crest with supplemental lag screws from the posterior inferior iliac spine (PIIS) into the sciatic buttress just above the greater notch. With smaller crescent fragments, the degree of SI joint instability increases and the injury behaves more like an SI dislocation; consideration must be given to supplemental fixation with SI screws or plates (**Figure 6**).

SI Joint Dislocations

The SI joint can be reduced from either an anterior or posterior direction. With significant vertical displace-

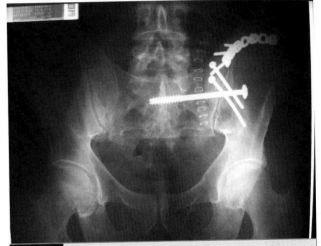

| Figure 6 | Radiograph demonstrating typical fixation construct for a crescent fracture associated with a small crescent fragment and SI joint instability. |

ment of the hemipelvis, forceful traction may be required, and recent studies have reported that rigidly stabilizing the patient to the operating room table using some form of table-skeletal fixation[24,25] helps considerably in achieving either open or indirect percutaneous closed reductions.

Although biomechanical studies[26] have not shown significant superiority of either iliosacral screw fixation, transiliac fixation, or anterior SI plating, iliosacral screws remain the workhorse for posterior pelvic ring stabilization because they can be applied in either the prone or supine position, and in open or percutaneous situations of severe soft-tissue damage when closed reduction is possible.[27,28]

Commonly used iliosacral screws are cannulated with diameters of 6.5, 7.3, or 8.0 mm made of titanium

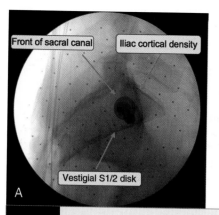
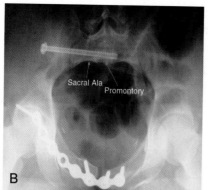
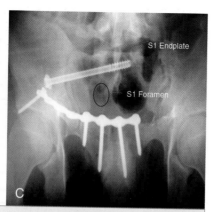

Front of sacral canal | Iliac cortical density

S1 Endplate

Sacral Ala
Promontory

S1 Foramen

Vestigial S1/2 disk

A

B

C

Figure 7 Lateral (**A**), inlet (**B**), and outlet (**C**) radiographic views demonstrating appropriate positioning and trajectory of an SI screw for an SI dislocation.

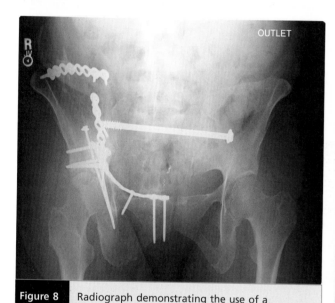

OUTLET

Figure 8 Radiograph demonstrating the use of a transsacral screw for fixation of a vertical sacral fracture.

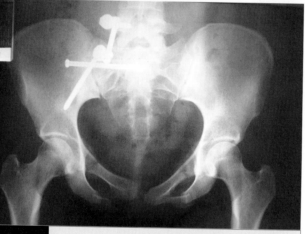

Figure 9 Radiograph demonstrating the use of triangular osteosynthesis for stabilization of a vertically unstable transforaminal sacral fracture.

or stainless steel. Long thread lengths with purchase in the sacral body and promontory offer the greatest resistance to pullout.[29] The SI screw should be directed as close to the superior end plate and anterior aspect of S1 to avoid the upper sacral nerve root tunnel (**Figure 7**). A second iliosacral screw can be placed into S1 or S2 if purchase of the first SI screw is thought to be suboptimal or considerable instability of the pelvic ring exists.[30] Currently available data from biomechanical studies suggest increased stability with a second iliosacral screw for SI dislocations, with a second screw into the S2 vertebral body being superior to a second screw into S1.[1,31]

Vertical Sacral Fractures

In addition to pelvic instability, vertical sacral fractures may result in varying degrees of neurologic deficit.[32] The indications for reduction and stabilization of vertical sa-

cral fractures include vertical or cephalad instability in the case of a vertical shear sacral fracture; comminuted, nonimpacted sacral alar fractures; and impacted sacral fractures from lateral compression injuries with excessive internal rotation and pelvic deformity.

Stabilization of most sacral fracture reductions is usually accomplished with one or two iliosacral screws placed posteriorly.[33] One study has shown that anatomic reduction of the fracture is important for improving fracture stability and increasing the diameter of the safe corridor for iliosacral screw placement.[34] Another recent publication has advocated the use of a "transsacral" screw that crosses the sacrum to gain purchase in the contralateral ilium[35] (**Figure 8**). There are no published biomechanical studies demonstrating superiority of transsacral screws over standard iliosacral screws.

An increased risk of loss of reduction in vertical sacral fractures treated with iliosacral screws alone when associated with severe comminution, osteoporotic

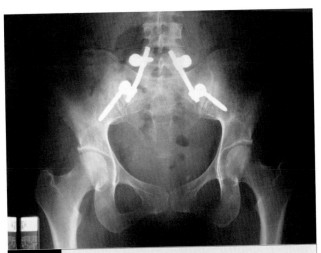

Figure 10 Radiograph demonstrating the use of a spinal-pelvic construct to stabilize an unstable U-shaped sacral fracture with spinal-pelvic dissociation.

Role of Surgical Navigation in the Treatment of Pelvic Fractures

Due to the inherent difficulties in fiducial positioning and obtaining image quality sufficient for tracking and navigation, surgical navigation systems for pelvic fixation have not had the same popularity and utility as pedicle screws and arthroplasty. Several preliminary reports have examined iliosacral screw placement in cadaver pelves demonstrating improved or equal accuracy with a substantial decrease in radiation exposure to the surgeon.[43,44] Surgical navigational systems still add considerable time to the procedure and should not be used in place of experience and knowledge of three-dimensional pelvic anatomy.

Internal Degloving Soft-Tissue Injuries

Serial drainage, débridement, and vacuum-assisted closure of the wound before formal open reduction and internal fixation is generally advocated by most trauma surgeons; however, percutaneous drainage and lavage may be appropriate in select cases.[45,46]

bone, or disruption of the L5/S1 facet joint has been noted by some authors.[36] Spinal-pelvic constructs, such as triangular osteosynthesis, have been implemented in these situations to help minimize the occurrence of late displacement and malunion. Spinal-pelvic constructs have been shown to be superior both biomechanically and clinically to SI screws alone for maintaining reduction in comminuted sacral fractures[37-39] (**Figure 9**). Patients are able to fully bear weight within a few weeks of surgery. Prominent and symptomatic fixation, delayed union and nonunion, lumbosacral scoliosis, and the need for later removal are the most commonly encountered problems.[40]

Sacral nerve root decompression may be required when the patient presents with sacral radiculopathy and the preoperative CT scan shows nerve root impingement. When necessary, decompression can be performed directly through the fracture and a sacral laminectomy is generally not required.[40]

U-Shaped Sacral Fractures: Spinal Pelvic Dissociation

U-shaped sacral fractures result in dissociation of the spine from the pelvic ring (spinal-pelvic dissociation), and pelvic ring stability is generally not affected. Rather than unilateral radiculopathy, these patients present neurologically with cauda equina lesions. Lateral pelvic or lumbosacral radiographs with sagittal and coronal CT reconstructions are critical in identifying this injury pattern. Some authors advocate in situ bilateral SI screw fixation alone for impacted, stable injuries without significant kyphosis or neurologic deficit.[41] However, U-shaped sacral fractures with spinal-pelvic dissociation and cauda equina syndrome commonly require reduction, decompression and some form of bilateral posterior spinal-pelvic fixation construct to control kyphotic deformity and allow early mobilization of the patient[42] (**Figure 10**).

Outcome Studies for Pelvic Fractures

Certain outcome studies[47,48] support the position that the long-term functional results are improved if reduction with less than 1 cm of combined displacement of the posterior ring is obtained, particularly with pure dislocations of the SI complex. Fractures of the posterior ring tend to have better postoperative function than dislocations that rely on scar formation and ligamentous healing.[49] However, pure dislocations of the SI joint that heal with a solid bony ankylosis have not demonstrated improved outcome over those without ankylosis.[50] Despite anatomic reduction, however, other studies have shown that a substantial number of patients continue to have poor outcomes, with chronic posterior pelvic pain.[51,52] Males frequently report erectile dysfunction and females frequently report dyspareunia, urinary difficulty, and pregnancy-related issues with an increase in the need for cesarean section.[53-56] Outcome after pelvic fracture is associated with significantly higher mortality in the elderly: 12.3% versus 2.3% in the younger age groups, despite equal need for transfusion and similar injury patterns.[57] Fewer than 50% of patients with severe pelvic fractures return to their previous level of function and work status and the majority of patients sustain persistent impairment in both the physical and mental components of the Short Form-36 questionnaire.

Current Issues and Controversies in the Treatment of Acetabular Fractures

Acetabular fractures are fairly rare injuries, with an annual incidence of approximately 0.003%.[58] Most of these injuries occur in a bimodal age distribution, with young adults more frequently suffering high-energy injuries (for example, motor vehicle accidents and falls from heights) and the elderly sustaining low-energy in-

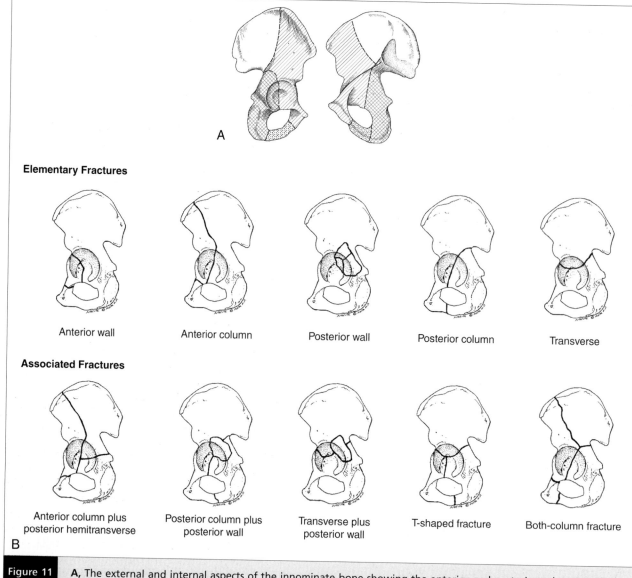

Elementary Fractures

Anterior wall Anterior column Posterior wall Posterior column Transverse

Associated Fractures

Anterior column plus posterior hemitransverse Posterior column plus posterior wall Transverse plus posterior wall T-shaped fracture Both-column fracture

Figure 11 **A,** The external and internal aspects of the innominate bone showing the anterior and posterior columns and ischiopubic rami. **B,** Schematic representation of the Letournel and Judet classification. (**A** reproduced with permission from Baumgaertner MR, Tornetta P III, eds: *Orthopaedic Knowledge Update: Trauma 3.* Rosemont, IL, American Academy of Orthopaedic Surgeons, 2005, pp 259–269. **B** reproduced with permission from Fischgrund JS, ed: *Orthopaedic Knowledge Update 9.* Rosemont, IL, American Academy of Orthopaedic Surgeons, 2008, pp 389–397.)

jury mechanisms (for example, falls from standing position).

Evaluation and Initial Management

Prior to deciding whether surgical treatment is indicated, an understanding of the local anatomy and radiographic portrayal of the fracture is required. The two-column concept was developed to elucidate a better understanding of the complex surrounding osseous anatomy and its radiographic corollaries responsible for supporting the asymmetric, hemispherical acetabulum. As a result, the Letournel classification of acetabular fractures was developed[59] (**Figure 11**) and has been shown to have substantial reliability (kappa >0.7) when used by surgeons who treat acetabular fractures regularly or who interpret images.[60] Plain radiographic analysis should include an AP pelvic radiograph with associated Judet views (45° obturator and iliac oblique views). A supplementary CT scan, often with coronal and sagittal or even three-dimensional reconstructions, can be very helpful. When combined with an AP radiograph, CT has been postulated to increase the interobserver reliability of classification over an AP radiograph combined with Judet views.[61] A recent analysis of 11 computer-reconstructed radiographs from CT scans determined that these radiographs were effective in supplying necessary data and more esthetically pleasing than standard plain radiographs. Computer-reconstructed radiographs have the potential to overcome patient-related factors (for example, discomfort, bowel gas, or overlying osseous structures) when positioning for standard radiographic views.[62]

The propensity for associated nonskeletal injury in patients with acetabular fractures, especially from high-energy mechanisms, should not be overlooked. A recent study indicated that when correlating Letournel classification of the fracture with the force vector most likely responsible for the fracture, a statistically significant higher association with retroperioneal hematomas, visceral injuries, and vascular injuries occurred with patterns that resulted from a lateral loading. Although posterior hip dislocations in isolation have a relatively impressive rate of osteonecrosis of the femoral head, those associated with an acetabular fracture do not necessarily correlate with a poor prognosis and have been shown to have a 71% rate of good to excellent results when appropriately managed.[63] Impaction fractures of the femoral head also can occur and can have implications on prognosis. These fractures often occur concomitantly with dislocation or with significant medialization of the femoral head to the ilioischial line (protrusio) as seen with many associated fracture patterns. The implication of injury to the femoral head is significant when considering prognosis.[63]

Surgical Timing and Bleeding

Assuming the patient is medically stable to undergo surgery, some authors have historically waited 3 to 5 days after injury to perform definitive treatment. Also, it has been anecdotally postulated that less bleeding occurs from fracture surfaces during surgery when delayed, but cessation of fracture bleeding most reliably occurs with reduction and fixation. No specific evidence exists to support that delayed fixation decreases intraoperative bleeding. Many surgeons incorporate the use of cell-saver technology in an effort to decrease the requirement of allogenic blood transfusion. In a recent analysis of 186 acetabular surgeries in which 60 of the patients had a cell-saver, a significant difference in the rates of intraoperative and postoperative transfusion received by patients was not determined. The cell-saver group averaged a 282% greater cost in blood-related charges.[64] Certain acetabular fractures have an increased need for blood transfusion within the first 24 hours after admission. In a retrospective review of 289 acetabular fractures, both-column, anterior column, anterior column/posterior hemitransverse, and T-type fractures had a 56% incidence of requiring transfusion within 24 hours of admission compared to 28% for other fracture types.[65]

It must be recognized that there has been variability within the literature when defining "early fixation" of acetabular fractures, which has ranged from 24 hours to 2 weeks.[66] Another recent series evaluated 68 patients with isolated injuries of the femur, pelvis/acetabulum, or spine. Preoperatively, those with femoral shaft fractures exhibited the highest levels of interleukin-6 and -8, but those with pelvic and acetab-

ular injuries exhibited similar levels of interleukin 24 hours after surgery as those with surgically treated femur fractures. This finding was not dependent on the duration of the procedure.[67]

Indications

If the patient is deemed medically and psychologically fit to undergo surgical treatment, the following questions must be answered when determining whether surgical treatment or nonsurgical management with or without skeletal traction is appropriate.

(1) Is there articular (wall or columnar) displacement, how much, and where in the acetabulum?
(2) If displaced, is there secondary congruence?
(3) Is the fracture stable?
(4) Can the fracture be appropriately fixed based on factors such as bone quality and excessive impaction?
(5) Does the surgeon or institution have the expertise and experience to adequately treat the fracture?

Many surgeons quantify the intact weight-bearing dome on radiographs by evaluating the roof-arc angle on the AP and Judet views. It has been postulated that a fracture that lies within a roof-arc of <45° on any of the three standard acetabular radiographs involves the weight-bearing dome. If displacement is unacceptable, reduction and fixation are required.[68] A recent study evaluating what CT findings correlate to this superior weight-bearing dome has determined that on the axial cuts, the superior 10 mm represents this area of importance.[69] Biomechanical analyses have suggested that the significance of the roof-arc angle is not the same on all three standard acetabular radiographs.[70,71] With certain both-column fractures that maintain secondary congruence, nonsurgical treatment may be considered with approximately 85% acceptable results.[72] It should be noted that with secondary congruence, the stress concentration during simulated single-leg stance increases substantially in the dome adjacent to the area of the fracture line.[73] The presence of articular displacement must be considered before nonsurgical treatment is undertaken. A recent review of 32 patients treated nonsurgically with more than 3 mm of articular incongruity yielded only 56% good to excellent results.[74]

Although posterior wall fractures are most common clinically,[59] they are often difficult to treat. Concomitant hip dislocation, femoral head injury, intra-articular fragments, patient age older than 55 years, and marginal impaction all have a significant effect on results and have only fair interobserver agreement when classifying these additional factors.[75-77] Determining displacement and potential instability also play a role when considering surgical management of posterior wall fractures. Gross instability after closed reduction with subluxation occurring with ≥40° of hip flexion, intra-articular osteochondral fragments that are not isolated small avulsions within the fovea, and fractures that involve more than 50% of the posterior wall are absolute indications for surgical intervention. A recent review of 10 years of acetabular fractures seen at a level

1 trauma center yielded a 26% rate of intra-articular osteochondral fragments when postreduction CT scan was evaluated.[78] When determining percentage of posterior wall involvement on axial CT scan to define instability, multiple measurement methods have been proposed, with the resultant conclusion that fractures involving less than 20% of the posterior wall are most likely stable, those involving 20% to 50% have intermediate risk of instability with justification for fluoroscopic stress examination, and those involving more than 50% are unstable. A recent study discusses a modified method that accounts for measurement at the level of the largest posterior wall defect and accounts for marginal impaction. When calculating the percentage of posterior wall involvement and tendency to be stable, intermediate risk, or unstable, there was a resultant 100% specificity, sensitivity, and positive predictive value.[79]

It is clear that anatomic reduction with stable fixation is the goal. The ability to accurately assess reduction quality does have variability between plain radiograph and CT scan. One study evaluated patients in whom received radiographs and CT scan were performed postoperatively to evaluate quality of reduction as well as interobserver and intraobserver agreement. Although plain radiography was only 75% sensitive at detecting residual articular displacement, the added cost and radiation exposure of postoperative routine CT scans could not be justified because altering postoperative management was not necessary in any of the 20 cases reviewed.[80]

Choices of Surgical Approach

Surgical treatment of acetabular fractures is with the Kocher-Langenbeck, ilioinguinal, or in selected cases, the extended iliofemoral approach. Variants to these as well as the option for percutaneous supplementary or definitive treatment may also be used. Direction of displacement, the ability to reduce the fracture and apply adequate fixation, and surgeon experience will dictate the approach chosen.

The Kocher-Langenbeck approach is recommended for posterior wall, posterior column, transverse, transverse-posterior wall, and some T-type fractures. It allows direct access to the posterior column and posterior wall safely from the superior aspect of the greater sciatic notch to the ischial tuberosity. Through the greater sciatic notch, reduction clamp access and digital palpation of the quadrilateral surface can be conducted. Care must be taken to surgically preserve any blood supply to the femoral head that has not been traumatized by the injury with preservation of the quadratus femoris.[81]

A modification of the Kocher-Langenbeck approach with the addition of a trochanteric digastric osteotomy will allow more superior and anterior exposure when addressing fracture patterns that require access for reduction and fixation that is proximal to the superior aspect of the greater sciatic notch and decrease the risk of affecting the neurovascular supply to the abductors

through inadvertent stretch injury. The ilioinguinal approach is advocated for anterior column, anterior wall, anterior column with associated posterior hemitransverse, both-column, and certain T-type or transverse fractures. Access to the pelvic brim, internal iliac fossa, iliac crest, and anterior SI joint are possible.[81] In an effort to directly buttress the quadrilateral plate and avoid the inadvertent potential complications of a hernia and external iliac vessel injury with the ilioinguinal approach, the modified Stoppa approach with or without the lateral window of the ilioinguinal approach has been advocated.[82,83] A retrospective review of 55 patients treated by two experienced pelvic/acetabular surgeons yielded an 89% good to excellent radiographic result, with a relatively low complication rate.[84] Another review of 25 patients yielded similar results with up to 95% satisfactory to anatomic reductions and highlighted the versatility of this approach to address acetabular and pelvic ring injuries[85] (**Figure 12**). The extended iliofemoral approach has been advocated for complex acetabular fractures that are being operated on more than 21 days after injury, fractures that have a transtectal transverse component or T-type fracture with dome involvement, both-column fractures with extension to the sacroiliac joint, or fractures requiring simultaneous anterior and posterior columnar exposure.[63,86,87] This seemingly morbid approach yields acceptable results based on quality of articular reduction, although heterotopic ossification can be more prevalent than with the other approaches discussed.[86,88,89]

New Technologies and Techniques

Recently, the ability to acquire three-dimensional (3-D) CT reconstructions, computer navigation, 3-D fluoroscopy, and improved visualization with two-dimensional fluoroscopy have contributed to better preoperative planning and percutaneous/limited open reduction and fixation techniques.[90-95] In an early series of limited open reduction with percutaneous fixation, acceptable reductions were obtained in all young patients, within an average of 3 mm of anatomic reduction in elderly patients. Surgical time averaged 75 minutes and blood loss averaged 50 mL. All of the younger patients went on to union with an average Harris hip score of 96. These techniques have also been used in elderly patients with minimally displaced acetabular fractures to improve early mobilization in an effort to avoid immobility-associated medical complications. A recent evaluation of 21 elderly patients with minimally or nondisplaced acetabular fractures underwent percutaneous fluoroscopically guided columnar screw fixation with no reported complications. Patients were allowed mobilization the first day after surgery and were bearing weight as tolerated at 4 weeks. At an average follow-up of 3.5 years, no radiographic evidence of degenerative changes, hardware failure, or fracture displacement was seen.[96] The use of these techniques requires a detailed understanding of the anatomy as well as a willingness and ability to convert to standard open

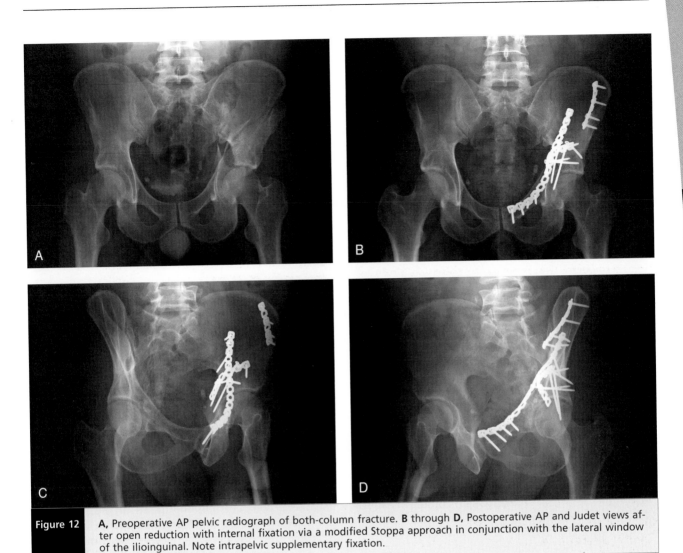

Figure 12   **A,** Preoperative AP pelvic radiograph of both-column fracture. **B** through **D,** Postoperative AP and Judet views after open reduction with internal fixation via a modified Stoppa approach in conjunction with the lateral window of the ilioinguinal. Note intrapelvic supplementary fixation.

surgery if appropriate reduction and stability is not attainable.

Specific Considerations
Construct Stability and Supplementation
Adequacy of fixation is always a concern. The ability to match the need for stable fixation with technical and anatomic limitations can be challenging. Each fracture pattern in conjunction with comminution, patient factors, and surgeon experience play a role in making this determination. A combination of fragment-specific 3.5-mm screws with reconstruction plates for buttress effect is commonly used. With plate fixation the concept of near-near and far-far screw positioning relative to the fracture site provides the greatest stability.[97]

Frequently, transverse acetabular fractures are approached through a single incision yet involve both columns. Therefore, fixation options are dictated by the surgical exposure with or without percutaneous screw supplementation. In terms of biomechanical stability, the combination of posterior column plating with anterior column screw fixation provides a significantly stiffer construct than posterior plate fixation alone or isolated

anterior and posterior column screw fixation or screw and wire fixation.[97,98] In some patients, anterior column width or fracture geometry may preclude anterior column screw fixation from the posterior approach. A recent evaluation of 35 patients with a minimum 18-month follow-up showed that isolated posterior column fixation with dual plating did not yield statistically different radiographic or clinical results when compared to posterior column plating combined with anterior column screw fixation.[99] An alternative to supplementing isolated posterior plating for transverse fractures is the use of locked plates, which have been shown to provide results similar to more traditional fixation methods in terms of resisting displacement under cyclical loading.[100] Locked plating may also be beneficial in the treatment of patients with osteopenia. In an effort to provide additional stability in the presence of marginal impaction that has been reduced, subchondral minifragment specific fixation has been used to supplement buttress plating with 93% good to excellent results at a mean follow-up of 35 months.[101] For smaller posterior wall fragments that are not amenable to lag screw fixation, spring plates have also been used.[102,103]

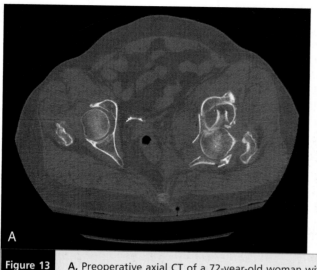
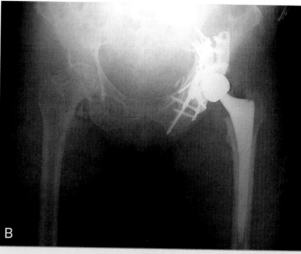

Figure 13 **A,** Preoperative axial CT of a 72-year-old woman with an acetabular fracture showing femoral head impaction, multiple intra-articular osteochondral fragments, osteopenia, and severe comminution. **B,** Postoperative AP pelvic radiograph of limited columnar fixation in conjunction with bone grafting and total arthroplasty with cage.

Dome Impaction/Arthroplasty

Osteopenia causes complications during acetabular fixation. Initial radiographic signs reveal known problems when treating these patients. Most significantly, superomedial dome impaction can result in a "gull wing" sign that precludes consistent long-term results with internal fixation.[104] Elderly patients and those with osteopenia, femoral head impaction, endogenous obesity, more than 40% cartilage abrasion, and extensive impaction may have better results with columnar fixation and total hip arthroplasty done acutely.[77] Outcome after early fixation and late hip arthroplasty is predictably poor.[105,106] Revision acetabular surgery delayed longer than 3 weeks when persistent instability concomitant with femoral head pathology is present yields poor results, especially in the elderly.[107] Limited fixation has been advocated in conjunction with these acute total hip arthroplasties to limit the undesired complication of significant superomedial migration of the hip center, which could result in premature loosening and poor results.[77] With a mean follow-up of 8.1 years and 79% good to excellent results, the average subsidence in one series was 3 mm medial and 2 mm vertical in the first 6 weeks. Ultimately, cup position stabilized and there were no instances of premature loosening using combined limited fixation and acute total hip arthroplasty.[108] A recent series of 18 patients using similar techniques, with an average age of 72 years and average follow-up of 3.9 years, yielded a mean Harris hip score of 88, minimal cup migration, no loosening, and one acute revision within 3 weeks.[76] Initial cup stability, when supplemented by limited fixation, may be an issue in certain situations. Combining limited fixation with cage reconstruction and cemented polyethylene liners may help achieve treatment goals (**Figure 13**). Elderly patients and those with osteopenia, acetabular fractures, and significant impaction remain challenging to treat.

Complications

Acetabular fracture surgery requires a detailed understanding of the local anatomy. Complications can be quite severe and such surgery should be performed by those who have had adequate training and experience. Appropriate prophylaxis can be implemented to limit the incidence of certain predictable complications. Wound infection, nerve injury, posttraumatic arthritis, osteonecrosis, heterotopic bone formation, and thromboembolic complications (discussed in the pelvis section) are most commonly associated with acetabular fractures.[63,109] Alterations in gait patterns affecting the hip, knee, and ankle, regardless of approach, have been discussed in the literature.[110]

Long-term single-surgeon series have shown infection rates between 2% and 5%.[63,111] Considerations of the surrounding soft tissues, approach, and timing play a significant role.[112] Obesity has been shown to contribute to the propensity for infection, thromboembolic events, and increased intraoperative blood loss.[113-115] Morbid obesity carries a relative risk of 2.6 when considering overall complication rate. A recent series showed a statistically significant increase in total surgical time, hospital stay, and complication rate (63%) in morbidly obese patients. Although not a statistically significant finding, morbidly obese patients also had increased positioning time and estimated intraoperative blood loss.[114]

Nerve injury can involve the sciatic, superior gluteal, femoral, ilioinguinal, lateral femoral cutaneous, and obturator nerves.[116] Large series rates of iatrogenically induced sciatic nerve injury have been shown to range from 2% to 6%.[63,117] Nerve injury may occur from the injury or surgical manipulation. Although fracture pattern or surgical approach may intuitively lead to suspicion of what nerve may be injured, these are not without deviation. A recent report of two cases with sciatic nerve palsy found entrapment in the posterior columnar component of a both-column fracture requiring release through a Kocher-Langenbeck approach and ultimate improvement of symptomatology.[118] Lower extremity positioning with the hip extended and knee flexed may decrease the incidence of sciatic nerve injury when undergoing a posterior approach to the acetabulum. Heterotopic ossification (HO) prophylaxis can help decrease the risk of delayed nerve entrapment. Electromyography has been shown to be superior to somatosensory-evoked potential monitoring in detecting intraoperative sciatic nerve compromise, but utility and consistent results in terms of decreasing iatrogenic intraoperative nerve injury are limited.[119-121]

HO is a known complication of acetabular fractures and their associated surgical interventions, which seem to be more prevalent after extended iliofemoral approaches compared to the Kocher-Langenbeck or ilioinguinal approach. HO has been shown to adversely affect outcome.[122,123] Necrotic gluteus minimus muscle has been postulated to contribute to HO. Débridement of necrotic gluteus minimus muscle has been suggested as a means of decreasing the incidence of HO after the Kocher-Langenbeck approach.[124] Prophylaxis with indomethacin or one low dose of irradiation (700 – 800 cGy) within 3 days of surgery has been shown to provide prophylaxis, but questions remain about the relative effectiveness of these treatments.[125] A recent meta-analysis yielded 5 appropriate prospective studies with a total of 384 patients, which showed a significantly lower incidence of HO in patients treated with radiation (3%) as opposed to indomethacin (9%) for prophylaxis.[126]

Posttraumatic arthritis can result from traumatic cartilage damage, osteochondral loss, intra-articular fragments or hardware, and imperfect surgical reductions. Also, development of arthritis, aside from causing pain, may be related to hip muscle weakness.[127] Detection of intra-articular hardware can be done with the aid of fluoroscopy and even adjunctive intraoperative auscultation with an esophageal stethoscope.[128] Clinical and radiographic results closely correlate. Anatomic reductions are considered to have less than 2 mm of displacement, imperfect reductions have 2 to 3 mm of displacement, and poor reductions have more than 3 mm of displacement. With anatomic reduction, an approximately 75% rate of good to excellent results can be expected. The rate of anatomic reduction decreases with increased fracture complexity, patient age, and the interval between the injury and the reduction.

Annotated References

1. Sagi HC, DiPasquale T: Biomechanical analysis of fixation for vertically unstable sacroiliac dislocations with iliosacral screws and symphyseal plating. *J Orthop Trauma* 2004;18(3):138-143.

2. Demetriades D, Karaiskakis M, Toutouzas K, Alo K, Velmahos G, Chan L: Pelvic fractures: Epidemiology and predictors of associated abdominal injuries and outcomes. *J Am Coll Surg* 2002;195(1):1-10.

3. Cass AS: The multiple injured patient with bladder trauma. *J Trauma* 1984;24(8):731-734.

4. Brenneman FD, Katyal D, Boulanger BR, Tile M, Redelmeier DA: Long-term outcomes in open pelvic fractures. *J Trauma* 1997;42(5):773-777.

5. American College of Surgeons Committee on Trauma: *Advanced Trauma Life Support for Doctors*, ed 6, 1997.

6. Hauschild O, Strohm PC, Culemann U, et al: Mortality in patients with pelvic fractures: Results from the German pelvic injury register. *J Trauma* 2008;64(2):449-455.

   The authors provide a review of more than 4,000 patients from 23 different hospitals over two segments of time, 1991-1993 (prior to well-organized prehospital and in-hospital resuscitative algorithms) and 1998-2000 (after establishment of such). Mortality directly attributable to the pelvic fracture decreased from 11% to 7% despite similar Injury Severity Scores.

7. DiGiacomo JC, Bonadies JA, Cole FJ, et al: Practice management guidelines for hemorrhage in pelvic fracture: Eastern Association for the Surgery of Trauma (EAST), Winston-Salem, North Carolina. 2001. http://www.east.org/tpg/pelvis.pdf. Accessed January 5, 2010.

8. Velmahos GC, Toutouzas KG, Vassiliu P, et al: A prospective study on the safety and efficacy of angiographic embolization for pelvic and visceral injuries. *J Trauma* 2002;53(2):303-308, discussion 308.

9. Cothren CC, Osborn PM, Moore EE, Morgan SJ, Johnson JL, Smith WR: Preperitonal pelvic packing for hemodynamically unstable pelvic fractures: A paradigm shift. *J Trauma* 2007;62(4):834-839, discussion 839-842.

   The authors describe the results of a team approach (critical care and orthopaedic trauma surgeons) to peritoneal and pelvic packing in hemodynamically unstable patients with pelvic fracture. In this series of 29 patients, blood loss and the need for both angiography and transfusion were decreased with preperitoneal pelvic packing.

10. Young JW, Burgess AR, Brumback RJ, Poka A: Pelvic fractures: Value of plain radiography in early assessment and management. *Radiology* 1986;160(2):445-451.

11. Pennal GF, Tile M, Waddell JP, Garside H: Pelvic disruption: Assessment and classification. *Clin Orthop Relat Res* 1980;151(151):12-21.

12. Garras DN, Carothers JT, Olson SA: Single-leg-stance (flamingo) radiographs to assess pelvic instability: How much motion is normal? *J Bone Joint Surg Am* 2008;90(10):2114-2118.

   Serial pelvic radiographs were taken in healthy men and multiparous and nulliparous women to identify the normal range of motion at the symphysis. Multiparous women had the most motion, and up to 5 mm of motion at the symphysis was considered within normal limits.

© 2011 American Academy of Orthopaedic Surgeons

13. Siegel J, Tornetta P III: Single-leg-stance radiographs in the diagnosis of pelvic instability. *J Bone Joint Surg Am* 2008;90(10):2119-2125.

    Radiographic examination of 38 patients with pelvic pain for greater than 6 weeks was done. The authors attempted to correlate radiographic findings of instability (>5 mm of motion using flamingo views) with visual analog scores; no correlation was found.

14. Mason WT, Khan SN, James CL, Chesser TJ, Ward AJ: Complications of temporary and definitive external fixation of pelvic ring injuries. *Injury* 2005;36(5):599-604.

15. Gänsslen A, Pohlemann T, Krettek C: [A simple supraacetabular external fixation for pelvic ring fractures]. *Oper Orthop Traumatol* 2005;17(3):296-312.

16. Archdeacon MT, Arebi S, Le TT, Wirth R, Kebel R, Thakore M: Orthogonal pin construct versus parallel uniplanar pin constructs for pelvic external fixation: A biomechanical assessment of stiffness and strength. *J Orthop Trauma* 2009;23(2):100-105.

    The authors present a biomechanical comparison of traditional iliac crest external fixators, supra-acetabular fixators, and orthogonal pin fixators (combination of iliac crest and supra-acetabular pins) in a cadaver study. Orthogonal constructs were stiffer in resisting flexion and extension, whereas supra-acetabular constructs were superior in resisting internal and external rotation.

17. Ponsen KJ, Joosse P, Van Dijke GA, Snijders CJ: External fixation of the pelvic ring: An experimental study on the role of pin diameter, pin position, and parasymphyseal fixator pins. *Acta Orthop* 2007;78(5):648-653.

    The authors present a cadaver biomechanical study that showed increased external fixation frame stiffness with pin diameters of 8 mm as well as the addition of supra-acetabular pins to an iliac crest construct.

18. Sagi HC, Papp S: Comparative radiographic and clinical outcome of two-hole and multi-hole symphyseal plating. *J Orthop Trauma* 2008;22(6):373-378.

    A retrospective review of 92 patients treated with multihole and two-hole symphyseal plates is presented. Two-hole symphyseal plates were associated with a higher rate of loss of reduction, pelvic malunion, and fixation failure.

19. Simonian PT, Schwappach JR, Routt ML Jr, Agnew SG, Harrington RM, Tencer AF: Evaluation of new plate designs for symphysis pubis internal fixation. *J Trauma* 1996;41(3):498-502.

20. Starr AJ, Nakatani T, Reinert CM, Cederberg K: Superior pubic ramus fractures fixed with percutaneous screws: What predicts fixation failure? *J Orthop Trauma* 2008;22(2):81-87.

    The authors describe a technique for retrograde ramus screws in pelvic fractures and report a 15% complication rate in 82 patients. Elderly female patients with fractures medial to the lateral border of the foramen were predicted to have the greatest chance of failure of retrograde ramus screws.

21. Switzer JA, Nork SE, Routt ML Jr: Comminuted fractures of the iliac wing. *J Orthop Trauma* 2000;14(4):270-276.

22. Charnley GJ, Dorrell JH: Small bowel entrapment in an iliac wing fracture. *Injury* 1993;24(9):627-628.

23. Borrelli J JR, Koval KJ, Helfet DL: Operative stabilization of fracture dislocations of the sacroiliac joint. *Clin Orthop Relat Res* 1996;329:141-146.

24. Lefaivre KA, Starr AJ, Reinert CM: Reduction of displaced pelvic ring disruptions using a pelvic reduction frame. *J Orthop Trauma* 2009;23(4):299-308.

    The authors present a technical description and report of 35 patient consecutive series for the use of pelvic reduction frame for closed or percutaneous reduction of displaced pelvic ring injuries.

25. Matta JM, Yerasimides JG: Table-skeletal fixation as an adjunct to pelvic ring reduction. *J Orthop Trauma* 2007;21(9):647-656.

    A technical description of table-skeletal fixation for applying greater amounts of traction in the reduction of pelvic ring injuries is presented.

26. Yinger K, Scalise J, Olson SA, Bay BK, Finkemeier CG: Biomechanical comparison of posterior pelvic ring fixation. *J Orthop Trauma* 2003;17(7):481-487.

27. Keating JF, Werier J, Blachut P, Broekhuyse H, Meek RN, O'Brien PJ: Early fixation of the vertically unstable pelvis: The role of iliosacral screw fixation of the posterior lesion. *J Orthop Trauma* 1999;13(2):107-113.

28. Carlson DA, Scheid DK, Maar DC, Baele JR, Kaehr DM: Safe placement of S1 and S2 iliosacral screws: The "vestibule" concept. *J Orthop Trauma* 2000;14(4):264-269.

29. Kraemer W, Hearn T, Tile M, Powell J: The effect of thread length and location on extraction strengths of iliosacral lag screws. *Injury* 1994;25(1):5-9.

30. Moed BR, Geer BL: S2 iliosacral screw fixation for disruptions of the posterior pelvic ring: A report of 49 cases. *J Orthop Trauma* 2006;20(6):378-383.

    A retrospective review of posterior pelvic fixation using iliosacral screws placed into the S2 vertebral segment is presented. All screws were safely placed and there were no iatrogenic nerve injuries. Loss of reduction occurred in 4%.

31. van Zwienen CM, van den Bosch EW, Snijders CJ, Kleinrensink GJ, van Vugt AB: Biomechanical comparison of sacroiliac screw techniques for unstable pelvic ring fractures. *J Orthop Trauma* 2004;18(9):589-595.

32. Denis F, Davis S, Comfort T: Sacral fractures: An important problem. Retrospective analysis of 236 cases. *Clin Orthop Relat Res* 1988;227:67-81.

33. Simonain PT, Routt C Jr, Harrington RM, Tencer AF: Internal fixation for the transforaminal sacral fracture. *Clin Orthop Relat Res* 1996;323(323):202-209.

34. Reilly MC, Bono CM, Litkouhi B, Sirkin M, Behrens FF: The effect of sacral fracture malreduction on the safe placement of iliosacral screws. *J Orthop Trauma* 2003;17(2):88-94.

35. Beaulé PE, Antoniades J, Matta JM: Trans-sacral fixation for failed posterior fixation of the pelvic ring. *Arch Orthop Trauma Surg* 2006;126(1):49-52.

36. Griffin DR, Starr AJ, Reinert CM, Jones AL, Whitlock S: Vertically unstable pelvic fractures fixed with percutaneous iliosacral screws: Does posterior injury pattern predict fixation failure? *J Orthop Trauma* 2003;17(6): 399-405.

37. Schildhauer TA, Ledoux WR, Chapman JR, Henley MB, Tencer AF, Routt ML Jr: Triangular osteosynthesis and iliosacral screw fixation for unstable sacral fractures: A cadaveric and biomechanical evaluation under cyclic loads. *J Orthop Trauma* 2003;17(1):22-31.

38. Sagi HC, Militano U, Caron T, Lindvall E: A comprehensive analysis with minimum 1-year follow-up of vertically unstable transforaminal sacral fractures treated with triangular osteosynthesis. *J Orthop Trauma* 2009; 23(5):313-319, discussion 319-321.

   A technical description and case series of 40 patients followed both clinically and radiographically are presented. The study shows the reliability of triangular fixation in maintaining reduction of comminuted sacral fractures, but complications such as iatrogenic nerve injury (13%), L5/S1 scoliosis (16%), delayed union (25%), and symptomatic fixation requiring removal (95%) were common.

39. Schildhauer TA, Josten C, Muhr G: Triangular osteosynthesis of vertically unstable sacrum fractures: A new concept allowing early weight-bearing. *J Orthop Trauma* 1998;12(5):307-314.

40. Sagi HC: Technical aspects and recommended treatment algorithms in triangular osteosynthesis and spinopelvic fixation for vertical shear transforaminal sacral fractures. *J Orthop Trauma* 2009;23(5):354-360.

   The author describes the technical aspects to applying the technique of spinal-pelvic fixation contructs relative to vertical shear sacral fractures, with the specific intent of maintaining reduction and avoiding potential complications and pitfalls.

41. Nork SE, Jones CB, Harding SP, Mirza SK, Routt ML Jr: Percutaneous stabilization of U-shaped sacral fractures using iliosacral screws: Technique and early results. *J Orthop Trauma* 2001;15(4):238-246.

42. Schildhauer TA, Bellabarba C, Nork SE, Barei DP, Routt ML Jr, Chapman JR: Decompression and lumbopelvic fixation for sacral fracture-dislocations with spino-pelvic dissociation. *J Orthop Trauma* 2006;20(7): 447-457.

43. Collinge C, Coons D, Tornetta P, Aschenbrenner J: Standard multiplanar fluoroscopy versus a fluoroscopically based navigation system for the percutaneous insertion of iliosacral screws: A cadaver model. *J Orthop Trauma* 2005;19(4):254-258.

44. Day AC, Stott PM, Boden RA: The accuracy of computer-assisted percutaneous iliosacral screw placement. *Clin Orthop Relat Res* 2007;463:179-186.

   The authors report on a cadaver accuracy study in 10 specimens during which iliosacral screws were placed using surgical navigation and conventional multiplanar fluoroscopy. Accuracy with navigation was as good as that of conventional methods, deviations in the intended path with navigation occurred only in dysmorphic sacra, and radiation exposure was decreased.

45. Hak DJ, Olson SA, Matta JM: Diagnosis and management of closed internal degloving injuries associated with pelvic and acetabular fractures: The Morel-Lavallée lesion. *J Trauma* 1997;42(6):1046-1051.

46. Tseng S, Tornetta P III: Percutaneous management of Morel-Lavallee lesions. *J Bone Joint Surg Am* 2006; 88(1):92-96.

47. Dujardin FH, Hossenbaccus M, Duparc F, Biga N, Thomine JM: Long-term functional prognosis of posterior injuries in high-energy pelvic disruption. *J Orthop Trauma* 1998;12(3):145-150, discussion 150-151.

48. Tornetta P III, Matta JM: Outcome of operatively treated unstable posterior pelvic ring disruptions. *Clin Orthop Relat Res* 1996;329(329):186-193.

49. Cole JD, Blum DA, Ansel LJ: Outcome after fixation of unstable posterior pelvic ring injuries. *Clin Orthop Relat Res* 1996;329(329):160-179.

50. Mullis BH, Sagi HC: Minimum 1-year follow-up for patients with vertical shear sacroiliac joint dislocations treated with iliosacral screws: Does joint ankylosis or anatomic reduction contribute to functional outcome? *J Orthop Trauma* 2008;22(5):293-298.

   Patients with pure SI dislocations treated with iliosacral screws were followed up after a minimum of 1 year for both functional outcome testing and CT. No correlation was made between the degree of ankylosis and functional outcome; however, magnitude of combined displacement was correlated with outcome, confirming some earlier studies.

51. Gustavo Parreira J, Coimbra R, Rasslan S, Oliveira A, Fregoneze M, Mercadante M: The role of associated injuries on outcome of blunt trauma patients sustaining pelvic fractures. *Injury* 2000;31(9):677-682.

52. Nepola JV, Trenhaile SW, Miranda MA, Butterfield SL, Fredericks DC, Riemer BL: Vertical shear injuries: Is there a relationship between residual displacement and functional outcome? *J Trauma* 1999;46(6):1024-1029, discussion 1029-1030.

53. Pohlemann T, Gänsslen A, Schellwald O, Culemann U, Tscherne H: Outcome after pelvic ring injuries. *Injury* 1996;27(suppl 2):B31-B38.

54. Ramirez JI, Velmahos GC, Best CR, Chan LS, Demetriades D: Male sexual function after bilateral internal iliac artery embolization for pelvic fracture. *J Trauma* 2004;56(4):734-739, discussion 739-741.

55. Copeland CE, Bosse MJ, McCarthy ML, et al: Effect of trauma and pelvic fracture on female genitourinary, sexual, and reproductive function. *J Orthop Trauma* 1997; 11(2):73-81.

56. Cannada LK, Barr J: Pelvic fractures in woment of childbearing age. *Clin Orthop Relat Res* 2010;468(7): 1781-1789.

    The authors completed a review of 71 women of childbearing age who sustained pelvic fractures. There was a high incidence of genitourinary complaints (49%) in this population; 38% of women had pain with sexual intercourse. Twenty-six women had children after their pelvic fracture: 38% delivered vaginally and 62% had a cesarean section. Four of the women who delivered vaginally had surgical fixation of their pelvic fracture. The rate of cesarean section was more than double standard norms, but the authors found that vaginal delivery after a pelvic fracture, even with surgical fixation sparing the public symphysis, is possible.

57. O'brien DP, Luchette FA, Pereira SJ, et al: Pelvic fracture in the elderly is associated with increased mortality. *Surgery* 2002;132(4):710-714, discussion 714-715.

58. Laird A, Keating JF: Acetabular fractures: A 16-year prospective epidemiological study. *J Bone Joint Surg Br* 2005;87(7):969-973.

59. Letournel E: Acetabulum fractures: Classification and management. *Clin Orthop Relat Res* 1980;151 :81-106.

60. Beaulé PE, Dorey FJ, Matta JM: Letournel classification for acetabular fractures: Assessment of interobserver and intraobserver reliability. *J Bone Joint Surg Am* 2003;85-A(9):1704-1709.

61. Ohashi K, El-Khoury GY, Abu-Zahra KW, Berbaum KS: Interobserver agreement for Letournel acetabular fracture classification with multidetector CT: are standard Judet radiographs necessary? *Radiology* 2006; 241(2):386-391.

62. Borrelli J Jr, Peelle M, McFarland E, Evanoff B, Ricci WM: Computer-reconstructed radiographs are as good as plain radiographs for assessment of acetabular fractures. *Am J Orthop (Belle Mead NJ)* 2008;37(9):455-459, discussion 460.

    This study evaluated 11 retrospectively identified patients with displaced acetabular fractures. Five orthopaedic surgeons with various trauma experience evaluated computer-generated radiographic acetabular series from information gathered on CT scan and overall were pleased with the provided information.

63. Matta JM: Fractures of the acetabulum: accuracy of reduction and clinical results in patients managed operatively within three weeks after the injury. *J Bone Joint Surg Am* 1996;78(11):1632-1645.

64. Scannell BP, Loeffler BJ, Bosse MJ, Kellam JF, Sims SH: Efficacy of intraoperative red blood cell salvage and autotransfusion in the treatment of acetabular fractures. *J Orthop Trauma* 2009;23(5):340-345.

    This recent analysis of 186 acetabular surgeries in which 60 of the patients had cell-saver could not yield a significant difference in the rates of intraoperative and postoperative transfusion received by patients. The cell-saver group averaged a 282% greater cost in blood-related charges.

65. Magnussen RA, Tressler MA, Obremskey WT, Kregor PJ: Predicting blood loss in isolated pelvic and acetabular high-energy trauma. *J Orthop Trauma* 2007;21(9): 603-607.

    In a retrospective review of 289 acetabular fractures, both-column, anterior column, anterior column posterior hemitransverse, and T-type fractures had a 56% incidence of receiving transfusion within 24 hours of admission compared to 28% for other fracture types.

66. Katsoulis E, Giannoudis PV: Impact of timing of pelvic fixation on functional outcome. *Injury* 2006;37(12): 1133-1142.

67. Pape HC, Griensven MV, Hildebrand FF, et al; Epoff Study group: Systemic inflammatory response after extremity or truncal fracture operations. *J Trauma* 2008; 65(6):1379-1384.

    This prospective multicenter, nonrandomized, cohort study evaluated 68 patients with truncal or extremity fractures. Patients were separated into three groups: spine fractures; pelvic or acetabular fractures; and femur fractures. Perioperative concentrations of IL-6 and IL-8 were evaluated during a 24-hour period and set in relation with the duration of surgery and degree of blood loss.

68. Matta JM, Anderson LM, Epstein HC, Hendricks P: Fractures of the acetabulum: A retrospective analysis. *Clin Orthop Relat Res* 1986;205:230-240.

69. Olson SA, Matta JM: The computerized tomography subchondral arc: A new method of assessing acetabular articular continuity after fracture (a preliminary report). *J Orthop Trauma* 1993;7(5):402-413.

70. Vrahas MS, Widding KK, Thomas KA: The effects of simulated transverse, anterior column, and posterior column fractures of the acetabulum on the stability of the hip joint. *J Bone Joint Surg Am* 1999;81(7):966-974.

71. Chuckpaiwong B, Suwanwong P, Harnroongroj T: Roof-arc angle and weight-bearing area of the acetabulum. *Injury* 2009;40(10):1064-1066.

    The purpose of this cadaver study was to identify exactly the medial, anterior, and posterior roof-arc angles that cross the weight bearing dome. Twenty cadaver hips had simulated transverse fractures created and radiographs obtained. The average medial, anterior, and posterior roof-arc angles were 46°, 52°, 61°, respectively.

72. Tornetta P III: Non-operative management of acetabular fractures. The use of dynamic stress views. *J Bone Joint Surg Br* 1999;81(1):67-70.

73. Levine RG, Renard R, Behrens FF, Tornetta P III: Biomechanical consequences of secondary congruence after both-column acetabular fracture. *J Orthop Trauma* 2002;16(2):87-91.

74. Sen RK, Veerappa LA: Long-term outcome of conservatively managed displaced acetabular fractures. *J Trauma* 2009;67(1):155-159.

   This review of 32 patients with displaced acetabular fractures (>3 mm) treated nonsurgically evaluated long-term follow-up (≥2 years). In 18 of 32 patients, fracture reduction was achieved along with a good to excellent clinical score.

75. Patel V, Day A, Dinah F, Kelly M, Bircher M: The value of specific radiological features in the classification of acetabular fractures. *J Bone Joint Surg Br* 2007;89(1): 72-76.

   Thirty sets of radiographs and CT scans were analyzed by six observers on two separate occasions with only a moderate interobserver and intraobserver agreement between description of associated issues with the acetabular fracture, as well as the fracture itself.

76. Boraiah S, Ragsdale M, Achor T, Zelicof S, Asprinio DE: Open reduction internal fixation and primary total hip arthroplasty of selected acetabular fractures. *J Orthop Trauma* 2009;23(4):243-248.

   This retrospective series of 18 patients using similar techniques, with an average age of 72 years and average follow-up of 3.9 years, yielded a mean Harris hip score of 88, minimal cup migration, no loosening, and one acute revision within 3 weeks.

77. Mears DC, Velyvis JH, Chang CP: Displaced acetabular fractures managed operatively: indicators of outcome. *Clin Orthop Relat Res* 2003;407:173-186.

78. Pascarella R, Maresca A, Reggiani LM, Boriani S: Intra-articular fragments in acetabular fracture-dislocation. *Orthopedics* 2009;32(6):402.

   Three hundred seventy-three acetabular fractures were reviewed over a 10-year period; 127 had a fracture-dislocation. In 45 cases, postreduction CT displayed intra-articular bony fragments that were not consistently defined on plain radiograph, thus, supporting postreduction CT scans in these patients.

79. Moed BR, Ajibade DA, Israel H: Computed tomography as a predictor of hip stability status in posterior wall fractures of the acetabulum. *J Orthop Trauma* 2009;23(1):7-15.

80. O'Shea K, Quinlan JF, Waheed K, Brady OH: The use-fulness of computed tomography following open reduction and internal fixation of acetabular fractures. *J Orthop Surg (Hong Kong)* 2006;14(2):127-132.

81. Templeman DC, Olson S, Moed BR, Duwelius P, Matta JM: Surgical treatment of acetabular fractures. *Instr Course Lect* 1999;48:481-496.

82. Qureshi AA, Archdeacon MT, Jenkins MA, Infante A, DiPasquale T, Bolhofner BR: Infrapectineal plating for acetabular fractures: A technical adjunct to internal fixation. *J Orthop Trauma* 2004;18(3):175-178.

83. Jakob M, Droeser R, Zobrist R, Messmer P, Regazzoni P: A less invasive anterior intrapelvic approach for the treatment of acetabular fractures and pelvic ring injuries. *J Trauma* 2006;60(6):1364-1370.

84. Cole JD, Bolhofner BR: Acetabular fracture fixation via a modified Stoppa limited intrapelvic approach: Description of operative technique and preliminary treatment results. *Clin Orthop Relat Res* 1994;305 :112-123.

85. Ponsen KJ, Joosse P, Schigt A, Goslings JC, Luitse JS: Internal fracture fixation using the Stoppa approach in pelvic ring and acetabular fractures: Technical aspects and operative results. *J Trauma* 2006;61(3):662-667.

86. Griffin DB, Beaulé PE, Matta JM: Safety and efficacy of the extended iliofemoral approach in the treatment of complex fractures of the acetabulum. *J Bone Joint Surg Br* 2005;87(10):1391-1396.

87. Johnson EE, Matta JM, Mast JW, Letournel E: Delayed reconstruction of acetabular fractures 21-120 days following injury. *Clin Orthop Relat Res* 1994;305 :20-30.

88. Alonso JE, Davila R, Bradley E: Extended iliofemoral versus triradiate approaches in management of associated acetabular fractures. *Clin Orthop Relat Res* 1994; 305:81-87.

89. Stöckle U, Hoffmann R, Südkamp NP, Reindl R, Haas NP: Treatment of complex acetabular fractures through a modified extended iliofemoral approach. *J Orthop Trauma* 2002;16(4):220-230.

90. Rommens PM: Is there a role for percutaneous pelvic and acetabular reconstruction? *Injury* 2007;38(4):463-477.

   This article reviews the indications and techniques as well as indications for incorporating percutaneous pelvic and acetabular reduction and fixation techniques into the complex algorithm of treating these injuries.

91. Starr AJ, Jones AL, Reinert CM, Borer DS: Preliminary results and complications following limited open reduction and percutaneous screw fixation of displaced fractures of the acetabulum. *Injury* 2001;32(Suppl 1): SA45-SA50.

92. Rosenberger RE, Dolati B, Larndorfer R, Blauth M, Krappinger D, Bale RJ: Accuracy of minimally invasive

4: Lower Extremity

navigated acetabular and iliosacral fracture stabilization using a targeting and noninvasive registration device. *Arch Orthop Trauma Surg* 2010;130(2):223-230.

The accuracy of guide pin placement was evaluated in 12 patients with a noninvasive targeting and registration device for treatment of acetabular fractures and iliosacral fractures. Accuracy of the target and starting and ending points was within 2.8 to 3.9 mm. The authors concluded that this method was effective in stabilizing the injuries described.

93. Kendoff D, Gardner MJ, Citak M, et al: Value of 3D fluoroscopic imaging of acetabular fractures comparison to 2D fluoroscopy and CT imaging. *Arch Orthop Trauma Surg* 2008;128(6):599-605.

In 24 cadaver acetabuli, the authors compared the accuracy of three-dimensional fluoroscopic imaging in evaluating acetabular fracture displacement and implant placement with fluoroscopy and CT scans. Its sensitivity and specificity for evaluating intraoperative hardware was greater than two-dimensional fluoroscopy and equivalent to CT scan.

94. Cimerman M, Kristan A: Preoperative planning in pelvic and acetabular surgery: The value of advanced computerised planning modules. *Injury* 2007;38(4):442-449.

Poperative planning of bone fragment reduction, plate contouring, and hardware placement using a computer-generated model from preoperative CT scans were helpful before pelvic and acetabular surgery in 10 cases.

95. Starr AJ, Reinert CM, Jones AL: Percutaneous fixation of the columns of the acetabulum: A new technique. *J Orthop Trauma* 1998;12(1):51-58.

96. Mouhsine E, Garofalo R, Borens O, et al: Percutaneous retrograde screwing for stabilisation of acetabular fractures. *Injury* 2005;36(11):1330-1336.

97. Shazar N, Brumback RJ, Novak VP, Belkoff SM: Biomechanical evaluation of transverse acetabular fracture fixation. *Clin Orthop Relat Res* 1998;352 :215-222.

98. Chang JK, Gill SS, Zura RD, Krause WR, Wang GJ: Comparative strength of three methods of fixation of transverse acetabular fractures. *Clin Orthop Relat Res* 2001;392 :433-441.

99. Giordano V, do Amaral NP, Pallottino A, Pires e Albuquerque R, Franklin CE, Labronici PJ: Operative treatment of transverse acetabular fractures: is it really necessary to fix both columns? *Int J Med Sci* 2009;6(4): 192-199.

This recent evaluation of 35 patients with a minimum 18-month follow-up showed that isolated posterior column fixation with dual plating did not yield statistically different radiographic or clinical results when compared to posterior column plating combined with anterior column screw fixation.

100. Mehin R, Jones B, Zhu Q, Broekhuyse H: A biomechanical study of conventional acetabular internal fracture fixation versus locking plate fixation. *Can J Surg* 2009;52(3):221-228.

In a biomechanical study, the authors found that locked plating provides similar strength when compared to conventional plating plus interfragmentary screw for fixing transverse acetabular fractures in terms of resisting displacement under cyclical loading.

101. Giannoudis PV, Tzioupis C, Moed BR: Two-level reconstruction of comminuted posterior-wall fractures of the acetabulum. *J Bone Joint Surg Br* 2007;89(4):503-509.

In an effort to provide further stability in the presence of marginal impaction that has been reduced, subchondral minifragment specific fixation was used by the authors in 29 acetabular fractures to supplement buttress plating, with 93% good to excellent results at a mean follow-up of 35 months.

102. Richter H, Hutson JJ, Zych G: The use of spring plates in the internal fixation of acetabular fractures. *J Orthop Trauma* 2004;18(3):179-181.

103. Mast JW: Techniques of open reduction and fixation of acetabular fractures, in Tile M, Helfet DL, Kellam JF, eds: *Fractures of the Pelvis and Acetabulum*, ed 3. Philadelphia, PA, Lippincott Williams & Wilkins, 2003, pp 632-633.

104. Anglen JO, Burd TA, Hendricks KJ, Harrison P: The "gull sign": A harbinger of failure for internal fixation of geriatric acetabular fractures. *J Orthop Trauma* 2003;17(9):625-634.

105. Mears DC: Surgical treatment of acetabular fractures in elderly patients with osteoporotic bone. *J Am Acad Orthop Surg* 1999;7(2):128-141.

106. Pagenkopf E, Grose A, Partal G, Helfet DL: Acetabular fractures in the elderly: Treatment recommendations. *HSS J* 2006;2(2):161-171.

107. Dean DB, Moed BR: Late salvage of failed open reduction and internal fixation of posterior wall fractures of the acetabulum. *J Orthop Trauma* 2009;23(3):180-185.

The outcome of late revision surgery was retrospectively reviewed in a series of four patients with posterior wall fractures having recurrent hip instability after failed initial open reduction and internal fixation. Three of four patients ultimately required arthroplasty.

108. Mears DC, Velyvis JH: Acute total hip arthroplasty for selected displaced acetabular fractures: Two to twelve-year results. *J Bone Joint Surg Am* 2002;84-A(1):1-9.

109. Letournel E, Judet R: *Fractures of the Acetabulum*, ed 2. New York, NY, Springer-Verlag, 1993, pp 535-562.

110. Engsberg JR, Steger-May K, Anglen JO, Borrelli J Jr: An analysis of gait changes and functional outcome in patients surgically treated for displaced acetabular fractures. *J Orthop Trauma* 2009;23(5):346-353.

According to a review of kinematic data, patients surgically treated for acetabular fractures, regardless of the open approach used, had alterations in gait patterns and strength at all joints of the affected extremity.

111. Letournel E, Judet R: *Fractures of the Acetabulum*, ed 2. New York, NY, Springer-Verlag, 1993, pp 535-537.

112. Hak DJ, Olson SA, Matta JM: Diagnosis and management of closed internal degloving injuries associated with pelvic and acetabular fractures: The Morel-Lavallée lesion. *J Trauma* 1997;42(6):1046-1051.

113. Russell GV Jr, Nork SE, Chip Routt ML Jr: Perioperative complications associated with operative treatment of acetabular fractures. *J Trauma* 2001;51(6):1098-1103.

114. Porter SE, Russell GV, Dews RC, Qin Z, Woodall J Jr, Graves ML: Complications of acetabular fracture surgery in morbidly obese patients. *J Orthop Trauma* 2008;22(9):589-594.

   Morbid obesity carries a relative risk of 2.6 when overall complication rate is considered. A recent series showed a statistically significant increase in total operative time, hospital stay, and complication rate (63%) in morbidly obese patients. Although not a statistically significant finding, morbidly obese patients also had increased positioning time and estimated intraoperative blood loss.

115. Karunakar MA, Shah SN, Jerabek S: Body mass index as a predictor of complications after operative treatment of acetabular fractures. *J Bone Joint Surg Am* 2005; 87(7):1498-1502.

116. Routt ML Jr: Surgical treatment of acetabular fractures, in Browner BD, Jupiter JB, Levine AM, Trafton PG, Krettek C, eds: *Skeletal Trauma*, ed 4. Philadelphia, PA, Saunders, 2009, pp 1207-1208.

117. Letournel E, Judet R: *Fractures of the Acetabulum* ed 2. New York, NY, Springer-Verlag, 1993. pp 537-539.

118. Dunbar RP Jr, Gardner MJ, Cunningham B, Routt ML Jr: Sciatic nerve entrapment in associated both-column acetabular fractures: A report of 2 cases and review of the literature. *J Orthop Trauma* 2009;23(1):80-83.

   This case report cites two cases in which the sciatic nerve was found entrapped in the posterior column component of a both-column fracture requiring surgical release. Both patients had return of nerve function after release.

119. Issack PS, Helfet DL: Sciatic nerve injury associated with acetabular fractures. *HSS J* 2009;5(1):12-18.

   This review outlines the potential causes of sciatic nerve injury from acetabular fractures, their treatment, and long-term sequelae. The authors discuss the superior results of sensory as opposed to motor function return with release.

120. Helfet DL, Anand N, Malkani AL, et al: Intraoperative monitoring of motor pathways during operative fixation of acute acetabular fractures. *J Orthop Trauma* 1997;11(1):2-6.

121. Haidukewych GJ, Scaduto J, Herscovici D Jr, Sanders RW, DiPasquale T: Iatrogenic nerve injury in acetabular fracture surgery: a comparison of monitored and unmonitored procedures. *J Orthop Trauma* 2002;16(5): 297-301.

122. Triantaphillopoulos PG, Panagiotopoulos EC, Mousafiris C, Tyllianakis M, Dimakopoulos P, Lambiris EE: Long-term results in surgically treated acetabular fractures through the posterior approaches. *J Trauma* 2007; 62(2):378-382.

   The authors reviewed results from 75 patients treated with open reduction and internal fixation of displaced acetabular fractures through a posterior approach. The patients' average follow-up was 12.5 years. Results were good to excellent in 80% and there was a definite correlation between radiographic and clinical results. The most frequent complication was HO (40%). Posttraumatic arthrosis was seen in 10.7% and osteonecrosis in 8%.

123. Murphy D, Kaliszer M, Rice J, McElwain JP: Outcome after acetabular fracture: Prognostic factors and their inter-relationships. *Injury* 2003;34(7):512-517.

124. Rath EM, Russell GV Jr, Washington WJ, Routt ML Jr: Gluteus minimus necrotic muscle debridement diminishes heterotopic ossification after acetabular fracture fixation. *Injury* 2002;33(9):751-756.

125. Burd TA, Lowry KJ, Anglen JO: Indomethacin compared with localized irradiation for the prevention of heterotopic ossification following surgical treatment of acetabular fractures. *J Bone Joint Surg Am* 2001; 83(12):1783-1788.

126. Blokhuis TJ, Frölke JP: Is radiation superior to indomethacin to prevent heterotopic ossification in acetabular fractures?: A systematic review. *Clin Orthop Relat Res* 2009;467(2):526-530.

   This meta-analysis of studies evaluating indomethacin in comparison with radiation for HO prophylaxis supports radiation therapy as the preferred method for preventing HO after surgical fixation of acetabular fractures.

127. Matta JM, Olson SA: Factors related to hip muscle weakness following fixation of acetabular fractures. *Orthopedics* 2000;23(3):231-235.

128. Anglen JO, DiPasquale T: The reliability of detecting screw penetration of the acetabulum by intraoperative auscultation. *J Orthop Trauma* 1994;8(5):404-408.

Hip Trauma

Brian H. Mullis, MD   Jeffrey Anglen, MD, FACS

4: Lower Extremity

Introduction

Injury to the hip, particularly fracture of the proximal femur, is a common and increasing cause of hospitalization, morbidity, and even mortality. In 2004, there were more than 320,000 hospital admissions in the United States because of hip fractures, with more than 500,000 hip fractures per year projected by 2040.[1] Approximately 4% of all deaths from injury in the United States are caused by hip fractures, and roughly 50% of fractures that lead to mortality are hip fractures.[2] In the younger population (generally defined as age younger than 65 years), hip fracture is usually caused by a high-energy injury, and mortality may result from associated injuries. The hip injury itself also can be a source of lifelong disability. In the elderly population, in whom hip fracture usually results from a low-energy mechanism such as a fall, mortality may ensue from associated medical comorbidities that are exacerbated by injury-related immobility or complications. In either population, the treatment decisions made by the orthopaedic surgeon may have a significant impact on the patient's outcome.

Hip trauma can consist of dislocation of the joint with or without associated fracture of the femur or acetabulum, or fracture of the proximal femur. Although fractures of the acetabulum are technically hip fractures, they will not be discussed in this chapter.

Hip Dislocations

Traumatic hip dislocations are high-energy injuries and are associated with other systemic and musculoskeletal

Dr. Mullis or an immediate family member serves as a board member, owner, officer, or committee member of Wishard Hospital and the Orthopaedic Trauma Association and has received research or institutional support from Amgen and Synthes. Dr. Anglen or an immediate family member serves as a board member, owner, officer, or committee member of the American Board of Orthopaedic Surgery, the American College of Surgeons, and the Orthopaedic Trauma Association; has received royalties from Biomet; serves as a paid consultant to or is an employee of Stryker; and has received research or institutional support from Stryker.

injuries in up to 75% of patients.[3] Dislocations may be simple (or not associated with a fracture), or may be more complex fracture-dislocations.[4] The rate of post-traumatic arthritis following a simple dislocation is up to 26% and can approach 90% in more complex fracture-dislocations.[5] This rate is particularly concerning because hip dislocation injuries often occur in young patients.

Given the inherent stability of the hip, a large force is needed to cause a dislocation. One of the more common mechanisms is a dashboard injury sustained during a motor vehicle collision in which the femoral head is driven posteriorly. There may also be an associated posterior wall or femoral head fracture. Other injury mechanisms include falls from a height, pedestrian–motor vehicle collisions, industrial accidents, and athletic injuries. Posterior dislocations accounts for 90% of all dislocations and are typically caused by a high-energy, axial load on the femur through a flexed and adducted hip.[6] Anterior dislocations are caused by an external rotation force in an abducted hip. A central dislocation describes protrusio of the femoral head associated with an acetabulum fracture.

Because there is a high association of other injuries in patients with hip dislocations, it is important that the Advanced Trauma Life Support (ATLS) protocols be followed before the focus turns to the musculoskeletal injuries. Up to 90% of patients will have visible swelling around the knee, with up to 25% of patients having significant internal knee derangement such as a cruciate or collateral ligament tear.[7]

A hip dislocation can typically be diagnosed based on the patient's physical examination. A patient with a posterior dislocation typically presents with a flexed, adducted, and internally rotated leg. An anterior dislocation results in an externally rotated leg with slight flexion and abduction. It is important to perform a detailed neurovascular examination before reduction is attempted. Typically, a plain radiograph of the pelvis is sufficient to make the diagnosis, but a cross-table lateral or frog-lateral radiograph should always be obtained in patients with pain and without an obvious dislocation or fracture based on the AP radiograph. A posterior dislocation is suggested by loss of congruency of the femoral head in the acetabulum, a lesser trochanter that is poorly visualized because of the internally rotated femur, and a femoral head that appears smaller than the contralateral side (**Figure 1**). Alternatively, a lesser trochanter seen in full profile with a larger femoral head suggests an anterior dislocation. If a femoral neck fracture is suspected, a CT scan before reduction is reasonable to prevent displacement of a possible fracture.

Closed reduction is typically achieved by traction in line with the deformity, with the patient under adequate sedation. Following reduction, an AP plain radiograph and CT scan of the pelvis are typically obtained to confirm a concentric reduction. A nonconcentric reduction indicates the presence of a loose body within the joint and warrants surgical removal. Ideally, this would be done urgently because of the pressure on the articular cartilage from the osteochondral loose body fragment. However, some surgeons believe that skeletal

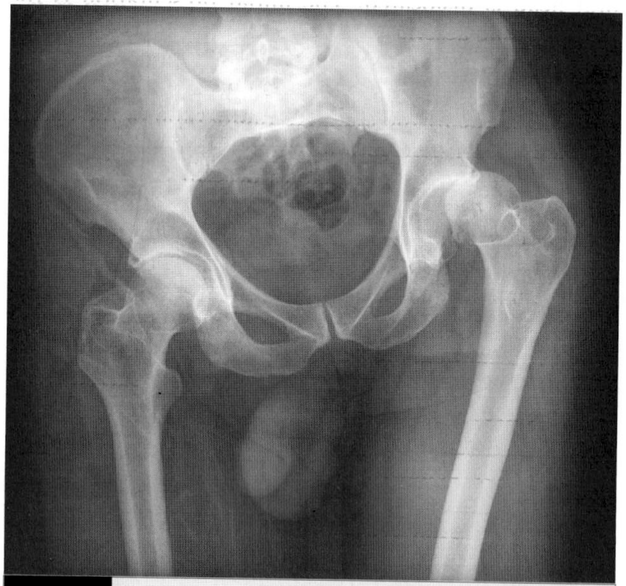

Figure 1   AP radiograph of the pelvis showing a posterior dislocation with the loss of profile of the lesser trochanter and the smaller femoral head.

traction is adequate to relieve pressure on the joint if surgery must be delayed. Even in the presence of a concentric reduction, loose bodies may be present that are too small to detect with CT.[8,9]

If closed reduction is unsuccessful, open reduction must be performed. Traditionally, the approach was determined by the direction of dislocation because of concern that an approach from the opposite direction would further disrupt the remaining blood supply to the femoral head.[10] However, it has been shown that it is safe to approach the hip opposite the direction of dislocation when such an approach is warranted because of associated injuries (for example, an anterior approach for a posterior dislocation if there is an associated femoral head or neck fracture).[11]

The critical time period from injury to reduction to prevent osteonecrosis is controversial. Based on studies showing lower rates of osteonecrosis in fractures reduced within 6 hours of injury, many surgeons use the 6-hour period as a guide.[12] The goal should be to achieve adequate sedation of the patient and to perform reduction as quickly as possible without putting the patient at risk for other life- or limb-threatening injuries. If osteonecrosis occurs, it will usually become apparent within the first year, but may not present until several years following injury.

After reduction, many surgeons restrict weight bearing by their patients to prevent possible femoral head collapse if osteonecrosis develops. Because no study has shown that prolonged non–weight-bearing restrictions impact the rate of osteonecrosis or femoral head collapse, consideration should be given to allowing patients to bear weight as tolerated immediately following reduction.[13]

Posterior Dislocations

The Thompson-Epstein and the Stewart-Milford classification systems (**Table 1**) have both been described in the literature,[4,5] and each essentially grades posterior

Table 1		
The Thompson-Epstein and the Stewart-Milford Classification Systems for Hip Dislocations		
Thompson-Epstein System		
Type I	Dislocation with or without minor fracture	
Type II	Posterior fracture-dislocation with a single, significant fragment	
Type III	Dislocation in which the posterior wall contains comminuted fragments with or without a major fragment	
Type IV	Dislocation with a large segment of posterior wall that extends into the acetabular floor	
Stewart-Milford System		
Type I	Simple dislocation with no fracture or an insignificant fracture	
Type II	Dislocation in a stable hip that has a significant single or comminuted element to the posterior wall	
Type III	Dislocation with a grossly unstable hip due to loss of bony support	
Type IV	Dislocation associated with femoral head fracture	

(Reproduced from Foulk DM, Mullis BH: Hip dislocation: Evaluation and management. *J Am Acad Orthop Surg* 2010;18:199-209.)

Chapter 31: **Hip Trauma**

hip dislocations as "simple" if there is no fracture, or as a more "complex" fracture-dislocation that is more likely to be unstable.[14,15] Small, posterior wall acetabulum fractures are frequently associated with posterior hip dislocations. Multiple studies have suggested that posterior wall fractures involving less than 20% of the wall are stable and may not necessarily warrant an examination under anesthesia if there is only a minor posterior wall fracture.[16,17] Posterior wall acetabulum fractures involving 20% to 50% of the wall are more likely to be unstable and warrant an examination under anesthesia. The examination is done by flexing the hip to 90° with slight adduction and internal rotation while applying a posteriorly directed force; fluoroscopy is used to determine if the femoral head maintains a concentric reduction.[18] If the hip is stable during examination under anesthesia and an open approach is not otherwise indicated because of a fracture of the posterior wall, femoral head, or femoral neck, hip arthroscopy is also a reasonable alternative with potentially less morbidity than a formal open approach. Posterior wall acetabulum fractures involving more than 50% of the wall require surgery.

Anterior Dislocations

Anterior hip dislocations account for less than 10% of hip dislocations and can be divided into three types (obturator, pubic, and iliac) based on the position of the femoral head as seen on the AP plain radiograph of the pelvis. Treatment is the same as for posterior dislocations, with reduction achieved by traction with abduction, and gentle internal and external rotation with slight flexion after adequate sedation is achieved.

The Role of Hip Arthroscopy

As advances have been made in hip arthroscopy, it has become a viable alternative to formal arthrotomies to remove loose bodies present within the hip.[8,9,19,20] Because the hip capsule has already been torn by the dislocation, hip arthroscopy is generally easier to perform in this setting because less force is needed to achieve distraction of the hip joint. Unfortunately, considerably more bleeding occurs during arthroscopy because it is typically done within several days of injury. Care must be taken to reduce surgical time to prevent complications from traction injuries or fluid extravasation because the hip capsule is torn.[9]

Complications

Because of the significantly increased risk of osteonecrosis and further articular injury, the most concerning complication is the missed or delayed diagnosis of a dislocation. The key to avoiding this complication is to obtain a good physical examination and to carefully review the AP plain radiograph of the pelvis. The risk of osteonecrosis following hip dislocation is 10% to 34% and usually occurs within 2 years of injury; however, osteonecrosis has been reported as many as 8 years following injury.[4,21] Posttraumatic arthritis is the most common complication following hip dislocation,

occurring in up to 20% of patients with simple dislocations and even higher rates in complex fracture-dislocations.[3,5,19,22] Sciatic nerve palsy is also common (15% occurrence rate) in posterior hip dislocations, with the peroneal division most affected.[14] Partial nerve recovery may be expected in 60% to 70% of patients.

Femoral Head Fractures

Femoral head fractures are relatively rare injuries that may present in up to 15% of posterior hip dislocations.[23] These fractures are usually associated with high-energy mechanisms such as motor vehicle collisions and are created by a shear mechanism as the femoral head is dislocated. The initial presentation is the same as that described for a posterior dislocation. The patient will typically present with an internally rotated, adducted, and flexed hip. Radiographic diagnosis is typically made by the plain AP radiograph of the pelvis. Because of the dislocation, emergent reduction is performed based on the principles described for posterior hip dislocations. Up to 10% of femoral head fracture-dislocations will be irreducible and should be treated as emergencies with open reduction in the surgical suite.[24] For the irreducible dislocation, it is reasonable to obtain an emergent CT scan because this may help with surgical planning; however, the scan should only be done if it will not unduly delay surgery. Delayed treatment of irreducible fracture-dislocations has been associated with higher rates of osteonecrosis.[24]

The most common classification used for femoral head fractures is still the Pipkin classification system (**Figure 2**). Pipkin type I fractures do not involve the weight-bearing portion of the femoral head. For this reason, if a concentric closed reduction can be achieved, nonsurgical management is acceptable. Pipkin type II fractures typically involve a large piece of the weight-bearing portion of the femoral head and are typically treated with open reduction and internal fixation. An anterior (Smith-Peterson) or anterolateral (Watson-Jones) approach provides the best visualization of the fracture. It has been shown that an anterior approach is safe following posterior dislocations and may allow shorter surgical time with less blood loss than a posterior approach for Pipkin type I and II fractures.[11] Pipkin type III fractures represent a more challenging injury because there is an associated femoral neck fracture. Reduction and fixation of the femoral head and neck can most easily be performed through an anterior or anterolateral approach. Pipkin type IV fractures have a posterior wall acetabulum fracture associated with the femoral head fracture. A posterior approach with a digastric osteotomy may afford the best visualization for both injuries and also protects the medial femoral circumflex artery from injury, thus preserving the blood supply to the femoral head[25,26] (**Figure 3**).

Fixation of a femoral head fracture has been described using a variety of implants. Two or more 3.5- or 2.7-mm lag screws are most commonly used with

4: Lower Extremity

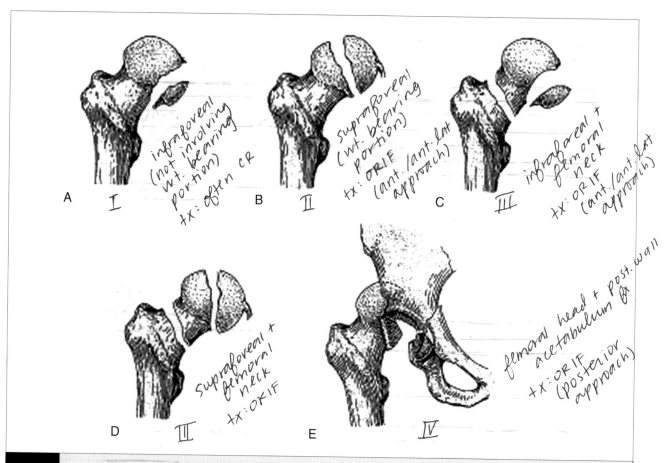

Figure 2 Illustration of the classification for femoral head fractures. **A,** Infrafoveal fracture, Pipkin type I. **B,** Suprafoveal fracture, Pipkin type II. Infrafoveal (**C**) or suprafoveal (**D**) femoral head fracture associated with a femoral neck fracture, Pipkin type III. **E,** Femoral head fracture associated with an acetabulum fracture, Pipkin type IV. (Reproduced with permission from Swiontkowski MF: Intrascapular hip fractures, in Browner BD, Jupiter JB, Levine AM, Trafton PF, eds: *Skeletal Trauma: Basic Science Management and Reconstruction*, ed 2. Philadelphia, PA, WB Saunders, 1992, p 1775.)

the heads of the screws countersunk to avoid prominence, but other implants, such as headless screws or bioabsorbable screws, are also available. The outcomes and complications of femoral head fractures mimic those of their associated injuries (hip dislocations and femoral neck fractures). A higher rate of osteonecrosis has been associated with the Kocher-Langenbeck approach, and worse outcomes with the use of 3.0-mm cannulated screws with washers.[27] There is a wide range (6% to 64%) in the reported incidence of heterotopic ossification.[12,23] In isolated hip injuries, consideration should be given to administering nonsteroidal anti-inflammatory drugs or radiation therapy if there is concern for heterotopic ossification, especially if the patient has an associated head injury.[28]

Hip Fractures

There are more than 2 million osteoporosis-related hip fractures in the United States annually, with an associated cost of more than $25 billion.[29] The annual inci-

dence is projected to increase to more than 3 million by 2025. Most patients with low-energy hip fractures are cared for at community hospitals. Patients treated by low-volume surgeons (fewer than 7 cases per year) and at low-volume hospitals (fewer than 57 cases per year) recently have been shown to have higher mortality rates, longer hospital stays, and higher complication rates.[30] This is not an indictment against community hospitals or surgeons, but does highlight the fact that even low-energy hip fractures should be not be considered "simple" fractures that are easily managed.

The adage, "never get sick in July," recently has been disproved with respect to hip fractures. Although some people believe that patients are placed at risk at academic centers in July because resident physicians take on new roles, the surgical mortality rate is no different in July for multiple procedures, including hip fractures.[31] Interestingly, there appears to be a higher rate of morbidity associated with hip fractures at academic centers following changes restricting the work hours of residents compared with historical controls before duty hours were limited.[32]

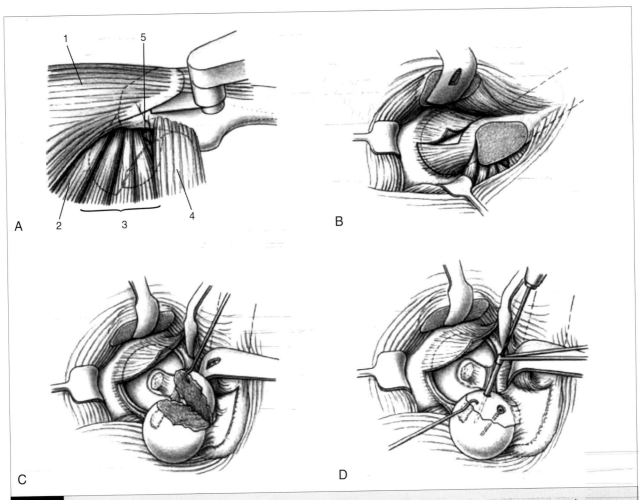

Figure 3 Illustration of digastric osteotomy to allow better visualization of a femoral head fracture from a posterior approach. **A,** Initial cut of the osteotomy (1: gluteus medius; 2: piriformis; 3: obturator internus and gemelli; 4: quadratus femoris; 5: deep branch of the medial circumflex femoral artery). **B,** Z-shaped capsular incision used for arthrotomy. **C** and **D,** Surgical dislocation with lag screw fixation of fracture. (Reproduced with permission from Henle P, Kloen P, Siebenrock KA: Femoral head injuries: Which treatment strategy can be recommended? *Injury* 2007;38(4):478-488. http://www.sciencedirect.com/science/journal/00201383.)

Femoral Neck Fractures

Classification

The type of femoral neck fracture is best determined with a traction, internal rotation, AP plain radiograph of the hip. The Garden classification is the most commonly used system for fractures in elderly patients, but could be further simplified to nondisplaced (Garden type I and II) and displaced (Garden type III and IV) fractures for treatment purposes[33,34] (**Figure 4**). The anatomic classification of basicervical, transcervical, and subcapital is also routinely used for low-energy fractures.

The Pauwels classification is more commonly used in describing high-energy fractures in young patients because this classification system is based on the angle of the fracture relative to a horizontal line (**Figure 5**). Type I fractures are less than 30°, type II are 30° to 50°, and type III fractures at greater than 50° are the most unstable fractures given the vertical orientation of the fracture line. Of note, the Pauwels classification system does not take into account fracture comminution, which is frequently present in high-energy fractures.

Treatment

Treatment principles differ for elderly patients with low-energy femoral neck fractures compared with younger patients with high-energy femoral neck fractures. Generally, elderly patients require appropriate medical risk stratification and management before surgery. Because delayed surgery has been shown to be an independent risk factor for mortality and other complications, every effort should be made to perform surgery within 2 to 4 days of the injury.[35-38] Young patients with high-energy fractures are generally considered to require more urgent treatment because of concern for vascular embarrassment of the femoral head with delayed surgery; however, excessive time should not be spent in the surgical suite when a patient in extremis with multiple injuries requires resuscitation.

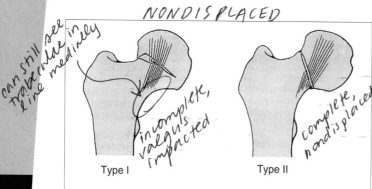

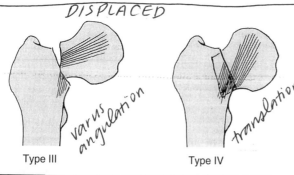

Handwritten annotations: NONDISPLACED; can still see trabecula in line medially; incomplete, valgus impacted; complete, nondisplaced; DISPLACED; varus angulation; translation

Type I   Type II

Type III   Type IV

Figure 4 Illustration of the Garden classification of femoral neck fractures. Type I: incomplete valgus impacted fracture. Type II: complete but nondisplaced fracture. Type III: displaced femoral neck fracture with varus malalignment. Type IV: displaced femoral neck fracture with trabeculae of the femoral head aligned with trabeculae of the acetabulum. (Reproduced with permission from Swiontkowski MF: Intrascapular hip fractures, in Browner BD, Jupiter JB, Levine AM, Trafton PF, eds: *Skeletal Trauma: Basic Science Management and Reconstruction*, ed 2. Philadelphia, PA, WB Saunders, 1992, p 1775.)

show if a fracture is present and the fracture propagation. Typically, a stress fracture involving only the compression (inferior) aspect of the neck is treated nonsurgically by limiting weight bearing for several weeks until symptoms improve. If the fracture extends throughout the entire length of the femoral neck or involves the tension (superior) side, surgery is usually recommended to prevent displacement.

In a young patient with a high-energy, displaced, femoral neck fracture, surgery is usually performed urgently unless the patient cannot tolerate surgery because of physiologic derangement or traumatic brain injury. An anatomic reduction must be obtained, which may require an open approach. This can be performed through either an anterior (Smith-Peterson) or anterolateral (Watson-Jones) surgical approach with direct visualization of the anterior neck. Cannulated screws may provide inadequate fixation for these fractures, which often have a high angle (Pauwels type III) and comminution because of the high-energy mechanism of injury.[43-45] A fixed-angle device such as a blade plate or cephalomedullary nail, or even newer implants such as a locked proximal femoral plate, provide more resistance to displacement.

Intertrochanteric Femoral Fractures

Classification
Radiographic diagnosis of an intertrochanteric femoral fracture is best made with an AP pelvic or hip radiograph. In addition to a lateral radiograph of the hip, internal rotation views are helpful in accurately identifying the fracture pattern. There are multiple classification systems for intertrochanteric femoral fractures, and essentially all of these systems help distinguish whether the fracture is stable or unstable. This determination can be misleading because all intertrochanteric femoral fractures are potentially unstable without fixation, but the fracture pattern is useful in choosing between different types of implants. The more stable fracture patterns are simple fracture patterns that run along the intertrochanteric ridge. Fractures that involve the lateral wall of the greater trochanter or that extend below the lesser trochanter with loss of the posteromedial buttress of the calcar are more unstable patterns. Reverse obliquity or low transverse pertrochanteric femoral fractures also represent more unstable patterns (**Figure 6**).

Treatment
Stable (or simple) intertrochanteric femoral fractures are best treated with a sliding hip screw. Although there are multiple other devices available, such as proximal femoral locking plates and cephalomedullary nails, there is no evidence that these more expensive devices provide added benefits for the patient, and there is overwhelming evidence that there is a higher complication rate with cephalomedullary nails.[46-50] A simple two-hole sliding hip screw has been shown to be bio-

Handwritten margin annotations: elderly; young; Stable Bx

Elderly patients with nondisplaced or valgus impacted fractures can typically be treated with percutaneous fixation with cannulated screws. Traditionally, the displaced fracture was treated with hemiarthroplasty and there was debate over whether the femoral stem should be cemented or cementless. Current literature supports the use of cemented over cementless stems because most of the evidence shows no difference in perioperative mortality but more pain and higher complication rates with the cementless stems.[39] More recent debate has centered over the use of hemiarthroplasty versus total hip arthroplasty for displaced femoral neck fractures. There is now considerable evidence to support total hip arthroplasty over hemiarthroplasty for highly functional elderly patients; however, there may still be a role for cemented unipolar hemiarthroplasty in bedridden or poorly functioning patients with limited life expectancy.[40-42]

In the young patient, an occult femoral neck fracture may occur without acute trauma in patients at risk for stress fracture such as amenorrheic women or marathon runners. Because these fractures typically are not seen on plain radiographs, a screening MRI may best

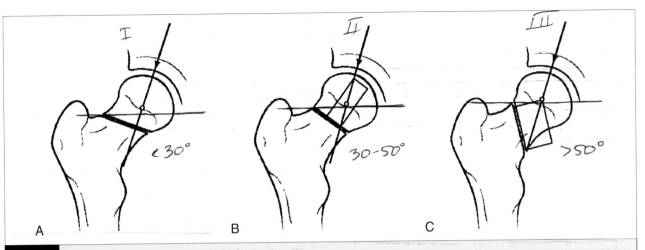

[handwritten: < 30°, 30-50°, >50°]

Figure 5	Illustration of the Pauwels classification for femoral neck fractures. **A,** Type I: the fracture angle is less than 30° from horizontal. **B,** Type II: the fracture angle is 30° to 50°. **C,** Type III: the fracture angle is greater than 50°. (Adapted with permission from Orthopaedic Trauma Association Classification, Database and Outcomes Committee: Fracture and Dislocation Classification Compendium, 2007. *J Orthop Trauma* 2007;21(suppl 10):S1-S163.)

mechanically stable for this fracture pattern, provides good clinical outcomes, and can be placed percutaneously.[51,52]

Fixation of unstable intertrochanteric femoral fractures is more controversial. There is a trend toward using cephalomedullary nails for these fractures among young practitioners.[53] The reason for this is unclear, but it has been postulated that this trend may reflect differences in reimbursement, the effect of marketing, or changes in training. There is evidence that supports the use of cephalomedullary nails in unstable fracture patterns.[49,54-56] Improved designs of newer-generation cephalomedullary nails and advances in techniques may have reduced the higher complication rate with these devices.[57] It is important to recognize fracture patterns that have a higher failure rate with traditional sliding hip screws, including fractures involving the lateral wall, reverse obliquity fractures, and low transverse peritrochanteric fractures. These fracture patterns should not be treated with a sliding hip screw; a cephalomedullary nail appears to be a better choice than a fixed-angle device for these fractures.[50]

Subtrochanteric Femoral Fractures

Classification

As with most fractures, there are multiple classification systems available to describe subtrochanteric femoral fractures. Most of these systems define the subtrochanteric fracture as a femoral fracture in which the major fracture line is within 5 cm of the lesser trochanter. As the fracture extends more proximally, the fracture is more difficult to control because of the deforming forces (flexion, abduction, and external rotation) on the proximal fragment and the greater distance of the fracture line from the isthmus of the femur.

[handwritten annotations: relatively stable; unstable; tx: sliding hip screw; tx: usually cephalo-medullary nail; most unstable; tx: cephalo-medullary nail]

Figure 6	AO/OTA classification of pertrochanteric femoral fractures. A1: relatively stable intertrochanteric femoral fracture; A2: relatively more unstable intertrochanteric femoral fracture because the fracture extends to lateral wall. A3: completely unstable pertrochanteric femoral fracture representing reverse obliquity or low transverse patterns. (Adapted with permission from Orthopaedic Trauma Association Classification, Database and Outcomes Committee: Fracture and Dislocation Classification Compendium, 2007. *J Orthop Trauma* 2007;21(suppl 10):S1-S163.)

[handwritten: narrowest part of bony canal; prox. frag. deforming f's: v. distal frag. adductors-prox. 1. ip-flex 2. gluteus-abduction 3. short rotators ext. rot. varus]

Treatment

Although fixed-angle devices have been described as treatment options for subtrochanteric femoral fractures,[58,59] most surgeons recommend the use of an intramedullary nail over an extramedullary device.[60] Although there has been a trend toward using the greater trochanter as a starting point for antegrade nailing for femoral fractures, the traditional piriformis fossa starting point still has a role, especially for subtrochanteric femoral fractures, because the piriformis fossa is coaxial with the rest of the femur, making it easier to achieve normal alignment. The disadvantage of using the trochanter as a starting point for nailing is that there can be a tendency to ream too laterally on the trochanter, which would lead to a varus deformity.[61] It is imperative to achieve an anatomic reduction before reaming a subtrochanteric femoral fracture. Many times this cannot be achieved by closed or percutaneous means, which may necessitate an open (or miniopen) reduction of the fracture to maintain alignment. It has been shown that judicious use of a cerclage wire placed to "maintain the reduction" is acceptable.[62] It should be noted that this technique should only be used if closed or percutaneous reduction fails; great care should be taken to avoid stripping the periosteum or overtightening the cable, which would lead to biologic insult to the periosteum.

Pathologic Fractures

Metastatic lesions of the proximal femur are common. It is necessary to proceed cautiously if the patient has a history of malignancy; it cannot be assumed that a pathologic lesion is a metastasis because it may represent a primary bone tumor. If there is concern that a lesion is a primary bone tumor, the patient is best referred to a musculoskeletal oncologist at a tertiary care center because of the high rate of errors (20%) that occur with biopsies obtained and analyzed at community medical centers.[63,64] Indications for surgery include pain with radiographic evidence of a lytic lesion in the proximal femur. Lesions of the femoral neck or femoral neck fractures are best treated with arthroplasty. Lesions or fractures in the intertrochanteric or subtrochanteric femur should be treated with a long cephalomedullary nail because of the possibility of skip lesions and future fracture if an extramedullary device is used. If there is significant lysis of the intertrochanteric region, a calcar-replacing prosthesis is also a reasonable treatment option.

Osteoporosis Evaluation and Treatment After Hip Fracture

Despite advances in medicine, the mortality rate following hip fracture in elderly patients is still 25% in the first year following injury, and may be higher in men than in women.[65] Ten million Americans have osteoporosis; one third of men and one half of women will have a fragility fracture in their lifetime. Involvement of orthopaedic surgeons in the identification, treatment, and referral of patients with osteoporosis has been shown to significantly reduce the risk of future fractures.[66] Active treatment of osteoporotic patients by the orthopaedic surgeon is more effective than referring patients to primary care clinics for treatment.[67] Treatment can be initiated while the patient is still an inpatient during his or her initial admission for the osteoporotic hip fracture. Although a multidisciplinary team is a good model for treating patients with osteoporosis, the orthopaedic surgeon should initiate therapy even if such a team has not been established at the physician's treatment facility. Prescribing calcium, vitamin D, and bisphosphonate therapy can significantly reduce the risk of a future hip fracture.[68,69] The American Orthopaedic Association's "Own the Bone" initiative offers orthopaedic surgeons tools to improve their communication with both patients who have had a hip fracture and their primary care physicians.[70]

Annotated References

1. ip fractures among older adults. Centers for Disease Control and Prevention Web site. http://www.cdc.gov/ncipc/factsheets/adulthipfx.htm. Accessed June 10, 2008.

   This online publication by the Centers for Disease Control and Prevention provides basic details regarding hip fractures in the United States.

2. Bergen G, Chen L, Warner M, Fingerhut L: Injury in the United States: 2007 chartbook. Hyattsville, MD, National Center for Health Statistics, 2008. http://www.cdc.gov/nchs/data/misc/injury2007.pdf. Accessed July 1, 2010.

   This US government online publication provides recent statistics regarding injuries in the United States.

3. Epstein HC: Traumatic dislocations of the hip. *Clin Orthop Relat Res* 1973;92:116-142.

4. Foulk DM, Mullis BH: Hip dislocation: Evaluation and management. *J Am Acad Orthop Surg* 2010;18(4):199-209.

   This review article focuses on recognition and management of traumatic hip dislocation and the role of newer technology such as hip arthroscopy in management.

5. Upadhyay SS, Moulton A: The long-term results of traumatic posterior dislocation of the hip. *J Bone Joint Surg Br* 1981;63B(4):548-551.

6. Dreinhöfer KE, Schwarzkopf SR, Haas NP, Tscherne H: Isolated traumatic dislocation of the hip: Long-term results in 50 patients. *J Bone Joint Surg Br* 1994;76(1):6-12.

7. Schmidt GL, Sciulli R, Altman GT: Knee injury in patients experiencing a high-energy traumatic ipsilateral

Chapter 31: Hip Trauma

hip dislocation. *J Bone Joint Surg Am* 2005;87(6):1200-1204.

8. Mullis BH, Dahners LE: Hip arthroscopy to remove loose bodies after traumatic dislocation. *J Orthop Trauma* 2006;20(1):22-26.

9. Yamamoto Y, Ide T, Ono T, Hamada Y: Usefulness of arthroscopic surgery in hip trauma cases. *Arthroscopy* 2003;19(3):269-273.

10. Epstein HC: Posterior fracture-dislocations of the hip: Long-term follow-up. *J Bone Joint Surg Am* 1974;56(6):1103-1127.

11. Swiontkowski MF, Thorpe M, Seiler JG, Hansen ST: Operative management of displaced femoral head fractures: Case-matched comparison of anterior versus posterior approaches for Pipkin I and Pipkin II fractures. *J Orthop Trauma* 1992;6(4):437-442.

12. Hougaard K, Thomsen PB: Coxarthrosis following traumatic posterior dislocation of the hip. *J Bone Joint Surg Am* 1987;69(5):679-683.

13. Sahin V, Karakaş ES, Aksu S, Atlihan D, Turk CY, Halici M: Traumatic dislocation and fracture-dislocation of the hip: A long-term follow-up study. *J Trauma* 2003;54(3):520-529.

14. Stewart MJ, Milford LW: Fracture-dislocation of the hip: An end-result study. *J Bone Joint Surg Am* 1954;36(A:2):315-342.

15. Thompson VP, Epstein HC: Traumatic dislocation of the hip: A survey of two hundred and four cases covering a period of twenty-one years. *J Bone Joint Surg Am* 1951;33(3):746-778, passim.

16. Keith JE Jr, Brashear HR Jr, Guilford WB: Stability of posterior fracture-dislocations of the hip: Quantitative assessment using computed tomography. *J Bone Joint Surg Am* 1988;70(5):711-714.

17. Moed BR, Ajibade DA, Israel H: Computed tomography as a predictor of hip stability status in posterior wall fractures of the acetabulum. *J Orthop Trauma* 2009;23(1):7-15.

    The authors report on their retrospective study showing that if the largest area of a posterior wall acetabulum fracture measures less than 20%, the hip is likely to be stable under fluoroscopic examination. Level of evidence: IV.

18. Tornetta P III: Non-operative management of acetabular fractures: The use of dynamic stress views. *J Bone Joint Surg Br* 1999;81(1):67-70.

19. Byrd JW, Jones KS: Diagnostic accuracy of clinical assessment, magnetic resonance imaging, magnetic resonance arthrography, and intra-articular injection in hip arthroscopy patients. *Am J Sports Med* 2004;32(7):1668-1674.

20. Philippon MJ, Kuppersmith DA, Wolff AB, Briggs KK: Arthroscopic findings following traumatic hip dislocation in 14 professional athletes. *Arthroscopy* 2009;25(2):169-174.

    This small retrospective series describes the results of hip arthroscopy for professional athletes with a simple (no fracture) hip dislocation. Level of evidence: IV.

21. Cash DJ, Nolan JF: Avascular necrosis of the femoral head 8 years after posterior hip dislocation. *Injury* 2007;38(7):865-867.

    This is a case report of a patient who had a simple posterior dislocation reduced within 3 hours of injury but did not develop osteonecrosis until 8 years after injury. Level of evidence: IV.

22. Upadhyay SS, Moulton A, Srikrishnamurthy K: An analysis of the late effects of traumatic posterior dislocation of the hip without fractures. *J Bone Joint Surg Br* 1983;65(2):150-152.

23. Droll KP, Broekhuyse H, O'Brien P: Fracture of the femoral head. *J Am Acad Orthop Surg* 2007;15(12):716-727.

    This review article discusses diagnosis and treatment of femoral head fractures.

24. Mehta S, Routt ML Jr: Irreducible fracture-dislocations of the femoral head without posterior wall acetabular fractures. *J Orthop Trauma* 2008;22(10):686-692.

    The authors report on a retrospective study reviewing seven patients with femoral head fracture-dislocations without an associated posterior wall fracture treated with open reduction and internal fixation using an anterior approach. The authors found just fewer than 10% of femoral head fractures at their institution (fracture-dislocations without posterior wall fracture) were of this variety and cautioned against attempts at closed reduction for this type of injury. They also noted those that were not treated as a surgical emergency were likely to develop osteonecrosis. Level of evidence: IV.

25. Henle P, Kloen P, Siebenrock KA: Femoral head injuries: Which treatment strategy can be recommended? *Injury* 2007;38(4):478-488.

    This restrospective review of 12 patients with femoral head fractures treated with a digastrics osteotomy (with illustrations and description of the technique) showed good or excellent results in over 80% of patients. Level of evidence: IV.

26. Solberg BD, Moon CN, Franco DP: Use of a trochanteric flip osteotomy improves outcomes in Pipkin IV fractures. *Clin Orthop Relat Res* 2009;467(4):929-933.

    This retrospective review of 12 patients with a combined femoral head and acetabulum fracture treated with a trochanteric flip osteotomy showed 10 of 12 patients had a good or excellent result. Level of evidence: IV.

27. Stannard JP, Harris HW, Volgas DA, Alonso JE: Functional outcome of patients with femoral head fractures associated with hip dislocations. *Clin Orthop Relat Res* 2000;377:44-56.

4: Lower Extremity

28. Webb LX, Bosse MJ, Mayo KA, Lange RH, Miller ME, Swiontkowski MF: Results in patients with craniocerebral trauma and an operatively managed acetabular fracture. *J Orthop Trauma* 1990;4(4):376-382.

29. Burge R, Dawson-Hughes B, Solomon DH, Wong JB, King A, Tosteson A: Incidence and economic burden of osteoporosis-related fractures in the United States, 2005-2025. *J Bone Miner Res* 2007;22(3):465-475.

    This study estimates the incidence of osteoporosis-related fractures in the United States in 2005 at 2 million fractures with a cost of $17 billion. The authors project both the cost and incidence of osteoporosis-related fractures to increase by 50% by the year 2025. Level of evidence: IV.

30. Browne JA, Pietrobon R, Olson SA: Hip fracture outcomes: Does surgeon or hospital volume really matter? *J Trauma* 2009;66(3):809-814.

    This review of just fewer than 100,000 hip fractures treated with surgery in the United States found that low-volume surgeons (those who operated on fewer than 7 hip fractures per year) had a higher mortality rate and higher rate of transfusions, pneumonia, and decubitus ulcers than high-volume surgeons (those who performed more than 15 hip surgeries for fractures per year). The review also found low-volume hospitals (those who performed fewer than 57 surgeries for hip fracture per year) were associated with higher rates of postoperative infection, pneumonia, transfusion, and nonroutine discharge, but were not associated with higher mortality. Both low-volume surgeons and low-volume hospitals had a longer length of stay for patients with hip fracture requiring surgery. Level of evidence: III.

31. Englesbe MJ, Fan Z, Baser O, Birkmeyer JD: Mortality in medicare patients undergoing surgery in July in teaching hospitals. *Ann Surg* 2009;249(6):871-876.

    This retrospective review of more than 300,000 patients having surgery for multiple conditions including hip fractures and others outside the field of orthopaedics showed no increased mortality in teaching hospitals in July (or any other month) relative to nonacademic hospitals. Level of evidence: III.

32. Browne JA, Cook C, Olson SA, Bolognesi MP: Resident duty-hour reform associated with increased morbidity following hip fracture. *J Bone Joint Surg Am* 2009; 91(9):2079-2085.

    The 80-hour workweek restrictions were made in July 2003. This retrospective review of more than 48,000 patients in the United States (those treated during 2001-2002 compared to 2004-2005) showed an increased rate of perioperative pneumonia, hematoma, transfusion, renal complications, nonroutine discharge, costs, and length of stay at teaching hospitals following the required changes to the resident work hours. There was no change seen with mortality. Level of evidence: III.

33. Beimers L, Kreder HJ, Berry GK, et al: Subcapital hip fractures: The Garden classification should be replaced, not collapsed. *Can J Surg* 2002;45(6):411-414.

34. Oakes DA, Jackson KR, Davies MR, et al: The impact of the garden classification on proposed operative treatment. *Clin Orthop Relat Res* 2003;409:232-240.

35. Hommel A, Ulander K, Bjorkelund KB, Norrman PO, Wingstrand H, Thorngren KG: Influence of optimised treatment of people with hip fracture on time to operation, length of hospital stay, reoperations and mortality within 1 year. *Injury* 2008;39(10):1164-1174.

    This retrospective study showed that surgical delay in treating hip fractures significantly increases mortality rates in some patients. Level of evidence: IV.

36. Moran CG, Wenn RT, Sikand M, Taylor AM: Early mortality after hip fracture: Is delay before surgery important? *J Bone Joint Surg Am* 2005;87(3):483-489.

37. Al-Ani AN, Samuelsson B, Tidermark J, et al: Early operation on patients with a hip fracture improved the ability to return to independent living: A prospective study of 850 patients. *J Bone Joint Surg Am* 2008; 90(7):1436-1442.

    This large prospective study showed that early fixation of hip fractures in elderly patients was significantly associated with a higher likelihood of return to independent living. Level of evidence: II.

38. Zuckerman JD, Skovron ML, Koval KJ, Aharonoff G, Frankel VH: Postoperative complications and mortality associated with operative delay in older patients who have a fracture of the hip. *J Bone Joint Surg Am* 1995; 77(10):1551-1556.

39. Miyamoto RG, Kaplan KM, Levine BR, Egol KA, Zuckerman JD: Surgical management of hip fractures: An evidence-based review of the literature. I: Femoral neck fractures. *J Am Acad Orthop Surg* 2008;16(10): 596-607.

    This article discusses the evidence supporting surgical treatment of hip fractures and outlining the evidence supporting different techniques and selection of implants.

40. Blomfeldt R, Törnkvist H, Eriksson K, Söderqvist A, Ponzer S, Tidermark J: A randomised controlled trial comparing bipolar hemiarthroplasty with total hip replacement for displaced intracapsular fractures of the femoral neck in elderly patients. *J Bone Joint Surg Br* 2007;89(2):160-165.

    This prospective randomized study of elderly patients with a displaced femoral neck fracture who were randomized to receive hemiarthroplasty versus total hip arthroplasty showed patients treated with total hip arthroplasty had higher function scores with no increased risk of complications as early as 1 year postoperatively. Level of evidence: I.

41. Goh SK, Samuel M, Su DH, Chan ES, Yeo SJ: Meta-analysis comparing total hip arthroplasty with hemiarthroplasty in the treatment of displaced neck of femur fracture. *J Arthroplasty* 2009;24(3):400-406.

    The authors report on their meta-analysis of randomized controlled trials comparing total hip arthroplasty to hemiarthroplasty. Patients treated with total hip arthro-

4: Lower Extremity

plasty had better function, less pain, and fewer repeat surgeries than those treated with hemiarthroplasty. Level of evidence: I.

42. Macaulay W, Nellans KW, Garvin KL, Iorio R, Healy WL, Rosenwasser MP; Other members of the DFACTO Consortium: Prospective randomized clinical trial comparing hemiarthroplasty to total hip arthroplasty in the treatment of displaced femoral neck fractures: Winner of the Dorr Award. *J Arthroplasty* 2008;23(6, Suppl 1): 2-8.

   In this prospective randomized study of patients treated with total hip arthroplasty versus hemiarthroplasty, the authors report that patients treated with total hip arthroplasty had better functional outcomes and less pain without a significantly increased risk of complication compared with patients treated with hemiarthroplasty. Level of evidence: I.

43. Aminian A, Gao F, Fedoriw WW, Zhang LQ, Kalainov DM, Merk BR: Vertically oriented femoral neck fractures: Mechanical analysis of four fixation techniques. *J Orthop Trauma* 2007;21(8):544-548.

   This biomechanical study of vertically unstable femoral neck fractures created in cadavers evaluated four treatment methods. Strongest fixation to weakest fixation was achieved with the following: a proximal femoral locking plate, a dynamic condylar screw, a dynamic hip screw, and cannulated screws.

44. Liporace F, Gaines R, Collinge C, Haidukewych GJ: Results of internal fixation of Pauwels type-3 vertical femoral neck fractures. *J Bone Joint Surg Am* 2008;90(8): 1654-1659.

   The authors present their findings in this retrospective review of vertical femoral neck fractures treated with a fixed-angled device versus cannulated screws. No difference in outcomes was found, although there was a trend toward a higher nonunion rate in the group treated with cannulated screw fixation. Level of evidence: IV.

45. Zlowodzki M, Brink O, Switzer J, et al: The effect of shortening and varus collapse of the femoral neck on function after fixation of intracapsular fracture of the hip: A multi-centre cohort study. *J Bone Joint Surg Br* 2008;90(11):1487-1494.

   This retrospective review of patients with displaced femoral neck fractures treated with cannulated screws showed that patients with varus collapse or shortening of the femoral neck had worse outcomes than those in whom reduction and length were maintained. Level of evidence: IV.

46. Adams CI, Robinson CM, Court-Brown CM, McQueen MM: Prospective randomized controlled trial of an intramedullary nail versus dynamic screw and plate for intertrochanteric fractures of the femur. *J Orthop Trauma* 2001;15(6):394-400.

47. Crawford CH, Malkani AL, Cordray S, Roberts CS, Sligar W: The trochanteric nail versus the sliding hip screw for intertrochanteric hip fractures: A review of 93 cases. *J Trauma* 2006;60(2):325-328, discussion 328-329.

48. Aros B, Tosteson AN, Gottlieb DJ, Koval KJ: Is a sliding hip screw or im nail the preferred implant for intertrochanteric fracture fixation? *Clin Orthop Relat Res* 2008;466(11):2827-2832.

   This case-control study reported longer length of hospital stay and higher costs associated with intramedullary nail versus sliding hip screw fixation for intertrochanteric femoral fractures. Level of evidence: III.

49. Haidukewych GJ: Intertrochanteric fractures: Ten tips to improve results. *J Bone Joint Surg Am* 2009;91(3): 712-719.

   This article provides technical tips and tricks on how to stay out of trouble when fixing intertrochanteric fractures. Level of evidence: V.

50. Parker MJ, Handoll HH: Gamma and other cephalocondylic intramedullary nails versus extramedullary implants for extracapsular hip fractures in adults. *Cochrane Database Syst Rev* 2008;3:CD000093.

   The authors report on their case-control study comparing the Gamma nail to sliding hip screws for extracapsular hip fractures in adults. Higher reoperation and complication rates were found with Gamma nails. Level of evidence: III.

51. Bolhofner BR, Russo PR, Carmen B: Results of intertrochanteric femur fractures treated with a 135-degree sliding screw with a two-hole side plate. *J Orthop Trauma* 1999;13(1):5-8.

52. McLoughlin SW, Wheeler DL, Rider J, Bolhofner B: Biomechanical evaluation of the dynamic hip screw with two- and four-hole side plates. *J Orthop Trauma* 2000;14(5):318-323.

53. Anglen JO, Weinstein JN; American Board of Orthopaedic Surgery Research Committee: Nail or plate fixation of intertrochanteric hip fractures: Changing pattern of practice. A review of the American Board of Orthopaedic Surgery Database. *J Bone Joint Surg Am* 2008; 90(4):700-707.

   A review of records of orthopaedic surgeons taking part II of the Board certification of the American Board of Orthopaedic Surgery showed an increasing use of cephalomedullary nail fixation for intertrochanteric femoral fractures. Level of evidence: IV.

54. Hardy DC, Descamps PY, Krallis P, et al: Use of an intramedullary hip-screw compared with a compression hip-screw with a plate for intertrochanteric femoral fractures: A prospective, randomized study of one hundred patients. *J Bone Joint Surg Am* 1998;80(5):618-630.

55. Kuzyk PR, Lobo J, Whelan D, Zdero R, McKee MD, Schemitsch EH: Biomechanical evaluation of extramedullary versus intramedullary fixation for reverse obliquity intertrochanteric fractures. *J Orthop Trauma* 2009; 23(1):31-38.

   A biomechanical study of reverse obliquity intertrochanteric femoral fractures showed that an intramedullary hip screw performed better than a 95° or 135° hip screw in a gap model. No differences in failure rates were seen when no gap existed at the fracture site.

56. Ruecker AH, Rupprecht M, Gruber M, et al: The treatment of intertrochanteric fractures: Results using an intramedullary nail with integrated cephalocervical screws and linear compression. *J Orthop Trauma* 2009;23(1): 22-30.

    This is a retrospective review of 48 patients treated with an InterTan (Smith and Nephew) cephalomedullary nail at a single institution. Level of evidence: IV.

57. Bhandari M, Schemitsch E, Jönsson A, Zlowodzki M, Haidukewych GJ: Gamma nails revisited: Gamma nails versus compression hip screws in the management of intertrochanteric fractures of the hip. A meta-analysis. *J Orthop Trauma* 2009;23(6):460-464.

    A meta-analysis of randomized trials comparing sliding hip screws to cephalomedullary nails for intertrochanteric femoral fractures showed the complications initially experienced with first-generation Gamma nails have improved over time. Recent trials suggest narrowing or a comparable complication rate with cephalomedullary nails of more recent design compared with compression hip screws. Level of evidence: I.

58. Madsen JE, Naess L, Aune AK, Alho A, Ekeland A, Strømsøe K: Dynamic hip screw with trochanteric stabilizing plate in the treatment of unstable proximal femoral fractures: A comparative study with the Gamma nail and compression hip screw. *J Orthop Trauma* 1998; 12(4):241-248.

59. Lee PC, Hsieh PH, Yu SW, Shiao CW, Kao HK, Wu CC: Biologic plating versus intramedullary nailing for comminuted subtrochanteric fractures in young adults: A prospective, randomized study of 66 cases. *J Trauma* 2007;63(6):1283-1291.

    The authors of this prospective, randomized, non-blinded study reported no higher failure rate in subtrochanteric femoral fractures treated with a dynamic condylar screw compared with a reconstruction nail; however, the hip screw was associated with more pain. Level of evidence: II.

60. Kuzyk PR, Bhandari M, McKee MD, Russell TA, Schemitsch EH: Intramedullary versus extramedullary fixation for subtrochanteric femur fractures. *J Orthop Trauma* 2009;23(6):465-470.

    This review of the literature showed grade B evidence that there is less operative time and a lower risk for loss of fixation when using intramedullary implants versus extramedullary implants for subtrochanteric femoral fractures.

61. Ostrum RF, Anglen JO, Archdeacon MT, Cannada LK, Herscovici D Jr: Prevention of complications after treatment of femoral shaft and distal femoral fractures. *Instr Course Lect* 2009;58:21-25.

    This article provides tips and tricks on how to stay out of trouble when treating femoral shaft and distal femoral fractures. Level of evidence: V.

62. Afsari A, Liporace F, Lindvall E, Infante A Jr, Sagi HC, Haidukewych GJ: Clamp-assisted reduction of high subtrochanteric fractures of the femur. *J Bone Joint Surg Am* 2009;91(8):1913-1918.

    In this retrospective review, subtrochanteric femoral fractures were treated with a limited open reduction if closed reduction could not be obtained. The reduction was held with a loosely applied cerclage cable. Acceptable union rates were achieved. Level of evidence: IV.

63. Mankin HJ, Lange TA, Spanier SS: The hazards of biopsy in patients with malignant primary bone and soft-tissue tumors. *J Bone Joint Surg Am* 1982;64(8):1121-1127.

64. Mankin HJ, Mankin CJ, Simon MA; Members of the Musculoskeletal Tumor Society: The hazards of the biopsy, revisited. *J Bone Joint Surg Am* 1996;78(5):656-663.

65. Yonezawa T, Yamazaki K, Atsumi T, Obara S: Influence of the timing of surgery on mortality and activity of hip fracture in elderly patients. *J Orthop Sci* 2009;14(5): 566-573.

    This retrospective study of more than 500 patients found increased mobility in those treated less than 24 hours, but higher mortality in a subset of sick patients treated less than 24 hours. The authors recommend otherwise healthy patients should have surgery within 24 hours but patients who have a medical condition which can be improved prior to surgery should be delayed. Level of evidence: III.

66. Dell R, Greene D, Schelkun SR, Williams K: Osteoporosis disease management: The role of the orthopaedic surgeon. *J Bone Joint Surg Am* 2008;90(Suppl 4):188-194.

    This study outlines how a dedicated program to identify and treat patients with osteoporosis was successful in a Kaiser HMO in California and estimates the reduction in hip fractures due to the program was 37%. The paper also discusses the role an orthopaedist can play in treating patients with osteoporosis.

67. Miki RA, Oetgen ME, Kirk J, Insogna KL, Lindskog DM: Orthopaedic management improves the rate of early osteoporosis treatment after hip fracture: A randomized clinical trial. *J Bone Joint Surg Am* 2008; 90(11):2346-2353.

    This randomized prospective study showed there was a significantly higher rate of pharmacologic treatment for osteoporosis when the treatment was initiated by the orthopaedist with referral to a specialized orthopaedic osteoporosis clinic rather than recommendation to the patient to follow up with primary care for osteoporosis treatment. Level of evidence: I.

68. Black DM, Cummings SR, Karpf DB, et al; Fracture Intervention Trial Research Group: Randomised trial of effect of alendronate on risk of fracture in women with existing vertebral fractures. *Lancet* 1996;348(9041): 1535-1541.

69. Harrington JT, Ste-Marie LG, Brandi ML, et al: Risedronate rapidly reduces the risk for nonvertebral fractures in women with postmenopausal osteoporosis. *Calcif Tissue Int* 2004;74(2):129-135.

70. Tosi LL, Gliklich R, Kannan K, Koval KJ: The American Orthopaedic Association's "own the bone" initiative to prevent secondary fractures. *J Bone Joint Surg Am* 2008;90(1):163-173.

This article reviews the American Orthopaedic Association's "Own the Bone" program and shows how it has significantly improved communication between orthopaedic surgeons, primary care, and patients. Level of evidence: II.

ACETABULUM

teardrop

- radiographic condensation of innominate bone at inferior end of acetabulum
- medial border: ilio-ischial line, aka Kohler's line
- lateral border: continuous superiorly c̄ floor of acetabulum
- wide teardrop assoc. with shallow acetabulum
- narrow teardrop assoc. with over-coverage of femoral head / coxa profunda

sourcil (note: fovea should not come into contact c̄ sourcil)

- radiodense subchondral bone of wt. bearing portion of acetabulum
- normally cover 80% of width of femoral head
- anterior center-edge of Wiberg measures amt. of acetabular coverage of femoral head
- slope measured by Tonnis angle; should be less than 10° b/c maintains jt. rxn F transmitted along primary compression trabeculae of femur to be ⊥ slope of sourcil → minimizes shear stresses btwn femoral head & acetabular roof
- ↑ in upslope of sourcil: lat. subluxation of femoral head
- down sloping sourcil: med. subluxation of femoral head and loading of fovea & acetabular fossa

version

- norm. acetabular anteversion 20°
- ant. wall: more horiz. v. post wall: more vertical & covers more of head
- norm. anteverted acetabulum: ant. & post. walls contact each other at lateral edge of sourcil & do NOT cross each other
- post. wall sign: if post. wall passes medial to center of head (norm. passes thru center of head)
- excessive anteversion: medial ant. wall / under coverage medially & overcoverage posteriorly
- crossover sign: anterior over coverage
- retroversion: post. under coverage + crossover sign + ischial spine on AP view

FEMUR

coxa vara <120°	coxa valga >135°	coxa breva (short neck)
- ↓ resting length of abductors	- ↑ resting length of abductors	- ↓ aB resting length
- Trendelenburg gait	- ↓ abductor lever arm	- ↓ aB lever arm
- ↑ aB lever arm, ↓ jt. rxn	- ↑ jt. rxn F	- ↑ jt rxn F
		- Trendelenburg gait

Chapter 32

Hip and Pelvic Reconstruction and Arthroplasty

Rafael J. Sierra, MD   Craig J. Della Valle, MD

Arthritis of the Hip

Epidemiology
Osteoarthritis
Arthritis and other rheumatologic conditions are the leading cause of disability among adults in the United States. In 2001 the estimated prevalence of arthritis among US adults was 33%, representing approximately 70 million adults. The prevalence increases with age. Women had a higher prevalence than men, and non-Hispanic whites and non-Hispanic blacks had a higher prevalence than Hispanics and people of other racial or ethnic backgrounds. The prevalence of self-reported, doctor-diagnosed arthritis is projected to increase to nearly 67 million by 2030.[1]

Inflammatory Arthritis
Rheumatoid arthritis (RA) affects 1.3 million adults older than 35 years of age in the United States.[1,2] In 2005, juvenile arthritis affected 294,000 children, spondyloarthritis affected 0.6 million to 2.4 million adults, systemic lupus erythematosus affected 161,000 to 322,000 adults, systemic sclerosis affected 49,000 adults, and primary Sjögrens syndrome affected 0.4 million to 3.1 million adults.

Dr. Sierra or an immediate family member serves as a paid consultant to or is an employee of Biomet; has received research or institutional support from DePuy, A Johnson & Johnson Company, Zimmer, and Stryker; and serves as a board member, owner, officer, or committee member of the Midamerica Orthopedic Society and Maurice Mueller Foundation. Dr. Della Valle or an immediate family member serves as a board member, owner, officer, or committee member of the American Association of Hip and Knee Surgeons and the Arthritis Foundation; serves as a paid consultant to or is an employee of Biomet, Kinamed, Smith & Nephew, and Zimmer; has received research or institutional support from Zimmer; and has received nonincome support (such as equipment or services), commercially derived honoraria, or other non-research–related funding (such as paid travel) from Stryker.

Posttraumatic Arthritis
The incidence of posttraumatic arthritis has been very difficult to calculate, but approximately 12% of overall prevalence of symptomatic osteoarthritis (OA) may be attributed to posttraumatic arthritis of the hip, knee, or ankle. This corresponds to approximately 5.6 million individuals in the United States.

Clinical Evaluation
History
The diagnosis of hip OA is usually straightforward and can be based on an appropriate history and physical examination. The pain associated with hip arthritis is commonly of insidious onset, unless there had been recent severe trauma. Pain is usually located in the groin and may be referred to the knee through a branch of the obturator nerve. The referral pattern for hip pathology is variable, and patients may have pain referred to the buttock and thigh. A patient may hold the hip with the hand, in a form of a "C," so-called "C-sign," that is commonly seen in patients with hip pathology. Pain that radiates past the knee, down the posterior thigh, and is associated with numbness or tingling is unlikely to be of hip origin. Articular pain is most commonly associated with groin pain and can be associated with diagnoses such as femoroacetabular impingement (FAI), hip dysplasia, osteonecrosis, OA, or femoral neck fractures. Buttock pain can be associated with posterior FAI, posterior acetabular wear, and OA, and piriformis or gluteus muscle problems.

Physical Examination
The examination of the arthritic hip is fairly simple and should focus on gait, measuring leg lengths, hip range of motion, provocative maneuvers and palpation, and a thorough neurovascular examination. Gait could be antalgic or related to limb-length discrepancy or muscle weakness (for example, Trendelenburg lurch). Pelvic obliquity and potential spine problems should be evaluated. The patient's foot progression angle should be annotated. Range of motion of the hip is usually painful, especially flexion and internal rotation, which are commonly the directions in which motion is first lost with hip arthritis. Provocative maneuvers such as an active straight leg with the patient supine (Stinchfield)

differentiate hip v. SI. v. spine

can be positive. Pain is elucidated by an increase in contact pressures within the acetabulum. The anterior impingement test may be positive in patients with anterior FAI, hip dysplasia with labral pathology, or OA. The posterior impingement test is positive in patients with posterior FAI and in those with posterior acetabular OA, and anterior apprehension is seen in patients with hip dysplasia, as a feeling that the hip were going to subluxate anteriorly from the acetabulum.

Radiographic Evaluation
Plain Radiographs
Plain radiographs are usually all that are needed for diagnosis of hip OA. The pattern of OA may vary. Most patients develop superolateral narrowing, which would then progress to global narrowing of the hip joint. A subgroup of patients, most commonly females, with underlying coxa profunda may develop a more medial pattern of OA with preservation of the superior and lateral joint space; this finding is commonly missed during evaluation.

[handwritten: Coxa profunda: floor of fossa acetabuli touching or overlapping ilioischial line medially]

Computed Tomography
CT is rarely required for the diagnosis of hip arthritis, but could be helpful in identifying the structural abnormality associated with precursor hip pathology, such as femoroacetabular impingement.

Magnetic Resonance Imaging
MRI with or without contrast is also useful in the diagnosis of early OA and in studying labral pathology associated with the underlying hip arthritis. Newer biochemical imaging techniques, such as the delayed gadolinium-enhanced MRI of cartilage (dGEMRIC), possibly assist in the early detection of articular cartilage damage because of the ability to detect the biochemical change of tissue that precedes tissue loss. These techniques are currently under study.[3]

[handwritten margin note: acetabular protrusio: intrapelvic protrusion of acetabulum]

Femoroacetabular Impingement

FAI has been defined as a prearthritic mechanism that occurs when the proximal femur abuts the acetabulum with range of motion.[4,5] Unrecognized and continued FAI can lead to cartilage degeneration and OA.[5]

Three types of FAI have been observed; cam, pincer, and combined. Femoral-side problems caused by abnormally shaped proximal femurs, which include hips affected by slipped capital femoral epiphysis (SCFE), femoral retroversion, and posttraumatic deformities, lead to cam impingement. Acetabular structural abnormalities caused by retroversion and coxa profunda or protrusio lead to pincer impingement. Up to 80% of hips may have a combined type of impingement with both femoral and acetabular structural abnormalities.[6]

Most patients who present with this condition are young and active and report groin pain in the affected hip during activity. Some patients report gluteal or trochanteric pain most commonly as the result of the ab-

errant gait mechanics associated with the abnormal hip morphology. Many other conditions can produce symptoms in or around the hip. Differential diagnoses should include an era of pathologies such as sacroiliitis, degenerative disk disease, abductor muscle tears and sprains, femoral head osteonecrosis, hip OA, psoas tendinitis, labral pathology, pubic ramus fractures, stress fracture of the proximal femur, or trochanteric bursitis.

Clinical Evaluation
Patients with post-SCFE deformities may ambulate with an externally rotated extremity and an open foot progression angle (greater than 10°). Hip range of motion is usually limited in patients with FAI, especially in flexion at 90° and internal rotation (<5°). Some female patients, however, may have greater than 20° to 25° of internal rotation at 90°; therefore, lack of internal rotation is not a universal finding. The anterior impingement test is usually positive in patients with rim and labral pathology. The posterior impingement sign may also be positive and may be seen in patients with posterior acetabular pathology and in patients with a "coup-contrecoup" lesion, a sign that both anterior and posterior acetabular damage has occurred, because of recurrent anterior impingement (**Figure 1**).

Radiographic Evaluation
Plain Radiographs

[handwritten: Dunn view: 45° flexion, max abd, neutral rotation → ant-sup head neck jx to fem anteversion]

Plain radiographs of the pelvis and hip are more commonly used for diagnosis of structural abnormalities about the hip. A cross-table lateral, frog-lateral, or Dunn view is commonly used for observing the proximal femoral deformity. It is now commonly accepted that a well-centered AP pelvic view is obtained when there is symmetry of the iliac wings and of the obturator foramina, and the coccyx is at a point in the midline within a distance of 0 to 2 cm above the symphysis pubis. With a well-centered radiograph, the borders of the acetabulum can be inspected for the absence of retroversion, coxa profunda, or protrusio (**Figure 2**). The radiographs should be examined for congruency of the femoral head and acetabulum, asphericity of the femoral head, and contour of the femoral head and neck junction. Asphericity of the femoral head or lateral head extension can be seen in patients with post-Perthes or post-SCFE deformities (**Figure 2, Table 1**). The grade of OA should be classified according to the criteria described by Tönnis (**Table 2**).

On the acetabular side, retroversion of the acetabulum should be diagnosed using the crossover sign or the ischial spine sign. Posterior wall coverage should be assessed using the posterior wall sign. A posterior wall sign indicates lack of posterior coverage; appropriate surgical treatment should be chosen (**Table 1, Figure 3**). Radiographic technique and assessment have been discussed in the literature.[7]

Computed Tomography
Conventional and three-dimensional CT scan of the hip is useful for assessing hip structural abnormalities and

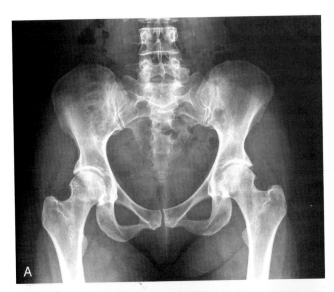

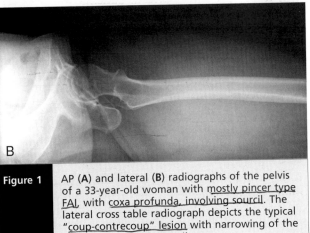

Figure 1 | AP (**A**) and lateral (**B**) radiographs of the pelvis of a 33-year-old woman with mostly pincer type FAI, with coxa profunda, involving sourcil. The lateral cross table radiograph depicts the typical "coup-contrecoup" lesion with narrowing of the posterior acetabular cartilage.

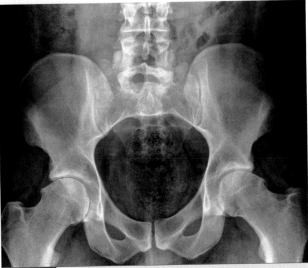

Figure 2 | AP radiograph of the pelvis of a 27-year-old man with advanced cam-type FAI. The patient has asphericity of the femoral head depicted by extension of the lateral aspect of the femoral head outside the red circle.

Table 1

Definitions of Radiographic Measurements Obtained in Patients With Structural Abnormalities Related to FAI

Coxa profunda	When the floor of the fossa acetabuli touches the ilioischial line.
Protrusio acetabulum	When the femoral head overlaps the ilioischial spine medially.
Aspheric head	When the epiphysis of the head protrudes laterally out of the circle around the head.
Pistol grip	Lateral contour of the femoral head extends into a convex shape to the base of the neck.
Double contour sign	Ossification of the rim caused by bone apposition resulting in a double projection of the anterior and posterior walls.

serves as a good tool for preoperative planning in patients undergoing hip arthroscopy and possible reconstructive procedures.

MRI-Arthrogram

Axial, coronal oblique, sagittal oblique, and radial sequences should be obtained. The radial sequence is a proton density–weighted sequence orthogonal to the femoral head and neck junction, and is a reconstruction of the true axial slice orthogonal to the acetabular plane and the sagittal oblique slice parallel to the acetabular plane.

Arthro-MRI is commonly used to diagnose labral pathology, articular cartilage degeneration, the presence or not of intraosseous ganglion formation, and femoral head and neck junction abnormalities. Adding a small field view to the arthro-MRI may increase sensitivity to diagnose labral tears as high as 92%. A ruptured labrum often shows increased signal intensity on T2-weighted images that extends to the articular surface (**Figure 4**). Acetabular cartilage degeneration can also be seen with arthro-MRI, but is less reliable than when assessing labral pathology. If on MRI the femoral head has migrated into the anterior-superior cartilage defect and the femoral head has lost its stable position, then joint-preserving surgery is usually contraindicated. The α angle has been described on axial MRI views to depict the grade of femoral head and neck junction abnormalities. A mean angle of 74° was seen in patients with FAI compared to 42° in control groups.[8]

Treatment Options

Surgical Dislocation

Surgical hip dislocation is currently considered the gold standard for management of FAI, with good to excel-

4: Lower Extremity

Handwritten annotations: coxa vara <120° | normal 130° 120-135° | coxa valga >135°

Table 2

Classification of OA as Described by Tönnis

Grade 0   No signs of OA

Grade 1   Increased <u>sclerosis</u> of the head and acetabulum

Grade 2   <u>Small cysts</u> in the head or acetabulum, <u>moderate joint space narrowing</u>, moderate loss of head sphericity

Grade 3   <u>Large cysts</u> in head or acetabulum, <u>severe joint space narrowing</u> or obliteration, severe deformity of femoral head, evidence of <u>necrosis</u>

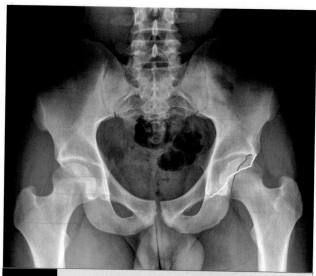

Figure 3   AP radiograph of the hip of a 19-year-old man with <u>isolated retroversion of the acetabulum.</u> The red line depicts the posterior wall, and the white line depicts the anterior wall. <u>The crossover between the anterior and posterior walls occurs more caudal than normal.</u> The <u>prominence of the ischial spine within the pelvic cavity</u> also gives an idea of the significant retroversion encountered in this patient.

---

lent results reported in over 80% to 90% of patients.[9-11] <u>Indications for surgery include preserved articular cartilage, correctable structural abnormality, and reasonable expectations.</u> <u>Surgery is usually not recommended</u> in patients in the fourth or fifth decade of life and in those with Tönnis grade 2 OA, or anterior translation of the femoral head into an anterior acetabular defect seen radiographically or on MRI, or a retroverted acetabulum with poor posterior coverage. A <u>periacetabular osteotomy [PAO]</u> would be a better treatment option for these patients. <u>Surgery is absolutely not recommended</u> for patients with grade 3 or higher OA, those with hip pain with an uncorrectable structural deformity, and the patient older than 60 years in whom total hip arthroplasty (THA) would be a better option if cartilage damage is detected.

<u>The dislocation is performed with preservation of all external rotators and protection of the medial circumflex artery.</u> The trochanter heals reliably and the operation allows direct visualization and protection of the superior femoral neck retinacular vessels at the time of surgery. The operation allows a <u>360° view of the acetabular and femoral heads</u> for inspection, diagnosis, and treatment of abnormalities associated with FAI. <u>Extra-articular components can also be corrected,</u> such as a reorientation of the proximal femur with flexion, valgus intertrochanteric osteotomies, or correction of coxa vara. The trochanter can also be advanced if necessary through this same approach. Studies have shown that <u>the best results are obtained in patients with early to no OA and when the labrum is preserved.</u> Complications can be minimized by understanding the anatomy and with good surgical technique.

Anterior Smith-Petersen or Heuter Approach

This procedure could be used as the sole management of FAI or combined with arthroscopic management of the intra-articular pathology. Advantages include a <u>smaller incision with minimal muscle damage and a fast recovery</u> when compared to surgical hip dislocation done through a trochanteric osteotomy. A disadvantage of the procedure is that <u>treatment of pathology is limited</u> and is mainly aimed at the <u>femoral side;</u> although both sides can be treated, <u>visualization is decreased</u> in comparison with the surgical hip dislocation.

To treat the acetabular side, the reflected head of the rectus may have to be taken down, and there are potential problems with traction of the superficial femoral cutaneous nerve. The results to date show that reasonable outcome can be achieved through this approach with an acceptable complication rate.[12]

Arthroscopy

The indications for hip arthroscopy in the setting of FAI are continually evolving. Central compartment arthroscopy allows management of labral pathology. Access to the peripheral compartment without traction allows treatment of mild to moderate cam FAI lesions of the anterior lateral femoral head and neck junction and can also be used to reattach the torn labrum. Limitations of hip arthroscopy are numerous. Hip arthroscopy is suitable in limited hands and has a <u>long learning curve.</u> It has a <u>limited role in assessing posterior FAI pathology.</u> The surgeon must have significant experience in hip arthroscopy to treat the acetabular rim with techniques that have been described for open surgery. <u>Arthroscopy is also difficult to perform in patients with coxa profunda or protrusio, those with severe acetabular retroversion, or in the obese patient.</u>

There has been a growing body of literature reporting the results of hip arthroscopy in FAI. The consensus of <u>recent literature is that satisfactory results can be obtained,</u> and that the outcomes are comparable to those of the open technique, although patient selection may play an important role in the outcomes between these two groups.[13-16]

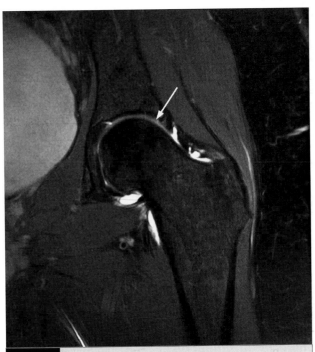

Figure 4   T2-weighted MRI with gadolinium shows an anterior-superior labral tear (*arrow*), seen as an increase in signal intensity that extends to the articular surface.

AP

False Profile view: anterior acetabular coverage of femoral head

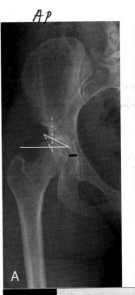
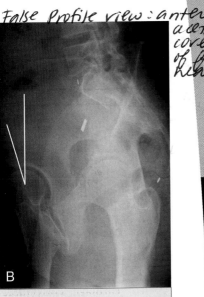

Figure 5   **A,** The right side of an AP pelvic radiograph showing the radiographic measurements used for hip dysplasia. The dotted line denotes the anterior center edge angle. The solid white line denotes the Tönnis angle. The black line denotes the medial clear space. **B,** A false-profile view showing measurement of the anterior center edge angle.

4: Lower Extremity

Developmental Dysplasia of the Hip in the Adult

History

Hip dysplasia is a structural hip disorder that can lead to degenerative arthritis in early adulthood if left untreated. Classic hip dysplasia has been well described in the literature and its pathologic features can vary substantially. It is common to see an increasing spectrum of abnormalities ranging from mild forms of dysplasia to severe cases in which the hip is completely dislocated from the acetabulum. In classic hip dysplasia, increased contact pressures on the small surface area between the acetabulum and femoral head can lead to degeneration of the superolateral cartilage, and early OA.

Physical Examination

Most patients with hip dysplasia are young and active and report groin pain during activity. Patients may also report pain over the trochanter. Patients usually do not specifically report loss of hip range of motion and actually may have increased range of motion. Patients with mild to moderate dysplasia report a knife-sharp pain in the groin and a sensation of catching or locking secondary to tearing of the labrum. Patients may ambulate with an antalgic gait; when weak abductors are present, they may have a Trendelenburg gait and a positive Trendelenburg test. Patients with classic dysplasia and increased femoral anteversion have more internal rotation than external rotation. With labral pathology an anterior impingement test will be positive. The ap-

prehension test may also be positive as patients feel that the hip subluxates anteriorly. Abduction strength is usually not affected except in extreme grades of hip dysplasia such as in the dislocated hip.

Radiographic Examination

Plain radiographs of the pelvis and hip are commonly used for diagnosis of hip dysplasia. All pertinent information is usually obtained from the AP pelvic radiograph, but additional studies such as a Lequesne false profile view, a cross-table lateral view, hip abduction views, and MRI-arthrogram of the hip are commonly used ancillary tests. Pelvic radiographs should be standardized as described previously in the section on FAI. The most commonly used methods to describe the grade of hip dysplasia are the lateral center edge angle of Wiberg, the acetabular index of the weight-bearing surface of Tönnis, the femoral head extrusion index, and the acetabular depth to width index of Stulberg and Harris (**Figure 5**). In addition, the Shenton line can be used to assess superior subluxation of the hip. Lateral subluxation should be quantified by measuring from the lateral side of the teardrop to the medial edge of the femoral head (**Table 3; Figure 5**). One study demonstrated that these radiographic parameters reliably predicted the outcome of the untreated dysplastic hip after age 65 years. In this study no patient had developed severe arthritic changes in the hip or had a Wiberg center edge angle of less than 16°, a Tönnis angle of more than 15°, an acetabular depth to width index of less than 38%, or an uncovered femoral head of more than 31%.[17]

An AP radiograph of the hip in maximal abduction

[handwritten: line from medial edge of sourcil to its lateral edge & horizontal line]

[handwritten: a measure of how much femoral head is needed to be covered by acetabulum]

Table 3

Radiographic Measurements Obtained in Patients With Hip Dysplasia

[handwritten: line from center of femoral head to outer edge of acetabular roof & vertical line]

Lateral Center Edge Angle	
>25°	Normal
Between 20-25	Borderline
<20°	Hip dysplasia
Tönnis Angle *[handwritten: aka inclination of wt.-bearing zone]*	
0-10°	Normal
>10°	Hip dysplasia
Femoral Extrusion Index	
>25%	Hip dysplasia
False Profile View (Anterior Center Edge Angle)	
>25°	Normal
<20°	Hip dysplasia
Between 20°-25°	Borderline

is commonly obtained at the time of surgical planning. The ideal candidate for the pelvic rotational osteotomy shows that the hip reduces and the femoral head is adequately covered and congruent and the joint space is preserved. Although the absence of these criteria is not a contraindication to pelvic osteotomy, it may indicate that a femoral osteotomy may also be necessary or that the procedure should be considered a salvage operation as the outcome would be less predictable.

[handwritten: pelvic rotational osteotomy]

Retroversion can also be seen in patients with hip dysplasia. It has been reported that up to one sixth of the hip dysplasias can have a retroverted acetabulum, and this has to be taken into account at the time of correction.[18]

A CT scan is not routinely used for diagnosing hip dysplasia. An MRI with gadolinium as described in the section on FAI can be used to assess labral pathology and/or early cartilage degeneration. The acetabular labrum, which is usually large, aids differentiation in borderline hips with both FAI and dysplastic features.

Treatment Options

Nonarthroplasty

Femoral osteotomy in itself is rarely used as sole management for acetabular hip dysplasia in the adult. The indications for concomitant femoral osteotomy in addition to a PAO are worth noting. Intertrochanteric osteotomy may be needed in approximately 10% of patients treated with PAO. There has been a significant association between a high extrusion index of the femoral head, abnormal femoral anteversion angles, a deformed femoral head, and radiographic signs of OA with the need for femoral osteotomy. Most importantly, a previous adduction osteotomy was highly predictive of the need for femoral osteotomy. Although these criteria can help in discerning which hips may need a femoral osteotomy preoperatively, consideration should be made at the time of the surgery if containment and congruency are not optimal after PAO.

Although there are multiple forms of acetabular osteotomy which are currently used for management of the patient with symptomatic hip dysplasia, PAO is the preferred pelvic osteotomy in many centers for treatment of the adult patient with hip dysplasia in the US. Surgical advantages include the ability to perform the osteotomy with a series of straight, relatively reproducible cuts through one incision preserving the abductors, the ability to permit a wide range of corrections medially, laterally, and anteriorly while maintaining adequate acetabular version, or the ability to perform isolated changes to acetabular version if needed, the need for minimal internal fixation and no external fixation as the posterior column is preserved, and the ability to perform a capsulotomy to assess the labrum and check for impingement without compromise to the acetabular fragment and blood supply. Patient-related advantages include the possibility of early mobilization and weight bearing because of the preserved posterior column and the ability to use the osteotomy in female patients who plan to become pregnant and deliver vaginally, as the pelvic ring and outlet are not changed after the correction.

The ideal patient for the osteotomy is younger than 40 years with little, if any, arthrosis (Tönnis grade 0 or 1); has a poorly covered femoral head with a lateralized hip center of rotation, a congruent hip joint with a round acetabulum, and a round femoral head, and is not obese. Contraindications to the procedure include complete dislocation and/or high subluxation of the femoral head articulating with the secondary acetabulum with arthritic changes, poor hip range of motion (flexion <105° and abduction <30°), and patient age younger than 12 years. Injury to the triradiate cartilage could result in acetabular retroversion.

The results of PAO have been reported in several studies.[14,19] The innovators of the osteotomy reported their long-term follow-up in 1999.[19] At an average 11.3 years after surgery, 58 of the 71 hips with the minimum follow-up of 10 years had a preserved hip joint. Thirteen hips had either a subsequent THA (12) or a hip fusion (1). Ninety percent of the patients who still had a preserved joint space at a minimum of 10 years had significant improvement in pain and functional scores. Including those hips in which treatment failed, 52 of 71 hips (73%) had a score of good or excellent. The association between grade of OA and surgical outcome has been studied.[20] At an average of 4 years of follow-up, patients with preoperative Tönnis grade 1 or 2 OA had mostly excellent or good results and those with grade 3 OA had mostly poor results. Five of nine patients with grade 3 arthritis required further major surgery.

Total Hip Arthroplasty

The technique of THA in patients with hip dysplasia varies according to the structural deformity. On the pelvic side the native acetabulum is typically shallow and open anterolaterally in excess (excessive anteversion), or it can be completely deficient anteriorly and superiorly, commonly resulting in a lateralized hip center. On

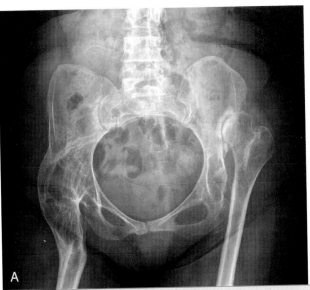
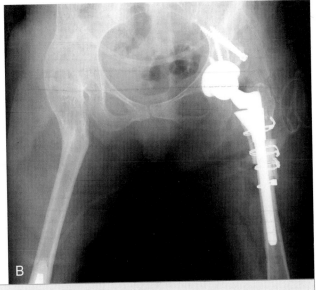

Figure 6 **A,** AP pelvic radiograph denoting a high dislocation with neoacetabulum formation. **B,** Radiograph obtained after THA. Acetabular autograft and subtrochanteric shortening osteotomy were required.

the femoral side, the neck is usually short with excessive anteversion and an increased neck shaft angle. The head is usually small. The greater trochanter is displaced posteriorly and the femoral canal is narrow. Most commonly, however, the changes of the femur are minor and it is the acetabulum that is dysplastic and the disproportionate contact between the two structures that produces symptoms. The classification of Crowe has been routinely used to describe the grade of subluxation of the hip.[21] Fifty percent subluxation is equal to translation of the medial head-neck junction superior to the interteardrop line by 10% of the pelvic height. Crowe I are hips with less than 50% subluxation, Crowe II are hips with 50% to 75% subluxation, Crowe III are hips with 75% to 100% subluxation, and Crowe IV are hips with more than 100% subluxation. For Crowe I hips, reconstruction of the anatomic hip center using an uncemented socket is usually the treatment of choice. Anterolateral structural autograft (femoral head) is used only if needed. The femoral component is either uncemented or cemented based on patient age, femoral anatomy, and surgeon philosophy. On the femoral side, the surgeon must try to avoid excessive anteversion of the stem. Distorted proximal anatomy suggests a role for modular stems or extensively coated stems that will obtain diaphyseal fixation and will allow for changes in femoral version. For Crowe II hips, the acetabulum is usually an uncemented socket in the anatomic or slightly high center; the goal is to optimize coverage with native bone and using autograft as needed. The femoral reconstruction is usually the same as for Crowe I hips. For Crowe III hips, the acetabulum reconstruction is the most difficult because of severe lateral deficiency; options include a high center with a small cup on native bone, or an anatomic hip center beneath a large autograft or metal augment. For Crowe IV, a completely dislocated hip,

the true acetabulum usually has thicker bone, is shallow and dysplastic, and has a thin anterior wall with a posterior wall that is adequately thick; therefore, restoration of anatomic hip center of rotation would be ideal. Graft is usually not needed. Because the bone is usually soft, care should be taken at the time of preparation of the socket. Patients with high hip dislocations may require either a trochanteric osteotomy with proximal shortening or a subtrochanteric shortening osteotomy. A subtrochanteric shortening osteotomy maintains proximal femoral anatomy, allows for an uncemented femur, and avoids trochanteric problems (**Figure 6**). One must be aware of overlengthening the dysplastic extremity. A good rule of thumb is to prevent lengthening the extremity greater than 3.5 cm.

Osteonecrosis of the Femoral Head

Epidemiology and Risk Factors
New cases of osteonecrosis of the femoral head are diagnosed at a rate of 10,000 to 20,000 per year, and the average age of these patients is 36 years.[22] Treatment of early osteonecrosis of the femoral head remains controversial. Late-stage osteonecrosis is commonly treated with arthroplasty with good results. In some instances the inciting event leading to osteonecrosis is clearly known, such as when direct injury or trauma has occurred. In other instances, the inciting event is unknown and can only be associated with risk factors that could predispose to the disease process, which include steroid use, alcohol abuse, smoking, HIV, blood clotting disorders, organ transplantation, and radiation (**Table 4**). There have been recent associations with inherited coagulopathies and with genetic polymorphisms that are potentially treatable pathophysiologic conditions.

Table 4

Risk Factors Associated With the Development of Osteonecrosis of the Femoral Head

Dysbaric (Caisson disease)

Gaucher disease

Sickle cell disease

Pancreatitis

Steroids

Alcohol

Vascular insult

Subacute bacterial endocarditis

Disseminated intravascular coagulation

Polycythemia rubra vera

Systemic lupus erythematosus

Polyarteritis nodosa

RA

Giant cell arteritis

Sarcoid metabolic diabetes

Hyperuricemia

Blood lipid disorders

Idiopathic

Table 5

The Steinberg Classification for Staging Osteonecrosis of the Femoral Head

Stage	
0	Normal or nondiagnostic radiograph, bone scan, and MRI
I[a]	Normal radiograph, abnormal bone scan and/or MRI
II[a]	Abnormal radiograph showing "cystic" and sclerotic changes in the femoral head
III[a]	Subchondral collapse producing a crescent sign
IV[a]	Flattening of the femoral head
V[a]	Joint narrowing with or without acetabular involvement
VI	Advanced degenerative changes

[a]The extent or grade of involvement should also be indicated as A, mild; B, moderate; or C, severe

It is currently believed that osteonecrosis is a multifactorial disease associated in some cases with a genetic predisposition and an exposure to one or more risk factors.

After the insult occurs, bone death follows and the reparative process (creeping substitution) ensues. The reparative process weakens the subchondral bone, resulting in collapse.

Radiographic Examination

There is no single diagnostic test that is 100% reliable. Plain radiographs including an oblique view of the hip (frog-leg) are normal initially. A frog-lateral view, however, is the radiographic test to confirm subchondral collapse and to make decisions regarding patient management. MRI has been shown to be approximately 98% sensitive and 98% specific. Bone scan in contrast is approximately 85% sensitive and 80% specific with an accuracy of about 85%.

MRI can become positive within 24 hours of insult, and can document the insult at a mean of 3.6 months after initiation of steroid use.

Classification

Staging of the disease progression is important because options and outcomes of nonreplacement treatment are predicated on these data. The classification of Ficat and Arlet is the most commonly used; however, the Steinberg classification is the most complete with its six subgroups[23] (**Table 5**). The classic radiographic finding of the so-called crescent sign is best demonstrated on the frog-lateral projection which represents subchondral fracture (**Figure 7**).

Treatment Options

The decision to proceed with one form of treatment modality should be based on patient symptoms and important radiographic findings that may portray outcome: evidence of precollapse or collapse involvement of the femoral head; the size of the necrotic lesion; the amount of femoral head depression; and acetabular involvement.

Nonsurgical

The natural history of the untreated osteonecrosis lesion is poor. Large lesions tend to progress while smaller (less than 10% involvement) may not.[24,25] Nonsurgical intervention may be warranted in small, precollapse lesions that are asymptomatic and that may have the better natural history. Protected weight bearing has demonstrated a failure rate of greater than 80% at a mean of 34 months and is not recommended as sole treatment.[26] Other nonsurgical interventions such as pulsed electromagnetic fields, hyperbaric oxygen, and extracorporeal shock wave therapy are not currently recommended. Pharmacologic treatment with lipid-lowering medications and/or bisphosphonates has shown some promising results in both animal models and early clinical series.[27,28] Pharmacologic treatment may be the treatment of choice in patients with multifocal osteonecrosis and in those who are not good candidates for surgical intervention.

Head-Sparing Procedures

Core decompression has traditionally been the treatment of choice during stages of precollapse. The results, however, continue to be conflicting in the literature. In a meta-analysis of outcomes of core decompression obtained from 24 published series before 1995, the best results were observed with core decompression in early stages. Eighty-four patients with Ficat stage 1 and 65% of patients with stage 2 had successful results.[26] The success of core decompression was higher than nonsurgical management in another study reporting 22 studies that compared core decompression versus nonsurgical management.

A recent study reports that vascularized fibular grafting can be performed even after subchondral collapse.[29] In early experience with follow-up ranging from 8 months to 6 years, only 3 of 50 patients had progressed to the point of requiring hip joint arthroplasty. Femoral head collapse did occur in three patients. Longer-term results of vascularized fibular graft have shown consistent successful results with good functional recovery and relief of pain. The results obtained in this study have not been shared by others.

Decompression of the femoral head and injection of mesenchymal stem cells into the necrotic lesion have gained some acceptance in the treatment of early osteonecrosis. A case series of 189 hips in 160 patients with ages ranging from 16 to 61 years old demonstrated slowing in the progression of osteonecrosis as well as a significant reduction in the need for total hip replacement.[30] Only 18% of hips and 20% of patients required total hip replacement in the 5- to 10-year follow-up period. These results were best for early osteonecrosis, and in select patients based on etiology of osteonecrosis.

Arthroplasty

Hemiarthroplasty is rarely indicated in patients with osteonecrosis of the femoral head. The disappointing results with an overall satisfactory rate of only 48% in 31 patients with 38 bipolar endoprostheses has led to the abandonment of this procedure for management of the young patient with osteonecrosis. Hemiresurfacing is another option for management of the young patient with osteonecrosis of the femoral head without acetabular involvement. The results in the literature have been contradictory, with some institutions reporting excellent results and others reporting disappointing results with an overall hip survivorship of around 60% at short-term follow-up. Poor results of hemiresurfacing could be related to patient selection. Continued groin pain was the leading cause of conversion to total hip arthroplasty in one study.[31]

The outcomes of total hip resurfacing for osteonecrosis are better than hemiresurfacing; however, the use of a metal-on-metal articulation in the young patient, especially female, is debatable. Newer data suggest that the results of total hip resurfacing are worse in patients with osteonecrosis than patients with OA.[32] The literature reports approximately an 86% to 92% survivorship at mid-term follow-up in patients who have undergone total hip resurfacing for osteonecrosis.[32] Total hip resurfacing should be performed in select patients with osteonecrosis, and evaluation of the lesion size, its loca-

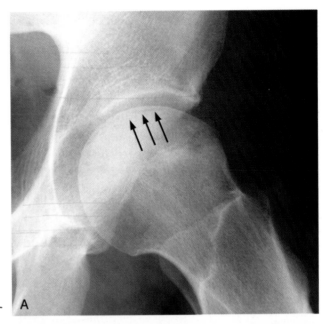

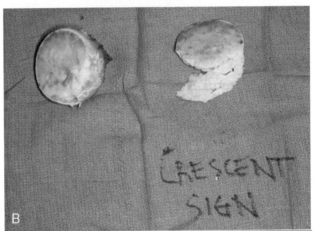

Figure 7   **A,** The crescent sign as depicted on the frog-lateral view (*arrows*). **B,** Intraoperative specimen of the same patient undergoing THA with evidence of subchondral collapse and a large necrotic segment.

tion, and bone quality is mandatory. THA provides the most reliable pain relief and good early clinical results for patients with advanced stages of osteonecrosis. Failure of THA in the treatment of osteonecrosis is related to age and activity level, and could be further limited by predisposing conditions that led to osteonecrosis. Because of the concern about higher failure rates of cemented THA in patients with osteonecrosis, biologically fixed implants have become popular in this patient population. When uncemented femoral components with a favorable track record are used, a high rate of success has been reported in patients with osteonecrosis.[33-35]

As in other young patient groups, the related problems of polyethylene wear and periprosthetic osteolysis have been reported in patients with osteonecrosis. The combination of good fixation achieved with uncemented sockets and newer bearing surfaces has the potential to markedly improve the durability of the acetabular component.

If radiation necrosis has occurred, either a reinforcement ring or highly porous metal socket is recommended, with overall good results. Higher dislocation rates in patients with osteonecrosis may be related to factors associated with the diagnoses that led to osteonecrosis or to structural factors such as less capsular hypertrophy in the patients with osteonecrosis compared to other diagnoses.

Patients with osteonecrosis and on immunosuppressive agents or those who are immunosuppressed because of their underlying disease probably are at high risk for prosthetic infection. These patients are at risk for numerous perioperative complications, such as sickle cell disease. Vaso-occlusive crises secondary to the stress of surgery may occur. This can be reduced with exchange transfusion before arthroplasty. Intraoperative bleeding in this group of patients is significant and a high reoperation rate has been seen in some studies.

Primary THA

Acetabular Reconstruction

Most acetabular components inserted in North America are cementless devices, with 20-year data that show durable fixation with a low risk of failure from aseptic loosening.[36] Optimal results seem to be associated with thinner walled, porous coated, titanium components. At longer-term follow-up, the prevalence of wear-related complications such as catastrophic wear and osteolysis increases, particularly in patients younger than 50 years, more active patients in whom standard polyethylene (non-highly cross-linked) was combined with a thinner liner (less than 7 mm),[37] and/or larger femoral heads[38] (which increase volumetric wear rates). As bearing surface technology improves along with better locking mechanisms for the liner to decrease backside wear, the prevalence of wear-related complications should decrease.[39] Although several manufacturers are now selling highly porous metal acetabular components that offer the theoretical benefits of better initial press-fit fixation and improved bone ingrowth, there are no data to suggest any clinical benefit in primary THA from the use of these materials over traditional porous titanium ingrowth surfaces.

Cemented acetabular components, although still used heavily outside of North America, have fallen out of favor secondary to a more demanding surgical technique, increased surgical time, lack of modularity, and a higher rate of aseptic loosening, particularly in younger, high-demand patient populations. They do, however, offer decreased implant costs, and in patients who are elderly and/or low demand, are an attractive option. They may also be useful for managing patients with poor acetabular bone quality (such as patients

with severe inflammatory arthritis) in whom the bony architecture may not be able to support a cementless device.

Femoral Reconstruction
Cemented Stems
Although long-term data suggest that some cemented femoral component designs (particularly trapezoidal-shaped stems that avoid sharp corners and have a smooth to matte finish) are associated with outstanding long-term survivorship,[40] the usage of cemented femoral components has decreased dramatically over the past decade in North America. Cemented stems are still used extensively in Europe, with excellent reported survivorship in the European registries. Concerns over greater technical difficulty, increased surgical time, and more variable results have contributed to this trend.

Cementless Stems
Early-generation cementless stems that were noncircumferentially porous coated proximally were associated with high rates of failed ingrowth leading to early revision.[36] If these stems did become ingrown, osteolysis developed later as the noncircumferential porous coating allowed for the egress of particles from the bearing surface to the femoral canal. Second-generation designs that incorporated proximal porous coating that was circumferential have fared much better,[41] with high rates of osseointegration and low rates of distal osteolyis; however, loosening secondary to osteolysis has been reported. Third-generation designs, even when designed to gain fixation primarily in the metaphysis, often now incorporate a roughened, biologically active surface that allows for ongrowth in the midsection of the stem to increase fixation.

Most cementless femoral components presently in use are made from titanium and gain their fixation primarily in the metaphysis. Stems may be metaphyseal filling or of a flat wedge taper design (**Figure 8**). Although outstanding survivorship has been reported with both designs at 10 years or more,[41,42] flat wedge taper designs have the theoretical benefits of increased ability to adjust version intraoperatively and easier removal if required. However, as the forces are more concentrated over a smaller surface area, the risk of intraoperative and early postoperative periprosthetic fractures may be higher. The addition of hydroxyapatite (HA) to the surface of the prosthesis does not seem to affect clinical or radiographic outcomes.[43]

Cylindrical, fully porous coated stems that are made from cobalt chromium and have a beaded surface are designed to gain fixation primarily in the diaphysis (**Figure 8**). Benefits of this design include a long track record of durable fixation beyond 20 years.[44] In addition, once bone is ingrown, there are no reports of late loosening. The major disadvantages include difficulty if removal of a well-fixed stem is required and proximal stress-shielding (relative osteopenia of the proximal femur seen secondary to stress transfer distally), which seems to be primarily a radiographic finding and has not been clearly linked to adverse clinical outcomes.

Modular femoral components, which allow for placement of a sleeve in the metaphysis for primary fixation and then independently allow for placement of the neck for anteversion, have been popular in some centers. Although reported results are excellent, these devices are generally reserved for treating patients with proximal femoral deformity or abnormal anteversion, such as patients with developmental hip dysplasia. In addition to increased surgical complexity and cost, some degree of corrosion occurs at the additional modular junction[45] that can lead to osteolysis. More recently, several manufacturers have introduced more traditionally shaped femoral components that use modular neck segments in addition to modular femoral heads. Although these stems allow for the increased ability to adjust leg length, version, and offset (in the hopes of better restoration of hip mechanics and avoiding dislocation), the additional modular junctions increase the risk of corrosion (and thus potentially osteolysis), breakage at this junction can occur and cost is higher. No studies as of yet report a clinical benefit to this design.

Hip Resurfacing

Metal-on-metal hip resurfacing has become more popular based on studies that show excellent durability, particularly in young active patients,[46] and the recent Food and Drug Administration approval of two devices. One review of 1,000 cases showed survivorship of 92% at 8 years, with most failures occurring early in the series when indications and techniques were developing.[47] Potential benefits of this approach include preservation of proximal femoral bone stock, better restoration of hip biomechanics (including a lower risk of limb length discrepancy), increased ability to engage in high-demand activities, and a lower risk of dislocation. The risk of fracture of the retained femoral neck and systemic and local effects of wear particles generated from the metal-on-metal bearing surface are cause for concern. Optimal results with a lower risk of complications have been reported for younger, larger, male patients with a diagnosis of OA[48] (as opposed to osteonecrosis), although the effect of sex may be more related to patient size and bone quality. Notching of the femoral neck and varus positioning of the femoral component seem to be associated with the occurrence of femoral neck fractures.[49] Prospective randomized trials have shown few differences between hip resurfacing and conventional, stemmed THA.[50]

Revision THA

Acetabular Reconstruction

The most commonly used classification for acetabular defects is that described by Paprosky.[51] This classification is based on evaluation of the AP pelvis radiograph and considers the quantity and quality of bone available for fixation of the revision component. It is impor-

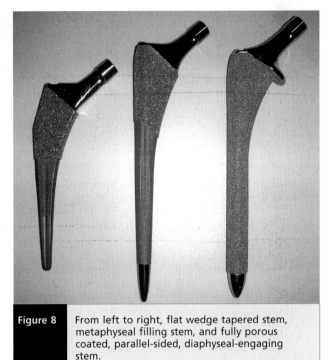

Figure 8   From left to right, flat wedge tapered stem, metaphyseal filling stem, and fully porous coated, parallel-sided, diaphyseal-engaging stem.

tant to recognize that the posterior column is the primary structure relied upon for fixation of a revision component.

In a type I defect, the architecture of the acetabulum is essentially normal and reconstruction can proceed as for a primary THA. This defect is rare, and is typically only seen when revising a hemiarthroplasty with isolated loss of articular cartilage.

In a type II defect, there is less than 3 cm of proximal migration of the component. A type IIa defect is associated with migration superomedially, whereas a type IIb defect is associated with superolateral migration and loss of the acetabular rim. A type IIc defect is associated with protrusion of the acetabular component medially, past the Kohler line (also known as the ilioischial line, which is drawn from the medial border of the ilium to the medial border of the ischium). Type II defects can normally be reconstructed using a cementless acetabular component with adjunctive screw fixation and morcellized cancellous bone grafting of contained defects.

A type III defect is characterized primarily by migration of the acetabular component of >3 cm. This is important, as it indicates damage to the acetabular columns that compromises fixation of the revision acetabular component. The use of a standard, cementless hemispherical component may not be possible, as the defect is often oblong and with progressive reaming of the acetabulum, the surgeon runs out of space front to back while the defect has not been filled from top to bottom. A type IIIA defect (**Figure 9**) is often referred to as an "up and out" defect where damage occurs primarily to the remaining acetabular rim superiorly and anteriorly; however, the posterior column is usually still

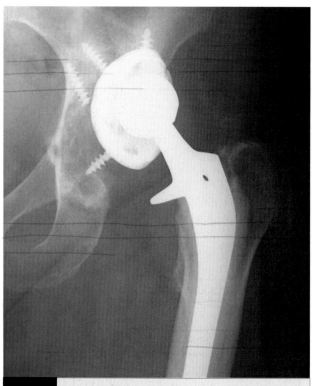

Figure 9 | Type IIIA acetabular defect with migration of more than 3 cm without migration medially.

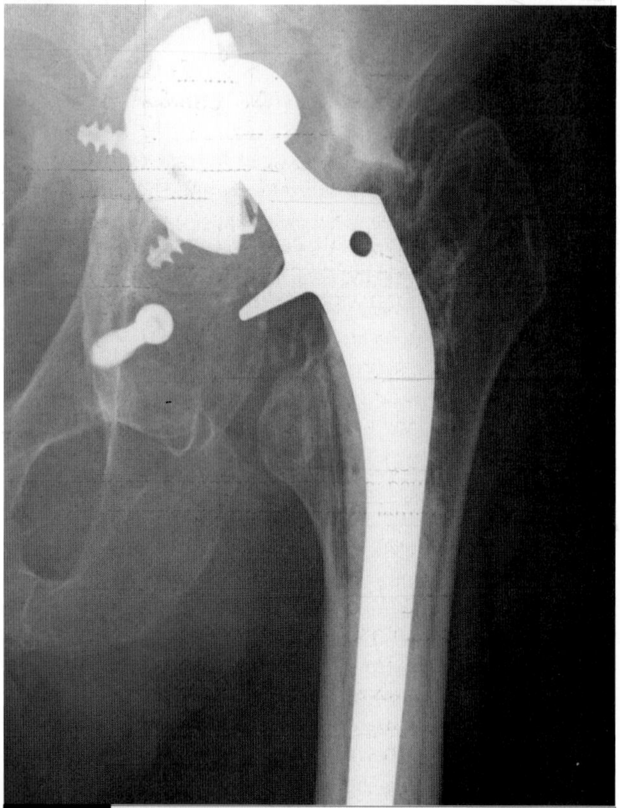

Figure 10 | Type IIIB acetabular defect with migration of more than 3 cm, disruption of the Kohler line, and ischial osteolysis.

intact. A type IIIB defect (**Figure 10**) is associated with further reconstructive complexity and is often referred to as an "up and in" defect where there is a large defect of the medial wall (indicated by disruption of the Kohler line) and associated severe osteolysis of the ischium indicating further damage to the posterior column.

A pelvic discontinuity refers to a separation of the superior and inferior halves of the hemipelvis.[52] This condition can occur acutely, but is typically chronic and associated with severe bone loss that greatly complicates subsequent reconstruction. Radiographic indicators include a transverse fracture line, medial translation of the inferior hemipelvis and often an asymmetry of the obturator foramen as seen on the AP pelvis radiograph. The best reported results in the literature for reconstruction have included stabilization of the posterior column with a plate, adjunctive bone grafting, and the use of either a cementless cup with multiple screws for adjunctive fixation or a cage that spans from the ilium to the ischium.

Hemispherical, Porous-Coated Acetabular Components
The use of a hemispherical, cementless acetabular component with adjunctive screw fixation is appropriate for most acetabular revisions. The surgical technique is straightforward, and durable fixation has been shown at 20 years postoperatively.[53]

Porous Metals
Several manufacturers presently offer highly porous metals (two to three times more porous than standard ingrowth surfaces) that not only offer the promise of greater bone ingrowth but higher frictional interference that may augment initial component stability. Case series have shown good clinical results;[54] however, comparative data on more traditional titanium ingrowth surfaces are lacking. An additional advantage of these materials is the availability of acetabular augments, which can be used in a manner similar to structural allograft for treating severe bony deficiency. Advantages of augments include decreased surgical time and complexity, while allowing for additional points for screw fixation and the potential for biologic ingrowth to occur without the risks of allograft resorption. The longer term results of this type of reconstruction are unknown.

Cages
The use of cages has decreased dramatically in the past decade. Without a surface for biologic ingrowth, these devices are mechanical in nature and are associated with a high rate of subsequent breakage. Devices that do not span from the ilium to the ischium (reconstruction "rings") are used infrequently by North American surgeons. The role of spanning devices seems limited to cases where biologic ingrowth is unlikely to occur (such as tumor or radiation necrosis of the pelvis) or as an adjunct to protect a cementless device (such as the cup-cage construct) or a strutural allograft.

Femoral Reconstruction

The most commonly used classification of femoral defects is that described by Paprosky et al.[55]

Type I defects are characterized by a supportive metaphysis and intact diaphysis and similar to a primary femur. They are unique in that there is intact cancellous bone present for fixation of the revision component with cement if desired. Revision can be performed as the surgeon would for a primary THA. This is typically only seen when revising a failed resurfacing or a cementless hemiarthroplasty without a porous ingrowth surface.

In type II defects, the metaphysis is supportive with an intact diaphysis; however, the cancellous bone of the proximal femur is not present. Because the metaphysis is supportive, it can be relied on for fixation; however, the use of a stem that gains primary fixation in the diaphysis is common.

In type III defects, the metaphysis is damaged and cannot be relied on for fixation; therefore, a stem that gains primary fixation in the diaphysis is used. If more than 4 cm of intact isthmus is available for distal fixation, the defect is classified as type IIIA (**Figure 11**), whereas if less than 4 cm is available it is classified as type IIIB. Type IIIA defects are most commonly reconstructed with a cylindrical, parallel-sided, fully porous coated stem. When less than 4 cm of isthmus is available for distal fixation, worse results have been reported with a fully porous coated device and thus a modular, titanium, tapered stem is typically used for type IIIB defects. Modular tapered stems are also used in the face of substantial femoral deformity (loose femoral components can cause the femur to remodel into varus and retroversion) and in cases where the diameter of the revision femoral component is larger than 18 mm.

In type IV defects, not only is the metaphysis unsupportive but there is no isthmus available for distal fixation and thus reconstruction is very difficult. If the "tube" of the femoral canal is intact, impaction grafting can be used. If it is not intact, a proximal femoral replacing prosthesis or a proximal femoral allograft-prosthetic composite can be used. Modular tapered stems can be used in some situations; however, as there is no isthmus available, stable fixation may be difficult to achieve.

Cylindrical Fully Porous-Coated Stems

These devices continue to be the workhorse for femoral revision surgery in North America. The surgical technique is relatively simple, and excellent initial component ingrowth and durable long-term fixation have been reported.[56] They have been shown to be particularly reliable for managing femoral defects when at least 4 cm of press-fit is obtained between the implant and the isthmus of the femur.

Modular Tapered Stems

With the introduction of bibody, modular systems that allow for placement of the distal tapered portion of the stem first, followed by the use of proximal body seg-

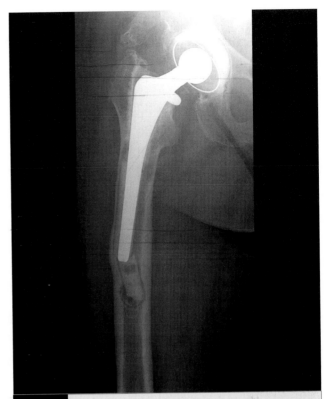

Figure 11 Type IIIA femoral defect. The metaphysis is nonsupportive; however, there is more than 4 cm of intact diaphysis for distal fixation.

ments that can be used to independently reconstruct leg length, offset, and version, the popularity of these stems has increased. Although the bibody concept has improved upon the problem of stem subsidence, which was common with earlier nonmodular tapered stems, breakage at the modular junction has been reported and corrosion at this modular junction is a concern. More recent designs seem to have addressed the problems of breakage; however, increased implant cost and surgical complexity are disadvantages. These stems do work well with a very short isthmus for distal fixation (even when less than 4 cm), and the ability to adjust version to optimize stability is attractive. One retrospective study suggested better outcomes among patients who received a modular, tapered titanium stem than when a parallel-sided, cobalt-chromium, fully porous coated stem was used.[57]

Impaction Grafting

Although still commonly used in Europe, this technique is infrequently used in North America because it is time and resource intensive, and higher rates of complications (particularly intraoperative and early postoperative periprosthetic fracture and stem subsidence) have been reported.[58]

Proximal Femoral Replacement

Although proximal femoral replacement (with an allograft prosthesic composite or a proximal femoral replacement) may be the only solution in the most complex situations, surgeons should note that these techniques can be associated with a substantial risk of complications. In particular, instability is common as reattachment of the abductors to the allograft or prosthetic proximal femur can be unreliable. The use of a constrained acetabular liner should be considered.

Cemented Stems

Cemented femoral revisions are performed infrequently because it can be difficult to obtain good cement interdigitation into viable cancellous bone in the revision femur with high rates of radiographic and repeat loosening requiring re-operation reported. The results of cementless revision femoral revision, particularly with stems that gain fixation primarily in the diaphysis, have been more consistent.

Complications of THA

Instability

A recent study has shown that recurrent instability is the most common reason for revision THA.[59] The risk of instability has been correlated with multiple factors, including surgeon experience, surgical approach (posterior approach higher risk than anterior or anterolateral approaches), and femoral head size. Larger femoral heads allow for increased range of motion before impingement, and component-to-component impingement is eliminated when they are larger than 36 mm. Large heads also eliminate the need for a skirt and increase the distance that the femoral head must travel (the so-called "jump distance") for a dislocation to occur, although this still requires appropriate component position. The use of larger-diameter femoral heads has become more commonplace with the routine use of more wear-resistant bearing surfaces.

When assessing the patient with recurrent instability, it is important to determine the cause of instability and also evaluate the patient for infection because not only may the two coexist, but infection may predispose to instability. A careful assessment of both femoral and acetabular component position is paramount with acceptable position being 15° of anteversion and 40° of abduction for the acetabular component (plus or minus 10°) and femoral component anteversion of 10° to 30°. Although acetabular component abduction is easy to determine on an AP radiograph of the hip or pelvis, anteversion of the femoral and acetabular components can be more difficult to measure. A CT scan of the pelvis can be used to determine acetabular component version as this can be difficult to assess accurately intraoperatively. A CT scan of the proximal femur including a cut through the ipsilateral epicondylar axis of the knee can reliably measure femoral component anteversion, although most surgeons find this relatively easy to assess at the time of revision surgery.

If component malposition is identified in a patient with recurrent instability, revision and component re-

orientation should be performed because other revision techniques (such as isolated head/liner exchange or use of a constrained liner) are unlikely to be successful. A search for soft-tissue and bony impingement is also undertaken to further optimize stability, and a large-diameter femoral head (typically larger than 36 mm) is used to decrease and potentially eliminate component-to-component impingement. Late instability has been associated with severe polyethylene wear and is typically treated with a modular head and liner exchange and a larger diameter femoral head.

The most challenging patients to manage are those whose instability is associated with damage to the abductor musculature or their attachment via the greater trochanter. In these cases, large femoral heads have been shown not to be particularly effective and a constrained liner is usually required.[60] Although devices such as a constrained liner are useful in the most complex of situations, it is important to recognize that these devices transmit strain to the bone-prosthesis interface and can lead to catastrophic failure and increased polyethylene wear. Finally, not all designs are the same, with variable rates of success reported in the literature.

Infection

All patients with a failed or painful THA should be screened for infection with an erythrocyte sedimentation rate (ESR) and C-reactive protein (CRP). Studies have shown that these tests are very sensitive and that they are rarely normal in the face of infection.[60] If the ESR and/or CRP are abnormal and the clinical suspicion for infection is high (such as less than 2 years after surgery or a history of prior infection or wound healing problems after the initial procedure), aspiration of the hip can be performed with fluoroscopic guidance; patients must refrain from antibiotics for a minimum of 2 weeks before aspiration to decrease the risk of a falsely negative aspiration.

A recent study found that the use of the synovial fluid white blood cell (WBC) count was the best perioperative test for identifying infection.[60] Aspiration can be performed either preoperatively or intraoperatively (before entering the hip capsule). The test is inexpensive, objective, and ubiquitous. Optimal cutoff values for the synovial fluid WBC count were found to be 3,000 /mm^3 if the ESR and CRP were both elevated and 9,000 /mm^3 if the ESR or CRP (but not both) was elevated. The synovial fluid WBC differential was also found to be helpful, with an optimal cutoff point of 80% polymorphonuclear cells. Intraoperative frozen sections have also been shown to be useful for diagnosing infection; however, the criteria for determining infection have been controversial and performance is dependent on a skilled pathologist and is subject to sampling error. Intraoperative Gram stains are not a useful test for identifying infection and while usually falsely negative, they can also be falsely positive and thus should not be routinely performed. For more information on the diagnosis of periprosthetic infection

Table 6

Vancouver Classification for Periprosthetic Fractures of the Femur

Type A	**Pertrochanteric fracture**
AL	Fracture of the lesser trochanter
AG	Fracture of the greater trochanter
Type B	**Fracture around the femoral component**
B1	Femoral component well-fixed → ORIF
B2	Femoral component loose
B3	Femoral component loose with severe loss of femoral bone stock
Type C	**Fracture distal to the femoral component**

(handwritten annotation: femoral component revision)

please see the AAOS clinical practice guideline, accessed at www.aaos.org/research/guidelines/guide.asp.

The mainstays of treatment of a chronic infection include removal of the components, insertion of an antibiotic-loaded cement spacer, and systemic antibiotics for 6 weeks followed by reimplantation once the infection has been cleared. Débridement and component retention has been shown to have a high rate of failure and seems only effective in the management of some early postoperative (infections occurring within the first 4 to 6 weeks) and acute hematogenous infections, although the presence of staphylococcal species in both of these scenarios seems to portend a worse prognosis for success.

Periprosthetic Fracture

The Vancouver classification is the most widely accepted for evaluation of periprosthetic fractures of the femur[61] (**Table 6**). This classification considers the location of the fracture and most importantly, the stability of the component. B1 fractures with a stable femoral component are treated with internal fixation. Periprosthetic fractures associated with a loose femoral component (B2 or B3) require femoral component revision, most commonly with the use of a cementless stem that bypasses the fracture site and gains fixation in the diaphysis distal to the fracture; however, proximal femoral replacement may be required for B3 fractures. The most common error in management is misclassifying a Vancouver B2 fracture as a B1 and treating it with internal fixation.

Deep Venous Thrombosis and Pulmonary Embolism

This topic is covered in chapter 12. Please refer to the AAOS Clinical Practice Guidelines on Pulmonary Embolism, which can be accessed at www.aaos.org/research/guidelines/guide.asp.

Annotated References

1. Helmick CG, Felson DT, Lawrence RC, et al; National Arthritis Data Workgroup: Estimates of the prevalence of arthritis and other rheumatic conditions in the United States: Part I. *Arthritis Rheum* 2008;58(1):15-25.

   The authors describe the prevalence of arthritis and other rheumatologic inflammatory conditions in the United States.

2. Lawrence RC, Felson DT, Helmick CG, et al; National Arthritis Data Workgroup: Estimates of the prevalence of arthritis and other rheumatic conditions in the United States. Part II. *Arthritis Rheum* 2008;58(1):26-35.

   The authors described the prevalence of arthritis and other rheumatologic inflammatory conditions in the United States.

3. Jessel RH, Zilkens C, Tiderius C, Dudda M, Mamisch TC, Kim YJ: Assessment of osteoarthritis in hips with femoroacetabular impingement using delayed gadolinium enhanced MRI of cartilage. *J Magn Reson Imaging* 2009;30(5):1110-1115.

   The authors found that the results of osteoplasty for FAI depend on the amount of preexisting OA in the hip joint. dGEMRIC can be used in the diagnosis and staging of OA.

4. Ganz R, Parvizi J, Beck M, Leunig M, Nötzli H, Siebenrock KA: Femoroacetabular impingement: A cause for osteoarthritis of the hip. *Clin Orthop Relat Res* 2003; 417(417):112-120.

5. Ganz R, Leunig M, Leunig-Ganz K, Harris WH: The etiology of osteoarthritis of the hip: An integrated mechanical concept. *Clin Orthop Relat Res* 2008;466(2): 264-272.

   The authors describe eloquently how FAI may lead to OA in the native hip.

6. Sierra RJ, Trousdale RT, Ganz R, Leunig M: Hip disease in the young, active patient: Evaluation and nonarthroplasty surgical options. *J Am Acad Orthop Surg* 2008;16(12):689-703.

   This is a review article describing physical examination findings, radiographic features, and surgical management of FAI.

7. Clohisy JC, Carlisle JC, Beaulé PE, et al: A systematic approach to the plain radiographic evaluation of the young adult hip. *J Bone Joint Surg Am* 2008;90(suppl 4):47-66.

   This is a description of the radiographic technique and evaluation of imaging findings in patients with FAI and hip dysplasia.

8. Notzli HP, Wyss TF, Stoecklin CH, Schmid MR, Treiber K, Hodler J: The contour of the femoral head-neck junction as a predictor for the risk of anterior impingement. *J Bone Joint Surg Br* 2002;84(4):556-560.

9. Ganz R, Gill TJ, Gautier E, Ganz K, Krügel N, Berle-

mann U: Surgical dislocation of the adult hip a technique with full access to the femoral head and acetabulum without the risk of avascular necrosis. *J Bone Joint Surg Br* 2001;83(8):1119-1124.

10. Espinosa N, Rothenfluh DA, Beck M, Ganz R, Leunig M: Treatment of femoro-acetabular impingement: Preliminary results of labral refixation. *J Bone Joint Surg Am* 2006;88(5):925-935.

11. Beck M, Leunig M, Parvizi J, Boutier V, Wyss D, Ganz R: Anterior femoroacetabular impingement: Part II. Midterm results of surgical treatment. *Clin Orthop Relat Res* 2004;418(418):67-73.

12. Laude F, Sariali E, Nogier A: Femoroacetabular impingement treatment using arthroscopy and anterior approach. *Clin Orthop Relat Res* 2009;467(3):747-752.

    The authors describe the treatment of FAI using an anterior approach combined with hip arthroscopy. There was a high rate of labral refixation failure in this study.

13. Byrd JW, Jones KS: Arthroscopic femoroplasty in the management of cam-type femoroacetabular impingement. *Clin Orthop Relat Res* 2009;467(3):739-746.

    The authors describe the arthroscopic treatment of cam FAI lesions with overall excellent results.

14. Ganz R, Klaue K, Vinh TS, Mast JW: A new periacetabular osteotomy for the treatment of hip dysplasias: Technique and preliminary results. *Clin Orthop Relat Res* 1988;232(232):26-36.

15. Philippon MJ, Briggs KK, Yen YM, Kuppersmith DA: Outcomes following hip arthroscopy for femoroacetabular impingement with associated chondrolabral dysfunction: Minimum two-year follow-up. *J Bone Joint Surg Br* 2009;91(1):16-23.

    The authors describe the arthroscopic management of FAI for both the acetabular and femoral sides. At a mean follow-up of 2.3 years, the results were satisfactory in most patients.

16. Stähelin L, Stähelin T, Jolles BM, Herzog RF: Arthroscopic offset restoration in femoroacetabular cam impingement: Accuracy and early clinical outcome. *Arthroscopy* 2008;24(1):51-57, e1.

    The authors report on 22 patients with symptomatic cam type femoroacetabular impingement treated with arthroscopic débridement and femoral osteochondroplasty. The results at 6 months were satisfactory with improvements in clinical scores.

17. Murphy SB, Ganz R, Müller ME: The prognosis in untreated dysplasia of the hip: A study of radiographic factors that predict the outcome. *J Bone Joint Surg Am* 1995;77(7):985-989.

18. Li PL, Ganz R: Morphologic features of congenital acetabular dysplasia: One in six is retroverted. *Clin Orthop Relat Res* 2003;416:245-253.

19. Siebenrock KA, Leunig M, Ganz R: Periacetabular osteotomy: The Bernese experience, in Sim H, ed: *Instructional Course Lectures.* Volume 50. Rosemont, IL, American Academy of Orthopaedic Surgeons, 2001, vol 50, pp 239-245.

20. Trousdale RT, Ekkernkamp A, Ganz R, Wallrichs SL: Periacetabular and intertrochanteric osteotomy for the treatment of osteoarthritis in dysplastic hips. *J Bone Joint Surg Am* 1995;77:73-85.

21. Crowe JF, Mani VJ, Ranawat CS: Total hip replacement in congenital dislocation and dysplasia of the hip. *J Bone Joint Surg Am* 1979;61:15-23.

22. Lavernia CJ, Sierra RJ, Grieco FR: Osteonecrosis of the femoral head. *J Am Acad Orthop Surg* 1999;7(4):250-261.

23. Steinberg ME, Hayken GD, Steinberg DR: A quantitative system for staging avascular necrosis. *J Bone Joint Surg Br* 1995;77(1):34-41.

24. Hernigou P, Habibi A, Bachir D, Galacteros F: The natural history of asymptomatic osteonecrosis of the femoral head in adults with sickle cell disease. *J Bone Joint Surg Am* 2006;88(12):2565-2572.

25. Hernigou P, Poignard A, Nogier A, Manicom O: Fate of very small asymptomatic stage-I osteonecrotic lesions of the hip. *J Bone Joint Surg Am* 2004;86(12):2589-2593.

26. Mont MA, Carbone JJ, Fairbank AC: Core decompression versus nonoperative management for osteonecrosis of the hip. *Clin Orthop Relat Res* 1996;324(324):169-178.

27. Ramachandran M, Ward K, Brown RR, Munns CF, Cowell CT, Little DG: Intravenous bisphosphonate therapy for traumatic osteonecrosis of the femoral head in adolescents. *J Orthop Surg* 2008;13(5):463-468.

    The authors evaluated the use of bisphosphonates in treating adolescents with osteonecrosis of the femoral head after trauma and found it to be a useful adjunct therapy.

28. Iwakiri K, Oda Y, Kaneshiro Y, et al: Effect of simvastatin on steroid-induced osteonecrosis evidenced by the serum lipid level and hepatic cytochrome P4503A in a rabbit model. *J Orthop Sci* 2008;13(5):463-468.

    In a study to determine the efficacy of lipid-lowering agents in the prevention of steroid-induced osteonecrosis in a rabbit model, the authors found that simvastatin and pravastatin substantially reduced the incidence of osteonecrosis, with simvastatin being more effective.

29. Korompilias AV, Lykissas MG, Beris AE, Urbaniak JR, Soucacos PN: Vascularised fibular graft in the management of femoral head osteonecrosis: Twenty years later. *J Bone Joint Surg Br* 2009;91(3):287-293.

    The authors discussed the advantages of vascularized fibular graft as a joint-preserving method in the treatment of femoral head osteonecrosis.

30. Hernigou P, Beaujean F: Treatment of osteonecrosis with autologous bone marrow grafting. *Clin Orthop Relat Res* 2002;405:14-23.

31. Cuckler JM, Moore KD, Estrada L: Outcome of hemiresurfacing in osteonecrosis of the femoral head. *Clin Orthop Relat Res* 2004;429(429):146-150.

32. Revell MP, McBryde CW, Bhatnagar S, Pynsent PB, Treacy RB: Metal-on-metal hip resurfacing in osteonecrosis of the femoral head. *J Bone Joint Surg Am* 2006; 88(suppl 3):98-103.

33. Fye MA, Huo MH, Zatorski LE, Keggi KJ: Total hip arthroplasty performed without cement in patients with femoral head osteonecrosis who are less than 50 years old. *J Arthroplasty* 1998;13(8):876-881.

34. Hungerford MW, Hungerford DS, Jones LC: Outcome of uncemented primary femoral stems for treatment of femoral head osteonecrosis. *Orthop Clin North Am* 2009;40(2):283-289.

    The authors report the results of uncemented primary total hip arthroplasty in patients with osteonecrosis with excellent results using an uncemented stem.

35. Steinberg ME, Lai M, Garino JP, Ong A, Wong KL: A comparison between total hip replacement for osteonecrosis and degenerative joint disease. *Orthopedics* 2008; 31(4):360.

    The authors studied 203 total hip replacements for osteonecrosis and compared them with 300 done for degenerative joint disease. Total hip replacement was found to be a good treatment for patients with advanced osteonecrosis.

36. Della Valle CJ, Mesko NW, Quigley L, Rosenberg AG, Jacobs JJ, Galante JO: Primary total hip arthroplasty with a porous-coated acetabular component: A concise follow-up, at a minimum of twenty years, of previous reports. *J Bone Joint Surg Am* 2009;91(5):1130-1135.

    At a minimum of 20 years, survivorship of the acetabular component was 96%. A modular polyethylene liner exchange was required or recommended in 19% of surviving hips. Level of evidence: IV.

37. Della Valle CJ, Berger RA, Shott S, et al: Primary total hip arthroplasty with a porous-coated acetabular component: A concise follow-up of a previous report. *J Bone Joint Surg Am* 2004;86(6):1217-1222.

38. Livermore J, Ilstrup D, Morrey B: Effect of femoral head size on wear of the polyethylene acetabular component. *J Bone Joint Surg Am* 1990;72(4):518-528.

39. Leung SB, Egawa H, Stepniewski A, Beykirch S, Engh CA Jr, Engh CA Sr: Incidence and volume of pelvic osteolysis at early follow-up with highly cross-linked and noncross-linked polyethylene. *J Arthroplasty* 2007; 22(6, suppl 2)134-139.

    Patients implanted with a highly cross-linked liner had a lower incidence of pelvic osteolysis than those implanted with a standard polyethylene liner that was not cross-linked as determined by pelvic CT scanning. Level of evidence: I.

40. Callaghan JJ, Liu SS, Firestone DE, et al: Total hip arthroplasty with cement and use of a collared matte-finish femoral component: Nineteen to twenty-year follow-up. *J Bone Joint Surg Am* 2008;90(2):299-306.

    At a minimum of 19 years, the matte-finish cemented femoral component had 85% survivorship with revision for aseptic loosening as the end point. Level of evidence: IV.

41. Lombardi AV Jr, Berend KR, Mallory TH, Skeels MD, Adams JB: Survivorship of 2000 tapered titanium porous plasma-sprayed femoral components. *Clin Orthop Relat Res* 2009;467(1):146-154.

    Survivorship of the tapered, titanium, porous plasma sprayed femoral component was 95.5% at 20 years with failure for any reason and 99.3% at 20 years with failure for aseptic loosening as the end point. Level of evidence: IV.

42. Teloken MA, Bissett G, Hozack WJ, Sharkey PF, Rothman RH: Ten to fifteen-year follow-up after total hip arthroplasty with a tapered cobalt-chromium femoral component (tri-lock) inserted without cement. *J Bone Joint Surg Am* 2002;84(12):2140-2144.

43. Kim YH, Kim JS, Oh SH, Kim JM: Comparison of porous-coated titanium femoral stems with and without hydroxyapatite coating. *J Bone Joint Surg Am* 2003; 85(9):1682-1688.

44. Belmont PJ Jr, Powers CC, Beykirch SE, Hopper RH Jr, Engh CA Jr, Engh CA: Results of the anatomic medullary locking total hip arthroplasty at a minimum of twenty years: A concise follow-up of previous reports. *J Bone Joint Surg Am* 2008;90(7):1524-1530.

    At a mean of 22 years, survivorship of the diaphyseal engaging, fully porous coated cobalt-chromium stem was 97.8%. Failure of the cementless acetabular component used was correlated with the presence of osteolysis. Level of evidence: IV.

45. Rodrigues DC, Urban RM, Jacobs JJ, Gilbert JL: In vivo severe corrosion and hydrogen embrittlement of retrieved modular body titanium alloy hip-implants. *J Biomed Mater Res B Appl Biomater* 2009;88(1):206-219.

    In this retrieval analysis of three different designs of modular body femoral components, some degree of corrosion was seen at the modular junction of all components studied.

46. Daniel J, Pynsent PB, McMinn DJ: Metal-on-metal resurfacing of the hip in patients under the age of 55 years with osteoarthritis. *J Bone Joint Surg Br* 2004;86(2): 177-184.

47. Amstutz HC, Le Duff MJ: Eleven years of experience with metal-on-metal hybrid hip resurfacing: A review of 1000 conserve plus. *J Arthroplasty* 2008;23(6, suppl 1): 36-43.

In this report of 1,000 consecutive resurfacings performed by a single surgeon, survivorship was 92% at 8 years, with most failures occurring early in the series. It is important to note that in general this series is a challenging group of young patients with abnormal femoral anatomy. Level of evidence: IV.

48. Buergi ML, Walter WL: Hip resurfacing arthroplasty: The Australian experience. *J Arthroplasty* 2007;22(7, suppl 3):61-65.

In this report of the Australian hip registry, early revision rates for hip resurfacing were shown to be higher than a conventional THA for all groups of patients other than males younger than 55 years. Level of evidence: IV.

49. Shimmin AJ, Back D: Femoral neck fractures following Birmingham hip resurfacing: A national review of 50 cases. *J Bone Joint Surg Br* 2005;87(4):463-464.

50. Lavigne M, Therrien M, Nantel J, Roy A, Prince F, Vendittoli PA: The John Charnley Award: The functional outcome of hip resurfacing and large-head THA is the same: A randomized, double-blind study. *Clin Orthop Relat Res* 2010;468:326-336.

In this prospective, blinded, randomized clinical trial, the functional outcomes of hip resurfacing and conventional THA were found to be similar. Level of evidence: I.

51. Paprosky WG, Perona PG, Lawrence JM: Acetabular defect classification and surgical reconstruction in revision arthroplasty: A 6-year follow-up evaluation. *J Arthroplasty* 1994;9(1):33-44.

52. Berry DJ, Lewallen DG, Hanssen AD, Cabanela ME: Pelvic discontinuity in revision total hip arthroplasty. *J Bone Joint Surg Am* 1999;81(12):1692-1702.

53. Park DK, Della Valle CJ, Quigley L, Moric M, Rosenberg AG, Galante JO: Revision of the acetabular component without cement: A concise follow-up, at twenty to twenty-four years, of a previous report. *J Bone Joint Surg Am* 2009;91(2):350-355.

At a minimum of 20 years, revision of the acetabulum with a cementless acetabular component showed survivorship of 95%. The most common reasons for repeat revision were infection and recurrent dislocation. Level of evidence: IV.

54. Nehme A, Lewallen DG, Hanssen AD: Modular porous metal augments for treatment of severe acetabular bone loss during revision hip arthroplasty. *Clin Orthop Relat Res* 2004;429:201-208.

55. Della Valle CJ, Paprosky WG: The femur in revision total hip arthroplasty evaluation and classification. *Clin Orthop Relat Res* 2004;420:55-62.

56. Weeden SH, Paprosky WG: Minimal 11-year follow-up of extensively porous-coated stems in femoral revision total hip arthroplasty. *J Arthroplasty* 2002;17(4, suppl 1):134-137.

57. Garbuz DS, Toms A, Masri BA, Duncan CP: Improved outcome in femoral revision arthroplasty with tapered fluted modular titanium stems. *Clin Orthop Relat Res* 2006;453:199-202.

58. Meding JB, Ritter MA, Keating EM, Faris PM: Impaction bone-grafting before insertion of a femoral stem with cement in revision total hip arthroplasty: A minimum two-year follow-up study. *J Bone Joint Surg Am* 1997;79(12):1834-1841.

59. Bozic KJ, Kurtz SM, Lau E, Ong K, Vail TP, Berry DJ: The epidemiology of revision total hip arthroplasty in the United States. *J Bone Joint Surg Am* 2009;91(1):128-133.

A review of 51,345 revision THAs from the nationwide inpatient sample database showed that instability and prosthetic loosening were the most common causes of revision THA. Level of evidence: II.

60. Kung PL, Ries MD: Effect of femoral head size and abductors on dislocation after revision THA. *Clin Orthop Relat Res* 2007;465:170-174.

This retrospective review of 230 patients undergoing revision THA showed that a 36-mm femoral head was associated with a significantly lower risk of dislocation than a 28-mm femoral head; however, the dislocation rate remained high if the abductor muscles were not intact. Level of evidence: IV.

61. Masri BA, Meek RM, Duncan CP: Periprosthetic fractures evaluation and treatment. *Clin Orthop Relat Res* 2004;420:80-95.

FEMUR

trochanteric ht: normally @ center of femoral head
version: 20° anteversion / internal torsion of condyles in relation to femoral head-neck axis
lateral offset: dist. btwn center of head & tip of trochanter = aBductor lever arm & inversely proportional to jt. rxn F in hip; norm. 2x width of head
head-neck offset: narrower neck relative to larger head = good for ROM
CONGRUITY OF HIP
medial space: btwn femoral head & Kohler's line, 10-15mm
shenton's line: continuation of superior obturator bordment & inferior femoral head-neck

Chapter 33

Femoral Fractures

Jodi Siegel, MD   Paul Tornetta III, MD

4: Lower Extremity

Introduction

Fractures of the femoral shaft occur in patients of all ages and result from a variety of mechanisms. These fractures tend to show a bimodal incidence, typically occurring as a result of high-energy trauma in younger patients or low-energy falls in elderly patients. The understanding of femoral shaft fractures and the effect of these fractures on patients has continued to grow over the past 60 years, allowing improvements in overall patient care and creating expectations of treatment success.

Classification

Femoral shaft fractures are often classified by location and geometry. The femoral shaft is often divided into thirds for descriptive purposes, with fractures reported in the proximal, middle, or distal portion of the shaft. Additionally, the fracture pattern is generally reported as transverse, short oblique, long spiral, or comminuted. The Winquist and Hansen classification more specifically quantifies the comminution of the fracture[1] (Table 1). This classification system helps to characterize axial stability; types I and II are axially stable and types III and IV are axially and rotationally unstable.

Mechanisms of Injury and Fracture Management

High-energy femoral shaft fractures occur from the usual trauma mechanisms: motor vehicle crashes, motorcycle crashes, pedestrian versus motor vehicle injuries, and falls from a height. Because patients often have other systemic injuries in addition to musculoskeletal injuries, a complete trauma examination must be performed.

The evaluation of patients with high-energy femoral shaft fractures must include a systematic assessment for associated injuries. Patients should be examined for head, chest, and abdominal injuries. Hemodynamic status must be monitored because clinically relevant blood loss can occur into the thigh.[2] The neurovascular status of the limb must be assessed in addition to the integrity of the skin. Although vascular compromise in association with closed femoral shaft fractures caused by blunt trauma is uncommon, it must not go undiagnosed. Restoration of general fracture alignment can unkink vessels and allow a more accurate examination. If there is any difficulty in examining the distal pulse, ankle-brachial index measurements should be obtained. Ankle-brachial values less than 0.9 are considered abnormal and may indicate clinically significant vascular compromise. A neurologic examination can be difficult because of the patient's inability to cooperate; however, attempts must be made to achieve an accurate examination.

Other musculoskeletal injuries are common. Bilateral femoral fractures occur in as many as 10% of patients and are associated with higher mortality and Injury Severity Scores.[3,4] Associated femoral neck fractures should be evaluated. Dedicated hip radiographs and a fine-cut CT scan through the femoral neck are recommended.[5] CT scans used to evaluate the abdomen and pelvis can be formatted to include fine cuts through the femoral neck to allow for a more thorough bony radiographic examination. Preoperative radiographs of the entire femur and dedicated radiographs of the hip and knee are necessary to look for

Table 1

Winquist and Hansen Classification of Femoral Shaft Fracture Comminution

Grade	Degree of Comminution
0	No comminution
I	Small butterfly fragment; ≥ 50% cortical contact
II	Large butterfly fragment; < 50% cortical contact
III	Larger butterfly fragment; minimal cortical abutment
IV	No cortical contact; segmentally comminuted

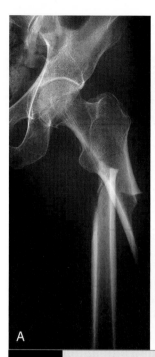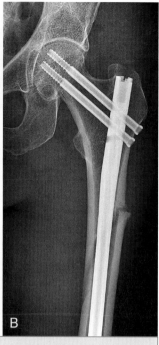

Figure 1 Radiographs showing unicortical beaking hypertrophy in a patient on prolonged bisphosphonate therapy. **A,** The injury is seen. **B,** Fixation with a cephalomedullary nail.

additional fractures that can affect the treatment plan. The stability of the knee can be evaluated after the femur has been stabilized.

Although elderly patients may present for treatment as a result of high-energy trauma, low-energy femoral fractures resulting from a fall from standing height are a common occurrence. Preexisting medical conditions complicate treatment in this patient cohort. The use of oral bisphosphonates for more than 4 years has recently been associated with simple transverse or short oblique femoral fractures in areas of diaphyseal cortical hypertrophy with a unicortical beak[6-9] (**Figure 1**). Pathologic femoral fractures can also present after trauma. Careful examination of the radiographs in addition to a thorough history should be completed for every patient to allow for appropriate treatment.

Treatment

Nonsurgical treatment for femoral fractures is rarely used in adult patients. Traction as a form of definitive treatment has limited indications, such as in patients with significant medical comorbidities. Traction is applicable for the temporary stabilization of femoral fractures until definitive internal fixation can be performed because it can reestablish limb length, prevent further injury to the soft tissues, and provide comfort to the patient. Traction is also useful when infection requires removal of all internal fixation devices. Both distal fem-

oral and proximal tibial skeletal traction can be used; however, proximal tibial traction is contraindicated in patients with knee dislocations.

External fixation as definitive treatment also has limited indications but is used more often as a temporizing measure. It provides bony stability while allowing for the care of multiple-trauma patients. Its application can also be beneficial in cases of vascular injury when fracture stability is urgent. External fixation also has a role in severely contaminated wounds, especially when the intramedullary canal is heavily soiled and would benefit from repeat débridements before definitive fixation.

Closed, locked, intramedullary nailing remains the treatment of choice for adult femoral shaft fractures. Union rates are reported as high as 99% and surgical complication rates are low.[1] Various techniques have been introduced, with support in the literature for the use of each technique.

Damage control orthopaedics has been advocated to avoid a "second hit" in multiple-trauma patients by delaying definitive fracture repair in favor of temporizing the fracture with traction or external fixation in physiologically unstable patients. Exacerbation of a systemic inflammatory response in an already compromised patient and of fat emboli released into a traumatized pulmonary system may be avoided by less invasive, temporizing measures in unstable patients and patients in extremis.[10] The borderline patient, especially with an associated chest injury, remains difficult to universally define[11] (**Table 2**). Multiple studies report acceptable pulmonary outcomes with early fixation, but there is concern that selection bias exists in those studies against patients with the most severe chest injuries.[12-14] Although thoracic trauma does not preclude fixation with an intramedullary nail, the exact timing of optimal stabilization in these patients is still being debated.[12,13,15-17]

Reamed intramedullary nailing is considered the gold standard of treatment.[13] The canal is filled by the insertion of a large-diameter nail, which is associated with greater union rates compared with smaller diameter nails. In patients with chest trauma, several investigators have examined whether reaming further compromises pulmonary function.[13,18,19] Initial reports expressed concern for worsening of pulmonary function with reaming, especially in the borderline patient.[18] More recent data report no difference ($P = 0.42$) in the incidence of acute respiratory distress syndrome using reamed nails (3 of 171 fractures) versus unreamed nails (2 of 151 fractures).[13] Additionally, delayed fixation compared with early fixation (within 24 hours of injury) was associated with higher rates of pneumonia in patients both with (48% versus 15%, respectively; $P = 0.002$) and without (38% versus 10%, respectively; $P = 0.07$) chest trauma. Mortality rates and the length of mechanical ventilation also tended to be higher in the delayed fixation groups.[19]

Table 2

Clinical Condition of Multiple-Trauma Patients[a]

	Parameter	Stable	Borderline	Unstable	In Extremis
Shock	Blood pressure	≥ 100	80-100	< 90	≤ 70
	Units blood over 2 hours	0-2	2-8	5-15	> 15
	Lactate	Normal	~2.5	> 2.5	Severe acidosis
	ATLS class	I	II-III	III-IV	IV
Coagulation	Platelets	> 110,000	90,000-110,000	< 70,000-90,000	< 70,000
	Factors II and IV	90-100	70-89	50-70	< 50
	Fibrinogen	> 1	~1	< 1	DIC
	D-dimer	Normal	Abnormal	Abnormal	DIC
Temperature	°C (°F)	< 33 (< 91.4)	33-35 (91.4-95.0)	30-32 (86.0-89.6)	≤ 30 (≤ 86.0)
Soft-tissue injury	Pao$_2$/FiO2	350-400	300-350	200-300	< 200
	AIS – chest	1 or 2	≥ 2	≥ 3	≥ 3
	Moore – abdomen	≤ II	≤ III	III	≥ III
	AO – pelvic fracture	A (none)	B or C	C	C
	External	AIS I-II	AIS II-III	AIS III-IV	Crush

[a]Three of four criteria must be met to classify for a certain grade.
ATLS = Advanced Trauma Life Support; AIS = Abbreviated Injury Score; Moore = classification for abdominal trauma; AO = pelvic trauma classification system; DIC = disseminated intravascular coagulation.

Antegrade Nailing

Insertion of an intramedullary nail from the hip is considered by many surgeons to be the gold standard for femoral fracture fixation. The piriformis fossa, which is colinear with the long axis of the intramedullary canal, has long been the preferred starting point for an antegrade nail. Using this site as the entry portal decreases the chances of fracture malalignment and iatrogenic comminution, particularly in proximal third fractures. However, precision in locating the piriformis fossa is important because an entry portal directed too anteriorly is associated with increased hoop stresses and iatrogenic femoral neck fracture.[20]

The greater trochanter is an attractive alternative to the piriformis fossa as an entry portal because of its more subcutaneous location. This entry portal facilitates access in patients with truncal obesity and may be preferred by a surgeon based on his or her experience. Nail designs have been altered to include a proximal lateral bend in an attempt to avoid varus malalignment with trochanteric entry.[21] Recent comparisons of trochanteric entry nails to piriformis entry nails have shown similar outcomes.[22,23] There was no difference in union (97% in trochanteric entry compared with 98% in piriformis entry), average surgical time (62 minutes versus 75 minutes, respectively; $P = 0.08$), number of infections (one in each group), or baseline and subsequent improvements in the Lower Extremity Measure score.

Hip abductor weakness and a Trendelenburg gait are common after antegrade nailing regardless of the entry portal used. Early postoperative lateral trunk lean correlates with poorer long-term patient-reported functional outcomes.[24] Even when there is no clinical evidence of a Trendelenburg gait, hip abductor muscles may still be significantly weak when compared with the uninjured extremity; this can lead to persistent mild to moderate pain.[25]

Retrograde Nailing

Proposed indications for retrograde nailing include patients with bilateral femoral fractures;[26] ipsilateral pelvic, acetabular, or hip fractures; multiple trauma; ipsilateral tibial fractures; and those who are pregnant or obese. Recently, retrograde nailing in obese patients was found to be associated with less surgical time and less radiation exposure compared with antegrade nailing.[27]

Many surgeons have expressed concerns for inserting femoral nails through the knee. The theoretical increased risk of joint sepsis, knee stiffness, or iatrogenic arthritis has not proven to be a problem. The effect on functional outcome of insertion site complications is unknown. In a randomized trial performed in the year 2000, proximal thigh and hip pain was reported in 10 of 46 patients (22%) treated with antegrade nailing.[28] Although knee pain and range of motion were similar in each group, 18 of 54 patients (33%) treated with retrograde nailing reported distal locking bolt pain. Lysholm knee scores and isokinetic knee measurements were similar between groups in a study of 71 patients randomized to either antegrade or retrograde nail.[29] Union rates and malalignment complications with newer techniques are similar between antegrade and retrograde nailing.[30]

Plating

Plate fixation of femoral shaft fractures is rarely used in adult patients secondary to the excellent union rates and limited complications associated with intramedullary nailing. Percutaneous techniques with indirect reduction methods and submuscular plating have decreased the morbidity of plate fixation. Nonetheless, periprosthetic fractures, fractures in patients with small intramedullary canals, and ipsilateral neck-shaft fractures may be more amenable to treatment with a plate.

Special Situations

Femoral Neck-Shaft Fractures

Ipsilateral femoral neck and femoral shaft fractures are believed to result from a longitudinal force directed through a flexed knee and hip. The incidence is reported to be as high as 10%, and as many as 30% of these injuries are not identified during the initial patient assessment.[31-34] Although femoral neck fractures that occur with an ipsilateral shaft fracture are associated with less risk of osteonecrosis than isolated femoral neck fractures because of the dissipation of force to the shaft,[35] the complications of nonunion of the femoral neck and osteonecrosis of the femoral head are time sensitive and more severe than those of femoral shaft fractures. Every effort should be used to prevent a delay in diagnosing femoral neck-shaft fractures. Because 25% to 60% of these femoral neck fractures are nondisplaced at the time of presentation, diagnosis can be difficult without adequate imaging studies. Various protocols have been reported to decrease the incidence of missed femoral neck fractures. A preoperative thin-cut CT scan of the femoral neck and postoperative 15° internal rotation AP image of the hip before waking the patient have been reported to reduce the delay in diagnosing an associated femoral neck fracture.[5]

Multiple treatment options exist for stabilizing these ipsilateral injuries. Prioritizing reduction and fixation of the femoral neck fracture is advocated. The pattern of femoral neck fracture tends to be a Pauwels type III vertical fracture. (See chapter 31, figure 5, for an illustration showing the Pauwels classification system.) A recent study reported that open reduction with internal fixation of the femoral neck followed by retrograde nailing for the shaft fracture allowed accurate reduction and uneventful union of both fractures.[36] The use of a cephalomedullary nail resulted in more malreductions of one of the fractures compared with the use of two devices. Thus, the current recommendation is using two devices for fixation, with accurate reduction of both fractures.

Open Fractures

Open femoral shaft fractures are much less common than open tibial shaft fractures because of the extensive soft-tissue envelope. Most open fractures are the result of high-energy trauma and are typically associated with significant soft-tissue injury and periosteal stripping.

These open fractures should be treated as soon as the patient is medically able and the appropriate resources are available. Wounds should be extended to débride all devitalized soft tissue and bone. Unless the intramedullary canal is grossly contaminated, immediate intramedullary nailing is acceptable. Low infection and nonunion rates have been reported.[1]

Gunshot Wounds

Femoral shaft fractures caused by low-velocity gunshot wounds are technically believed to be open injuries but can be treated like closed fractures; local débridement of the skin and subcutaneous tissues at the entry and exit sites without deep débridement is adequate.[37,38] Immediate, reamed, locked intramedullary nailing is associated with similar union and infection rates as those in closed femoral fractures.[39,40] Higher-energy gunshot wounds, such as those caused by shotgun blasts and high-velocity guns, should be treated with standard open fracture care because of the increased amount of soft-tissue injury.[41]

Bilateral Fractures

Patients with bilateral fractures of the femur have a higher mortality rate and overall worse prognosis. There is an increased risk of adult respiratory distress syndrome. The mortality rate ranges from 5% to 25%, compared with 1.5% to 11% for patients with unilateral femoral fractures.[3,4,26] This increase is related to the associated injuries and physiologic parameters as opposed to the fractures themselves.[3] Treatment with bilateral reamed intramedullary nails is recommended.[4,26]

Vascular Injury

Femoral shaft fractures with vascular or neurologic injury are typically caused by penetrating trauma. Bony stability and prompt revascularization is the goal but the sequence of these events is controversial.[42,43] The timing of the injury in relationship to presentation is vital because revascularization within 6 hours will decrease complications. External fixation is the simplest way to achieve immediate bony stability. In the absence of infected pin sites, external fixation can be converted safely to an intramedullary nail within 2 weeks without an increased risk of deep infection.[44] An alternative treatment method is to use a temporary vascular shunt to reestablish blood flow and then perform definitive internal fixation and vascular repair.[45] A shunt decreased total ischemia time in a group of patients with blunt popliteal injury treated with a temporary intraluminal arterial shunt compared with a group of patients treated without a shunt.[45] The shunt group had less total ischemic time, which decreased the fasciotomy rate, the need for repeat operations, and the overall complication rate.

Complications

Although surgical complication rates with locked intramedullary nail treatment of femoral shaft fractures is low, the rate of other minor complications, including hip and knee pain, hardware-related pain, and the presence of a limp, is as high as 40%.[30]

Malunion

Malalignment of femoral shaft fractures can be prevented by obtaining an adequate reduction before reaming and nail insertion. Obtaining an accurate entry portal is also essential to preventing malalignment because lateralized starting portals with antegrade nailing cause varus malalignment.[1,23,46,47] Fractures involving the isthmus rarely (2% of cases) result in unacceptable alignment (2%). Proximal (30%), distal (10%), and unstable (12%) shaft fractures are at higher risk for malunion.[48] Rotational alignment can be difficult to judge intraoperatively. Careful assessment and positioning can prevent unacceptable reductions. By using the intact, contralateral femur as the template, fluoroscopy can be used to judge rotational alignment based on the femoral neck anteversion, the position of the lesser trochanter, and the cortical thickness[49] (**Figure 2**). The surgically treated limb should be compared clinically with the contralateral side for any malrotation or length discrepancies, and these should be corrected before leaving the operating theater. Prepping both lower extremities into the surgical field may facilitate this evaluation.

Nonunion

Regardless of the technique used, the nonunion rate of femoral shaft fractures after reamed, locked intramedullary nailing is less than 10%. When nonunion occurs, the first step in treatment should include a thorough evaluation for deep infection and metabolic abnormalities. Infection rates in closed fractures treated with intramedullary nails is 1%; open fracture infection rates are higher and correlate with the associated soft-tissue injury. In general, the most common metabolic or endocrine abnormality associated with fracture nonunion is vitamin D deficiency; correction of this abnormality has been reported to lead to union without further surgery with medical treatment alone.[50] A recent, large, case-controlled study reported that risk factors for nonunion include tobacco use, the presence of an open fracture, and delayed weight bearing (defined as more than 6 weeks after surgery).[51] Previous investigations identified nonsteroidal anti-inflammatory drug use and unreamed nail insertion as other risk factors.[52,53] Dynamization as a treatment method has questionable support in the literature. Patients must be followed closely because of the risk of significant limb shortening. Success rates are variable, with one study reporting a decrease in the nonunion rate from 16% to 4% with early dynamization.[54] The success rate of exchange nailing has been reported only in poorly controlled, small, retrospective studies, with failure rates approaching 50%.[55] A recent study reported fracture union in 36 of 42 patients (86%) 4 months after exchange nailing.[56] Plate fixation of nonunions, with or without bone grafting, has a more reliable union rate;

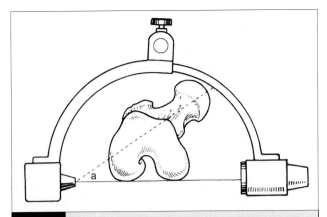

| **Figure 2** | Illustration of a C-arm used to obtain a perfect lateral fluoroscopic image of the femoral neck of the uninjured femur. The C-arm is then rotated until the posterior condyles of the femur are aligned for a perfect lateral image of the distal femur. This angle (a) is the true anteversion; it can then be applied to the fractured femur before interlocking to prevent rotational malalignment. (Adapted with permission from Tornetta P III, Ritz G, Kantor A: Femoral torsion after interlocked nailing of unstable femoral fractures. *J Trauma* 1995;38:213-219.) |

however, protected weight bearing is required after surgery.

Other Complications

Painful hardware in association with femoral nailing is most commonly encountered with distal locking bolts and retrograde femoral nails.[28] Because of the trapezoidal anatomy of the femoral condyles, if the length of the locking bolts is determined radiographically, the bolts will be proud and cause irritation. Additionally, nails that are left even 1 mm proud in the intercondylar notch can irritate the patellar cartilage, especially in knee flexion. Care must be taken when inserting the nails to use accurate fluoroscopic views to avoid these complications. A direct examination by palpation should be performed if there is concern for nail protrusion.

Patient positioning and the surgical table used affect the risk of complications. Antegrade nailing on a fracture table with a peroneal post can cause pudendal nerve compression and neurapraxia. Symptoms resolve in most patients by 6 months. The magnitude of intraoperative traction is implicated more than the duration of traction.[57] Genitoperineal skin necrosis can result from prolonged traction against the post. A recent report describes six patients who required surgical débridement of partial-thickness necrosis involving the perineum and scrotum.[58] The hemilithotomy position of the well leg can cause compartment syndrome, especially in instances of prolonged nailing or when there are contralateral leg injuries. Using a heel support instead of a calf sling to allow the calf to hang freely has been reported to significantly decrease the intramuscular pressures.[59]

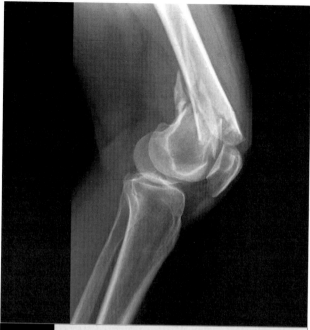

Figure 3   Lateral radiograph showing a typical deformity in a supracondylar femoral fracture.

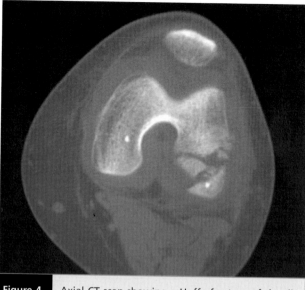

Figure 4   Axial CT scan showing a Hoffa fracture of the distal femoral condyle.

Fat embolism is often discussed as a complication of intramedullary nailing of femoral fractures in the patient with multiple traumatic injuries with an associated chest injury. Patients with pathologic fractures are also at risk. Severe embolization and large coagulative masses have been shown to occur with reaming of pathologic femurs.[60] Venting of the femur may decrease the risk of fat embolism during prophylactic nailing of intact femurs.

Distal Femoral Fractures

Fractures at the distal end of the femur can also be categorized into high-energy injuries in trauma patients and low-energy injuries in elderly patients. The high-energy fractures can include significant damage to the articular surface and can potentially result in long-term disability and posttraumatic arthritis.

Mechanism of Injury

Most distal femoral fractures are the result of an axial load on the knee. Motor vehicle crashes or falls from a height are typical injury mechanisms. In the elderly population, a fall from standing height onto a flexed knee is a common cause of distal femoral fractures.

The resulting deformity is characteristic and caused by the anatomy in the region. The muscle pull of the quadriceps and hamstrings shortens the femur. The shaft is shortened and anterior. The gastrocnemius muscles pull the distal fragment posteriorly (**Figure 3**). The gastrocnemius, quadriceps, and hamstring muscle groups provide this deforming force. An intercondylar split can further displace, with each condyle being pulled by a head of the gastrocnemius muscle. Open injuries typically occur anteriorly through the distal quadriceps, just proximal to the patella.

Many musculoskeletal injuries can occur with an axial load along the femoral shaft. Radiographic assessment of the pelvis, acetabulum, hip, and femoral shaft must be included in the initial evaluation. If any concern exists for an intra-articular component to the fracture, a CT scan will assist in delineating the complexity of the fracture, aid in detecting a coronal place fracture (**Figure 4**), and allow maximal preparation for an anatomic reduction.[61]

Classification

The AO/Orthopaedic Trauma Association classification of distal femur fractures is often used. Type A fractures are extra-articular, supracondylar fractures. Type B fractures include partial articular, condylar fractures (either medial or lateral) in the sagittal plane or the so-called Hoffa fracture in the coronal plane (**Figure 5**). Intra-articular fractures with metadiaphyseal dissociation are classified as type C fractures.

Supracondylar Fractures

Supracondylar fractures are rarely treated nonsurgically. Indications for nonsurgical treatment include nondisplaced fractures and fractures in nonambulating patients or in those who are poor surgical candidates.

Surgical treatment includes either intramedullary nail or plate fixation depending on the characteristics of the fracture. The more distal the fracture and the more extensive the intra-articular component, the less likely the fracture will be amenable to intramedullary nailing rather than fixation with plating.

The basic principles of articular fixation apply in these fractures. Surgical goals are anatomic reduction and stable fixation of the joint surface followed by re-

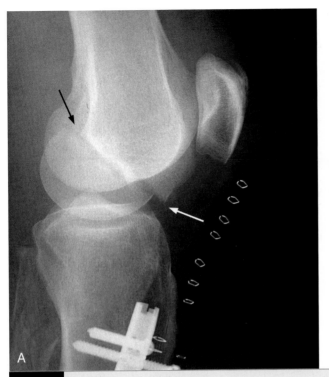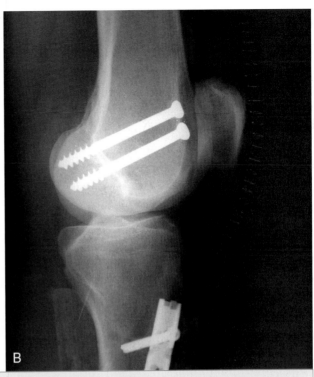

Figure 5 **A,** Radiograph of a Hoffa fracture (*arrows*) of the distal femoral condyle. **B,** Radiograph showing the fracture stabilized with lag screws.

duction to the intact shaft while maintaining physiologic valgus. Modern plating techniques allow open reduction of the joint with direct visualization, passing a plate submuscularly while using indirect fracture reduction techniques, and then fixing the joint to the shaft percutaneously. Locked plating technology has almost completely replaced 95° condylar screws and blade plates in fixing these difficult fractures. Fixed-angle plates have eliminated the need for a medial buttress plate in all but the most comminuted fractures.

Biologically sound percutaneous plating of distal femoral fractures with locked plates is associated with a union rate of approximately 93% at between 11 and 14 weeks.[62,63] Malreduction rates have decreased as surgeons have become more experienced with newer techniques but approaches 20% in some studies.[64] Reported knee range of motion averages 105° to 110° of flexion.[62,63]

Periprosthetic Fractures

Periprosthetic supracondylar fractures about a stable total knee arthroplasty are similar to extra-articular fractures. If the arthroplasty implant allows, these fractures can be treated with either an intramedullary nail or a fixed-angle plate depending on the amount of bone remaining intact to the distal fragment. Posterior-stabilized total knee implants will not allow passage of an intramedullary implant unless the knee implant is cut. If an intramedullary nail is to be used with posterior cruciate-sparing implants, it is vital to determine the size of the intercondylar distance that would accept

the nail. If the information is unavailable, a CT scan will allow radiographic measurement of the distance. A recent report on 15 patients with 16 supracondylar periprosthetic fractures treated with intramedullary nails reported 100% union at an average of 16 weeks with return to preinjury function in 11 of 13 patients.[65]

Minimally invasive locked plating for periprosthetic supracondylar fractures also provides satisfactory results. The authors of a 2006 study reported union in 19 of 22 patients (86%) and postoperative alignment within 5° of the contralateral limb in 20 of 22 patients.[66]

Hoffa Fractures

Coronal plane condylar fractures (Hoffa fractures) have been reported to occur in 38% of distal femoral fractures.[61] These fractures are 2.8 times more likely in open fractures, with the lateral condyle more commonly involved. CT scans should be obtained preoperatively to reliably evaluate the distal femur for these fractures (**Figure 4**). Because nonsurgical treatment is associated with poor functional outcomes, surgical fixation is generally recommended. These fractures can be difficult to reduce and stabilize because of their size, shape, and location. Often the optimal location for placement of the lag screws is in the articular surface (**Figure 5**). Headless screws or countersunk screws can be used in those situations.

Unicondylar Fractures

Unicondylar fractures are articular and require anatomic reduction with stable fixation to avoid posttrau-

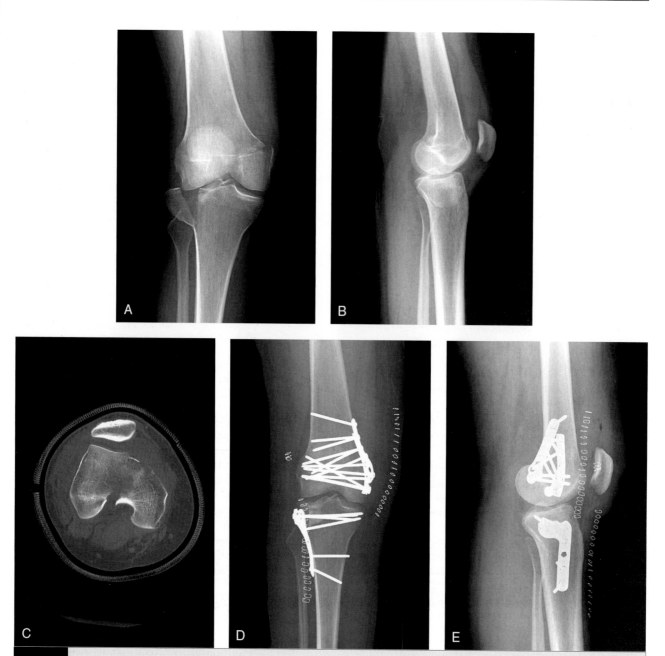

Figure 6 AP (**A**) and lateral (**B**) preoperative radiographs of a distal femoral condylar fracture. **C**, Axial CT scan of the fracture showing the intercondylar split. Postoperative AP (**D**) and lateral (**E**) radiographs showing the fracture stabilized with a buttress plate and lag screws.

matic arthritis. Open reduction with lag screw fixation can maintain the fracture reduction in patients with good bone quality. Large varus and valgus shear stresses on the knee in the plane of these fractures can exceed the ability of lag screws to maintain the reduction; therefore, a buttress plate is recommended, especially if there is any question regarding bone quality (**Figure 6**).

Complications

Partial articular type B fractures are more likely to result in nonunion because of the shearing forces across the fracture and often are associated with inadequate

fixation. Nonunion of the metaphyseal portion of distal fractures, with or without intra-articular extension, is reported to be as high as 17% and is most common in open fractures with associated bone loss.[67] Fortunately, the articular extension, if present, typically heals. Rigid stability with compression of the metaphyseal fracture site either with lag screws and a neutralization plate or with a compression plate is often all that is necessary to achieve union in fractures without a large defect. If there is a defect, then grafting is needed. The need for grafting is often overlooked when using locked plates for fixation of distal femoral fractures; however, this can lead to plate failure. If necessary, a medial plate or intramedullary augmentation with a plate or fibula allograft may also be used.

Annotated References

1. Winquist RA, Hansen ST Jr, Clawson DK: Closed intramedullary nailing of femoral fractures. A report of five hundred and twenty cases. *J Bone Joint Surg Am* 1984;66(4):529-539.

2. ATLS Subcommittee, eds: *Advanced Trauma Life Support for Doctors: Student Course Manual*, ed 8. Chicago, IL, American College of Surgeons, 2008.

3. Copeland CE, Mitchell KA, Brumback RJ, Gens DR, Burgess AR: Mortality in patients with bilateral femoral fractures. *J Orthop Trauma* 1998;12(5):315-319.

4. Nork Se, Agel J, Russell GV, Mills WJ, Holt S, Routt ML Jr: Mortality after reamed intramedullary nailing of bilateral femur fractures. *Clin Orthop Relat Res* 2003;415(415):272-278.

5. Tornetta P III, Kain MS, Creevy WR: Diagnosis of femoral neck fractures in patients with a femoral shaft fracture: Improvement with a standard protocol. *J Bone Joint Surg Am* 2007;89(1):39-43.

   The authors present a standardized protocol, including a preoperative fine-cut CT scan of the femoral necks and a dedicated postoperative 15° internal rotation hip radiograph to reduce the delay in diagnosing a femoral neck fracture in association with an ipsilateral femoral shaft fracture. A 91% reduction in the risk of a delayed diagnosis was reported.

6. Lenart BA, Neviaser AS, Lyman S, et al: Association of low-energy femoral fractures with prolonged bisphosphonate use: A case control study. *Osteoporos Int* 2009;20(8):1353-1362.

   The authors present a retrospective case-control study comparing 41 postmenopausal women with low-energy subtrochanteric or femoral shaft fractures with women who sustained low-energy intertrochanteric or femoral neck fractures. Bisphosphonate use was higher in the subtrochanteric/shaft fracture group compared with the intertrochanteric/femoral neck fracture groups. Of the 15 subtrochanteric/shaft fracture patients using bisphosphonates, 10 had the characteristic radiographic pattern termed "simple with thick cortices."

7. Goh SK, Yang KY, Koh JS, et al: Subtrochanteric insufficiency fractures in patients on alendronate therapy: A caution. *J Bone Joint Surg Br* 2007;89(3):349-353.

   This retrospective review, over a 10-month period, of 13 women with low-energy subtrochanteric femoral fractures identified alendronate therapy in 9 of those women within the year before the fracture. Five of those patients reported prodromal pain compared with none of the patients in the nonalendronate group. Cortical hypertrophy was identified in six patients in the alendronate group. The patients in the alendronate group were younger (mean age, 66.9 years) compared with the nonalendronate patients (mean age, 80.3 years).

8. Kwek EB, Goh SK, Koh JS, Png MA, Howe TS: An emerging pattern of subtrochanteric stress fractures: A long-term complication of alendronate therapy? *Injury* 2008;39(2):224-231.

   The authors retrospectively reviewed patients admitted to their institution with a low-energy subtrochanteric femur fracture over a 20-month period. Seventeen patients with an average age of 66 years were identified. All patients had been on bisphosphonate therapy; 13 patients reported prodromal pain before the fracture. All patients had characteristic radiographic findings of cortical thickening laterally and a transverse fracture line with a medial cortical spike.

9. Neviaser AS, Lane JM, Lenart BA, Edobor-Osula F, Lorich DG: Low-energy femoral shaft fractures associated with alendronate use. *J Orthop Trauma* 2008;22(5):346-350.

   The authors describe a characteristic low-energy femur fracture pattern in elderly patients (mean age, 75 years). The study included 70 patients, 25 of whom were being treated with alendronate therapy. A simple transverse fracture pattern with unicortical beaking in an area of cortical diaphyseal hypertrophy was discovered in 19 of the 25 patients (76%). The average duration of alendronate use in this group was 6.9 years.

10. Pape HC, Hildebrand F, Pertschy S, et al: Changes in the management of femoral shaft fractures in polytrauma patients: From early total care to damage control orthopedic surgery. *J Trauma* 2002;53(3):452-461, discussion 461-462.

11. Pape HC, Giannoudis PV, Krettek C, Trentz O: Timing of fixation of major fractures in blunt polytrauma: Role of conventional indicators in clinical decision making. *J Orthop Trauma* 2005;19(8):551-562.

12. Bosse MJ, MacKenzie EJ, Riemer BL, et al: Adult respiratory distress syndrome, pneumonia, and mortality following thoracic injury and a femoral fracture treated either with intramedullary nailing with reaming or with a plate: A comparative study. *J Bone Joint Surg Am* 1997;79(6):799-809.

13. Canadian Orthopaedic Trauma Society: Reamed versus unreamed intramedullary nailing of the femur: Comparison of the rate of ARDS in multiple injured patients. *J Orthop Trauma* 2006;20(6):384-387.

14. Pape HC, Aur'm'Kolk M, Paffrath T, Regel G, Sturm JA, Tscherne H: Primary intramedullary femur fixation in multiple trauma patients with associated lung contusion—a cause of posttraumatic ARDS? *J Trauma* 1993;34(4):540-547, discussion 547-548.

15. Bone LB, Johnson KD, Weigelt J, Scheinberg R: Early versus delayed stabilization of femoral fractures: A prospective randomized study. *J Bone Joint Surg Am* 1989;71(3):336-340.

16. Morshed S, Miclau T III, Bembom O, Cohen M, Knudson MM, Colford JM Jr: Delayed internal fixation of femoral shaft fracture reduces mortality among patients with multisystem trauma. *J Bone Joint Surg Am* 2009; 91(1):3-13.

The authors present a retrospective cohort study (level III) of the National Trauma Data Bank to evaluate the timing of internal fixation on mortality in patients with multisystem trauma and a femoral shaft fracture. A delay in internal fixation greater than 12 hours to allow for appropriate resuscitation reduced mortality by approximately 50%.

17. Pape HC, Rixen D, Morley J, et al; EPOFF Study Group: Impact of the method of initial stabilization for femoral shaft fractures in patients with multiple injuries at risk for complications (borderline patients). *Ann Surg* 2007;246(3):491-499, discussion 499-501.

Ten European trauma centers randomized 165 multiply injured patients with femoral shaft fractures to immediate (< 24 hours) intramedullary nail fixation or external fixation, with later conversion to intramedullary nail fixation. The patients were evaluated for an increased incidence of acute lung injuries. After accounting for the differences in initial injury severity between the groups, the odds of developing an acute lung injury were 6.7 times greater ($P < 0.05$) in the borderline patients treated with immediate intramedullary nailing compared with those treated with external fixation.

18. Pape HC, Regel G, Dwenger A, et al: Influences of different methods of intramedullary femoral nailing on lung function in patients with multiple trauma. *J Trauma* 1993;35(5):709-716.

19. Charash WE, Fabian TC, Croce MA: Delayed surgical fixation of femur fractures is a risk factor for pulmonary failure independent of thoracic trauma. *J Trauma* 1994;37(4):667-672.

20. Johnson KD, Tencer AF, Sherman MC: Biomechanical factors affecting fracture stability and femoral bursting in closed intramedullary nailing of femoral shaft fractures, with illustrative case presentations. *J Orthop Trauma* 1987;1(1):1-11.

21. Ricci WM, Devinney S, Haidukewych G, Herscovici D, Sanders R: Trochanteric nail insertion for the treatment of femoral shaft fractures. *J Orthop Trauma* 2005; 19(8):511-517.

22. Ricci WM, Schwappach J, Tucker M, et al: Trochanteric versus piriformis entry portal for the treatment of femoral shaft fractures. *J Orthop Trauma* 2006;20(10):663-667.

23. Starr AJ, Hay MT, Reinert CM, Borer DS, Christensen KC: Cephalomedullary nails in the treatment of high-energy proximal femur fractures in young patients: A prospective, randomized comparison of trochanteric versus piriformis fossa entry portal. *J Orthop Trauma* 2006;20(4):240-246.

24. Archdeacon M, Ford KR, Wyrick J, et al: A prospective functional outcome and motion analysis evaluation of the hip abductors after femur fracture and antegrade nailing. *J Orthop Trauma* 2008;22(1):3-9.

The authors report on eight patients with isolated femoral shaft fractures treated with an antegrade nail and evaluated with motion analysis, clinical examination, radiography, and patient-reported functional outcomes. Early lateral trunk lean was correlated to longer-term, poorer, self-reported functional outcomes. A significant improvement in the dysfunction index (21.3 ± 15.0 versus 6.5 ± 8.9; $P = 0.08$) was reported over time.

25. Helmy N, Jando VT, Lu T, Chan H, O'Brien PJ: Muscle function and functional outcome following standard antegrade reamed intramedullary nailing of isolated femoral shaft fractures. *J Orthop Trauma* 2008;22(1):10-15.

The authors retrospectively reviewed 21 patients with isolated femoral shaft fractures treated with a reamed, piriformis entry intramedullary nail. Lower peak hip abductor torque was present compared with the contralateral side (89.6 Nm versus 106.4 Nm: $P = 0.003$) despite a normal gait pattern.

26. Cannada LK, Taghizadeh S, Murali J, Obremskey WT, DeCook C, Bosse MJ: Retrograde intramedullary nailing in treatment of bilateral femur fractures. *J Orthop Trauma* 2008;22(8):530-534.

The authors retrospectively report data on a cohort of 111 patients with bilateral femoral fractures of whom 89 were treated with retrograde reamed intramedullary nails within 48 hours of injury. Associated injuries were present in 85 of 89 patients (96%), including 35 of 89 (39%) with thoracic injuries. The mortality rate was 5.6% (5 of 89 patients).

27. Tucker MC, Schwappach JR, Leighton RK, Coupe K, Ricci WM: Results of femoral intramedullary nailing in patients who are obese versus those who are not obese: A prospective multicenter comparison study. *J Orthop Trauma* 2007;21(8):523-529.

In a prospective, multicenter study, the authors report longer surgical time (94 minutes versus 62 minutes; $P < 0.003$) and increased radiation exposure (247 seconds versus 135 seconds; $P < 0.03$) for femoral intramedullary antegrade nailing in obese patients compared with nonobese patients. With respect to obese patients, retrograde nailing required less surgical time (67 minutes versus 94 minutes; $P < 0.02$) and less radiation exposure (76 seconds versus 247 seconds; $P < 0.002$) compared with antegrade nailing.

28. Ostrum RF, Agarwal A, Lakatos R, Poka A: Prospective comparison of retrograde and antegrade femoral intramedullary nailing. *J Orthop Trauma* 2000;14(7):496-501.

29. Daglar B, Gungor E, Delialioglu OM, et al: Comparison of knee function after antegrade and retrograde intramedullary nailing for diaphyseal femoral fractures: Results of isokinetic evaluation. *J Orthop Trauma* 2009;23(9):640-644.

Seventy patients with 71 femoral shaft fractures were randomized by surgeon to treatment with either antegrade or retrograde femoral nailing. Patients were followed for at least 1 year. Lysholm knee scores and isokinetic knee measurements were obtained at least 6 months after fracture union, and 30 patients had a minimum follow-up of 24 months. These were no differences in Lysholm knee scores, isokinetic measurements, or time to union between the groups.

30. Ricci WM, Bellabarba C, Evanoff B, Herscovici D, DiPasquale T, Sanders R: Retrograde versus antegrade nailing of femoral shaft fractures. *J Orthop Trauma* 2001;15(3):161-169.

31. Cannada LK, Viehe T, Cates CA, et al; Southeastern Fracture Consortium: A retrospective review of high-energy femoral neck-shaft fractures. *J Orthop Trauma* 2009;23(4):254-260.

The authors reviewed data from eight level I trauma centers to report the incidence of missed femoral neck fractures in association with ipsilateral shaft fractures and to evaluate the timing of the diagnosis. In a database that included 2,897 femoral shaft fractures, there were 91 ipsilateral neck-shaft fractures. Sixty-seven of the neck fractures were discovered preoperatively; of the 24 identified late, 11 fractures were discovered in the operating room, 10 were diagnosed during the hospital stay, and 3 were found at the follow-up visit. Sixteen of the 24 patients with a missed fracture had preoperative CT scans; 12 were read as negative for neck fracture and 4 showed fractures but the diagnosis was not made preoperatively.

32. Wolinsky PR, Johnson KD: Ipsilateral femoral neck and shaft fractures. *Clin Orthop Relat Res* 1995;318:81-90.

33. Alho A: Concurrent ipsilateral fractures of the hip and shaft of the femur: A systematic review of 722 cases. *Ann Chir Gynaecol* 1997;86(4):326-336.

34. Riemer BL, Butterfield SL, Ray RL, Daffner RH: Clandestine femoral neck fractures with ipsilateral diaphyseal fractures. *J Orthop Trauma* 1993;7(5):443-449.

35. Swiontkowski MF, Winquist RA, Hansen ST Jr: Fractures of the femoral neck in patients between the ages of twelve and forty-nine years. *J Bone Joint Surg Am* 1984;66(6):837-846.

36. Bedi A, Karunakar MA, Caron T, Sanders RW, Haidukewych GJ: Accuracy of reduction of ipsilateral femoral neck and shaft fractures—an analysis of various internal fixation strategies. *J Orthop Trauma* 2009;23(4):249-253.

Accurate reductions and uneventful union with open reduction and fixation of femoral neck fractures followed by retrograde nailing were reported by the authors of this study. The use of cephalomedullary nails resulted in fracture malreduction of one fracture in 3 of 9 patients compared with no malreductions in 28 patients treated with two devices. Two patients who had good to excellent reductions and who were treated with two devices went on to femoral neck nonunion and required secondary procedures.

37. Dickey RL, Barnes BC, Kearns RJ, Tullos HS: Efficacy of antibiotics in low-velocity gunshot fractures. *J Orthop Trauma* 1989;3(1):6-10.

38. Wiss DA, Brien WW, Becker V Jr: Interlocking nailing for the treatment of femoral fractures due to gunshot wounds. *J Bone Joint Surg Am* 1991;73(4):598-606.

39. Bergman M, Tornetta P, Kerina M, et al: Femur fractures caused by gunshots: Treatment by immediate reamed intramedullary nailing. *J Trauma* 1993;34(6):783-785.

40. Nowotarski P, Brumback RJ: Immediate interlocking nailing of fractures of the femur caused by low- to mid-velocity gunshots. *J Orthop Trauma* 1994;8(2):134-141.

41. Patzakis MJ, Harvey JP Jr, Ivler D: The role of antibiotics in the management of open fractures. *J Bone Joint Surg Am* 1974;56(3):532-541.

42. McHentry TP, Holcomb JB, Aoki N, Lindsey RW: Fractures with major vascular injuries from gunshot wounds: Implications of surgical sequence. *J Trauma* 2002;53(4):717-721.

43. Starr AJ, Hunt JL, Reinert CM: Treatment of femur fracture with associated vascular injury. *J Trauma* 1996;40(1):17-21.

44. Harwood PJ, Giannoudis PV, Probst C, Krettek C, Pape HC: The risk of local infective complications after damage control procedures for femoral shaft fracture. *J Orthop Trauma* 2006;20(3):181-189.

45. Hossny A: Blunt popliteal artery injury with complete lower limb ischemia: Is routine use of temporary intraluminal arterial shunt justified? *J Vasc Surg* 2004;40(1):61-66.

46. French BG, Tornetta P III: Use of an interlocked cephalomedullary nail for subtrochanteric fracture stabilization. *Clin Orthop Relat Res* 1998;348(348):95-100.

47. Kempf I, Grosse A, Beck G: Closed locked intramedullary nailing. Its application to comminuted fractures of the femur. *J Bone Joint Surg Am* 1985;67(5):709-720.

48. Ricci WM, Bellabarba C, Lewis R, et al: Angular malalignment after intramedullary nailing of femoral shaft fractures. *J Orthop Trauma* 2001;15(2):90-95.

49. Tornetta P III, Ritz G, Kantor A: Femoral torsion after interlocked nailing of unstable femoral fractures. *J Trauma* 1995;38(2):213-219.

50. Brinker MR, O'Connor DP, Monla YT, Earthman TP: Metabolic and endocrine abnormalities in patients with nonunions. *J Orthop Trauma* 2007;21(8):557-570.

The authors present their data on a subset of nonunion patients who were referred to an endocrinologist for an underlying metabolic or endocrine abnormality. Vitamin D deficiency was the most common abnormality identified (25 of 37 patients). Eight patients who received treatment of the newly diagnosed metabolic or endocrine disorder went on to union without surgical intervention.

51. Taitsman LA, Lynch Jr, Agel J, Barei DP, Nork SE: Risk factors for femoral nonunion after femoral shaft fracture. *J Trauma* 2009;67(6):1389-1392.

The authors evaluated risk factors for nonunion after femoral nailing in a case-controlled study based on cases in their trauma database. There were 1,126 femoral shaft fractures treated with intramedullary nails during the study period with 46 (4.1%) going on to nonunion. Independent variables and a regression model predictive of nonunion were open fracture, delay to weight bearing (> 6 weeks), and tobacco use.

52. Giannoudis PV, MacDonald DA, Matthews SJ, Smith RM, Furlong AJ, De Boer P: Nonunion of the femoral diaphysis: The influence of reaming and non-steroidal anti-inflammatory drugs. *J Bone Joint Surg Br* 2000; 82(5):655-658.

53. Canadian Orthopaedic Trauma Society: Nonunion following intramedullary nailing of the femur with and without reaming: Results of a multicenter randomized clinical trial. *J Bone Joint Surg Am* 2003;85(11):2093-2096.

54. Moed BR, Watson JT, Cramer KE, Karges DE, Teefey JS: Unreamed retrograde intramedullary nailing of fractures of the femoral shaft. *J Orthop Trauma* 1998; 12(5):334-342.

55. Weresh MJ, Hakanson R, Stover MD, Sims SH, Kellam JF, Bosse MJ: Failure of exchange reamed intramedullary nails for ununited femoral shaft fractures. *J Orthop Trauma* 2000;14(5):335-338.

56. Shroeder JE, Mosheiff R, Khoury A, Liebergall M, Weil YA: The outcome of closed, intramedullary exchange nailing with reamed insertion in the treatment of femoral shaft nonunions. *J Orthop Trauma* 2009;23(9):653-657.

Exchange nailing in 42 patients with femoral shaft nonunions, which were initially managed with an intramedullary nail, were retrospectively evaluated. Thirty-six of 42 patients (86%) went on to union without further intervention. There were six failures (three aseptic and three septic), which all went on to union with further interventions. Treatment failures were associated with lack of immediate weight bearing, open fractures, atrophic/oligotrophic nonunions, and infection.

57. Brumback RJ, Ellison TS, Molligan H, Molligan DJ, Mahaffey S, Schmidhauser C: Pudendal nerve palsy complicating intramedullary nailing of the femur. *J Bone Joint Surg Am* 1992;74(10):1450-1455.

58. Coelho RF, Gomes CM, Sakaki MH, et al: Genitoperineal injuries associated with the use of an orthopedic table with a perineal posttraction. *J Trauma* 2008; 65(4):820-823.

The authors report on six patients, followed over a 2-year period, with perineal and scrotal complications attributed to the use of intraoperative traction on a fracture table. Partial-thickness necrosis developed in all patients necessitating surgical débridement. Infection developed in three patients. Five of six wounds healed by secondary intention and one was closed primarily.

59. Meyer RS, White KK, Smith JM, Groppo ER, Mubarak SJ, Hargens AR: Intramuscular and blood pressures in legs positioned in the hemilithotomy position: Clarification of risk factors for well-leg acute compartment syndrome. *J Bone Joint Surg Am* 2002;84(10):1829-1835.

60. Christie J, Robinson CM, Pell AC, McBirnie J, Burnett R: Transcardiac echocardiography during invasive intramedullary procedures. *J Bone Joint Surg Br* 1995; 77(3):450-455.

61. Nork SE, Segina DN, Aflatoon K, et al: The association between supracondylar-intercondylar distal femoral fractures and coronal plane fractures. *J Bone Joint Surg Am* 2005;87(3):564-569.

62. Weight M, Collinge C: Early results of the less invasive stabilization system for mechanically unstable fractures of the distal femur (AO/OTA types A2, A3, C2, and C3). *J Orthop Trauma* 2004;18(8):503-508.

63. Kregor PJ, Stannard JA, Zlowodzki M, Cole PA: Treatment of distal femur fractures using the less invasive stabilization system: Surgical experience and early clinical results in 103 fractures. *J Orthop Trauma* 2004;18(8): 509-520.

64. Schandelmaier P, Partenheimer A, Koenemann B, Grün OA, Krettek C: Distal femoral fractures and LISS stabilization. *Injury* 2001;32(suppl 3):SC55-SC63.

65. Chettiar K, Jackson MP, Brewin J, Dass D, Butler-Manuel PA: Supracondylar periprosthetic femoral fractures following total knee arthroplasty: Treatment with a retrograde intramedullary nail. *Int Orthop* 2009; 33(4):981-985.

66. Ricci WM, Loftus T, Cox C, Borrelli J: Locked plates combined with minimally invasive insertion technique for the treatment of periprosthetic supracondylar femur fractures above a total knee arthroplasty. *J Orthop Trauma* 2006;20(3):190-196.

67. Bellabarba C, Ricci WM, Bolhofner BR: Indirect reduction and plating of distal femoral nonunions. *J Orthop Trauma* 2002;16(5):287-296.

Chapter 34

Fractures About the Knee

Michael J. Gardner, MD

Tibial Plateau Fractures

Tibial plateau fractures involve the proximal tibial articular surface. These injuries are extremely heterogeneous, ranging from minimally displaced fractures with mild soft-tissue injuries to highly comminuted fractures of both tibial condyles and the metaphysis, which are often associated with significant soft-tissue injury. Many injury- and patient-specific factors influence treatment decisions.

Classification

Several classification systems for tibial fractures have been proposed. Historically, the Schatzker classification has been used most frequently.[1] In this system, types I, II, and III are lateral plateau pure split, split-depressed, and pure depressed fractures, respectively. These fractures commonly result from lower-energy injuries. Type I patterns occur in younger patients with good bone quality. Type II fractures are the most common, and account for up to 75% of all tibial plateau fractures. Type III fractures are extremely rare, occurring in patients with severe osteoporosis (**Figure 1**). Types IV, V, and VI are medial plateau, bicondylar plateau, and metaphyseal dissociation fractures, respectively. These three types of fractures most often occur following high-energy mechanisms. Unfortunately, many fracture patterns do not fall into one of these categories. Additional variables that influence treatment, such as the presence of a fracture-dislocation and coronal obliquity of the medial plateau fracture, are not accounted for with the Schatzker classification system (**Figure 2**). Nevertheless, the Schatzker system is useful in providing clinicians with general fracture descriptions.

The Orthopaedic Trauma Association (OTA) classification was devised as a more comprehensive classification system. The proximal tibia is number 41, and A, B, or C denotes extra-articular, partial articular, or complete articular fractures, respectively. Each category has many additional subtypes. Because of the large

number of fracture types delineated, the OTA classification is the most useful system for research purposes.[2]

Mechanisms of Injury

The specific details of the injury mechanism are extremely important aspects of the evaluation and treatment planning process. The first consideration is whether the injury occurred from a low- or high-energy mechanism. Although this can be somewhat subjective, attempts should be made to quantify the energy involved. A fall from a standing height is a typical low-energy mechanism. Motorcycle or motor vehicle collisions often impart greater energy to the injury. The soft-tissue status reveals significant and clinically relevant information, particularly when fracture blisters, nonwrinkling skin, open lacerations, tense compartments, or ecchymosis is present. The fracture pattern itself often contributes to the "personality" of the injury. Fracture-dislocations, involvement of the medial tibial plateau, and metaphyseal comminution all indicate high-energy mechanisms. In general, the bony injury is static and the soft-tissue injury is dynamic and can evolve.

Evaluation

Prior to evaluating the injured limb, a thorough trauma evaluation should be performed on the patient when warranted. Many tibial plateau fractures occur in multiply injured patients, and Advanced Trauma Life Support protocols must be initiated in this setting. After the airway and ventilation have been secured and hemodynamic stability has been assessed and managed, attention is turned to the extremity. Visual inspection focuses on soft-tissue swelling, open lacerations, and limb deformity. A complete neurologic examination is performed. Because of the close proximity of the common peroneal nerve to the fibular neck, this nerve is at particular risk for injury. Tibial plateau fractures can be associated with a knee dislocation, especially with medial tibial plateau fractures. Thus, a vascular examination is critical and should include distal pulse palpation, assessment of the color and temperature of the foot, and obtaining ankle-brachial indices. An ankle-brachial index of less than 0.9 warrants more invasive vascular studies.[3] Even though these are periarticular fractures, because of the low fascial compliance and abundant muscular tissue in the proximal tibia, a high index of suspicion should be maintained for compartment syndrome.

Dr. Gardner or an immediate family member serves as a paid consultant to or is an employee of Synthes, Amgen, and DGIMed and has received research or institutional support from AO, Synthes, Smith & Nephew, Wright Medical Technologies, and the Foundation for Orthopaedic Trauma.

4: Lower Extremity

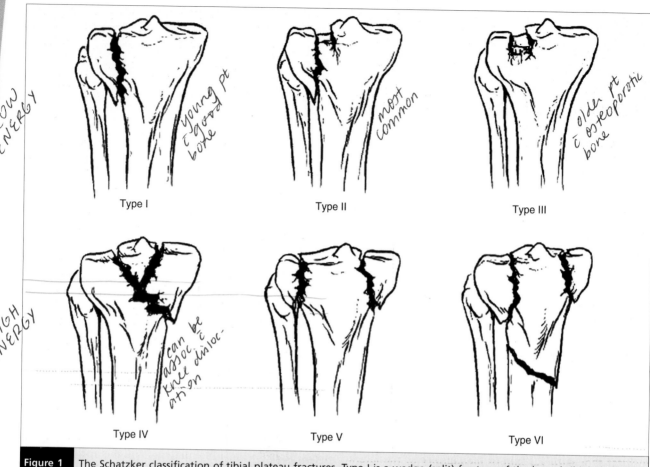

[Handwritten annotations: "LOW ENERGY", "young pt c̄ good bone", "most common", "older pt c̄ osteoporotic bone", "HIGH ENERGY", "can be assoc c̄ knee dislocation"]

Figure 1 The Schatzker classification of tibial plateau fractures. Type I is a wedge (split) fracture of the lateral tibial plateau. Type II is a split-depression fracture of the lateral plateau. Type III is a pure central depression fracture of the lateral plateau without an associated split. Type IV is a fracture of the medial tibial plateau, usually involving the entire condyle. Type V is a bicondylar fracture, which typically consists of split fractures of both the medial and lateral plateaus without articular depression. Type VI is a tibial plateau fracture with an associated proximal shaft fracture. (Adapted from Koval KJ, Helfet DL: Tibial plateau fractures: Evaluation and treatment. *J Am Acad Orthop Surg* 1995;3:86-94).

Radiographic evaluation typically includes two or four radiographic views of the knee and the entire tibia. CT scans are also extremely helpful for delineating specific fracture lines and fragments. MRI may also provide adequate bony detail, and additionally shows structural injuries to soft tissues, such as meniscal tears, displacement, and ligament injuries.[4] Both CT and MRI provide more information when obtained after closed reduction and external fixation; therefore, if provisional external fixation is necessary, these studies should be deferred until external fixation is performed.

Treatment

Indications

Although tibial plateau fractures are intra-articular injuries, some fractures can effectively be treated nonsurgically. For fractures that are stable to varus and valgus stress, those that do not affect the coronal plane limb alignment, and those with minimal articular displacement, initial nonsurgical treatment is appropriate. Additionally, nonambulatory or medically unstable patients should be considered for nonsurgical treatment. The necessity of anatomic articular reduction has been questioned because of a lack of data,[5] and the knee joint may tolerate greater levels of incongruity because of the protective effects of the meniscus. Historically, a threshold for acceptable articular step-off of up to 10 mm had been recommended.[6-8] However, many of these early studies included older implant and fixation techniques with total meniscectomies; involved a long period of postoperative casting; and were based on nonvalidated, physician-based, outcome scores.

Over the past several decades, the understanding of many aspects of these injuries has improved. The importance of early joint motion to minimize stiffness and improve the nutrition and health of the injured cartilage has been stressed. It is now clear that meniscal preservation is critical for long-term joint maintenance.[7] Many patient-based outcomes scores have been developed and validated that accurately capture functional outcomes after injury and treatment. A recent large series of bicondylar tibial plateau fractures reported that a more accurate articular reconstruction

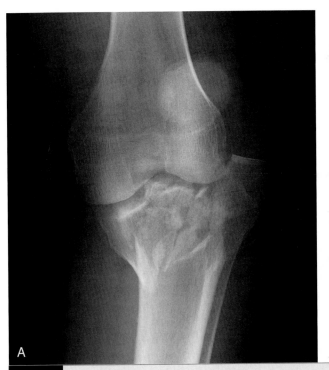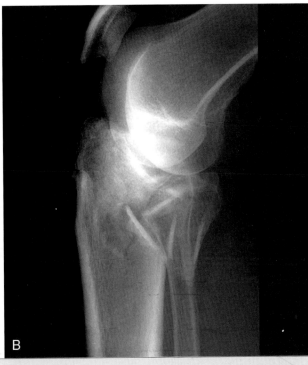

| Figure 2 | AP (**A**) and lateral (**B**) radiographs showing a tibial plateau fracture with an associated dislocation of the knee joint, as well as a coronal plane fracture of the medial tibial plateau, neither of which are accounted for with current classification systems. |

improved functional outcomes.[9] Laboratory data also indicate that with 1.5 mm of incongruity of the lateral tibial plateau, the contact stresses on the adjacent cartilage are approximately doubled.[10] Currently, in most centers, a threshold of 2 mm of articular step-off is used for surgical indications and for intraoperative reductions.

Urgent and Provisional Treatments

Tibial plateau fractures with axial instability, metaphyseal comminution, associated dislocations, and substantial soft-tissue swelling are usually indicated for closed reduction and provisional spanning external fixation until soft-tissue swelling permits definitive treatment. This regimen achieves multiple goals, including bone stabilization, and realignment and healing of the soft-tissue injury, before definitive open reduction and internal fixation.[11] It is important to achieve an accurate closed reduction, particularly length restoration, to achieve appropriate soft-tissue relationships. As a result, patient comfort is improved, useful postoperative imaging can be obtained, definitive open reduction is facilitated, and the overall complication rate is minimized. Typically, two Schanz half pins are placed in the femur, and two pins are placed in the tibia. These pins are connected with multiple clamps and bars in the region of the knee. Care should be taken to avoid placing the clamp directly over the knee to allow radiographic visualization. The tibial pins should be placed sufficiently distal to the knee joint to avoid interference with the definitive incisions and implants. Additionally,

joint overdistraction may be detrimental to neurovascular structures.

Compartment syndrome should be ruled out in all patients with a tibial plateau fracture. Leg compartment fullness associated with pain that is disproportionate to the injury severity, and increased pain with passive flexion and extension of the toes and ankle, should alert the clinician to the development of compartment syndrome. Direct compartment pressure measurements can then be used to confirm the diagnosis, and immediate decompressive fasciotomies should be performed through dual incisions or a single lateral incision.[12] If a vascular lesion is suspected, consultation with a vascular surgeon is warranted.

Definitive Surgical Treatment

When the skin wrinkles and the fracture blisters have resolved and epithelialized, surgical intervention is planned. The goal of surgery is to restore bony anatomy, achieve bone and soft-tissue healing without complications, and impart adequate fixation stability to allow early knee motion to minimize stiffness. Most tibial plateau fractures involve the lateral plateau and are amenable to treatment through an anterolateral incision. A femoral distractor may be useful to distract the joint to allow space and visualization during elevation of depressed osteochondral fragments. A transverse submeniscal arthrotomy can be performed for direct articular visualization and instrument palpation. Displaced articular fragments may be accessed using elevators through fracture lines, or with tamps through

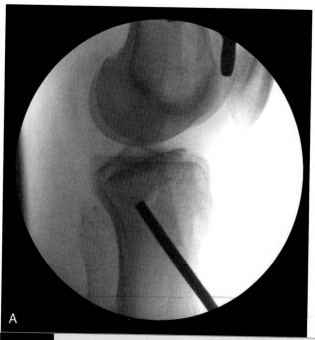
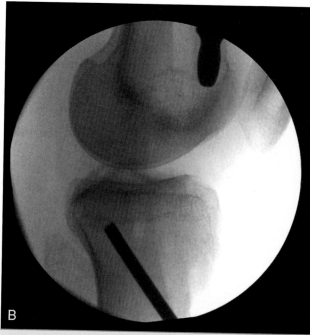

| **Figure 3** | In these lateral fluoroscopic views, a bone tamp is inserted through a small window created with osteotomes (**A**) and is used to elevate the impacted articular fragment (**B**). |

separate bone "windows" created using osteotomes (**Figure 3**). The lateral plateau may also be externally rotated and displaced to improve access. Some fractures involving the medial tibial plateau are best treated with a separate posteromedial approach for direct reduction and fixation.[13,14]

Subchondral screws placed through the lateral plate are anchored in strong medial bone, and nonlocking screws provide adequate fixation in most patients. Nonlocking screws allow for lag compression, which is important to maintain anatomic plateau width and for stabilization. The strongest subchondral support is achieved using multiple 3.5-mm cortical screws and small fragment fixation.[15,16] In severely osteoporotic patients, locking screws may be considered after lag screws have been placed. The lateral plate in most fracture patterns needs to provide buttress or an antiglide function; therefore, in all OTA type B (partial articular) fractures, locking fixation is unnecessary, more costly, and may be counterproductive.

Much attention has recently been focused on the morphology of the medial tibial plateau fracture fragments.[17,18] Important fracture characteristics include the amount of articular surface comprised by the fragment and its coronal plane obliquity. Locking screws placed through a lateral plate, even if angled posteriorly, are not ideally suited to obtain stable fixation of medial coronal plane fractures (**Figure 4**). Both clinical and biomechanical studies have shown the low complication rate of a posteromedial approach, the low incidence of fixation failure, and the mechanical advantage with dual plating of these patterns.[9,13,19,20]

Conversely, some bicondylar patterns involve mainly metaphyseal fracture lines and result in a large medial plateau fragment that involves little or none of the articular surface. Although evidence is somewhat unclear, these patterns may be more amenable to stabilization using a lateral locking plate (**Figure 5**). Several studies have reported substantial rates of reduction loss using this technique, although no distinction between medial fracture patterns was made.[21,22] A more recent study found no difference in reduction loss between lateral locked and dual plating but found a higher incidence of proximal tibial malalignment with lateral locked plating.[23] Other authors have reported the efficacy of lateral locked plating for metaphyseal bicondylar fractures.[24,25]

In many fractures, additional compressive support of the articular surface is provided using bone graft or biologic cement in the residual metaphyseal defect.[26] A recent prospective, randomized, multicenter trial compared the use of calcium phosphate cement with autologous cancellous bone graft for subarticular defects.[26] A significantly higher rate of articular fragment subsidence occurred in the bone graft group. A meta-analysis of various fractures (including tibial plateau fractures) concluded that calcium phosphate cement to fill a defect leads to less fracture site pain compared with results in patients managed without defect grafting, and results in improved articular support compared with cancellous bone graft.[27]

Aside from traditional open reduction and internal fixation, other methods have been used to definitively treat tibial plateau fractures. Circular thin-wire frames

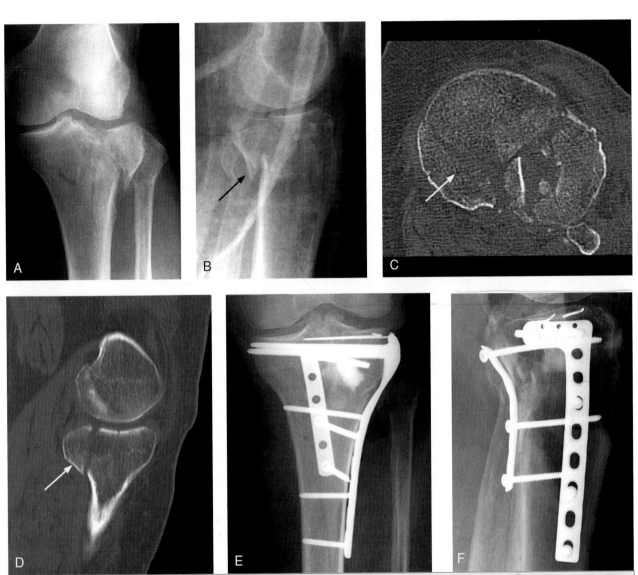

Figure 4 **A,** Radiograph showing a bicondylar tibial plateau fracture. **B,** On the lateral injury radiograph, the coronal plane nature of the medial tibial plateau fragment (*arrow*) is suggested. The axial (**C**) and sagittal (**D**) CT scans demonstrate the coronal obliquity of the medial plateau (*arrows*). This fragment is not amenable to lateral locked plate fixation. AP (**E**) and lateral (**F**) radiographs show a posterior buttress plate is applied through a supine posteromedial approach to buttress the medial plateau fragment.

(with or without hybrid-type fixation) may be effective, particularly in patients with severe soft-tissue defects.[28] Arthroscopy can also be used to assist in articular visualization during reduction.[29] In arthroscopically assisted techniques, no fluid or low pressure fluid should be used to minimize extravasation through the fracture into the leg compartments, which could potentially cause compartment syndrome.

Outcomes

Outcomes following tibial plateau fractures depend on patient characteristics and the extent of the bone and soft-tissue injuries. In a series of elderly patients, older age and the need for provisional spanning external fixation were predictors of worse functional outcomes.[30]

A clinical analysis of 83 bicondylar tibial plateau fractures also reported that older patients and those with multiple injuries had worse outcomes.[9] In this series, 55% of patients had articular reductions within 2 mm; this correlated strongly with improved outcomes. In a Canadian study of patients with tibial plateau fractures treated with open reduction and internal fixation and followed for an average of 8.3 years, Medical Outcomes Study 36-Item Short Form scores were no different than in the normal population.[31] However, only 57% of patients older than 40 years returned to normal function. A large, long-term study of 109 patients with tibial plateau fractures treated with open reduction and internal fixation and followed for an average of 14 years reported that overall results were excellent and were independent of age.[32]

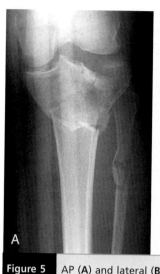
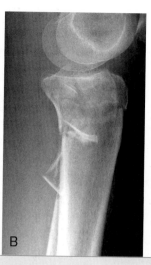
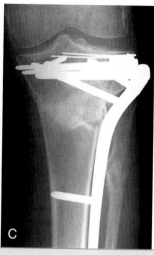
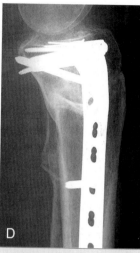

Figure 5 AP (**A**) and lateral (**B**) radiographs showing a tibial plateau fracture. The articular component of the tibial plateau fracture was treated with open reduction and rigid lag screw compression. The medial plateau was a large extra-articular fragment, and the metaphyseal component was treated successfully with a lateral locked plate (**C** and **D**).

Extensor Mechanism Injuries

The extensor mechanism is considered the quadriceps, the patella, and the patellar tendon. Any of these structures can be traumatically disrupted, leading to incompetence of the extensor mechanism and the inability to actively extend the knee. Secure fixation of a fracture or tendon disruption is imperative for restoration of function.

Patellar Fractures

Patellar fractures typically occur following either direct impact, such as a dashboard injury, or from an indirect mechanism, such as eccentric quadriceps contraction with sudden knee flexion. Other less common causes include insufficiency fractures following graft harvesting for anterior cruciate ligament reconstruction and total knee arthroplasty. The patient history and physical examination typically lead to the diagnosis. Following a direct impact mechanism, a superficial abrasion or ecchymosis is often present along with a large hemarthrosis in the knee. Rupture of the medial and lateral retinacula are common, and the patient is unable to actively extend the knee. A straight leg raise leads to a substantial extensor lag, and often a defect is palpable. It is imperative to ensure any regional lacerations do not communicate with the joint or the fracture site; injection of normal saline will assist with this diagnosis.

AP and lateral radiographs are obtained for fracture evaluation. The displacement is clearly seen on a true lateral radiograph. Common patterns include transverse noncomminuted, stellate, or avulsion fractures. Transverse fractures frequently occur in younger patients with healthy bone. Stellate fractures are multifragmentary and range from widely displaced to minimally displaced fractures. Superior and inferior pole avulsion fractures are functionally equivalent to quad-

riceps and patellar tendon bone–tendon junction disruptions, respectively. Elderly patients frequently have occult comminution and coronal plane splits, particularly of the inferior pole, and these should be actively sought as the presence of these fracture lines impacts fixation techniques.

Fractures with minimal articular displacement and with an intact extensor mechanism can be managed with a trial of nonsurgical treatment. A period of weight bearing with the knee supported in extension with a cylinder cast, a locked knee brace, or a knee immobilizer is initiated for 4 to 6 weeks. For displaced fractures, or those with extensor mechanism dysfunction, surgical treatment is warranted. Supine positioning with a longitudinal midline incision allows full access for fracture reduction and fixation. Full-thickness flaps are raised medially and laterally for articular digital access through retinacular rents, and for retinacular repair following internal fixation. Most midaxial transverse fracture patterns have sufficient intact bone in the proximal and distal fracture fragments to permit longitudinal fixation. Many fixation constructs have been described. The historic workhorse of fixation constructs is the modified tension band, which involves longitudinal 0.062-inch Kirchner wires across the fracture, with a figure-of-8 wire passed deep to the ends of the longitudinal wires and joined and tensioned on the dorsal patellar surface. This construct acts as a tension band, converting dorsal distraction forces to articular compressive forces during knee motion. Other options include placing a cerclage wire circumferentially around the patella; independent minifragment lag screw fixation for individual fragments; or placing longitudinal cannulated screws, with the dorsal tension band wire passed through the screw cannulations.

Biomechanical data indicate that wire fixation alone is inferior to tension band techniques.[33] Modified tension band constructs using longitudinal cannulated

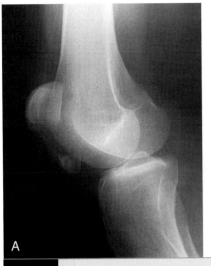
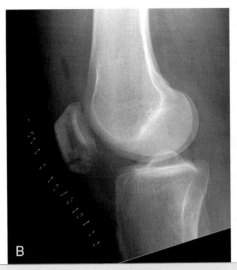
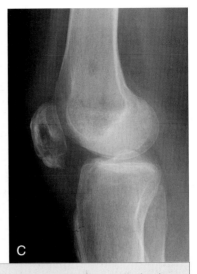

Figure 6 | A through **C**, Radiographs demonstrating treatment of an inferior pole patellar fracture. **A**, The fracture is clearly seen (**A**). The patellar tendon was repaired through drill holes in the superior patellar fragment (**B**). The inferior pole bone fragments were not excised, allowing for bone-to-bone healing at 10 weeks (**C**).

screws combined with anterior tension band wires function better than using wires alone.[34,35] Consideration should also be given to using a braided cable instead of a monofilament wire for the anterior tension band.[36] When comminution exists, the addition of a cerclage wire can add to fixation stability.[37]

Inferior pole patellar fractures, or those with highly comminuted inferior fragments, are often treated with partial patellectomy and advancement with repair to the patellar tendon. Three longitudinal drill holes are made through the superior pole. Several braided nonabsorbable sutures are then placed as locking stitches along the patellar tendon, leaving the free ends proximally. The suture ends are then passed through the drill holes and tied over the superior pole. Because the patellar tendon originates from the dorsal half of the patella, the drill holes should be made dorsally to avoid a patellar extension deformity. Alternatively, when using this technique, the comminuted fragments need not be completely excised to allow for bone-to-bone healing at the injury site (**Figure 6**).

The incidence of patellar fracture fixation failure using current techniques is significant.[38] Fixation failure, symptomatic implants, anterior knee pain, and revision surgery have frequently been reported. One study reported that 22% of 49 patellar fractures treated with modified tension band wiring and early motion showed displacement in the early postoperative period.[39] Long-term functional outcomes have not been reliably excellent, although most clinical series have not used validated outcome scales.[40-45] In a review of 68 patients with patellar fractures, only 72% were satisfied with the result.[42] Thirty-seven percent of patients had broken implants and 15% required revision procedures. Böstrom reported that more than 50% of patients have long-term symptoms following a displaced patellar fracture, more than 33% have functional impairment, and 21% require additional surgery.[46] In more recent

studies, 34 of 203 fractures (17%) had fair or poor results,[47] 9 of 20 patients (45%) had moderate or poor results,[48] and 12 of 68 elderly patients (18%) failed to return to their preinjury functional status.[38,49]

Tendon Disruptions

Traumatic disruptions of the quadriceps and patellar tendons occur by mechanisms similar to patellar fractures, although indirect, eccentric quadriceps contraction predominates. Quadriceps ruptures most commonly occur at the musculotendinous junction in older patients (typically older than 40 years).[50] Patellar tendon ruptures are more often "weekend warrior" injuries, occurring in patients approximately 40 years of age. Physical examination is notable for ecchymosis and knee effusion, as well as a palpable defect and the inability to complete a straight leg raise. Because of the substantial contribution of the retinacula to extensor mechanism stability, the inability to perform a straight leg raise implies tears in the retinacula.[51]

Lateral knee radiographs are valuable for diagnosing extensor mechanism tendon injuries based on the relationship of the patella to the tibial tubercle. The Insall-Salvati ratio quantifies the relationship between the patellar height and the patellar tendon length (**Figure 7**). A difference of greater than 20% between these measurements indicates potential tendon disruption.[52] The drawbacks of this threshold have been noted because of the high variability of patellar morphology; a difference of 100% has been suggested as a more accurate measurement for detecting acute injuries.[53] MRI is useful for confirming lesions and can help delineate associated injuries.

Treating acute tendon disruptions with direct suture repair leads to reliable tendon reapproximation, stability, and healing. Through a midline incision, a technique using large nonabsorbable sutures with locking

4: Lower Extremity

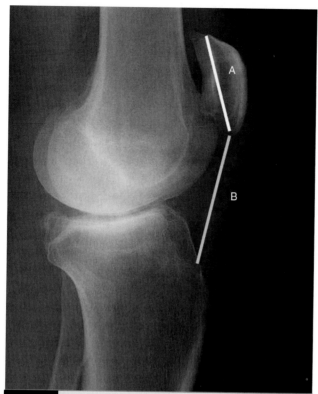

Figure 7 Lateral knee radiograph used to calculate the Insall-Salvati ratio. The ratio of patellar height (A) to patellar tendon length (B) should be approximately 1. A difference of at least 20% (for example, ratio A/B < 0.8 or > 1.2) indicates likely quadriceps or patellar tendon disruption, respectively.

stitches longitudinally on either side of the tear, with at least four suture strands crossing the tendon, is preferable.[54]

Following repair of a bony or tendinous extensor mechanism disruption, rehabilitation protocols must be carefully tailored to the individual patient and fracture characteristics. Early motion is desirable for cartilage health and for minimizing adhesion formation; however, it also increases the risk of fixation failure. Maintaining knee extension in an immobilizer brace or cylinder cast for the first 4 to 6 weeks allows early healing and may decrease repair failure rates.[39] Weight bearing may be instituted during this time in compliant and able patients. Subsequently, supervised passive knee extension and gentle active-assisted flexion exercises are initiated; acceptable range of motion is usually attainable.

Annotated References

1. Schatzker J, McBroom R, Bruce D: The tibial plateau fracture: The Toronto experience 1968--1975. *Clin Orthop Relat Res* 1979;138:94-104.

2. Walton NP, Harish S, Roberts C, Blundell C: AO or Schatzker? How reliable is classification of tibial plateau fractures? *Arch Orthop Trauma Surg* 2003;123(8): 396-398.

3. Mills WJ, Barei DP, McNair P: The value of the ankle-brachial index for diagnosing arterial injury after knee dislocation: a prospective study. *J Trauma* 2004;56(6): 1261-1265.

4. Gardner MJ, Yacoubian S, Geller D, et al: The incidence of soft tissue injury in operative tibial plateau fractures: A magnetic resonance imaging analysis of 103 patients. *J Orthop Trauma* 2005;19(2):79-84.

5. Marsh JL, Buckwalter J, Gelberman R, et al: Articular fractures: Does an anatomic reduction really change the result? *J Bone Joint Surg Am* 2002;84-A(7):1259-1271.

6. Lucht U, Pilgaard S: Fractures of the tibial condyles. *Acta Orthop Scand* 1971;42(4):366-376.

7. Rasmussen PS: Tibial condylar fractures: Impairment of knee joint stability as an indication for surgical treatment. *J Bone Joint Surg Am* 1973;55(7):1331-1350.

8. Lansinger O, Bergman B, Körner L, Andersson GB: Tibial condylar fractures: A twenty-year follow-up. *J Bone Joint Surg Am* 1986;68(1):13-19.

9. Barei DP, Nork SE, Mills WJ, Coles CP, Henley MB, Benirschke SK: Functional outcomes of severe bicondylar tibial plateau fractures treated with dual incisions and medial and lateral plates. *J Bone Joint Surg Am* 2006;88(8):1713-1721.

10. Brown TD, Anderson DD, Nepola JV, Singerman RJ, Pedersen DR, Brand RA: Contact stress aberrations following imprecise reduction of simple tibial plateau fractures. *J Orthop Res* 1988;6(6):851-862.

11. Egol KA, Tejwani NC, Capla EL, Wolinsky PL, Koval KJ: Staged management of high-energy proximal tibia fractures (OTA types 41): the results of a prospective, standardized protocol. *J Orthop Trauma* 2005;19(7): 448-455, discussion 456.

12. Maheshwari R, Taitsman LA, Barei DP: Single-incision fasciotomy for compartmental syndrome of the leg in patients with diaphyseal tibial fractures. *J Orthop Trauma* 2008;22(10):723-730.

    The authors present a detailed surgical technique and case series on using a single-incision, four-compartment fasciotomy for leg compartment releases. Of 58 leg fasciotomies performed, no patient required additional fasciotomies because of incomplete compartment releases.

13. Barei DP, Nork SE, Mills WJ, Henley MB, Benirschke SK: Complications associated with internal fixation of high-energy bicondylar tibial plateau fractures utilizing a two-incision technique. *J Orthop Trauma* 2004; 18(10):649-657.

14. Weil YA, Gardner MJ, Boraiah S, Helfet DL, Lorich DG: Posteromedial supine approach for reduction and fixation of medial and bicondylar tibial plateau fractures. *J Orthop Trauma* 2008;22(5):357-362.

    A case series and surgical technique of the posteromedial approach for tibial plateau fractures performed in the supine position is described. Twenty-seven fractures were analyzed. Fracture reductions were excellent overall, and a low complication rate was reported.

15. Patil S, Mahon A, Green S, McMurtry I, Port A: A biomechanical study comparing a raft of 3.5 mm cortical screws with 6.5 mm cancellous screws in depressed tibial plateau fractures. *Knee* 2006;13(3):231-235.

16. Karunakar MA, Egol KA, Peindl R, Harrow ME, Bosse MJ, Kellam JF: Split depression tibial plateau fractures: A biomechanical study. *J Orthop Trauma* 2002;16(3):172-177.

17. Barei DP, O'Mara TJ, Taitsman LA, Dunbar RP, Nork SE: Frequency and fracture morphology of the posteromedial fragment in bicondylar tibial plateau fracture patterns. *J Orthop Trauma* 2008;22(3):176-182.

    The results of large clinical series of bicondylar tibial plateau fractures are presented with analyses of the anatomy of the posteromedial fracture fragment. A posteromedial fragment was present in 29% of all bicondylar fractures and in 74% of those with medial articular involvement.

18. Higgins TF, Kemper D, Klatt J: Incidence and morphology of the posteromedial fragment in bicondylar tibial plateau fractures. *J Orthop Trauma* 2009;23(1):45-51.

    An analysis of 111 bicondylar tibial plateau fractures, in which 59% included a posteromedial fragment, is presented. Most fractures had a sagittally oriented fracture line, indicating vertical instability and potentially requiring buttress plate fixation for adequate stabilization.

19. Higgins TF, Klatt J, Bachus KN: Biomechanical analysis of bicondylar tibial plateau fixation: How does lateral locking plate fixation compare to dual plate fixation? *J Orthop Trauma* 2007;21(5):301-306.

    The authors describe a biomechanical cadaver study comparing lateral locked plating with dual plating for bicondylar tibial plateau fractures. After cyclic loading, significantly more medial fracture subsidence occurred in the group treated with lateral locked plating.

20. Eggli S, Hartel MJ, Kohl S, Haupt U, Exadaktylos AK, Röder C: Unstable bicondylar tibial plateau fractures: A clinical investigation. *J Orthop Trauma* 2008;22(10):673-679.

    A small clinical series of bicondylar tibial plateau fractures using direct open reduction and plate fixation both medially and laterally is described. This treatment led to excellent fracture reduction and stabilization, low complications, and good functional outcomes.

21. Gosling T, Schandelmaier P, Muller M, Hankemeier S, Wagner M, Krettek C: Single lateral locked screw plating of bicondylar tibial plateau fractures. *Clin Orthop Relat Res* 2005;439:207-214.

22. Phisitkul P, McKinley TO, Nepola JV, Marsh JL: Complications of locking plate fixation in complex proximal tibia injuries. *J Orthop Trauma* 2007;21(2):83-91.

    Clinical series of lateral locked plates for treating proximal tibial bicondylar fractures is described. A high complication rate was reported, including an 8% loss of reduction.

23. Jiang R, Luo CF, Wang MC, Yang TY, Zeng BF: A comparative study of Less Invasive Stabilization System (LISS) fixation and two-incision double plating for the treatment of bicondylar tibial plateau fractures. *Knee* 2008;15(2):139-143.

    The authors of this clinical case series analyzed 84 bicondylar tibial plateau fractures treated with lateral locked plating or dual buttress plating. Although most outcomes were similar between groups, postoperative malalignment was greater in the group treated with lateral locked plating.

24. Egol KA, Su E, Tejwani NC, Sims SH, Kummer FJ, Koval KJ: Treatment of complex tibial plateau fractures using the less invasive stabilization system plate: clinical experience and a laboratory comparison with double plating. *J Trauma* 2004;57(2):340-346.

25. Stannard JP, Wilson TC, Volgas DA, Alonso JE: The less invasive stabilization system in the treatment of complex fractures of the tibial plateau: short-term results. *J Orthop Trauma* 2004;18(8):552-558.

26. Russell TA, Leighton RK; Alpha-BSM Tibial Plateau Fracture Study Group: Comparison of autogenous bone graft and endothermic calcium phosphate cement for defect augmentation in tibial plateau fractures: A multicenter, prospective, randomized study. *J Bone Joint Surg Am* 2008;90(10):2057-2061.

    In this clinical trial, 120 tibial plateau fractures were randomized to autograft versus calcium phosphate cement for defect grafting and subchondral support. Autografting led to a significantly greater articular subsidence compared with biologic cement.

27. Bajammal SS, Zlowodzki M, Lelwica A, et al: The use of calcium phosphate bone cement in fracture treatment: A meta-analysis of randomized trials. *J Bone Joint Surg Am* 2008;90(6):1186-1196.

    The authors describe a meta-analysis of the evidence for using calcium phosphate cement to fill a defect during fracture fixation. Clinical evidence suggests that calcium phosphate leads to less fracture site pain and less loss of reduction compared with other traditional methods.

28. Canadian Orthopaedic Trauma Society: Open reduction and internal fixation compared with circular fixator application for bicondylar tibial plateau fractures: Results of a multicenter, prospective, randomized clinical trial. *J Bone Joint Surg Am* 2006;88(12):2613-2623.

29. Chan YS, Chiu CH, Lo YP, et al: Arthroscopy-assisted surgery for tibial plateau fractures: 2- to 10-year follow-up results. *Arthroscopy* 2008;24(7):760-768.

    In a case series of 54 tibial plateau fractures treated with an arthroscopy assisted technique with a mean follow-up of 7 years, no nonunions, no complications related to arthroscopy, and good overall outcomes were reported.

30. Su EP, Westrich GH, Rana AJ, Kapoor K, Helfet DL: Operative treatment of tibial plateau fractures in patients older than 55 years. *Clin Orthop Relat Res* 2004; 421:240-248.

31. Stevens DG, Beharry R, McKee MD, Waddell JP, Schemitsch EH: The long-term functional outcome of operatively treated tibial plateau fractures. *J Orthop Trauma* 2001;15(5):312-320.

32. Rademakers MV, Kerkhoffs GM, Sierevelt IN, Raaymakers EL, Marti RK: Operative treatment of 109 tibial plateau fractures: Five- to 27-year follow-up results. *J Orthop Trauma* 2007;21(1):5-10.

    The results of a long-term outcome study of more than 100 tibial plateau fractures followed for an average of 14 years is described. Unicondylar fractures had better outcomes compared with bicondylar fractures. Malalignment was a predictor of radiographic arthritis. Overall, results were excellent.

33. Benjamin J, Bried J, Dohm M, McMurtry M: Biomechanical evaluation of various forms of fixation of transverse patellar fractures. *J Orthop Trauma* 1987; 1(3):219-222.

34. Carpenter JE, Kasman RA, Patel N, Lee ML, Goldstein SA: Biomechanical evaluation of current patella fracture fixation techniques. *J Orthop Trauma* 1997;11(5):351-356.

35. Burvant JG, Thomas KA, Alexander R, Harris MB: Evaluation of methods of internal fixation of transverse patella fractures: A biomechanical study. *J Orthop Trauma* 1994;8(2):147-153.

36. Scilaris TA, Grantham JL, Prayson MJ, Marshall MP, Hamilton JJ, Williams JL: Biomechanical comparison of fixation methods in transverse patella fractures. *J Orthop Trauma* 1998;12(5):356-359.

37. Curtis MJ: Internal fixation for fractures of the patella. A comparison of two methods. *J Bone Joint Surg Br* 1990;72(2):280-282.

38. Gardner MJ, Griffith MH, Lawrence BD, Lorich DG: Complete exposure of the articular surface for fixation of patellar fractures. *J Orthop Trauma* 2005;19(2):118-123.

39. Smith ST, Cramer KE, Karges DE, Watson JT, Moed BR: Early complications in the operative treatment of patella fractures. *J Orthop Trauma* 1997;11(3):183-187.

40. Böstman O, Kiviluoto O, Nirhamo J: Comminuted displaced fractures of the patella. *Injury* 1981;13(3):196-202.

41. Levack B, Flannagan JP, Hobbs S: Results of surgical treatment of patellar fractures. *J Bone Joint Surg Br* 1985;67(3):416-419.

42. Hung LK, Chan KM, Chow YN, Leung PC: Fractured patella: Operative treatment using the tension band principle. *Injury* 1985;16(5):343-347.

43. Gosal HS, Singh P, Field RE: Clinical experience of patellar fracture fixation using metal wire or non-absorbable polyester—a study of 37 cases. *Injury* 2001; 32(2):129-135.

44. Wu CC, Tai CL, Chen WJ: Patellar tension band wiring: A revised technique. *Arch Orthop Trauma Surg* 2001; 121(1-2):12-16.

45. Böstman O, Kiviluoto O, Santavirta S, Nirhamo J, Wilppula E: Fractures of the patella treated by operation. *Arch Orthop Trauma Surg* 1983;102(2):78-81.

46. Boström A: Fracture of the patella: A study of 422 patellar fractures. *Acta Orthop Scand Suppl* 1972;143:1-80.

47. Mehdi M, Husson JL, Polard JL, Ouahmed A, Poncer R, Lombard J: [Treatment results of fractures of the patella using pre-patellar tension wiring: Analysis of a series of 203 cases]. *Acta Orthop Belg* 1999;65(2):188-196.

48. Ozdemir H, Ozenci M, Dabak K, Aydin AT: [Outcome of surgical treatment for patellar fractures]. *Ulus Travma Derg* 2001;7(1):56-59.

49. Shabat S, Mann G, Kish B, Stern A, Sagiv P, Nyska M: Functional results after patellar fractures in elderly patients. *Arch Gerontol Geriatr* 2003;37(1):93-98.

50. Clayton RA, Court-Brown CM: The epidemiology of musculoskeletal tendinous and ligamentous injuries. *Injury* 2008;39(12):1338-1344.

    A demographic analysis of a large series of patients who sustained a variety of soft-tissue injuries is presented.

51. Powers CM, Chen YJ, Farrokhi S, Lee TQ: Role of peripatellar retinaculum in transmission of forces within the extensor mechanism. *J Bone Joint Surg Am* 2006;88(9): 2042-2048.

52. Insall J, Salvati E: Patella position in the normal knee joint. *Radiology* 1971;101(1):101-104.

53. Grelsamer RP, Meadows S: The modified Insall-Salvati ratio for assessment of patellar height. *Clin Orthop Relat Res* 1992;282:170-176.

54. Konrath GA, Chen D, Lock T, et al: Outcomes following repair of quadriceps tendon ruptures. *J Orthop Trauma* 1998;12(4):273-279.

Chapter 35

Soft-Tissue Injuries About the Knee

Scott G. Kaar, MD   Michael J. Stuart, MD   Bruce A. Levy, MD

4: Lower Extremity

Anterior Cruciate Ligament Injuries

Anterior cruciate ligament (ACL) injuries commonly occur from a noncontact, twisting, or landing event during sports activities. Video analysis has shown that athletes tear their ACL with the foot flat, the knee in relative abduction, and the hip in relative flexion.[1]

Participation in high-risk activities is the main predisposing factor for an ACL injury; another notable factor is female sex. Females are more likely to sustain an ACL tear than males with similar sports activity involvement. Possible explanations include neuromuscular control differences of the trunk and the lower extremities. Females land from a height with the knee in a position of relative extension and apparent increased valgus due to hip internal rotation. Other possible factors include the size of the ACL, dimensions of the intercondylar notch, and cyclic hormonal levels. According to a systematic review, the ACL is at greater risk for injury during the first half (preovulatory phase) of the menstrual cycle.[2] There is also a possible genetic predisposition for female athletes to sustain ACL ruptures. Female athletes with a CC genotype of the COL5A1 *BstUI RFLP* gene that encodes for the α1 chain of type V collagen have a decreased risk of ACL rupture.[3]

The ACL has two bundles that are not distinct from one another but rather are confluences of the ligament that function at slightly different knee flexion angles. The anteromedial and posterolateral bundles are named for the location of their tibial insertions between the tibial spines. The femoral insertion of both bundles is distal to the lateral intercondylar ridge and the bundles are separated by the bifurcate ridge.[4] The antero-

Neither Dr. Kaar nor any immediate family member has received anything of value from or owns stock in a commercial company or institution related directly or indirectly to the subject of this chapter. Dr. Stuart or an immediate family member serves as a paid consultant to Arthrex and Fios; has received research or institutional support from Stryker; and serves as a board member, owner, officer, or committee member of the American Academy of Orthopaedic Surgeons and the American Orthopaedic Society for Sports Medicine. Dr. Levy or an immediate family member has received royalties from VOT Solutions and serves as a paid consultant to Arthrex.

medial bundle is taut in relative knee flexion whereas the posterolateral bundle is taut in knee extension. The anatomic location of the ACL bundle insertions has important implications for reconstruction techniques.

The main function of the ACL is to prevent a pivot shift of the knee during activities that may cause injury. Instrumented knee evaluation of anterior tibial laxity can also be performed with a KT-1000 arthrometer or other similar device.[5] These tools are commonly used in research data collection; however, most surgeons do not use them routinely. The ACL has much less of a role in knee stability during activities of daily living such as walking, running on a flat surface, and biking. Therefore, a patient's activity level must be taken into account when deciding whether to reconstruct the ACL, especially in middle-aged and elderly patients.[6,7] An active patient with no arthritic changes in their 40s or 50s may be a candidate for an ACL reconstruction to treat symptoms of instability. On the other hand, that same patient who is not involved in athletics or any high-risk activities may be better treated nonsurgically.

Lateral meniscus tears are more common following an acute ACL disruption and medial meniscus tears in the chronic ACL-deficient knee. Studies have shown that the risk of cartilage lesions and meniscus tears increases over time.[8,9] Recurrent instability episodes caused by ACL insufficiency are associated with the development of arthritis. However, patients who have undergone ACL reconstruction also are prone to develop arthritic changes in the tibiofemoral joint and it is not clear whether or not reconstruction alters this degenerative process.[10,11] Young patients, high-demand athletes, and patients who experience instability symptoms should be considered candidates for ACL reconstruction. Middle-aged or elderly patients who lead a more sedentary lifestyle, especially those with preexisting arthritic changes, are best treated nonsurgically.

Primary repair of the ACL leads to high failure rates.[12] The exact reason is unknown; however, it may be because of a poor blood supply to the ligament or inhibitory factors in the synovial fluid. Therefore, ACL reconstruction is the treatment of choice and may be performed with various techniques using different graft options. Arthroscopic surgery, either by drilling tunnels in the tibia or the femur through a transtibial or a medial portal technique, is common. The transtibial femoral tunnel drilling method was initially developed during conversion from a two-incision to a single-incision

Table 1

Evidence for Postoperative ACL Protocol

Protocol	Evidence (For or Against)
Continuous passive motion	No evidence for or against the use of a continuous passive motion device
Bracing	No difference in ACL failure rates or laxity[26]
Regional pain management	No benefit to femoral nerve block compared with single intra-articular bupivacaine injection[27]
Open vs closed chain quadriceps rehabilitation exercises	Closed chain exercises may produce less pain, decreased laxity, and better subjective outcomes, although improved and more comprehensive studies are needed[28]

arthroscopic technique. Recently, there has been a focus on the ACL femoral insertion anatomy. There is evidence that transtibial femoral tunnel drilling does not allow anatomic placement of the femoral tunnel on the medial wall of the lateral femoral condyle. Also, the reconstructed ACL fibers have a relatively vertical orientation in comparison with the native ligament.[13] Drilling the femoral tunnel through a medial portal allows for independent access to the anatomic femoral insertion. Also, the fiber orientation can more closely resemble that of the native ligament.[14] One study demonstrated similar rotational stability in a comparision of patients who had a low femoral tunnel drilled through a medial portal with those who had a double-bundle reconstruction.[15]

Recent attempts to duplicate native ACL anatomy have led to the development of double-bundle ACL reconstruction techniques. Laboratory data have suggested that a double-bundle reconstruction provides improved rotational stability.[16,17] Patient outcome studies to date have not shown a consistent improvement in outcomes between single- and double-bundle techniques.[18,19]

There are many different graft options for ACL reconstruction, but they mainly consist of quadrupled hamstring autograft, bone-patellar tendon-bone autograft, and a variety of allografts. Allografts allow for quicker surgical techniques without patient morbidity associated with graft harvest and a slightly more cosmetic incision. Disadvantages include a small risk of viral transmission (1 in 1.6 million), increased surgical costs, and slower graft incorporation that may translate into a higher rate of graft failure.[20,21] Studies comparing autograft and allograft ACL reconstruction have a variety of outcomes, with some showing similar failure rates and others demonstrating a significantly higher percentage of failures in the allograft groups.[22] With the variety of allograft types used and the heterogeneity of surgical techniques, it is unclear which graft type is best. Likewise, comparative studies of autograft choices

do not consistently favor one type over another.[23,24] A 10-year comparative study showed similar functional outcomes of four-strand hamstrings and patellar tendon grafts.[25]

Recent advances in ACL reconstruction surgical techniques have mirrored improvements in postoperative rehabilitation protocols[26-28] (Table 1). Most surgeons encourage early range of motion immediately after surgery, with added emphasis on closed chain quadriceps strengthening. Guidelines for return to athletics vary from surgeon to surgeon but usually involve a quantitative measure of quadriceps strength and functional status. The recommended return to full sports participation ranges from 4 to 9 months after surgery.[29] Currently there is evidence based on randomized controlled trials that postoperative bracing has no benefit with regard to re-tear rates.[26]

Medial Collateral Ligament Injuries

Recent cadaver work has led to a greater understanding of the anatomy of the medial collateral ligament (MCL) and posteromedial corner (PMC).[30] The MCL consists of a superficial band that originates just proximal and posterior to the medial femoral epicondyle and attaches distally approximately 6 cm below the joint line at the midportion of the proximal tibia. The deep layer has both a meniscofemoral ligament and a meniscotibial ligament, both of which adhere to the peripheral meniscocapsular region. The posterior oblique ligament (POL) runs posterior to the superficial MCL and has multiple bands that attach to the posteromedial capsule, the semimembranosus, and the proximal tibia (Figure 1, *A*). A greater understanding of the specific anatomic locations of these structures has led to the development of newer anatomic reconstruction techniques.[31]

Stability examination is performed by applying a valgus stress to the knee at 0° and 30° of flexion. Greater than 10 mm of valgus opening in full extension is consistent with injury to the ACL, PCL, MCL, and POL. A thorough clinical examination of both knees is critical to truly appreciate the amount of clinical laxity.

Standard AP and supine lateral radiographs often give clues to an injury to the MCL/PMC. Subtle amounts of medial joint space opening, subtle tibiofemoral subluxation, and bony avulsions off the femur in particular can often be seen. At times, fluoroscopic bilateral stress examination may be necessary to truly appreciate the amount of laxity. MRI is the diagnostic imaging modality of choice. MRI is advantageous because of its ability to identify the injury, its specific tear pattern, and location. Additionally, all other associated injuries can be readily identified.

Treatment of isolated MCL injuries is typically nonsurgical, with bracing for 6 weeks. Because most of the injuries occur at the proximal femoral attachment site, healing rates are predictable and usually lead to complete return to preinjury function. However, distal injuries, including the Stener lesion of the knee in which the

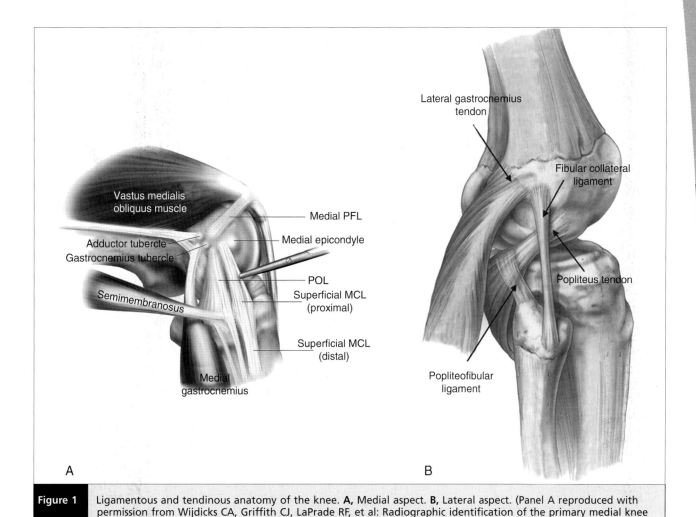

| Figure 1 | Ligamentous and tendinous anatomy of the knee. **A,** Medial aspect. **B,** Lateral aspect. (Panel A reproduced with permission from Wijdicks CA, Griffith CJ, LaPrade RF, et al: Radiographic identification of the primary medial knee structures. *J Bone Joint Surg Am* 2009;91:521-529. Panel B reproduced with permission from LaPrade RF, Ly TV, Wentorf FA, Engebretsen L: The posterolateral attachments of the knee: A qualitative and quantitative morphologic analysis of the fibular collateral ligament, popliteus tendon, popliteofibular ligament, and lateral gastrocnemius tendon *Am J Sports Med* 2003;31:854-860.) |

superficial MCL fibers displace superficial to the pes anserine tendons, prevent anatomic healing. Those MCL injuries in the setting of a multiligament knee injury usually require surgery.

The decision to repair or reconstruct the MCL/PMC in the multiligament-injured knee is a subject of debate. A recent systematic review of the literature[32] found only eight papers in the English literature that met inclusion criteria and found no advantage of one technique over the other. The decision to repair is also dependent on the tissue quality; repair can usually be accomplished in the acute setting. Typically, suture anchors as well as suture/washer post constructs are used for repair. However, when the tissue is difficult to identify and mobilize, reconstruction appears to be a better choice. Several authors have reported excellent outcomes with MCL/PMC reconstructions in the rare instance of combined instability.[33,34] A recent study reported on the anatomic reconstruction of the MCL/PMC with the use of hamstring autograft in patients with chronic MCL instability.[34] This series included pa-

tients treated with isolated reconstruction as well as combined ligament injuries; results were satisfactory in 91%.

Fibular Collateral Ligament and Posterolateral Corner Injuries

The posterolateral corner (PLC) of the knee consists of static and dynamic stabilizers. The three main static stabilizers include the fibular collateral ligament (FCL), the popliteofibular ligament (PFL), and the posterolateral capsule. The popliteus tendon serves as both a dynamic and static stabilizer. The FCL is the primary restraint to varus stress. It attaches to the femur just proximal and posterior to the lateral epicondyle, and to the anterior third of the fibular head. The PFL arises from the musculotendinous junction of the popliteus and attaches to the posterior aspect of the fibular head and has both anterior and posterior divisions. The PFL acts as the main restraint to external rotation of the

Table 2

Examination Techniques for PCL and FCL/PLC Injuries[a]

PCL injury (isolated)

    Posterior drawer at 90° of knee flexion (grade I/II)

    Posterior sag sign at 90° of knee flexion (grade I/II)

    Positive quadriceps active test

FCL/PLC injury (isolated)

    Positive varus stress test at 30° knee flexion

    Positive dial test at 30°, negative at 90° of knee flexion

    Positive external rotation posterior drawer test at 90° of knee flexion

PCL and FCL/PLC injuries

    Posterior drawer at 90° of knee flexion (grade III)

    Posterior sag sign at 90° of knee flexion (grade III)

    Positive dial test at 30° and 90° of knee flexion

[a]Grade I: < 5 mm translation; grade II: 5-10 mm translation; grade III: > 10 mm translation. Degree of laxity is measured in comparison to the unaffected contralateral knee.

tibia. The popliteus tendon attaches on the anterior fifth of the popliteal sulcus on the femur approximately 2 cm anterior and distal to the FCL femoral attachment site (**Figure 1, B**).

Physical examination for ligamentous stability includes the varus stress test at 0° and 30° of flexion. Recently, a biomechanical cadaver study[35] demonstrated that greater than 2.5 mm of side-to-side difference in varus at 30° of flexion was consistent with isolated injury to the FCL, whereas greater than 4 mm side-to-side difference was consistent with an injury to both the FCL and remaining posterolateral corner structures. To assess for rotational stability of the posterolateral corner, the dial test is performed at 30° and 90° of knee flexion. An increase in external rotation of greater than 10° to 15° side-to-side comparison at 30° of flexion is consistent with an injury to the PLC. If this side-to-side difference persists at 90° of flexion, then injuries are present to both PLC and posterior cruciate ligament (PCL). More specific physical examination tests, including the external rotation recurvatum test and the external rotation drawer test, can aid in the diagnosis of PLC injury. The external rotation recurvatum test is a side-to-side comparison with both legs in fully extended positions. The examiner picks up the limbs by the great toe, and the test is positive when the tibia falls into external rotation in the recurvatum position relative to the femur. The external rotation drawer test is

performed at 90° of flexion with the foot in an externally rotated position. A positive test is when the medial step-off becomes absent when a posterior drawer is applied to the tibia. Grading is similar to a standard posterior drawer test (Table 2).

It is important to recognize that isolated injuries to the FCL/PLC are extremely rare, and in most instances, concomitant ACL and/or PCL injuries are present. A recent study of 20 cadaver knees examined by posterior drawer and stress radiography was performed.[36] The knees were tested intact and retested after sequential testing of the PCL and PLC. Posterior stress radiography demonstrated an average posterior displacement of 10 mm with sectioning of the PCL, and an increase of approximately 20 mm with sectioning of the PCL and PLC structures. The authors concluded that a grade III posterior drawer or a side-to-side difference on stress radiography of greater than 10 mm implied a combined injury to both the PCL and PLC.

Because most FCL/PLC injuries occur in the setting of the multiligament-injured knee, surgical management is most often recommended. The decision to repair rather than reconstruct remains controversial. A recently presented series from the Mayo Clinic demonstrated a failure rate of 45% with repair compared to 4% with reconstruction in 44 multiligament-injured knees.[37] Although neither of these studies was randomized, the authors cautioned against repair alone of the FCL/PLC in the multiligament-injured knee.

Numerous reconstruction techniques have been developed with varying degrees of success. The anatomic reconstruction involves a two-tailed reconstruction of the FCL, PFL, and popliteus tendon. Although no clinical data are available, this anatomic reconstruction has been shown to biomechanically replicate the stability of the native ligaments. Other variations of anatomic reconstructions have shown satisfactory outcomes. One study described a single soft-tissue graft reconstruction of the FCL and PLC in 16 knees.[38] At 2-year follow-up, no patients required revision reconstruction. This series showed no significant differences in clinical and functional outcomes between two-ligament and multiligament PLC-based reconstructions. The authors describe the importance of the posterolateral capsular shift in addition to reconstruction of the ligaments.

PCL Injuries

The PCL consists of the anterolateral and posteromedial bundles. The PCL is a robust ligament, 30% larger than the ACL, and measures approximately 33 mm × 13 mm wide. The anterolateral bundle is the strongest bundle and is taut in flexion, whereas the posteromedial bundle is taut in extension. Most reconstruction techniques in the past have focused on reconstruction of the anterolateral bundle. Difficulties arise in identifying the isometric point of the anterolateral bundle on the femur, as the insertion is crescent-shaped. Recent cadaver studies have helped to elucidate the anatomic characteristics and specific insertion points of the PCL

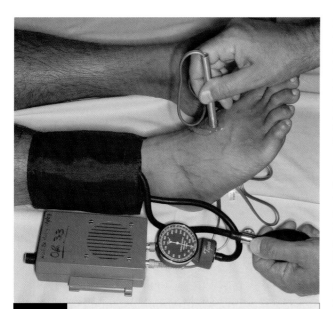

Figure 2 Measurement of systolic blood pressure in the dorsalis pedis artery using ultrasound. (Reproduced with permission from Levy BA, Fanelli GC, Whelan DB, et al: Controversies in the treatment of knee dislocations and multiligament reconstruction. *J Am Acad Orthop Surg* 2009;17: 197-206.)

bundles,[39,40] and numerous double-bundle reconstruction techniques are now available.[41,42]

The posterior drawer test, performed with the knee at 90° of flexion, is the primary tool for assessment of PCL stability. The normal tibial step-off is approximately 1 cm (10 mm). Degree of laxity graded as I, II, and III injuries are defined as ≤ 5 mm, ≤ 10 mm, and > 10 mm of posterior translation, respectively. When applying a posterior drawer, if the tibia moves posterior to sit flush with the femoral condyles, this would imply approximately 10 mm of posterior translation, consistent with a grade II injury. If the tibia moves posterior to the femoral condyles, this would imply a grade III injury (**Table 2**).

Radiographic assessment, in particular a supine lateral view, is helpful in assessing posterior tibiofemoral subluxation. Radiographic or fluoroscopic posterior stress views with bilateral comparison are often helpful in diagnosing and grading the PCL injury. MRI is the imaging modality of choice, although it can lead to falsely positive results. Often, substantial signal change may be seen; however, clinical examination may be completely normal. Therefore, it is important to correlate physical findings, MRI findings, and stress views to confirm the presence and extent of a clinically relevant PCL injury.

Recent biomechanical evidence suggests that a grade III posterior drawer is indicative of a combined PCL/PLC injury.[36] This has important ramifications for management of the isolated PCL tear. For example, an isolated grade I or grade II PCL injury can be successfully treated with quadriceps rehabilitation and PCL brac-

ing, if necessary. An isolated grade III PCL injury, now thought to be a combined ligament injury, may best be treated with surgical reconstruction of both PCL and PLC ligamentous structures. This underscores the importance of differentiating between grade II and grade III injuries. A special circumstance is PCL avulsion injuries of the tibia. These injuries in isolation can be successfully treated surgically with open reduction and internal fixation with satisfactory results.

Reconstruction of the PCL can be approached by transtibial or tibial inlay techniques. Several biomechanical and clinical studies have failed to demonstrate an advantage of one technique over the other.[43] Current controversy persists regarding single-bundle versus double-bundle techniques. One study demonstrated in a cadaver model that a single-bundle anterolateral graft best reproduced normal PCL force profiles and that the double-bundle graft did slightly reduce posterior laxity at 0° to 30° of flexion but at the expense of higher than normal graft forces on the posteromedial bundle.[44] The long-term ramification of these excess graft forces is unknown. A more recent cadaver sectioning study demonstrated that in the setting of a combined PCL/PLC injury, the double-bundle technique offered better rotational control when only the PCL was reconstructed.[45] The authors concluded that because PLC reconstruction techniques tend to stretch out over time, there may be an advantage to the double-bundle PCL reconstruction technique in this particular injury combination.

Clinically, no studies to date have demonstrated an advantage of the double-bundle technique over the single-bundle anterolateral reconstruction. Further prospective randomized trials will be necessary to answer this question.

Multiligament Knee Injuries/Traumatic Knee Dislocation

The dislocated knee is a limb-threatening injury, with a significant rate of neurovascular compromise. It is imperative to recognize that a knee dislocation has occurred; most of these injuries are seen after spontaneous reduction. Normal radiographs and substantial soft-tissue swelling with gross instability in a patient who presents to the emergency department should alert the physician to the possibility of a knee dislocation.

Thorough vascular assessment is probably the most important first step in the management of these injuries. Recently, it has been demonstrated that serial physical examination alone is safe. However, it is also recognized that normal and symmetric pulses may be present with a complete popliteal artery occlusion secondary to collateral flow. Measurement of the ankle-brachial index (ABI) is recommended for every patient who presents to the emergency department with a diagnosis or presumption of a knee dislocation. The ABI is a noninvasive screening tool that is easy to perform in the acute setting[46] (**Figure 2**).

The ABI has shown excellent sensitivity and specificity for detecting clinically relevant vascular injury with

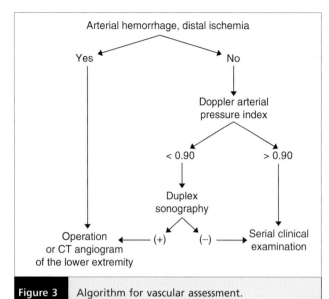

Arterial hemorrhage, distal ischemia

Yes   No

Doppler arterial
pressure index

< 0.90   > 0.90

Duplex
sonography

Operation
or CT angiogram   (+)   (−)   Serial clinical
examination
of the lower extremity

| **Figure 3** | Algorithm for vascular assessment. |

Table 3	

Modified Schenck Classification System for Multiligament Knee Injury

Classification	Pattern of Injury
KD-I	Multiligamentous injury with involvement of only one cruciate ligament
KD-II	Injury to ACL and PCL only
KD-III	Injury to ACL, PCL, and either PMC or PLC
KD-IV	Injury to ACL, PCL, PMC, and PLC
KD-V	Multiligamentous injury with periarticular fracture

a negative predictive value of 100% if the ABI is greater than 0.9. If patients have an abnormal ABI, then further vascular screening with arterial duplex ultrasound is warranted. If the ultrasound is equivocal or nondiagnostic, conventional arteriography or CT arteriography is recommended (**Figure 3**). The advantage of CT arteriography compared to conventional arteriography is that the contrast material is injected into the antecubital fossa as opposed to the groin and requires less than one fourth the radiation.[47]

A thorough neurologic examination is also important because the risk of peroneal nerve injury is approximately 25%. Chronic peroneal nerve palsy, even after a successful multiligament knee reconstruction, can cause significant functional impairment. Conventional treatment consists of neurolysis, nerve grafting, and tibial tendon transfers, all with moderate success. A technique for direct nerve transfer from a healthy motor branch of the tibial nerve to the healthy distal portion of the injured peroneal nerve has been described,[48] although no clinical data are currently available.

The modified Schenck classification system for multiligament knee injury (**Table 3**) has achieved popularity as a means of more precisely communicating patterns of ligament injury. Although this system does not offer a scheme for decision making with regard to management, it helps standardize research results. In this system, a multiligament injury involving only one cruciate ligament is defined as a KD-I. A KD-II describes injury to both cruciate ligaments only. Injury to both cruciate ligaments and either of the collateral ligaments is a KD-III, whereas injury to both cruciate and both collateral ligaments is a KD-IV. A KD-V injury describes damage to two or more ligaments with periarticular fracture.

Optimal treatment strategies for the acutely dislocated knee remain highly debated. There are a paucity of data in the literature to help guide treatment strate-

gies with regard to ligament repair/reconstruction. Current controversies include surgical versus nonsurgical management, early versus delayed surgery, graft selection, repair versus reconstruction of the collateral ligaments, and postoperative rehabilitation. Once a reduction is maintained, the knee must be held stable in the reduced position, often with a long leg splint or cast. Care must be taken to obtain new radiographs with the knee in the splint or cast to verify reduction. Rarely, when the knee is too unstable to maintain a reduction in a splint or if there is a vascular injury, a temporary spanning external fixator can be placed in the acute setting.

A recent evidence-based systematic review was reported, specifically addressing three areas: surgical versus nonsurgical treatment, repair versus reconstruction of injured ligamentous structures, and early versus late surgery of damaged ligaments. This review demonstrated that early surgical treatment (usually defined as within the first 3 weeks following injury) of the multiligament-injured knee led to improved functional and clinical outcomes compared with nonsurgical management or delayed surgery.[49]

Performing research studies with high levels of evidence for these complex injuries is extremely difficult, predominantly because of the heterogeneity of the study group and wide variation of injury patterns/combinations.

Meniscus Tears

The menisci are fibrocartilage structures interposed between the medial and lateral tibiofemoral joints. They are attached to the capsule at their periphery and to the tibia at their anterior and posterior horns. The lateral meniscus is more C-shaped and mobile than its medial counterpart. The menisci function to increase tibiofemoral surface contact area and therefore decrease joint forces. They perform a dampening mechanism for articular cartilage from excessive loads. Joint compressive forces are dissipated by the meniscus when they are converted to outwardly directed radial oriented forces. The radial forces are ultimately borne by meniscus fibers oriented parallel to its macroscopic semicircular structure. Outward forces on the parallel meniscus fibers are resisted by perpendicularly oriented radial tie fibers. A meniscectomized knee demonstrates significantly higher joint forces and leads to progressive tibiofemoral compartment arthritis.

The outer 25% to 30% of each meniscus has a sufficient blood supply suitable for healing (the red-red zone). The middle third of the meniscus is termed the red-white zone because it is at the junction of the vascular outer third and the avascular central third. This central zone, which has no healing potential, is termed the white-white zone. With age, the meniscus becomes further devascularized and it also loses water content.

A meniscus tear can be classified based on shape, size, chronicity, vascularity, and whether the tear is degenerative or acutely traumatic. A patient's age is also important because there is some evidence that meniscus repair healing rates decrease with older age. The shape of a tear can be longitudinal, radial, horizontal, flap, or bucket-handle (a large, unstable, longitudinal tear). Degenerative and chronic tears often have more complex shapes and are often located more centrally. These tears are usually irreparable because of the complex nature of their shape, their chronicity, their avascular location, and the older age of most patients. Tears of the root of the meniscus also can occur and cause a significant decrease in meniscus function, leading to higher tibiofemoral contact forces more often than a tear not involving the root. Cadaver studies have shown that a posterior horn medial meniscus root tear increased medial joint contact pressures equivalent to a total meniscectomy, and those values were restored to normal following repair.[50,51]

The natural history of meniscus tear progression depending on treatment is not known. Also, it is clear that many tears may exist in asymptomatic patients. In a young symptomatic patient with an acute meniscus tear that is longitudinal in shape and displaceable, repairing the meniscus is clearly indicated. Also, a symptomatic meniscus root tear in a patient without degenerative changes should undergo repair. Nondisplaceable acute tears less than 1 cm in length and those that are seen during knee arthroscopy in patients without symptoms should not undergo repair.

Symptomatic meniscus tears cause mechanical symptoms of catching and locking due to displacement of the tear between the femoral condyle and the tibial plateau, or within the intercondylar notch. These tears should be treated with partial meniscectomy or repair. Meniscus tears that are avascular, complex degenerative in shape, found in elderly patients, and that are otherwise irreparable should undergo partial meniscectomy to a stable rim. Normal meniscus should be left intact to preserve some force-dissipating function in the remaining tissue.

Repairable meniscus tears are repaired with one of three techniques: outside-in, inside-out, and all-inside.

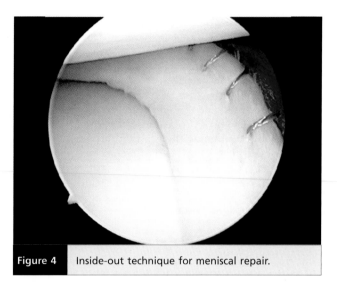

Figure 4 | Inside-out technique for meniscal repair.

The inside-out technique with vertical mattress nonabsorbable suture configuration is the gold standard for meniscus repair and is the strongest repair technique (**Figure 4**). However, with recent advances in arthroscopic repair instrumentation, all-inside techniques have become more popular. All-inside repair techniques now approach the strength of inside-out repairs and outcomes have been largely successful. Disadvantages of inside-out repair are related to the increased morbidity and neurologic injury risk of the medial or lateral meniscus approach required to retrieve and tie sutures over capsule. Although all-inside techniques decrease this morbidity, there is still a risk of neurovascular injury following capsular penetration of all-suture passing devices.[52]

Healing rates of meniscus repairs are generally good.[53,54] The main determinant of healing rates, in addition to the tear pattern, is the location of the tear within the vascularized zone. Meniscus repairs in the setting of a concurrent ACL reconstruction have higher healing rates.[55] This may be due to intra-articular bleeding that occurs from the injury or with bone tunnel preparation.

Postoperative rehabilitation following a meniscus repair often involves a period of no or limited weight bearing as well as limitation of deep knee flexion. This is an attempt to decrease the shear forces across the repaired meniscus while it heals. One advantage of a partial meniscectomy is that immediate weight-bearing is possible, and therefore postoperative recovery is easier.

A young patient who has had a meniscectomy may develop symptoms related to his or her lack of meniscus function (recurrent tibiofemoral joint pain and an effusion). When there are minimal degenerative cartilage changes, the patient may be a candidate for meniscus allograft transplantation. The patient's lower extremity alignment must be taken into account and a high tibial or distal femoral osteotomy may be indicated before or concurrent with the transplantation. Medial meniscus transplantation can be performed with either a single bone plug containing both the anterior and posterior roots or with independent bone plugs for each root. This procedure is possible because there is sufficient distance between the anterior and posterior horn meniscus roots. Because the lateral meniscus roots are very close together, a single plug is usually used on this side. Leaving the allograft bone attached to the meniscus root during the transplantation is critical to maintaining the graft's ability to withstand compressive forces. Outcomes of meniscus transplantation are generally good; however, the rate of meniscus extrusion is approximately 33% and usually occurs in the first year postoperatively.[56] A 10-year follow-up of meniscus transplants found an improvement in subjective outcome scores; however, 55% of grafts had failed and most had radiographic progression of tibiofemoral degenerative changes.[57]

Articular Cartilage Injury

Articular cartilage is mainly composed of type II collagen. Its main function is to dissipate forces within the tibiofemoral and patellofemoral joints. Compression of articular cartilage leads to extrusion of water normally contained within the cartilage matrix loosely bound to negatively charged proteoglycan molecules. Damage to articular cartilage occurs with various arthritides, most commonly osteoarthritis. Focal defects can lead to higher forces in the surrounding intact cartilage and lead to its subsequent breakdown.

Focal injury to knee articular cartilage can occur with any injury to the knee that leads to excessive compression or shear forces from momentary impact of two surfaces. This type of injury can be isolated or seen at the time of concurrent cruciate ligament injury. The natural history of a focal traumatic lesion is unclear. A loose body produced by a cartilage injury may enlarge and become a source of mechanical locking. Cartilage defects in any compartment of the knee can also produce mechanical symptoms in some cases, although they are often asymptomatic once the initial injury subsides. There is evidence that with overloading forces to surrounding intact articular cartilage, the natural history might involve progressive cartilage deterioration and arthritis. However, other studies, including those in patients with concurrent ACL injuries, suggest a relatively benign natural history of untreated cartilage lesions.[58]

Indications for treatment of focal articular cartilage lesions include pain with mechanical symptoms or recurrent swelling. Initial nonsurgical management of patients without true mechanical locking includes range of motion and quadriceps strengthening exercise as well as treatment of the knee effusion. Those patients with mechanical symptoms or with symptoms that persist despite nonsurgical treatment are candidates for surgical intervention. In general, patients younger than 50 years could be considered for cartilage repair whereas older patients are more likely candidates for an arthroplasty procedure.

Surgical options for cartilage repair include chondral débridement, marrow-stimulating techniques such as microfracture and drilling, osteochondral transfer (autograft and allograft), and autologous chondrocyte implantation (ACI). These techniques have all been well studied, and it is unclear which is superior. The size of the lesion is important in determining what graft options are appropriate. Small lesions less than 1 to 2 cm² can be treated with any of these options. Larger lesions that are greater than 2 cm are likely too large for an autograft osteochondral transfer. When there is subchondral bone loss present, the bone void can be filled with the bone plug of an osteochondral transfer or grafting beneath an ACI procedure.

Débridement or a marrow-stimulating technique is a first-line treatment of most small and many medium-sized lesions.[59] In recent randomized controlled trials comparing microfracture and ACI, there was no difference found in outcomes.[60] There is some evidence that second-generation ACI techniques involving a hyaluronic acid scaffold may have better midterm results than microfracture.[61] Patients with large lesions and those in whom simpler procedures have failed are candidates for osteochondral transfer or ACI.[62-64] There is some evidence that removing the calcified cartilage layer during a previous microfracture adversely affects the outcomes of ACI later.

Postoperative rehabilitation from cartilage repair in general emphasizes range of motion, often with a continuous passive motion machine and a period of no weight bearing, usually around 6 to 8 weeks. Weight-bearing exercises and deep bending weight training exercises are introduced gradually.

A patient's coronal plane alignment is extremely important in treating cartilage lesions and has a significant effect on tibiofemoral contact pressures.[65] The weight-bearing line as measured on a full-length standing AP lower extremity radiograph must not go through the affected compartment. If it does, then a realignment procedure, either a high tibial osteotomy or distal femoral osteotomy, is indicated concurrent with or before cartilage repair. If alignment is not corrected, the failure rate of cartilage procedures is higher.

Patellar Instability

Many factors contribute to patellofemoral stability and include both local and distant anatomic etiologies. Factors related to knee anatomy include the medial patellofemoral ligament (MPFL), which is the primary restraint to lateral patellar translation in the first 20° of knee flexion and guides the patella into the trochlear groove. The bony structures of the patella and trochlea account for most patellofemoral stability in deeper knee flexion. Soft-tissue restraints include the medial and lateral patellofemoral retinacula and the quadriceps muscle-tendon unit. Patella alta can also lead to instability before the patella engages the trochlear groove.

Factors that contribute to patellofemoral stability include those that can increase the lateral moment of the patella, such as increased femoral anteversion, internal tibial torsion, core and hip abductor weakness, and pes planus. Static coronal plane alignment of the extensor mechanism, the Q angle, has considerable influence on patellar stability. Generalized ligamentous laxity can contribute to patellofemoral instability.

Patellofemoral instability is lateral in most instances. Medial dislocations occur mainly from iatrogenic causes such as a failed prior procedure for lateral instability. Lateral instability may be due to a single traumatic event causing an MPFL tear or a combination of the aforementioned pathology that has lead to chronic recurrent instability with minor or even no trauma.

Treatment of patellofemoral instability is complex and depends on the exact pathoanatomy present in each case. Each abnormal structure or pathology must be addressed to ensure successful treatment. In atraumatic instability, initial treatment usually consists of physical therapy and bracing. With a first-time traumatic patellar lateral dislocation there is some controversy regarding treatment. The benefit of acute surgical repair has not been definitively established although some studies recommend this approach.[66-68] Significant loose bodies should be removed arthroscopically. Residual lateral tilting or subluxation of the patella may be considered an indication for early MPFL repair. In most cases, however, initial treatment consists of a period of immobilization to allow the MPFL to heal, followed by physical therapy to regain motion and strength, including quadriceps control and hip abductor strengthening. Later transition to a J-brace resists lateral patellar translation.

Surgical management for most patients is reserved for recurrence of instability. Most procedures are categorized as proximal-distal and combined realignment. Proximal realignment procedures mainly repair or reconstruct the MPFL and may address the retinaculum and/or the vastus medialis. These procedures are done for deficient soft-tissue structures that cause the patella to not consistently engage the trochlear groove in early flexion. The radiographic MPFL femoral attachment site for its reconstruction has been defined.[69] Other common procedures include lateral retinacular lengthening and vastus medialis advancement. Distal realignment procedures are performed when there is an increased Q angle documented by a trochlear groove to tibial tubercle distance of more than 20 mm on axial CT scan. In most cases, this consists of an anteromedialization tibial tubercle osteotomy. The amount of anterior and medial displacement of the osteotomy can be tailored to the specific patient's pathology. Combined procedures are reserved for when a patient has deficient soft-tissue restraints as well as increased extensor mechanism valgus alignment. When a patient has a dysplastic trochlear groove, this may have to be specifically addressed with a trochlear groove deepening procedure.[70] Also, patella alta can be treated with a patellar tendon imbrication or tibial tubercle distalization.

Annotated References

1. Boden BP, Torg JS, Knowles SB, Hewett TE: Video analysis of anterior cruciate ligament injury: Abnormalities in hip and ankle kinematics. *Am J Sports Med* 2009; 37(2):252-259.

   This video analysis of ACL injuries found that landing ground contact with a flatfoot or heel first, knee abduction, and hip flexion may be risk factors for injury.

2. Hewett TE, Zazulak BT, Myer GD: Effects of the menstrual cycle on anterior cruciate ligament injury risk: A systematic review. *Am J Sports Med* 2007;35(4):659-668.

   This systematic review of the effect of the menstrual cycle and hormone levels found that female athletes may be more predisposed to ACL injuries during the preovulatory phase of the menstrual cycle.

3. Posthumus M, September AV, O'Cuinneagain D, van der Merwe W, Schwellnus MP, Collins M: The COL5A1 gene is associated with increased risk of anterior cruciate ligament ruptures in female participants. *Am J Sports Med* 2009;37(11):2234-2240.

   This case-control study of 345 patients demonstrated an underrepresentation of the CC genotype of a *COL5A1* gene sequence in females with ACL ruptures, demonstrating for the first time a genetic predisposition for ACL rupture in female athletes.

4. Ferretti M, Ekdahl M, Shen W, Fu FH: Osseous landmarks of the femoral attachment of the anterior cruciate ligament: An anatomic study. *Arthroscopy* 2007;23(11): 1218-1225.

   This anatomic study found that the ACL femoral attachment has a unique topography with a constant presence of the lateral intercondylar ridge and often an osseous ridge between anteromedial and posterolateral femoral attachments, the lateral bifurcate ridge.

5. Pugh L, Mascarenhas R, Arneja S, Chin PY, Leith JM: Current concepts in instrumented knee-laxity testing. *Am J Sports Med* 2009;37(1):199-210.

   This systematic review of the literature suggested that the KT-1000 knee arthrometer and the Rolimeter were most reliable for testing anterior laxity in the knee, whereas the Telos device was determined to best discern posterior laxity.

6. Arbuthnot JE, Brink RB: The role of anterior cruciate ligament reconstruction in the older patients, 55 years or above. *Knee Surg Sports Traumatol Arthrosc* 2010; 18(1):73-78.

   This case series of ACL reconstruction in 14 patients older than 55 years showed a significant improvement in postoperative clinical outcomes with decreased anterior laxity in all but one patient, demonstrating the safety of this procedure in this population.

7. Khan RM, Prasad V, Gangone R, Kinmont JC: Anterior cruciate ligament reconstruction in patients over 40 years using hamstring autograft. *Knee Surg Sports Traumatol Arthrosc* 2010;18(1):68-72.

Clinical outcomes of arthroscopically assisted ACL reconstruction with four-stranded hamstring autograft were retrospectively evaluated in 21 patients older than 40 years at mean 2-year follow-up. Satisfactory results were observed in Lysholm, International Knee Documentation Committee, Tegner, and KT-1000 arthrometer measurements.

8. Granan LP, Bahr R, Lie SA, Engebretsen L: Timing of anterior cruciate ligament reconstructive surgery and risk of cartilage lesions and meniscal tears: A cohort study based on the Norwegian National Knee Ligament Registry. *Am J Sports Med* 2009;37(5):955-961.

    This study evaluated a cohort of patients undergoing ACL reconstructions in the Norwegian National Knee Ligament Registry. The odds of a cartilage lesion in the adult knee increased by nearly 1% for each month that elapsed from the injury date until the surgery date, and that of cartilage lesions were nearly twice as frequent if there was a meniscal tear, and vice versa.

9. Tayton E, Verma R, Higgins B, Gosal H: A correlation of time with meniscal tears in anterior cruciate ligament deficiency: Stratifying the risk of surgical delay. *Knee Surg Sports Traumatol Arthrosc* 2009;17(1):30-34.

    This retrospective review of patients who underwent ACL reconstruction found that those patients with no meniscal damage at the time of diagnosis and who had no further damage at surgery had a median time to surgery of 6 months. This time was significantly different from those with no meniscal damage at diagnosis, but who were found subsequently to have sustained damage to one meniscus, when the median time was 11 months ($P = 0.0017$), or both menisci, when the median time was 32 months ($P = 0.0184$).

10. Lebel B, Hulet C, Galaud B, Burdin G, Locker B, Vielpeau C: Arthroscopic reconstruction of the anterior cruciate ligament using bone-patellar tendon-bone autograft: A minimum 10-year follow-up. *Am J Sports Med* 2008;36(7):1275-1282.

    This was a retrospective study of patients undergoing ACL reconstruction using bone–patellar tendon–bone autograft. The authors found high patient satisfaction levels and good clinical results after 10 years. Moreover, a high percentage of patients remained involved in sports activities, and ACL reconstruction protected the meniscus from a secondary tear. However, knee osteoarthritis developed in 17.8% of patients so treated.

11. Lidén M, Sernert N, Rostgård-Christensen L, Kartus C, Ejerhed L: Osteoarthritic changes after anterior cruciate ligament reconstruction using bone-patellar tendon-bone or hamstring tendon autografts: A retrospective, 7-year radiographic and clinical follow-up study. *Arthroscopy* 2008;24(8):899-908.

    This retrospective review found at a median of 7 years after ACL reconstruction with either bone–patellar-tendon–bone or hamstring tendon autografts, the prevalence of osteoarthritis as seen on standard weight-bearing radiographs and the clinical outcome were comparable. The presence of meniscal injuries increased the prevalence of osteoarthritis.

12. Taylor DC, Posner M, Curl WW, Feagin JA: Isolated tears of the anterior cruciate ligament: Over 30-year follow-up of patients treated with arthrotomy and primary repair. *Am J Sports Med* 2009;37(1):65-71.

    At more than 30-year follow-up, patients have decreased activity levels and an equal mix of acceptable and unacceptable outcomes. The authors were unable to identify any predictive factors that correlated with the results; however, subsequent meniscal surgery did correlate with poor results. The results at greater than 30 years reinforce the 5-year results that showed unsatisfactory results after the open evaluation and treatment of ACL injuries with or without repair.

13. Stanford FC, Kendoff D, Warren RF, Pearle AD: Native anterior cruciate ligament obliquity versus anterior cruciate ligament graft obliquity: An observational study using navigated measurements. *Am J Sports Med* 2009;37(1):114-119.

    This laboratory study compared transtibial ACL reconstruction to the native anatomy. The sagittal and coronal plane obliquity of well-functioning grafts placed using the transtibial technique were more vertical than anatomic fibers.

14. Harner CD, Honkamp NJ, Ranawat AS: Anteromedial portal technique for creating the anterior cruciate ligament femoral tunnel. *Arthroscopy* 2008;24(1):113-115.

    The authors describe the technique of using an anteromedial portal for femoral tunnel drilling in ACL reconstruction.

15. Kanaya A, Ochi M, Deie M, Adachi N, Nishimori M, Nakamae A: Intraoperative evaluation of anteroposterior and rotational stabilities in anterior cruciate ligament reconstruction: Lower femoral tunnel placed single-bundle versus double-bundle reconstruction. *Knee Surg Sports Traumatol Arthrosc* 2009;17(8):907-913.

    This prospective, randomized trial evaluated stability after single- versus double-bundle ACL reconstruction with hamstring tendons in 26 patients with anteroposterior knee laxity. No differences were found in AP displacement or tibial rotation at 30° and 60° of flexion between groups.

16. Markolf KL, Park S, Jackson SR, McAllister DR: Simulated pivot-shift testing with single and double-bundle anterior cruciate ligament reconstructions. *J Bone Joint Surg Am* 2008;90(8):1681-1689.

    The authors' cadaver model of ACL reconstruction found that a single-bundle reconstruction was sufficient to restore intact knee kinematics during a simulated pivot-shift event. The higher graft forces with some double-bundle graft-tensioning protocols reduced the coupled rotations and displacements from an applied valgus moment to less than the intact levels. This overcorrection should theoretically make the knee less likely to pivot but could have unknown clinical consequences.

17. Markolf KL, Park S, Jackson SR, McAllister DR: Anterior-posterior and rotatory stability of single and double-bundle anterior cruciate ligament reconstructions. *J Bone Joint Surg Am* 2009;91(1):107-118.

The authors' cadaver model of ACL reconstruction found that the single-bundle reconstruction produced graft forces, knee laxities, and coupled tibial rotations that were closest to normal. Adding a posterolateral graft to an anteromedial graft tended to reduce laxities and tibial rotations, but the reductions were accompanied by markedly higher forces in the posterolateral graft near 0° that occasionally caused it to fail during tests with internal torque or anterior tibial force.

18. Lewis PB, Parameswaran AD, Rue JP, Bach BR Jr: Systematic review of single-bundle anterior cruciate ligament reconstruction outcomes: A baseline assessment for consideration of double-bundle techniques. *Am J Sports Med* 2008;36(10):2028-2036.

This systematic review of one single-bundle anterior cruciate ligament reconstruction demonstrates it to be a safe, consistent surgical procedure affording reliable results.

19. Meredick RB, Vance KJ, Appleby D, Lubowitz JH: Outcome of single-bundle versus double-bundle reconstruction of the anterior cruciate ligament: A meta-analysis. *Am J Sports Med* 2008;36(7):1414-1421.

This meta-analysis of single-bundle and double-bundle reconstruction found that double-bundle reconstruction does not result in clinically significant differences in KT-1000 arthrometer or pivot shift testing. The pivot shift results have particular clinical relevance because the test is designed to evaluate knee rotational instability; the results do not support the theory that double-bundle reconstruction better controls knee rotation.

20. Cohen SB, Sekiya JK: Allograft safety in anterior cruciate ligament reconstruction. *Clin Sports Med* 2007;26(4):597-605.

This review article discusses the risks and benefits of using allograft tissue for ACL reconstruction and advocates providing this information to patients before their procedure.

21. Borchers JR, Pedroza A, Kaeding C: Activity level and graft type as risk factors for anterior cruciate ligament graft failure: A case-control study. *Am J Sports Med* 2009;37(12):2362-2367.

This case-control study compared activity level and graft selection in 21 patients with ACL graft failure to a 2:1 age- and sex-matched control group, determining a roughly 5.5 odds ratio for higher activity levels and allograft versus autograft for failure.

22. Prodromos C, Joyce B, Shi K: A meta-analysis of stability of autografts compared to allografts after anterior cruciate ligament reconstruction. *Knee Surg Sports Traumatol Arthrosc* 2007;15(7):851-856.

This meta-analysis found that allografts had significantly lower normal stability rates than autografts. The allograft abnormal stability rate, which usually represents graft failure, was significantly higher than that of autografts: nearly three times greater. It would therefore appear that autografts are the graft of choice for routine ACL reconstruction with allografts better reserved for multiple ligament–injured knees where extra tissue may be required.

23. Maletis GB, Cameron SL, Tengan JJ, Burchette RJ: A prospective randomized study of anterior cruciate ligament reconstruction: A comparison of patellar tendon and quadruple-strand semitendinosus/gracilis tendons fixed with bioabsorbable interference screws. *Am J Sports Med* 2007;35(3):384-394.

The authors found that the bone–patellar tendon–bone group had better flexion strength in the operated leg than in the nonoperated leg (102% versus 90%, P = 0.0001), fewer patients reporting difficulty jumping (3% vs 17%, P = 0.03), and a greater number of patients returning to preinjury Tegner level (51% vs 26%, P = 0.01). The quadruple-strand semitendinosus/gracilis group had better extension strength in the operated leg than in the nonoperated leg (92% versus 85%, P = 0.04), fewer patients with sensory deficits (14% versus 83%, P = 0.0001), and fewer patients with difficulty kneeling (6% versus 20%, P = 0.04). Both groups showed significant improvement in KT-1000 arthrometer manual maximum difference, Lysholm score, Tegner activity level, International Knee Documentation Committee grade, and patient knee rating score.

24. Poolman RW, Abouali JA, Conter HJ, Bhandari M: Overlapping systematic reviews of anterior cruciate ligament reconstruction comparing hamstring autograft with bone-patellar tendon-bone autograft: Why are they different? *J Bone Joint Surg Am* 2007;89(7):1542-1552.

The currently available best evidence, derived from a methodologically sound meta-analysis, suggests that hamstring tendon autografts are superior for preventing anterior knee pain, and there is limited evidence that bone-–atellar tendon–bone autografts provide better stability.

25. Pinczewski LA, Lyman J, Salmon LJ, Russell VJ, Roe J, Linklater J: A 10-year comparison of anterior cruciate ligament reconstructions with hamstring tendon and patellar tendon autograft: A controlled, prospective trial. *Am J Sports Med* 2007;35(4):564-574.

The authors found it possible to obtain excellent results with both hamstring tendon and patellar tendon autografts. They recommend hamstring tendon reconstructions because of decreased harvest-site symptoms and radiographic osteoarthritis.

26. Birmingham TB, Bryant DM, Giffin JR, et al: A randomized controlled trial comparing the effectiveness of functional knee brace and neoprene sleeve use after anterior cruciate ligament reconstruction. *Am J Sports Med* 2008;36(4):648-655.

This randomized controlled trial of functional knee bracing versus neoprene sleeve in 150 patients after ACL reconstruction with hamstring autograft demonstrated no significant differences in functional or clinical outcomes at 1- and 2-year follow-up visits.

27. Matava MJ, Prickett WD, Khodamoradi S, Abe S, Garbutt J: Femoral nerve blockade as a preemptive anesthetic in patients undergoing anterior cruciate ligament reconstruction: A prospective, randomized, double-blinded, placebo-controlled study. *Am J Sports Med* 2009;37(1):78-86.

This randomized controlled trial evaluated the effectiveness of preemptive femoral nerve blockade versus placebo for pain control after patellar tendon ACL reconstruction in 56 patients. No significant differences in postoperative pain, narcotic use, or hospital stay data were noted.

28. Andersson D, Samuelsson K, Karlsson J: Treatment of anterior cruciate ligament injuries with special reference to surgical technique and rehabilitation: An assessment of randomized controlled trials. *Arthroscopy* 2009; 25(6):653-685.

   This systematic review of the literature found 70 articles dealing with surgical technique and rehabilitation after ACL reconstruction, determining from these that closed kinetic chain exercises promote better subjective outcomes, decreased laxity, and less pain compared to open chain exercises.

29. Shelbourne KD, Gray T, Haro M: Incidence of subsequent injury to either knee within 5 years after anterior cruciate ligament reconstruction with patellar tendon autograft. *Am J Sports Med* 2009;37(2):246-251.

   The authors found that women have a higher incidence of ACL injury to the contralateral knee than men after reconstruction. The incidence of injury to either knee after reconstruction is associated with younger age and higher activity level, but returning to full activities before 6 months postoperatively does not increase the risk of subsequent injury.

30. LaPrade RF, Engebretsen AH, Ly TV, Johansen S, Wentorf FA, Engebretsen L: The anatomy of the medial part of the knee. *J Bone Joint Surg Am* 2007;89(9):2000-2010.

   Anatomic dimensions and attachment sites for the main medial knee structures were recorded in eight cadaver knees, confirming a consistent attachment pattern for these structures.

31. Kim SJ, Lee DH, Kim TE, Choi NH: Concomitant reconstruction of the medial collateral and posterior oblique ligaments for medial instability of the knee. *J Bone Joint Surg Br* 2008;90(10):1323-1327.

   This article describes a surgical technique for and clinical outcomes of concomitant reconstruction of the MCL and POL with semitendinosus autograft in 24 patients at mean 52.6-month follow-up, demonstrating satisfactory improvement in medial-side stability.

32. Kovachevich R, Shah JP, Arens AM, Stuart MJ, Dahm DL, Levy BA: Operative management of the medial collateral ligament in the multi-ligament injured knee: An evidence-based systematic review. *Knee Surg Sports Traumatol Arthrosc* 2009;17(7):823-829.

   This systematic review examined evidence in the literature comparing outcomes of repair versus reconstruction of the MCL in multiligament knee injuries. Satisfactory results were observed with both techniques. Treatment decisions should be made on a case-by-case basis.

33. Hayashi R, Kitamura N, Kondo E, Anaguchi Y, Tohyama H, Yasuda K: Simultaneous anterior and posterior cruciate ligament reconstruction in chronic knee instabilities: Surgical concepts and clinical outcome. *Knee Surg Sports Traumatol Arthrosc* 2008;16(8):763-769.

   This case series of 19 patients with chronic multiligament knee injuries demonstrated single-stage reconstruction of two or more knee ligaments with autograft to be safe and effective, with satisfactory postoperative outcomes at a mean 42-month follow-up.

34. Lind M, Jakobsen BW, Lund B, Hansen MS, Abdallah O, Christiansen SE: Anatomical reconstruction of the medial collateral ligament and posteromedial corner of the knee in patients with chronic medial collateral ligament instability. *Am J Sports Med* 2009;37(6):1116-1122.

   This case series of 61 patients with medial-sided knee instability described satisfactory clinical, functional, and subjective outcomes at a minimum of 2 years after MCL/PMC reconstruction using an anatomic technique.

35. LaPrade RF, Heikes C, Bakker AJ, Jakobsen RB: The reproducibility and repeatability of varus stress radiographs in the assessment of isolated fibular collateral ligament and grade-III posterolateral knee injuries: An in vitro biomechanical study. *J Bone Joint Surg Am* 2008;90(10):2069-2076.

   This study of 10 cadaver knees measured lateral compartment opening on varus stress radiography after PLC sectioning, determining that an isolated FCL injury or grade III PLC injury was likely if 2.7 mm or 4.0 mm of opening was found, respectively.

36. Sekiya JK, Whiddon DR, Zehms CT, Miller MD: A clinically relevant assessment of posterior cruciate ligament and posterolateral corner injuries: Evaluation of isolated and combined deficiency. *J Bone Joint Surg Am* 2008;90(8):1621-1627.

   Twenty cadaver knees underwent sectioning of the PCL and PLC structures. A grade 3 posterior drawer test and >10 mm of posterior tibial translation on stress radiography were associated with PLC injury in addition to complete disruption of the PCL.

37. Levy BA, Dajani KA, Morgan JA, Shah JP, Dahm DL, Stuart MJ: Repair versus reconstruction of the fibular collateral ligament and posterolateral corner in the multiligament-injured knee. *Am J Sports Med* 2010; 38(4):804-809.

   The authors found a statistically significant higher rate of failure for repair compared with reconstruction of the FCL and PLC. Level of evidence: III.

38. Schechinger SJ, Levy BA, Dajani KA, Shah JP, Herrera DA, Marx RG: Achilles tendon allograft reconstruction of the fibular collateral ligament and posterolateral corner. *Arthroscopy* 2009;25(3):232-242.

   FCL and PLC reconstruction via a single Achilles tendon allograft construct was evaluated in 16 knees (minimum 2-year follow-up). No significant difference in clinical or functional outcomes was observed between two-ligament and multiligament PLC-based reconstructions. Level of evidence: IV.

39. Lopes OV Jr, Ferretti M, Shen W, Ekdahl M, Smolinski P, Fu FH: Topography of the femoral attachment of the posterior cruciate ligament. *J Bone Joint Surg Am* 2008; 90(2):249-255.

This study of 20 cadaver knees described the dimensions and anatomy of the femoral footprints of each bundle of the PCL using gross observation and three-dimensional laser photography. A medial intercondylar ridge and medial bifurcate ridge are described.

40. Moorman CT III, Murphy Zane MS, Bansai S, et al: Tibial insertion of the posterior cruciate ligament: A sagittal plane analysis using gross, histologic, and radiographic methods. *Arthroscopy* 2008;24(3):269-275.

This study of 14 cadaver knees describes the anatomy of the tibial attachment site of the posterior cruciate ligament and recommends measurement for tunnel placement along the posterior cruciate ligament facet seen on a lateral radiographic view.

41. Forsythe B, Harner C, Martins CA, Shen W, Lopes OV Jr, Fu FH: Topography of the femoral attachment of the posterior cruciate ligament: Surgical technique. *J Bone Joint Surg Am* 2009;91(suppl 2 pt 1):89-100.

This study of 20 cadaver knees describes the anatomic dimensions and femoral attachment sites of both bundles of the PCL as well as a related surgical technique for double-bundle PCL reconstruction.

42. Lee YS, Ahn JH, Jung YB, et al: Transtibial double bundle posterior cruciate ligament reconstruction using TransFix tibial fixation. *Knee Surg Sports Traumatol Arthrosc* 2007;15(8):973-977.

A transtibial double-bundle PCL reconstruction technique is described using TransFix tibial fixation.

43. Fanelli GC, Edson CJ: Arthroscopically assisted combined anterior and posterior cruciate ligament reconstruction in the multiple ligament injured knee: 2- to 10-year follow-up. *Arthroscopy* 2002;18(7):703-714.

44. Markolf KL, Feeley BT, Jackson SR, McAllister DR: Biomechanical studies of double-bundle posterior cruciate ligament reconstructions. *J Bone Joint Surg Am* 2006;88(8):1788-1794.

45. Whiddon DR, Zehms CT, Miller MD, Quinby JS, Montgomery SL, Sekiya JK: Double compared with single-bundle open inlay posterior cruciate ligament reconstruction in a cadaver model. *J Bone Joint Surg Am* 2008;90(9):1820-1829.

Posterior tibial translation and external rotation after single- and double-bundle PCL tibial-inlay reconstruction were compared in nine cadaver knees with a deficient and repaired posterolateral corner. The double-bundle technique resulted in significantly greater rotational and anterior-posterior stability.

46. Levy BA, Zlowodzki MP, Graves M, Cole PA: Screening for extremity arterial injury with the arterial pressure index. *Am J Emerg Med* 2005;23(5):689-695.

47. Redmond JM, Levy BA, Dajani KA, Cass JR, Cole PA: Detecting vascular injury in lower-extremity orthopedic

trauma: The role of CT angiography. *Orthopedics* 2008;31(8):761-767.

CT angiography demonstrates excellent sensitivity and specificity as a screening tool for vascular injury in the setting of trauma to the lower extremity and has several advantages compared to conventional arteriography.

48. Bodily KD, Spinner RJ, Bishop AT: Restoration of motor function of the deep fibular (peroneal) nerve by direct nerve transfer of branches from the tibial nerve: An anatomical study. *Clin Anat* 2004;17(3):201-205.

49. Levy BA, Dajani KA, Whelan DB, et al: Decision making in the multiligament-injured knee: An evidence-based systematic review. *Arthroscopy* 2009;25(4):430-438.

This systematic review suggested that early surgical treatment of the multiligament-injured knee produces improved functional and clinical outcomes compared with nonsurgical management or delayed surgery, and that repair of the PLC yields higher revision rates compared with reconstruction.

50. Allaire R, Muriuki M, Gilbertson L, Harner CD: Biomechanical consequences of a tear of the posterior root of the medial meniscus: Similar to total meniscectomy. *J Bone Joint Surg Am* 2008;90(9):1922-1931.

This laboratory study found significant changes in contact pressure and knee joint kinematics due to a posterior root tear of the medial meniscus. Root repair was successful in restoring joint biomechanics to within normal conditions.

51. Marzo JM, Gurske-DePerio J: Effects of medial meniscus posterior horn avulsion and repair on tibiofemoral contact area and peak contact pressure with clinical implications. *Am J Sports Med* 2009;37(1):124-129.

This laboratory study found that posterior horn medial meniscal root avulsion leads to deleterious alteration of the loading profiles of the medial joint compartment and results in loss of hoop stress resistance, meniscus extrusion, abnormal loading of the joint, and early knee medial compartment degenerative changes.

52. Chen NC, Martin SD, Gill TJ: Risk to the lateral geniculate artery during arthroscopic lateral meniscal suture passage. *Arthroscopy* 2007;23(6):642-646.

This laboratory study found that the lateral geniculate artery is in close proximity to the lateral meniscus and is punctured often during in vitro inside-out meniscal repair in the embalmed cadaver model.

53. Logan M, Watts M, Owen J, Myers P: Meniscal repair in the elite athlete: Results of 45 repairs with a minimum 5-year follow-up. *Am J Sports Med* 2009;37(6): 1131-1134.

This retrospective review found that meniscal repair and healing are possible, and most elite athletes can return to their preinjury level of activity.

54. Pujol N, Panarella L, Selmi TA, Neyret P, Fithian D, Beaufils P: Meniscal healing after meniscal repair: A CT arthrography assessment. *Am J Sports Med* 2008;36(8): 1489-1495.

4: Lower Extremity

This retrospective review found that using all-inside fixation or outside-in sutures provided good clinical and anatomic outcomes. No statistically significant effect of ACL reconstruction or laterality (medial versus lateral) on overall healing after meniscal repair was identified. Partial healing occurred often, with a stable tear on a narrowed and painless meniscus. The posterior segment healing rate remained low, suggesting a need for further technical improvements.

55. Feng H, Hong L, Geng XS, Zhang H, Wang XS, Jiang XY: Second-look arthroscopic evaluation of bucket-handle meniscus tear repairs with anterior cruciate ligament reconstruction: 67 consecutive cases. *Arthroscopy* 2008;24(12):1358-1366.

This retrospective review found that for large bucket-handle meniscus tears involving red-red and red-white zones, an arthroscopic hybrid suture technique with ACL reconstruction achieves high anatomic healing results, with an overall meniscal healing rate of 89.6%, including 82.1% completely healed and 7.5% incompletely healed. The failure rate was 10.4% in the average 26-month follow-up period.

56. Lee DH, Kim TH, Lee SH, Kim CW, Kim JM, Bin SI: Evaluation of meniscus allograft transplantation with serial magnetic resonance imaging during the first postoperative year: Focus on graft extrusion. *Arthroscopy* 2008;24(10):1115-1121.

This retrospective review found that a meniscus that extrudes early remains extruded and does not progressively worsen, whereas one that does not extrude early is unlikely to extrude within the first postoperative year.

57. Hommen JP, Applegate GR, Del Pizzo W: Meniscus allograft transplantation: Ten-year results of cryopreserved allografts. *Arthroscopy* 2007;23(4):388-393.

This retrospective review found that transplantation of cryopreserved allografts improved knee pain and function, and the average knee function was fair at long-term follow-up. Fifty-five percent of allografts failed when failure criteria for second-look surgery, knee improvement surveys, and MRI were added to Lysholm and pain score failure rates. The protective benefits of meniscus allografts remain debatable, and inferences cannot be made from this study.

58. Widuchowski W, Widuchowski J, Koczy B, Szyluk K: Untreated asymptomatic deep cartilage lesions associated with anterior cruciate ligament injury: Results at 10- and 15-year follow-up. *Am J Sports Med* 2009;37(4):688-692.

The authors found that untreated deep cartilage lesions found during ACL reconstruction do not appear to affect clinical outcome at 10- to 15-year follow-up. Level of evidence: III.

59. Mithoefer K, McAdams T, Williams RJ, Kreuz PC, Mandelbaum BR: Clinical efficacy of the microfracture technique for articular cartilage repair in the knee: An evidence-based systematic analysis. *Am J Sports Med* 2009;37(10):2053-2063.

This systematic analysis shows that microfracture provides effective short-term functional improvement of knee function but insufficient data are available on its long-term results. Shortcomings of the technique include limited hyaline repair tissue, variable repair cartilage volume, and possible functional deterioration. The quality of the currently available data on microfracture is still limited by the variability of results and study designs.

60. Knutsen G, Drogset JO, Engebretsen L, et al: A randomized trial comparing autologous chondrocyte implantation with microfracture. Findings at five years. *J Bone Joint Surg Am* 2007;89(10):2105-2112.

This randomized controlled trial found that both methods provided satisfactory results in 77% of the patients at 5 years. There was no significant difference in the clinical and radiographic results between the two treatment groups and no correlation between the histologic findings and the clinical outcome. One third of the patients had early radiographic signs of osteoarthritis 5 years after the surgery.

61. Kon E, Gobbi A, Filardo G, Delcogliano M, Zaffagnini S, Marcacci M: Arthroscopic second-generation autologous chondrocyte implantation compared with microfracture for chondral lesions of the knee: Prospective nonrandomized study at 5 years. *Am J Sports Med* 2009;37(1):33-41.

This nonrandomized trial found that both methods have shown satisfactory clinical outcome at medium-term follow-up. Better clinical results and sports activity resumption were noted in the group treated with second-generation autologous chondrocyte transplantation.

62. Marcacci M, Kon E, Delcogliano M, Filardo G, Busacca M, Zaffagnini S: Arthroscopic autologous osteochondral grafting for cartilage defects of the knee: Prospective study results at a minimum 7-year follow-up. *Am J Sports Med* 2007;35(12):2014-2021.

This retrospective review found that the results of this technique at medium- to long-term follow-up are encouraging. This arthroscopic one-step surgery appears to be a valid solution for treatment of small grade III to IV cartilage defects.

63. Williams RJ III, Ranawat AS, Potter HG, Carter T, Warren RF: Fresh stored allografts for the treatment of osteochondral defects of the knee. *J Bone Joint Surg Am* 2007;89(4):718-726.

This prospective study found that fresh osteochondral allografts that were hypothermically stored between 17 and 42 days were effective in the short term both structurally and functionally in reconstructing symptomatic chondral and osteochondral lesions of the knee.

64. Zaslav K, Cole B, Brewster R, et al; STAR Study Principal Investigators: A prospective study of autologous chondrocyte implantation in patients with failed prior treatment for articular cartilage defect of the knee: Results of the Study of the Treatment of Articular Repair (STAR) clinical trial. *Am J Sports Med* 2009;37(1):42-55.

This prospective study found that patients with moderate to large chondral lesions with failed prior cartilage treatments can expect sustained and clinically meaningful improvement in pain and function after ACI. The subsequent surgical procedure rate observed in this study (49% overall; 40% related to autologous chondrocyte implantation) appears higher than generally reported after autologous chondrocyte implantation.

65. Agneskirchner JD, Hurschler C, Wrann CD, Lobenhoffer P: The effects of valgus medial opening wedge high tibial osteotomy on articular cartilage pressure of the knee: A biomechanical study. *Arthroscopy* 2007; 23(8):852-861.

    This cadaver study found that a medial opening wedge high tibial osteotomy (HTO) maintains high medial compartment pressure despite the fact that the loading axis has been shifted into valgus. Only after complete release of the distal fibers of the MCL does the opening wedge HTO produce a decompression of the medial joint compartment.

66. Christiansen SE, Jakobsen BW, Lund B, Lind M: Isolated repair of the medial patellofemoral ligament in primary dislocation of the patella: A prospective randomized study. *Arthroscopy* 2008;24(8):881-887.

    This randomized controlled trial found that delayed primary repair of the MPFL by use of an anchor-based reattachment to the adductor tubercle without vastus medialis obliquus repair after primary patella dislocation does not reduce the risk of redislocation nor does it produce any significantly better subjective functional outcome based on the Kujala knee score. Only the specific subjective patella stability score was improved by MPFL repair compared with conservative treatment.

67. Palmu S, Kallio PE, Donell ST, Helenius I, Nietosvaara Y: Acute patellar dislocation in children and adolescents: A randomized clinical trial. *J Bone Joint Surg Am* 2008;90(3):463-470.

    This randomized controlled trial found that long-term subjective and functional results after acute patellar dislocation are satisfactory in most patients. Initial surgical repair of the medial structures combined with lateral release did not improve the long-term outcome, despite the very high rate of recurrent instability. A positive family history is a risk factor for recurrence and for contralateral patellofemoral instability. Routine repair of the torn medial stabilizing soft tissues is not advocated for the treatment of acute patellar dislocation in children and adolescents.

68. Sillanpää PJ, Mattila VM, Mäenpää H, Kiuru M, Visuri T, Pihlajamäki H: Treatment with and without initial stabilizing surgery for primary traumatic patellar dislocation: A prospective randomized study. *J Bone Joint Surg Am* 2009;91(2):263-273.

    This randomized controlled trial found that in a study of young, mostly male adults with primary traumatic patellar dislocation, the rate of redislocation for those treated with surgical stabilization was significantly lower than the rate for those treated without surgical stabilization. However, no clear subjective benefits of initial stabilizing surgery were seen at the time of long-term follow-up.

69. Schöttle PB, Schmeling A, Rosenstiel N, Weiler A: Radiographic landmarks for femoral tunnel placement in medial patellofemoral ligament reconstruction. *Am J Sports Med* 2007;35(5):801-804.

    This cadaver study found that a reproducible anatomic and radiographic point, 1 mm anterior to the posterior cortex extension line, 2.5 mm distal to the posterior origin of the medial femoral condyle, and proximal to the level of the posterior point of the Blumensaat line on a lateral radiograph with both posterior condyles projected in the same plane, shows the mean femoral MPFL center.

70. Koëter S, Pakvis D, van Loon CJ, van Kampen A: Trochlear osteotomy for patellar instability: Satisfactory minimum 2-year results in patients with dysplasia of the trochlea. *Knee Surg Sports Traumatol Arthrosc* 2007; 15(3):228-232.

    This retrospective review found that anterior femoral osteotomy of the lateral condyle appears to be a satisfactory and safe method for treating patients with patellofemoral joint instability caused by trochlear dysplasia.

Chapter 36

Knee Reconstruction and Replacement

Raymond H. Kim, MD   Bryan D. Springer, MD   Douglas A. Dennis, MD

Introduction

Arthritic conditions of the knee remain one of the most common reasons for disability. With the aging population, the number of patients with arthritis is expected to reach 67 million Americans by the year 2030.[1] Demographic projections estimate a 673% increase in the number of total knee arthroplasties (TKAs) and a 60.1% increase in revision TKAs by the year 2030.[2]

Clinical Evaluation

History and Physical Examination

The clinical evaluation of the patient with a painful knee begins with a thorough history and physical examination. The history includes the duration of symptoms, previous trauma, and any prior surgeries on the affected extremity. In addition, any medical conditions that may affect the limb such as rheumatoid arthritis, childhood musculoskeletal conditions (such as Blount disease), or blood dyscrasias (sickle cell anemia) should be ascertained. The location of the pain along with the exacerbating activities may be an important indicator of the underlying pathology. It is important to remember that referred pain from both the lumbar spine as well as the ipsilateral hip may also present as knee pain. Anterior knee pain that is exacerbated with squatting or stair climbing may indicate patellofemoral involvement. Pain located at the joint line associated with mechanical symptoms may indicate meniscal pathology. Additionally, it is important to assess the impact of the patient's pain and disability on quality of life.

The physical examination should begin with an evaluation of gait, including assessment of antalgia, stride length, and muscle weakness (Trendelenburg gait). Overall standing limb alignment (varus or valgus) should be noted along with the contribution of this alignment from the hip, knee, and foot. To rule out referred pain, the contribution of the spine and hip as part of the examination should be assessed. The knee examination should always include a comparison with the opposite side and any discrepancy noted. Range of motion, patellar alignment (Q angle), and joint line tenderness should be noted. Tenderness over soft-tissue structures such as pes anserine bursae, patellar tendon, or iliotibial band should also be evaluated. Ligamentous stability should be tested with varus stress (fibular collateral ligament), valgus stress (medial collateral ligament), anteriorly with the Lachman or anterior drawer test (anterior cruciate ligament), or posteriorly with the posterior drawer test (posterior cruciate ligament).

Radiographic Evaluation

A proper evaluation of the knee begins with plain radiographs. Standard radiographs should include standing AP, lateral, and Merchant views. It is important that these views be obtained with the patient in a standing position; otherwise; the amount of joint space narrowing and deformity may be minimized (**Figure 1, *A***). These radiographs should be evaluated for bone quality, alignment, and joint space narrowing. Additional plain radiographs may be indicated when standard films are equivocal or to further assess pathology. A 45° PA flexion view is useful to evaluate the posterior aspect of the medial compartment. Stress radiographs may be obtained to assess ligamentous instability or as an indirect measure of cartilage thickness or deformity correction in the medial or lateral compartment in patients with arthritic knees (**Figure 1, *B***). MRI provides a detailed evaluation of soft-tissue structures, including tendons, ligaments, meniscus, articular cartilage, and bone marrow. Newer delayed gadolinium-enhanced MRI of cartilage (dGEMRIC) allows for detailed evaluation of articular cartilage and associated lesions.[3]

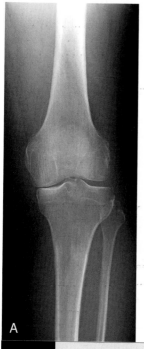
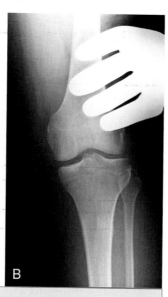

Figure 1 **A,** Standing weight-bearing AP radiograph demonstrating medial compartment narrowing. **B,** Stress radiograph demonstrating passive correction of varus deformity.

Nonsurgical Treatment

Nonsurgical treatment is generally indicated for patients with knee pain. Initial management may include the use of analgesics such as acetaminophen or nonsteroidal anti-inflammatory drugs (NSAIDs), ice, activity modification, and physical therapy.[4] In December 2008, the American Academy of Orthopaedic Surgeons (AAOS) released the clinical practice guidelines for the treatment of osteoarthritis of the knee[5] based on the best available scientific evidence. **Table 1** summarizes these guidelines for the nonsurgical management of osteoarthritis.

Joint-Preserving Procedures

Arthroscopic Débridement

Controversy exists over whether arthroscopy for degenerative knee arthritis provides palliative relief.[6-8] The authors of one study conducted a prospective, randomized study comparing arthroscopic lavage, débridement, and a sham procedure; no significant therapeutic benefit was shown.[6] Careful assessment of the study design, however, revealed poor preoperative disease classification with inadequate radiographic assessment, and concerns with patient selection criteria and selection bias.[9] In another study, long-term results of patients undergoing arthroscopic knee débridement in the context of degenerative arthritis were reviewed. Sixty-seven percent of patients at a mean 13.2 years postoperatively had not undergone arthroplasty, and satisfaction scores rating the success of the arthroscopic procedure was 8.6 on a scale of 0 to 10.[10] In a prospective study done

Table 1

AAOS Clinical Practice Guideline on the Treatment of Osteoarthritis of the Knee

Treatment	Recommendation	Level of Evidence
Self-management and education programs	Yes	II B
Promotion of self-care	Yes	IV C
Weight loss with diet and exercise	Yes	I A
Low-impact exercise	Yes	I A
Patellar taping	Yes	II B
NSAIDs or acetaminophen	Yes	II B
Intra-articular cortisone injection	Yes	II B
Heel wedges	No	II B
Glucosamine and/or chondroitin sulfate	No	I A
Needle lavage of joint	No	I and II B
Medial or lateral unloader braces	Inconclusive	
Accupuncture therapy	Inconclusive	
Intra-articular hyaluronic acid injection	Inconclusive	

(Adapted from American Academy of Orthopaedic Surgeons: Clinical Practice Guideline on the Treatment of Osteoarthritis (OA) of the Knee. Rosemont, IL, American Academy of Orthopaedic Surgeons, December 2008.)

on patients older than 50 years, surgical (partial meniscectomy, débridement of loose articular cartilage, and loose body removal) and nonsurgical treatment of limited degenerative knee arthritis were compared.[11] At follow-up of 1 to 3 years, 75% of the group that had surgery obtained symptomatic improvement, compared to 16% of the nonsurgical group.

Proximal Tibial Osteotomy

Proximal tibial osteotomy remains a reasonable option for a particular subset of patients. Patients younger than 55 to 60 years with medial compartment degenerative arthritis associated with malalignment, or malalignment in conjunction with ligamentous reconstruction, meniscal transplantation, or cartilage transplantation may obtain pain relief and functional improvement with a proximal tibial osteotomy. Contraindications for proximal tibial osteotomy include diffuse knee pain, patellofemoral pain, instability, previous meniscectomy or arthrosis in the lateral compartment, inflammatory disease, obesity (1.3 times ideal body weight), and unrealistic patient expectations.

Proximal tibial osteotomy can be performed with either a medial opening wedge or a lateral closing wedge technique. Advantages of the opening wedge technique include avoidance of the proximal tibiofibular joint, anterior compartment, and peroneal nerve; and better control of multiplanar deformity correction. Disadvantages include the need for bone grafting, slower progression to union compared to the closing wedge technique, and limitations to mild to moderate corrections. A closing wedge provides the advantages of allowing accelerated weight bearing postoperatively and no required bone grafting. Disadvantages include violation of the tibiofibular joint and alteration of patellar height.

Most clinical studies reviewing proximal tibial osteotomy results reveal modest clinical outcomes. One study revealed a 57% satisfactory outcome with 15-year follow-up.[12] According to another study, there was a 75% rate of survival free of failure with 10-year follow-up, with failure defined as arthroplasty.[13] In a review of 106 high tibial valgus osteotomies, improved survivorship was noted with careful selection of patients younger than 50 years who also had preoperative flexion greater than 120°.[14] Properly performed proximal tibial osteotomy yields satisfactory clinical results with appropriate patient selection.

Total Knee Arthroplasty

TKA is an effective procedure that has been shown to relieve pain and restore function to most patients with advanced arthritis of the knee, and is indicated for these patients when nonsurgical measures have failed. Multiple studies have demonstrated excellent outcomes for TKA. In one study, a 98.1% survival rate at 14 years was observed for a cemented posterior cruciate substituting (PS) TKA design.[15] Similar excellent survivorship of 96.8% at 15 years for a modular cemented

PS TKA with mechanical failure as an end point has been noted.[16]

Disease Variables Affecting Outcome

Diabetes
Following surgery, patients with diabetes have been shown to have a statistically significant increased risk of pneumonia, stroke, and blood transfusion compared to nondiabetic patients.[17] In addition to systemic complications, patients with poorly controlled diabetes have an increased likelihood of superficial and deep periprosthetic infections.[18] Measures should be taken to ensure adequate control of blood glucose before surgery (Hgb A1C) and appropriate management in the postoperative period.

Obesity
Obese patients have a higher incidence of osteoarthritis and tend to be a younger cohort of patients requiring TKA. The clinical and mechanical survival of TKA in obese patients, however, has been shown to be comparable to that of a nonobese population.[19] Superficial and deep periprosthetic infection following TKA in the obese population remains a concern. Studies in the literature indicate a sixfold to eightfold increase in the incidence of superficial and deep infection in patients with a body mass index above 35.[20,21] There are no data to suggest that obese patients tend to lose weight or increase activity level after successful TKA.[22]

Systemic Risk Factors for Infection

In addition to obesity and diabetes, several other systemic factors increase a patient's risk for deep periprosthetic infection following TKA,[23] such as rheumatoid arthritis and chronic steroid use. The contribution of disease-modifying drugs used to treat inflammatory arthritis remains uncertain. These drugs that alter the immune system may affect wound healing and increase the risk for development of infection. No set guidelines are available regarding the discontinuation of these drugs before surgery or resumption after surgery.

Surgical Technique

Because malalignment and instability are two common causes of TKA failure, careful attention to surgical technique is critical to optimize clinical outcome. Key principles include achieving adequate exposure while respecting the soft tissues, restoration of the mechanical alignment, and proper balancing of the soft tissues.

Despite significant enthusiasm for minimally invasive TKA, there are no data that show improved long-term clinical results with minimally invasive surgical exposures. The short-term benefits of improved function, less pain, and better cosmetic appearance of incisions should be tempered by data that demonstrate increased complication risks due to inadequate exposure.[24] The ability to adequately visualize component positioning, alignment, and soft-tissue balancing should never be compromised by a limited exposure.

Restoration of the mechanical axis can be achieved

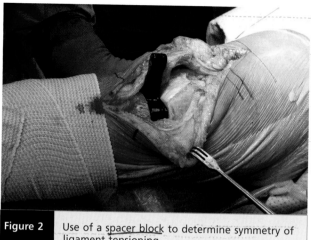

Figure 2 | Use of a spacer block to determine symmetry of ligament tensioning.

using contemporary instrumentation to make the appropriate distal femoral and proximal tibial cuts. Intramedullary referencing is commonly used for the distal femoral cut, whereas extramedullary jigs are more commonly used for the proximal tibial cut. Once the distal femur and proximal tibia are resected, attention can then be turned to ligament balancing in extension. A titrated release of soft tissues may be performed on the medial or lateral side of the knee to accommodate for a fixed varus or valgus deformity, respectively. Use of spacer blocks or tensioning devices is helpful to determine symmetry of ligament tension (**Figure 2**).

The method of determining femoral component rotation remains controversial. The measured resection technique references one of several axes defined by bony landmarks on the femur: the posterior condylar axis, the transepicondylar axis, or the AP axis. Because of anatomic variations in the osseous anatomy, advocates of the gap-balancing method reference the tibial cut surface to establish the femoral component rotation with the use of a flexion gap–tensioning device.

Design Issues
PS Compared With Cruciate-Retaining TKA

Advantages of using a PS design include ease of technique, minimization of tibial resection, restoration of knee kinematics, improved motion, potential reduction in polyethylene wear due to ability to use a more conforming bearing surface, and ease of deformity correction. Disadvantages include potential post wear caused by post impingement, fixation stresses due to post constraint, removal of intercondylar bone stock, and patellar clunk or crepitus complications. Specific indications for the use of a PS design over a cruciate-retaining (CR) design include severe deformity, severe flexion contracture, preoperative ankylosis of the knees, previous patellectomy, and revision of a TKA. When comparing CR to PS designs, a meta-analysis that reviewed eight randomized controlled trials noted no differences in function, patient satisfaction, and survivorship.[25] However, 8.1° higher range of motion was noted for the PS group compared to the CR group ($P = 0.01$).

Mobile-Bearing Design

Mobile-bearing TKA designs offer the advantage of allowing increased implant conformity and contact area without dramatically increasing stresses transmitted to the fixation interface. The incorporation of polyethylene bearing mobility, such as in a rotating platform TKA design, allows rotation through the tibial tray-polyethylene articulation and effectively minimizes the transfer of torsional stresses to the fixation interface that have been associated with fixed-bearing TKA implants. This is supported by the excellent long-term clinical results with minimal loosening reported in numerous studies of mobile-bearing TKA. The 9- to 12-year results of the Low Contact Stress (LCS) rotating platform design (DePuy, Warsaw, IN) were evaluated; 100% survivorship was reported.[26] Survivorship of the cementless LCS rotating platform system with loosening as the end point was determined to be 99.4% at 20 years.[27] Various studies evaluating primary TKA using the rotating platform system reported no evidence of radiographic loosening, even at 20-year radiographic follow-up; revision TKA reportedly was required in up to 0.2% of patients because of aseptic loosening.[26,27]

Patellar Resurfacing

Patellar resurfacing has remained a source of controversy with varying trends across countries. Advantages of patellar resurfacing in TKA include reduced anterior knee pain, removal of articular cartilage antigens in rheumatoid arthritis patients, decreased reoperation rates, and functional improvement with stair climbing. Disadvantages include extensor mechanism complications (rupture, patellar osteonecrosis, patellar fracture), component failure (polyethylene wear, aseptic loosening, osteolysis), and mechanical complications (overstuffing the patellofemoral compartment limiting flexion, patellar clunk). The authors of one study performed a meta-analysis of 14 studies and observed a higher incidence of anterior knee pain and an 8.7% incidence of secondary resurfacing in nonresurfaced knees.[28] In a meta-analysis of 10 randomized controlled trials, a 40% reduction in anterior knee pain and a 48% lower reoperation rate in the resurfacing group were noted.[29] In contrast, a 2007 study reviewed 32 patients who underwent bilateral TKA and were randomized to have the first knee resurfaced or nonresurfaced and the second knee received the opposite treatment. With minimum follow-up of 10 years, no difference in range of motion, Knee Society clinical scores, satisfaction, revision rates, or anterior knee pain was observed.[30] The differing reported results mirror the lack of consensus within the arthroplasty community regarding patellar resurfacing.

Computer-Assisted Surgery and Patient-Specific Instruments

Recent technology has sought to improve the accuracy and precision of component alignment and position. Based on intraoperative registered data, computer-assisted surgery allows the surgeon to understand the three-dimensional morphology of the knee and its relative position to the overall alignment of the entire extremity. Bone cuts can be planned and checked with improved accuracy and precision compared to traditional instrumentation. Although multiple studies have demonstrated improved radiographic alignment and component positioning, no articles have suggested any improvement in the clinical outcome of patients undergoing TKA using computer navigation.

Patient-specific instruments are similar in concept while allowing the surgeon to establish the desired component position and alignment based on preoperative imaging (MRI or CT). Two drastically different philosophies have been developed to "custom fit" TKA components. Anatomic shape fitting identifies kinematic axes, which can be defined by the articular surface of the femoral condyles based on an individual patient's MRI, and templates the position of the femoral component using a single-radius TKA design. Custom jigs are then manufactured to allow the surgeon to carry out the planned bone resection. Critics of this technology have observed malalignment of the components, particularly the tibial component,[31] whereas advocates describe its ease of application, the avoidance of ligament balancing, and a better functioning knee.[32] No data are available to discern the clinical differences in functional outcome.

The alternative form of patient-specific instrumentation holds to the traditional principle that mechanical alignment is paramount. Intraoperative registration of the anatomic morphology of the knee allows the surgeon to position and align the components to restore the limb to a neutral mechanical axis. Multiple studies have confirmed the improved component position and alignment with fewer outliers while using computer navigation.[33] Additional benefits include reduced blood loss,[33] reduced embolic phenomenon,[34] and advantages in complex situations/conditions such as severe deformity, retained hardware, previous osteomyelitis, and obesity.[35]

High-Flexion Designs

A popular trend in TKA design has been the advent of "high-flexion" knees. The designs by multiple companies permit greater flexion without increasing polyethylene contact stresses at high flexion. Despite the hope that the high-flexion designs would improve motion, studies demonstrate no significant difference in motion between standard and high-flexion prostheses. A meta-analysis of high-flexion TKAs reviewed 9 studies that included 399 TKAs.[36] Although five studies reported greater motion, the methodology of these studies was criticized for inadequate blinding, flawed patient selection, and short follow-up. It was concluded that there was inadequate evidence for improved motion or function with high-flexion designs. Several recent studies also revealed no significant differences between motion comparing high-flexion with standard knee designs.[37,38]

Unicompartmental Knee Arthroplasty

Classic indications for unicompartmental knee arthroplasty (UKA) include isolated unicompartmental arthrosis in low-demand patients older than 60 years, weighing less than 82 kg (180 lb), with a range-of-motion arc of greater than 90° and flexion contracture less than 5°, and having a minimal deformity of less than 15° that is passively correctable.[39] Controversy currently exists regarding specific contraindications related to age, presence of patellofemoral degenerative changes, anterior cruciate ligament deficiency, and obesity. Clinical results of both fixed-bearing and mobile-bearing knees have demonstrated excellent long-term results. One study reviewed 49 knees with a minimum 10-year follow-up using a fixed-bearing metal-backed modular tibial component, and a 98% 10-year survivorship was reported.[40] Mobile-bearing UKAs have also demonstrated excellent clinical results. One study reviewed 439 knees, and a 93% 15-year survivorship using the Oxford knee (Biomet, Warsaw, IN), a mobile-bearing UKA, was observed.[41] Failure of UKA commonly occurs due to polyethylene wear, component loosening, and progression of arthritis. Revision procedures may be relatively straightforward with minimal complexity.[42,43] However, if failure occurs because of collapse of the medial tibial plateau, revision is technically more demanding to address significant bony defects.[44]

Patellofemoral Arthroplasty

Patellofemoral arthroplasty is a surgical option for the treatment of isolated patellofemoral arthritis with variable success rates. Outcomes of early designs were complicated by patellar instability and mechanical catching.[45,46] More recent designs have demonstrated improved clinical outcomes. A 95.8% 5-year survivorship was reported after a review of 109 patellofemoral arthroplasties.[47] In a longer term series 66 patients were reviewed at an average follow-up of 16.2 years (range, 12 to 20 years) and a 58% survivorship at 16 years was noted.[48]

Infection in TKA

Treatment of infection following TKA depends on timing of the infection, the condition of the patient, the fixation of the components, and the infecting organism. Acute infections (less than 3 weeks of symptom duration) can occur in the early postoperative period or secondary to hematogenous seeding. In these situations, open irrigation and débridement with complete synovectomy and polyethylene exchange may be considered. A successful outcome is dependent on well-fixed and functioning components, the absence of immunocompromise, and a susceptible organism. Regardless of timing of the infection, the presence of drug-resistant organisms has a negative impact on the outcome of component retention.

For patients with chronic infections (present longer than 3 to 4 weeks), two-stage exchange arthroplasty has the highest rate of success with regard to eradication of infection (88% to 93% in most studies).[49,50] The procedure consists of removal of all components, a thorough débridement, and placement of a high-dose antibiotic cement spacer. Both articulating and static spacers have been used with success. Articulating spacers that allow for motion between surgeries may have a better functional outcome with technically easier exposure at the time of reimplantation.[51] Following the initial resection arthroplasty, patients are generally treated with a course of intravenous antibiotics. The resolution of infection is based on clinical examination, trend in serologic markers, and joint aspiration.

Deep Venous Thrombosis and Pulmonary Embolism

This topic is discussed in chapter 12. Please refer to the AAOS clinical practice guideline on pulmonary embolism. The guideline can be accessed at www.aaos.org/research/guidelines/guide.asp.

Revision TKA

Evaluation of the Patient With a Painful TKA

Evaluation should proceed in a stepwise and systemic manner. A thorough history, physical examnation, radiographic evaluation, and appropriate ancillary testing should be used to evaluate the patient with a painful TKA. Whenever possible, old radiographs should be obtained and evaluated. Serial radiographic evaluation can provide clues to progression of radiolucencies that may indicate loosening and polyethylene wear and osteolysis. In most instances plain radiographs are sufficient to make or confirm the diagnosis. Other tests may include fluoroscopic views to assess the bone-implant interface to look for subtle lucencies, stress views to evaluate for instability, or CT to evaluate for femoral or tibial component malrotation.[52] Metal suppression MRI techniques may be useful to evaluate the size and extent of osteolytic lesions that are not readily apparent on plain radiographs.[53] Serologic tests and joint aspiration are important, cost-effective assessments to rule out infection in the patient with a painful TKA. No single serologic test is 100% sensitive or specific for the diagnosis of infection. When used in combination, the erythrocyte sedimentation rate and C-reactive protein level are useful screening tests in the initial evaluation of the patient with a painful TKA. Other serologic markers such as interleukin-6, tumor necrosis factor, and procalcitonin are being evaluated as other potential markers for infection.[54] Joint aspiration should be performed in any patient with elevated serologic markers or when there is high clinical suspicion for infection. A synovial leukocyte count greater than 1,700 with a differential neutrophil count greater than 65% is considered diagnostic of deep periprosthetic infection.[55]

Surgical Management

Adequate surgical exposure is essential for successful surgery in revision TKA. Exposure begins with the incision. The vascular anatomy of the knee must be understood by the surgeon. The blood supply to the anterior aspect of the knee is medially based, with the vessels traveling in the subcutaneous layer. A patient often may have multiple incisions about the knee from previous surgeries. It is generally advised to use the lateralmost incision to maintain the blood supply to the medial flap.

The goal of the exposure in revision TKA is to allow easy access to the components and bony anatomy without jeopardizing the ligaments or extensor mechanism. Exposure should occur in a stepwise manner. Rarely is there a need to evert the patella during revision. Reestablishment of the medial and lateral gutters of the femur and the suprapatellar pouch along with an early lateral release will provide adequate exposure in most instances. A multitude of other exposure options exist that may be used in the difficult knee, including a quadriceps snip, V-Y turndown, and tibial tubercle osteotomy.

Component Removal

Component removal should be methodical and proceed in a stepwise fashion. The goal of component removal is to extract the components with minimal bone loss. In general, the polyethylene is removed first, followed by the femoral and tibial components. Meticulous technique is required to disrupt the bone-cement interface. Proper tools such as osteotomes and microsagittal saws can help to facilitate this process.

Dealing With Bone Loss and Component Fixation

Dealing with bone loss at the time of revision can be challenging. Options include cement augmentation for small defects, modular metal augments, and allografts.[56] Tibial and femoral porous cones and sleeves are available to deal with segmental bone defects (Figure 3). These augments have highly porous surfaces that allow for rapid ingrowth in addition to providing mechanical support of the implants. Recent data at short-term follow-up show promising results with these materials.[57,58] The patella may be retained in many cases if it is well fixed, has minimal wear, and a congruent tracking with the new implants. When the patella is removed, adequate bone should be available for reconstruction. In general, thickness below 12 mm increases the risk of patella fracture. If severe patellar bone loss is present, the patella may be left unresurfaced or augmented with bone graft or porous tantalum augmentation.[59] A patellectomy is rarely indicated.

In the revision setting, condylar bone loss on both the femur and tibia make these surfaces inadequate alone for support of the revision components. Stem fixation should be used to bypass defects and unload the deficient condylar bone. Both cemented and cementless press-fit stems can be used with success.[60,61] Cementless

The demand for primary TKA is projected to grow by 673% to 3.48 million procedures. The demand for knee revisions is expected to grow by 601% by the year 2030.

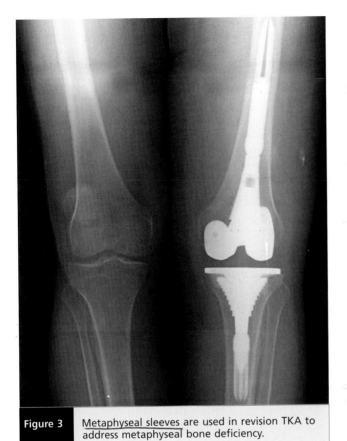

Figure 3 Metaphyseal sleeves are used in revision TKA to address metaphyseal bone deficiency.

stems, when used, should engage the diaphysis of both the femur and tibia to allow for adequate fixation.

Constraint in Revision TKA

Constraint in revision TKA should be viewed as a spectrum from standard posterior stabilized to hinged arthroplasty. In most revision settings with proper component position and ligament balancing, a standard posterior stabilized insert can be used. Constraint is indicated when there is collateral ligament compromise or the inability to obtain proper flexion and extension balance. Results of constrained TKA in the revision setting have demonstrated excellent survivorship.[62] A hinged prosthesis is indicated in patients with global instability, a deficient extensor mechanism, or severe bone loss from fracture, tumor, or multiple surgeries.

Annotated References

1. Hootman JM, Helmick CG: Projections of US prevalence of arthritis and associated activity limitations. *Arthritis Rheum* 2006;54(1):226-229.

2. Kurtz S, Ong K, Lau E, Mowat F, Halpern M: Projections of primary and revision hip and knee arthroplasty in the United States from 2005 to 2030. *J Bone Joint Surg Am* 2007;89(4):780-785.

3. Miller TT: MR imaging of the knee. *Sports Med Arthrosc* 2009;17(1):56-67.

   This article provides an excellent review of MRI of the knee, including the role of dGEMRIC imaging.

4. Richmond J, Hunter D, Irrgang J, et al; American Academy of Orthopaedic Surgeons: Treatment of osteoarthritis of the knee (nonarthroplasty). *J Am Acad Orthop Surg* 2009;17(9):591-600.

   This article provides clinical guidlelines for less invasive treatments than knee arthroplasty for symptomatic knee osteoarthritis.

5. American Academy of Orthopaedic Surgeons Clinical Practice Guideline on the Treatment of Osteoarthritis of the Knee. American Academy of Orthopaedic Surgeons (AAOS), Rosemont, Illinois. 2008. http://www.aaos.org/research/guidelines/GuidelineOAKnee.asp

   This clinical practice guideline is published on the Website of the AAOS (www.aaos.org). It provides a comprehensive review of the literature and guidelines for the nonsurgical and nonarthroplastic treatment of knee arthritis.

6. Moseley JB, O'Malley K, Petersen NJ, et al: A controlled trial of arthroscopic surgery for osteoarthritis of the knee. *N Engl J Med* 2002;347(2):81-88.

7. Kirkley A, Birmingham TB, Litchfield RB, et al: A randomized trial of arthroscopic surgery for osteoarthritis of the knee. *N Engl J Med* 2008;359(11):1097-1107.

   A randomized controlled study comparing arthroscopic lavage and debridement with optimized physical and medical therapy to physical and medical therapy alone for patients with moderate to severe knee osteoarthritis demonstrated no additional benefit with arthroscopic surgery. Level of evidence: I.

8. Marx RG: Arthroscopic surgery for osteoarthritis of the knee? *N Engl J Med* 2008;359(11):1169-1170.

   This is an editorial in response to the study by Kirkley et al stating that although knee osteoarthritis is not an indication for arthroscopic surgery, it is not a contraindication for arthroscopic surgery in specific situations such as a symptomatic meniscal tear.

9. Johnson LL: A controlled trial of arthroscopic surgery for osteoarthritis of the knee. *Arthroscopy* 2002;18(7):683-687.

10. McGinley BJ, Cushner FD, Scott WN: Debridement arthroscopy: 10-year followup. *Clin Orthop Relat Res* 1999;367(367):190-194.

11. Merchan EC, Galindo E: Arthroscope-guided surgery versus nonoperative treatment for limited degenerative osteoarthritis of the femorotibial joint in patients over 50 years of age: A prospective comparative study. *Arthroscopy* 1993;9(6):663-667.

4: Lower Extremity

12. Aglietti P, Buzzi R, Vena LM, Baldini A, Mondaini A: High tibial valgus osteotomy for medial gonarthrosis: A 10- to 21-year study. *J Knee Surg* 2003;16(1):21-26.

13. Coventry MB, Ilstrup DM, Wallrichs SL: Proximal tibial osteotomy: A critical long-term study of eighty-seven cases. *J Bone Joint Surg Am* 1993;75(2):196-201.

14. Naudie D, Bourne RB, Rorabeck CH, Bourne TJ: Survivorship of the high tibial valgus osteotomy: A 10- to -22-year followup study. *Clin Orthop Relat Res* 1999; 367:18-27.

15. Colizza WA, Insall JN, Scuderi GR: The posterior stabilized total knee prosthesis: Assessment of polyethylene damage and osteolysis after a ten-year-minimum follow-up. *J Bone Joint Surg Am* 1995;77(11):1713-1720.

16. Lachiewicz PF, Soileau ES: Fifteen-year survival and osteolysis associated with a modular posterior stabilized knee replacement: A concise follow-up of a previous report. *J Bone Joint Surg Am* 2009;91(6):1419-1423.

    This is a follow-up study of a previous report on a consecutive series of patients with a modular posterior stabilized TKA. With reoperation for mechanical failure as the end point, 15-year survival rate was 96.8%. Level of evidence: IV.

17. Marchant MH Jr, Viens NA, Cook C, Vail TP, Bolognesi MP: The impact of glycemic control and diabetes mellitus on perioperative outcomes after total joint arthroplasty. *J Bone Joint Surg Am* 2009;91(7):1621-1629.

    The goal of the present study was to determine whether the quality of preoperative glycemic control affected the prevalence of in-hospital perioperative complications following lower extremity total joint arthroplasty.

18. Yang K, Yeo SJ, Lee BP, Lo NN: Total knee arthroplasty in diabetic patients: A study of 109 consecutive cases. *J Arthroplasty* 2001;16(1):102-106.

19. Krushell RJ, Fingeroth RJ: Primary total knee arthroplasty in morbidly obese patients: A 5- to 14-year follow-up study. *J Arthroplasty* 2007;22(6, suppl 2):77-80.

    This retrospective study examined the results of 39 TKAs in morbidly obese patients with 5- to 14-year follow-up compared with a case-controlled group of nonobese patients. Although there was a somewhat higher rate of minor wound complications, suboptimal alignment, and late revision (5%) in the morbidly obese group compared with the case-controlled group overall, the problems in morbidly obese patients have been relatively few thus far. The substantial improvement in scores and high rate of patient satisfaction (85%) suggests that TKA should continue to be offered to morbidly obese patients. Level of evidence: III.

20. Namba RS, Paxton L, Fithian DC, Stone ML: Obesity and perioperative morbidity in total hip and total knee arthroplasty patients. *J Arthroplasty* 2005;20(7, suppl 3):46-50.

21. Rajgopal V, Bourne RB, Chesworth BM, MacDonald SJ, McCalden RW, Rorabeck CH: The impact of morbid obesity on patient outcomes after total knee arthroplasty. *J Arthroplasty* 2008;23(6):795-800.

    Five hundred fifty patients who underwent primary TKA between 1987 and 2004 with a primary diagnosis of osteoarthritis and 1-year outcome data (Western Ontario and McMaster Osteoarthritis Index [WOMAC]) were evaluated. Patients were stratified into body mass index categories based on the World Health Organization classification of obesity. Although 1-year outcomes were worse for morbidly obese patients ($P < 0.05$), they showed greater improvement in function compared with non–morbidly obese patients. Morbid obesity does not affect 1-year outcomes in patients who have had a TKA. Level of evidence: IV.

22. Lachiewicz AM, Lachiewicz PF: Weight and activity change in overweight and obese patients after primary total knee arthroplasty. *J Arthroplasty* 2008;23(1):33-40.

    A prospective study of changes in mean weight, body mass index (BMI), and physical activity over 2 years in 188 consecutive overweight or obese patients. Weight, BMI, and physical activity, evaluated using the Lower Extremity Activity Scale (LEAS), were assessed preoperatively and at 1 and 2 years. At 2 years, no significant weight change was found ($P = 0.80$), but BMI increased by 0.46 kg/m^2 ($P = 0.049$). The LEAS score increased from preoperatively to 2 years ($P < 0.001$). Preoperative LEAS score was not associated with weight or BMI at 2 years. This finding has implications for patient expectations and preoperative counseling. Level of evidence: IV.

23. Jämsen E, Huhtala H, Puolakka T, Moilanen T: Risk factors for infection after knee arthroplasty: A register-based analysis of 43,149 cases. *J Bone Joint Surg Am* 2009;91(1):38-47.

    The purpose of the present study was to determine the risk factors for infection following primary and revision TKA in a large register-based series. There was an increased risk of deep postoperative infection in male patients and in patients with rheumatoid arthritis or a fracture around the knee as the underlying diagnosis for TKA. The results of the present study suggest that the infection rate is similar after partial revision and complete revision TKA. Combining intravenous antibiotic prophylaxis with antibiotic-impregnated cement seems advisable in revision arthroplasty. Level of evidence: III.

24. Dalury DF, Dennis DA: Mini-incision total knee arthroplasty can increase risk of component malalignment. *Clin Orthop Relat Res* 2005;440:77-81.

25. Jacobs WC, Clement DJ, Wymenga AB: Retention versus removal of the posterior cruciate ligament in total knee replacement: A systematic literature review within the Cochrane framework. *Acta Orthop* 2005;76(6):757-768.

26. Callaghan JJ, O'Rourke MR, Iossi MF, et al: Cemented rotating-platform total knee replacement: A concise follow-up, at a minimum of fifteen years, of a previous report. *J Bone Joint Surg Am* 2005;87(9):1995-1998.

27. Buechel FF Sr: Long-term followup after mobile-bearing total knee replacement. *Clin Orthop Relat Res* 2002; 404(404):40-50.

28. Parvizi J, Rapuri VR, Saleh KJ, Kuskowski MA, Sharkey PF, Mont MA: Failure to resurface the patella during total knee arthroplasty may result in more knee pain and secondary surgery. *Clin Orthop Relat Res* 2005; 438:191-196.

29. Pakos EE, Ntzani EE, Trikalinos TA: Patellar resurfacing in total knee arthroplasty: A meta-analysis. *J Bone Joint Surg Am* 2005;87(7):1438-1445.

30. Burnett RS, Boone JL, McCarthy KP, Rosenzweig S, Barrack RL: A prospective randomized clinical trial of patellar resurfacing and nonresurfacing in bilateral TKA. *Clin Orthop Relat Res* 2007;464:65-72.

A randomized trial was performed to study the outcomes of patella resurfacing versus nonresurfacing in patients undergoing bilateral TKA. No differences were noted with regard to range of motion, Knee Society Clinical Rating Score, satisfaction, revision rates, or anterior knee pain. Level of evidence: I.

31. Klatt BA, Goyal N, Austin MS, Hozack WJ: Custom-fit total knee arthroplasty (OtisKnee) results in malalignment. *J Arthroplasty* 2008;23(1):26-29.

A case series of four patients who underwent TKA with the OtisKnee system resulted in malalignment of the components more than 3° off of a neutral mechanical axis. Level of evidence: IV.

32. Howell SM, Kuznik K, Hull ML, Siston RA: Results of an initial experience with custom-fit positioning total knee arthroplasty in a series of 48 patients. *Orthopedics* 2008;31(9):857-863.

A series of TKAs utilizing a custom-fit positioning system in 48 patients demonstrated rapid return to function, restoration of motion, restoration of alignment, and high patient satisfaction. Level of evidence: IV.

33. Chauhan SK, Scott RG, Breidahl W, Beaver RJ: Computer-assisted knee arthroplasty versus a conventional jig-based technique: A randomised, prospective trial. *J Bone Joint Surg Br* 2004;86(3):372-377.

34. Kalairajah Y, Cossey AJ, Verrall GM, Ludbrook G, Spriggins AJ: Are systemic emboli reduced in computer-assisted knee surgery? A prospective, randomised, clinical trial. *J Bone Joint Surg Br* 2006;88(2):198-202.

35. Fehring TK, Mason JB, Moskal J, Pollock DC, Mann J, Williams VJ: When computer-assisted knee replacement is the best alternative. *Clin Orthop Relat Res* 2006;452: 132-136.

36. Murphy M, Journeaux S, Russell T: High-flexion total knee arthroplasty: A systematic review. *Int Orthop* 2009;33(4):887-893.

This systematic literature review identified nine studies representing 399 high-flexion TKAs in 370 patients. It was concluded that there was not sufficient evidence demonstrating improved range of motion or functional outcome with high-flexion designs.

37. Kim YH, Choi Y, Kim JS: Range of motion of standard and high-flexion posterior cruciate-retaining total knee prostheses: A prospective randomized study. *J Bone Joint Surg Am* 2009;91(8):1874-1881.

This randomized study compared standard cruciate-retaining total knees to high-flexion posterior cruciate-retaining total knees in bilateral TKA patients and found no significant differences in range of motion or any clinical or radiographic parameters. Level of evidence: I.

38. Seon JK, Park SJ, Lee KB, Yoon TR, Kozanek M, Song EK: Range of motion in total knee arthroplasty: A prospective comparison of high-flexion and standard cruciate-retaining designs. *J Bone Joint Surg Am* 2009; 91(3):672-679.

The range of motion was found to be similar in 50 knees treated with a standard cruciate-retaining TKA compared to 50 knees treated with a high-flexion cruciate-retaining design under both non–weight-bearing and weight-bearing conditions. Level of evidence: II.

39. Kozinn SC, Scott R: Unicondylar knee arthroplasty. *J Bone Joint Surg Am* 1989;71(1):145-150.

40. Berger RA, Meneghini RM, Jacobs JJ, et al: Results of unicompartmental knee arthroplasty at a minimum of ten years of follow-up. *J Bone Joint Surg Am* 2005; 87(5):999-1006.

41. Price AJ, Waite JC, Svard U: Long-term clinical results of the medial Oxford unicompartmental knee arthroplasty. *Clin Orthop Relat Res* 2005;435:171-180.

42. McAuley JP, Engh GA, Ammeen DJ: Revision of failed unicompartmental knee arthroplasty. *Clin Orthop Relat Res* 2001;392(392):279-282.

43. Levine WN, Ozuna RM, Scott RD, Thornhill TS: Conversion of failed modern unicompartmental arthroplasty to total knee arthroplasty. *J Arthroplasty* 1996;11(7): 797-801.

44. Aleto TJ, Berend ME, Ritter MA, Faris PM, Meneghini RM: Early failure of unicompartmental knee arthroplasty leading to revision. *J Arthroplasty* 2008;23(2): 159-163.

This retrospective review of 32 consecutive revisions from UKA to TKA revealed the predominant mode of failure was medial tibial collapse (47%). Those knees that failed by medial tibial collapse required more complex reconstructions due to more significant bone defects. Level of evidence: IV.

45. Krajca-Radcliffe JB, Coker TP: Patellofemoral arthroplasty: A 2- to 18-year followup study. *Clin Orthop Relat Res* 1996;330(330):143-151.

46. Lonner JH: Patellofemoral arthroplasty: Pros, cons, and design considerations. *Clin Orthop Relat Res* 2004; 428(428):158-165.

4: Lower Extremity

47. Ackroyd CE, Newman JH, Evans R, Eldridge JD, Joslin CC: The Avon patellofemoral arthroplasty: Five-year survivorship and functional results. *J Bone Joint Surg Br* 2007;89(3):310-315.

A retrospective review of 109 consecutive patellofemoral arthroplasties in 85 patients with a minimum follow-up of 5 years revealed a 95.8% 5-year survivorship with revision as the end point. The main complication was radiographic progression of arthritis in other compartments in 28% of patients. Level of evidence: IV.

48. Argenson JN, Flecher X, Parratte S, Aubaniac JM: Patellofemoral arthroplasty: An update. *Clin Orthop Relat Res* 2005;440:50-53.

49. Hofmann AA, Goldberg T, Tanner AM, Kurtin SM: Treatment of infected total knee arthroplasty using an articulating spacer: 2- to 12-year experience. *Clin Orthop Relat Res* 2005;430:125-131.

50. Haleem AA, Berry DJ, Hanssen AD: Mid-term to long-term followup of two-stage reimplantation for infected total knee arthroplasty. *Clin Orthop Relat Res* 2004; 428:35-39.

51. Freeman MG, Fehring TK, Odum SM, Fehring K, Griffin WL, Mason JB: Functional advantage of articulating versus static spacers in 2-stage revision for total knee arthroplasty infection. *J Arthroplasty* 2007;22(8):1116-1121.

Seventy-six two-stage reimplantation procedures met the study inclusion criteria. There were 28 static spacers and 48 articulating spacers. The eradication rate was 94.7% in the articulating group compared with 92.1% in the static group (P = 0.7). There were no significant differences in postoperative Knee Society pain scores. There were 28 (58%) good to excellent function scores in the articulating group and 10 (36%) in the static group (P = 0.05). Interim use of an articulating spacer maintains excellent infection eradication rates and may improve function over the use of static spacers.

52. Berger RA, Crossett LS, Jacobs JJ, Rubash HE: Malrotation causing patellofemoral complications after total knee arthroplasty. *Clin Orthop Relat Res* 1998;356: 144-153.

53. Vessely MB, Frick MA, Oakes D, Wenger DE, Berry DJ: Magnetic resonance imaging with metal suppression for evaluation of periprosthetic osteolysis after total knee arthroplasty. *J Arthroplasty* 2006;21(6):826-831.

54. Di Cesare PE, Chang E, Preston CF, Liu CJ: Serum interleukin-6 as a marker of periprosthetic infection following total hip and knee arthroplasty. *J Bone Joint Surg Am* 2005;87(9):1921-1927.

55. Trampuz A, Hanssen AD, Osmon DR, Mandrekar J, Steckelberg JM, Patel R: Synovial fluid leukocyte count and differential for the diagnosis of prosthetic knee infection. *Am J Med* 2004;117(8):556-562.

56. Bush JL, Wilson JB, Vail TP: Management of bone loss in revision total knee arthroplasty. *Clin Orthop Relat Res* 2006;452:186-192.

57. Radnay CS, Scuderi GR: Management of bone loss: Augments, cones, offset stems. *Clin Orthop Relat Res* 2006;446:83-92.

58. Meneghini RM, Lewallen DG, Hanssen AD: Use of porous tantalum metaphyseal cones for severe tibial bone loss during revision total knee replacement: Surgical technique. *J Bone Joint Surg Am* 2009;91(suppl 2 pt 1): 131-138.

The purpose of this study was to determine the initial results obtained with a unique reconstructive implant, the porous tantalum metaphyseal cone, designed as an alternative treatment of severe tibial bone loss following TKA. The porous tantalum metaphyseal tibial cones effectively provided structural support for the tibial implants in this series. The potential for long-term biologic fixation may provide durability for these tibial reconstructions. Level of evidence: IV.

59. Nelson CL, Lonner JH, Lahiji A, Kim J, Lotke PA: Use of a trabecular metal patella for marked patella bone loss during revision total knee arthroplasty. *J Arthroplasty* 2003;18(7, suppl 1):37-41.

60. Wood GC, Naudie DD, MacDonald SJ, McCalden RW, Bourne RB: Results of press-fit stems in revision knee arthroplasties. *Clin Orthop Relat Res* 2009;467(3):810-817.

The aim of this study was to report the authors' experience with press-fit uncemented stems and metaphyseal cement fixation in a selected series of patients undergoing revision TKA. One hundred twenty-seven patients (135 knees) who underwent revision TKA using a press-fit technique (press-fit diaphyseal fixation and cemented metaphyseal fixation) were reviewed. Minimum follow-up was 2 years. Survivorship analysis revealed a probability of survival free of revision for aseptic loosening of 98% at 12 years. Survivorship of press-fit stems for revision TKA is comparable to reported survivorship of cemented stem revision TKA.

61. Whaley AL, Trousdale RT, Rand JA, Hanssen AD: Cemented long-stem revision total knee arthroplasty. *J Arthroplasty* 2003;18(5):592-599.

62. Kim YH, Kim JS: Revision total knee arthroplasty with use of a constrained condylar knee prosthesis. *J Bone Joint Surg Am* 2009;91(6):1440-1447.

A retrospective review of a case series of revision TKA with a constrained condylar prosthesis by a single surgeon was performed to ascertain the role of this prosthesis and to determine whether it provided satisfactory results. Kaplan-Meier survivorship analysis, with revision or radiographic failure as the end point, revealed that the 10-year rate of survival of the components was 96% (95% confidence interval, 94% to 100%). Revision TKA with use of a constrained condylar knee prosthesis had reproducible clinical success, but a complication rate of up to 9% can be expected at intermediate-term follow-up.

Chapter 37

Tibial Shaft Fractures

Brett D. Crist, MD   Rahul Banerjee, MD

Introduction

Tibia fractures affect patients of all ages. Nonsurgical management is typically reserved for stable, low-energy fractures and requires close observation and immobilization. Unstable and high-energy fractures are typically managed surgically with either intramedullary nailing, external fixation (uniplanar and multiplanar), or plate fixation. Historically, surgically treated tibial shaft fractures have the benefits of faster functional return and lower risk of malunion. However, each surgical technique has its potential associated complications. Open tibial shaft fractures continue to be debilitating and problematic due to an increased risk of infection and nonunion and the need to address the associated bone and soft-tissue loss. Because multiple treatment options are available and each has advantages and disadvantages, surgeons must individualize their treatment strategy based on the patient's injury, functional demands, and healing potential.

Clinical Examination

Tibia fractures may occur from direct or indirect trauma. Simple falls, twisting injuries, and sports injuries result in low-energy closed tibia fractures. High-energy mechanisms of injury such as motor vehicle or motorcycle crashes frequently cause more severe, or open, tibia fractures.

Patients with tibia fractures present with leg pain, swelling, deformity, and an inability to bear weight. Evaluation should begin with a primary survey and assessment of airway, breathing, and circulation. Details of the injury or accident, if available from the patient or emergency medical services, should be obtained to raise suspicion of associated injuries and/or risk of compartment syndrome.

On physical examination, careful circumferential examination of the patient's skin is necessary to assess for abrasions, ecchymosis, or open wounds. Gross defor-

Dr. Crist has received research or institutional support from Synthes, KCI, Medtronic, and Pfizer. Dr. Banerjee or an immediate family member has received research or institutional support from Synthes, Smith & Nephew, Medtronic, Stryker, and Zimmer.

mity of the extremity may be evident in the presence of displaced fractures. Careful neurovascular examination is imperative and should include documentation of motor function, sensory examination, and pulses distal to the injury. Examination of the ipsilateral hip, knee, and ankle is important to identify associated injuries.

High-energy tibia fractures may present with concomitant vascular injuries. On examination, vascular injuries may manifest with signs such as diminished or absent pulses, decreased capillary refill, or gross bleeding. Suspected vascular compromise should prompt the surgeon to realign and splint the limb, and reassess the vascular status. In addition, if an associated vascular injury is suspected, ankle-brachial indices should be performed. Identification of vascular injury requires early vascular surgery consultation.

Tibia fractures may present with associated compartment syndrome. Younger patients and patients with diaphyseal tibia fractures are more likely to develop compartment syndrome.[1] Compartment syndrome occurs as a result of increased pressure within the limited space of the myofascial compartments of the leg. Ultimately, this increased pressure leads to vascular compromise. The anterior and deep posterior compartments are most susceptible to injury from associated compartment syndrome.

Patients with tibia fractures and associated compartment syndrome may have severe pain, tense swelling of the leg, and pain with passive stretch of the ankle or toes. These so-called "cardinal signs" are often difficult to assess in patients with tibia fractures, as similar symptoms and signs may result from the fracture. Although the diagnosis of compartment syndrome is a clinical diagnosis, assessment may be aided by the measurement of intracompartmental pressures when the diagnosis is unclear or when the ability to obtain a physical examination is limited (such as in an obtunded or pediatric patient, or in the presence of neurologic impairment). If intracompartmental pressures are used, the difference between the patient's diastolic blood pressure and the compartment pressure (delta P) should be calculated. Compartment pressures should not be measured after the induction of anesthesia because a spuriously low value for the diastolic blood pressure and a consequently high value for delta P may result.[2]

Compartment syndrome is treated with four-compartment fasciotomy of the affected leg. A delta P less than or equal to 30 mm Hg indicates the need for fasciotomy.[3] It is imperative to verify release of all four

4: Lower Extremity

Table 1

Gustilo and Anderson Classification of Open Fractures

Fracture Type	Characteristics
Type I	Wounds less than 1 cm; minimal contamination and soft-tissue injury; simple fracture pattern
Type II	Wounds 1 to 10 cm; moderate comminution and contamination
Type IIIA	Minimal periosteal stripping and soft-tissue coverage required
Type IIIB	Significant periosteal stripping at the fracture site; soft-tissue coverage required
Type IIIC	Indicates an associated repairable vascular injury

Table 2

Oestern and Tscherne Soft-Tissue Injury Classification of Closed Fractures

Grade	Characteristics
Grade 0	Minimal soft-tissue injury; typically associated with a simple fracture pattern secondary to an indirect force
Grade 1	Superficial abrasions or contusions apparent; may range from a mild to moderately severe fracture pattern
Grade 2	Include deep contaminated abrasions associated with localized skin or muscle contusion; severe fracture pattern and impending compartment syndrome
Grade 3	Extensive skin contusion or crush with significant underlying muscle damage, compartment syndrome, and severe fracture pattern

compartments because incomplete release may result in ongoing muscle necrosis and irreversible injury. The anterior compartment is most frequently incompletely released.[4]

Radiographic examination of patients with suspected tibia fractures includes anteroposterior and lateral radiographs of the entire tibia, along with radiographs of the ipsilateral knee and the ankle to assess for associated injuries.

Tibial shaft fractures are frequently associated with other musculoskeletal injuries. Intra-articular knee injuries (cruciate or collateral ligament injuries, meniscal tears, and cartilage injuries) are often unrecognized. Tibial shaft fractures may occur in conjunction with tibial plateau fractures or ankle fractures.[5] There is a high association of spiral tibia fractures with isolated fractures of the posterior malleolus.[6,7]

Classification

The soft-tissue injury associated with tibial shaft fractures can be the main determinant of the patient's outcome. For open fractures, the Gustilo and Anderson classification is typically used to communicate the amount of soft-tissue injury and fracture severity.[8,9] This system is mainly based on the size of the open wound, amount of contamination, and the fracture severity and is outlined in **Table 1**. This system has been used to determine antibiotic prophylaxis, surgical management strategies and the risk of complications such as infection and nonunion. The Oestern and Tscherne classification is used to classify the amount of soft-tissue injury severity associated with closed fractures in an effort to predict outcome and associated complications[10] and is outlined in **Table 2**.

Fracture classification has been used to compare patient populations from different clinical studies. The AO/Orthopaedic Trauma Association fracture classification is commonly used.[11]

Indications for Surgery

Absolute indications for surgery include open fractures, the presence of concomitant vascular injuries or compartment syndrome, irreducible or unstable fractures, or failure of closed treatment. Relative indications for surgical treatment include fractures with concomitant intra-articular fractures that will require surgery, displaced fractures with an intact fibula, fractures with soft tissue injuries that require surgical management, the presence of multiple injuries, or fractures that require frequent monitoring of soft tissues that may be obscured in a cast.

Nondisplaced, low-energy tibia fractures may be treated nonsurgically. Although no studies have defined the amount of displacement that precludes nonsurgical treatment, fractures with displacement of more than 50% of the shaft, angulation greater than 5° to 10°, rotation greater than 10°, and greater than 1 cm of shortening may be best treated surgically.[12]

Nonsurgical Treatment

Nonsurgical treatment of tibial shaft fractures is best reserved for closed low-energy, isolated, nondisplaced, or minimally displaced fractures that may be reduced and immobilized effectively. Absence of an ipsilateral fibula fracture is a relative contraindication. Initial immobilization is best achieved with long leg splinting that allows for swelling. After reduction of swelling, the patient's leg is placed into a new well-padded long leg cast. Physical examination should demonstrate decreased or minimal tenderness at the fracture site. The long leg cast is then replaced with a short leg patellar tendon bearing cast or a functional fracture brace; progressive weight bearing is initiated. The patellar tendon bearing cast or functional brace may be discontinued when there is evidence of bridging callus on radiographs.

Closed treatment with functional bracing has been shown to achieve high union rates with angulation and shortening that may be comparable to surgical treatment.[12,13] With functional bracing, most fractures heal with less than 12 mm of shortening and less than 8° of angulation in either the frontal or sagittal plane. Although malunion and shortening are the primary associated complications, a small prospective randomized trial also revealed that patients undergoing nonsurgical treatment had a slower return to work, healing rate, return of knee, ankle, and hindfoot motion, and a higher rate of hindfoot stiffness.[14] No study has commented on the risk of rotational malunion.

Surgical Treatment

External Fixation

External fixation is a minimally invasive method of treatment that allows for relative stability of the fracture and can be used for either temporary or definitive management. With the success of other methods of treatment, however, external fixation is typically used for patients who cannot tolerate more extensive surgery because of medical or soft-tissue conditions, or osseous defect. Another relative indication may be a medullary canal too small for placement of an intramedullary nail.

As a temporary form of fixation used during damage control techniques, uniplanar external fixation allows for relatively rapid application and stability of the extremity. It allows for easier soft-tissue evaluation and wound care, patient mobility, and typically more patient comfort than skeletal traction or splinting until definitive management can be performed. In patients with open fractures, this type of fixation allows for repeat débridement of the bone ends during subsequent débridements.

Depending on the level of the tibial shaft fracture and any associated articular involvement, uniplanar external fixator pins should be placed in a near-far configuration on either side of the fracture to provide the most stable construct. Typically the pins are placed along the anteromedial surface of the tibia to avoid neurovascular or tendinous structures. If the fracture extends close to either the knee or ankle, caution should be used when placing pins to avoid penetrating the articular surface or joint capsule. For the knee, pins should be placed greater than 14 mm distal to the subchondral bone of the tibia.[15] If there is any question about proximity to the joint or if there is articular fracture extension, joint-spanning external fixation should be performed.

Because of the success of intramedullary nailing and patient dissatisfaction with long-term external fixator use, definitive uniplanar or circular external fixation for acute fractures is typically reserved for open tibia fractures that have significant soft-tissue injury or bone loss.

Plate Fixation

Plate fixation of tibial shaft fractures may be achieved with either an open surgical approach with direct fracture visualization and reduction or by indirect reduction and minimally invasive percutaneous plating. Wound-healing problems and prominent hardware plague plate fixation of tibial shaft fractures; therefore, this technique is best reserved for specific indications such as tibial shaft fractures with ipsilateral articular fractures of the tibial plateau or pilon (**Figure 1**), periprosthetic fractures, open physes, too small of a medullary canal for an intramedullary nail, previous cruciate ligament reconstruction, fracture where external fixators are already present (**Figure 1**), or open fractures where the open fracture wound provides the surgical exposure.

Open reduction and internal fixation may be achieved through three different surgical approaches. Anteromedial incisions and exposure of the fracture often results in wound-healing problems and prominent hardware; therefore, posteromedial or anterolateral exposure and plate application is preferred. Although open reduction and internal fixation is an alternative to intramedullary nailing, plating of tibial shaft fractures (particularly open fractures) is associated with higher rates of complications (19% to 30%) and worse outcomes.[16]

Minimally invasive or percutaneous plating is another alternative. Medial or anteromedial plating using this technique is advantageous because of the subcutaneous location of the tibia; however, the use of medial plates may still result in symptomatic hardware, risk of wound breakdown, and saphenous vein and nerve injury.[17] Anterolateral percutaneous plating allows for submuscular plate placement that decreases the risk of symptomatic hardware, but injury to the superficial peroneal nerve may occur during placement of distal screws.[18,19] Regardless of the plate location, minimally invasive plating of the tibia must still follow the principles of open plating, including achieving optimal fracture reduction (alignment, length, and rotation) and promoting bone healing through compression for simple fracture patterns. For comminuted fractures, bridge plating techniques are used where indirect fracture reduction techniques are used to maintain length, overall alignment, and rotation. The area of fracture comminution is spanned using longer plates with screw fixation on either side of the zone of comminution in an effort to minimize disruption of the fracture blood supply.

Intramedullary Nailing

Intramedullary nailing continues to be the gold standard for treating displaced tibial shaft fractures. Despite this success, long-term follow-up shows that patients may have persistent sequelae after fracture healing. At 14 years, patients with isolated tibial shaft fractures have similar functional outcomes to population norms but approximately 73% continue to have moderate knee pain with activity, 42% have decreased ankle motion, and 35% have radiographic evidence of either knee or ankle arthrosis.[20]

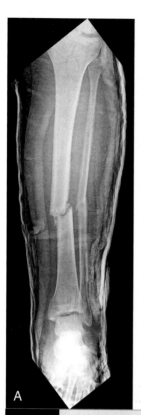
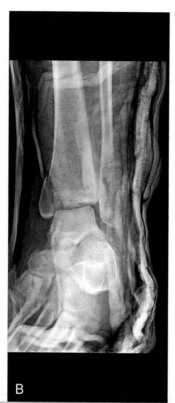
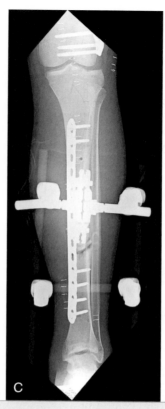
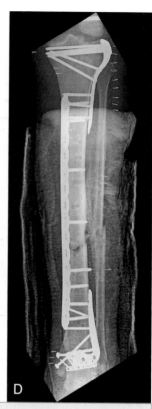

Figure 1 A closed left tibial shaft fracture with ipsilateral fractures of the left tibial plateau (**A**) and left tibial pilon (**B**) is treated with initial plate fixation of the shaft fracture and spanning external fixation of the periarticular injuries with delayed open reduction and internal fixation of the plateau and pilon fractures after the soft-tissue injury resolved (**C** and **D**).

Controversies that still exist with intramedullary nailing of tibia fractures include the high incidence of knee pain, the need for reaming, and managing proximal and distal metadiaphyseal fractures. Anterior knee pain is the most common complication associated with nailing of tibial shaft fractures, but no definitive reason exists for the up to 67% incidence.[21] Iatrogenic injury during creation of the starting point and during nail insertion, nail prominence, quadriceps weakness, and use of a transpatellar tendon surgical approach have all been proposed.[22-24] Relatively small prospective randomized controlled trials, including one with up to 8-year follow-up, have shown that there is no increased incidence with a transpatellar tendon approach.[21,25] When discussing the risk of chronic anterior knee pain with patients, it is encouraging to note that knee pain is not usually severe and may continue to improve up to 8 years after surgery.[22,25]

Although reaming is controversial, its benefits have long been thought to outweigh any disadvantages such as nonunion and incidence of secondary procedures.[26] The Study to Prospectively Evaluate Reamed Intramedullary Nails in Patients with Tibial Fractures (SPRINT) randomized 1,319 patients with open and closed tibia fractures to either reamed or unreamed nails and potentially challenged how substantial a difference reaming makes. At 1-year follow-up, closed fractures treated with reamed nails had a lower risk of autodynamization (locking bolt bending or breakage), but actual re-

operation rates for bony union were not statistically different. There was no significant difference for open fractures. The authors believe that not much of a substantial effect of reaming was seen because of the study's rigorous design, including waiting 6 months before allowing reoperation for nonunion—although this prerequisite was followed for only 55% of cases and equal in both reamed and unreamed groups.

Proximal and distal metadiaphyseal tibia fractures can be very challenging to manage. Fractures with simple articular fracture extension can be addressed with simple lag screw fixation before the nailing procedure. Deforming forces created by the patellar tendon and iliotibial band have contributed to the incidence of malunion (up to 84%) of proximal metadiaphyseal tibia fractures.[27] Both surgical techniques and nail designs have been modified to decrease the risk of malunion. Several authors have proposed technical modifications that include the semiextended position;[28] a starting point just medial to the lateral tibial spine and at the anterior margin of the articular surface and placing the guidewire parallel to the anterior cortex;[29] use of provisional fixation to maintain fracture reduction during nailing including an external fixator or femoral distractor,[30] or a medial unicortical plate;[29,31] and blocking or Pöller screws to narrow the potential path of the nail, which leads to improved reduction[32] (**Figure 2**). Nail designs with a more proximal bend[33]

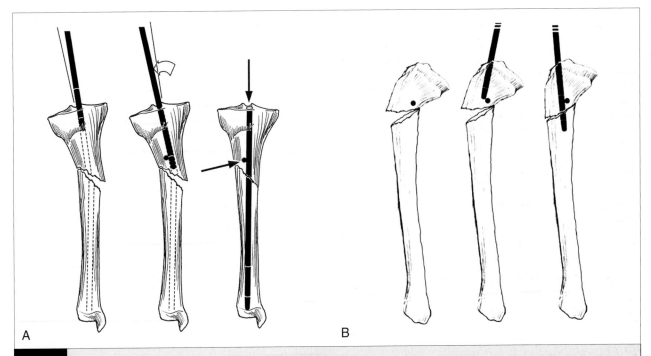

Figure 2 Illustration showing the use of a posterior blocking screw (**A**) and a lateral blocking screw (**B**) to help maintain alignment of the tibia in both coronal and sagittal planes during nailing of a proximal-third tibia fracture. By keeping the nail against the medial (**A**) and anterior (**B**) cortices, deformity is prevented. (Reproduced with permission from Stannard J, Schmidt A, Kregor P: *Surgical Treatment of Orthopaedic Trauma*. New York, NY, Thieme Medical Publishers, 2007, pp 767-791.)

and oblique locking bolt options have also minimized the risk of fracture malreduction during nail placement and improved biomechanical stability.

Although the malunion rate is lower (up to 58%) in distal metadiaphyseal fractures,[34] similar surgical technique modifications and nail design changes have led to improved alignment and biomechanical stability. Technical tricks to improve alignment during intramedullary nailing include ensuring that the guidewire is centered in the distal tibia on all fluoroscopic views; open reduction and internal fixation of the ipsilateral fibula fracture; limited open reduction; fracture reduction with the use of percutaneous reduction forceps, joysticks, femoral distractor or external fixator (**Figure 3**); provisional fixation with unicortical plates; and use of blocking screws to create a pseudocortex to help direct the nail and improve biomechanical stability.[30,35-38] Nail designs with locking bolts within 3 mm of the end of the nail, oblique locking bolt options, and modified locking bolts[39] have improved fixation options and biomechanical stability for intramedullary nailing of distal tibia fractures.

Plating Compared With Nailing of Proximal and Distal Metadiaphyseal Tibia Fractures

The desire to decrease the incidence of malunion and the development of percutaneous plating techniques have led some surgeons to turn to plating of extra-articular proximal and distal metadiaphyseal fractures. A recent small retrospective cohort study comparing plating and nailing of proximal fractures revealed that apex anterior malreduction was twice as common in the nail group, additional surgical techniques for reduction were used substantially more often in the nail group, and hardware removal was three times more common in the plating group.[40] A meta-analysis of treatment of extra-articular proximal tibia fractures (intramedullary nail, external fixator, plating) revealed that nailing was associated with a lower rate of infection and a higher incidence of malunion.[41]

Distal tibia fractures are challenging to treat because of the short segment available for nail fixation; however, the risk of surgical wound breakdown and prominent hardware has contributed to resistance in using plate fixation. A retrospective review of 113 open and closed distal tibia fractures 4 to 11 cm proximal to the plafond that were either nailed (76) or plated (37) revealed that the nail group had a higher risk of delayed or nonunion (12% versus 2.7%), especially if the fibula was fixed, and malunion (29% versus 5.4%). Although there may be a higher risk of delayed or nonunion with ipsilateral fibula fracture fixation, the risk of postoperative loss of the initial tibial fracture reduction is lower.[38] A systematic review of retrospective studies from 1975-2005 of extra-articular distal tibia fractures revealed that there has been no prospective trial comparing nailing with plating of these fractures; although no conclusions can be made, the limited number of small case series show that nailing leads to a higher risk of nonunion and malunion.[42]

4: Lower Extremity

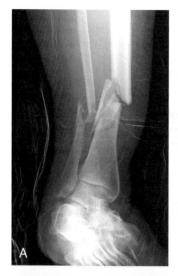

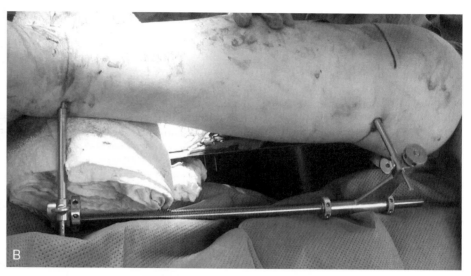

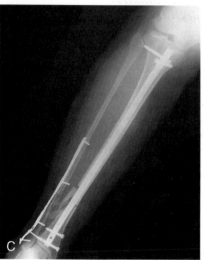

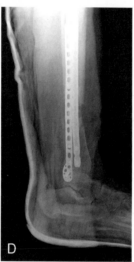

Figure 3 **A,** Radiograph of a distal one-third closed tibia and ipsilateral fibula fracture. **B,** A femoral distractor was used to provisionally reduce the tibia and fibula fractures. Radiographs showing percutaneous plating of the distal fibula were obtained to aid in reduction of the tibia. Reamed intramedullary nailing was then performed with a tibial nail with very distal locking bolt options. AP **(C)** and lateral **(D)** radiographs show restoration of length, rotation, and coronal and sagittal alignment.

Open Tibia Fractures

Open tibial shaft fractures are the most common significant open fracture. Treatment should consist of early antibiotic administration, coverage of the wound with a sterile but nontoxic dressing, tetanus prophylaxis, surgical débridement, and stabilization of the fracture.

Open fractures are described by the Gustilo-Anderson classification, which classifies wounds based on severity, size, contamination, and associated vascular injury. The classification is useful in determining choice of antibiotic treatment. However, final determination of the Gustilo-Anderson grade should be performed by the treating surgeon in the operating room.

Early administration (within 3 hours of injury) of the appropriate antibiotics decreases the risk of infection following open fractures.[43] For Gustilo-Anderson type 1 or 2 open fractures, patients are given a first- or second-generation cephalosporin to treat the causative infectious organisms, which are most frequently gram-positive bacteria. For type 3 open fractures, the addition of an aminoglycoside is necessary to address gram-

negative bacteria. With soil contamination, penicillin should be added to cover gram-positive anaerobes. Although the duration of antibiotic treatment following open fractures is also controversial because no benefit has been shown with prolonged antibiotic administration, 24 to 72 hours of antibiotic coverage has been recommended following initial surgical débridement of the open fracture and 24 hours after each subsequent débridement until the wound is closed.[44]

The timing of surgical débridement has recently been debated. The previously held dogma of early débridement within 6 hours has been disproven by numerous studies.[43,45,46] Currently, no level I evidence exists to direct timing of débridement. However, open fractures should nonetheless be treated urgently and efficiently to optimize patient care.

Skillful surgical débridement remains the most important factor in the optimal treatment of open tibia fractures. All devitalized and contaminated tissue, including bone, should be sharply excised from the wound. Débridement should proceed systematically, beginning with the skin and progressing to the bone. Depending on the severity of the injury and level of contamination, some open fractures may be managed with primary closure. However, this is best determined by the experience of the treating surgeon and routine primary closure should not be performed. In wounds with severe contamination, serial débridements to reassess the wound and tissue viability after 48 to 72 hours may be beneficial.

If primary closure is not chosen, wounds should be dressed and left undisturbed between débridements. Negative pressure wound therapy (NPWT) may be useful in the management of these wounds. Antibiotic-impregnated beads may also be placed in open fracture wounds. The concentration of local antibiotics achieved with antibiotic beads far exceeds that achieved with intravenous antibiotics.

Stabilization of the open fracture is essential because it provides an optimal environment for soft-tissue healing and prevention of infection. Primary definitive stabilization with intramedullary nailing or plating may be performed depending on the severity of the injury and the level of contamination. Definitive fixation should only be performed when the open fracture bed, including the soft tissues, has been thoroughly débrided and is clean and viable. Immediate nailing of open tibia fractures has been supported in up to type IIIB fractures using both reamed and unreamed nails. Plating of open fractures is associated with a higher rate of infection.[47] External fixation provides an excellent alternative to nailing or plating in the face of severe injury or contamination. External fixation may be followed by definitive treatment (intramedullary nail or plate) once soft tissues have recovered. Conversion to an intramedullary nail is best performed less than 2 weeks after application of the external fixator.[48,49]

If primary wound closure is not possible, alternative means of soft-tissue coverage must be sought. NPWT may be useful in decreasing the size and depth of the wound that will ultimately require coverage. Split-thickness skin grafts may be used to cover skin defects over muscle or subcutaneous tissue. For coverage of bone, nerves, or blood vessels, flaps may be required. Acute shortening of the tibia during definitive fixation to allow for local soft-tissue coverage has been successful in small retrospective series. Depending on the amount of acute shortening, bone transport or subsequent lengthening can be done, typically using external fixation methods.[50]

Flap coverage for open tibia fractures is determined by the severity and location of the wound. Proximal wounds are best covered with rotational gastrocnemius flaps. Wounds in the middle third of the tibia may be covered with a soleus flap. Distal defects are best covered with a sural island pedicle flap or free tissue transfer. Local rotational flaps are often compromised by the trauma that resulted in the open tibia fracture and are therefore suboptimal for soft-tissue coverage. The Lower Extremity Assessment Project study revealed that there is a higher rate of wound complications requiring reoperation when rotational flaps were used instead of free flaps in open fractures with more complex osseous injury (AO/Orthopaedic Trauma Association

type C fractures).[51] NPWT may decrease the need for rotational or free flap reconstructive surgeries for severe open wounds; if flap coverage is required, delaying definitive coverage beyond 7 days substantially increases the risk of infection.[52,53]

Acceleration of Fracture Healing and Management of Osseous Defects

Tibial shaft fractures are a targeted area for orthobiologics. Tibial nonunions and open fractures, especially with bone loss, can lead to significant morbidity and loss of function. Although several multicenter trials are ongoing to evaluate the effects of different orthobiologics on tibial shaft fractures, the only data from prospective trials (level I evidence) that are currently available involve recombinant human bone morphogenetic protein-2 (rhBMP-2) and rhBMP-7.

In the United States, the only current Food and Drug Administration (FDA)–approved use in acute fractures is for rhBMP-2 in open tibia fractures treated within 14 days of injury. The BMP-2 Evaluation in Surgery for Tibial Trauma (BESTT) trial revealed that open tibia fractures treated with an intramedullary nail and 1.5 mg/mL of rhBMP-2 on a collagen sponge implanted at the time of definitive closure required fewer secondary procedures and had a faster time to union and lower rates of nonunion and infection.[54] Further subgroup analysis of types IIIA and IIIB open fractures treated with rhBMP-2 had fewer bone grafting procedures and secondary interventions and a lower infection rate.[55]

For tibial nonunions, rhBMP-7 is FDA approved as a humanitarian device exemption. One study prospectively compared rhBMP-7 with autogenous bone grafting for tibial nonunions; results showed similar rates of clinical and radiographic union.[56]

Managing osseous defects in open tibia fractures, nonunions, and infected fractures continues to be challenging. The use of rhBMP-2 for management of osseous defects has been evaluated in a small prospective randomized controlled trial.[57] RhBMP-2 combined with allograft bone graft was compared with autogenous bone grafting alone in open and closed tibia fractures without signs of infection initially managed with either intramedullary nailing or external fixation. Fractures with 1- to 7-cm osseous defects and at least 50% circumferential bone loss were included. Both groups had similar union rates and need for secondary interventions. Although circular wire external fixation and bone transport has been successful in managing acute and chronic osseous defects,[58] the use of a two-staged technique incorporating the use of an antibiotic-impregnated cement spacer (which leads to development of a biologic membrane) in managing large osseous defects up to 25 cm in combination fixation and soft-tissue coverage procedures has been successful.[59]

The role that bone stimulators may play in the management of acute fracture and nonunion management is still a topic for debate. Although some studies support the use of low-intensity ultrasound in acute fractures

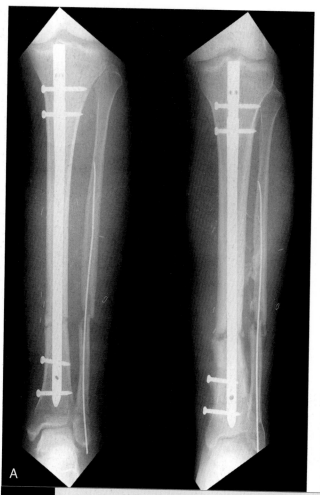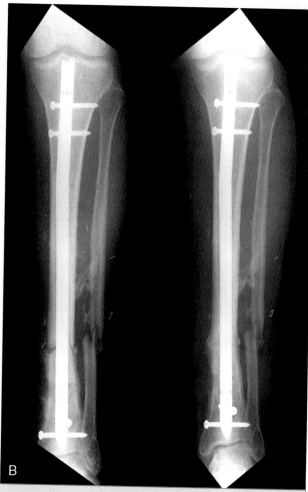

Figure 4 AP and lateral radiographs showing treatment of a tibial shaft fracture. **A,** An open tibial shaft fracture initially treated with reamed intramedullary nailing that eventually became an infected nonunion.) A staged exchange nailing was performed with interval débridement, external fixator placement, and culture-specific antibiotic therapy. **B,** Three months after exchange nailing, the fracture was healed and the patient was pain free.

and nonunions[60] and electromagnetic stimulation in nonunions,[61] comparative studies without methodological flaws are required to truly support their use.

Tibial Malunion

Most tibial shaft malunions result from either nonsurgical management or technical errors in surgical management. Proximal and distal metadiaphyseal fractures treated surgically have historically had high rates of malunion. Surgically treated diaphyseal fractures have a much lower rate of malunion unless they are managed with external fixation.

Without restoration of the mechanical axis, malunion of the tibial shaft affects both the ankle and knee and can lead to exacerbation of ligamentous instability, and progressive pain and arthritis. Although the definition of malunion varies in trials, retrospective trials have shown that greater than 5° to 10° of coronal or sagittal plane alignment, 10° of rotation, and 1 cm of shortening leads to poor outcomes.[62] If malunions are symptomatic, full-length weight-bearing lower extremity radiographs should be used to evaluate angular deformity and limb-length discrepancies. A CT scan may be helpful to evaluate rotational deformities. Corrective osteotomies and lengthening procedures may be performed to address symptomatic malunions.

Tibial Nonunion

Nonunion of tibial shaft fractures may occur as a result of the injury, patient factors such as smoking or medical comorbidities (for example, diabetes), or treatment. Historically, there has been an absence of a well-accepted definition of a time frame for nonunion, but typically a fracture that has not healed at 6 months or shows no progressive healing for 3 consecutive months is considered a nonunion.

Other patient factors that may increase the risk of nonunion are poor nutrition and a history of previous nonunion. Many patients with a nonunion have an underlying metabolic or endocrine disorder.[63] Surgeon factors that may increase the risk of nonunion include distraction of the fracture site while performing intramedullary nailing or plating, excessive soft-tissue stripping with open reduction and internal fixation, or excessive reaming resulting in injury to the endosteal blood supply. In the case of open fractures, the injury itself may result in ultimate nonunion.

The SPRINT trial demonstrated a lower risk of reoperation with reamed intramedullary nailing, particularly in closed tibial shaft fractures, but most of these events were related to autodynamization and not reoperation for bony union.[26] In addition, in patients with a suspected nonunion, delaying reoperation for 6 months decreased the need for the procedure.

Preoperative evaluation for tibial nonunions should include a history of the original injury and the subsequent treatment. Radiographs and a CT scan are useful to categorize the nature and extent of the nonunion. The potential for infection should be addressed by obtaining a white blood cell count with differential, erythrocyte sedimentation rate, and C-reactive protein levels. Screening for metabolic and endocrine disorders is also helpful.

Tibial shaft nonunions, like most nonunions, may be broadly categorized into hypertrophic or atrophic nonunions. Hypertrophic nonunions may be treated with improved surgical stabilization of the fracture, whereas atrophic nonunions will also require biologic enhancement (through bone graft or orthobiologics) to achieve union.

Tibial shaft nonunions may be treated by a variety of surgical methods. Exchange nailing for previously nailed tibial shaft fractures is effective (**Figure 4**). Open treatment with posterolateral or direct lateral (central) bone grafting may also achieve union.[64] Ring (Ilizarov) external fixation provides a powerful method to treat nonunions but is often poorly tolerated by patients. Infected nonunions may be best treated with ring (Ilizarov) external fixation. Tissue culture from the nonunion site should be sent at the time of surgical treatment to determine if prolonged antibiotic therapy is required.

Annotated References

1. Park S, Ahn J, Gee AO, Kuntz AF, Esterhai JL: Compartment syndrome in tibial fractures. *J Orthop Trauma* 2009;23(7):514-518.

   Four hundred fourteen patients with tibial fractures were retrospectively reviewed for the incidence and risk factors for compartment syndrome. The rate of compartment syndrome was highest for diaphyseal tibia fractures (8.1%). Patients who developed compartment syndrome were of younger age (average 27.5 years) than those who did not (average 39 years). Level of evidence: III.

2. Kakar S, Firoozabadi R, McKean J, Tornetta P III: Diastolic blood pressure in patients with tibia fractures under anaesthesia: Implications for the diagnosis of com-

partment syndrome. *J Orthop Trauma* 2007;21(2):99-103.

   In this prospective cohort study, preoperative, intraoperative, and postoperative diastolic blood pressures (DBP) were measured in patients undergoing intramedullary nailing of the tibia. Preoperative DBP correlated with postoperative DBP, but intraoperative DBP was significantly lower (average, 18 mm Hg lower). Therefore, reliance of intraoperative DBP for measurement of delta P to determine compartment syndrome may result in a spuriously low value and therefore in a missed diagnosis of compartment syndrome. Level of evidence: II.

3. McQueen MM, Court-Brown CM: Compartment monitoring in tibial fractures. The pressure threshold for decompression. *J Bone Joint Surg Br* 1996;78(1):99-104.

4. Ritenour AE, Dorlac WC, Fang R, et al: Complications after fasciotomy revision and delayed compartment release in combat patients. *J Trauma* 2008;64(2, suppl):S153-S161, discussion S161-S162.

   Three hundred thirty-six combat casualties from the wars in Iraq and Afghanistan were retrospectively reviewed to evaluate outcomes and complications of fasciotomies. The anterior compartment of the lower leg was most commonly missed during surgical compartment release. Patients who underwent delayed fasciotomies had twice the rate of major amputation and a threefold higher mortality. Level of evidence: III.

5. Stuermer EK, Stuermer KM: Tibial shaft fracture and ankle joint injury. *J Orthop Trauma* 2008;22(2):107-112.

   Forty-three of 214 patients with tibia fracture (20.1%) were found to have associated ankle joint injury including distal fibula fractures, Maissoneuve injuries, syndesmotic injuries, posterior malleolus fractures, and medial malleolus fractures. Level of evidence: II.

6. Hou Z, Zhang Q, Zhang Y, Li S, Pan J, Wu H: A occult and regular combination injury: The posterior malleolar fracture associated with spiral tibial shaft fracture. *J Trauma* 2009;66(5):1385-1390.

   A retrospective study of 28 of 288 tibial shaft fractures (9.7%) had ipsilateral posterior malleolar fractures (PMF). None of the PMFs were identified preoperatively and only 10 were identified intraoperatively. Nine of the fractures displaced postoperatively. Thirty-four additional tibial shaft fractures were evaluated prospectively with CT and MRI if plain films were negative for PMF. Thirty out of 34 PMFs were identified–3 by plain film, 23 by CT scan, and 4 by MRI. Level of evidence: III.

7. Boraiah S, Gardner MJ, Helfet DL, Lorich DG: High association of posterior malleolus fractures with spiral distal tibial fractures. *Clin Orthop Relat Res* 2008;466(7):1692-1698.

   Sixty-two patients with distal third tibial shaft fractures were retrospectively evaluated for posterior malleolar fractures. Twenty-four of 62 patients (39%) had associated posterior malleolus fractures. A protocol was instituted, after two fractures were missed, to obtain CT of the ankle on all patients with distal third tibial shaft

4: Lower Extremity

fractures. Twenty-three patients were evaluated prospectively and 11 (48%) had posterior malleolar fractures and none were missed. Level of evidence: II.

8. Gustilo RB, Anderson JT: Prevention of infection in the treatment of one thousand and twenty-five open fractures of long bones: Retrospective and prospective analyses. *J Bone Joint Surg Am* 1976;58(4):453-458.

9. Gustilo RB, Mendoza RM, Williams DN: Problems in the management of type III (severe) open fractures: A new classification of type III open fractures. *J Trauma* 1984;24(8):742-746.

10. Tscherne HG: *Fractures Associated with Soft Tissue Injuries*. New York, NY: Springer-Verlag; 1984.

11. Marsh JL, Slongo TF, Agel J, et al: Fracture and dislocation classification compendium - 2007: Orthopaedic Trauma Association classification, database and outcomes committee. *J Orthop Trauma* 2007;21(10, suppl): S1-S133.

    This supplement presents the OTA Fracture and Dislocation Classification, the revisions made since it was originally published in 1996, and reviews the fracture classification literature published since 1996.

12. Sarmiento A, Latta LL: 450 closed fractures of the distal third of the tibia treated with a functional brace. *Clin Orthop Relat Res* 2004;428:261-271.

13. Sarmiento A, Latta LL: Fractures of the middle third of the tibia treated with a functional brace. *Clin Orthop Relat Res* 2008;466(12):3108-3115.

    In a retrospective review, 434 closed fractures of the middle third of the tibial shaft were evaluated for angular deformity and final shortening. Ninety-seven percent of fractures healed with 8° or less of angulation in the mediolateral plane. Nonunion occurred in 0.9% of fractures. Mean final shortening of these fractures was 4.3 mm. Level of evidence: IV

14. Hooper GJ, Keddell RG, Penny ID: Conservative management or closed nailing for tibial shaft fractures: A randomised prospective trial. *J Bone Joint Surg Br* 1991;73(1):83-85.

15. Reid JS, Van Slyke MA, Moulton MJ, Mann TA: Safe placement of proximal tibial transfixation wires with respect to intracapsular penetration. *J Orthop Trauma* 2001;15(1):10-17.

16. Bilat C, Leutenegger A, Rüedi T: Osteosynthesis of 245 tibial shaft fractures: Early and late complications. *Injury* 1994;25(6):349-358.

17. Ozsoy MH, Tuccar E, Demiryurek D, et al: Minimally invasive plating of the distal tibia: Do we really sacrifice saphenous vein and nerve? A cadaver study. *J Orthop Trauma* 2009;23(2):132-138.

    Minimally invasive plating of the distal tibia was performed on cadavers using two different precontoured medial distal tibia plates using a medial approach. Post-

18. Pichler W, Grechenig W, Tesch NP, Weinberg AM, Heidari N, Clement H: The risk of iatrogenic injury to the deep peroneal nerve in minimally invasive osteosynthesis of the tibia with the Less Invasive Stabilisation System: A cadaver study. *J Bone Joint Surg Br* 2009;91(3): 385-387.

    Minimally invasive plating of the tibia was performed on 18 cadavers using the Less Invasive Stabilization System through an anterolateral approach. The deep peroneal nerve was at most risk between the 11th and 13th holes. Because the nerve was in contact with the plate in all specimens, the authors recommend either not using a longer than 10-hole plate, or using a larger distal approach to ensure that the nerve is not injured.

19. Cole PA, Zlowodzki M, Kregor PJ: Less Invasive Stabilization System (LISS) for fractures of the proximal tibia: Indications, surgical technique and preliminary results of the UMC Clinical Trial. *Injury* 2003;34(Suppl 1):A16-A29.

20. Lefaivre KA, Guy P, Chan H, Blachut PA: Long-term follow-up of tibial shaft fractures treated with intramedullary nailing. *J Orthop Trauma* 2008;22(8):525-529.

    A prospective cohort study was conducted in 56 patients who underwent locked intramedullary nailing for isolated tibial shaft fractures. Median follow-up was 14 years. Mean normalized Short Form-36 scores demonstrated that these patients' functional outcomes were comparable to referenced population norms. However, many patients experienced significant sequelae, including persistent knee pain (73.2%), swelling (33.9%), and restricted ankle range of motion (42.4%). Level of evidence: II.

21. Väistö O, Toivanen J, Paakkala T, Järvelä T, Kannus P, Järvinen M: Anterior knee pain after intramedullary nailing of a tibial shaft fracture: An ultrasound study of the patellar tendons of 36 patients. *J Orthop Trauma* 2005;19(5):311-316.

22. Väistö O, Toivanen J, Kannus P, Järvinen M: Anterior knee pain and thigh muscle strength after intramedullary nailing of a tibial shaft fracture: An 8-year follow-up of 28 consecutive cases. *J Orthop Trauma* 2007;21(3):165-171.

    Forty patients who underwent nailing for a tibial shaft fracture were evaluated at an average of 3.2 years. Twenty-eight of these patients were evaluated at 8 years. Anterior knee pain symptoms resolved in these patients between 3 to 8 years after surgery. Patients with persistent anterior knee pain at 8 years had significantly weaker quadriceps strength and lower functional knee scores. Level of evidence: IV.

23. Orfaly R, Keating JE, O'Brien PJ: Knee pain after tibial nailing: Does the entry point matter? *J Bone Joint Surg Br* 1995;77(6):976-977.

24. Keating JF, Orfaly R, O'Brien PJ: Knee pain after tibial nailing. *J Orthop Trauma* 1997;11(1):10-13.

25. Väistö O, Toivanen J, Kannus P, Järvinen M: Anterior knee pain after intramedullary nailing of fractures of the tibial shaft: An eight-year follow-up of a prospective, randomized study comparing two different nail-insertion techniques. *J Trauma* 2008;64(6):1511-1516.

A prospective randomized study comparing transtendinous versus paratendinous incision techniques for intramedullary nailing was conducted with 42 patients followed for an average of 3 years; 28 patients (14 paratendinous, 14 transtendinous) were reexamined at an average of 8 years after surgery. Four patients (29%) of each group reported anterior knee pain at 8-year follow-up. Lysholm, Tegner, and Iowa knee scores demonstrated no difference in the two groups. Level of evidence: II.

26. Bhandari M, Guyatt G, Tornetta P III, et al; Study to Prospectively Evaluate Reamed Intramedullary Nails in Patients with Tibial Fractures Investigators: Randomized trial of reamed and unreamed intramedullary nailing of tibial shaft fractures. *J Bone Joint Surg Am* 2008; 90(12):2567-2578.

A multicenter, blinded prospective randomized trial of 1,226 patients with tibial shaft fractures was performed. Six hundred twenty-two patients were randomized to reamed intramedullary nailing and 604 patients were randomized to unreamed nailing. Reoperation for nonunion before 6 months was disallowed. At 1-year follow-up, only 57 patients (4.6%) required reoperation for nonunion. In patients with closed fractures, 45 of 416 patients (11%) in the reamed nailing group and 68 of 410 patients (17%) in the unreamed nailing group experienced a primary outcome event (relative risk, 0.67; 95% confidence interval, 0.47 to 0.96; $P = 0.03$), suggesting that there may be an advantage to reamed intramedullary nailing in these patients due to less risk of screw breakage (autodynamization). In patients with open fractures, there was no difference between the two groups. Level of evidence: I.

27. Cannada LK, Anglen JO, Archdeacon MT, Herscovici D Jr, Ostrum RF: Avoiding complications in the care of fractures of the tibia. *J Bone Joint Surg Am* 2008;90(8): 1760-1768.

The authors discuss surgical techniques to avoid complications in acute fracture care as well as the treatment of infections and nonunions.

28. Tornetta P III, Collins E: Semiextended position of intramedullary nailing of the proximal tibia. *Clin Orthop Relat Res* 1996;328:185-189.

29. Nork SE, Barei DP, Schildhauer TA, et al: Intramedullary nailing of proximal quarter tibial fractures. *J Orthop Trauma* 2006;20(8):523-528.

30. Wysocki RW, Kapotas JS, Virkus WW: Intramedullary nailing of proximal and distal one-third tibial shaft fractures with intraoperative two-pin external fixation. *J Trauma* 2009;66(4):1135-1139.

This retrospective case series reviewed the use of a two-pin external fixator (traveling traction) used as a reduction aid during intramedullary nailing of proximal (15) and distal (27) extra-articular tibia fractures. Fourteen

of 15 proximal and 25 of 27 distal tibia fractures healed with less than 5° of angulation and less than 1 cm of shortening. Level of evidence: IV.

31. Archdeacon MT, Wyrick JD: Reduction plating for provisional fracture fixation. *J Orthop Trauma* 2006;20(3): 206-211.

32. Ricci WM, O'Boyle M, Borrelli J, Bellabarba C, Sanders R: Fractures of the proximal third of the tibial shaft treated with intramedullary nails and blocking screws. *J Orthop Trauma* 2001;15(4):264-270.

33. Henley MB, Meier M, Tencer AF: Influences of some design parameters on the biomechanics of the unreamed tibial intramedullary nail. *J Orthop Trauma* 1993;7(4): 311-319.

34. Vallier HA, Le TT, Bedi A: Radiographic and clinical comparisons of distal tibia shaft fractures (4 to 11 cm proximal to the plafond): Plating versus intramedullary nailing. *J Orthop Trauma* 2008;22(5):307-311.

In this retrospective review, 111 patients with 113 distal tibial fractures (4 to 11 cm proximal to the tibial plafond) were treated either with an intramedullary nail (76) or a medial plate (37). Nine patients had delayed union or nonunion after nailing. One patient had a nonunion after plating. Nonunion was more common if the fibula was fixed at the time of tibial fixation. Angular malunion greater than or equal to 5° occurred in 22 patients with nails and 2 with plates. Delayed union, malunion, and secondary procedures were more frequent after nailing. Level of evidence: III.

35. Krettek C, Miclau T, Schandelmaier P, Stephan C, Möhlmann U, Tscherne H: The mechanical effect of blocking screws ("Pöller screws") in stabilizing tibia fractures with short proximal or distal fragments after insertion of small-diameter intramedullary nails. *J Orthop Trauma* 1999;13(8):550-553.

36. Tang P, Gates C, Hawes J, Vogt M, Prayson MJ: Does open reduction increase the chance of infection during intramedullary nailing of closed tibial shaft fractures? *J Orthop Trauma* 2006;20(5):317-322.

37. Nork SE, Schwartz AK, Agel J, Holt SK, Schrick JL, Winquist RA: Intramedullary nailing of distal metaphyseal tibial fractures. *J Bone Joint Surg Am* 2005; 87(6):1213-1221.

38. Egol KA, Weisz R, Hiebert R, Tejwani NC, Koval KJ, Sanders RW: Does fibular plating improve alignment after intramedullary nailing of distal metaphyseal tibia fractures? *J Orthop Trauma* 2006;20(2):94-103.

39. Horn J, Linke B, Höntzsch D, Gueorquiev B, Schwieger K: Angle stable interlocking screws improve construct stability of intramedullary nailing of distal tibia fractures: A biomechanical study. *Injury* 2009;40(7):767-771.

A cadaver distal third extra-articular gap model was created to compare conventional distal locking bolts

4: Lower Extremity

and "angle stable" locking bolts. Axial stiffness, maximal load to failure, and interfragmentary motion were measured. The "angle stable" group was significantly stiffer and had significantly less interfragmentary motion compared to the conventional group.

40. Lindvall E, Sanders R, Dipasquale T, Herscovici D, Haidukewych G, Sagi C: Intramedullary nailing versus percutaneous locked plating of extra-articular proximal tibial fractures: Comparison of 56 cases. *J Orthop Trauma* 2009;23(7):485-492.

    In this retrospective review, 56 patients with extra-articular proximal tibia fractures were treated with an intramedullary nail (22) or percutaneous locked plating (34) and evaluated at an average of 3.4 years of follow-up (nail group) or 2.7 years of follow-up (locked plate group). There was no difference in final union rates. Implant removal in the locked plate group was three times greater than in the nail group. An apex anterior deformity was the most prevalent form of malreduction in both groups. Level of evidence: III.

41. Bhandari M, Audige L, Ellis T, Hanson B; Evidence-Based Orthopaedic Trauma Working Group: Operative treatment of extra-articular proximal tibial fractures. *J Orthop Trauma* 2003;17(8):591-595.

42. Zelle BA, Bhandari M, Espiritu M, Koval KJ, Zlowodzki M; Evidence-Based Orthopaedic Trauma Working Group: Treatment of distal tibia fractures without articular involvement: A systematic review of 1125 fractures. *J Orthop Trauma* 2006;20(1):76-79.

43. Patzakis MJ, Wilkins J: Factors influencing infection rate in open fracture wounds. *Clin Orthop Relat Res* 1989;243:36-40.

44. Okike K, Bhattacharyya T: Trends in the management of open fractures: A critical analysis. *J Bone Joint Surg Am* 2006;88(12):2739-2748.

45. Harley BJ, Beaupre LA, Jones CA, Dulai SK, Weber DW: The effect of time to definitive treatment on the rate of nonunion and infection in open fractures. *J Orthop Trauma* 2002;16(7):484-490.

46. Skaggs DL, Friend L, Alman B, et al: The effect of surgical delay on acute infection following 554 open fractures in children. *J Bone Joint Surg Am* 2005;87(1):8-12.

47. Clifford RP, Beauchamp CG, Kellam JF, Webb JK, Tile M: Plate fixation of open fractures of the tibia. *J Bone Joint Surg Br* 1988;70(4):644-648.

48. Della Rocca GJ, Crist BD: External fixation versus conversion to intramedullary nailing for definitive management of closed fractures of the femoral and tibial shaft. *J Am Acad Orthop Surg* 2006;14(10 Spec No.):S131-S135.

49. Nowotarski PJ, Turen CH, Brumback RJ, Scarboro JM: Conversion of external fixation to intramedullary nailing for fractures of the shaft of the femur in multiply injured patients. *J Bone Joint Surg Am* 2000;82(6):781-788.

50. El-Rosasy MA: Acute shortening and re-lengthening in the management of bone and soft-tissue loss in complicated fractures of the tibia. *J Bone Joint Surg Br* 2007;89(1):80-88.

    Ten type III open tibia fractures within 6 weeks of injury and 11 established tibial nonunions with bone or soft-tissue loss of more than 3 cm were managed with acute shortening and relengthening through a tibial metaphyseal osteotomy using either an Ilizarov or monolateral external fixator. Average amount of bone loss addressed was 4.7 cm. Nine of 10 acute fractures healed without bone grafting. Only 1 of 10 acute fractures had a residual limb-length discrepancy. No deep infections occurred. Level of evidence: IV.

51. Pollak AN, McCarthy ML, Burgess AR; The Lower Extremity Assessment Project (LEAP) Study Group: Short-term wound complications after application of flaps for coverage of traumatic soft-tissue defects about the tibia. *J Bone Joint Surg Am* 2000;82A(12):1681-1691.

52. Bhattacharyya T, Mehta P, Smith M, Pomahac B: Routine use of wound vacuum-assisted closure does not allow coverage delay for open tibia fractures. *Plast Reconstr Surg* 2008;121(4):1263-1266.

    In patients with grade IIIB open tibia fractures, the infection rate was significantly decreased if coverage occurred within 7 days even with utilization of NPWT (wound vacuum-assisted closure). Level of evidence: IV.

53. Dedmond BT, Kortesis B, Punger K, et al: The use of negative-pressure wound therapy (NPWT) in the temporary treatment of soft-tissue injuries associated with high-energy open tibial shaft fractures. *J Orthop Trauma* 2007;21(1):11-17.

    The authors present a retrospective review of 49 patients with 50 grade III open tibia fractures treated with NPWT before definitive wound closure or coverage. There was a 30% infection rate. Seventeen patients required free tissue transfer or rotational muscle flap for coverage. Level of evidence: IV.

54. Govender S, Csimma C, Genant HK, et al; BMP-2 Evaluation in Surgery for Tibial Trauma (BESTT) Study Group: Recombinant human bone morphogenetic protein-2 for treatment of open tibial fractures: A prospective, controlled, randomized study of four hundred and fifty patients. *J Bone Joint Surg Am* 2002;84(12):2123-2134.

55. Swiontkowski MF, Aro HT, Donell S, et al: Recombinant human bone morphogenetic protein-2 in open tibial fractures: A subgroup analysis of data combined from two prospective randomized studies. *J Bone Joint Surg Am* 2006;88(6):1258-1265.

56. Friedlaender GE, Perry CR, Cole JD, et al: Osteogenic protein-1 (bone morphogenetic protein-7) in the treatment of tibial nonunions. *J Bone Joint Surg Am* 2001;83(pt 2, suppl 1):S151-S158.

57. Jones AL, Bucholz RW, Bosse MJ, et al; BMP-2 Evaluation in Surgery for Tibial Trauma-Allograft (BESTT-ALL) Study Group: Recombinant human BMP-2 and allograft compared with autogenous bone graft for reconstruction of diaphyseal tibial fractures with cortical defects. A randomized, controlled trial. *J Bone Joint Surg Am* 2006;88(7):1431-1441.

58. Rozbruch SR, Pugsley JS, Fragomen AT, Ilizarov S: Repair of tibial nonunions and bone defects with the Taylor Spatial Frame. *J Orthop Trauma* 2008;22(2):88-95.

 A retrospective review of 38 tibial nonunions treated with the Taylor Spatial Frame is presented. Seventy-one percent achieved bony union after initial treatment. Infection correlated with initial failure of treatment and persistent nonunion. Functional outcome inversely correlated with the number of previous surgeries. Level of evidence: IV.

59. Masquelet AC: Muscle reconstruction in reconstructive surgery: Soft tissue repair and long bone reconstruction. *Langenbecks Arch Surg* 2003;388(5):344-346.

60. Busse JW, Kaur J, Mollon B, et al: Low intensity pulsed ultrasonography for fractures: Systematic review of randomised controlled trials. *BMJ* 2009;338:b351.

 A systematic review of 13 randomized trials examining the efficacy of low-intensity pulsed ultrasound for fractures suggests that the evidence is moderate to very low in quality and provides conflicting results. Level of evidence: II.

61. Mollon B, da Silva V, Busse JW, Einhorn TA, Bhandari M: Electrical stimulation for long-bone fracture-healing: A meta-analysis of randomized controlled trials. *J Bone Joint Surg Am* 2008;90(11):2322-2330.

 A meta-analysis of randomized controlled trials investigating the efficacy of electromagnetic stimulation on delayed unions or nonunions suggested no significant impact of this modality. Level of evidence: II.

62. Schmidt A, Finkemeier CG, Tornetta P: Treatment of closed tibia fractures, in: Tornetta P, ed: *Instructional Course Lectures Trauma.* Rosemont, IL, American Academy of Orthopaedic Surgeons, 2006, 215–229.

63. Brinker MR, O'Connor DP, Monla YT, Earthman TP: Metabolic and endocrine abnormalities in patients with nonunions. *J Orthop Trauma* 2007;21(8):557-570.

 Thirty-seven patients with nonunions were referred to endocrinologists and evaluated. Eighty-four percent of patients had one or more new diagnoses of metabolic or endocrine abnormalities. The most common newly diagnosed abnormality was vitamin D deficiency. Eight patients underwent no surgical intervention for nonunion, but achieved bony union following the diagnosis and treatment of a new metabolic or endocrine abnormality. Level of evidence: IV.

64. Ryzewicz M, Morgan SJ, Linford E, Thwing JI, de Resende GV, Smith WR: Central bone grafting for nonunion of fractures of the tibia: A retrospective series. *J Bone Joint Surg Br* 2009;91(4):522-529.

 In a retrospective cohort study, 23 out of 24 tibial nonunions united after undergoing autogenous bone grafting through lateral approach and anterior to the fibula and interosseous membrane. A tibiofibular synostosis was created upon union. These 24 patients were compared to a cohort of 20 tibial nonunions treated with posterolateral bone grafting procedures. The central bone graft patients healed faster and required fewer procedures to achieve union. Level of evidence: III.

Chapter 38

Ankle Fractures

Matt Graves, MD

4: Lower Extremity

Ankle Fractures

Ankle fractures are among the most common injuries treated by an orthopaedic surgeon.[1] As with other fractures, the treatment goal is expedient return to optimal function in the absence of complications. This goal typically requires an anatomic reduction of the ankle mortise with maintenance of ankle joint stability during early, active mobilization. With nondisplaced, stable fractures, function can be achieved nonsurgically. With displaced, unstable fractures, surgical treatment is necessary. It logically follows that a clear understanding of displacement and stability is required. More than 50 years after the popularization of surgical treatment, the understanding of these concepts is still being refined. Over the past 5 years, understanding has improved significantly. These changes will be covered as they relate to the clinical and radiographic evaluation, currently used classification systems, recent modifications of surgical treatment, and the complications and expected outcomes of treatment.

Initial Evaluation

Clinical

The patient history focuses on the mechanism and timing of injury, as these provide clues to associated injuries and progression of swelling. Specific findings in the history noted to have an adverse effect on outcome include advanced age, osteoporosis, diabetes mellitus, peripheral vascular disease, female sex, and high American Society of Anesthesiologists (ASA) class.[2-4] The effect of obesity is controversial, as it has had differing effects depending on the study.[5,6] Social factors such as smoking, alcohol use, and lower levels of education have been noted as independent predictors of lower physical function postoperatively.[7] The presence of these findings should not prevent surgical treatment of unstable, displaced ankle fractures but instead should (1) allow for a more candid preoperative discussion regarding potential complications and outcome, (2) encourage more careful soft-tissue handling and attention

Dr. Graves or an immediate family member is a member of a speakers' bureau or has made paid presentations on behalf of Synthes or is a paid consultant for product development and has received research or institutional support from Synthes.

to construct stability, and (3) encourage treatment of modifiable risk factors during the perioperative period. The physical examination should include a neurovascular examination of the leg and focus on the soft tissue in line with proposed surgical incisions. Dislocations and subluxations should be reduced expediently to take pressure off of the skin and neurovascular bundle and prevent point loading of articular cartilage. This can be accomplished by using intra-articular analgesic injections, intravenous narcotics, or conscious sedation. A recent study compared the efficacy of an intra-articular block to conscious sedation for the closed reduction of ankle fracture-dislocations.[8] The intra-articular lidocaine block provided a similar degree of analgesia that was adequate for reduction, and a decreased time to reach the reduced, splinted position.

Radiographic

Plain radiographs are the standard imaging modality for the evaluation of ankle fractures. Quality imaging is essential and consists of the AP, mortise, and lateral radiographs. Each view provides insight into the pathoanatomy of the injury complex. Classic studies have shown that reproducible radiographic measurements can be used to quantify the extent of injury and help predict clinical outcome.[9,10]

The AP view is defined by placing the long axis of the foot in the true vertical position. In addition to viewing the cortical margins of the malleoli and the talus, it is necessary to evaluate the relationship between the talus and the distal tibial subchondral surface. The tibiotalar joint space should be symmetric with no signs of talar tilt. Markers for syndesmotic injury include the tibiofibular overlap and the tibiofibular clear space (**Figure 1, A**).

The mortise view is defined by internally rotating the leg so that the medial and lateral malleoli are parallel to the tabletop. This typically requires approximately 10° of internal rotation of the fifth metatarsal with respect to the vertical position.[11] This rotation is required because the coronal plane of the ankle joint is externally rotated with respect to the coronal plane of the knee joint. It provides the true AP view of the tibiotalar articulation. In addition to evaluating cortical margins and the tibiotalar joint space, specific radiographic parameters should be noted (**Figure 1, B**). The tibiofibular overlap is also used in this view to evaluate syndesmotic injury. The medial clear space is considered to be representative of the status of the deep deltoid liga-

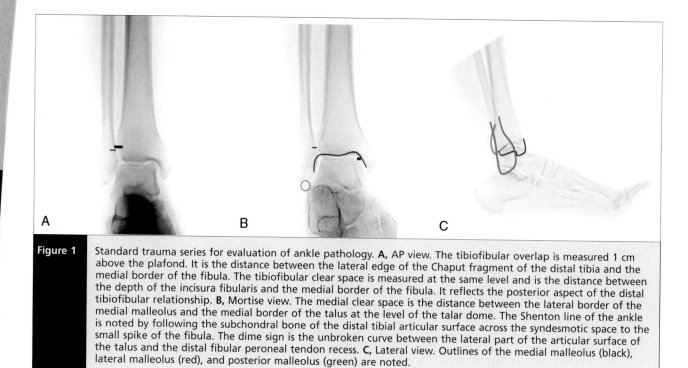

Figure 1 Standard trauma series for evaluation of ankle pathology. **A,** AP view. The tibiofibular overlap is measured 1 cm above the plafond. It is the distance between the lateral edge of the Chaput fragment of the distal tibia and the medial border of the fibula. The tibiofibular clear space is measured at the same level and is the distance between the depth of the incisura fibularis and the medial border of the fibula. It reflects the posterior aspect of the distal tibiofibular relationship. **B,** Mortise view. The medial clear space is the distance between the lateral border of the medial malleolus and the medial border of the talus at the level of the talar dome. The Shenton line of the ankle is noted by following the subchondral bone of the distal tibial articular surface across the syndesmotic space to the small spike of the fibula. The dime sign is the unbroken curve between the lateral part of the articular surface of the talus and the distal fibular peroneal tendon recess. **C,** Lateral view. Outlines of the medial malleolus (black), lateral malleolus (red), and posterior malleolus (green) are noted.

ment. Markers for fibular length include the talocrural angle, the Shenton line of the ankle, and the dime sign.[12,13]

The lateral view is defined by placing the radiographic beam perpendicular to the long axis of the ankle joint (**Figure 1, C**). It provides for evaluation of the cortical margins of the malleoli, with improved visualization of the posterior malleolus. The tibiotalar joint space should be symmetric with no signs of talar subluxation. The relationship of the posterior border of the distal fibula to the tibia provides information regarding syndesmotic competency. Associated or occult injuries are also noted, including fractures of the lateral process of the talus, posterior tubercle of the talus, and anterior process of the calcaneus.

The indications for additional imaging modalities such as CT and MRI are unclear. CT has provided for an improved understanding of posterior malleolar fracture patterns, articular impaction, and syndesmotic reduction.[14-17] MRI has been used to evaluate the competency of the syndesmosis and deep deltoid ligament, as well as to better view osteochondral talar lesions associated with ankle fractures.[18-20]

Classification

Danis and Weber/AO

The Danis and Weber/AO classification of malleolar fractures focuses on the height of the fibular fracture (**Figure 2**). The rationale is based on the relationship between the height of the fibula fracture and the associated damage to the tibiofibular ligaments. The higher the fibula fracture, the more extensive the damage to the syndesmosis, and thus the greater degree of ankle joint instability. A recently published study has sup-

ported the reproducibility of this classification system, revealing substantial interobserver and intraobserver agreement using an AP and lateral view of the ankle.[21] Although this classification system still is commonly used, some have taken issue with prioritizing the fibula in evaluation of ankle joint stability, as many recent studies have convincingly established the primacy of the deep deltoid and medial malleolus in determining ankle joint stability.[22] In addition to this, an MRI study has recently questioned the relationship of the level of fibula fracture to the integrity of the interosseous membrane.[18]

Lauge-Hansen

The Lauge-Hansen classification system is an extensive mechanistic system based on a cadaver study that attempted to improve the understanding of ankle fracture patterns.[23] The first word in the classification system refers to the position of the foot at the time of injury; the second word refers to the direction of the deforming force (**Figure 2**). The system is imperfect. All ankle fractures do not fit neatly into the different classes. The proposed mechanism of injury has been refuted and the interobserver and intraobserver reliability have been questioned; nevertheless, the system is still commonly used.[24,25] Much of the recent literature devoted to ankle fractures has used the Lauge-Hansen system; recent treatment advances will therefore be described with respect to this system.

Treatment Advances

Supination-Eversion

Supination-eversion (also called supination-external rotation) ankle fractures are the most common type seen

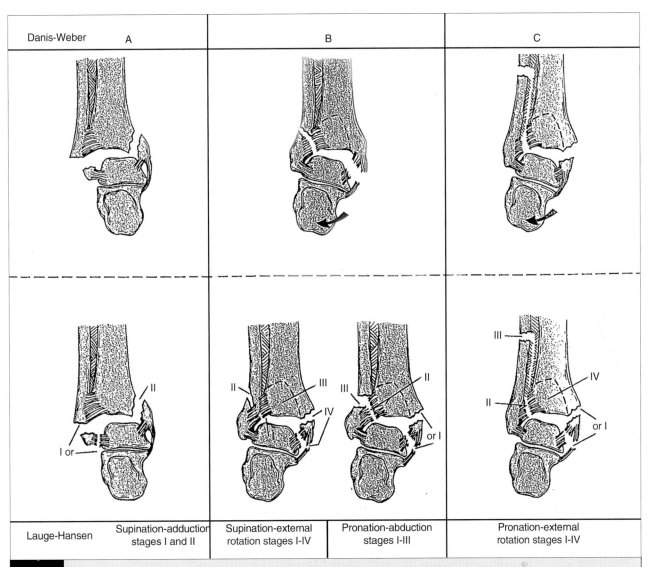

Danis-Weber	A	B	C

| Lauge-Hansen | Supination-adduction stages I and II | Supination-external rotation stages I-IV | Pronation-abduction stages I-III | Pronation-external rotation stages I-IV |

Figure 2 The Danis and Weber and Lauge-Hansen classification systems of ankle fractures. (Reproduced with permission from Carr JB, Trafton PG: Malleolar fractures and soft tissue injuries of the ankle, in Browner BD, Jupiter JB, Levine AM, Trafton PG: *Skeletal Trauma*, ed 2. Philadelphia, PA, WB Saunders, 1998, pp 2327-2404.)

clinically, accounting for nearly 70% of all malleolar fractures. The fibular fracture pattern is oblique and oriented from posterosuperior to anteroinferior, typically at the level of the syndesmotic ligaments (Weber B). If there is no associated medial injury, the ankle mortise is thought to be stable, with closed treatment leading to successful long-term outcomes.[26] If there is an associated medial malleolar fracture, the ankle mortise is thought to be unstable, and surgical fixation is the treatment of choice.

Recent literature has centered on the determination of instability in the absence of a medial malleolar fracture. Historically, clinical signs and symptoms have been used as a correlate for deep deltoid instability. The presence of these findings, in addition to a radiograph revealing the typical fibular fracture pattern, led to surgical management. More recently, findings such as medial tenderness, medial swelling, and medial ecchymosis have been identified as inaccurate predictors of instability.[27,28] These soft-tissue findings can be present secondary to superficial deltoid injury in the absence of deep deltoid compromise. Because of this, radiographic stress examinations have been used to more accurately demonstrate dynamic instability that is not apparent on static radiographs. With the applied stress, a mortise radiographic view is used and the medial clear space is evaluated for widening. This widening represents talar subluxation and is evidence of deep deltoid instability (**Figure 3**). Both the gravity stress view and the manual stress view have been proposed for differentiating between supination-eversion type II and ligamentous supination-eversion type IV fractures.[27-29] Although both views seem to be reliable, the gravity stress view requires less radiation exposure for the surgeon and has been perceived as more comfortable for the patient.[30] Most recently, the assumption that a positive ankle

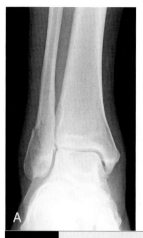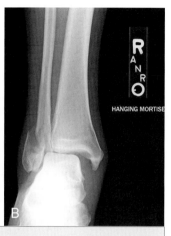

Figure 3 Evaluation of the medial clear space in the presence of an isolated fibular fracture. **A,** Mortise view of ankle fracture without stress. **B,** Mortise view of ankle fracture with stress. Widening of the medial clear space reveals a nonfunctional deep deltoid ligament and ankle joint instability.

stress test represents a complete deep deltoid transection has been questioned.[20] In this study, MRI was used as a decision tool in the treatment of ankle fractures. Patients with a positive stress test after an isolated Weber B lateral malleolus fracture were further evaluated using MRI to determine the status of the deep deltoid. If the deep deltoid is partially intact, the extremity was placed in a walking boot and weight bearing with ambulation was allowed as tolerated. At short-term follow-up, there was no evidence of residual medial clear space widening, posttraumatic arthrosis, or poor outcomes in this group. Further work will be necessary to clearly define the role of MRI as a decision-making tool in the treatment of ankle fractures.

Controversy also exists as to the ideal type of lateral malleolar fixation in this fracture pattern. Lag screw fixation has been efficacious in noncomminuted oblique fractures in patients younger than 50 years, when the fracture was long enough to accept two lag screws at least 1 cm apart.[31] Smaller incisions and fewer reports of hardware prominence were noted. More commonly, the implant decision is between the dorsal antiglide plate and the lateral neutralization plate. Although dorsal plating provides the potential advantages of improved biomechanical strength, less soft-tissue dissection, less palpable hardware, and longer screw placement, it provides the potential disadvantage of peroneal tendon irritation.[32,33] Lateral neutralization plating provides the potential advantage of avoidance of the peroneal tendons. To date, no clinical study comparing the two techniques has statistically shown one to be superior.[34]

To summarize, isolated oblique Weber B lateral malleolar fractures can be treated nonsurgically with the expectation of a good outcome. When this form of fibula fracture is associated with a medial malleolar fracture, surgical treatment is recommended to reduce and

stabilize the ankle mortise. In the absence of a medial malleolar fracture, evidence of deep deltoid incompetence can be reached through stress views by examining the medial clear space. If instability is present, surgical treatment is recommended. Syndesmotic stability should always be examined via a stress examination while visualizing the tibiofibular clear space and tibiofibular overlap after fixing other components of the injury.

Supination-Adduction
Supination-adduction ankle fractures are characterized by a transverse, tension-based fibula fracture below the level of the syndesmotic ligaments (Weber A level) with an associated vertical medial malleolar fracture. Because the medial-sided injury is compression based, articular impaction is often present at the anteromedial corner of the tibial plafond. Evidence of this associated marginal impaction was noted in early descriptions of the Weber A fracture, and highlighted in a more recent case series of supination-adduction ankle fractures.[16]

Radiographic visualization of this impaction is noted at the medial gutter on the AP and/or mortise view and at the anterior aspect of the plafond on the lateral view. Although cortical reduction reads are often used to ensure articular reduction in malleolar fractures, the associated impaction present in these injuries makes this technique less than ideal. Because of this, an anteromedial approach that allows direct visualization of the articular surface is a logical choice with this fracture pattern. Reduction of the articular surface with possible grafting of the impaction defect is possible. Stabilization of this medial reduction can take many forms. A recent biomechanical study revealed that a properly applied buttress plate offers a significant mechanical advantage over screw-only constructs. This advantage must be weighed against the disadvantages of greater soft-tissue dissection and more prominent hardware.[35]

Pronation-Abduction
Pronation-abduction fractures are characterized by a tension-based medial-sided injury (deltoid disruption and/or transverse medial malleolar fracture) in association with a compression-based, comminuted Weber B fibula fracture. More severe pronation-abduction injuries often present with transverse medial tension failure soft tissue injuries with extrusion of the plafond. As in the supination-adduction variant of ankle fractures, the compression gutter should be evaluated for plafond impaction. In the pronation-abduction pattern, the compression gutter is the anterolateral corner of the tibial plafond. Because of the primacy of the medial side of the ankle in controlling talar displacement—and the simple transverse fracture noted on the medial side with this pattern—it is logical to fix the medial malleolus first if a fracture is present. Through the pull of the deep deltoid, the talus typically returns to its anatomic position in the mortise and indirectly reduces the fibula via the intact lateral ligamentous complex. Extraperiosteal plating is then possible, decreasing the risk of

fibular nonunion associated with excessive soft-tissue dissection.[36] If length is not adequately restored indirectly through the pull of the lateral ligamentous complex, direct manipulation of the distal fragment and a length-stable fibular construct is required. A stress examination of the syndesmosis is then completed, with fixation recommended if instability is noted upon visualization of the distal tibiofibular clear space and overlap.

Pronation-External Rotation

Pronation-external rotation injuries are the most unstable of all ankle fracture patterns. Pathoanatomy begins on the medial side with a deltoid disruption and/or a medial malleolar fracture. After disrupting the anterior inferior tibiofibular ligament, a Weber C fibula fracture takes the form of a spiral or oblique pattern. Posterior malleolar injuries are occasionally noted. A syndesmotic disruption is present until proven otherwise and should be addressed if any instability is present. Treatment requires an anatomic reduction of the malleolar fractures and the syndesmotic disruption. Outcomes are generally not as good as with other malleolar fracture patterns. These deficiencies are likely related to problems with the distal tibiofibular syndesmosis. This specific injury component requires further discussion.

Specific Fracture Components Requiring Further Delineation

Distal Tibiofibular Syndesmosis

The distal tibiofibular syndesmosis is a fibrous articulation connecting the tibia and fibula that consists of five parts: (1) interosseous membrane, (2) interosseous ligament, (3) anterior inferior tibiofibular ligament, (4) posterior inferior tibiofibular ligament, and (5) inferior transverse tibiofibular ligament. It functions to resist external rotation, axial translation, and lateral translation of the talus. The mechanism of injury is typically severe external rotation of the ankle and foot relative to the position of the tibia. Clinical signs and symptoms of injury include ecchymosis proximal to the ankle joint, pain over the anterior inferior tibiofibular ligament, pain created while squeezing the tibia and fibula together ("squeeze test"), and pain with an external rotation stress test. Classic radiographic signs of injury on the AP view include a tibiofibular clear space of greater than 5 mm and a tibiofibular overlap of less than 10 mm. On the mortise radiograph, a tibiofibular overlap of less than 1 mm is suggested to be pathologic.[10] These numbers have been questioned in multiple studies, as there is considerable variability in the absolute values among uninjured patients as well as variability within the same patient based on radiographic positioning. Radiographic subtleties can be clarified with stress views. Standard stress mechanisms include an external rotation stress view or directly manipulating the fibula intraoperatively (after fixation) via a clamp.

If instability is present, surgical treatment is recommended. Obtaining and maintaining an accurate reduction improves Short Musculoskeletal Functional Assess-

ment Index scores.[37] The understanding of what constitutes an accurate reduction is changing. A recent study using axial CT to evaluate reduction after standard fixation techniques noted that radiographic measurements did not accurately reflect the status of the syndesmotic reduction.[17] Alternative techniques such as open visualization of the syndesmosis and radiographic imaging in multiple planes have been described to improve reduction.[38,39] Assuming an accurate reduction has been established, there is little consensus as to what is necessary to maintain that reduction. There is general agreement that weight bearing should be delayed and syndesmotic fixation should remain in place for at least 3 months. There is no general agreement on the use of 3.5- or 4.5-mm screws, one screw or two, tricortical screws or quadricortical screws, or screw removal over leaving the screw in place.

Posterior Malleolus

The posterior malleolus has three important functions: resisting posterior translation of the talus, enhancing syndesmotic stability through the attachment of the posterior inferior tibiofibular and inferior transverse tibiofibular ligaments, and distributing weight-bearing forces by increasing the surface area of the ankle joint. The classic indication for fixation is based on size. Measurements are made on the lateral radiograph, with fragments greater than 25% of the articular surface requiring surgical treatment.[40] This indication has been questioned, as posterior malleolar fracture patterns are variable and rarely oriented purely in the coronal plane. A recent CT study clarified the typical pathoanatomy of the posterior malleolus and divided fracture patterns into three basic types (**Figure 4**). Because of fracture pattern variability, the authors encouraged preoperative CT to assist with surgical planning. Clearer surgical indications revolve around the function of the posterior malleolus. Dynamic intraoperative stress radiographs allow testing of posterior talar translation and syndesmotic stability after the remainder of the osseous ankle pathology has been stabilized. Decision making based on distributing weight-bearing forces is more complicated. Biomechanical studies reveal changes in peak pressure distribution with larger fragments that could potentially lead to posttraumatic arthrosis, but guidelines for treatment based on these studies are lacking. If surgical stabilization is chosen, visualization of the reduction can be enhanced radiographically via the external rotation lateral view and clinically via a posterolateral approach exploiting the interval between the flexor hallucis longus and the peroneal tendons.[41] Occasionally an adjunctive posteromedial approach is helpful.[15]

When a posterior malleolar fracture is combined with a lateral malleolar fracture, the order of fixation should be considered. Advantages of fixing the lateral malleolus before the posterior malleolus include indirectly improving the reduction of the posterior malleolus via the posterior inferior tibiofibular ligament attachment, and allowing for dynamic intraoperative

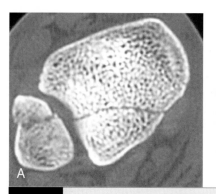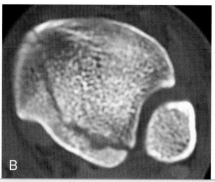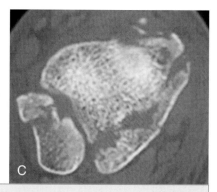

Figure 4   The three common patterns of posterior malleolar fractures. **A,** Posterolateral oblique type. **B,** Medial extension type. **C,** Small shell type. (Reproduced with permission from Haraguchi N, Haruyama H, Toga H, Kato F: Pathoanatomy of posterior malleolar fractures of the ankle. *J Bone Joint Surg Am* 2006;88:1085-1092.)

stress radiographs that isolate the function of the posterior malleolus after all other ankle fracture components have been treated. A potential advantage of fixation of the posterior malleolus before the lateral malleolus includes improved visualization of the posterior malleolar reduction by looking through the displaced fibula fracture.

Fixation of the posterior malleolus takes one of three forms. The choice among the three forms revolves around the compromise between increasing stability and increasing exposure. Screws oriented from anterior to posterior (typically anteromedial to posterolateral secondary to the most common position of the posterior malleolar fragment and orientation of the fracture line) are a common method of fixation. The advantage is limiting the exposure to the fracture site; the consequence is fixation that relies on a limited number of screw threads in the posterior malleolar fragment. Screws oriented from posterior to anterior require an increased exposure at the fracture site, but provide the advantage of screw heads buttressing the malleolar fragment. Antiglide or buttress plating maximizes stability at the cost of a larger exposure of the posterior malleolar fragment. No single technique is proved to be superior; therefore, the choice should be made based on deliberate thought about the size of the posterior malleolar fragment and the pattern and degree of instability.

Isolated Medial Malleolar Fractures

Medial malleolar fractures typically occur as a component of bimalleolar or trimalleolar fractures, or in association with a distal tibiofibular syndesmotic disruption. The importance of regaining stability of the medial malleolus in these scenarios is rarely questioned. Other surgical indications include open fractures, a compromised skin envelope secondary to fragment displacement, articular dome impaction, and tendon subluxation into the fracture plane. In the absence of all of these findings, isolated medial malleolar fractures can be treated nonsurgically with the expectation of good functional results and lower extremity specific outcome scores most of the time.[42]

Outcomes and Complications

Local complications are varied and include wound healing problems, infection, nerve injury, intra-articular hardware, prominent hardware, complex regional pain syndrome, chronic swelling, hardware failure, malunion, nonunion, and posttraumatic arthrosis. Short-term outcomes are affected by comorbid conditions, social factors, and surgical technique.[3,7,43] As mentioned earlier in the discussion on initial evaluation, findings noted to have an adverse effect on outcome include advanced age, osteoporosis, diabetes mellitus, peripheral vascular disease, female sex, and high ASA class.[2-4] Social factors such as smoking, alcohol use, and lower levels of education have been noted as independent predictors of lower physical function postoperatively.[7] Although outcomes begin to stabilize at the 6-month mark postoperatively, recovery does continue up to 1 year.[3] In the absence of complications, patients are generally functioning well, with little pain and few restrictions at 1 year. Long-term outcomes are not always excellent. Fracture type and severity, complications during healing, and patient-related factors such as age are associated with the likelihood and timing of posttraumatic ankle arthritis.[44]

Diabetic Ankle Fractures

One particular comorbid condition deserves further discussion both for its frequency and treatment challenges. Diabetes mellitus is a common medical condition that is increasing in prevalence.[45] Both closed and open management of ankle fractures in diabetic patients are associated with higher complications rates.[46] Despite the higher complication rates with treatment, the indications and goals remain the same. Unstable ankle fractures in diabetic patients are best treated with anatomic restoration of the ankle mortise and stable internal fixation. Because the soft-tissue complication rate is higher, increased focus should be placed on using atraumatic soft-tissue techniques. Because the osseous complication rate is higher, increased focus should be placed on empowering fracture fixation constructs.

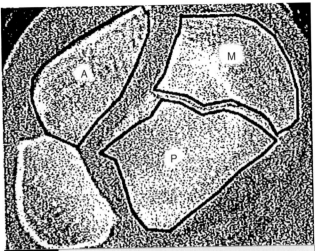

Figure 5 Primary fracture lines are outlined, creating common fragments in complete articular fractures. A is the anterolateral or Chaput fragment. M denotes the medial malleolar fragment. P is the posterior malleolar or Volkmann fragment. The size of the common fragments varies and additional articular pieces are created via secondary fracture lines. Reproduced from Topliss CJ, Jackson M, Atkins RM: Anatomy of pilon fractures of the distal tibia. *J Bone Joint Surg* 2005;87:692-697.

Postoperative care varies in that non–weight-bearing status is typically prolonged, and protected weight bearing takes a longer course.[45]

Tibial Plafond Fractures

Although ankle fractures typically occur from lower energy rotational mechanisms, have minor articular damage, are surrounded by a reasonable soft-tissue envelope, and have a low complication rate with surgical treatment, tibial plafond fractures are very different. The difference is related to the energy and direction of the mechanism of injury. Tibial plafond fractures typically occur from higher energy mechanisms with a component of axial load, have significant articular damage in the weight-bearing zone, are surrounded by more compromised soft-tissue envelopes, and present a historically high complication rate with surgical treatment. Because of these differences, tibial plafond fractures must be approached with an understanding of the small margin for error and a great respect for the complication profile.

Emergency Department Evaluation: Clinical and Radiographic

Clinical evaluation begins with a search for associated systemic injuries. The level of energy associated with these injury mechanisms demands a thorough patient evaluation. Associated musculoskeletal injuries include those created by axial load, such as fractures of the calcaneus, tibial plateau, supracondylar femur, femoral

neck, acetabulum, and spine. The lower extremity should be evaluated for neurologic or vascular compromise and signs of compartment syndrome. Recent evidence suggests that abnormalities of the arterial tree of the distal leg are noted in a significant percentage of high-energy tibial plafond fractures.[47] Despite this finding, the routine use of CT angiograms is not currently recommended. Specific attention should be placed on the soft-tissue envelope surrounding the ankle joint. Energy is manifested via swelling, abrasions, ecchymosis, fracture blister formation, and open wounds. Subluxations and dislocations should be urgently reduced in the emergency department. The initial reduction should be maintained with the use of a well-padded splint to alleviate pressure on the skin from displaced fragments and decrease the secondary injury created by fragment instability.

Initial radiographic evaluation includes AP, mortise, and lateral views of the ankle. High-quality radiographs provide clear evidence of the pattern of instability and the requisite forces that must be negated with the fixation construct, but are typically inadequate to provide a clear understanding of the articular injury. Because of this, additional imaging studies are common. CT provides useful information that often alters surgical decision making.[48] The timing of CT is variable and depends on the injury characteristics and the treatment plan. In complex articular injuries with axial instability, the information provided from CT scans is most useful after the ligamentotaxis provided by spanning external fixation.

Classification

Ruedi and Allgöwer System and the AO/OTA System
Multiple classification systems have been developed for tibial plafond fractures. The two most widely used are the Ruedi and Allgöwer system and the AO/OTA system. The Ruedi and Allgöwer system differentiates pilon fractures based on the presence of articular displacement and the degree of articular comminution. The AO/OTA system is first based on the degree of continuity of the articular surface to the tibial shaft, creating a division between extra-articular, partial articular, and complete articular fractures. Further subdivisions relate to the degree of fragmentation noted in the metaphyseal and articular regions. Problems have been noted with interobserver agreement beyond the initial division of the classification system.[49]

Articular Surface
Although the previously mentioned classification systems differentiate between pilon fractures based on the degree of articular comminution, they do not denote the commonly encountered articular fracture lines. Although the articular fracture pattern varies from case to case, typical fragments and primary fracture lines are present (**Figure 5**). The primary fracture line begins at the anterolateral portion of the articular surface at the level of the distal tibiofibular joint. This fracture line extends medially and splits near the central portion of

the plafond, exiting anteriorly and posteriorly. This creates three typical fragments in complete articular fractures: a medial malleolar fragment, a posterior malleolar (Volkmann) fragment, and an anterolateral joint (Chaput) fragment. Variability in the size of these fragments and further articular comminution is created via secondary fracture lines. In addition to noting the size and position of the typical articular fragments, care should be taken to evaluate articular impaction. Impaction occurs in both complete articular and partial articular fractures. In partial articular fractures, the talus acts as a pestle during axial loading, impinging on the leading edge of the intact articular surface before escaping through the fractured fragments.

Evolution of Treatment

Immediate Open Reduction and Internal Fixation

Because of the inconsistent and often poor outcomes associated with closed treatment of these complex injuries, other treatment options were evaluated. With the advent of improved instrumentation and surgical technique, a classic study described the fundamental principles of surgical management. These principles included reconstruction of the fibula, primarily in simple fibular fracture patterns and secondarily in complex fibular fracture patterns; anatomic reconstruction of the tibial articular surface; cancellous grafting of defects resulting from the reduction of impacted pieces; and plate osteosynthesis via the medial aspect of the tibia. These principles required atraumatic surgical technique and allowed for early, active pain-free mobilization. Following these principles led to remarkable results, with 75% of the patients in the series being pain free with good functional outcomes.[50]

Multiple series of patients treated with immediate open reduction and internal fixation (ORIF) in the United States showed equally remarkable but very different results.[51-53] Wound dehiscence, postsurgical infections, and hardware failure were commonly noted after ORIF of Ruedi and Allgöwer type III fractures. It was postulated that the difference in results was related to the energy associated with the injury and the experience of the operating surgeons. Most patients in the Swiss series[50] were injured during lower energy skiing accidents, whereas most in the North American series[51-53] were injured via higher energy mechanisms such as falls from heights, motor vehicle collisions, and motorcycle crashes. The system of health care also differed with fewer, more experienced surgeons treating pilon fractures in the Swiss series. This high complication rate led to a change in management techniques and management principles. If an anatomic reduction and stable fixation without soft-tissue compromise could not be predicted based on the injury pattern, alternative methods of treatment were chosen. The complication profile began to drive surgical decision making.

External Fixation With/Without Limited ORIF

With the goal of preventing major complications, external fixation began to replace ORIF as the definitive treatment modality for complex pilon fractures.[54,55] Avoiding or limiting surgical approaches logically limited wound complications; it also limited the surgeon's ability to directly see the articular surface and achieve an anatomic reduction. Another compromise included the inability to allow for postoperative motion with joint-spanning, nonhinged frames. Further experience with the technique led to improved radiographic reductions. Alternative frame types (joint-spanning articulated frames and hybrid frames that did not span the joint) were popularized because they allowed for earlier ankle motion.[56] Despite the improvements, many surgeons still thought that the technique did not consistently allow for the same quality of reduction that could be achieved with direct visualization through an open approach. Different management strategies were developed in an attempt to limit the compromises created by avoiding open approaches.

Staged ORIF

Staged surgical management strategies were developed to maximize the advantages of an open approach while minimizing the disadvantages.[57,58] Temporizing joint-spanning external fixation in axially unstable fractures decreased the secondary soft-tissue trauma created by fragment instability. Additionally it allowed for improved initial pain control via increased stability, improved provisional reductions via ligamentotaxis, and improved soft-tissue evaluation by eliminating the need for splinting. After the initial stage of treatment, time was allowed for restoration of healthy soft tissue. Although not preventing the need for careful soft-tissue handling, the delay provided a larger margin of error for the definitive surgical treatment.

Currently, open approaches are described for anterolateral, anteromedial, medial, posteromedial, posterolateral, and lateral access. The choice of approach is related to many factors, including articular fracture pattern, metadiaphyseal fracture pattern, direction of talar displacement, soft-tissue quality, necessity of fibular fixation, and surgeon preference. If multiple approaches are used, maximizing the interval between the approaches is ideal. Despite this recommendation, incisions may be safely placed less than 7 cm apart if careful attention is given to soft-tissue technique and surgical timing.[59] Plate osteosynthesis through open approaches in a delayed fashion has substantially decreased wound healing complications and secondary surgical infections (**Figure 6**).

Complications and Determinants of Outcome

High-energy pilon fracture management has been fraught with complications. The injured soft-tissue envelope and traumatic surgical soft-tissue handling have led to wound-healing complications and subsequently deep infections. Comminuted metaphyseal areas with limited inherent stability and marginal muscle coverage have led to malunions and nonunions. Severe articular cartilage damage and unsuccessful articular reconstructive efforts have led to posttraumatic arthritis. The

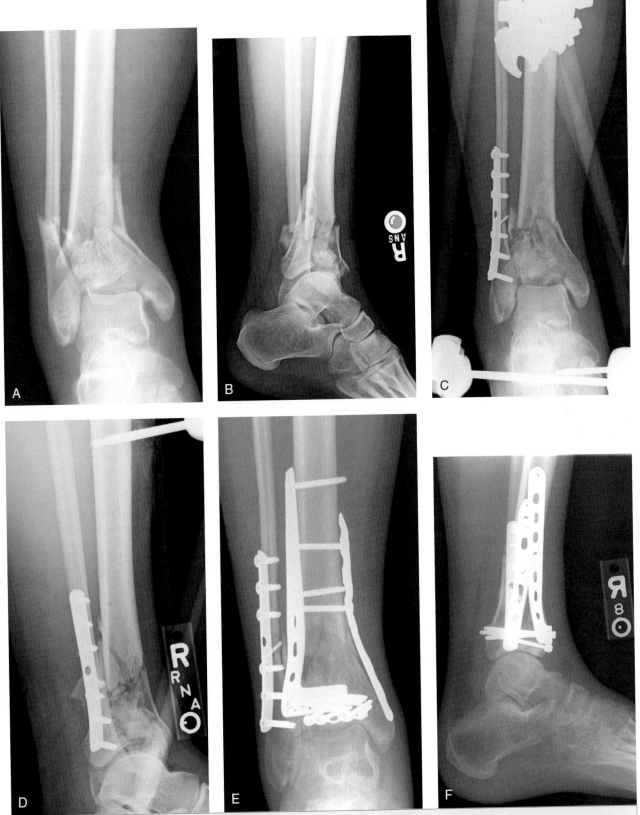

Figure 6   Staged management using initial spanning external fixation and fibular fixation followed by an interval for soft-tissue recovery before definitive treatment. **A** and **B,** Injury AP and lateral radiographs. **C** and **D,** AP and lateral radiographs following the first stage of management. **E** and **F,** Six-month follow-up radiographs after the definitive surgical treatment.

damage to the soft-tissue envelope created by the initial injury, surgical intervention, and joint immobilization has led to postoperative scarring and stiffness. The limited soft-tissue envelope and bulky implants have led to hardware prominence.

Changes in treatment techniques and implant design have decreased but not eliminated the incidence of complications. Staged management, improved soft-tissue handling, less extensile approaches, indirect reduction techniques, definitive external fixation, and lower profile plates have all likely played a role. Honest assessments of individual interest and capabilities as well as improvements in referral networks will likely continue to decrease the incidence of complications. Outcome instruments vary greatly and both clinician-based and patient-reported outcome instruments have been used to describe function after pilon fracture treatment. General health-related instruments have revealed that patients with pilon fractures continue to experience physical and psychosocial impairment long after the initial injury.[60-63] Patient-specific and fracture-specific variables are linked to the overall outcome. Preexisting medical comorbidities, male sex, work-related injuries, lower income levels, and lower education levels are noted to negatively affect scores.[60,62,63] The severity of the injury and the quality of the reduction have been correlated with the development of arthrosis, but not always with the clinical outcome.[60,63] Despite the high incidence of posttraumatic ankle arthritis, the rate of ankle arthrodesis remains low and patients continue to improve for many years after the index procedure.[63] Optimizing outcome requires achieving the best possible reduction in the absence of postoperative complications, with attention also placed on the recognition of and assistance with patient-specific variables.

Annotated References

1. Court-Brown CM, McBirnie J, Wilson G: Adult ankle fractures—an increasing problem? *Acta Orthop Scand* 1998;69(1):43-47.

2. Ganesh SP, Pietrobon R, Cecílio WA, Pan D, Lightdale N, Nunley JA: The impact of diabetes on patient outcomes after ankle fracture. *J Bone Joint Surg Am* 2005; 87(8):1712-1718.

3. Egol KA, Tejwani NC, Walsh MG, Capla EL, Koval KJ: Predictors of short-term functional outcome following ankle fracture surgery. *J Bone Joint Surg Am* 2006; 88(5):974-979.

4. SooHoo NF, Krenek L, Eagan MJ, Gurbani B, Ko CY, Zingmond DS: Complication rates following open reduction and internal fixation of ankle fractures. *J Bone Joint Surg Am* 2009;91(5):1042-1049.

   California's discharge database was queried for patients who had undergone ORIF of an ankle fracture over a 10-year period with complications reviewed and dis-cussed. Open injuries, diabetes, and peripheral vascular disease were strong risk factors for short-term complications. Level of evidence: II.

5. Böstman OM: Body-weight related to loss of reduction of fractures of the distal tibia and ankle. *J Bone Joint Surg Br* 1995;77(1):101-103.

6. Strauss EJ, Frank JB, Walsh M, Koval KJ, Egol KA: Does obesity influence the outcome after the operative treatment of ankle fractures? *J Bone Joint Surg Br* 2007; 89(6):794-798.

   The authors present a retrospective review evaluating the number of comorbidities, incidence of complications, time to fracture union, fracture type, and level of function between obese and nonobese patients with ankle fractures. At 2 years after surgery, obesity did not seem to have an effect on the incidence of complications, time to fracture union, or level of function.

7. Bhandari M, Sprague S, Hanson B, et al: Health-related quality of life following operative treatment of unstable ankle fractures: A prospective observational study. *J Orthop Trauma* 2004;18(6):338-345.

8. White BJ, Walsh M, Egol KA, Tejwani NC: Intra-articular block compared with conscious sedation for closed reduction of ankle fracture-dislocations: A prospective randomized trial. *J Bone Joint Surg Am* 2008; 90(4):731-734.

   The authors discuss a prospective, randomized trial comparing conscious sedation and intra-articular block for analgesia and the ability to allow for ankle fracture reduction and application of a splint. No difference in analgesia or allowance for reduction was noted. The intra-articular block allowed for a shorter average time for reduction and splinting. Level of evidence: I.

9. Joy G, Patzakis MJ, Harvey JP Jr: Precise evaluation of the reduction of severe ankle fractures. *J Bone Joint Surg Am* 1974;56(5):979-993.

10. Pettrone FA, Gail M, Pee D, Fitzpatrick T, Van Herpe LB: Quantitative criteria for prediction of the results after displaced fracture of the ankle. *J Bone Joint Surg Am* 1983;65(5):667-677.

11. Goergen TG, Danzig LA, Resnick D, Owen CA: Roentgenographic evaluation of the tibiotalar joint. *J Bone Joint Surg Am* 1977;59(7):874-877.

12. Weber BG, Simpson LA: Corrective lengthening osteotomy of the fibula. *Clin Orthop Relat Res* 1985;199:61-67.

13. Sarkisian JS, Cody GW: Closed treatment of ankle fractures: A new criterion for evaluation - a review of 250 cases. *J Trauma* 1976;16(4):323-326.

14. Haraguchi N, Haruyama H, Toga H, Kato F: Patho-anatomy of posterior malleolar fractures of the ankle. *J Bone Joint Surg Am* 2006;88(5):1085-1092.

15. Weber M: Trimalleolar fractures with impaction of the posteromedial tibial plafond: Implications for talar stability. *Foot Ankle Int* 2004;25(10):716-727.

16. McConnell T, Tornetta P III: Marginal plafond impaction in association with supination-adduction ankle fractures: A report of eight cases. *J Orthop Trauma* 2001;15(6):447-449.

17. Gardner MJ, Demetrakopoulos D, Briggs SM, Helfet DL, Lorich DG: Malreduction of the tibiofibular syndesmosis in ankle fractures. *Foot Ankle Int* 2006; 27(10):788-792.

18. Nielson JH, Gardner MJ, Peterson MG, et al: Radiographic measurements do not predict syndesmotic injury in ankle fractures: An MRI study. *Clin Orthop Relat Res* 2005;436:216-221.

19. Boraiah S, Paul O, Parker RJ, Miller AN, Hentel KD, Lorich DG: Osteochondral lesions of talus associated with ankle fractures. *Foot Ankle Int* 2009;30(6):481-485.

    In this retrospective case series, the incidence and effect of osteochondral lesions of the talus in ankle fractures that were surgically treated were evaluated. All patients were assessed preoperatively by MRI and functional outcome was measured at a minimum of 6 months using Foot and Ankle Outcome Scoring. Osteochondral lesions were noted in 17% of cases but showed no statistically significant effect on outcome. Level of evidence: IV.

20. Koval KJ, Egol KA, Cheung Y, Goodwin DW, Spratt KF: Does a positive ankle stress test indicate the need for operative treatment after lateral malleolus fracture? A preliminary report. *J Orthop Trauma* 2007;21(7): 449-455.

    The authors present a retrospective review of patients who had a positive ankle stress test after an isolated Weber B lateral malleolar fracture. An MRI was ordered to evaluate the status of the deep deltoid ligament. If the deep deltoid was partially torn, patients were treated nonsurgically. At a minimum 12-month follow-up, all fractures had united without evidence of medial clear space widening or posttraumatic arthritis.

21. Malek IA, Machani B, Mevcha AM, Hyder NH: Interobserver reliability and intra-observer reproducibility of the Weber classification of ankle fractures. *J Bone Joint Surg Br* 2006;88(9):1204-1206.

22. Michelson JD, Magid D, McHale K: Clinical utility of a stability-based ankle fracture classification system. *J Orthop Trauma* 2007;21(5):307-315.

    To test the hypothesis that ankle fracture prognosis is dependent on initial biomechanical stability, an alternative classification system created using stability-based treatment criteria was developed on the basis of a structured analysis of the ankle fracture literature. Results supported the hypothesis that a stability-based ankle classification system could be prognostic.

23. Lauge-Hansen N: Fractures of the ankle. II. Combined experimental-surgical and experimental-roentgenologic investigations. *Arch Surg* 1950;60(5):957-985.

24. Michelson J, Solocoff D, Waldman B, Kendell K, Ahn U: Ankle fractures: The Lauge-Hansen classification revisited. *Clin Orthop Relat Res* 1997;345:198-205.

25. Gardner MJ, Demetrakopoulos D, Briggs SM, Helfet DL, Lorich DG: The ability of the Lauge-Hansen classification to predict ligament injury and mechanism in ankle fractures: An MRI study. *J Orthop Trauma* 2006; 20(4):267-272.

26. Kristensen KD, Hansen T: Closed treatment of ankle fractures. Stage II supination-eversion fractures followed for 20 years. *Acta Orthop Scand* 1985;56(2): 107-109.

27. McConnell T, Creevy W, Tornetta P III: Stress examination of supination external rotation-type fibular fractures. *J Bone Joint Surg Am* 2004;86(10):2171-2178.

28. Egol KA, Amirtharajah M, Tejwani NC, Capla EL, Koval KJ: Ankle stress test for predicting the need for surgical fixation of isolated fibular fractures. *J Bone Joint Surg Am* 2004;86(11):2393-2398.

29. Michelson JD, Varner KE, Checcone M: Diagnosing deltoid injury in ankle fractures: the gravity stress view. *Clin Orthop Relat Res* 2001;387:178-182.

30. Schock HJ, Pinzur M, Manion L, Stover M: The use of gravity or manual-stress radiographs in the assessment of supination-external rotation fractures of the ankle. *J Bone Joint Surg Br* 2007;89(8):1055-1059.

    Gravity and manual stress tests were compared in supination-external rotation ankle fractures. Gravity stress was determined to be as reliable and perceived as more comfortable than manual stress.

31. Tornetta P III, Creevy W: Lag screw only fixation of the lateral malleolus. *J Orthop Trauma* 2001;15(2):119-121.

32. Weber M, Krause F: Peroneal tendon lesions caused by antiglide plates used for fixation of lateral malleolar fractures: The effect of plate and screw position. *Foot Ankle Int* 2005;26(4):281-285.

33. Schaffer JJ, Manoli A II: The antiglide plate for distal fibular fixation: A biomechanical comparison with fixation with a lateral plate. *J Bone Joint Surg Am* 1987; 69(4):596-604.

34. Lamontagne J, Blachut PA, Broekhuyse HM, O'Brien PJ, Meek RN: Surgical treatment of a displaced lateral malleolus fracture: The antiglide technique versus lateral plate fixation. *J Orthop Trauma* 2002;16(7):498-502.

35. Dumigan RM, Bronson DG, Early JS: Analysis of fixation methods for vertical shear fractures of the medial

malleolus. *J Orthop Trauma* 2006;20(10):687-691.

36. Siegel J, Tornetta P III: Extraperiosteal plating of pronation-abduction ankle fractures. *J Bone Joint Surg Am* 2007;89(2):276-281.

    A retrospective review of consecutive patient series managed with extraperiosteal plating of fibular fractures in pronation-abduction type injuries is presented. Extraperiosteal plating was found to be an effective method of stabilization that led to predictable union. Level of evidence: IV.

37. Weening B, Bhandari M: Predictors of functional outcome following transsyndesmotic screw fixation of ankle fractures. *J Orthop Trauma* 2005;19(2):102-108.

38. Candal-Couto JJ, Burrow D, Bromage S, Briggs PJ: Instability of the tibio-fibular syndesmosis: Have we been pulling in the wrong direction? *Injury* 2004;35(8):814-818.

39. Miller AN, Carroll EA, Parker RJ, Boraiah S, Helfet DL, Lorich DG: Direct visualization for syndesmotic stabilization of ankle fractures. *Foot Ankle Int* 2009;30(5):419-426.

    An established protocol for treatment of ankle fractures with syndesmotic injury was evaluated retrospectively. Patients who underwent stabilization of the syndesmosis with direct visualization were compared with historic control subjects who underwent indirect fluoroscopic syndesmotic visualization. Postoperative CT scans were obtained in all patients. Based on the definition of an anatomic syndesmotic reduction, malreductions were significantly decreased in the direct visualization group. Level of evidence: III.

40. Hartford JM, Gorczyca JT, McNamara JL, Mayor MB: Tibiotalar contact area: Contribution of posterior malleolus and deltoid ligament. *Clin Orthop Relat Res* 1995;320:182-187.

41. DeCoster TA: External rotation-lateral view of the ankle in the assessment of the posterior malleolus. *Foot Ankle Int* 2000;21(2):158.

42. Herscovici D Jr , Scaduto JM, Infante A: Conservative treatment of isolated fractures of the medial malleolus. *J Bone Joint Surg Br* 2007;89(1):89-93.

    Patients who had nonsurgical treatment of isolated medial malleolar fractures were evaluated retrospectively. High rates of union and good functional results were noted with nonsurgical treatment.

43. Mont MA, Sedlin ED, Weiner LS, Miller AR: Postoperative radiographs as predictors of clinical outcome in unstable ankle fractures. *J Orthop Trauma* 1992;6(3):352-357.

44. Horisberger M, Valderrabano V, Hintermann B: Posttraumatic ankle osteoarthritis after ankle-related fractures. *J Orthop Trauma* 2009;23(1):60-67.

    The etiologies, pathomechanisms, and predisposing factors that lead to the development and progression of posttraumatic ankle arthritis after ankle related fractures were analyzed in a retrospective cohort study. Fracture type and severity, occurrence of complications, and patient-related factors were associated with the latency time between injury and the development of arthritis.

45. Wukich DK, Kline AJ: The management of ankle fractures in patients with diabetes. *J Bone Joint Surg Am* 2008;90(7):1570-1578.

    This article discusses treatment options for ankle fractures in patients with diabetes, along with complications associated with diabetes.

46. Chaudhary SB, Liporace FA, Gandhi A, Donley BG, Pinzur MS, Lin SS: Complications of ankle fracture in patients with diabetes. *J Am Acad Orthop Surg* 2008;16(3):159-170.

    The authors discuss issues related to open or closed treatment of ankle fractures in patients with diabetes.

47. LeBus GF, Collinge C: Vascular abnormalities as assessed with CT angiography in high-energy tibial plafond fractures. *J Orthop Trauma* 2008;22(1):16-22.

    CT angiography was added to a routine staged treatment protocol for ORIF of tibial plafond fractures. In more than half of high-energy tibial plafond fractures, CT angiography identified significant abnormalities of the arterial tree of the distal leg.

48. Tornetta P III, Gorup J: Axial computed tomography of pilon fractures. *Clin Orthop Relat Res* 1996;323:273-276.

49. Swiontkowski MF, Sands AK, Agel J, Diab M, Schwappach JR, Kreder HJ: Interobserver variation in the AO/OTA fracture classification system for pilon fractures: Is there a problem? *J Orthop Trauma* 1997;11(7):467-470.

50. Ruedi T: Fractures of the lower end of the tibia into the ankle joint: Results 9 years after open reduction and internal fixation. *Injury* 1973;5(2):130-134.

51. Dillin L, Slabaugh P: Delayed wound healing, infection, and nonunion following open reduction and internal fixation of tibial plafond fractures. *J Trauma* 1986;26(12):1116-1119.

52. McFerran MA, Smith SW, Boulas HJ, Schwartz HS: Complications encountered in the treatment of pilon fractures. *J Orthop Trauma* 1992;6(2):195-200.

53. Teeny SM, Wiss DA: Open reduction and internal fixation of tibial plafond fractures: Variables contributing to poor results and complications. *Clin Orthop Relat Res* 1993;292:108-117.

54. Bonar SK, Marsh JL: Unilateral external fixation for severe pilon fractures. *Foot Ankle* 1993;14(2):57-64.

55. Bone L, Stegemann P, McNamara K, Seibel R: External fixation of severely comminuted and open tibial pilon

fractures. *Clin Orthop Relat Res* 1993;292:101-107.

56. Tornetta P III, Weiner L, Bergman M, et al: Pilon fractures: Treatment with combined internal and external fixation. *J Orthop Trauma* 1993;7(6):489-496.

57. Patterson MJ, Cole JD: Two-staged delayed open reduction and internal fixation of severe pilon fractures. *J Orthop Trauma* 1999;13(2):85-91.

58. Sirkin M, Sanders R, DiPasquale T, Herscovici D Jr: A staged protocol for soft tissue management in the treatment of complex pilon fractures. *J Orthop Trauma* 1999;13(2):78-84.

59. Howard JL, Agel J, Barei DP, Benirschke SK, Nork SE: A prospective study evaluating incision placement and wound healing for tibial plafond fractures. *J Orthop Trauma* 2008;22(5):299-305, discussion 305-306.

    The authors of a prospective observational cohort study tested the validity of the recommendation that a 7-cm skin bridge represents the minimum safe distance between surgical incisions in the treatment of tibial plafond fractures. With careful attention to soft- tissue management and surgical timing, incisions for tibial plafond fractures can be placed less than 7 cm apart.

60. Williams TM, Nepola JV, DeCoster TA, Hurwitz SR, Dirschl DR, Marsh JL: Factors affecting outcome in tibial plafond fractures. *Clin Orthop Relat Res* 2004;423:93-98.

61. Harris AM, Patterson BM, Sontich JK, Vallier HA: Results and outcomes after operative treatment of high-energy tibial plafond fractures. *Foot Ankle Int* 2006;27(4):256-265.

62. Pollak AN, McCarthy ML, Bess RS, Agel J, Swiontkowski MF: Outcomes after treatment of high-energy tibial plafond fractures. *J Bone Joint Surg Am* 2003;85(10):1893-1900.

63. Marsh JL, Weigel DP, Dirschl DR: Tibial plafond fractures. How do these ankles function over time? *J Bone Joint Surg Am* 2003;85(2):287-295.

4: Lower Extremity

Chapter 39

Foot Trauma

Brad J. Yoo, MD   Eric Giza, MD

4: Lower Extremity

Introduction

The human foot is a complex assembly of irregularly shaped bones interwoven with stout ligaments and muscle-tendon units. It represents a defining characteristic of the human species, enabling erect bipedal motion and releasing the upper extremities from the responsibilities of locomotion. The foot must be durable enough to withstand seemingly endless repetitive loads of up to seven times body weight. As further testament to its incredible design, the foot exhibits contradictory motion within the span of a single gait cycle. One moment, the foot is a rigid platform, serving as an effective lever to propel the body forward. Immediately afterward, the foot becomes flexible, yielding under the body's weight, dispersing load, and conforming to uneven walking surfaces.

The foot's versatile behavior is made possible through the intimate interactions of more than 28 asymmetrically-shaped bones and 31 articulations. The hindfoot, being most proximal to the ankle, consists of the talus and calcaneus. These two bones comprise most of the diarthrodial subtalar joint, which enables hindfoot supination and pronation. The midfoot consists of the navicular bone, three keystone-shaped cuneiforms, and the trapezoidal cuboid. These bones articulate via flat, relatively immobile rigid joints that form a Roman arch in the transverse plane. Like water under an arch, the space created by the arcade of the midfoot bones allows neurovascular and tendinous structures to pass underneath without being compressed by the body's weight. Most distally, the forefoot is composed of the metatarsals and phalanges. Motion via diarthrodial joints occurs at the metatarsophalangeal and interphalangeal articulations.

Flexibility is obtained through the ankle, subtalar, talonavicular, and metatarsophalaneal joints. To a lesser extent, the calcaneocuboid and the flat tarsometatarsal articulations of the fourth and fifth digits also require some mobility to allow for normal foot

mechanics. Other articulations, such as the naviculocuneiform joints or the tarsometatarsal joints of the first, second, and third columns, demand rigidity and often cause painful symptoms when instability is induced from fracture or ligament injury.

From a functional standpoint, the foot may be compared to a three-legged stool. The calcaneus, the great hallux, and the lesser metatarsal heads comprise each of the legs while the talus represents the seat. The tripod has stability only when the position of each of its legs are in their correct anatomic relationships. Shortening of the foot's medial column will create a cavus deformity. Shortening of the foot's lateral column will create a planovalgus deformity. The calcaneus, when fractured, will shorten and angulate. All components of the foot must be spatially oriented in their proper position in order for the foot to function properly. This crucial concept must be kept close in mind while reconstructing fractures of the foot. Advances in fracture fixation and the recognition of the importance of an anatomic reduction have helped to dramatically improve functional outcomes following injury.

Initial Evaluation

The foot remains a commonly overlooked aspect of the secondary musculoskeletal survey. Metatarsal and foot phalanx fractures remain as one of the most frequently unnoticed fractures during the initial evaluation. A high level of suspicion is the first step toward an accurate diagnosis and prevention of missed injuries. Evaluation begins with a detailed history of the traumatic event. The mechanism, magnitude, duration, and location of the traumatic event will raise the index of suspicion, prompt the examiner to inquire further, and aid in the diagnosis. A complete review of systems should include additional mitigating factors that may impact treatment. Identifying the presence of diabetes mellitus, previous bony or soft tissue injury, or existing arthritic conditions is helpful. The ambulatory status of the patient should be documented. Questions regarding current or previous nicotine use should not be neglected, as a positive history may influence surgical decision making. Occupational status and patient expectations are additional important pieces of information.

Patients frequently are vague with reports of foot pain. If the patient is cooperative during the interview, it is helpful to obtain specific information regarding the

Dr. Yoo or an immediate family member has received research or institutional support from the AO and Smith & Nephew. Dr. Giza or an immediate family member serves as a paid consultant to or is an employee of Arthrex and has received research or institutional support from the Orthopaedic Scientific Research Foundation.

point of maximal pain. Pain localized at the medial midfoot will increase the suspicion for a Lisfranc injury and simultaneously decrease concern for a lateral talar process or calcaneus fracture. Both feet and ankles should be completely exposed and visually inspected for swelling, ecchymoses, and deformity. Puncture wounds or lacerations should increase vigilance for the presence of open fractures. The web spaces are often overlooked and should be individually examined for skin injury, along with the posterior heel. Open fractures should be treated with sterile gauze dressing and the prompt administration of a first-generation cephalosporin and tetanus toxoid. It is generally not advisable to probe wounds or attempt débridement in the emergency department, especially if a formal inspection and surgical débridement are planned during surgical treatment. Formal wound cultures typically are not helpful unless obtained after thorough débridement and irrigation in a sterile environment. A detailed neurovascular examination must be performed. Vascular assessment is still possible if the patient is not awake. A cursory examination is not sufficient because subtle dysesthesias are frequently present despite the patient reporting "intact sensation."[1] These sensory disturbances can frequently result in postinjury neuropathic pain. All sensory nerves to the foot should be examined, including the deep peroneal, superficial peroneal, medial plantar, lateral plantar, sural, and saphenous nerves. Motor function also should be assessed. The dorsalis pedis and posterior tibial arteries should be palpated and the quality, cadence, and amplitude of the pulses documented. Ankle-brachial indices are objective measurements to evaluate the vascular competency of the limb compared with the contralateral side.

High-quality radiographs are obtained, preferably without the area being obscured by articles of clothing or plaster. It is crucial that orthogonal radiographs with true AP, oblique, and lateral projections include the joint above and the joint below the suspected injury. Based on plain radiographic findings, a CT scan may be obtained. Upon completion of the assessment, the foot and ankle are placed into a well-padded, durable splint to improve pain control and allow easy soft-tissue inspection if warranted.

Skin blistering has a correlation with the degree of soft-tissue shearing at the time of trauma.[2] Blisters may emerge immediately or over the course of hours, sometimes days. Two main subtypes of fracture blister have been identified (serous or hemorrhagic), based on the depth of dermal-epidermal injury. Proponents of the deroofing of blister skin argue that epithelialization of the blister bed is hastened with this technique. Those against deroofing of blisters argue that the intact blister skin serves as biologic dressing that keeps the blister bed sterile. Deroofing or application of silver-based topical ointments have been shown to confer no statistical difference in patient outcomes.[3] Surgery should be delayed until blister beds have been re-epithelialized, and incisions across unepithelialized or hemorrhagic blister beds should be avoided.[3]

Compartment syndrome of the foot is a frequently overlooked clinical entity. Suspicion should be especially heightened in the presence of a high-energy crushing event; however, isolated compartment syndromes of the foot without fracture have been reported. Some authors suggest that compartment syndrome develops in up to 10% of calcaneal fractures.[4] The presence of an open injury does not preclude compartment syndrome, as small fascial defects may not be sufficient to significantly alter compartment volume.[5] A missed compartment syndrome results in treatable "curly toes," and is associated with well-documented disabling sequelae such as toe clawing, stiffness, aching, weakness and atrophy, sensory disturbances, and fixed deformities of the forefoot.[6] Compartment syndrome is clinically challenging to diagnose because foot trauma is an especially painful event, and often patients are experiencing considerable discomfort even at rest. Despite this nebulous presentation, patients with compartment syndrome frequently describe a severe, relentless, burning pain involving the entire foot. The skin often is shiny and taut. Toe abduction and adduction specifically provoke compartments within the foot and help confirm the diagnosis. In one series, up to 85% of patients with foot compartment syndrome experienced pain with passive motion, making this the most sensitive clinical finding.[7] If pathologic pain, swelling, numbness, or vascular status worsen, the patient should be reassessed and invasive pressure monitoring performed if necessary. All nine foot compartments should be measured. The medial compartment is confluent with the deep posterior compartment of the leg. The calcaneal compartment is especially susceptible to involvement with calcaneal fractures. This compartment contains the quadratus plantae, the lateral plantar nerve, and occasionally the medial plantar nerve. This frequently overlooked compartment must be recognized as a possible offending factor, especially in the setting of a calcaneus fracture.[8] Surgical release is performed by way of a dorsal medial and dorsal lateral incision to decompress the four interossei and the deeper adductor compartment. A medial longitudinal incision will release the medial, calcaneal, superficial, and lateral compartments. Negative pressure dressings may aid with postoperative wound care, and delayed closure is performed in a staged manner as is typical for compartment syndromes elsewhere in the body.

Calcaneus Fractures

With the development of internal fixation principles the patient with calcaneus fracture is no longer incapacitated. Despite these advances, the definitive treatment of calcaneus fractures and the indications for surgical intervention remain controversial.[9-11]

Mechanism of Injury and Fracture Characteristics

Calcaneus fractures result from a complex interaction of axial, angulatory, and torsional loads. The injury mechanism can be likened to an axe cleaving a block of wood. The most lateral portion of the talar lateral process acts as the axe, with the critical angle of Gissane serving as the strike point. This latter region is more clearly defined as the dense cortical bone on the lateral superior calcaneal surface, just anterior to the posterior facet. The resulting fracture line travels anterolaterally and posteromedially. The anterolateral fracture exit point typically is at the critical angle of Gissane, but frequently may be located as anterior as the calcaneocuboid facet. The posteromedial fracture line exit point is posterior to the sustentaculum. As a result, two main fragments are created by the primary fracture line. The posterior fragment consists of the posterolateral tuberosity and portions of the posterior facet. The anterior fragment consists of the anterior process, the middle facet, and typically the most medial regions of the posterior facet.[12] Depending on the magnitude of injury, additional fracture lines may emanate from the strike point. These secondary fracture lines split the anterior process in the sagittal plane. Posterior-directed secondary fracture lines may cleave the posterior facet in a predominantly sagittal plane, creating a joint depression fracture pattern. In this scenario, a variable portion of the superolateral posterior facet is rotated distally and caudally into the trabeculae sparse region known as the neutral triangle. Both elevation and rotation of this fragment are required to properly reduce the posterior facet. The posterior-directed secondary fracture line may similarly travel in the coronal plane, cleaving the tuberosity in half when viewed from the lateral projection. A tongue-type injury can be identified by the presence of an intact cephalad tuberosity cortex that is confluent with portions of the posterior facet.[13] In this setting, tuberosity displacement is further exacerbated by the attachment of the gastrocnemius-soleus complex.

With the primary and secondary fracture lines thus formed, the calcaneus adopts a typical posture of vertical height loss, widening with lateral wall expulsion, length loss when viewed from the lateral projection, and varus positioning of the heel. There is commonly a separate medial sustentacular fragment of varying size, also termed the "constant fragment" because of the tendency of discovering this fragment in its correct anatomic relationship with the talus due to the competency of the talocalcaneal interosseous ligament. This fragment may be used as the starting point for reconstructive efforts. The pathologic posturing of the fractured calcaneus also causes the talus to rest in a more horizontal position, which eventually will result in tibiotalar impingement and the inability to dorsiflex the ankle.

If the energy absorbed is extreme, open fractures may result. The caudal extent of the sustentaculum is frequently the offender, piercing the medial soft tissues. A severe eversion moment of the foot at the time of axial load may precipitate further tension failure of the medial soft tissues. As expected, more severe open fractures are associated with high rates of osteomyelitis and wound complications.[14-16] These injury patterns should be approached with great caution.

Imaging

All patients with suspected calcaneus fractures should undergo a plain radiographic evaluation including high-quality AP, oblique, and lateral projections of the foot. The diagnosis is most evident on the lateral projection, which will demonstrate the degree of calcaneal compression quantified by the Bohler angle. The degree of height loss has prognostic implications, with a smaller Bohler angle correlating with poorer function outcomes.[17] Shortening of the calcaneus and degree of involvement of the posterior facet may also be appreciated with a lateral radiograph. The AP foot radiograph examines for anterior process fracture lines commonly oriented in the sagittal plane. A separate Harris axial heel view will depict the amount of varus tuberosity angulation, lateral wall displacement, and lateral tuberosity displacement. The degree of fibular abutment is also appreciated on this radiograph. Because calcaneal fractures are typically involved with high-energy events, additional imaging is warranted for concomitant injuries including the ipsilateral ankle, knee, or lumbar spine.

CT is frequently performed primarily before surgery. Each fracture line and fragment are clearly discernable. Axial sections define the size of the sustentacular fragment, extension to the calcaneocuboid facet, and the status of the posterior facet. Reformats in the lateral and coronal planes parallel the findings in the lateral and Harris axial views, respectively. Three-dimensional reformats may help the surgeon crystallize these multiple sequences as a readily comprehensible modeled simulation.

Classifications of CT are widely accepted, helping in preoperative identification of those patterns associated with poorer outcomes or more technically challenging surgery. The most common, the Sanders classification, uses the coronal plane reformats to identify the widest portion of the talar inferior facet. The number and location of posterior facet fracture lines have been demonstrated to correlate with outcomes following surgical fixation, with poorer outcome measures associated with more comminuted patterns.[17,18]

Decision Making for Treatment

Optimal treatment of calcaneus fractures remains controversial and varies according to each individual fracture and patient. Nonsurgical treatment is indicated for patients with nondisplaced fractures, those unable to tolerate surgery, and those unable to walk. Nonsurgical treatment should be considered for patients with documented psychiatric, organic brain, or substance abuse disorders because they may not comply with a postoperative weight-bearing protocol. Factors that affect the local microcirculation and threaten wound healing should be considered in the decision to treat surgically. Relative contraindications include a history of smoking, diabetes mellitus, or peripheral vascular disease.

Improved outcomes following surgical fixation are associated with smoking cessation, age younger than 40 years, and a simple fracture pattern found on CT. Surgically treated patients who have poor physiologic

4: Lower Extremity

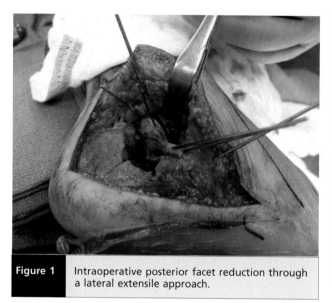

Figure 1 Intraoperative posterior facet reduction through a lateral extensile approach.

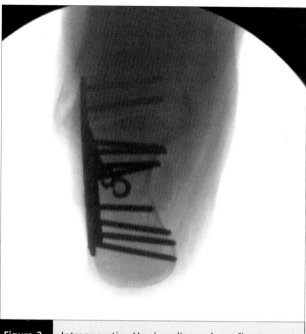

Figure 2 Intraoperative Harris radiograph confirms restoration of heel alignment as well as length and position of screw fixation.

status, a heavy physical workload, workers' compensation claims, comminuted fracture patterns, and those who smoke do not demonstrate statistically different functional outcome scores than those treated nonsurgically.[18] Women, males younger than 40 years, those patients with a light physical workload, or those with simple articular fracture patterns have a better prognosis with surgical intervention. Recent literature suggests that despite comminution of the posterior facet, open surgical treatment to restore calcaneal morphology will facilitate later fusion procedures. Patients treated with staged fusion had improved long-term functional outcome scores compared with patients initially treated without surgery and then with staged calcaneal osteotomy and fusion.[19]

Surgical Treatment

Most displaced intra-articular calcaneal fractures are treated with direct visualization and open reduction and internal fixation. Once the decision for surgical treatment has been made, the foot must achieve soft-tissue quiescence before incisions, which is indicated by the disappearance of turgidity from the lateral calcaneal soft tissue and the appearance of fine skin wrinkles. Generalized swelling should not be confused with the pathologically widened foot due to tuberosity displacement and angulation. Extreme tuberosity displacement can affect skin perfusion directly over the medial sustentaculum. Full-thickness ulcerations can result from this pressure-induced necrosis. Fracture blisters may be deroofed and treated with a dry bandage until epithelialization. Although typically on the medial side, some blisters may appear laterally. Planned incisions should avoid blister beds, especially hemorrhagic blisters. Incisions that cross these types of blister beds have demonstrated an increased risk of postoperative wound complications.[3] A perisurgical sciatic nerve blockade, an analgesic technique, has been correlated with a significant decrease in the amount of postoperative nar-

cotics required to achieve pain control and is a safe intervention because postoperative foot compartment syndrome in this setting is rare.[20]

Surgical intervention is typically performed as a lateral extensile approach.[16] The developed flap is nourished by branches of the lateral calcaneal artery. Injury to this feeding vessel during exposure may compromise the viability of the flap and increase the risk of apical flap necrosis.[21] Exposure of the lateral aspect of the calcaneus allows for direct reduction of the anterior process, the posterior facet, and the tuberosity (**Figure 1**). Key elements in the reduction are anatomic congruity of articular surfaces, especially the posterior facet; medialization and compression of the calcaneal tuberosity; restoration of calcaneal height (Bohler angle); and ensuring the three talocalcaneal articulations are aligned anatomically with respect to each other, thus enabling subtalar motion. Appropriate valgus positioning of the tuberosity may be confirmed with the use of Harris radiographs (**Figure 2**). The reduction may be held and compressed by any number of prefashioned calcaneal plates. Without these plates, effective internal fixation may be accomplished with a series of strategically placed small fragment plates. Screws may be directed toward regions with the highest bone density available: the sustentaculum, the subchondral region of the posterior facet, the superior anterior process, and the calcaneal tuberosity deep to the Achilles insertion. If screw purchase is ineffective or severe osteopenia is present, a locked implant may be considered. The clinical ramifications of using a mechanically stronger locked implant remains unclear and warrants further investigation.[13]

The use of bone graft or bone graft substitutes continues to be a source of debate when treating calcaneus

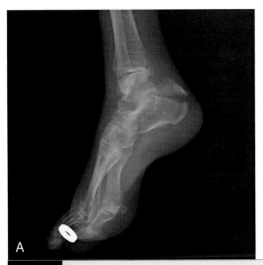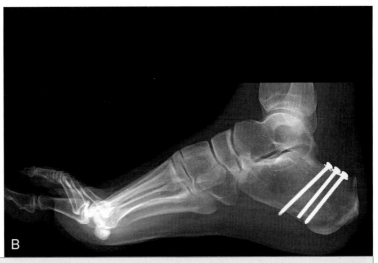

Figure 3	Displaced tongue-type fracture (**A**) with skin at risk over the posterior heel. Percutaneous fixation of the displaced tuberosity fragment (**B**).

fractures. The graft functions as a supplement to internal fixation, supporting the elevated posterior facet from below and as an osteoconductive matrix to facilitate bony ingrowth. In this regard, autograft bone has not been shown to improve functional outcome. Allograft bone may be used largely as scaffolding, with little supportive power. In contrast, injectable calcium phosphate cement as a fixation adjunct has been shown to permit early weight bearing without loss of the articular reduction. Though early weight bearing may be possible with these fractures, the literature does not demonstrate superior outcome scores with respect to the use of bone graft substitutes compared with allograft or no graft at all.

Wound closure is a crucial element in surgical treatment. The flap periosteum is annealed to the periosteum of the calcaneus. Placement of accurate sutures is crucial and is aided by the passage of all the sutures before knot-tying. A tension-free closure is then performed using a modified Allgöwer-Donati mattress suture. This technique has the least impact upon cutaneous blow flow compared with simple, vertical mattress, or horizontal mattress configurations.[22] A well-padded splint is applied with the ankle in neutral position to prevent equinus posture. After wound healing has been documented, the foot is placed in a removable orthosis and subtalar motion is initiated under the supervision of a physical therapist. Weight bearing may be initiated at the surgeon's discretion, typically once bony consolidation has occurred (between 6 to 12 weeks).

Results of Surgical Treatment

An investigation performed by the Evidence-based Orthopaedic Trauma Group examined the difference between surgically and nonsurgically treated calcaneal fractures. Level II data, two meta-analyses, and one economic analysis abstract determined no statistical difference existed with respect to pain and functional outcome.[17] Surgical treatment was considered superior to nonsurgical treatment concerning return to work and the ability to wear shoes of the same size before injury. When data were separated for subgroup analysis, a potential benefit was identified for women and young males, those patients with a single, simple displaced intra-articular fracture, and patients with light physical occupations. Arthrodesis rates were significantly reduced compared with nonsurgical treatment. From an economic perspective, surgical treatment was less costly than nonsurgical care. Potential benefits for nonsurgical treatment were seen in patients older than 50 years, those receiving workers' compensation, and those with demanding physical occupations. It was concluded that large, randomized, controlled trials are required to validate the conclusions generated by the subgroup analysis.[17]

Fractures Involving the Calcaneal Tuberosity

Depending on the nature of the axial load, a fracture line may allow cephalad and rotational migration of the calcaneal tuberosity. The fracture fragment may be purely extra-articular or involve extension into the posterior facet, a tongue type-fracture. Chronic tightness of the gastrocnemius-soleus complex may contribute to this pattern. Whether intra-articular or extra-articular, the displaced tuberosity segment is pulled proximally by the gastrocnemius-soleus tendon with a variable degree of rotation. This fracture pattern has the potential of tenting the posterior heel skin, leading to soft-tissue compromise. If this fracture is left without intervention, skin necrosis and subsequent open fracture status may result. A recent study evaluating 139 patients with tongue type fractures revealed that 21% of patients had some degree of posterior skin compromise at presentation. The authors concluded that early recognition of the threatened posterior skin and emergent treatment with percutaneous fixation effectively minimized progression to soft-tissue compromise[23] (**Figure 3**).

Talus Fractures

The talus articulates with the tibia, fibula, calcaneus, and navicular, and 60% of its surface is covered in cartilage. Talar body cartilage is thickest on the medial side and ranges from 0.8 to 2.0 mm on average. It thins at the proximal and distal portions of the curved dome. The talar radius of curvature is flattest in the center and matches the radius of curvature and cartilage thickness of the medial and lateral edges of the femoral trochlea.

The talus serves as a link to transmit load to the foot and absorbs up to six times body weight with each step. A recent study of 25 tali identified consistent sets of lamellae of the talus, including vertical plates from the posterior two thirds of the lateral part of the trochlear surface onto the posterior facet, and sagittal plates from the medial body extending through the neck in continuity with curved plates of the head.[22] Although the talus has no tendinous attachments, the unique bony architecture affords pronation-supination and dorsiflexion-plantar flexion through multiple facets and multiple ligament attachments. The body of the talus and the neck are not coaxial, with an average medial angulation of 24°.[23] Varus malposition of the talus by 2 mm can prevent hindfoot eversion by locking the transverse tarsal joints, which leads to forefoot adduction.[24]

Branches of the peroneal, posterior tibial, and anterior tibial arteries supply the talus, with most of the vascular supply from an anastomosis at the inferior talar neck. The extraosseous contributions of the surrounding arteries and tarsal canal are particularly important for healing. The artery of the tarsal canal, a branch of the posterior tibial artery, is considered the primary blood supply contributing to the lateral two thirds of the body.[25]

An anteromedial approach (between the tibialis anterior and posterior) and an anterolateral approach (lateral to the peroneus tertius) are often combined with a posterolateral approach (between the peroneal and Achilles tendons) to gain adequate exposure of the fracture. Understanding of the blood supply is important when considering exposure of the talus, and a medial or lateral malleolar osteotomy can improve visualization while minimizing soft-tissue dissection and disruption of the bloody supply.[26]

Plain AP, lateral, and oblique radiographs of the ankle as well as a Canale view (foot internally rotated 15° with the beam tilted 15° cephalad) are appropriate in the initial evaluation of a talus fracture. CT can add valuable information about fracture pattern and amount of preoperative comminution, and has been found to be the most accurate method to measure postoperative malunion and rotation.[24] A cadaver study demonstrated that posteromedial fractures of the talus could be reliably identified on plain radiographs by implementing a 30° external rotation view.[27]

Talar Neck Fractures

Fractures of the talar neck occur after dorsiflexion of the ankle. The pattern of comminution and articular involvement depends on the deforming force and position of the limb at the time of injury. The Hawkins classification continues to be the standard preoperative grading system that correlates with postoperative osteonecrosis of the talar body.[28,29] It has been suggested that delay in fixation of the fracture does not adversely affect outcome as much as the initial degree of displacement and association with an open injury.[30] Initial treatment includes reduction of the fracture, if displaced, via knee flexion, ankle plantar flexion, and ankle distraction. The reduced fracture should be placed in a well-padded splint with careful monitoring of the soft tissues. Open fractures require emergent surgical treatment.

Type I are nondisplaced, whereas type II are displaced fractures where the body stays reduced in the ankle mortise and the subtalar joint is dislocated. Type III fractures involve talar neck displacement with dislocation of both the ankle and subtalar joints. Type IV fractures are type III with a corresponding talonavicular dislocation.

Hawkins type I fractures can be treated nonsurgically but require strict adherence to no weight bearing and recurrent radiographs to ensure that displacement does not develop. Displaced fractures (types II through IV) require open fixation to restore talus anatomy and function. Union has been reported in 88% of fractures.[30] Fixation of the fracture depends on the fracture pattern and presence of comminution, which commonly occurs in the medial neck. Spanning plates are frequently necessary to maintain talar neck length and may be used as an adjunct to screw fixation.[31] Posterior to anterior screw fixation has improved strength over anterior screws alone.[32] However, posterior fixation can be technically difficult and adds another potential insult to the tenuous blood supply of the talus when combined with anteromedial/lateral incisions. A recent cadaver study demonstrated that a mini-blade plate combined with an anterior screw provided equivalent stability to posterior fixation.[33] Patients may begin range of motion if stable fixation was obtained postoperatively; however, strict adherence to no weight bearing is necessary until radiographic union is confirmed.

Functional outcomes following talar neck fractures vary and depend on the development of complications such as osteonecrosis, malunion, and arthritis of the tibiotalar and talocalcaneal joints. Posttraumatic arthritis is more common than osteonecrosis[30,34,35] (**Figure 4**). In one study of 70 patients, approximately half required secondary reconstructive procedures 10 years following fixation of talar neck fractures.[36] Rates of osteonecrosis range from 10% to 20% for Hawkins type I fractures, 20% to 50% for type II, and 60% to 100% for type III. A positive Hawkins sign is characterized by radiolucency of the subchondral bone in the talar body on mortise radiographs and represents localized osteopenia as bone resorption occurs during the revascu-

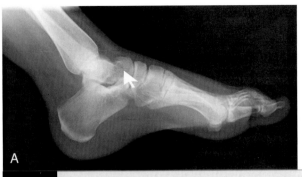
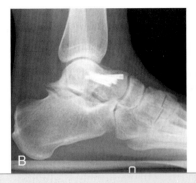
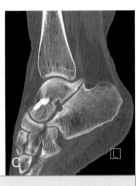

Figure 4   Displaced talar neck fracture (*arrow*) (**A**) that underwent open reduction and internal fixation and complete healing (**B**). Five years postoperatively, the patient complained of subtalar discomfort; a sagittal CT demonstrates progressive degenerative change (**C**).

larization and remodeling process. The prognostic reliability of the Hawkins sign was evaluated in 41 patients with displaced talar fractures, and was found to have a sensitivity of 100% and a specificity of 58%.[35] It most commonly appears between 6 and 9 weeks after fixation.[35]

Talar Body Fractures

Fractures of the talar body are uncommon and account for 13% to 23% of talus fractures. An anatomic reduction and fixation is necessary to lessen the potential for posttraumatic arthritis, which has been reported in 88% of patients.[37] Body fractures are often the result of high-energy trauma and cause caudal compression when the hindfoot is supinated or pronated.[38] Fracture patterns include coronal and sagittal split as well as articular crush. Specialized radiographs, such as a 30° external rotation view,[27] and CT are needed to identify the fracture pattern so that proper exposure can be planned via a medial, lateral, or posterior malleolar osteotomy.[39] Fixation with cannulated, headless screws can allow for solid fixation of the fracture fragments below the articular surface.

One study reported the retrospective results of 19 patients with displaced fractures of the talar body treated by internal fixation with an average follow-up of 26 months.[38] Results were excellent in four patients, good in six, fair in four, and poor in five. Complications included superficial wound problems, delayed union or malunion, and osteonecrosis in seven patients. It was concluded that talar body crush fractures and fractures associated with open injuries or talar neck fractures have a less favorable outcome.[38]

Lateral Process and Posteromedial Fractures

The lateral process of the talus forms the talofibular joint on its superolateral margin and the most lateral portion of the posterior subtalar facet on its inferolateral margin. Fractures of the lateral process of the talus most commonly occur from forced dorsiflexion and axial loading with eversion. According to one study, lateral process fractures represent 10.4% of all talus fractures at a level I trauma center.[40] The awareness of this

fracture type has grown along with the popularity of snowboarding, as it comprises 34% of ankle fractures in snowboarders. Type I involves a nonarticular fragment, type II involves the talofibular and subtalar joints, and type III involves comminution. The fracture can often be a source of chronic pain and is commonly misdiagnosed as an ankle sprain. The long-term sequelae of lateral process fractures include malunion, nonunion, and degenerative subtalar arthritis. CT is often necessary to visualize the entire fragment, but the fracture can sometimes be seen on an AP ankle radiograph. Nonsurgical treatment with limited weight bearing is recommended for nondisplaced fractures; however, surgical intervention with open reduction and internal fixation or excision of the fragment is suggested for displaced or large fractures.

One study evaluated the clinical and radiologic outcome after unilateral fracture of the lateral process of the talus in 23 snowboarders with a mean follow-up of 3.5 years treated either surgically or nonsurgically.[41] Subtalar osteoarthritis was present in 45% of patients; outcome after fracture of the lateral process of the talus in snowboarders is favorable with early diagnosis and prompt treatment.

Posteromedial fractures are often associated with high-energy trauma and medial subtalar dislocations. CT or an external rotation radiograph is usually needed to identify the amount of displacement.[27] Larger, displaced fragments require fixation via a direct posterior or medial malleolus osteotomy in order restore the articulations of the ankle and subtalar joint.

Subtalar Dislocations

Subtalar dislocations often result from high-energy injuries with the medial or lateral clinical appearance of the foot demonstrating the direction of the dislocation. Medial dislocation is more common and occurs via plantar flexion and inversion. Prevention of reduction results from buttonholing through the extensor digitorum brevis. Lateral dislocation occurs with plantar flexion and eversion, and prevention of reduction results from buttonholing through the medial talonavicular capsule and dorsal subluxation of the posterior tibial tendon. Plain radiographs will reveal the disloca-

4: Lower Extremity

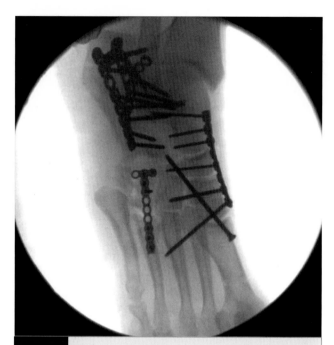

Figure 5 Radiograph showing a medial column plate for temporary stabilization of navicular dislocations.

tion, and early closed reduction is advised. Postreduction CT is advised to ensure joint congruency and to evaluate for subtalar debris or osteochondral injury. Up to 89% of patients will develop radiographic signs of subtalar arthritis.[42]

Fractures of the Tarsal Navicular

The tarsal navicular is a rectangular bone that articulates with the talar head, calcaneus, cuboid, and each cuneiform. On the concave side exists a synovial ball and socket joint with the talar head. This articulation is a major component of subtalar motion. This mobile region is contrasted by the relatively immobile planar naviculocuneiform articulations, a rigid complex that forms the midfoot arch. Fractures of the navicular may either be intra-articular body fractures, ligamentous avulsion fractures, or chronic stress fractures.

Acute fractures of the tarsal navicular body commonly occur after axial loading injuries to the medial column of the forefoot. Variable amounts of navicular articular impaction may be seen. Untreated subluxation and instability leads to abnormal contact stresses and the subsequent propensity for posttraumatic arthritis. Isolated talonavicular arthrosis is a particularly difficult condition to treat, as attempts at solitary fusion of this articulation are associated with high rates of nonunion. The resultant arthrodesis, if successful, significantly limits subtalar motion and imparts increased stress upon adjacent joints.

Navicular body fractures have been classified into three types. Type 1 fractures exist in the coronal plane, without resulting angulation of the forefoot. In type 2

fractures, the fracture line is from dorsolateral to plantar-medial and the forefoot is displaced medially. In type 3 injuries, there is sagittal plane comminution and the forefoot is displaced laterally. In type 3 fractures, which are increasingly observed following high-speed motor vehicle accidents, the head of the talus is forced in a plantar-lateral direction, resulting in talonavicular subluxation and instability. There is often impaction and comminution of the plantar-lateral navicular body, which contributes to further instability and joint incongruity. This classification system separates simpler patterns from more complex types. As expected, simpler fracture patterns and those patterns where anatomic reduction was possible were associated with high clinical outcome scores.[43]

If the patient is an acceptable surgical candidate, surgical fixation of displaced intra-articular navicular body fractures is indicated. Surgical goals include restoration of a congruous talonavicular articular surface and permission of early subtalar motion, if possible. Nondisplaced navicular fracture may be treated in a non–weight-bearing cast for 6 to 8 weeks. Simple fracture patterns may be treated with lag screw or plate fixation, confirming the articular reduction visually and radiographically. Temporary joint distraction with the use of an external fixator will permit better visualization of the articular surface. It is important to avoid exposing the complete cephalad surface of the navicular body for concern of jeopardizing the blood supply. Type 3 fractures are challenging to treat surgically. As mentioned previously, there is often joint impaction plantarly, which must be disimpacted to reestablish the normal arcade of the talar facet. The normal curvature of the tarsal navicular must not only be restored from a medial to lateral dimension, but also from a dorsal to plantar dimension. Unfortunately, the plantar-lateral comminution present in these injuries can be difficult to see. Often, the fragmentation is so extensive that internal fixation is impossible. Despite these surgical challenges, the instability must be addressed if the talar head remains persistently subluxated. In these instances, a temporary medial column plate may be applied. An 8- to 10-hole, 2.7-mm reconstruction plate with fixation points in the first metatarsal, cuneiforms, and talar head creates a medial column scaffold. Once appropriately reduced, screw fixation will permit a durable construct while bony and soft-tissue healing occurs[44] (**Figure 5**). Plate removal is typically possible after 3 to 4 months. Another option for these challenging injuries is a transarticular screw across the talonavicular articulation to maintain the reduction. This screw must be removed once bony healing has occurred to allow some talonavicular motion.

Avulsion fractures of the navicular body are also common, representing up to half of all navicular fractures.[45] Fractures involving the dorsal lip result from foot eversion and pull of the deltoid ligament attachments. Injury to the medial or plantar navicular results from the attachments of the posterior tibial tendon or the spring ligament. Nonsurgical treatment typically results in excellent functional results. The foot is placed in a rigid shoe for 3 to 6 weeks. Larger fragments associated with the posterior tibial tendon insertion may undergo reduction and internal fixation if significant retraction and subsequent concern for healing exists.

Stress fractures of the tarsal navicular are insidious conditions that are often initially overlooked. The fracture line is characteristic, oriented in the sagittal plane in the central third of the bone.[9] This overuse injury frequently seen in athletes may be exacerbated by preexisting foot deformities such as cavovarus posture. The diagnosis may be confirmed with the use of either technetium bone scan or CT. Initial treatment is strict adherence to no weight bearing in a short leg cast for 6 to 8 weeks. Progressive weight bearing is permitted once the patient is clinically symptom free. Patients who do not respond to nonsurgical treatment are candidates for lag screw fixation, which should be augmented with autogenous grafting.

Fractures of the Cuboid

The cuboid represents a key element in the lateral column of the foot. It is the only bone in the foot that articulates with both the tarsometatarsal joint (Lisfranc complex) as well as the midtarsal joint (Chopart joint). The cuboid also connects the lateral column to the transverse plantar arch, thus providing rigid inherent stability to the foot. Fractures of the cuboid typically result from an axial load or abduction moment of the forefoot. The injury may be subtle and is often difficult to detect with plain radiographs alone. A slight break in the cuboid cortical line or double density of the calcaneal facet may be the only finding. When evaluating for cuboid fractures, it is essential to consider the foot as two separate but linked medial and lateral columns. Like the pelvic ring, injury to one column frequently creates injury to the other. For example, compression of the cuboid is accompanied by tension failure of the medial column, typically through capsuloligamentous structures. Though the only radiographically evident injury is a cuboid fracture, there may be global ligamentous instability of the forefoot, which predisposes to lateral subluxation or frank midfoot dislocation.

The diagnosis of a cuboid fracture requires a high index of suspicion. Lateral swelling or tenderness should prompt a careful physical examination as well as high-quality views of the foot. Loss of cuboid height and intra-articular involvement of the calcaneal facet is best appreciated on the oblique view. Articular impaction may also be appreciated on the lateral view. CT will help clarify each individual fracture line to aid in preoperative assessment. Currently, no consensus exists regarding surgical indications of these fractures. Nondisplaced fractures of the cuboid may be closely observed in a non–weight-bearing short leg cast for evidence of early fracture displacement. If no displacement occurs, treatment should continue until the fracture is healed in approximately 6 to 8 weeks. Extra-articular fractures that result in forefoot deformity should be considered for surgical treatment. Loss of lateral column height

with accompanying medial capsuloligamentous incompetence allows the foot to assume a pathologic planovalgus position and creates the potential for long-term disability. This so-called nutcracker injury can be treated with a lateral distraction frame to regain the appropriate cuboid height, followed by bone grafting and internal fixation to secure the reduction. Depending on the quality of the fixation, the distraction frame may be left in place as additional support for the lateral column lengthening. It is important to avoid overdistraction of the lateral column, as this may create a paradoxical cavus foot. Preoperative planning using the contralateral limb as a template will prevent this surgical error. Displaced intra-articular fractures should also be considered for surgical fixation. The calcaneocuboid joint is a mobile planar synovial joint and articular incongruity results in abnormal contact force distribution, joint irritation, and subsequent arthrosis. In addition, distal impaction of the articular facet results in an osseous defect into which the calcaneal anterior process may subside, effectively creating dynamic lateral column instability. Progressive weight bearing may occur once fracture consolidation has been achieved, typically at 6 to 8 weeks.

Tarsometatarsal Injuries

Injury to the tarsometatarsal joints (Lisfranc injuries) represents approximately 0.2% of all fractures; however, the injuries are missed in approximately 20% to 30% of multitrauma patients, so the actual incidence may be underestimated.[46] The proximal intermetatarsal ligaments create a strong connection in the midfoot, but are absent between the first and second metatarsals. The plantar ligaments between the base of the second metatarsal and the medial cuneiform are the strongest component of the Lisfranc ligament. The inherent stability of the tarsometatarsal joints creates a rigid lever arm of the medial column of the foot during push-off in the gait cycle, and is maintained through an anatomic Roman arch in the coronal plane and recessed base of the second metatarsal in the axial plane. A recent study comparing preoperative MRI to intraoperative findings of Lisfranc injuries identified the important role of the intercuneiform ligaments for midfoot stability.[47] Normal tarsometatarsal joints allow for only 2 to 4 mm of motion in the first tarsometatarsal joint and no motion in the second and third joints, while the fourth and fifth tarsometatarsal joints allow up to 10° of plantar flexion and dorsiflexion.[46]

Trauma often results from direct crushing or indirect axial loading combined with a twisting mechanism. Patients will report pain with weight bearing and midfoot rotation. Patients with more subtle or purely ligamentous injuries have midfoot pain when the second metatarsal is depressed and elevated. Care must be taken to examine for a compartment syndrome or neurovascular injury and to document decreased dorsal sensation. AP, lateral, and oblique radiographs will often reveal a fleck sign at the base of the second metatarsal, which

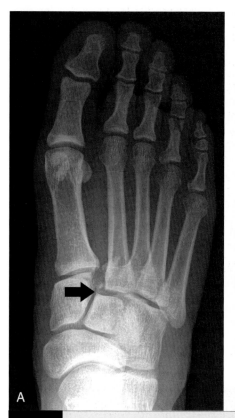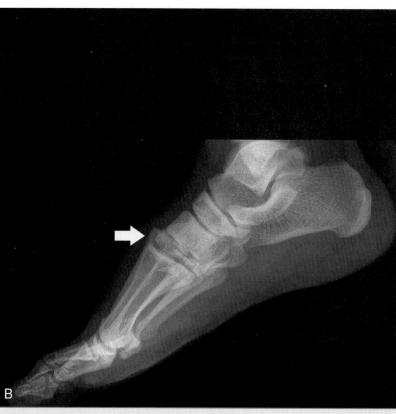

Figure 6 AP (**A**) and lateral (**B**) foot radiographs demonstrating a fleck sign (*arrows*) of the base of the second metatarsal in a patient with an unstable Lisfranc fracture-dislocation.

represents the plantar attachment of Lisfranc ligament (**Figure 6**). For injuries associated with lower energy trauma, weight-bearing or simulated weight-bearing AP views of the bilateral feet are needed to evaluate for widening. MRI is helpful to delineate the involvement of the ligament complex in cases where the plain radiographs are negative with a positive clinical examination.[47] CT can be useful in patients with comminution to better define the extent of injury. Various classification schemes have been proposed and are based on the presence of a lateral column disruption or the divergence of the lateral and medial columns.[48]

Surgical intervention is recommended for any displaced injury and outcomes demonstrate that improved function is associated with anatomic reduction and minimal delay in treatment.[48,49] Anatomic restoration of the second tarsometatarsal articulation should be performed first and secured with Kirschner wires. Care must be taken to then assess the remaining tarsometatarsal joints and intercuneiform joints for instability. Fixation of the first and third tarsometatarsal joints as well as the intercuneiform joints can be performed with screws or bridging plates. In the absence of comminution and shortening of the lateral column, the fourth and fifth tarsometatarsal joints can be pinned. Removal of hardware is recommended 8 to 16 weeks after initial surgery. Disruption of the articular surface with multiple passes of wires and drills may be associated with late arthritis, and one recent cadaver study demon-

strated a significant increase in articular damage with multiple repositioning of the guidewire during fixation.[50] Another cadaver study demonstrated that a suture-button fixation device has similar stability to screw fixation for Lisfranc injuries.[51] To date, there have been no clinical studies that investigate the use of the suture-endobutton compared with traditional screw fixation.

Even with immediate fixation, 25% to 50% of patients can develop chronic midfoot pain and posttraumatic arthritis requiring subsequent procedures.[52] A prospective, randomized study of 41 patients comparing open reduction and internal fixation to primary fusion of tarsometatarsal fracture-dislocations found a statistical improvement in American Orthopaedic Foot and Ankle Society scores and return to function in the primary arthrodesis group.[53] Another prospective study compared the results of 22 patients treated with delayed fusion after nonsurgical treatment to those of 22 patients who had immediate open reduction and internal fixation and found improved functional results with early surgical treatment.[54]

Fifth Metatarsal Fractures

Fractures of the fifth metatarsal are classified by anatomic location of the fracture. Classification of proximal fractures includes proximal tubercle fractures in-

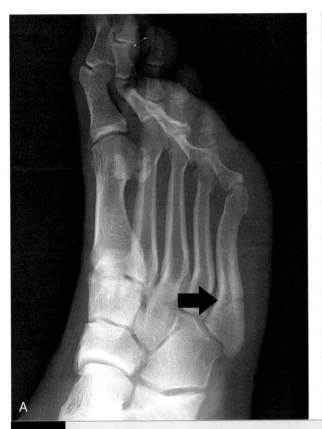
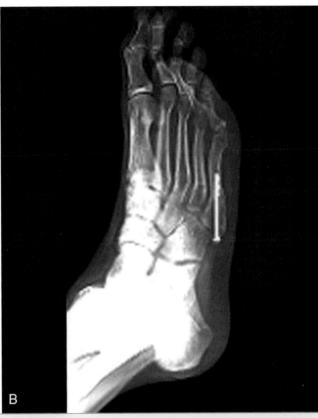

Figure 7   Oblique radiographs of the foot of a professional American football player with a stress fracture of the fifth metatarsal (*arrow*) before (**A**) and after (**B**) intramedullary fixation with a 5.5-mm screw and calcaneal bone grafting.

volving the metatarsocuneiform joint (type I), Jones fractures involving the proximal watershed metaphyseal-diaphyseal region (type II), and diaphyseal stress fractures (type III).[55] The blood supply to the proximal fifth metatarsal is composed of metaphyseal arteries that enter at the base of the fifth metatarsal and a nutrient artery that enters at the proximal diaphysis. This perfusion pattern has a correlation to the risk of delayed union or nonunion due to an avascular zone created by the watershed area. One study reviewed 21 type II proximal fifth metatarsal fractures that underwent open reduction and internal fixation and found that 18 of 21 patients had clinical and radiographic evidence of a varus hindfoot.[56]

For all foot fractures, AP, lateral, and oblique radiographs should be obtained. Type I fractures can initially be treated with protected weight bearing in a removable boot, with increasing activity as tolerated by pain. Type II and III fractures should be treated with 6 to 8 weeks of no weight bearing until signs of radiographic union have occurred. One prospective study of 52 fifth metatarsal proximal avulsion fractures treated with a stiff-soled shoe demonstrated that patients returned to work after an average of 22 days, but full recovery could take at least 6 months.[57] A univariate and regression analysis on the factors predicting outcome of fifth metatarsal avulsion fractures performed on 38 patients showed that prolonged absence of weight bearing was associated with stiffness and a poor global outcome.[58] In individuals with high physical demands, or those with a type II delayed union or nonunion, open reduction and internal fixation of the fifth metatarsal is warranted. Percutaneous or limited open reduction and internal fixation with a solid or cannulated screw can be performed under fluoroscopy (**Figure 7**). Full fracture healing can take up 12 weeks.[59] One study investigated the fixation of proximal fifth metatarsal fractures using 5.5-mm screws and compared them to a retrospective group of patients whose fractures were fixed with 4.5-mm screws. More of the 4.5-mm screws experienced bending, whereas more of the 5.5-mm screws penetrated the cortex distally; however, no clinical difference was noted between the screws.[60] Another study followed 14 athletes for an average of 42 months after open reduction and internal fixation of a proximal fifth metatarsal fracture; 13 patients returned to the same level of activity and good to excellent results were achieved in all patients.[61]

Metatarsophalangeal Dislocations

Due to the thick plantar ligamentous attachments, metatarsophalangeal dislocations are uncommon and usually the result of high-energy injuries. Treatment includes closed reduction and assessment of stability under fluoroscopy to confirm stability and cast or boot immobilization to prevent dorsiflexion of the toes for 4 to 6 weeks. First metatarsophalangeal dislocation can be classified into type I, where the plantar plate buttonholes over the first metatarsal head proximal to the sesamoids; type IIA, where the intersesamoid ligament ruptures and the plantar plate buttonholes with separation of the sesamoids; and type IIB, where the sesamoid fractures in a transverse direction. Irreducible dislocations or proximal migration of the plantar plate and sesamoids warrant surgical intervention and repair.

Metatarsal Fractures

The metatarsals have dense proximal ligamentous attachments as well as strong distal intermetatarsal ligaments at the level of the metatarsal neck. Therefore, isolated metatarsal fractures do not displace because of soft-tissue connections. Multiple metatarsal fractures are usually the result of direct trauma from a crush or fall, whereas isolated fractures of the fifth metatarsal usually occur from torsion creating an oblique fracture.

Nondisplaced or minimally displaced lesser metatarsal shaft and neck fractures can often be treated in a cam walker boot with frequent early follow-up to ensure that displacement does not occur. Isolated fractures often heal uneventfully, but multiple fractures can displace. Metatarsal neck fractures that heal in plantar flexion of the metatarsal head can create metatarsophalangeal overload, metatarsalgia, and hammering of the lesser toes. A single dorsal incision can be used for the second, third, and fourth metatarsals, and fixation can be accomplished with Kirschner wires of dorsal plating. Surgical intervention is usually indicated for first metatarsal fractures due to the higher loads transmitted through the first ray for the medial column. Complications include malunion, nonunion, and synostosis, which can lead to alteration in gait from a change in the biomechanics of the weight-bearing surface of the foot. A review of 23 open metatarsal fractures in 10 patients with clinical follow-up of 6 to 122 months (mean, 53 months) found that injuries with minimal soft-tissue damage had improved outcomes compared to those with Gustilo type IIIB injuries.[62]

Annotated References

1. Trepman E, Nihal A, Pinzur MS: Current topics review: Charcot neuroarthropathy of the foot and ankle. *Foot Ankle Int* 2005;26(1):46-63.

2. Giordano CP, Scott D, Koval KJ, Kummer F, Atik T, Desai P: Fracture blister formation: A laboratory study. *J Trauma* 1995;38(6):907-909.

3. Strauss EJ, Petrucelli G, Bong M, Koval KJ, Egol KA: Blisters associated with lower-extremity fracture: Results of a prospective treatment protocol. *J Orthop Trauma* 2006;20(9):618-622.

Treatment of fracture blisters with silver sulfadiazine (Silvadene) promoted epithelialization and reduced soft-tissue complications in nondiabetic patients with fracture blisters. Hemorrhagic blisters involve a higher risk of complications than serous blisters, presumably because hemorrhagic blisters represent a more severe tissue disruption.

4. Myerson M, Manoli A: Compartment syndromes of the foot after calcaneal fractures. *Clin Orthop Relat Res* 1993;290:142-150.

5. Matsen FA III: Compartmental syndrome: An unified concept. *Clin Orthop Relat Res* 1975;113:8-14.

6. Fulkerson E, Razi A, Tejwani N: Review: acute compartment syndrome of the foot. *Foot Ankle Int* 2003; 24(2):180-187.

7. Myerson M: Diagnosis and treatment of compartment syndrome of the foot. *Orthopedics* 1990;13(7):711-717.

8. Manoli A II, Weber TG: Fasciotomy of the foot: An anatomical study with special reference to release of the calcaneal compartment. *Foot Ankle* 1990;10(5):267-275.

9. Miric A, Patterson BM: Pathoanatomy of intra-articular fractures of the calcaneus. *J Bone Joint Surg Am* 1998; 80(2):207-212.

10. Heier KA, Infante AF, Walling AK, et al: Open fractures of the calcaneus: Soft-tissue injury determines outcome. *J Bone Joint Surg Am* 2003;85(12):2276-2282.

11. Berry GK, Stevens DG, Kreder HJ, et al: Open fractures of the calcaneus: A review of treatment and outcome. *J Orthop Trauma* 2004;18(4):202-206.

12. Benirschke SK, Kramer PA: Wound healing complications in closed and open calcaneal fractures. *J Orthop Trauma* 2004;18(1):1-6.

13. Gardner MJ, Nork SE, Barei DP, Kramer PA, Sangeorzan BJ, Benirschke SK: Secondary soft tissue compromise in tongue-type calcaneus fractures. *J Orthop Trauma* 2008;22(7):439-445.

A high incidence of wound complications (21%) exists with displaced tongue-type calcaneus fractures. Urgent closed reduction, plantar flexion splinting, and wound observation are essential.

14. Buckley R, Tough S, McCormack R, et al: Operative compared with nonoperative treatment of displaced intra-articular calcaneal fractures: A prospective, randomized, controlled multicenter trial. *J Bone Joint Surg Am* 2002;84(10):1733-1744.

15. Sanders R: Displaced intra-articular fractures of the calcaneus. *J Bone Joint Surg Am* 2000;82(2):225-250.

16. Radnay CS, Clare MP, Sanders RW: Subtalar fusion after displaced intra-articular calcaneal fractures: Does

initial operative treatment matter? *J Bone Joint Surg Am* 2009;91(3):541-546.

Improved functional outcome and fewer wound complications were associated with subtalar fusion for symptomatic posttraumatic subtalar arthritis after initial open reduction and internal fixation for displaced intra-articular calcaneus fractures compared with subtalar arthrodesis for the treatment secondary to calcaneal malunion following initial nonsurgical management. Level of evidence: III.

17. Cooper J, Benirschke S, Sangeorzan B, Bernards C, Edwards W: Sciatic nerve blockade improves early postoperative analgesia after open repair of calcaneus fractures. *J Orthop Trauma* 2004;18(4):197-201.

18. Borrelli J Jr, Lashgari C: Vascularity of the lateral calcaneal flap: A cadaveric injection study. *J Orthop Trauma* 1999;13(2):73-77.

19. Richter M, Gosling T, Zech S, et al: A comparison of plates with and without locking screws in a calcaneal fracture model. *Foot Ankle Int* 2005;26(4):309-319.

20. Schildhauer TA, Bauer TW, Josten C, Muhr G: Open reduction and augmentation of internal fixation with an injectable skeletal cement for the treatment of complex calcaneal fractures. *J Orthop Trauma* 2000;14(5):309-317.

21. Sagi HC, Papp S, Dipasquale T: The effect of suture pattern and tension on cutaneous blood flow as assessed by laser Doppler flowmetry in a pig model. *J Orthop Trauma* 2008;22(3):171-175.

   As tension was increased across a porcine wound model, the modified Allgöwer-Donati suture configuration had the least effect on cutaneous blood flow compared with sutures made in a simple, vertical mattress, or horizontal mattress fashion.

22. Athavale SA, Joshi SD, Joshi SS: Internal architecture of the talus. *Foot Ankle Int* 2008;29(1):82-86.

   Twenty-five pairs of dry adult human tali were sectioned in various planes and dissected grossly to study the internal architecture of the talus. Two sets of lamellae were observed in the body of the talus. One set was descending from the posterior two thirds of the lateral part of trochlear surface onto the posterior calcaneal facet of the talus. These lamellae were in the form of vertical perforated interconnected plates. The second set of trabeculae originated from the medial part of the trochlear surface and the anterior third of the lateral part.

23. Sarrafian S: Osteology, in *Anatomy of the Foot and Ankle*. Philadelphia, PA, JB Lippincott, 1983, pp 40-80.

24. Chan G, Sanders DW, Yuan X, Jenkinson RJ, Willits K: Clinical accuracy of imaging techniques for talar neck malunion. *J Orthop Trauma* 2008;22(6):415-418.

   Eight cadaveric tali were evaluated to compare the ability of plain radiographs, CT, and radiostereometric analysis (RSA) to detect changes in talus fracture fragment position and alignment. The fragments were then displaced and rotated to create a varus and supination deformity, and screw fixation was repeated in nonanatomic alignment. Displacement and rotation were directly measured. The most accurate imaging technique to measure displacement in talar neck malunion is CT scan. RSA was less useful as an imaging technique in this study.

25. Mulfinger GL, Trueta J: The blood supply of the talus. *J Bone Joint Surg Br* 1970;52(1):160-167.

26. Ziran BH, Abidi NA, Scheel MJ: Medial malleolar osteotomy for exposure of complex talar body fractures. *J Orthop Trauma* 2001;15(7):513-518.

27. Ebraheim NA, Karkare N, Gehling DJ, Liu J, Ervin D, Werner CM: Use of a 30-degree external rotation view for posteromedial tubercle fractures of the talus. *J Orthop Trauma* 2007;21(8):579-582.

   The investigators evaluated the use of the 30° external rotation view for the diagnosis of fractures of the posteromedial tubercle of the talus using cadaver specimens. On the 30° external rotation view of the ankle, all fractures of the posteromedial tubercle of the talus were revealed. In contrast, the fracture was visualized in only two cases using the standard lateral radiograph of the ankle, and not once in the anteroposterior or mortise views.

28. Hawkins LG: Fractures of the neck of the talus. *J Bone Joint Surg Am* 1970;52(5):991-1002.

29. Canale ST, Kelly FB Jr: Fractures of the neck of the talus: Long-term evaluation of seventy-one cases. *J Bone Joint Surg Am* 1978;60(2):143-156.

30. Lindvall E, Haidukewych G, DiPasquale T, Herscovici D Jr, Sanders R: Open reduction and stable fixation of isolated, displaced talar neck and body fractures. *J Bone Joint Surg Am* 2004;86(10):2229-2234.

31. Fleuriau Chateau PB, Brokaw DS, Jelen BA, Scheid DK, Weber TG: Plate fixation of talar neck fractures: Preliminary review of a new technique in twenty-three patients. *J Orthop Trauma* 2002;16(4):213-219.

32. Swanson TV, Bray TJ, Holmes GB Jr: Fractures of the talar neck: A mechanical study of fixation. *J Bone Joint Surg Am* 1992;74(4):544-551.

33. Attiah M, Sanders DW, Valdivia G, et al: Comminuted talar neck fractures: A mechanical comparison of fixation techniques. *J Orthop Trauma* 2007;21(1):47-51.

   Thirty human cadaver tali were osteotomized across the talar neck. The specimens were randomized to one of three fixation groups: three anterior-to-posterior screws, two cannulated screws inserted from posterior to anterior, and one screw from anterior to posterior and a medially applied blade plate. No statistically significant difference was found between the fixation methods, even when variations in age and sex were considered.

34. Vallier HA, Nork SE, Barei DP, Benirschke SK, Sangeorzan BJ: Talar neck fractures: Results and outcomes. *J Bone Joint Surg Am* 2004;86(8):1616-1624.

35. Tezval M, Dumont C, Stürmer KM: Prognostic reliability of the Hawkins sign in fractures of the talus. *J Orthop Trauma* 2007;21(8):538-543.

 In a retrospective study of the prognostic reliability of the Hawkins sign, 31 patients with displaced, surgical talar fractures were followed for more than 36 months. The Hawkins sign was absent in the five patients who developed osteonecrosis of the talus. In the remaining 26 patients who did not develop osteonecrosis, a positive (full) Hawkins sign was observed 11 times, a partially positive Hawkins sign 4 times, and a negative Hawkins sign 11 times. The Hawkins sign thus showed a sensitivity of 100% and a specificity of 57.7%. Therefore, the Hawkins sign is a good indicator of talus vascularity following fracture.

36. Sanders DW, Busam M, Hattwick E, Edwards JR, McAndrew MP, Johnson KD: Functional outcomes following displaced talar neck fractures. *J Orthop Trauma* 2004;18(5):265-270.

37. Vallier HA, Nork SE, Benirschke SK, Sangeorzan BJ: Surgical treatment of talar body fractures. *J Bone Joint Surg Am* 2004;86(Pt 2, suppl 1)180-192.

38. Ebraheim NA, Patil V, Owens C, Kandimalla Y: Clinical outcome of fractures of the talar body. *Int Orthop* 2008;32(6):773-777.

 Nineteen patients with talar body fractures were studied retrospectively to assess outcome after surgical treatment with an average follow-up of 26 months. Talar injuries are serious because they can compromise motion of the foot and ankle and result in severe disability. Crush fractures of the talar body and those associated with open injuries and talar neck fractures are associated with a less favorable outcome.

39. Muir D, Saltzman CL, Tochigi Y, Amendola N: Talar dome access for osteochondral lesions. *Am J Sports Med* 2006;34(9):1457-1463.

40. Langer P, DiGiovanni C: Incidence and pattern types of fractures of the lateral process of the talus. *Am J Orthop (Belle Mead NJ)* 2008;37(5):257-258.

 A retrospective review at a level I trauma center over 3 years identified the respective incidence and variation in fracture configuration of all isolated lateral process injuries. The incidence was 10.4%. The fractures were most commonly single large fragments closely followed in frequency by nonarticular chip patterns.

41. von Knoch F, Reckord U, von Knoch M, Sommer C: Fracture of the lateral process of the talus in snowboarders. *J Bone Joint Surg Br* 2007;89(6):772-777.

 The authors present a study of the clinical and radiologic outcome after unilateral fracture of the lateral process of the talus in 23 snowboarders with a mean follow-up of 3.5 years. The outcome after fracture of the lateral process of the talus in snowboarders is favorable provided an early diagnosis is made and adequate treatment, which is related to the degree of displacement and associated injuries, is undertaken.

42. Bibbo C, Anderson RB, Davis WH: Injury characteristics and the clinical outcome of subtalar dislocations: A clinical and radiographic analysis of 25 cases. *Foot Ankle Int* 2003;24(2):158-163.

43. Sangeorzan BJ, Benirschke SK, Mosca V, Mayo KA, Hansen ST Jr: Displaced intra-articular fractures of the tarsal navicular. *J Bone Joint Surg Am* 1989;71(10):1504-1510.

44. Schildhauer TA, Nork SE, Sangeorzan BJ: Temporary bridge plating of the medial column in severe midfoot injuries. *J Orthop Trauma* 2003;17(7):513-520.

45. Eichenholtz SN, Levine DB: Fractures of the tarsal navicular bone. *Clin Orthop Relat Res* 1964;34:142-157.

46. Desmond EA, Chou LB: Current concepts review: Lisfranc injuries. *Foot Ankle Int* 2006;27(8):653-660.

47. Raikin SM, Elias I, Dheer S, Besser MP, Morrison WB, Zoga AC: Prediction of midfoot instability in the subtle Lisfranc injury: Comparison of magnetic resonance imaging with intraoperative findings. *J Bone Joint Surg Am* 2009;91(4):892-899.

 MRIs of 21 feet in 20 patients were evaluated with regard to the integrity of the dorsal and plantar bundles of the Lisfranc ligament, the plantar tarsal-metatarsal ligaments, and the medial-middle cuneiform ligament. Nineteen (90%) of the 21 Lisfranc joint complexes were correctly classified on MRI; therefore, MRI is accurate for detecting traumatic injury of the Lisfranc ligament and for predicting Lisfranc joint complex instability.

48. Myerson MS, Fisher RT, Burgess AR, Kenzora JE: Fracture dislocations of the tarsometatarsal joints: End results correlated with pathology and treatment. *Foot Ankle* 1986;6(5):225-242.

49. Calder JD, Whitehouse SL, Saxby TS: Results of isolated Lisfranc injuries and the effect of compensation claims. *J Bone Joint Surg Br* 2004;86(4):527-530.

50. Gaines RJ, Wright G, Stewart J: Injury to the tarsometatarsal joint complex during fixation of Lisfranc fracture dislocations: An anatomic study. *J Trauma* 2009;66(4):1125-1128.

 The purpose of this study was to determine whether the involved joint surface area increased with repositioning of the guidewire before screw placement. Nine matched pairs of cadaver feet were dissected after cannulated screws were placed after a single pass across the joint for right feet and two passes across the joint for left feet. The mean injury area for the first metatarsal (MT1) was 0.106 cm² for one pass and 0.168 cm² for two passes of the guidewire before screw advancement (P = 0.003) The mean injury area for the second metatarsal (MT2) was 0.123 and 0.178 cm² for one and two passes, respectively (P = 0.018). The authors concluded that changing the placement of the guidewire across the mid-foot significantly increased the joint surface affected by screw placement.

51. Panchbhavi VK, Vallurupalli S, Yang J, Andersen CR: Screw fixation compared with suture-button fixation of isolated Lisfranc ligament injuries. *J Bone Joint Surg Am* 2009;91(5):1143-1148.

This cadaver study of 14 paired specimens was performed to compare the stability provided by a suture button with that provided by a screw when used to stabilize the diastasis associated with Lisfranc ligament injury. The authors found no significant difference in displacement between specimens fixed with the suture button and those fixed with the screw.

52. Kuo RS, Tejwani NC, Digiovanni CW, et al: Outcome after open reduction and internal fixation of Lisfranc joint injuries. *J Bone Joint Surg Am* 2000;82(11):1609-1618.

53. Coetzee JC, Ly TV: Treatment of primarily ligamentous Lisfranc joint injuries: Primary arthrodesis compared with open reduction and internal fixation. Surgical technique. *J Bone Joint Surg Am* 2007;89(suppl 2 pt 1): 122-127.

Forty-one patients with an isolated acute or subacute primarily ligamentous Lisfranc joint injury were enrolled in a prospective, randomized clinical trial comparing primary arthrodesis with traditional open reduction and internal fixation. The patients were followed for an average of 42.5 months. The patients who had been treated with a primary arthrodesis estimated that their postoperative level of activities was 92% of their preinjury level, whereas the open reduction group estimated that their postoperative level was only 65% of their preoperative level. A primary stable arthrodesis of the medial two or three rays appears to have a better short- and medium-term outcome than open reduction and internal fixation of ligamentous Lisfranc joint injuries.

54. Rammelt S, Schneiders W, Schikore H, Holch M, Heineck J, Zwipp H: Primary open reduction and fixation compared with delayed corrective arthrodesis in the treatment of tarsometatarsal (Lisfranc) fracture dislocation. *J Bone Joint Surg Br* 2008;90(11):1499-1506.

This comparative cohort study conducted over a period of 5 years compared primary open reduction and internal fixation in 22 patients with secondary corrective arthrodesis in 22 patients who presented with painful malunion at a mean of 22 months after injury. It was concluded that primary treatment by open reduction and internal fixation of tarsometatarsal fracture-dislocations leads to improved functional results, earlier return to work, and greater patient satisfaction than secondary corrective arthrodesis.

55. Torg JS, Balduini FC, Zelko RR, Pavlov H, Peff TC, Das M: Fractures of the base of the fifth metatarsal distal to the tuberosity: Classification and guidelines for non-surgical and surgical management. *J Bone Joint Surg Am* 1984;66(2):209-214.

56. Raikin SM, Slenker N, Ratigan B: The association of a varus hindfoot and fracture of the fifth metatarsal metaphyseal-diaphyseal junction: The Jones fracture. *Am J Sports Med* 2008;36(7):1367-1372.

The objective of the study was to assess the utility of MRI for the diagnosis of an injury to the Lisfranc and adjacent ligaments in 21 patients and to determine whether conventional MRI is a reliable diagnostic tool, with manual stress radiographic evaluation with the patient under anesthesia and surgical findings being used as a reference standard. The authors found that intraoperatively, 17 unstable and 4 stable Lisfranc joints were identified. The strongest predictor of instability was disruption of the plantar ligament between the first cuneiform and the bases of the second and third metatarsals. Nineteen (90%) of the 21 Lisfranc joint complexes were correctly classified on MRI. They concluded that MRI is accurate for detecting traumatic injury of the Lisfranc ligament and for predicting Lisfranc joint complex instability when the plantar Lisfranc ligament bundle is used as a predictor.

57. Egol K, Walsh M, Rosenblatt K, Capla E, Koval KJ: Avulsion fractures of the fifth metatarsal base: A prospective outcome study. *Foot Ankle Int* 2007;28(5):581-583.

Fifty-two patients who sustained an avulsion fracture of the fifth metatarsal base and presented to the outpatient clinic of the hospital system were followed prospectively with a standardized protocol. An average of 22 days were lost from work, and although patients can be expected to return to their preinjury level of function, recovery may take 6 months or longer.

58. Vorlat P, Achtergael W, Haentjens P: Predictors of outcome of non-displaced fractures of the base of the fifth metatarsal. *Int Orthop* 2007;31(1):5-10.

The purpose of this study was to identify those factors that influence the outcome after nonsurgical treatment of undisplaced fractures of the fifth metatarsal on 38 patients who were treated with plaster and periods of no weight bearing (NWB). The most significant predictor of poor functional outcome was longer NWB, which was strongly associated with worse global outcome, discomfort, and reported stiffness. The authors concluded that NWB should be kept to a minimum for acute avulsions of the tuberosity of the fifth metatarsal.

59. Clapper MF, O'Brien TJ, Lyons PM: Fractures of the fifth metatarsal: Analysis of a fracture registry. *Clin Orthop Relat Res* 1995;315:238-241.

60. Porter DA, Rund AM, Dobslaw R, Duncan M: Comparison of 4.5- and 5.5-mm cannulated stainless steel screws for fifth metatarsal Jones fracture fixation. *Foot Ankle Int* 2009;30(1):27-33.

61. Leumann A, Pagenstert G, Fuhr P, Hintermann B, Valderrabano V: Intramedullary screw fixation in proximal fifth-metatarsal fractures in sports: Clinical and biomechanical analysis. *Arch Orthop Trauma Surg* 2008;128(12):1425-1430.

Fourteen active patients with fifth metatarsal fracture were followed for an average of 42 months with clinical, radiologic, and biomechanical evaluation. Thirteen of 14 patients were highly satisfied and returned to full activity.

62. Hoxie S, Turner NS III, Strickland J, Jacofsky D: Clinical course of open metatarsal fractures. *Orthopedics* 2007;30(8):662-665.

This case series examined the outcome of 10 patients with open metatarsal fractures. Six sustained Gustilo grade I or II injuries, and all healed without the need for additional soft-tissue coverage. Four patients with Gustilo grade IIIB developed complications and all eventually required amputation. Level of evidence: IV.

Chapter 40

Foot and Ankle Reconstruction

Mark D. Perry, MD   Arthur Manoli II, MD

Introduction

Foot and ankle reconstruction is taking an increasingly more important role as patient expectations, survivability of injuries, and patient demands increase overall. The goal of surgery, whether because of elective, acquired, or traumatic issues, is to align the foot in a neutral position without pain on weight bearing and provide the mobility and support desired. More than $3 billion a year is spent on the treatment of posttraumatic arthritis.[1] This chapter will focus on the traditional treatments used in reconstructing the foot and ankle secondary to arthritis, malalignment, or tendon issues with emphasis on emerging treatments.

Arthritis and Malposition

A broad area of reconstruction is related to arthritis/malalignment. This involves arthrosis resulting from cartilage injury or incongruent surfaces. Ankle stability is provided by a combination of bony architecture and ligament integrity. Either bone loss or joint subluxation results in malalignment of the foot or ankle. Issues regarding the medial column of the foot are traditionally treated with arthrodesis because this is the more rigid and stable column. Issues involving the lateral aspect of the foot tend to focus on joint preservation to help maintain mobility.

Anatomic Areas of Injury

Syndesmosis

Injury to the syndesmosis is treated with a realignment procedure. To hold the ankle mortise in position, a combination of bony stability as well as ligamentous stability needs to be achieved. A stable syndesmosis can be achieved by restoring the proper anatomy between the fibula and the tibia incisura[2] (Figure 1). When the syndesmosis can be reconstructed, there is adequate restoration of function. When the mortise cannot be held with stability, such as fractures of the Chaput tubercle or comminution resulting in the loss of the anterolateral aspect of the distal tibia, then treatment with syndesmosis fusion can be attempted.

Ankle

Traumatic arthritis of the tibiotalar joint occurs as a result of articular injuries resulting from rotational injuries about the ankle, typically valgus impaction fractures (Figure 2). These injuries also occur as direct-impact loading through the tibiotalar joint (pilon fractures) or as a result of osteochondral injuries of the talar dome. Treatment options for ankle arthritis are resection, arthroplasty, and arthrodesis.

Resection

Tibiotalar joints with significant bony impingement may require excision of the protruding bone (Figure 3). Ligament realignment and calcaneal osteotomy may provide symptomatic relief in ankles with mild arthritis but mechanical overloading secondary to talar tilt.[3] Fresh osteochondral total ankle allograft transplantation is not currently a feasible treatment option.[4]

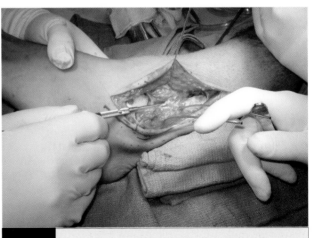

Figure 1 Intraoperative photograph showing unrecognized syndesmotic injury with interposed soft tissue.

Dr. Perry or an immediate family member serves as a board member, owner, officer, or committee member of the American Academy of Orthopaedic Surgeons resolutions committee. Dr. Manoli or an immediate family member has received royalties from DJ Orthopaedics; is a member of a speakers' bureau or has made paid presentations on behalf of Stryker and Synthes; and serves as a board member, owner, officer, or committee member of the Michigan Orthopaedic Society.

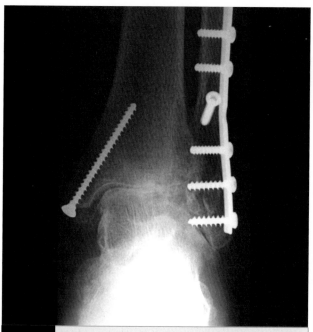

Figure 2 | AP radiograph showing loss of lateral tibiotalar joint space after a valgus impaction fracture.

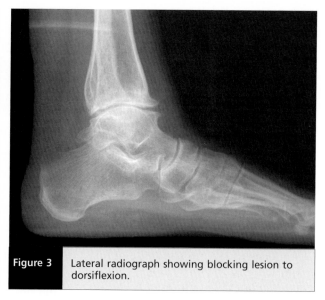

Figure 3 | Lateral radiograph showing blocking lesion to dorsiflexion.

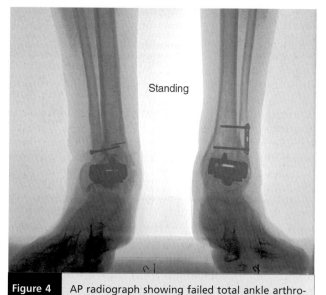

Figure 4 | AP radiograph showing failed total ankle arthroplasty in a patient with severe bilateral pain.

Arthroplasty

Appropriate patient selection is critically important for good outcomes of total ankle athroplasty[5] (Figure 4). Proponents of ankle arthroplasty cite preservation of the subtalar joint as a benefit to arthroplasty. However, more recent ankle replacement designs are incorporating fixation into the calcaneus through the subtalar joint.[6] Ankle replacement must be performed with bony alignment and soft-tissue tensions restored to normal. The deltoid ligament may need its length shortened to restore soft-tissue balance. Arthroplasties placed in a varus or valgus position will fail.[7] At 2-year follow-up

of Hintegra prosthesis (Integra Life Sciences, Plainsboro, NJ) placement, there was no difference in results for patients with severe varus deformity compared to control subjects.[8] Varus deformity correction was accomplished by a medial release and, if necessary, a lateral plication of tissues.

Although the concept of total ankle replacement is simple, in actuality the results depend on implant design and surgical expertise. Currently there are more than 10 different implants available for use in Europe, with an increasing number in the United States. Each design has specific and unique consequences that may result in the need for revision.

It is anticipated that "over the next few years as indications and techniques are refined, total ankle replacement will also become as reliable as knee replacement."[9] Proprioception does not significantly change after total ankle arthroplasty.[10] The motion achieved after total ankle replacement is similar to preoperative range of motion. However, the improvement of a measured 5° resulted in a clinically greater perception of motion, perhaps because of the additional motion being "pain free."[11]

In a 2009 study of the Scandinavian Total Ankle Replacement (STAR; Small Bone Innovations, New York, NY), there was a 50% decrease in secondary minor and major surgeries when comparing surgeons who performed an average of 16 versus 43 total ankle replacements. Component size was adapted to smaller implants as the "learning curve" was refined. The overall reoperation rate in this series was 11%.[12]

A third-generation total ankle implant demonstrated good pain relief and improved function with a 95% survival rate at 6 years. However, this implant was withdrawn by the manufacturer because of significant osteolysis issues.[13]

It is difficult to make a broad statement that total ankle replacement is preferable to arthrodesis. It is possible that each implant design will have different short-, medium-, and long-term function and survivorship with different necessary secondary surgeries (such as syndesmotic fusion). The learning curve for these procedures is not insignificant. Although total ankle replacement may be a powerful tool in the treatment of ankle arthritis, many factors must be considered before treatment of tibiotalar arthritis.

Arthrodesis

The traditional attitudes concerning the role of arthrodesis are being challenged. The functional results of arthrodesis in general have been an elimination of painful ambulation with known limitations in mobility. The outcomes, however, with resultant loss of joint motion are resulting in the design of procedures and techniques to salvage joint motion. Whether significant differences in outcomes are seen is unclear.[14]

Although a salvage procedure, ankle arthrodesis currently has broader surgical indications and remains the primary treatment of ankle arthritis.[15] Shoe wear with an appropriate rocker bottom and increased subtalar joint motion provide restorative aspects of gait after arthrodesis.[15] Arthrodesis of the tibiotalar joint can be successfully treated with compression screws,[16] external frames,[17] or plates used in combination. Plate fixation has been shown to increase stability.[18] Failed arthrodesis can be treated with arthroplasty[19] if there is intrinsic coronal plane stability, which can be facilitated by wider talar components. Repeat arthrodesis is warranted if failure was the result of poor fixation technique or other correctable issues. Failed arthroplasty can be treated with arthrodesis;[20] however, significant replacement bone stock and rigid fixation are required.

Hindfoot and Midfoot

Painful arthritis of the hindfoot and midfoot is treated with fusion of the symptomatic joints. The results of subtalar fusion are better after failed surgical treatment than in nonsurgically treated intra-articular calcaneal fractures[21] because of the restoration of bone morphology. Talonavicular arthritis as a result of a trauma requires fusion. Similar to the lateral column of the foot, the talonavicular joint provides significant sagittal and coronal plane motion to the foot. However, there is no alternative to a talonavicular fusion or a talonavicular cuneiform fusion where there is significant talonavicular arthritis. Incorporation of a subtalar fusion with an isolated talonavicular fusion can increase fusion rates, although this results in even more restrictive foot motion. Midfoot posttraumatic arthritis occurs as a result of fractures of the cuneiforms as a sequelae of injury to the tarsometatarsal joints. The first, second, and third tarsometatarsal joints are treated collectively by arthrodesis to eliminate arthritic pain to the medial column of the midfoot with no significant functional limitations. Fusions between the tarsal navicular and intercuneiform joints provide effective, asymptomatic support to a previously arthritic medial column of the midfoot.

The lateral tarsometatarsal joints, the fourth and fifth metatarsals, and their articulation to the cuboid are qualitatively different from the first, second, and

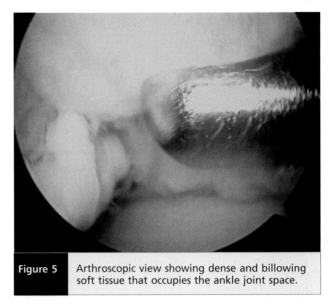

| Figure 5 | Arthroscopic view showing dense and billowing soft tissue that occupies the ankle joint space. |

third medial tarsometatarsal joints. This relatively rigid column of the midfoot requires significant mobility. Tarsometatarsal arthrodesis relieves the symptoms of arthritis but provides an undesirable rigid foot. This condition can be resolved with either tissue arthroplasty or joint arthroplasty.[22]

Os Trigonum

Fractures of the os trigonum occur in the region of incomplete coalescence of the posterior talus ossicle to the rest of the talar body. This posteromedial region of the talar body is where the flexor hallucis longus slides into the groove. This area is impinged in maximal plantar flexion and also may have symptoms with flexor hallucis longus gliding. Removal of the os trigonum will eliminate the acute symptoms.

Treatment of Foot and Ankle Pain

Patients who have continued pain after routine ankle fractures or twisting injuries will often have symptomatic impingement in the anterolateral or anteromedial aspect of the tibiotalar joint. Arthroscopy in this setting reveals significant areas of fibrosis and fibrous bands that impinge during normal ankle joint motion (**Figure 5**). Arthroscopy also can be used to remove cartilage from the distal tibia and talus as mentioned for arthroscopically assisted arthrodesis. Therapeutic indications for subtalar arthroscopy include arthrodesis[23] and minimally invasive calcaneal reconstruction.

Osteochondral Lesions

Cartilage lesions of the talus can be more accurately described as osteochondral lesions (OCLs). Osteochondritis dissecans is a subtype of OCL. The current classification system uses the four-stage Berndt and Harty 1959 classification system.[24] Stage I is an intact carti-

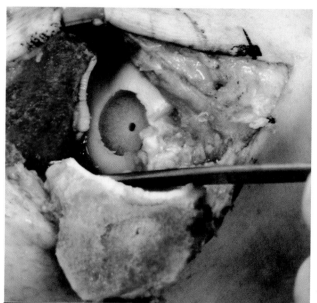

| Figure 6 | Intraoperative photograph showing talar dome preparation after a medial malleolar osteotomy. (Courtesy of Al Pearsall, MD, Mobile, AL.) |

lage lesion with a bone injury. Stage II and III lesions are nondisplaced cartilage injuries that are incomplete (stage II) or complete (stage III). Stage IV is a detached OCL. Clinically these injuries present as ankle joint effusions with periarticular tenderness. Nonsurgical treatment consists of rest and ice with temporary reduction of weight bearing.

The most common areas of OCLs are the central medial aspect followed by the central lateral talus. Central medial lesions tend to be the largest. Injuries that do not penetrate the subchondral bone have no stimulus for healing. Therefore, initial treatment is aimed at revascularizing the bony defect. The healing response induces a fibrocartilage, not hyaline cartilage. For intact cartilage, retrograde drilling provides revascularization of the bone without introducing chondral injury. Microfracture and microdrilling similarly seek to stimulate fibrocartilage development for stage II and III lesions. For lesions with small cartilage damage (less than 6 mm), microfracture/microdrilling is the preferred treatment of chondral injuries. When chondral injury is greater than 15 mm, the efficacy of microfracture/microdrilling is questionable.

Tissue transplantation becomes the treatment modality for larger chondral injuries of the talus or failed microfracture. Most of the talar dome is accessible without a medial malleolar osteotomy. If required, three-screw fixation of the osteotomy is preferable to two-screw fixation to prevent proximal migration. Most authors consider osteochondral autograft tissue transplantation to be a salvage procedure unless the lesion is larger than 6 mm in diameter.

In the osteochondral autologous transfer system, the tissue is taken from the non–weight-bearing aspect of the ipsilateral distal femur. Often the lesion can be

treated with one core (Figure 6). Large defects are treated with multiple transplantations or plugs. Reproduction of a smooth articular surface is technically challenging and may result in an "organ pipe" arrangement of cartilage plugs. Sometimes this results in a catching sensation for large lesions. Osteochondral allograft transplantation using either fresh osteochondral allografts or fresh-frozen grafts has been described. Allograft has a risk of resorption and fragmentation of the graft. Autologous chondrocyte implantation is a technique in which autologous chondrocytes are cultured and injected into the prepared lesion. Although this hyaline-like cartilage regeneration is a possible treatment method, there is considerable cost, and additional surgical procedures are necessary. Although interarticular hyaluronic acid derivative injections are used in the treatment of knee arthritis, treatment of compromised ankle joint cartilage currently is not standard practice but may prove to be a useful adjunctive therapy.[24]

Major Acquired Deformities

Hallux Valgus
Hallux valgus, the main deformity of the forefoot, has more than 130 described procedures.[25-32] More than 80% of patients have family history and bilaterality, with surgery improving quality of life.[33,34] The classification of bunions and their subsequent treatment is based on the intermetatarsal angle (IMA; normal <9°) and the hallux valgus angle (HVA; normal <15°). Other considerations are the distal metatarsal articular angle (normal <10°) and the hallux interphalangeal angle (normal <10°).

Nonsurgical treatment of symptomatic bunions is a shoe with a soft leather upper and a high and wide toe box to accommodate the foot. The current position of the American Orthopaedic Foot and Ankle Society asserts that cosmesis is not a valid surgical indication. Bunion deformities are classified according to HVA and IMA as mild (HVA <30°, IMA <13°), moderate (HVA <40°, IMA >13°), or severe (HVA >40°, IMA >20°).

Moderate to severe bunion deformities require proximal intervention using either arthrodesis of the first tarsometatarsal joint or a proximal osteotomy. Working proximally allows significant correction of the increased IMA. The Lapidus procedure also addresses hypermobility of the first ray (the first tarsometatarsal joint). In addition to being an effective primary procedure, the Lapidus procedure has been shown to be a good salvage procedure for failed hallux valgus surgeries.[35] Once the tarsometatarsal fusion is established, recurrence of the deformity is unlikely.[36]

Distal soft-tissue releases and tightenings will need to be done to improve the HVA. The medial capsulorrhaphy is enhanced with a suture anchor closure. Soft-tissue procedures that release the adductor may result in an iatrogenic adduction deformity of the great toe (hallux varus).

For moderate hallux valgus deformities an osteotomy closer to the metatarsophalangeal joint is performed. The standard osteotomy is a chevron where the metatarsal head is slid laterally and held in position by fixation. The plantar osteotomy should be proximal to the joint capsule.[37] If first metatarsophalangeal joint arthritis is present, a fusion alone may decrease the IMA in patients with moderate disease.[38] Lesser bunion deformities may be treated with distal soft-tissue releases. However, it is more likely that the bunion will respond to nonsurgical intervention for these minor deformities.

Pes Planus

Peritalar subluxations are responsible for two main types of deformities. The dorsilateral peritalar subluxation is most recognized because of the adult-acquired flatfoot. This condition results in abduction of the forefoot and the development of a hindfoot valgus deformity (Figure 7). There is a spectrum of tendon involvement that begins as a tendinitis of the posterior tibial tendon and ends with an incompetent and painful tendon with significant tendinosis, lack of tendon excursion, and fixed deformity of the subtalar, talonavicular, and calcaneocuboid joints. A tenolysis may be appropriate early treatment; later during the course of the disease when the deformity is not reducible and an arthrosis has occurred, a triple arthrodesis is appropriate treatment.

Adult acquired flatfoot deformity is most often caused by posterior tibial tendon dysfunction. Stage I is characterized by early degeneration of the tendon with medial focal pain or a peritendinitis. Stage II is distinguished by a passively correctable deformity. Stage IIA is defined to be less than 30% of the talar head and coverage on the standing AP radiograph. Stage IIB is associated with more deformity. Initial nonsurgical treatment is with nonsteroidal anti-inflammatory drugs and immobilization, although this treatment has not been shown to prevent or decrease the progression of deformity. Stage III is a fixed valgus deformity of the hindfoot. In stage IV, a valgus deformity of the tibiotalar joint has formed.[39]

Surgical treatment of stage I involves a tenosynovectomy and tendon repair for intrasubstance or longitudinal tears. Stage II has more surgical options. A calcaneal medial slide and tendon transfer are performed for stage IIA deformity. For stage IIB deformity, lateral column lengthening is often required.

The reconstruction of a stage IIB adult acquired flatfoot deformity requires multiple significant surgeries at different locations throughout the foot. Temporary fixation of the osteotomies and arthrodesis allow better control of the final alignment.[40] There is concern that the addition of a lateral column lengthening increases lateral pressure. Increased lateral pressure was not the result of excessive lengthening of the lateral column when fluoroscopy was used to assess the reduction of the talonavicular joint.[41] The increase in lateral pressure may be negated/improved by a medial tarsometa-

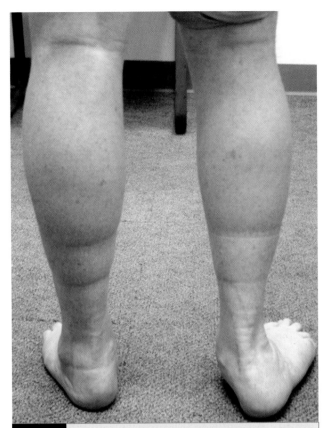

Figure 7 | Clinical photograph showing right heel valgus deformity displaying "too many toes."

tarsal arthrodesis or medial cuneiform osteotomy.[42] Tarsometatarsal arthrodesis may also correct resulting supination deformity occurring after lateral column lengthening.

Subtle Cavus Foot

A plantar-medial peritalar subluxation results in a subtle cavus foot, which is radiographically determined by the Meary angle, which must be greater than zero. The angle is formed by a line drawn through the talus and by another line directed down the first metatarsal on a lateral weight-bearing radiograph. The subtle cavus foot is supinated with a varus heel, resulting in an inflexible, stiff foot. If the deformity is not passively correctable, osteotomies are required to provide a normal plantigrade foot. A heel slide is performed to incur hindfoot valgus and a closing wedge osteotomy is performed on the dorsal surface of the first metatarsal to provide a predictable correction with resolution of symptoms.

Minor Acquired Deformities

Progressive deformities are a result of an inbalance of foot invertors and evertors. Similarly, an imbalance between the intrinsic muscles and the long dorsiflexors and plantar flexors results in claw toe deformities.

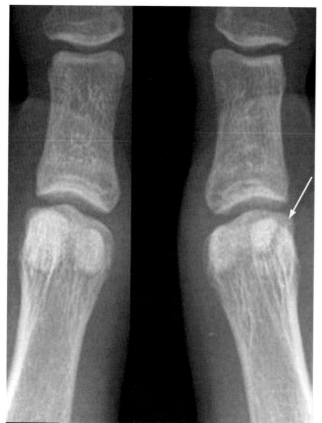

Figure 8 Radiograph showing right foot lateral sesamoid disruption (*arrow*) with the left side as comparison.

an avascular condition (**Figure 8**). Treatment initially consists of unloading the sesamoid using offloading splints and stretching of the gastrocnemius-soleus complex. If the medial sesamoid is involved, downward shaving of the sesamoid may be appropriate for symptom relief. Conditions involving the lateral sesamoid that are unresponsive to nonsurgical treatment may require resection, and frequently can be confused with a bipartite sesamoid. Sesamoiditis, however, tends to be associated with more stellate sesamoids and is more indicative of nonhealing.

Tendinopathy

Peroneal tendinopathy results from either acute trauma or microtrauma as opposed to a watershed vascular area of the posterior tibial tendon. The peroneal tendons frequently develop with longitudinal splits to the brevis (**Figure 9**) or the longus. When seen early, primary repair of the tendons have good functional outcomes. A predisposing factor for tears of the brevis is the presence of space-occupying lesions in the fibular groove at the tip of the lateral malleolus. The brevis muscle, which protrudes distally onto the tendon, needs to be resected such that the retrofibular groove is clear. Acute injuries to the peroneal tendon frequently involve a rupture of the superior peroneal retinaculum that can often be seen on plain radiographs as an avulsion of the lateral malleolus. Subluxating or dislocating peroneal tendons have been described following calcaneal fractures or other lower extremity trauma. Multiple Kirschner wires can percutaneously hold the reduced tendons.[44]

The peroneus brevis tendon is an important structure in defining forefoot anatomy. If torn beyond repair, tenodesis may be done by sacrificing the longus or secondary repair involving autograft or allograft tendon. Primary repair and tubularization are indicated for tears involving less than 50% of the tendon, and tenodesis is indicated for tears involving more than 50% of the tendon.[45]

Lateral ankle pain may also present secondary to an accessory peroneal tendon, which is often poorly visualized on MRI. The most common is the peroneus tertius, which runs in the anterior compartment of the leg. Other accessory peroneal tendons, however, run behind the fibula in the retinaculum and attach to either tendons or the calcaneus itself (**Figure 10**).

The region of the Achilles tendon has several areas of pathology: between the tendon and the cortex of the calcaneus (bursitis), tendinitis, or tendinosis in the distal tendon. Initially for tendinitis or retrocalcaneal bursitis, nonsurgical treatment consisting of stretching with focus on the gastrocnemius tendon, or possibly a release of the tendon[46] and modalities to control inflammation has been successful.[47] With persistent pain due to tendinosis, a posterior midline incision[48] is recommended to detach the Achilles tendon insertion, débride diseased tendon and bursae,[49] and reattach the Achilles tendon.[50]

These conditions are common in tall patients or those with neurovascular issues. The denervation of the small nerves of the foot intrinsics results in overpull of the longus muscles. Nonsurgical management consists of a sling to hold the proximal phalanx parallel to the ground. Surgical management is reserved for painful deformities at the distal tips of the toes or proximal interphalangeal joint symptoms or ulcerations from the shoe rubbing against the toes. After surgery the toe should be straight and not interfere with other toes. The metatarsophalangeal joint will have appropriate passive plantar flexion and dorsiflexion, accomplished through a combination of tendon transfers and bony resection.

Crossover toe is caused by a traumatic injury to the metatarsophalangeal joint capsule, with development of fibrosis and contractures causing the toe to deviate into another toe.[43] This condition typically will cause impingement of the second toe onto the great toe. Because of the absence of a flexion contracture, bone shortening does not need to be performed. Instead, a dorsal capsulotomy and a tendon transfer of the brevis over the dorsum of the proximal phalanx holds the toe in the reduced position.

Sesamoiditis is a painful condition of the sesamoids at the level of the first metatarsophalangeal joint and is the result of overpressure similar to a metatarsalgia or

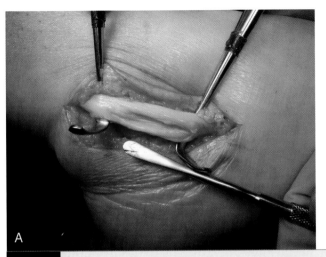

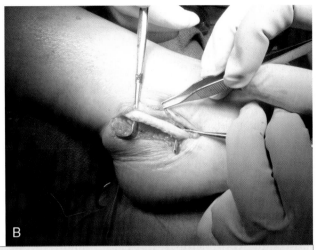

Figure 9 | **A,** Longitudinal tear with cavitation. **B,** The tendon after repair is shown.

Achilles tendon lacerations are always surgically repaired. Ruptures may be treated surgically or nonsurgically. Achilles tendon repairs have approximately 10% complication rates (wound problems in 5% and rerupture in 5%). Without surgery, there are 10% reruptures. Posterior ankle incisions require great care with tissue handling. The presence of a palpable gap is a contraindication to nonsurgical treatment. The AAOS Clinical Practice Guideline on Achilles Tendon Ruptures (www.aaos.org/research/guidelines/atrsummary.pdf) recommends early postoperative protected weight bearing.

Ligamentous Issues

The anterior talofibular ligament is most frequently sprained. Continued lateral instability following nonsurgical management is an indication for lateral reconstruction of the ankle. The repairs fall into two main categories: anatomic and nonanatomic. Anatomic repair of the ligament ends is preferred. If the ligament is avulsed from bone, it is anchored appropriately into the fibular origin or talar insertion. Often this repair is augmented with fibular periosteum[51] and extensor tendon retinaculum. The anterior talofibular repair is often done in conjunction with ankle arthroscopy, and appropriate placement of restricting tape during the arthroscopy enables the repair to be performed without significant fluid extravasation. When a primary repair cannot be performed, the use of a gracilis graft[52] has been described. Using the native peroneal brevis tendon for ankle ligament reconstruction is rarely considered given the importance of the brevis tendon.

Nerve Pain

Patients with foot and ankle injuries often have persistent pain after nonsurgical or surgical treatment. Oc-

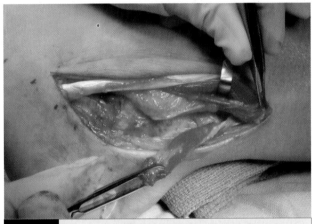

Figure 10 | Photograph showing the accessory peroneal in a 20-year-old woman who plays soccer and has lateral ankle pain. The aberrant tendon/muscle was reflected off the calcaneus.

cult fractures or dislocations may be responsible for persistence of symptoms, which is common with nondisplaced tarsometatarsal dislocations and lateral process of the talus fractures. Additionally, tarsal tunnel syndrome should be anticipated and expected in patients with crush injuries (Figure 11). Studies of release of the tarsal tunnel per se show mixed results.[53] The best surgical results are found when there is a space-occupying lesion within the tarsal tunnel. The inability to abduct the small toe is consistent with poor functioning of the lateral plantar nerve. Patients with complex regional pain syndrome should be referred to appropriate providers for medical management.

Surgical neuromas are a common complication following foot and ankle surgery; the density of sensory nerves in the region may be a contributing factor. Surgery on the lateral aspect of the foot often requires traction of a branch of the sural nerve. Surgical incisions on the anteromedial aspect of the ankle often involve iatrogenic injury to the saphenous nerve. Diagnostic blocks with lidocaine can help differentiate the location of these neuromas. The neuromas or nerve irritation may occur proximal to the obvious orthopaedic injury, for example, the superficial peroneal nerve as it crosses from posteriorly to anteriorly in the lower leg.

Diabetic Neuropathy

Diabetes has particular influence on foot and ankle reconstruction, beyond that of poor bone quality. The persistent microtrauma that develops in patients with diabetes results in deformities of the midfoot and hindfoot. Additionally, the insensate foot is susceptible to pressure ulcers.

Forefoot ulcers occur as a result of skin breakdown secondary to increasing pressure. Because the patient has lost protective sensation there is an absence of appropriate unloading of the offending areas, resulting in skin ulcerations. Forefoot pressure is exacerbated by a plantar-flexed ankle position secondary to either a tight Achilles tendon or a gastrocnemius tendon. Although ulcers may develop infections that necessitate amputation, the pressure ulcers can be successfully treated by unloading the affected area. Total contact casting is a useful tool in dispersing the overall forefoot pressure to a broad area. Additionally, correction of the plantar flexion contracture is successful in relieving forefoot pressure. Total contact casting is effective in treating Wagner grade 1 and 2 ulcers (absence of osteomyelitis) and after 4 weeks substantial healing should be apparent.[54]

Ulcerations in the hindfoot tend to be vascular in nature and more difficult to heal. Ulcerations in the midfoot are caused by increased pressure secondary to architectural collapse. The offending bone (cuneiform or cuboid) needs to be resected, often by a separate incision from the area of ulceration to remove the bony prominence that is causing increasing pressure.

Midfoot Charcot deformities in patients with diabetes require surgical intervention if there is an unbraceable deformity, a persistent or recurring ulceration, or an inability to provide support. Realignment fusions of the midfoot often require surgical implants that use locking plate technology or the addition of adjuvants to bone healing.

Hindfoot involvement in diabetes is associated with severe bone loss and malalignment. Tibiotalar fusions in this setting often include the calcaneus[55] (Figure 12). Implant fixation in patients with severe deformity and poor bone quality can be challenging.[56] Nails for a calcaneotalar tibial fusion have a significant incidence of tibial stress fractures, if the nail is contained in the distal third of the tibia. Formal joint preparation of the subtalar joint may not be necessary.[57]

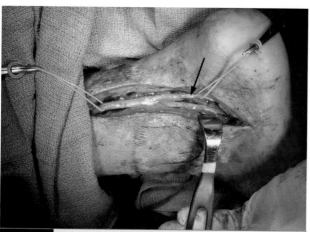

Figure 11 Photograph showing nerve release from scar. Note the constriction of the calcaneal branch.

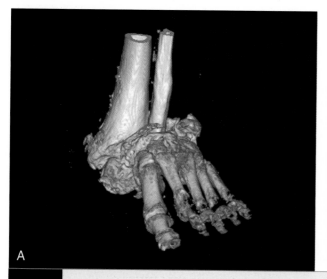

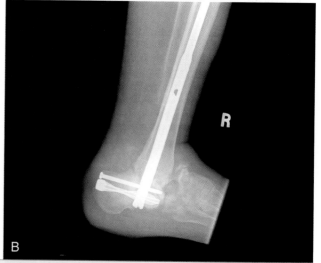

Figure 12 Charcot deformity of the tibiotalar joint and hindfoot. **A,** CT reconstruction AP view. **B,** Postoperative lateral radiograph.

Chronic and Persistent Deforming Forces

Neuromuscular issues affect the ability of the foot to transfer force more proximally into the lower extremity. A persistent plantar-flexed deformity will result in a functionally lengthened limb and make gait difficult. If the deformity has been present for a short to moderate time, then lengthening the gastrocnemius tendon or the Achilles tendon may allow the foot to be placed into a neutral position. For a long-term deformity, release of the tibiotalar posterior capsule may be necessary. Additionally, shortened flexor tendons without excursion that are also contracted will need to be released.

If there is no fixed plantar contracture but a loss of active dorsiflexion, then a transfer of the posterior tibial tendon from the posterior aspect of the ankle into the anterior midfoot can provide successful treatment of a foot drop. The surgical goal is to allow the ankle to dorsiflex such that the leg is able to swing unobstructed during the gait cycle and to provide eccentric contraction that will prevent "foot slap." Additionally, acute ruptures or lacerations of the tibialis anterior are treated with repair or reattachment of the anterior tibial tendon into the navicular.

Neuromuscular diseases such as Charcot-Marie-Tooth have predictable malalignments. With the weakened peroneus brevis, the foot develops a varus heel and posterior tibial tendon overpull. A weakened anterior tibial tendon results in plantar flexion of the first ray by the action of the peroneus longus. As previously discussed for the subtle cavus foot, a valgus heel slide and a dorsiflexion osteotomy of the first ray are required to place the foot into a position that can better facilitate the transfer of force from the ground to the lower extremity. The peroneus longus can be transferred to the brevis in conjunction with a heel slide to strengthen weak ankle evertors during stance phase.[58]

Annotated References

1. Brown TD, Johnston RC, Saltzman CL, Marsh JL, Buckwalter JA: Posttraumatic osteoarthritis: A first estimate of incidence, prevalence, and burden of disease. *J Orthop Trauma* 2006;20(10):739-744.

2. Weber BG, Simpson LA: Corrective lengthening osteotomy of the fibula. *Clin Orthop Relat Res* 1985; 199(199):61-67.

3. Lee HS, Wapner KL, Park SS, Kim JS, Lee DH, Sohn DW: Ligament reconstruction and calcaneal osteotomy for osteoarthritis of the ankle. *Foot Ankle Int* 2009; 30(6):475-480.

   The authors studied clinical and radiologic results of calcaneal osteotomy, joint débridement, and ligament reconstruction in the treatment of osteoarthritis of the ankle.

4. Jeng CL, Kadakia A, White KL, Myerson MS: Fresh osteochondral total ankle allograft transplantation for the treatment of ankle arthritis. *Foot Ankle Int* 2008;29(6): 554-560.

   The authors studied 169 patients with crossover second toe. The predominant incidence occurs in women older than 50 years. There was no correlation between crossover toe and second metatarsal length or IMA. Level of evidence: IV.

5. Chou LB, Coughlin MT, Hansen S Jr, et al: Osteoarthritis of the ankle: The role of arthroplasty. *J Am Acad Orthop Surg* 2008;16(5):249-259.

   A focused discussion on ankle arthritis and its treatment including total ankle arthroplasty is presented. The authors are encouraged by the improvements of total ankle arthroplasty but highlight the need for long-term studies not performed by surgeons involved in the implant's design. Level of evidence: V.

6. DeOrio JK, Easley ME: Total ankle arthroplasty. *Instr Course Lect* 2008;57:383-413.

   A comprehensive description of total ankle arthroplasty is presented, including contraindications, specific manufactured implants, costs, and future developments. Level of evidence: V.

7. Coetzee JC: Management of varus or valgus ankle deformity with ankle replacement. *Foot Ankle Clin* 2008; 13(3):509-520.

8. Kim BS, Choi WJ, Kim YS, Lee JW: Total ankle replacement in moderate to severe varus deformity of the ankle. *J Bone Joint Surg Br* 2009;91(9):1183-1190.

   Total ankle arthroplasty in 22 uninjured patients and 23 patients with varus deformity were compared. No significant difference in outcomes at 27 months was noted. Numerous charts depict surgical planning/interventions. Level of evidence: IV.

9. Wood PL, Prem H, Sutton C: Total ankle replacement: Medium-term results in 200 Scandinavian total ankle replacements. *J Bone Joint Surg Br* 2008;90(5):605-609.

   Two hundred STAR total ankle replacements were seen at a minimum of 5 years after surgery. Nineteen ankles were forward facing and 39 were backward facing; 68% had good relief from pain. American Orthopaedic Foot and Ankle Society score did not change compared to that of the 2-year study. The authors anticipate that total ankle replacement will be as reliable as knee replacement.

10. Conti SF, Dazen D, Stewart G, et al: Proprioception after total ankle arthroplasty. *Foot Ankle Int* 2008; 29(11):1069-1073.

    Thirteen patients (mean age, 57 years) who received an ankle replacement were studied 2 years later for proprioceptive differences; none were noted. Level of evidence: III.

11. Coetzee JC, Castro MD: Accurate measurement of ankle range of motion after total ankle arthroplasty. *Clin Orthop Relat Res* 2004;424:27-31.

12. Saltzman CL, Mann RA, Ahrens JE, et al: Prospective controlled trial of STAR total ankle replacement versus ankle fusion: Initial results. *Foot Ankle Int* 2009;30(7): 579-596.

    This article discusses the initial STAR total ankle replacement compared with ankle fusion and results and an additional 448 total ankle arthroplasties 24 months after surgery. At 2 years, total ankle arthroplasty led to better function and pain relief. Patients weighing more than 250 lb were excluded. There is a significant learning curve. Level of evidence: II.

13. Morgan SS, Brooke B, Harris NJ: Total ankle replacement by the Ankle Evolution System: Medium-term outcome. *J Bone Joint Surg Br* 2010;92(1):61-65.

    Thirty-eight consecutive patients received a three-part prosthesis with a mobile bearing component. Twenty-eight patients were able to walk unaided; however, within the first year, nine patients underwent revision because of edge loading. Despite an American Orthopaedic Foot and Ankle Society score of 88.1, the device was removed from the market because of high rates of osteolysis. Level of evidence: III.

14. Haddad SL, Coetzee JC, Estok R, Fahrbach K, Banel D, Nalysnyk L: Intermediate and long-term outcomes of total ankle arthroplasty and ankle arthrodesis: A systematic review of the literature. *J Bone Joint Surg Am* 2007;89(9):1899-1905.

    Of 460 citations studied, there were 10 articles on pertinent total ankle arthroplasties and 39 on ankle fusion for comparison. The study showed both procedures yield satisfactory results. The authors postulate that the poor connotations associated with total ankle arthroplasty are caused by failures in first-generation implants. Level of evidence: IV.

15. Sealey RJ, Myerson MS, Molloy A, Gamba C, Jeng C, Kalesan B: Sagittal plane motion of the hindfoot following ankle arthrodesis: A prospective analysis. *Foot Ankle Int* 2009;30(3):187-196.

    In 4 years, 48 patients were identified for a prospective study of sagittal plane motion following ankle fusion. A significant increase in hindfoot sagittal motion was noted as well as an uncoupling of the subtalar joint to the talonavicular joint. Patients with greater residual motion had better clinical outcomes. Level of evidence: II.

16. Gentchos CE, Bohay DR, Anderson JG: Technique tip: A simple method for ankle arthrodesis using solid screws. *Foot Ankle Int* 2009;30(4):380-383.

    A simple and effective tip to using solid screws is provided for ankle fusion. Radiation exposure and implant cost are minimized. This technique is easily performed by orthopaedic residents.

17. Eylon S, Porat S, Bor N, Leibner ED: Outcome of Ilizarov ankle arthrodesis. *Foot Ankle Int* 2007;28(8): 873-879.

    Seventeen patients were treated with Ilizarov ankle arthrodesis. The American Orthopaedic Foot and Ankle Society score was 65 of 86 possible (14 points were for motion that is not attainable). Weight bearing began on the third day and the patients were fully weight bearing by 6 weeks. Average follow-up was 6 years. No deterioration of results over time was noted. Level of evidence: IV.

18. Tarkin IS, Mormino MA, Clare MP, Haider H, Walling AK, Sanders RW: Anterior plate supplementation increases ankle arthrodesis construct rigidity. *Foot Ankle Int* 2007;28(2):219-223.

    Six cadaver ankles (four matched pairs) were tested. Anterior plate supplementation increased the stiffness of the tibiotalar interface by minimizing micromotion to the prepared joints. There was substantial variability in the specimens. This result may support the use of anterior plating in clinically osteoporotic bone.

19. Hintermann B, Barg A, Knupp M, Valderrabano V: Conversion of painful ankle arthrodesis to total ankle arthroplasty. *J Bone Joint Surg Am* 2009;91(4):850-858.

    The authors discuss minimum 3-year follow-up on 30 arthrodeses converted to total ankle arthroplasty using a three-component system. Indications were painful malunion or osteoarthritis of adjacent joints. Three-component systems are superior to the historically used two-component system. Level of evidence: IV.

20. Culpan P, Le Strat V, Piriou P, Judet T: Arthrodesis after failed total ankle replacement. *J Bone Joint Surg Br* 2007;89(9):1178-1183.

    Sixteen patients with failed total ankle arthroplasty underwent arthrodesis with screw fixation and an additional anterior bridging plate if necessary for stable fixation. Corticocancellous iliac crest graft was used to fill the void. This technique works best in patients with posttraumatic arthritis. One instance of nonunion occurred in a patient with juvenile rheumatoid arthritis. Level of evidence: IV.

21. Radnay CS, Clare MP, Sanders RW: Subtalar fusion after displaced intra-articular calcaneal fractures: Does initial operative treatment matter? *J Bone Joint Surg Am* 2009;91(3):541-546.

    Seventy-five calcaneal fractures underwent subtalar fusion; 36 were treated initially with surgery and 39 were treated closed. The American Orthopaedic Foot and Ankle Society score was better for the initial surgery group (87 versus 74). Postoperative wound compliations were also lower. Level of evidence: III.

22. Shawen SB, Anderson RB, Cohen BE, Hammit MD, Davis WH: Spherical ceramic interpositional arthroplasty for basal fourth and fifth metatarsal arthritis. *Foot Ankle Int* 2007;28(8):896-901.

    Thirteen patients with failed resection arthroplasty underwent ceramic ball interposition. The average American Orthopaedic Foot and Ankle Society score increased from 28.1 to 52.5. An extensive discussion of lateral midfoot arthrosis is presented. Level of evidence: IV.

23. Lee K-B, Saltzman CL, Suh J-S, Wasserman L, Amendola A: A posterior 3-portal arthroscopic approach for isolated subtalar arthrodesis. *Arthroscopy* 2008;24(11): 1306-1310.

Ten feet with subtalar arthritis and no deformity were fused in the prone position using an extra (third) portal. Fusion was achieved in 10 weeks. There were no complications with the posteromedial portal with the patient prone. Level of evidence: IV.

24. O'Loughlin PF, Heyworth BE, Kennedy JG: Current concepts in the diagnosis and treatment of osteochondral lesions of the ankle. *Am J Sports Med* 2010;38(2): 392-404.

    This review article discusses the authors' preferred technique and thoroughly discusses the history and current treatment strategies for osteochondral lesions. Level of evidence: V.

25. Sammarco VJ: Surgical correction of moderate and severe hallux valgus: Proximal metatarsal osteotomy with distal soft-tissue correction and arthrodesis of the metatarsophalangeal joint. *Instr Course Lect* 2008;57:415-428.

    Various methods of proximal metatarsal osteotomy are discussed (chevron, scarf, Ludloff, Mau, and crescentic), including the author's preferred technique of fusion: cup-in-cone. Diagrams of intrinsically stable and unstable osteotomies are presented. Level of evidence: V.

26. Trnka HJ, Hofstaetter SG, Easley ME: Intermediate-term results of the Ludloff osteotomy in one hundred and eleven feet: Surgical technique. *J Bone Joint Surg Am* 2009;91(Suppl 2 Pt 1):156-168.

    One hundred eleven feet underwent a Ludloff osteotomy for moderate to severe hallux valgus. American Orthopaedic Foot and Ankle Society scores increased from 53 to 88. This is a poor procedure for osteoporotic bone. The first metatarsal shortened 2.2 mm. Excellent clinical photographs and diagrams of the technique are presented. Level of evidence: IV.

27. Pinney S, Song K, Chou L: Surgical treatment of mild hallux valgus deformity: The state of practice among academic foot and ankle surgeons. *Foot Ankle Int* 2006; 27(11):970-973.

28. Pinney SJ, Song KR, Chou LB: Surgical treatment of severe hallux valgus: The state of practice among academic foot and ankle surgeons. *Foot Ankle Int* 2006; 27(12):1024-1029.

29. Murawski DE, Beskin JL: Increased displacement maximizes the utility of the distal chevron osteotomy for hallux valgus deformity correction. *Foot Ankle Int* 2008; 29(2):155-163.

    Thirty-nine feet were followed for an average of 34 months; American Orthopaedic Foot and Ankle Society score was 93. The lateral displacement of the chevron was 50% of the diaphysis. Postoperative American Orthopaedic Foot and Ankle Society hallux valgus score averaged 93, with a 7.9° improvement in intermetatarsal angle. Level of evidence: IV.

30. Deenik A, van Mameren H, de Visser E, de Waal Malefijt M, Draijer F, de Bie R: Equivalent correction in scarf and chevron osteotomy in moderate and severe hallux valgus: A randomized controlled trial. *Foot Ankle Int* 2008;29(12):1209-1215.

    Chevron osteotomy was at least as effective as a scarf osteotomy in treating moderate and severe hallux valgus. Three of 70 patients receiving chevron osteotomy developed osteonecrosis, and 1 developed complex regional pain syndrome. Seven of 66 scarf osteotomy patients developed complex regional pain syndrome. Level of evidence: I.

31. Coughlin MJ, Smith BW: Hallux valgus and first ray mobility: Surgical technique. *J Bone Joint Surg Am* 2008;90(suppl 2, pt 2):153-170.

    One hundred twenty-two feet were reviewed 27 months after surgical repair consisting of a proximal crescentic osteotomy. Hypermobility of the first ray was not noted after surgery. Level of evidence: IV.

32. Tai CC, Ridgeway S, Ramachandran M, Ng VA, Devic N, Singh D: Patient expectations for hallux valgus surgery. *J Orthop Surg (Hong Kong)* 2008;16(1):91-95.

    One hundred fifty-three patients were questioned concerning surgical expectations. The expectations differed in three age groups: younger than 40 years, 40 to 60 years, and older than 60 years. A 10-minute questionnaire allows the surgeon to address specific expectations during preoperative counseling. Level of evidence: II.

33. Coughlin MJ, Jones CP: Hallux valgus: Demographics, etiology, and radiographic assessment. *Foot Ankle Int* 2007;28(7):759-777.

    One hundred twenty-two feet with moderate or severe hallux valgus were demographically studied. Constricting shoes were implicated in 34% of patients. Magnitude of deformity was not associated with Achilles tendon or gastrocnemius tightness or first ray mobility. Level of evidence: IV.

34. Saro C, Jensen I, Lindgren U, Felländer-Tsai L: Quality-of-life outcome after hallux valgus surgery. *Qual Life Res* 2007;16(5):731-738.

    Ninety-four Swedish women with hallux valgus were evaluated 1 year after surgery with the Medical Outcomes Study 36-Item Short Form. Quality of life was improved after surgery. The degree of radiologic correction does not correlate with quality of life. Level of evidence: IV.

35. Coetzee JC, Resig SG, Kuskowski M, Saleh KJ: The Lapidus procedure as salvage after failed surgical treatment of hallux valgus: Surgical technique. *J Bone Joint Surg Am* 2004;86(suppl 1):30-36.

36. Coetzee JC, Wickum D: The Lapidus procedure: A prospective cohort outcome study. *Foot Ankle Int* 2004; 25(8):526-531.

37. Malal JJ, Shaw-Dunn J, Kumar CS: Blood supply to the first metatarsal head and vessels at risk with a chevron osteotomy. *J Bone Joint Surg Am* 2007;89(9):2018-2022.

    Ten cadaver limbs were dissected to study the blood supply to the distal first metatarsal head. The dorsal aspect of the neck had minor supply; the main supply to the capital fragment was the distal plantar-lateral corner. Therefore, a chevron osteotomy using a long plantar limb may decrease osteonecrosis.

38. Cronin JJ, Limbers JP, Kutty S, Stephens MM: Inter-metatarsal angle after first metatarsophalangeal joint arthrodesis for hallux valgus. *Foot Ankle Int* 2006;27(2): 104-109.

39. Squires NA, Jeng CL: Posterior tibial tendon dysfunction. *Operative Techniques in Orthopaedics* 2006; 16(1):44-52.

40. Deland JT: Adult-acquired flatfoot deformity. *J Am Acad Orthop Surg* 2008;16(7):399-406.

    A review of the literature with the author's preferred treatments is presented. Level of evidence: V.

41. Ellis SJ, Yu JC, Johnson AH, Elliott A, O'Malley M, Deland J: Plantar pressures in patients with and without lateral foot pain after lateral column lengthening. *J Bone Joint Surg Am* 2010;92(1):81-91.

    Ten patients 2 years after lateral column lengthening and hardware removal were compared for the presence of lateral column pain. Those with pain had higher lateral midfoot pressure. These increased pressures were not as a result of excessive lengthening. Level of evidence: III.

42. Logel KJ, Parks BG, Schon LC: Calcaneocuboid distraction arthrodesis and first metatarsocuneiform arthrodesis for correction of acquired flatfoot deformity in a cadaver model. *Foot Ankle Int* 2007;28(4):435-440.

    Ten cadaver specimens were loaded in two-legged stance after lengthening the lateral column by 10 mm. Lateral pressure increased from 24.2 to 30.4 after lengthening and then decreased to 26.2 after the first tarsometatarsal joint fusion. No calcaneal slide was performed.

43. Kaz AJ, Coughlin MJ: Crossover second toe: Demographics, etiology, and radiographic assessment. *Foot Ankle Int* 2007;28(12):1223-1237.

    One hundred sixty-nine patients with crossover second toe were studied. A prominent incidence in women older than 50 years was noted. There was no correlation between crossover toe and second metatarsal length or intermetatarsal angle. Level of evidence: IV.

44. Summers H, Kramer PA, Benirschke SK: Percutaneous stabilization of traumatic peroneal tendon dislocation. *Foot Ankle Int* 2008;29(12):1229-1231.

    Nine patients were treated with an indirect, manual reduction of peroneal tendons and stabilization percutaneously. None had recurrence or tendon pathology. Level of evidence: IV.

45. Heckman DS, Reddy S, Pedowitz D, Wapner KL, Parekh SG: Operative treatment for peroneal tendon disorders. *J Bone Joint Surg Am* 2008;90(2):404-418.

    A review of peroneal tendon disorders is presented. Level of evidence: V.

46. Gentchos CE, Bohay DR, Anderson JG: Gastrocnemius recession as treatment for refractory achilles tendinopathy: A case report. *Foot Ankle Int* 2008;29(6):620-623.

    After 2 years of chronic, progressive pain with 5 cm of tendinopathy, a patient underwent a modified Vulpius gastrocnemius lengthening with complete resolution of pain. Level of evidence: V.

47. Nicholson CW, Berlet GC, Lee TH: Prediction of the success of nonoperative treatment of insertional Achilles tendinosis based on MRI. *Foot Ankle Int* 2007;28(4): 472-477.

    Four hundred eighty-eight patients over a 3-year period were refined to 157 patients with Achilles tendinitis. An MRI classification system based on short-tau inversion recovery images was developed. MRI type II and III tears required surgery (91% and 70%, respectively). Only 2 of 16 of type I tendons had unsuccessful nonsurgical treatment. Level of evidence: IV.

48. Hammit MD, Hobgood ER, Tarquinio TA: Midline posterior approach to the ankle and hindfoot. *Foot Ankle Int* 2006;27(9):711-715.

49. McGarvey WC, Palumbo RC, Baxter DE, Leibman BD: Insertional Achilles tendinosis: Surgical treatment through a central tendon splitting approach. *Foot Ankle Int* 2002;23(1):19-25.

50. Wagner E, Gould JS, Kneidel M, Fleisig GS, Fowler R: Technique and results of Achilles tendon detachment and reconstruction for insertional Achilles tendinosis. *Foot Ankle Int* 2006;27(9):677-684.

51. Kirk KL, Schon LC: Technique tip: periosteal flap augmentation of the Brostrom lateral ankle reconstruction. *Foot Ankle Int* 2008;29(2):254-255.

    The authors present a technique tip accompanied by clinical photographs.

52. Boyer DS, Younger AS: Anatomic reconstruction of the lateral ligament complex of the ankle using a gracilis autograft. *Foot Ankle Clin* 2006;11(3):585-595.

53. Sung KS, Park SJ: Short-term operative outcome of tarsal tunnel syndrome due to benign space-occupying lesions. *Foot Ankle Int* 2009;30(8):741-745.

    The authors discussed clinical results after surgical treatment for tarsal tunnel syndrome caused by benign space-occupying lesions and found significant improvement in average visual analog scale and American Orthopaedic Foot and Ankle Society scores, but subjective satisfaction was less favorable (54%) than expected.

54. Coerper S, Beckert S, Küper MA, Jekov M, Königsrainer A: Fifty percent area reduction after 4 weeks of treatment is a reliable indicator for healing—analysis of a single-center cohort of 704 diabetic patients. *J Diabetes Complications* 2009;23(1):49-53.

    A cohort of 704 diabetic patients were treated with initial sharp débridement and adequate pressure offloading over a 10-year period. Wounds that do not reduce by half after 4 weeks require a modification of the patient's treatment regimen. Level of evidence: IV.

55. Chodos MD, Parks BG, Schon LC, Guyton GP, Campbell JT: Blade plate compared with locking plate for tibiotalocalcaneal arthrodesis: A cadaver study. *Foot Ankle Int* 2008;29(2):219-224.

Nine matched pairs of cadavers were treated with either a locking proximal humerus plate or a blade plate. The locking plate was found to be mechanically superior in providing fixation under cyclical loads.

56. Ahmad J, Pour AE, Raikin SM: The modified use of a proximal humeral locking plate for tibiotalocalcaneal arthrodesis. *Foot Ankle Int* 2007;28(9):977-983.

Sixteen of 17 patients with significant medical comorbidities healed at 21 weeks; 15 had osteoporosis. The plate was placed laterally; American Orthopaedic Foot and Ankle Society scores increased from 15 to 77 (maximum, 86). Level of evidence: IV.

57. Boer R, Mader K, Pennig D, Verheyen CC: Tibiotalocalcaneal arthrodesis using a reamed retrograde locking nail. *Clin Orthop Relat Res* 2007;463:151-156.

The authors present a retrospective multicenter study with one implant and a technique that differed only on débridement of the ankle joint (osteotome or drill bit). Both groups had a 100% tibiotalar union rate and American Orthopaedic Foot and Ankle Society scores of 70 (out of 86) at a mean of 51 months. The subtalar joint was débrided only by the reamer. Only 2 of 50 subtalar joints developed symptomatic nonunions. Level of evidence: IV.

58. Younger AS, Hansen ST Jr: Adult cavovarus foot. *J Am Acad Orthop Surg* 2005;13(5):302-315.

4: Lower Extremity

myodesis: suture muscle to bone for distal muscle stabilization
myoplasty: suture muscle to muscle, then place over end of
bone before wound closure
myodesis provides better distal muscle stabilization,
but myoplasty better if poor vascular health

Chapter 41

Lower Extremity Amputations

Michael T. Mazurek, MD   Scott Helmers, MD

Background

Traditionally, the main indications for amputation have been to preserve life by removing a badly damaged limb or for the treatment of malignancy. Amputation surgery currently is known as a refined reconstructive procedure intended to prepare the residual limb for motor functions of locomotion as well as for sensory feedback and cosmesis.[1] Common reasons for lower limb amputation are trauma, vascular pathology, neoplasm, infectious conditions, and congenital abnormalities.

In developed countries, most lower extremity amputations are performed for peripheral vascular disease secondary to atherosclerosis and/or diabetes mellitus (DM). In developing countries, the main indications are for trauma and infection. Although the pathophysiology of traumatic amputation may be different than dysvascular amputation, rehabilitation strategies and prosthetic component prescriptions for both should maximize function and quality of life. One of the many challenges in managing individuals requiring a trauma-related amputation is addressing the wide variety of comorbid injuries common in the multiply injured patient. In war-related amputations, additional injuries to peripheral nerves, retained shrapnel, heterotopic ossification, contaminated wounds, burns, grafted skin, and fractures require modified rehabilitation strategies to maximize the performance of activities of daily living (ADL) and ambulation.

The decision to amputate should be made by a surgeon comfortable with selection of level of amputation, muscle balancing, and wound closure[2] and in conjunction with the patient and their needs. In the presence of trauma, careful consideration should be made with respect to the acute decision between limb salvage and amputation,[3,4] especially in light of recent literature demonstrating that none of the currently used injury severity scores is predictive of outcome.[5] When considering amputation in the setting of neoplasm, an orthopaedic oncologist should be involved in the decision-making process.

Preoperative Management

The medical status of a patient undergoing an amputation should be optimized to facilitate the best surgical and rehabilitative outcomes. This includes managing any comorbidities present before proceeding with amputation; these will be reviewed later in the chapter. When possible, appropriate rehabilitation interventions should be initiated while the patient is awaiting amputation to maximize present function and prevent secondary complications.

Amputation Level

Level of amputation often dictates rehabilitation, functional outcome, and long-term quality of life. Several factors are important in determining level of amputation, including patient goals, the patient's general medical condition, associated injuries, risks associated with additional surgeries, physiologic healing potential, surgeon experience, the soft-tissue zone of injury, and predicted functional outcome.

Amputation should preserve as much of the limb as possible because a longer residual limb allows for better prosthetic control. If possible, the knee should be salvaged to decrease the energy consumption required for ambulating. In transtibial amputations, the energy expenditure in walking is 25% to 40% above normal, whereas in transfemoral amputations, it is 68% to 100% above normal.[6,7] This increased energy expenditure may result in a lower level of function in patients with cardiovascular or pulmonary comorbidities, rendering some patients nonambulatory.[7] Level of amputation is more predictive of mobility than any other patient factor, including age, sex, diabetes, emergency admission, indication for amputation, and prior vascular surgery.[8] The amount of residual limb needed varies with level of amputation.

With transtibial amputation, an optimal residual limb allows adequate space for the prosthetic foot and sufficient muscle padding over the residual limb. The ideal location of amputation is the middle of the tibia. At a minimum, amputation should be performed at the

Dr. Mazurek is deceased. At the time of publication, Dr. Mazurek or an immediate family member had received research or institutional support from the Orthopaedic Trauma Extremity Research Program, a federally funded project. Neither Dr. Helmers nor any immediate family member has received anything of value from or owns stock in a commercial company or institution related directly or indirectly to the subject of this chapter.

myodesis: suture muscle to bone for distal muscle stabilization
myoplasty: suture muscle to muscle, then place over end of bone before wound closure
myodesis provides better distal muscle stabilization, but myoplasty better if poor vascular health

junction of the middle third and proximal third of the tibia, just below the flare of the tibial plateau, preserving the tibial tubercle (which allows sufficient tibia for weight bearing).

With transfemoral amputation, an optimal residual limb allows space for an uncompromised knee system. The ideal location of amputation is typically just above the condylar flare at the level of the adductor tubercle. At a minimum, amputation should be performed at the junction of the middle third and proximal third of the femur (below the level about the lesser trochanter) to allow for a sufficient lever arm to operate the prosthesis. If there is uncertainty about the optimal length of the residual limb, preoperative consultation with an experienced physiatrist or prosthetist should be considered.

The ultimate functional desires and expectations of the patient must be included in the decision-making process. A desire to return to high-level athletic activities may influence the ultimate level of ambulation in an attempt to preserve a longer limb with a lower chance of healing. Conversely, in the presence of severe medical conditions, amputation at a more proximal level with a greater chance of healing may be more reasonable.

The potential for wound healing is another factor that must be included in surgical decision making. Healing potential may be determined by noninvasive tests to assess for vascular competency.[9-11] The most reliable and sensitive test for wound healing is transcutaneous oxygen pressure measurement, which assesses the partial pressure of oxygen diffusing through the

transfemoral

skin.[12-14] Values greater than 40 mg Hg indicate acceptable wound healing potential. Values less than 30 mm Hg indicate poor wound healing potential.[12] The ischemic index, a ratio of Doppler pressure at the level being tested compared to the brachial systolic pressure, has been advocated as another noninvasive method to determine wound healing potential. An ischemic index of 0.5 or greater at the surgical level has been shown to be necessary to support healing. These tests are useful adjuncts to the clinical decision-making process.

The amputation level may ultimately be determined by the site of injury and damaged tissues. In addition to preserving length, it is important to ensure that the residual limb is adequately covered with muscle and sensate skin that is free of scar tissue.[15] Although some authors have advocated the use of a through-knee amputation as an alternative, suggesting the benefits of a weight-bearing end, the Lower Extremity Assessment Project study suggested through-knee amputations have a worse Sickness Impact Profile (SIP) score than transfemoral amputations.[16]

General Principles

The handling of the bone, muscles, and nerves during the surgical amputation can have a profound impact on the patient's prosthetic fitting and rehabilitation. Bone cuts should be made transverse and beveled to avoid bony prominence. No periosteal stripping should be performed to avoid heterotopic bone formation. Bony prominences and heterotopic bone may complicate prosthetic fabrication and wear. Muscle should be divided distal to the bone resection to ensure adequate soft-tissue coverage. Myodeses may be performed in patients with good healing potential to facilitate muscle tone, balance, and strength in the residual limb. A balanced myoplasty can also be performed, approximating the antagonistic muscles together, centering the bone. Nerves should be individually identified, placed under gentle traction, sharply transected, and allowed to retract proximally. This will place the nerve in a scarless area in an attempt to reduce the risk of neuroma stimulation. When closing the wound, there should be no tension on the skin. The surgery flaps developed should be closed in a location that will not affect prosthetic fitting. It is a good idea to leave the sutures in longer than the usual 2-week period because when the patient lifts the stump, tension is placed on the wound. Sutures should be removed after adequate skin healing.

Creating a bone bridge between the tibia and fibula can be considered in traumatic, nondysvascular transtibial amputations[1] (**Figure 1**). Proponents of this technique argue that the creation of a bone bridge allows for weight bearing on the end of the residual limb. Others believe that although the technique does increase the surface area for distributing mechanical load and prevent pain from pathologic motion of the fibula, it should be reserved for young, active amputees whose potential to benefit from a better terminal weight-bearing surface offsets the morbidity of additional sur-

neuroma: nerve endings form neuromas when transected, but if not in an area subject to pressure, less likely to become stimulated → impt to let nerves retract proximally

gery.[17] One study examined a cohort of 20 consecutive patients who had a unilateral transtibial amputation with distal tibiofibular bone bridging following lower extremity trauma.[17] These patients were compared to a historical control group of 15 highly functional patients with a traditional transtibial amputation. The groups were compared using the Prosthesis Evaluation Questionnaire, a validated outcomes measure that quantifies the effect of lower extremity amputation on quality of life. No significant difference was found between the groups,[17] suggesting that distal tibiofibular bone bridging may not lead to improved outcomes, particularly when it requires an additional operation. The study also further highlights the need for prospective research to facilitate further understanding of the residual limb as an end-bearing surface in patients with transtibial amputation.[18]

Postoperative Dressing

The appropriate postoperative dressing should be planned preoperatively. A proper dressing should protect the residual limb, decrease edema, and facilitate wound closure. There is inconclusive evidence for the use of any specific postoperative dressing, with or without an immediate postoperative prosthesis. Current protocols and decisions are based on local practice, skill, and intuition with the primary goal of maintaining the integrity of the residual limb.

Pain Management

Pain should be assessed at all phases of rehabilitation, preferably with a tool specifically designed for use in lower extremity amputees (**Tables 1** and **2**). Pain after amputation may occur in the phantom limb, the residual limb, the contralateral limb, or the lower back. The intensity of pain should be assessed separately at each significant site to achieve a thorough assessment of pain-related impairment. During the immediate postoperative phase, liberal narcotic analgesics should be considered. With progression through the rehabilitation process, a gradual transition to a nonnarcotic pharmacologic regimen combined with physical, psychological, and mechanical modalities should be used. Treatment should target pain related to the residual/phantom limb and address pain in other body parts. There is no consistent evidence to support any specific type of analgesia. Available modalities include pharmacologic agents such as antiseizure medications (gabapentin), tricyclic antidepressants (TCAs), selective serotonin reuptake inhibitors (SSRIs), nonsteroidal anti-inflammatory drugs (NSAIDs), N-methyl-D-aspartic acid (NMDA) receptor antagonists, and long-acting narcotics; epidural analgesia (patient-controlled analgesia [PCA] or regional analgesia); and nonpharmacologic agents such as transcutaneous electrical nerve stimulation (TENS), desensitization, scar mobilization, relaxation, acupuncture, biofeedback, and mirror therapy. Mirror therapy con-

sisted of the patient placing their intact limb into a box with a mirror down the midline, so that when viewed from slightly off center, it would give the appearance of having two intact limbs. By using a series of limb movement exercises, some patients experienced a reduction in phantom limb pain. The exact mechanism behind mirror therapy's effect is unknown, but it is thought to reverse this cortical remapping and alleviate pain.[19]

Two recent studies have examined the development and treatment of pain following amputation. The first study examined the potential mechanisms for origin of phantom limb pain in a study of 96 upper limb amputees.[20] A questionnaire was used to assess preamputation pain and the presence or absence of phantom pain, phantom sensation, stump pain, and stump sensation, with a median duration of follow-up of 3.2 years (range, 0.9 to 3.8 years). The authors concluded that stump pain/sensation is the initial predominating source of patient discomfort and that phantom pain/sensation is a long-term consequence with some patients noting an onset almost a year after surgery.

The second study examined modalities for the management of persistent pain following lower extremity amputation in a double-blind, randomized trial evaluating the effect of ketamine on pain and sensory processing in amputees.[21] Fifty-three patients undergoing lower limb amputation participated. After receiving a combined intrathecal-epidural anesthetic for surgery, patients either received an epidural infusion of racemic ketamine and bupivacaine (group K) or saline solution and bupivacaine (group S). In the immediate postoperative period, group K patients had substantially lower pain scores than group S patients. After discontinuation of the epidural anesthetic until the time of the 1-year follow-up, the rates of stump and phantom pain did not differ between the two groups (21% and 50%, respectively, for group K compared with 33% and 40%, respectively, for group S). The levels of depression and anxiety were found to decrease significantly in group K patients during the course of the study, whereas a similar decrease was not seen in group S patients. This is believed to be due to the NMDA receptor antagonist effects of ketamine.

Medical Cormorbidity Management

The cardiovascular demands of ambulation with a residual limb are significant, as are the risks that cardiovascular disease imparts on patients undergoing amputation. It has been estimated that the mean oxygen consumption is 9% to 40% higher in patients with unilateral transtibial amputations, 49% to 100% higher in unilateral transfemoral amputations, and 280% percent higher in bilateral transfemoral amputations.[6,22] Cardiac risk may impact the survival risk from the amputation surgery and thus may play a role in the decision regarding the level of amputation.[23] Additionally, exercise tolerance testing may be warranted during the rehabilitation phase to help establish clear guidelines for cardiac precautions in therapy.

Table 1

Pain Diagnosis and Treatment Options for Phantom and Sensational Limb Pain

Etiology	Key History or Examination Features	Evaluation	Treatment	
			Nonpharmacologic	Pharmacologic
Phantom Limb Pain (Pain distal to the end of the residual limb)				
Primary phantom limb pain	Onset usually later in postamputation period. Often nocturnal .Gradually reduced in intensity and frequency over time. Can be excacerbated by residual limb pain.	Diagnosis of exclusion once other causes of phantom limb pain have been ruled out.	Desensitization Mirror therapy Residual limb compressive devices Prosthetic use TENS Acupuncture Alternative and complementary medicine Mental health evaluation and treatment (depression, PTSD)	TCAs Anticonvulsants Antispasmodics SSRIs NMDA receptor antagonists
Referred pain from proximal neurologic or musculoskeletal source	Consider symptoms of typical musculo-skeletal, radicular, causes.	Imaging as appropriate. EMG/nerve conduction velocity studies.	Treat underlying cause as appropriate	Pharmacologic Rx as appropriate
Referred pain from a neuroma	Aggravated by prosthetic use. Local tinel or tenderness at the end of the nerve.	Diagnostic injection Ultrasound or MRI.	Prosthetic modification to reduce mechanical loads Corticosteroid injection Phenol ablation Surgical resection	Consider pharmacologic Rx if nonresponsive to other treatments: TCAs Anticonvulsants Antispasmodics SSRIs NMDA receptor antagonists
Phantom Limb Sensation (Nonpainful sensations distal to the residual limb; wide spectrum of sensory experiences that vary in intensity, frequency, and severity)				
If mild and not functionally limiting		None	Educate and reassure patient	None
If of adequate severity that is perceived as uncomfortable or distressing	Onset in early postamputation period. Often nocturnal. Gradually reduced in intensity and frequency over time.	No specific	Desensitization Mirror therapy Residual limb compressive devices Prosthetic use TENS Acupuncture Alternative and complementary medicine	Consider pharmacologic Rx if nonresponsive to other treatments: TCAs Anticonvulsants Antispasmodics SSRIs NMDA receptor antagonist

Evidence indicates that individuals undergoing amputation have an incidence of deep venous thrombosis (DVT) ranging from 11% to 50%.[24,25] Complications of venous thrombus formation may include thrombophlebitis, pulmonary embolism, or death. DVT prophylaxis is, therefore, warranted in all patients with amputation as per institutional and/or consensus guidelines. Considerable debate exists as to which prophylactic method is best. A recent study found equal efficacy of low-molecular-weight heparin (enoxaparin) with unfractionated heparin in this patient population.[26] Care should be taken when using anticlotting agents in multiple-trauma patients, especially those with suspected intracranial hemorrhage.

Patients with conditions such as hyperlipidemia, hypertension, obesity, and diabetes should also be monitored carefully throughout the continuity of care. These health care concerns are the leading causes of morbidity and mortality. In the United States, 75% of amputations occur in people age 65 years or older, and 95% are performed because of peripheral vascular disease, with or without diabetes.[27] Malnourished patients are

Table 2

Pain Diagnosis and Treatment Options for Residual Limb Pain

Etiology	Key History or Examination Features	Evaluation	Treatment Nonpharmacologic	Pharmacologic
Residual Limb Pain (Pain in the limb between the end of the residual limb and the next most proximal joint)				
Mechanical	Excacerbated by use of the prosthesis Associated with residual limb findings of redness, callous, or ulceration	Evaluate prosthetic fit and alignment	Refer to prosthetist	Acetaminophen NSAIDs
Neuroma	Pain with prothetic use Local tinel sign Possible palpable mass	Diagnostic injection Ultrasound or MRI	Prosthetic modification to reduce mechanical loads Corticosteroid injection Phenol ablation Surgical resection	Consider pharmacologic Rx if nonresponsive to other treatments: TCAs Anticonvulsants Antispasmodics SSRIs NMDA receptor antagonist
Ischemic	Claudication with ambulation	Vascular evaluation	Treat as appropriate	
Infection Cellulitis Abcess Osteomyelitis	Classical examination features Unexplained poor glucose control Pain unexplained by other causes	Laboratory evaluation WBC CRP/ESR Glucose Imaging studies as appropriate	Treat as appropriate	
Neuropathic Central (CRPS) Peripheral	Hypersensitivity Autonomic features	Consider triple phase bone scan	Desensitization Residual limb compressive devices Prosthetic use TENS Acupuncture Alternative and complementary medicine Mental health evaluation and treatment (depression, PTSD)	Consider pharmacologic Rx if nonresponsive to other treatments: TCAs Anticonvulsants Antispasmodics SSRIs NMDA receptor antagonists

at greater risk for delayed wound healing, decubitus ulcer formation, infection, congestive heart failure, progressive weakness, apathy, and death. Evidence suggests that malnourishment is common in patients with amputations and that supplementary nutrition may improve healing.[28]

Behavioral Health / Psychological Management

Assessment

Assessment of the amputee should focus on current psychiatric symptoms, with a particular focus on depressive and anxiety symptoms, including posttraumatic stress symptoms. Posttraumatic stress symptoms may include re-experiencing of the trauma (flashbacks), avoidance to the point of having a phobia of places, people, and experiences that remind the sufferer of the trauma, and chronic physical signs of hyperarousal (sleep problems, trouble concentrating, irritability, anger, poor concentration, blackouts, or difficulty remembering things). There is evidence that a relatively high percentage of patients experience such problems.[29-32] Posttraumatic stress disorder (PTSD) symptoms are more common and severe for individuals whose trauma involves combat-related injury.[32] Levels of depression and anxiety appear to be relatively high for up to 2 years after amputation and then decline to normal pop-

4: Lower Extremity

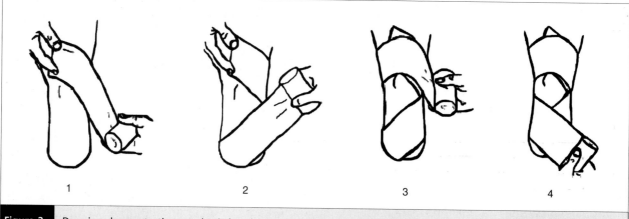

1   2   3   4

Figure 2 Drawing demonstrating an elastic bandaging technique. (Copyright Alvin L. Muilenburg and A. Bennett Wilson Jr, Houston, TX, 1996. http://www.oandp.com/resources/patientinfo/manuals/5.htm)

ulation levels.[30] There is good evidence that depression and posttraumatic stress can be effectively treated with both pharmacologic and psychotherapeutic interventions.

Postoperative depression and anxiety can, therefore, resolve in a period of a few months, much more rapidly than was previously believed.[33] During the immediate postoperative course, inpatient rehabilitation should be focused on teaching skills that can improve patient function by the time of discharge as such function is correlated with less depression even in patients who are in severe distress. Furthermore, patients at greater risk for postamputation depression (those with comorbidities or living alone) can be identified such that additional support be given both preoperatively and postoperatively.

Assessment should also address major life stressors as well as a patient's familial/social network, as these factors are likely to influence rehabilitation. Several studies indicate that social support enhances psychosocial adjustment, overall functioning, and pain management after amputation.[30,31,34] Effective coping strategies may also enhance psychosocial adjustment and pain management, wheras ineffective strategies may diminish these characteristics.

At later phases of rehabilitation (after the amputation), the provider should assess social and body image anxiety/discomfort, which is not uncommon, particularly among younger and female patients.[30,35,36] The loss of a limb distorts the body image; lowers self-esteem; and increases social isolation, discomfort, and dependence on others, resulting in activity restriction (which may be a mediating factor for depression).[30]

Advances in the cosmetic appearance of prostheses have led to the development of cosmetic covers that are remarkably similar in appearance to the contralateral limb. The appearance of the prosthesis affects the patient's ability to disguise the disability and reduces the amputation-related body image concerns and perceived social stigma.[37] Overall activity level, including the presence of excessive activity restriction, and satisfac-

tion with the prosthesis should be assessed. Activity level is reciprocally related to depressive and anxiety symptoms, and excessive activity restriction compromises functional outcomes.

Residual Limb Management

Edema Control

Edema control through compressive therapy is the foundation of limb shaping and will reduce pain and improve mobility. Edema can be controlled by rigid dressings with or without an attached pylon, residual limb shrinkers, or soft dressings such as an elastic wrap. Proper wrapping techniques are essential whenever soft dressings are used to reduce complications from poor application (**Figure 2**).

Contracture Prevention

Several passive strategies are available to prevent contractures at both the hip and the knee. Knee immobilizers and rigid dressings attempt to address the goal of knee flexion contracture prevention in the patient with a transtibial amputation. Active strategies to prevent contractures are well documented for the patient with a transtibial or transfemoral amputation and include bed positioning, prone activities, various stretching techniques, and knee and hip joint mobilization by therapists. A seemingly innocuous and caring gesture of placing a pillow under the residual limb actually encourages development of hip and knee flexion contractures. A pillow or rolled towel along the lateral aspect of the thigh, however, may help prevent a hip abduction contracture and should be considered as a preventive technique.

Heterotopic Ossification in the Residual Limbs of Individuals With Traumatic and Combat-Related Amputations

Reports on the occurrence and treatment of heterotopic ossification in patients with amputations are rare. Heterotopic ossification in the residual limbs of patients with amputation may cause pain and skin breakdown and complicate or prevent optimal prosthetic fit (**Figure 3**). The recent experience of the military amputee centers with traumatic and combat-related amputations has demonstrated a surprisingly high prevalence of heterotopic ossification in residual limbs (up to 63%). Occurrence rates are related to amputations through the initial zone of injury and those that are caused by blast injuries.[38] Primary prophylactic regimens, such as NSAIDs and local irradiation, which have proved to be effective in preventing or limiting heterotopic ossification in other patient populations, have not been studied in patients with amputations and generally are not feasible in the setting of acute traumatic amputation. Many patients are asymptomatic or can be successfully managed with modification of the prosthesis. For patients with refractory symptoms, surgical excision is associated with low recurrence rates and decreased medication requirements with acceptable complication rates.[38]

unknown whether NSAIDs or irradiation works for HO prevention

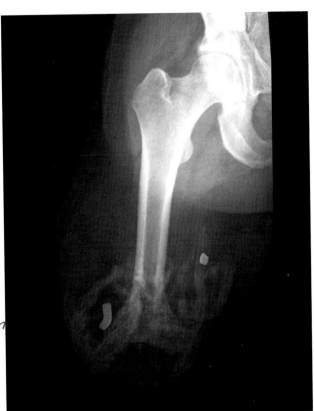

Figure 3 | Radiograph showing posttraumatic heterotopic bone formation.

Patient Education

Patients who are active participants in their rehabilitation and maintain positive interactions with team members are more likely to have successful outcomes after amputation. Patients should be given appropriate advice and adequate information on rehabilitation programs, prosthetic options, and possible outcomes with realistic rehabilitation goals.[39]

Prosthetic Management

Amputees have wide-ranging personal, social, and professional demands. Their ability to meet these demands will be mediated by several factors, including residual limb characteristics, overall health, fitness, and other medical conditions. Based upon these factors, a best estimate of future activities needs to be made so that the patient may receive the most appropriate prosthetic prescription (**Table 3**).

The Centers for Medicare and Medicaid Services, formerly known as the Health Care Financing Administration, requires a determination of functional level with certificates of medical necessity for a prosthesis. These are known as "K" levels.

Prostheses are described at this phase as either preparatory (preliminary) or definitive. The preparatory prosthesis is fitted while the residual limb is still remodeling. This allows the patient to commence the rehabilitation program of donning and doffing, transfer training, building wear tolerance, improving balance, and ambulating with the prosthesis several weeks earlier. A preparatory prosthesis often allows a better fit in the final prosthesis as the preparatory socket can be used to decrease edema and shape the residual limb.[40]

Technologic advances have led to vastly improved prostheses for amputees. With the changing nature of military combat, there have been an increasing number of young men and women who have sustained traumatic amputations, leading to to increased interest and research in the development of upper and lower extremity prostheses.[41-45] Unfortunately, despite several well-designed gait analysis studies and many subjective observations by patients and clinicians, there are few objective data to guide the use of various high-technology knee and foot systems.

Rehabilitation

The goal of rehabilitation is to achieve maximum independence and function. The individual's rehabilitation program takes into account preamputation lifestyle, expectations, and medical limitations. The following areas of interventions include a suggested step approach, indicating the key elements in each area during progression throughout the rehabilitation process.

Range of Motion

An amputation results in an inherent weakness of the residual limb due to the new attachments of the cut distal muscles to either bone or other muscle. The patient with a transfemoral amputation has a greater propensity for hip flexion and abduction contracture because of the relative weakness of the adductor magnus muscle, which normally is a strong hip adductor and exten-

Table 3

Prosthetic Prescription

Functional Level	Transtibial	Transfemoral
Unlimited household ambulatory (K1) - The patient has the ability or potential to use the prosthesis for transfers or ambulation on level surfaces at a fixed cadence.	• Patella tendon bearing (PTB) or total surface bearing (TSB) • Sleeve or pin/shuttle • Soft foam or gel liner • Flexible keel foot • Endoskeletal or exoskeletal pylon	• Modified quadrilateral (quad) (improve sitting comfort) • Silesian/pin/ shuttle/lanyard/total elastic suspension (TES) • Gel liner or frame socket • Knee systems[a] • Flexible keel or single-axis foot • Endoskeletal pylon
Limited community ambulatory (K2) - The patient has the ability or potential for ambulation with the ability to traverse low-level environmental barriers such as curbs, stairs, or uneven surfaces.	• PTB or TSB • Sleeve or pin/shuttle or suction • Soft foam or gel liner or hard socket • Flexible keel, multi-axial, or energy storage foot • Endoskeletal or exoskeletal pylon	• Quad, modified quad, or ischial containment • Pin/shuttle/lanyard/silesian/suction/TES • Gel liner or frame socket • Knee systems[a] • Flexible keel or single-axis foot • Endoskeletal pylon
Community ambulatory (K3) - The patient has the ability or potential for ambulation with variable cadence, has the ability to traverse most environmental barriers, and may have vocational, therapeutic, or exercise activity that demands prosthetic utilization beyond simple locomotion.	• PTB or TSB • Sleeve, pin/shuttle, suction, or vacuum • Soft foam or gel liner or hard socket • Flexible keel, multi-axial foot • Torsion and/or vertical shock pylon • Endoskeletal or exoskeletal pylon	• Quad, modified quad, or ischial containment • Pin/shuttle, suction, silesian/suction/TES • Gel liner or frame socket • Knee systems[a] • Flexible keel, multi-axial, or energy storage foot • Torsion and/or vertical shock pylon • Endoskeletal pylon
Exceeds basic ambulation (K4) - Exhibiting high impact, stress, or energy levels typical of the prosthetic demands of the child, active adult, or athlete	• PTB or TSB • Pin/shuttle/sleeve/suction • Soft foam or gel liner • Flexible, multiaxial, or energy storage foot • Specialty foot (running) • Torsion and/or vertical shock pylon • Endoskeletal or exoskeletal pylon	• Ischial containment • Suction/pin/shuttle/silesian/ suction/combo • Gel liner or frame socket • Knee systems[a] • Quad, modified quad • Flexible keel or specialty foot (running) • Torsion and/or vertical shock pylon • Endoskeletal pylon

[a] With variable specifications.

sor. Some hip and knee flexion contractures can be accommodated by modifications in the prosthesis. However, normal range of motion of all joints should be pursued.

Proper positioning will decrease the risk of developing joint contractures, particularly at the hip and knee of the involved limb. Contractures at these joints may adversely affect prosthetic fitting and subsequent mobility and function. The authors of one study used a clinically relevant regression model to demonstrate the effectiveness of early inpatient rehabilitation. Contractures were aggressively addressed and preventive strategies, such as prone lying, side lying, and aggressive pain control, were implemented to decrease the risk of contracture. The investigators found that these strategies, combined with the initiation of prosthetic gait training, led to a higher rate of successful prosthetic use.[46] Another study found similar results when similar strategies were focused on the proximal joints.[47]

Strengthening

It has been found that ambulating with a prosthesis results in an increase in energy expenditure.[48] In addition, higher metabolic costs were found in patients with higher levels of amputation, advanced age, or a history of peripheral vascular disease.[22] The amputee must, therefore, improve strength and cardiovascular endurance to maximize function.

Mobility and Equipment

The key to independence and reintegration after amputation is personal mobility, which comprises both ease and freedom of movement. Only walking provides freedom of movement and is indispensable for independence.[49] Several studies describe a positive association between a patient's mobility and his or her quality of life. Authors of one study used the Nottingham Health Profile in 1993 to determine that persons with amputations rated their overall quality of life as poor compared to a control group. They found that mobility was the only significant factor that impacted this rating.[50] Another study emphasized that regaining ambulation is a key to returning patients to their previous lifestyles, roles, activities, and socialization.[51] These studies suggest that the major focus of a rehabilitation program should be improving patient mobility.

Long-term outcomes are assessed in relation to the ultimate rehabilitation goals. Successful long-term rehabilitation outcomes must take into account not only the success of prosthetic fitting but also an individual's overall level of function in a community setting.[52]

Prosthetic Rehabilitation

Prosthetic training follows the preprosthetic rehabilitation phase. Once a patient is deemed a candidate for a prosthesis, provisions are made for a prosthetic prescription, basic rehabilitation, prosthetic management, and gait training based on identified goals. If the patient is not a candidate for a prosthesis, the team will perform basic rehabilitation and provide durable medical equipment. At the conclusion of the prosthetic phase, the goal is to attain maximal functional independence and mobility with the artificial limb. Also desired are prosthetic fitting and intensive gait training interventions to reduce the occurrence of phantom pain and improve long-term outcomes, including returning to work. During this phase, patients are given advice on employment, recreational activity, driving, and vocational rehabilitation. The continuation of care at the community level should be promoted and arranged. A recent study has shown little benefit of early walking aids during this phase of rehabilitation.[53]

Community Reintegration

Reintegration into a normal, preamputation level of work and physical activity is generally poor for the patient with an amputation in the areas of community mobility, work, and recreation. Return to work after severe lower extremity trauma remains a challenge. One study found that 75% of patients in the working-age group considered their integration into work unsuccessful, despite rating their perceptions of self-worth, home mobility, and psychosocial adjustment as satisfactory. Dependent factors were prior education, type of employment (sedentary compared with manual work), underlying medical condition, level of amputation, the availability of retraining assistance, the attitudes of employers and associates, and their own attitudes toward work. Emphasis should be placed on these aspects in rehabilitation.[54]

Follow-up Care

Follow-up care for all patients with amputations is needed to ensure continued optimal function in the home and community. Without scheduled follow-up care, patients may not recognize problems with the fit of their prosthesis, a change in their gait pattern, or changes in their contralateral or residual limb.[55] As a result, major or minor secondary complications may arise. Given the importance of optimal socket fit, the patient must also be monitored for volumetric and anatomic changes, alignment adjustments, component replacement, and continuing education. A lifelong consultation with other health care providers regarding the interaction between other disease processes and the function of patients with an amputation may be required to prevent amputations of the contralateral limb or ipsilateral limb more proximally (with a rate reportedly as high as 21% within the first 18 months after amputation).[56] For the patient with vascular disease or diabetes, long-term follow-up care should include appropriate foot care and patient education at every patient visit.

In addition, the level of independent walking decreases with time. One third of persons who were young (average age of 24 years, with standard deviation of 10 years) at the time of amputation were successfully rehabilitated; however, in subsequent follow-up (average age of 54 years, with standard deviation of 15 years) were noted to have limitations in mobility. Reevaluations should be conducted as needed for modification of a prosthesis to accommodate changes in functional status.[57] Reassessment of the available advancements in medical science and prosthetic technology will continue for the patient's lifetime.

There are no clinical trials that provide evidence of the need for lifelong care. Patients need to have access to primary care and amputation teams, but there is no evidence to indicate how often that follow-up should occur. However, follow-up visits to assess and modify the prosthesis become important because of changes that occur in amputees during the aging process.[58]

The loss of a limb provides ongoing stress to other areas of the body. Musculoskeletal problems may arise in the residual and contralateral limbs, spine, and upper extremities.

Approximately 65% of the amputations in people older than 50 years are due to vascular disease or the effects of diabetes. Of this population, 30% will lose a second limb to the same disease. Therefore, as much emphasis should be placed on preserving the contralateral limb as is placed on recovering from the amputation.[59]

Changes associated with aging, changes in the residual limb, prosthetic wear, and new technologies are all reasons to order a new prosthesis. Better technology has provided more responsive components and lighter materials, allowing for increased mobility in older amputees.

Annotated References

1. Pinzur MS, Gottschalk F, Pinto MA, Smith DG: Controversies in lower extremity amputation. *Instr Course Lect* 2008;57:663-672.

   The authors discuss the history, decision making, and techniques in amputation surgery.

2. Smith D; Clinical Standards of Practice Consensus Conference: Assessing outcomes and the future. *J Prosthet-*

ics Orthotics 2004;16(3S). http://www.oandp.org/jpo/library/index/2004_03S.asp. Accessed February 2007.

3. Bosse MJ, MacKenzie EJ, Kellam JF, et al: A prospective evaluation of the clinical utility of the lower-extremity injury-severity scores. *J Bone Joint Surg Am* 2001;83(1):3-14.

4. Bosse MJ, McCarthy ML, Jones AL, et al; Lower Extremity Assessment Project (LEAP) Study Group: The insensate foot following severe lower extremity trauma: An indication for amputation? *J Bone Joint Surg Am* 2005;87(12):2601-2608.

5. Ly TV, Travison TG, Castillo RC, Bosse MJ, MacKenzie EJ; LEAP Study Group: Ability of lower-extremity injury severity scores to predict functional outcome after limb salvage. *J Bone Joint Surg Am* 2008;90(8):1738-1743.

   This study examined the clinical utility of the five commonly used lower-extremity injury severity scoring systems as predictors of final functional outcome in 407 patients from the Lower Extremity Assessment Project (LEAP) study group: the Mangled Extremity Severity Score; the Limb Salvage Index; the Predictive Salvage Index; the Nerve Injury, Ischemia, Soft-Tissue Injury, Skeletal Injury, Shock, and Age of Patient Score; and the Hannover Fracture Scale-98. The analysis showed that none of the scoring systems were predictive of the SIP outcomes or patient recovery at 6 or 24 months. *[handwritten: sickness impact profile]*

6. Czerniecki JM: Rehabilitation in limb deficiency: 1. Gait and motion analysis. *Arch Phys Med Rehabil* 1996;77(3, suppl)S3-S8.

7. Volpicelli LJ, Chambers RB, Wagner FW Jr: Ambulation levels of bilateral lower-extremity amputees: Analysis of one hundred and three cases. *J Bone Joint Surg Am* 1983;65(5):599-605.

8. Turney BW, Kent SJ, Walker RT, Loftus IM: Amputations: No longer the end of the road. *J R Coll Surg Edinb* 2001;46(5):271-273.

9. Apelqvist J, Castenfors J, Larsson J, Stenström A, Agardh CD: Prognostic value of systolic ankle and toe blood pressure levels in outcome of diabetic foot ulcer. *Diabetes Care* 1989;12(6):373-378.

10. Wagner FW: Transcutaneous Doppler ultrasound in the prediction of healing and the selection of surgical level for dysvascular lesions of the toes and forefoot. *Clin Orthop Relat Res* 1979;142:110-114.

11. Barnes RW, Shanik GD, Slaymaker EE: An index of healing in below-knee amputation: Leg blood pressure by Doppler ultrasound. *Surgery* 1976;79(1):13-20.

12. Pinzur MS, Sage R, Stuck R, Ketner L, Osterman H: Transcutaneous oxygen as a predictor of wound healing in amputations of the foot and ankle. *Foot Ankle* 1992;13(5):271-272.

13. Burgess EM, Matsen FA III, Wyss CR, Simmons CW: Segmental transcutaneous measurements of PO2 in patients requiring below-the-knee amputation for peripheral vascular insufficiency. *J Bone Joint Surg Am* 1982;64(3):378-382.

14. Lalka SG, Malone JM, Anderson GG, Hagaman RM, McIntyre KE, Bernhard VM: Transcutaneous oxygen and carbon dioxide pressure monitoring to determine severity of limb ischemia and to predict surgical outcome. *J Vasc Surg* 1988;7(4):507-514.

15. Kostuik J: Indications, levels and limiting factors in amputation surgery of the lower extremity, in Kostuik J, ed: *Amputation Surgery and Rehabilitation: The Toronto Experience.* New York, NY, Churchill Livingstone, 1981, pp 17–25.

16. Bosse MJ, MacKenzie EJ, Kellam JF, et al: An analysis of outcomes of reconstruction or amputation after leg-threatening injuries. *N Engl J Med* 2002;12;347(24):1924-1931.

17. Pinzur MS, Beck J, Himes R, Callaci J: Distal tibiofibular bone-bridging in transtibial amputation. *J Bone Joint Surg Am* 2008;90(12):2682-2687.

    This study examined 20 patients who underwent a unilateral traumatic transtibial amputation, with a distal tibiofibular bone-bridging technique performed by a single surgeon. Using a Prosthesis Evaluation Questionnaire (PEQ), a validated outcomes instrument designed to measure patient self-reported health-related quality of life after a lower-extremity amputation, the authors compared their responses to those of a previously reported control group of nondiabetic patients who had undergone transtibial amputation with the use of a traditional technique. No difference in scores between the bone-bridge group and those in the control group were noted.

18. Hosalkar H, Pandya NK, Hsu J, Keenan MA: What's new in orthopaedic rehabilitation. *J Bone Joint Surg Am* 2009;91(9):2296-2310.

19. Hanling SR, Wallace SC, Hollenbeck KJ, Belnap BD, Tulis MR: Preamputation mirror therapy may prevent development of phantom limb pain: A case series. *Anesth Analg* 2010;110(2):611-614.

    The authors found that preamputation mirror therapy may lead to improved postamputation compliance and decrease the incidence of phantom limb pain. Four patients were studied for 2 weeks before elective limb amputation.

20. Schley MT, Wilms P, Toepfner S, et al: Painful and nonpainful phantom and stump sensations in acute traumatic amputees. *J Trauma* 2008;65(4):858-864.

    This study examined 96 patients with upper extremity amputations to look for factors in the formation, prevalence, intensity, course, and predisposing factors for phantom limb pain. The prevalence of phantom pain was 44.6%, phantom sensation 53.8%, stump pain 61.5%, and stump sensation 78.5%. After its first appearance, phantom pain had a decreasing course in

48%, was stable in 38%, and worsened in 7% of patient with amputations. Stump pain had a decreasing course in 48% but was stable in 30% of patients with amputations. Phantom pain occurred immediately after amputation in 28%, between 1 and 12 months in 10%, and after 12 months or more in 41% of patients with amputations.

21. Wilson JA, Nimmo AF, Fleetwood-Walker SM, Colvin LA: A randomised double blind trial of the effect of pre-Emptive epidural ketamine on persistent pain after lower limb amputation. *Pain* 2008;135(1-2):108-118.

    This study examined the effect of preemptively modulating sensory input with epidural ketamine (an NMDA antagonist) on postamputation pain and sensory processing on 53 patients undergoing lower limb amputation. Patients were randomized to receive epidural infusion (group K received racemic ketamine and bupivacaine; group S received saline and bupivacaine). At 1 year, there was no significant difference between groups (group K=21% and 50%; and group S=33% and 40% for stump and phantom pain, respectively). Postoperative analgesia was significantly better in group K, with reduced stump sensitivity which may reflect acute effects of ketamine on central sensitization.

22. Huang CT, Jackson JR, Moore NB, et al: Amputation: Energy cost of ambulation. *Arch Phys Med Rehabil* 1979;60(1):18-24.

23. Fleisher LA, Beckman JA, Brown KA, et al; American College of Cardiology/American Heart Association Task Force on Practice Guidelines Writing Committee to Update the 2002 Guidelines on Perioperative Cardiovascular Evaluation for Noncardiac Surgery; American Society of Echocardiography; American Society of Nuclear Cardiology; Heart Rhythm Society; Society of Cardiovascular Anesthesiologists; Society for Cardiovascular Angiography and Interventions; Society for Vascular Medicine and Biology: ACC/AHA 2006 guideline update on perioperative cardiovascular evaluation for noncardiac surgery: Focused update on perioperative beta-blocker therapy. A report of the American College of Cardiology/American Heart Association Task Force on Practice Guidelines (Writing Committee to Update the 2002 Guidelines on Perioperative Cardiovascular Evaluation for Noncardiac Surgery): Developed in collaboration with the American Society of Echocardiography, American Society of Nuclear Cardiology, Heart Rhythm Society, Society of Cardiovascular Anesthesiologists, Society for Cardiovascular Angiography and Interventions, and Society for Vascular Medicine and Biology. *Circulation* 2006;113(22):2662-2674.

24. Burke B, Kumar R, Vickers V, Grant E, Scremin E: Deep vein thrombosis after lower limb amputation. *Am J Phys Med Rehabil* 2000;79(2):145-149.

25. Yeager RA, Moneta GL, Edwards JM, Taylor LM Jr, McConnell DB, Porter JM: Deep vein thrombosis associated with lower extremity amputation. *J Vasc Surg* 1995;22(5):612-615.

26. Lastória S, Rollo HA, Yoshida WB, Giannini M, Moura R, Maffei FH: Prophylaxis of deep-vein thrombosis after lower extremity amputation: comparison of low molecular weight heparin with unfractionated heparin. *Acta Cir Bras* 2006;21(3):184-186.

27. Leonard JA: The elderly amputee, in Felsenthal G, Garrison SJ, Stienberg FU, eds: *Rehabilitation of the Aging and Elderly Patient.* Baltimore, MD, Williams & Wilkins, 1994, pp 397-406.

28. Eneroth M, Apelqvist J, Larsson J, Persson BM: Improved wound healing in transtibial amputees receiving supplementary nutrition. *Int Orthop* 1997;21(2):104-108.

29. Cansever A, Uzun O, Yildiz C, Ates A, Atesalp AS: Depression in men with traumatic lower part amputation: A comparison to men with surgical lower part amputation. *Mil Med* 2003;168(2):106-109.

30. Horgan O, MacLachlan M: Psychosocial adjustment to lower-limb amputation: A review. *Disabil Rehabil* 2004;26(14-15):837-850.

31. Jensen MP, Ehde DM, Hoffman AJ, Patterson DR, Czerniecki JM, Robinson LR: Cognitions, coping and social environment predict adjustment to phantom limb pain. *Pain* 2002;95(1-2):133-142.

32. Koren D, Norman D, Cohen A, Berman J, Klein EM: Increased PTSD risk with combat-related injury: A matched comparison study of injured and uninjured soldiers experiencing the same combat events. *Am J Psychiatry* 2005;162(2):276-282.

33. Singh R, Hunter J, Philip A: The rapid resolution of depression and anxiety symptoms after lower limb amputation. *Clin Rehabil* 2007;21(8):754-759.

34. Williams RM, Ehde DM, Smith DG, Czerniecki JM, Hoffman AJ, Robinson LR: A two-year longitudinal study of social support following amputation. *Disabil Rehabil* 2004;26(14-15):862-874.

35. Fukunishi I: Relationship of cosmetic disfigurement to the severity of posttraumatic stress disorder in burn injury or digital amputation. *Psychother Psychosom* 1999;68(2):82-86.

36. Rybarczyk BD, Nyenhuis DL, Nicholas JJ, Schulz R, Alioto RJ, Blair C: Social discomfort and depression in a sample of adults with leg amputations. *Arch Phys Med Rehabil* 1992;73(12):1169-1173.

37. Donovan-Hall MK, Yardley L, Watts RJ: Engagement in activities revealing the body and psychosocial adjustment in adults with a trans-tibial prosthesis. *Prosthet Orthot Int* 2002;26(1):15-22.

38. Potter BK, Burns TC, Lacap AP, Granville RR, Gajewski DA: Heterotopic ossification following traumatic and combat-related amputations. Prevalence, risk factors, and preliminary results of excision. *J Bone Joint Surg Am* 2007;89(3):476-486.

This study examined the prevalence of and risk factors for heterotopic ossification following trauma-related amputation as well as the preliminary results of surgical excision in 187 patients with a total of 213 traumatic and combat-related amputations. Heterotopic ossification was present in 63% of residual limbs. A final amputation level within the zone of injury and blast mechanism were risk factors for the development of heterotopic ossification. For 25 patients with refractory symptoms (12%), surgical excision is associated with low recurrence rates (8%) and decreased medication requirements, with acceptable complication rates (32%). There was a significant decrease in the use of pain medication following surgery.

39. Pandian G, Kowalske K: Daily functioning of patients with an amputated lower extremity. *Clin Orthop Relat Res* 1999;361(361):91-97.

40. Bodeau VS: Lower limb prosthetics. http://www.emedicine.com/pmr/topic175.htm. Accessed February 12, 2007.

41. Adderson JA, Parker KE, Macleod DA, Kirby RL, McPhail C: Effect of a shock-absorbing pylon on transmission of heel strike forces during the gait of people with unilateral trans-tibial amputations: A pilot study. *Prosthet Orthot Int* 2007;31(4):384-393.

This study examined the effects on walking with a shock-absorbing pylon (SAP) in seven patients with unilateral transtibial amputations. The SAP provided no significant shock absorption as indicated by either the mean peak proximal accelerations of 3.19 g and 2.82 g without and with the SAP, respectively, or the mean difference between the peak proximal and distal accelerometers, 0.16 g and 0.19 g. Unfortunately, variances were high and the study was likely underpowered to determine the efficacy of SAPs.

42. Raichle KA, Hanley MA, Molton I, et al: Prosthesis use in persons with lower- and upper-limb amputation. *J Rehabil Res Dev* 2008;45(7):961-972.

This study examined factors related to prosthesis use in 107 patients with upper limb amputation (ULA) and 752 patients with lower limb amputation (LLA) and the effect of phantom limb pain (PLP) and residual limb pain (RLP) on prosthesis use. Factors related to greater use (hours per day) for persons with LLA included younger age, full- or part-time employment, marriage, a distal amputation, an amputation of traumatic etiology, and an absence of PLP. Less use was associated with reports that prosthesis use worsened RLP, and greater prosthesis use was associated with reports that prosthesis use did not affect PLP. Having a proximal amputation and reporting lower average PLP were related to greater use in hours per day for persons with a ULA, while having a distal amputation and being married were associated with greater use in days per month. Participants with LLA were significantly more likely to wear a prosthesis than those with ULA.

43. Sansam K, Neumann V, O'Connor R, Bhakta B: Predicting walking ability following lower limb amputation: A systematic review of the literature. *J Rehabil Med* 2009;41(8):593-603.

This systematic literature review examined factors that predict walking with a prosthesis after lower limb amputation in 57 studies. Predictors of good walking ability following lower limb amputation include cognition, fitness, ability to stand on one leg, independence in activities of daily living and preoperative mobility. Longer time from surgery to rehabilitation and stump problems are predictors of poor outcome. In general, unilateral and distal amputation levels, and younger age were predictive of better walking ability.

44. Tang PC, Ravji K, Key JJ, Mahler DB, Blume PA, Sumpio B: Let them walk! Current prosthesis options for leg and foot amputees. *J Am Coll Surg* 2008;206(3):548-560.

45. Versluys R, Beyl P, Van Damme M, Desomer A, Van Ham R, Lefeber D: Prosthetic feet: State-of-the-art review and the importance of mimicking human ankle-foot biomechanics. *Disabil Rehabil Assist Technol* 2009;4(2):65-75.

This review discussed the numerous prosthetic feet currently on the market for individuals with a transtibial amputation, each device aimed at raising the 3C-level (control, comfort and cosmetics) with emphasis on energy-storing-and-returning feet and the recent so-called bionic feet.

46. Munin MC, Espejo-De Guzman MC, Boninger ML, Fitzgerald SG, Penrod LE, Singh J: Predictive factors for successful early prosthetic ambulation among lower-limb amputees. *J Rehabil Res Dev* 2001;38(4):379-384.

47. Davidson JH, Jones LE, Cornet J, Cittarelli T: Management of the multiple limb amputee. *Disabil Rehabil* 2002;24(13):688-699.

48. Waters RL, Perry J, Antonelli D, Hislop H: Energy cost of walking of amputees: The influence of level of amputation. *J Bone Joint Surg Am* 1976;58(1):42-46.

49. Collin C, Collin J: Mobility after lower-limb amputation. *Br J Surg* 1995;82(8):1010-1011.

50. Pell JP, Donnan PT, Fowkes FG, Ruckley CV: Quality of life following lower limb amputation for peripheral arterial disease. *Eur J Vasc Surg* 1993;7(4):448-451.

51. Esquenazi A, DiGiacomo R: Rehabilitation after amputation. *J Am Podiatr Med Assoc* 2001;91(1):13-22.

52. Purry NA, Hannon MA: How successful is below-knee amputation for injury? *Injury* 1989;20(1):32-36.

53. Barnett C, Vanicek N, Polman R, et al: Kinematic gait adaptations in unilateral transtibial amputees during rehabilitation. *Prosthet Orthot Int* 2009;33(2):135-147.

This randomized study examined the use of two different early walking aids (EWAs) in individuals who have recently undergone unilateral transtibial amputation on kinematic gait patterns during early rehabilitation. Patients were randomly assigned to use the Amputee Mobility Aid or the Pneumatic Postamputation Aid prior to receiving their functional prosthesis. A three-dimensional motion capture system recorded kinematic data from their first steps up to discharge from rehabilitation. The results from this study would suggest that neither EWA was more beneficial for gait retraining during rehabilitation.

54. Nissen SJ, Newman WP: Factors influencing reintegration to normal living after amputation. *Arch Phys Med Rehabil* 1992;73(6):548-551.

55. Gailey R, Allen K, Castles J, Kucharik J, Roeder M: Review of secondary physical conditions associated with lower-limb amputation and long-term prosthesis use. *J Rehabil Res Dev* 2008;45(1):15-29.

    The authors discussed the musculoskeletal imbalances or pathologies that often develop into secondary physical conditions or complications that may affect the mobility and quality of life of people with lower limb amputation. They reviewed the literature on secondary complications among people with lower limb loss who are long-term prosthesis wearers.

56. Skoutas D, Papanas N, Georgiadis GS, et al: Risk factors for ipsilateral reamputation in patients with diabetic foot lesions. *Int J Low Extrem Wounds* 2009;8(2): 69-74.

    This study examined the rates and risk factors for ipsilateral reamputation in 121 patients with diabetic foot and prior amputation. The authors found that 21.5% of patients required reamputation during a mean follow-up of 18 months. Most reamputations were performed within the first 6 months of the initial amputation. Patients older than 70 years and those with heel lesions are at greatest risk for reamputation.

57. Burger H, Marincek C, Isakov E: Mobility of persons after traumatic lower limb amputation. *Disabil Rehabil* 1997;19(7):272-277.

58. Frieden RA: The geriatric amputee. *Phys Med Rehabil Clin N Am* 2005;16(1):179-195.

59. Jeffries GE: Aging americans and amputation. In Motion 1996 Apr-May;6(2). http://www.amputee-coalition.org/inmotion/apr_may_96/aging_amputees.pdf. Accessed October 28, 2010.

4: Lower Extremity

Section 5

Spine

SECTION EDITOR:

JEFFREY C. WANG, MD

Chapter 42

Spinal Tumors

Scott D. Daffner, MD

Introduction

Primary spinal tumors are relatively rare, typically representing less than 5% of all spinal tumors;[1] however, the spine is the most common site for skeletal metastases. Initial symptoms may be subtle, leading to a delay in diagnosis. As treatment algorithms continue to evolve, survival rates for patients with many types of cancer have improved, underlying the importance of early detection and treatment. However, patients with spinal tumors are challenging to treat; questions remain about which patients should have surgery, the timing of surgery, and the optimal surgical procedure.

Epidemiology

Lesions of the spine may affect patients of any age. Benign lesions are more commonly seen in children and tend to localize to the posterior elements, whereas malignant tumors are more common in adults and more frequently affect the vertebral body.[1] The spine is the most common site for skeletal metastases, which have a predilection for the thoracic region. Autopsy studies suggest that between 30% and 80% of patients with cancer have evidence of bony metastases.[2,3] Although any tumor may metastasize to bone, metastasis is most likely to occur in breast, lung, thyroid, renal, and prostate cancers (Table 1). Although the different prevalence of cancer types in men and women leads to variable rates of skeletal metastases, the distribution of primary bony tumors of the spine is almost equal between men and women. Malignant primary tumors are more common in males and benign tumors are more common in females.[1]

Evaluation

A thorough history and physical examination are of utmost importance in evaluating a patient with a suspected spinal tumor. Pain is the most common presenting complaint, occurring in approximately 85% of patients with spinal tumors. This pain is typically axial in nature and of insidious onset. Night pain is common and may be unrelated to activity, but may be caused by the normal variation of endogenous steroid secretion, which decreases at night but helps mitigate inflammatory mediators released by tumors when present. Mechanical pain, pain with activity, or pain with changing positions suggests spinal instability. Acute onset or worsening of axial pain is suggestive of a fracture. Although axial pain is more common, patients may also present with symptoms of neurologic impingement. In this population, approximately 61% present with radicular pain, 37% present with a motor deficit, and 2% have an isolated sphincter dysfunction.[4] Neurologic impairment may have an acute onset in 28% of patients.[4]

Patients should be questioned to determine history of cancer, no matter how remote. The presence of constitutional symptoms such as weight changes, fatigue, and changes in appetite should be noted. Adult patients should be asked whether their primary care provider has performed age-appropriate screening studies (such as colonoscopy or mammography). In addition, the social history should include documentation of any tobacco usage or possible occupational exposure to carcinogens; a family history of cancer also should be probed. A thorough physical examination should be performed with particular attention to details such as focal spinal tenderness, limited range of motion, or subtle neurologic deficits.

Table 1

Common Spinal Tumors

Metastatic	Breast
	Gastrointestinal
	Lung
	Kidney
	Prostate
	Thyroid
Primary benign	Aneurysmal bone cyst
	Eosinophilic granuloma
	Giant cell tumor
	Hemangioma
	Neurofibroma
	Osteoid osteoma
	Osteoblastoma
	Osteochondroma
Primary malignant	Chondrosarcoma
	Chordoma
	Ewing sarcoma
	Multiple myeloma
	Osteosarcoma

Plain radiographs are the initial study of choice and allow an assessment of overall spinal alignment, general bone quality, and localization of the lesion. Because lesions typically cannot be seen on plain radiographs until 30% to 50% of the bone has been destroyed, a negative plain radiograph cannot exclude the presence of a tumor. CT provides excellent bony detail, and MRI provides soft-tissue detail and is of great benefit in demonstrating neurologic impingement. MRI should be performed with intravenous gadolinium contrast when a tumor is suspected because more vascular regions will be highlighted. Metastatic tumors typically have decreased signal on T1-weighted MRI, with surrounding hyperintense fatty marrow. Whole-body technetium-99 bone scans performed with or without single photon emission CT (SPECT) can identify remote lesions and assist in staging the disease as well as potentially locating a lesion that may be more easily biopsied.

Laboratory evaluation is helpful in establishing a differential diagnosis, particularly in patients with no known primary tumor. A complete blood count with differential, serum and urine electrolytes, erythrocyte sedimentation rate, and C-reactive protein can be a useful starting point. Other tests may be ordered depending on the suspected primary cancer; for example, thyroid-stimulating hormone and thyroxine (free T4) if thyroid cancer is suspected, prostate-specific antigen in patients who may have prostate cancer, or liver function tests and carcinoembryonic antigen for gastrointestinal cancers. Serum and urine protein electrophoresis typically demonstrate a monoclonal gammopathy in multiple myeloma.

Diagnosis, Staging, and Surgical Planning

When taken together, the patient history, physical examination, laboratory studies, and imaging should provide most of the needed information for a diagnosis. Definitive diagnosis, however, is provided by biopsy. The workup may demonstrate remote sites of tumor that may be more amenable to biopsy than the spine. When necessary, CT- or MRI-guided transpedicular fine-needle aspiration or core biopsies are the study of choice.[5-7] The accuracy of CT-guided biopsy has been reported at approximately 89%, with better yield from lytic lesions (93%) than sclerotic lesions (76%).[8] The tract of the needle biopsy should be tattooed to allow resection at the time of definitive surgery. On occasion, open excisional biopsy may be required. If this is the case, meticulous surgical technique to reduce the risk of contamination should be followed. Open biopsy can be performed at the time of definitive surgical treatment (resection, decompression, and/or stabilization); however, new drapes and instruments should be used after the biopsy is obtained to minimize potential seeding of unaffected tissue. Image-guided biopsies should be performed by the interventional neuroradiologist or musculoskeletal radiologist in consultation with the treating surgeon. Open biopsy, when necessary, should be performed by the surgeon performing definitive treatment.

Staging of spinal tumors can aid in surgical planning. The Enneking classification of musculoskeletal tumors is useful in oncologic staging; however, because its applicability to the surgical staging of spinal lesions is limited, it will not be discussed. This is because performing a true en bloc resection of a spinal tumor would frequently require excision of the spinal cord. The most widely accepted staging system for spinal tumors is the Weinstein, Boriani, and Biagini (WBB) system[9] (**Figure 1**). This system divides the axial plane of the involved vertebral body into 12 zones resembling a clock face. Additionally, the spine is divided into five layers (A to E) moving from peripherally centrally, from the paraspinal extraosseous soft tissues to the intradural space. Based on this system, a vertebrectomy can be performed when the tumor is isolated to the vertebral body and at least one pedicle is free of tumor. A sagittal resection can be performed for tumors involving one side of the vertebral body, a pedicle, and transverse process, and resection of the posterior arch alone can be performed for lesions isolated to the posterior elements with tumor-free pedicles.[9]

Primary Benign Lesions

Aneurysmal Bone Cyst

Aneurysmal bone cysts (ABCs) most frequently arise in the second decade of life. Approximately 20% of ABCs occur within the spine, predominantly in the posterior elements. Radiographs typically demonstrate an expansile, lytic lesion with a rim of reactive bone. The fluid-fluid levels seen on MRI are virtually pathognomonic. Treatment options include radiation therapy, selective arterial embolization, curettage, and en bloc resection. Recently, selective arterial embolization has become the first-line treatment of choice.[10] Larger lesions can cause compression of the neural elements or instability of the spine resulting from bony destruction. In such cases, en bloc resection (if limited to posterior elements) or intralesional extracapsular excision followed by reconstruction and fusion is appropriate. Similarly, surgical treatment is recommended for local recurrence or failure of embolization. Preoperative embolization to reduce blood loss is recommended.

Eosinophilic Granuloma

Eosinophilic granuloma (also known as Langerhans cell histiocytosis) affects the vertebral body during the first and second decades of life. Vertebra plana is commonly seen on plain radiographs. Because multiple other benign and malignant tumors may also cause this deformity, a histologic diagnosis is critical. Intralesional injection of corticosteroid at the time of biopsy (once histologically confirmed) can be helpful.[11] Most lesions will spontaneously resolve, with near-complete restoration of vertebral body height.[12]

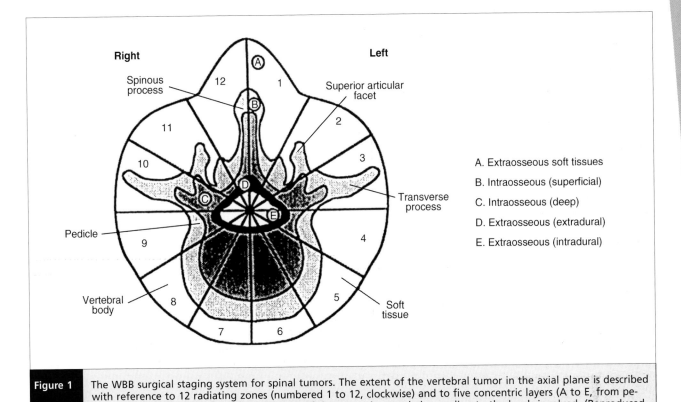

Right — Left

Spinous process
Superior articular facet
Transverse process
Pedicle
Vertebral body
Soft tissue

A. Extraosseous soft tissues
B. Intraosseous (superficial)
C. Intraosseous (deep)
D. Extraosseous (extradural)
E. Extraosseous (intradural)

Figure 1	The WBB surgical staging system for spinal tumors. The extent of the vertebral tumor in the axial plane is described with reference to 12 radiating zones (numbered 1 to 12, clockwise) and to five concentric layers (A to E, from peripheral to central). The longitudinal extent of the tumor is recorded according to the levels involved. (Reproduced with permission from Boriani S, Weinstein JN, Biagini R: Primary bone tumors of the spine. *Spine* 1997;22:1036-1044.)

Giant Cell Tumor

Although histologically benign, giant cell tumors can be locally aggressive. They typically occur in adults (third decade of life) and occur most commonly in the vertebral body. The sacrum is most frequently affected. Radiographically, a giant cell tumor appears as an expansile, lytic lesion, frequently with an associated soft-tissue mass. In the mobile spine, en bloc excision is curative.[13] Certain lesions may not be amenable to this because of adjacent neurologic or vascular structures; therefore, intralesional, extracapsular excision is the next choice of management. Preoperative embolization reduces intraoperative blood loss. Adjuvant radiation therapy may increase the success rate, but with a 5% to 15% risk of developing a high-grade sarcoma. Recurrence rates can be high (83%), but are significantly lower (18%) if patients are treated at a tertiary tumor referral center.[13]

Hemangioma

Asymptomatic hemangiomas are frequent incidental findings seen on MRI scans. Larger lesions may cause instability, pathologic fractures, or compression of neural elements. On radiographs, larger lesions typically demonstrate vertical striations within the vertebral body; these lesions have a speckled appearance on CT. On MRI, hemangiomas have increased signal intensity on both T1- and T2-weighted images. In the setting of impending pathologic fracture, percutaneous cement

augmentation of the vertebral body is recommended.[14] Lesions causing neurologic compromise should be treated with surgical decompression and stabilization, which may also include the use of cement augmentation.

Neurofibroma

Intraspinal neurofibromas are associated with neurofibromatosis and should be suspected in any patients with typical skin lesions of this condition (café-au-lait spots, cutaneous neurofibromas). They typically occur within the dura, although they may occur within the neuroforamen and have a classic dumbbell shape. Radiographic findings may include penciling of the rib heads, enlarged neuroforamina, or scalloping of the vertebra. Symptomatic lesions should be treated with a marginal excision. Neurofibromas can be associated with rapidly progressive scoliosis, which should be treated aggressively with spinal fusion.

Osteoid Osteoma

Typically occurring in the second decade of life, osteoid osteoma frequently presents with pain unrelated to activity that is worse at night and resolves with the use of nonsteroidal anti-inflammatory drugs (NSAIDs). It may also cause painful scoliosis. CT demonstrates a nidus of bone surrounded by a sclerotic rim and bone scan shows a very "hot" lesion, most in the posterior elements of the lumbar spine. First-line treatment is long-term use of NSAIDs. Resolution of symptoms is good, but takes an average of 36 months.[15] Radiofrequency ablation has been used to treat osteoid osteoma elsewhere in the body but is not routinely used in the spine because of the proximity of neural elements. For lesions that are safely away from neurologic structures, radiofrequency ablation can provide excellent relief, whereas lesions close to neurologic structures are best treated with percutaneous or open excision.[16] Associated scoliosis will spontaneously resolve following en bloc resection if performed within 15 months of onset of the curvature.

Osteoblastoma

Approximately 40% of osteoblastomas occur in the spine, most frequently affecting the posterior elements of the cervical or lumbar regions. It generally affects the same patient population as osteoid osteoma and has similar presenting symptoms, although pain is not as reliably controlled with NSAIDs and neurologic symptoms may also be present. Painful scoliosis also may be present. Although histologically indistinguishable from osteoid osteoma, osteoblastoma is larger (diameter > 2 cm) and may include expansion into the soft tissue. Radiographs show an expansile, lytic lesion. Well-defined lesions confined to the bone can be treated with intralesional curettage; en bloc resection (when feasible) can be curative.[17]

Osteochondroma

Most frequently affecting the posterior elements of the cervical and upper thoracic spine, osteochondromas are frequently asymptomatic. Plain radiographs may demonstrate a pedunculated mass, although CT or MRI will better show the cartilaginous cap. Asymptomatic lesions require no treatment other than observation. En bloc excision is recommended for persistently painful lesions or those that cause neurologic compromise. A single lesion has an approximately 1% risk of malignant transformation into a chondrosarcoma, although that risk is up to 25% in patients with multiple hereditary exostoses.[18]

Primary Malignant Lesions

Chondrosarcoma

Chondrosarcomas typically present in the fifth decade of life. When occurring in the posterior elements of the spine, they may represent malignant transformation of a preexisting osteochondroma. When they occur in the vertebral body, they are more likely a primary lesion. A lytic lesion with poor margins and stippled calcifications is seen radiographically, although plain radiographs typically underestimate the size because of the cartilaginous cap and associated soft-tissue mass. En bloc excision is the treatment of choice as curettage is associated with higher recurrence and mortality.[19] Proton and photon beam radiation therapy may prove useful in treating lesions that are not amenable to complete resection with clean margins.[20]

Chordoma

Although rare, chordomas are the most common primary malignant spinal tumor in adults and are typically diagnosed in the fifth or sixth decade. They are most commonly found in the sacrum but may occur elsewhere in the spine, with the upper cervical spine being the second most common location. Because they evolve from remnants of the notochord, they have a midline location. Plain radiographs show a lytic or mixed lytic-blastic lesion. CT or MRI will demonstrate the large degree of soft-tissue extension. Because they are slow growing, onset of symptoms may be subtle (constipation, tenesmus, low back pain). A mass is usually palpable on digital rectal examination in sacral lesions.

En bloc resection is the treatment of choice, and survival is directly related to the quality of margins obtained.[21,22] Surgical treatment of sacral lesions places patients at extremely high risk for bowel and bladder incontinence and sexual dysfunction after total or partial sacrectomy. Whenever possible, efforts to save either the bilateral S2 nerve roots or the unilateral S2, S3, and S4 roots should be made to possibly allow retention of near-normal bowel and bladder function. Functional outcome, however, should be carefully weighed against the need for negative surgical margins, and nerve roots may have to be sacrificed to help ensure a more favorable long-term outcome. Frequently, extensive bony and soft-tissue reconstruction follows resection of the tumor.

Long-term outcomes vary depending on the surgical margins, the time of diagnosis, and the location of the tumor. Survival in patients with sacral lesions may average 8 to 10 years, whereas those with lesions at other sites have a 5-year average survival. Although once believed to be highly resistant to both chemotherapy and radiation therapy, recent evidence suggests a possible role for proton-photon beam radiation, particularly in cases of recurrence.[23] In addition, chordomas have been found to respond favorably to chemotherapeutic agents targeted against molecular tyrosine kinase and angiogenesis pathways.[24]

Ewing Sarcoma

Ewing sarcoma presents in the second decade of life, typically with pain, swelling, and constitutional symptoms. Within the spine, Ewing sarcoma most often affects the sacrum. Neurologic symptoms are common. The radiographic appearance is of moth-eaten permeative destruction with poor margins. MRI may demonstrate significant soft-tissue extension. A multimodal treatment approach is essential. Current treatment recommendations are neoadjuvant chemotherapy followed by radiation therapy or en bloc excision.[25] Neoadjuvant chemotherapy can substantially reduce the size of the tumor. The use of radiation for definitive treatment, however, is associated with progressive kyphosis and radiation-induced myelopathy; therefore, en bloc excision may offer a better long-term solution. Radiation should be used when en bloc resection is not feasible or if surgical margins are positive.

Multiple Myeloma

Multiple myeloma is the most common primary malignancy of bone and is the result of malignant transformation of plasma cells causing destruction of bone locally and abnormal immunoglobulin production. It typically affects older individuals in the sixth or seventh decade of life. Initial presentation may be a painful vertebral compression fracture. On occasion, patients may present with a neurologic deficit. Radiographs demonstrate punched-out discrete lytic lesions, although the spine may also simply appear as diffusely osteopenic. Lesions are "cold" on bone scans. MRI may show diffuse involvement at multiple levels not readily seen on plain radiographs. Laboratory testing shows a monoclonal gammopathy on serum and/or urine electrophoresis.

Chemotherapy and radiation therapy are the standard treatments.[26] Bracing is indicated for pain control in patients with compression fractures. In the setting of epidural compression and neurologic deficit, administration of corticosteroids may help decrease symptoms. Bisphosphonates can help allay the effects of bony destruction.[27] Combined therapy with thalidomide and dexamethasone has had better response and longer time to progression than dexamethasone alone and has become the regimen of choice in patients with newly diagnosed multiple myeloma.[28] Patients with continued back pain caused by bony destruction or compression fractures may benefit from percutaneous cement augmentation (vertebroplasty or kyphoplasty).[29,30]

Multiple myeloma may represent the progression of a solitary plasmacytoma. These lesions occur as single, isolated plasma cell neoplasms. Up to 50% of these lesions will progress to multiple myeloma. Although radiographically they may appear to be a single lesion, MRI should be performed to evaluate for occult lesions elsewhere. They are highly radiosensitive. Surgery is indicated in cases of spinal instability or severe neurologic compromise. The median survival of patients with plasmacytoma is more than 60 months, whereas that of patients with multiple myeloma is 28 months.

Osteosarcoma

Osteosarcoma affects younger individuals, typically in the second decade of life. It rarely affects the spine; however, neurologic symptoms are fairly common when it does. Lesions are usually in the vertebral body, but frequently extend to cause compression of the spinal cord. The radiographic appearance can be lytic, blastic, or mixed. A biopsy should be performed (preferably by the treating surgeon) to establish the diagnosis. Once established, staging studies including a whole-body bone scan, chest CT, and CT and MRI of the lesion should be performed.

Neoadjuvant chemotherapy with subsequent en bloc excision and postoperative chemotherapy is the treatment of choice. Local recurrence is significantly more common if clean margins are not obtained at the time of resection.[31] Radiation therapy is not recommended postoperatively unless there is concern for tumor con-tamination at the time of resection. Survival rates correlate with the percentage of tumor death accomplished with preoperative chemotherapy; if tumor kill is greater than 90%, the 5-year survival is 85%, whereas it is only 25% if tumor kill is less than 90%. In general, spinal osteosarcoma portends a worse prognosis than an isolated extremity lesion.

Metastatic Disease

Most spinal column tumors are metastatic, and the spine is the most common site of bony metastases. Between 30% and 80% of patients who die of cancer have evidence of spinal metastases on autopsy.[2,3] Frequently, metastatic tumors include those of the lung, prostate, breast, kidney, and gastrointestinal system.[32] The vertebral body is the most affected site, and the intervertebral disk spaces are usually spared. In patients with a known history of cancer, new onset of back pain should be assumed to be caused by spinal metastases until proven otherwise. Radiographic evidence of bony destruction only becomes visible when 30% to 50% of the vertebra has been affected. Any patient with a known history of cancer, or those with persistent back pain despite 4 to 6 weeks of appropriate nonsurgical management should undergo spinal imaging. A simplified algorithm for evaluating patients for spinal tumors is shown in **Figure 2**. As discussed earlier, plain radiographs offer a starting point, with CT and MRI providing added information as to the degree of bony destruction and soft-tissue involvement or neural compression. Imaging studies should also evaluate for systemic metastases (**Table 2**).

Treatment of spinal metastases depends on the individual patient's overall health, ambulatory status, tumor type, tumor load, spinal level involved, presence of neurologic compromise, and spinal stability. The modified Tokuhashi scoring system for patients with metastatic spinal tumors can guide treatment based on the prognosis.[33] This system allows a total of 15 points for various degrees of severity of six main patient characteristics: general medical condition, number of extraspinal bone metastases, number of spinal metastases, metastases to internal organs, primary site of cancer, and neurologic impairment (**Table 3**). Patients scoring 8 points or less have a prognosis of less than 6 months and are offered conservative or palliative treatments. Those with scores of 9 to 11 points have a predicted prognosis of greater than 6 months and are offered palliative surgery, although a single lesion without visceral metastases may be treated with excisional surgery. Patients scoring 12 or more points have a predicted survival greater than 1 year and are treated with excisional surgery. This system showed consistency of 82% to 86% comparing the predicted to actual survival.[33] It has recently been shown to correlate well with neurologic outcome in cases of metastatic spinal cord compression.[34] Age is also an important predictor of neurologic outcome and survival in patients with spinal metastases. Authors of a 2009 study found that as age

5: Spine

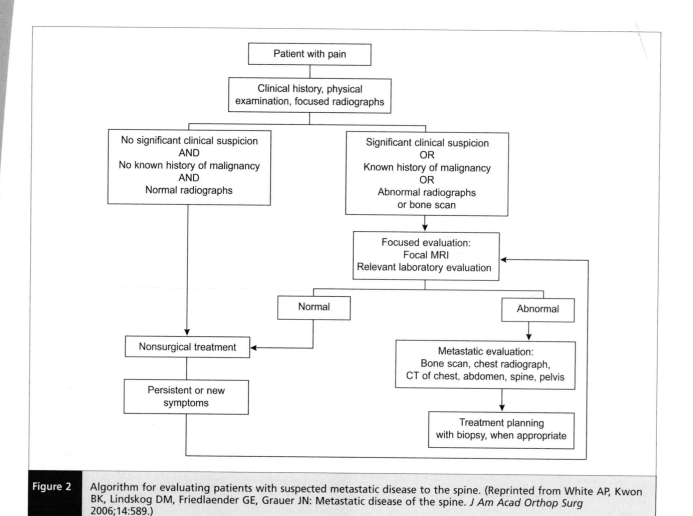

Figure 2 Algorithm for evaluating patients with suspected metastatic disease to the spine. (Reprinted from White AP, Kwon BK, Lindskog DM, Friedlaender GE, Grauer JN: Metastatic disease of the spine. *J Am Acad Orthop Surg* 2006;14:589.)

Table 2

Metastatic Imaging Evaluation

Whole-body bone scan

Chest radiograph

CT of the chest, abdomen, or pelvis

CT of the head

CT of the spine (cervical, thoracic, lumbar)

Long-bone series

increased, the benefits of surgery over radiation alone narrowed; while the ability to ambulate was preserved for a longer duration following surgery in patients younger than 65 years, for older patients there was no difference in outcome regardless of treatment type.[35]

The presence of a neurologic deficit represents a challenge in treatment. Deficits of rapid onset or complete paraplegia have a less favorable prognosis than deficits with insidious onset. Up to one third of deficits may be caused by multifocal spinal lesions; therefore,

MRI of the entire spine is recommended in patients with any neurologic symptoms. Radiation therapy is appropriate for patients with neurologic deficit who are not surgical candidates or for patients with radiosensitive tumors such as lymphoma or myeloma. Administration of systemic corticosteroids may slow the progression of neurologic deficits.

One useful decision-making tool for the treatment of patients with spinal metastases is the NOMS (neurologic, oncologic, mechanical instability, systemic disease) system[36] (**Figure 3**). Evaluation of neurologic impairment includes assessment of function (myelopathy or radiculopathy) as well as radiographic spinal cord compression. Oncologic evaluation refers primarily to the radiosensitivity of the tumor. Mechanical instability focuses on motion-related pain, which is to be differentiated from baseline biologic tumor pain (for example, night pain). Mechanical pain is reflective of bony destruction and potentially heralds structural failure. Systemic disease includes an assessment of the patient's overall medical condition, including not only the extent of tumor burden but also other medical comorbidities. In general, patients with significant spinal cord compression from radioresistant tumors or those who demonstrate mechanical instability should be offered surgery (assuming their systemic disease will allow it). Those with radiosensitive tumors should be offered radiation therapy. Patients with radioresistant tumors without significant spinal cord compression may benefit from treatment with newer, more focused radiation treatment such as image-guided intensity modulated radiation therapy (IGIMRT).[36]

IGIMRT offers potential advantages over traditional external beam radiation, particularly in its potential for treating what have been believed to be radioresistant tumors (Table 4). Traditional therapy, while focused around the general region of a tumor, also exposed a substantial three-dimensional radius of normal tissue to radiation. Advanced imaging techniques now allow more sophisticated, geographic treatment planning. Image guidance techniques and procedures to focus or adapt radiation therapy have evolved to allow more precise delivery of radiation to tumors (**Figure 4**). It was recently reported that use of IGIMRT for palliative care in patients not responding to other treatments can be performed efficiently.[37] Although potentially effective, a 39% rate of vertebral fracture progression was noted after just a single fraction of IGIMRT, particularly for lytic lesions involving greater than 40% of the vertebral body and located caudal to T10.[38] Patients with low-grade spinal cord compression caused by radioresistant tumors probably benefit from IGIMRT treatment, whereas those with high-grade compression should be offered surgical decompression followed by IGIMRT.[36]

As previously mentioned, the role of surgical excision depends on many factors. Data suggest that among patients with epidural compression caused by metastatic disease (of nonradiosensitive tumors), decompressive surgery combined with radiation therapy proved superior to radiotherapy alone.[39] In a randomized, prospective study, more patients in the surgical group maintained (84%) or regained (62%) the ability to ambulate after treatment than patients in the radiotherapy group (57% and 19%, respectively).[39] Another recent study showed that en bloc resection of metastatic lesions results in lower local recurrence rates than debulking procedures. The median survival time was 41 months for en bloc resection compared with 25 months for debulking, a substantial, but not statistically significant, difference.[40]

Patients with painful vertebral body compression fractures caused by metastases may also be treated with percutaneous cement augmentation. Pain relief can be dramatic and sustained over the long term, with the additional benefit of spinal stability.[41] Because the procedure is performed in a percutaneous, minimally invasive fashion and does not rely on the need for bone fusion or wound healing, chemotherapy or radiation therapy may be instituted without the necessary delay recommended for open procedures.

Surgical treatment of spinal metastases can lead to improved quality of life with low complication rates.[42] One recent study found that surgery, whether en bloc excision, debulking, or palliative, led to improvement in pain in 71% of patients, return or maintenance of in-

Table 3

Modified Tokuhashi Scoring System[a]

Characteristic	Score
General Condition	
Poor	0
Moderate	1
Good	2
Number of extraspinal bone metastases	
≥ 3	0
1-2	1
0	2
Number of vertebral body metastases	
≥ 3	0
2	1
1	2
Metastases to major internal organs	
Unresectable	0
Resectable	1
No metastases	2
Primary site of cancer	
Lung, osteosarcoma, stomach, bladder, esophagus, pancreas	0
Liver, gallbladder, unidentified	1
Other	2
Kidney, uterus	3
Rectum	4
Thyroid, breast, prostate, carcinoid	5
Palsy	
Complete (Frankel A, B)	0
Incomplete (Frankel C, D)	1
None (Frankel E)	2

[a] Patients are assigned points based on general condition, number of extraspinal bony metastases, number of spinal metastases, metastases to major visceral organs, type of primary tumor, and neurologic status. A total of 15 points is possible. Point totals are prognostic: ≥12 points predicts survival >12 months, 9 to 11 points predicts survival > 6 months, and ≤8 points predicts survival < 6 months.

dependent mobility in 53% of patients, and return of urinary control in 39% of patients.[43] Functional improvement and survival was highest among those patients undergoing en bloc excision and lowest among those who received palliative surgery. Although surgical treatment offers potentially improved quality of life, it is not without complications. Among those admitted for surgical management of spinal metastases, in-hospital mortality is 5.6%, and the overall complication rate is nearly 22% with pulmonary complications and bleeding or hematoma the most common.[44] Complications are more likely in older patients and those with two or more comorbidities.

5: Spine

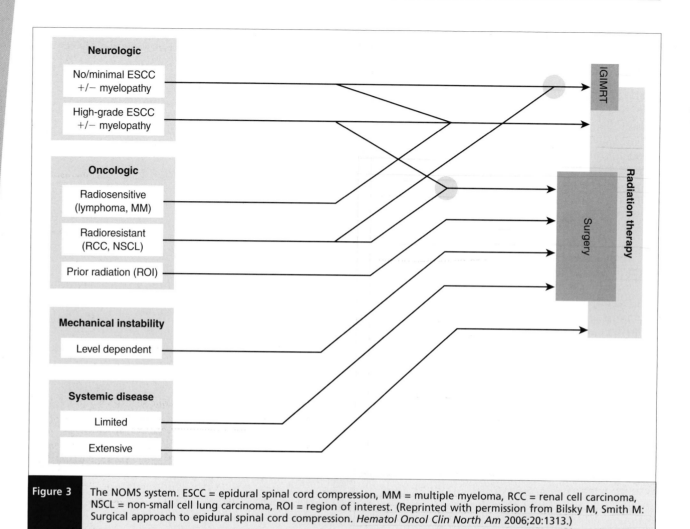

Figure 3 The NOMS system. ESCC = epidural spinal cord compression, MM = multiple myeloma, RCC = renal cell carcinoma, NSCL = non-small cell lung carcinoma, ROI = region of interest. (Reprinted with permission from Bilsky M, Smith M: Surgical approach to epidural spinal cord compression. *Hematol Oncol Clin North Am* 2006;20:1313.)

Table 4

Radiosensitivity of Common Metastatic Spinal Tumors

Radiosensitive	Myeloma
	Lymphoma
Moderately radiosensitive	Breast
	Prostate
Radioresistant	Lung
	Colon
	Renal cell
	Sarcoma
	Melanoma

Following treatment, whether radiation or surgery, the patient must be followed closely for potential recurrence. One of the earliest presentations of tumor recurrence is pain. Serum tumor markers (when appropriate) should be monitored intermittently as a potential sign of recurrence. Routine MRI may show recurrent masses. Reoperation may be considered based on the patient's potential for meaningful recovery.

Surgical Technique

Tumor type and location are the prime determinants of the type of surgical treatment performed. En bloc excision with negative margins is ideal, but not always practical. This can be performed on lesions contained entirely within the anterior vertebral body, the posterior elements, or the distal sacrum. Tumors that lie adjacent to or involve critical neurovascular structures (for example, tumors extending into the bilateral vertebral artery foramina) and tumors that extend from vertebral body through the pedicle into the lamina are best managed with intralesional extracapsular excision. When possible, functionally important nerve roots should be spared. This makes true en bloc resection in the cervical spine virtually impossible; typically a combined anteroposterior approach is required. However, tumors located from T2 to T12 are amenable to en bloc resection because sacrifice of nerve roots has minimal functional impact. This can be done from a posterior only approach. In the lumbar spine, the nerve roots can usually be spared during en bloc resection, although this may require a combined posteroanterior approach. Proximal sacral lesions also typically require a com-

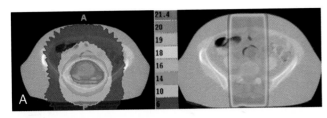

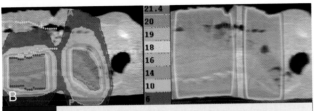

Figure 4   IGIMRT allows radiation to be focused on the specific target organ, significantly reducing the exposure of surrounding tissues to high-dose radiation. **A,** IGIMRT (*left*) and traditional field radiation therapy (*right*) of a sacral lesion. **B,** Treatment of two adjacent sites of vertebral metastases with IGIMRT (*left*) versus traditional field radiation (*right*). Numbers and colors on the center bar represent radiation dosage (Gy); colors on the images correlate with dosage and radiation field. (Reproduced with permission from Samant R, Gerig L, Montgomery L, et al: The emerging role of IG-IMRT for palliative radiotherapy: A single-institution experience. *Curr Oncol* 2009;16:43.)

bined approach, whereas those below S2 can be excised through a posterior approach. As mentioned earlier, accurate surgical staging can help direct treatment.[9] The use of titanium implants is favored as they have less ferromagnetic artifact if postoperative MRI is required to assess for recurrence.

Summary

Obtaining a comprehensive history, detailed physical examination, and relevant radiographic studies will help the surgeon determine the optimal treatment of patients with primary or metastatic tumors of the spine. The suspected diagnosis should be confirmed by biopsy. The treating surgeon should be competent and comfortable with both conservative and aggressive surgical management of tumors. Patients should be presented with a realistic assessment of their prognosis, well-defined goals of treatment, potential outcomes, and different treatment options. Both surgical and nonsurgical management can lead to improved quality of life in terms of pain control and functional independence.

Annotated References

1. Kelley SP, Ashford RU, Rao AS, Dickson RA: Primary bone tumours of the spine: A 42-year survey from the Leeds Regional Bone Tumour Registry. *Eur Spine J* 2007;16(3):405-409.

In a retrospective review of a tumor registry, the authors identified 2,750 cases of primary osseous tumors, of which only 126 (4.6%) occurred in the spine. Multiple myeloma and plasmacytoma were most common, followed by osteosarcoma. Pain was the most common presenting symptom.

2. Ortiz Gómez JA: The incidence of vertebral body metastases. *Int Orthop* 1995;19(5):309-311.

3. Wong DA, Fornasier VL, MacNab I: Spinal metastases: The obvious, the occult, and the impostors. *Spine (Phila Pa 1976)* 1990;15(1):1-4.

4. Constans JP, de Divitiis E, Donzelli R, Spaziante R, Meder JF, Haye C: Spinal metastases with neurological manifestations: Review of 600 cases. *J Neurosurg* 1983;59(1):111-118.

5. Carrino JA, Khurana B, Ready JE, Silverman SG, Winalski CS: Magnetic resonance imaging-guided percutaneous biopsy of musculoskeletal lesions. *J Bone Joint Surg Am* 2007;89(10):2179-2187.

In this retrospective case series, the authors review the results of MRI-guided biopsies for musculoskeletal lesions in 45 consecutive patients. They report that overall, 91% of samples taken contained sufficient material for diagnostic purposes. For bone lesions, this number was 95%, with a sensitivity of 0.92, specificity of 1.00, positive predictive value of 1.00, and negative predictive value of 0.86.

6. Nourbakhsh A, Grady JJ, Garges KJ: Percutaneous spine biopsy: A meta-analysis. *J Bone Joint Surg Am* 2008;90(8):1722-1725.

The authors report a meta-analysis of adequacy and accuracy of percutaneously obtained spinal biopsies, noting that adequacy, accuracy, and complications increased as needle inner diameter increased and that CT guidance was associated with a lower complication rate (3.3%) than fluoroscopically assisted biopsy (5.3%).

7. Ogilvie CM, Torbert JT, Finstein JL, Fox EJ, Lackman RD: Clinical utility of percutaneous biopsies of musculoskeletal tumors. *Clin Orthop Relat Res* 2006;450:95-100.

8. Lis E, Bilsky MH, Pisinski L, et al: Percutaneous CT-guided biopsy of osseous lesion of the spine in patients with known or suspected malignancy. *AJNR Am J Neuroradiol* 2004;25(9):1583-1588.

9. Boriani S, Weinstein JN, Biagini R: Primary bone tumors of the spine: Terminology and surgical staging. *Spine (Phila Pa 1976)* 1997;22(9):1036-1044.

10. Boriani S, De Iure F, Campanacci L, et al: Aneurysmal bone cyst of the mobile spine: Report on 41 cases. *Spine (Phila Pa 1976)* 2001;26(1):27-35.

11. Yasko AW, Fanning CV, Ayala AG, Carrasco CH, Murray JA: Percutaneous techniques for the diagnosis and treatment of localized Langerhans-cell histiocytosis (eo-

5: Spine

sinophilic granuloma of bone). *J Bone Joint Surg Am* 1998;80(2):219-228.

12. Garg S, Mehta S, Dormans JP: Langerhans cell histiocytosis of the spine in children: Long-term follow-up. *J Bone Joint Surg Am* 2004;86(8):1740-1750.

13. Hart RA, Boriani S, Biagini R, Currier B, Weinstein JN: A system for surgical staging and management of spine tumors: A clinical outcome study of giant cell tumors of the spine. *Spine (Phila Pa 1976)* 1997;22(15):1773-1782, discussion 1783.

14. Jones JO, Bruel BM, Vattam SR: Management of painful vertebral hemangiomas with kyphoplasty: A report of two cases and a literature review. *Pain Physician* 2009;12(4):E297-E303.

    The authors report on two patients with painful vertebral hemangiomas unresponsive to conservative care who were successfully treated with cement augmentation (kyphoplasty).

15. Kneisl JS, Simon MA: Medical management compared with operative treatment for osteoid-osteoma. *J Bone Joint Surg Am* 1992;74(2):179-185.

16. Hadjipavlou AG, Tzermiadianos MN, Kakavelakis KN, Lander P: Percutaneous core excision and radiofrequency thermo-coagulation for the ablation of osteoid osteoma of the spine. *Eur Spine J* 2009;18(3):345-351.

    The authors report a case series of four patients who underwent percutaneous radiofrequency ablation and three patients who underwent percutaneous core excision of osteoid osteoma. The overall success rate was 85.7%, with improved pain scores for both groups. The authors concluded that the former treatment is safe and effective when intact cortex separated the nidus from the neural elements, but that the latter technique reduces the risk of thermal damage when lesions are in close proximity to neurologic structures.

17. Boriani S, Capanna R, Donati D, Levine A, Picci P, Savini R: Osteoblastoma of the spine. *Clin Orthop Relat Res* 1992;278:37-45.

18. Sharma MC, Arora R, Deol PS, Mahapatra AK, Mehta VS, Sarkar C: Osteochondroma of the spine: An enigmatic tumor of the spinal cord. A series of 10 cases. *J Neurosurg Sci* 2002;46(2):66-70, discussion 70.

19. Boriani S, De Iure F, Bandiera S, et al: Chondrosarcoma of the mobile spine: Report on 22 cases. *Spine (Phila Pa 1976)* 2000;25(7):804-812.

20. Wagner TD, Kobayashi W, Dean S, et al: Combination short-course preoperative irradiation, surgical resection, and reduced-field high-dose postoperative irradiation in the treatment of tumors involving the bone. *Int J Radiat Oncol Biol Phys* 2009;73(1):259-266.

    The authors evaluated a regimen of preoperative radiation, surgical resection, and reduced-field high-dose postoperative radiation in 48 patients with tumors of the spine and pelvis. They found that the 5-year overall survival rate was 65%, disease-free survival was 53.8%, and the local control rate was 72% with this regimen. This effect was most pronounced with treatment of primary disease rather than recurrence.

21. Fourney DR, Rhines LD, Hentschel SJ, et al: En bloc resection of primary sacral tumors: Classification of surgical approaches and outcome. *J Neurosurg Spine* 2005; 3(2):111-122.

22. Fuchs B, Dickey ID, Yaszemski MJ, Inwards CY, Sim FH: Operative management of sacral chordoma. *J Bone Joint Surg Am* 2005;87(10):2211-2216.

23. Park L, Delaney TF, Liebsch NJ, et al: Sacral chordomas: Impact of high-dose proton/photon-beam radiation therapy combined with or without surgery for primary versus recurrent tumor. *Int J Radiat Oncol Biol Phys* 2006;65(5):1514-1521.

24. Tamborini E, Miselli F, Negri T, et al: Molecular and biochemical analyses of platelet-derived growth factor receptor (PDGFR) B, PDGFRA, and KIT receptors in chordomas. *Clin Cancer Res* 2006;12(23):6920-6928.

25. Marco RA, Gentry JB, Rhines LD, et al: Ewing's sarcoma of the mobile spine. *Spine (Phila Pa 1976)* 2005; 30(7):769-773.

26. Rao G, Ha CS, Chakrabarti I, Feiz-Erfan I, Mendel E, Rhines LD: Multiple myeloma of the cervical spine: Treatment strategies for pain and spinal instability. *J Neurosurg Spine* 2006;5(2):140-145.

27. Berenson JR, Hillner BE, Kyle RA, et al; American Society of Clinical Oncology Bisphosphonates Expert Panel: American Society of Clinical Oncology clinical practice guidelines: The role of bisphosphonates in multiple myeloma. *J Clin Oncol* 2002;20(17):3719-3736.

28. Rajkumar SV, Rosiñol L, Hussein M, et al: Multicenter, randomized, double-blind, placebo-controlled study of thalidomide plus dexamethasone compared with dexamethasone as initial therapy for newly diagnosed multiple myeloma. *J Clin Oncol* 2008;26(13):2171-2177.

    The authors conducted a randomized, double-blind, placebo-controlled study comparing the use of thalidomide and dexamethasone versus dexamethasone alone for treatment of multiple myeloma. A total of 235 patients were randomized to each group. The authors reported a better overall response rate (63% versus 46%), longer time to progression (22.6 versus 6.5 months), but higher rates of adverse events (30.3% versus 22.8%) with the thalidomide-dexamethasone group.

29. Masala S, Anselmetti GC, Marcia S, Massari F, Manca A, Simonetti G: Percutaneous vertebroplasty in multiple myeloma vertebral involvement. *J Spinal Disord Tech* 2008;21(5):344-348.

    The authors describe treatment of 64 patients with painful spinal lesions associated with multiple myeloma who underwent percutaneous vertebroplasty, reporting excellent early and sustained pain relief.

30. McDonald RJ, Trout AT, Gray LA, Dispenzieri A, Thielen KR, Kallmes DF: Vertebroplasty in multiple myeloma: Outcomes in a large patient series. *AJNR Am J Neuroradiol* 2008;29(4):642-648.

The authors conducted a retrospective review of 64 patients with multiple myeloma who had undergone percutaneous vertebroplasty. Activity-related pain, pain during rest, and functional outcomes demonstrated early and sustained improvement.

31. Rao G, Suki D, Chakrabarti I, et al: Surgical management of primary and metastatic sarcoma of the mobile spine. *J Neurosurg Spine* 2008;9(2):120-128.

In this retrospective review of 80 patients who underwent 110 intralesional or en bloc resections of spinal sarcomas, the authors report a mean survival time of 20.6 months (40.2 for primary lesions and 17.3 for metastatic lesions). There was no significant difference in survival rate or local recurrence rate between intralesional or en bloc resections, although there were fewer resections (12) in the latter group.

32. Destombe C, Botton E, Le Gal G, et al: Investigations for bone metastasis from an unknown primary. *Joint Bone Spine* 2007;74(1):85-89.

The authors retrospectively reviewed 152 patients who presented with metastatic lesions to the spine from an unknown primary tumor. The most common primary tumor site was the lung (37 patients), followed by prostate (26), breast/female genital tract (24), urologic system (11), gastrointestinal tract (11), head and neck (6), and other sites (4).

33. Tokuhashi Y, Matsuzaki H, Oda H, Oshima M, Ryu J: A revised scoring system for preoperative evaluation of metastatic spine tumor prognosis. *Spine (Phila Pa 1976)* 2005;30(19):2186-2191.

34. Putz C, Wiedenhöfer B, Gerner HJ, Fürstenberg CH: Tokuhashi prognosis score: An important tool in prediction of the neurological outcome in metastatic spinal cord compression. A retrospective clinical study. *Spine (Phila Pa 1976)* 2008;33(24):2669-2674.

In a retrospective review of 35 patients who underwent surgical treatment of vertebral metastases with associated incomplete spinal cord injury, the authors reported that patients with a Tokuhashi score of 9 showed improved motor scores, those with a score of 8 showed no change, and those with a score of 7 deteriorated.

35. Chi JH, Gokaslan Z, McCormick P, Tibbs PA, Kryscio RJ, Patchell RA: Selecting treatment for patients with malignant epidural spinal cord compression: Does age matter? Results from a randomized clinical trial. *Spine (Phila Pa 1976)* 2009;34(5):431-435.

The authors analyzed data from a randomized clinical trial of surgical treatment versus radiation therapy for malignant epidural spinal cord compression and reported that as age increases, the likelihood of outcomes from surgery being equal to those of radiation alone also increases. There was no difference in outcomes between treatments in patients older than 65 years, whereas the ability to preserve ambulation was significantly improved in those younger than 65 years.

36. Bilsky M, Smith M: Surgical approach to epidural spinal cord compression. *Hematol Oncol Clin North Am* 2006;20(6):1307-1317.

37. Samant R, Gerig L, Montgomery L, et al: The emerging role of IG-IMRT for palliative radiotherapy: A single-institution experience. *Curr Oncol* 2009;16(3):40-45.

The authors report a single-institution experience over 2 years in the use of IGIMRT for short-course palliative therapy, describing its use in four general scenarios. It was concluded that for patients not responding to other therapies, palliative IGIMRT is feasible and efficient.

38. Rose PS, Laufer I, Boland PJ, et al: Risk of fracture after single fraction image-guided intensity-modulated radiation therapy to spinal metastases. *J Clin Oncol* 2009;27(30):5075-5079.

The authors followed 62 patients who underwent single fraction IGIMRT and noted a 39% rate of fracture progression following treatment. Lytic lesions were 6.8 times more likely to fracture than sclerotic or mixed lesions; lesions caudal to T10 were 4.6 times more likely to fracture.

39. Patchell RA, Tibbs PA, Regine WF, et al: Direct decompressive surgical resection in the treatment of spinal cord compression caused by metastatic cancer: A randomised trial. *Lancet* 2005;366(9486):643-648.

40. Li H, Gasbarrini A, Cappuccio M, et al: Outcome of excisional surgeries for the patients with spinal metastases. *Eur Spine J* 2009;18(10):1423-1430.

The authors report on 131 patients who underwent either en bloc resection or debulking procedures. The local recurrence rate was significantly less in en bloc resection. En bloc resection resulted in a mean survival time of 41 months compared to 25 months for debulking (not statistically significant).

41. Lim BS, Chang UK, Youn SM: Clinical outcomes after percutaneous vertebroplasty for pathologic compression fractures in osteolytic metastatic spinal disease. *J Korean Neurosurg Soc* 2009;45(6):369-374.

The authors performed vertebroplasty procedures at 185 levels (102 patients) with painful spinal lesions caused by metastases (81%) and multiple myeloma (19%). They report nearly immediate pain relief from a visual analog scale score of 8.24 preoperatively to 3.59 at 1 day postoperatively. The relief was sustained with a mean visual analog scale score of 5.22 at 1 year.

42. Falicov A, Fisher CG, Sparkes J, Boyd MC, Wing PC, Dvorak MF: Impact of surgical intervention on quality of life in patients with spinal metastases. *Spine (Phila Pa 1976)* 2006;31(24):2849-2856.

43. Ibrahim A, Crockard A, Antonietti P, et al: Does spinal surgery improve the quality of life for those with extradural (spinal) osseous metastases? An international multicenter prospective observational study of 223 patients. Invited submission from the Joint Section Meeting on Disorders of the Spine and Peripheral Nerves, March 2007. *J Neurosurg Spine* 2008;8(3):271-278.

5: Spine

The authors report on outcomes of 223 patients undergoing surgical treatment (en bloc resection, debulking, or palliative decompression) for spinal lesions, noting that pain was improved in 71% of patients, mobility was improved in 53%, and urinary sphincter control was regained in 39%. Patients undergoing excisional procedures demonstrated significantly increased survival rates and functional improvement than those undergoing palliative surgery.

44. Patil CG, Lad SP, Santarelli J, Boakye M: National inpatient complications and outcomes after surgery for spinal metastasis from 1993-2002. *Cancer* 2007;110(3): 625-630.

The authors used the National Inpatient Sample to identify 26,233 patients who underwent surgical treatment of spinal metastases and found that the overall in-hospital mortality rate was 5.6% with an overall complication rate of 22%. Pulmonary and bleeding complications were most common. Postoperative complications substantially increased both length of stay and mortality; risk of complications was highest in patients with medical comorbidities.

Chapter 43

Spinal Infections

Thomas E. Mroz, MD   Michael P. Steinmetz, MD

Introduction

There are various types of infections that can involve the spine, and each is unique with regard to epidemiology, natural history, and treatment. Biomechanical variations in different regions of the spinal column should be taken into account when designing a rational treatment.

Most infections occurring in developed countries are caused by pyogenic bacteria, whereas nonpyogenic pathogens such as *Mycobacteriae, Brucella* species, and fungi are important pathogens in underdeveloped regions of the world and in immunocompromised patients.

Pyogenic Vertebral Osteomyelitis

Pathophysiology

Two vascular theories have been proposed to explain the evolution of vertebral osteomyelitis (VO). An arteriole theory was proposed, in which bacteria become entrapped in the end arteriole system near the vertebral end plate.[1] In Batson's[2] venous theory, bacteria gain entry into the perivertebral venous system via retrograde flow from the pelvic venous plexus.

Whichever vascular theory is responsible, bacteria become entrapped in the rich vascularity of the vertebral bodies near the end plates, which have a relatively poor vascular supply. The total action of the pyogenic enzymes and the host immune response result in progressive loss of osseous integrity of the body and destruction of the intervertebral disk. The destruction of the intervertebral disk can result in involvement of the adjacent body. As a focal consideration, the loss of structural integrity can result in pathologic fracture, which has serious implications for overall spinal alignment and for the neural elements. Abscess formation can occur focally within the disk space, the vertebral body, and/or the spinal canal. In rare instances, bacterial meningitis can result. Spread of the infection can occur via the prevertebral fascia in the cervical spine to spread to other levels of the prevertebral space, including the mediastinum inferiorly. Infection in the lumbar spine can spread via the anterior longitudinal ligament and psoas muscle fascia to result in abscess formation in the piriformis fossa, perianal region, and psoas muscle.

Biomechanical characteristics and neural anatomy of the spinal region must be considered when treating spinal infections. The cervical and thoracic columns have narrower canal diameters, and this has serious implications in the case of epidural abscess and/or VO management. The cervical, thoracic, and lumbar columns are anatomically and biomechanically unique, and this must be taken into account during both nonsurgical and surgical treatment.

Epidemiology

Hematogenous VO is a serious infection that is associated with a mortality rate of up to 15%.[3-5] In developed countries, *Staphylococcus aureus* accounts for approximately 50% of cases of VO; however, gram-negative (for example, *Escherichia coli, Enterococcus*) and other gram-positive (for example, *Proteus* species) bacteria, mycobacteria, and fungi also should be considered. Patients with diabetes and penetrating injuries are prone to developing anaerobic infections. *Pseudomonas* infections have a higher incidence among intravenous drug abusers. VO is more common in males and in the fifth and sixth decades of life.[2,5] The lumbar spine is affected in about 50% of cases of VO; thoracic involvement is second, followed by the cervical spine (approximately 5%). Although patients with VO often will have an identifiable source of infection (for example, complicated urinary tract infection, infected central line, cutaneous infection) or an immunocompromised state (for example, history of organ transplant, dialysis, HIV, intravenous drug use, recent dental procedure, diabetes mellitus, or chemotherapy), healthy patients without any risk factor may also present with spontaneous VO.

Dr. Mroz or an immediate family member has stock or stock options held in PearlDiver and is a member of a speakers' bureau or has made paid presentations on behalf of Stryker and AO Spine. Dr. Steinmetz or an immediate family member serves as a board member, owner, officer, or committee member of the Congress of Neurological Surgeons AANS/CNS Section on Disorders of the Spine and Peripheral Nerves Council of State Neurosurgical Societies; is a member of a speakers' bureau or has made paid presentations on behalf of Stryker; and has received research or institutional support from DePuy, a Johnson & Johnson Company, Stryker, and Synthes.

5: Spine

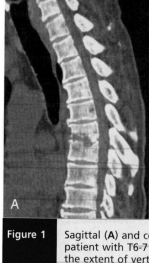
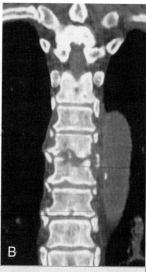

Figure 1   Sagittal (**A**) and coronal (**B**) CT reconstruction of a patient with T6-7 pyogenic osteomyelitis. Note the extent of vertebral body destruction.

Clinical Presentation

Pain in the affected region, which occurs in 90% of patients with VO, is the most common complaint and is associated with paraspinal muscle spasm. The pain may be described as dull or sharp, constant or intermittent. As the process progresses with loss of structural integrity, the pain worsens and becomes more mechanical in nature. Constitutional signs and symptoms including fever and malaise occur in about half of affected patients. Range of motion may become limited by pain, and focal tenderness can be present. The physician must be alert to meningeal symptoms and signs. In patients with psoas involvement, resisted hip flexion or passive hip extension may exacerbate pain. Upper cervical involvement may result in torticollis.

Neurologic impairment occurs in approximately 17% of cases of VO, and it is more common with cervical and thoracic involvement because of a smaller space available for the spinal cord in these areas. Neurologic involvement can result from pathologic fracture with retropulsion of material into the canal or from epidural abscess/phlegmon formation in the canal. Neurologic involvement is a surgical emergency and requires prompt surgical treatment. The neurologic picture will depend on the region of the spine affected. Lumbar spine VO can present with radiculopathy or cauda equine syndrome (rarely), whereas involvement of the cervical or thoracic spine result in myelopathy or myeloradiculopathy.

Imaging

Plain radiography is helpful in the evaluation of infection and if possible should be performed with the patient standing to detect structural changes under physiologic loading. The typical changes of disk space narrowing, end plate irregularity, and end plate sclerosis take several weeks to appear on radiographs. Stand-

ing radiographs may demonstrate angular and/or translational instability in cases of diskitis or osteomyelitis. A thorough assessment must be made of the prevertebral soft-tissue shadows in the cervical spine and mediastinal width, and soft-tissue gas must be ruled out in cases of anaerobic infection. CT with coronal and sagittal reconstructions is very useful in delineating psoas abscess and the pattern and extent of structural degradation, and should be a part of any workup in patients with advanced VO (**Figure 1**).

MRI with gadolinium is a standard imaging technique and has a sensitivity of 96% and a specificity of 93% in diagnosing VO. T1-weighted images demonstrate hypointense signal intensity in the disk space and adjacent vertebral bodies. Conversely, the same regions appear hyperintense on T2-weighted images. Contrasted images are helpful in identifying abscess formation and in delineating neoplasm (**Figure 2**). Serial MRIs obtained during the course must be carefully interpreted because the scans will often look worse despite clinical improvement. Thus, serial scanning is not typically necessary. **Figure 3** demonstrates an illustrative case of T12-L1 osteomyelitis treated nonsurgically.

Radionuclide scans can be a useful tool in patients with infection. Technetium Tc-99m scintigraphy has a sensitivity of approximately 90% but lacks specificity. It is dependent on blood flow, and cases of enhanced perfusion (degeneration) or diminished flow (extremes of patient age) decrease the utility of the test. Gallium Ga-67 citrate scan, when performed with bone scan, has a sensitivity of 92%, specificity of 100%, and accuracy of 94% in detecting VO.[6] Gallium scans normalize with resolution of the infection and can be useful for following the response to treatment.

Laboratory Assessment

All patients should have a complete white blood cell (WBC) count with differential, Westergren erythrocyte sedimentation rate (ESR), and C-reactive protein (CRP) level. It is important to note that WBC count is often normal in patients with VO, particularly with indolent organisms. CRP level and ESR are elevated in more than 90% of patients with pyogenic VO. CRP level will rise and fall more quickly than ESR and should be used serially to judge the effectiveness of treatment. The nutritional status should also be assessed by checking the total lymphocyte count and prealbumin and transferrin levels.

Blood cultures should be obtained in all patients with suspected VO and will yield a positive culture in 85% of patients.[7] If blood cultures do not identify an organism, then a CT-guided biopsy is indicated and will be successful in organism identification in 50% to 75% of patients.[7] The avoidance of antibiotic treatment before cultures is extremely important because the likelihood of a positive culture is substantially diminished; this detail should be made known to all involved in the care of the patient.

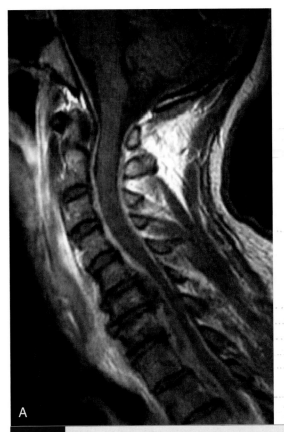
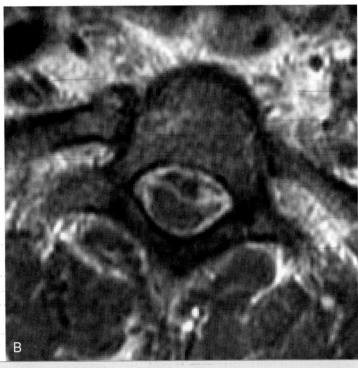

Figure 2 Imaging studies of a 45-year-old man with incomplete quadriplegia due to a large epidural abscess from a C6-7 osteomyelitis. **A,** Midsagittal T1-weighted cervical spine image with gadolinium enhancement. **B,** Axial T1-weighted image with gadolinium demonstrating a well-circumscribed enhancing epidural abscess.

Nonpyogenic Osteomyelitis

Epidemiology

Multiple organisms including *Mycobacterium* species (*M tuberculosis*, *M avium-intracellulare*), *Nocardia*, *Brucella*, *Actinomyces* and fungi (*Candida*, *Aspergillus*, *Coccidioides*, *Petrillidium*, and *Spirochaetes*) induce a granulomatous immune response and can result in nonpyogenic VO. Tuberculosis, caused by *M tuberculosis*, is the most common cause of granulomatous spinal VO (Potts disease).[8] There has been a resurgence of the disease worldwide because of the increase in immunocompromising states (such as AIDS, chemotherapy regimens, and immunosuppressive therapy [for example, for organ transplants]). Systemic tuberculosis results in spine involvement in approximately 50% of patients, and it is thought that hematogenous seeding from the lungs or genitourinary tract is the primary route. Peak ages are the fourth and fifth decades. Neurologic involvement varies widely from 10% to 47%, and in large part is due to the time to diagnosis and treatment and the degree of kyphotic deformity. In contrast to pyogenic VO, tuberculosis occurs more commonly in the thoracic spine, followed by the lumbar spine, and rarely occurs in the cervical spine.

Pathogenesis

M tuberculosis is an acid-fast bacteria that causes a unique pattern of infection. The disk space is resistant to infection, and thus is typically spared. Hence the radiographic hallmark is osseous destruction with preservation of the disk space. Tuberculosis of the spine is an indolent infection that is often diagnosed late, and this underscores why many patients present with large kyphotic deformities. Three types of body involvement have been defined: anterior, peridiskal, and central. Anterior involvement refers to progression of the infection along the dorsal side of the anterior longitudinal ligament resulting in scalloping of the ventral vertebral bodies. Peridiskal involvement involves the metaphyseal portion of the vertebral bodies and can result in substantial collapse and deformity. The infection may be confined to the central body (central pattern) and is often confused with malignancy.

Clinical Presentation and Laboratory Diagnosis

The clinical presentations of pyogenic and nonpyogenic VO share similarities. Both result in pain due to loss of structural integrity, which occurs later in nonpyogenic VO and is a result of the indolent pathogenesis. Fever

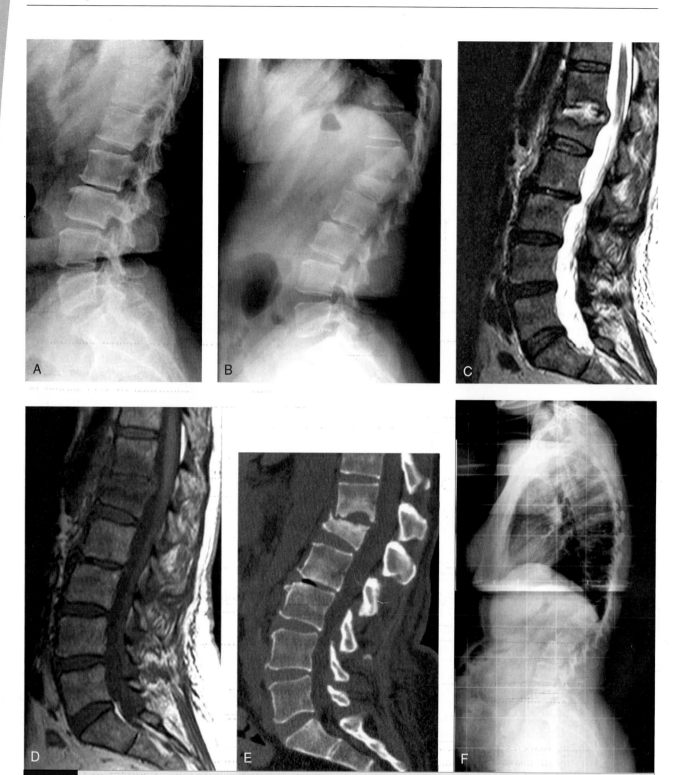

Figure 3 Imaging studies of a 59-year-old woman with a 3-week history of progressive thoracolumbar pain. **A,** Lateral radiograph demonstrating spondylotic changes at L2-3. Nine weeks after symptom onset, the patient was treated nonsurgically for 6 weeks, but pain worsened, prompting another radiograph (**B**) that showed loss of veterbral height of L1 and T12, irregularity of the end plates, and a focal kyphosis. **C,** MRI showing diskitis and osteomyelitis at T12-L1. A CT-guided biopsy yielded *Staphylococcus aureus*. The patient was started on antibiotics and placed in a thoracolumbosacral orthosis. Seventeen weeks after onset of symptoms, the patient's pain was improved after 7 weeks on parenteral antibiotics and brace management. **D,** T1-weighted midsagittal MRI at 17 weeks after symptom onset. The image demonstrates vertebral end plate and body erosion typical of diskitis and osteomyelitis. **E,** Midsagittal CT demonstrates findings typical of osteomyelitis: loss of structural integrity, sclerosis of the adjacent bone, and focal kyphosis. The patient was treated with 6 weeks of parenteral antbiotics, 6 weeks of oral antiobiotics, and 3 months in the brace. **F,** Eight months after symptom onset, the patient was pain free. Full-length radiograph shows a focal thoracolumbar kyphosis but overall acceptable sagittal balance.

may or may not be present. Patients with nonpyogenic VO often have a history and appearance of chronic illness and malnourishment (characterized by weight loss, fatigue, night sweats, temporal wasting, and depletion of nutritional markers). Tuberculosis should be suspected in patients with this presentation and coexisting risk factors (for example, immunocompromised state, travel to or residence in underdeveloped countries or the southwest United States [prevalence of coccidioidomycosis], history of tuberculosis). In patients with advanced stages of tuberculosis, a kyphotic or gibbus deformity is often present.

Like pyogenic disease, ESR and CRP levels in nonpyogenic VO will be elevated, and the WBC count is often normal. A tuberculin skin test should be performed, but a false-negative test can occur in anergic patients who have advanced immunoincompetency. In patients with tuberculosis, a biopsy specimen positive for acid-fast bacillus is ideal; however, this identification method has a sensitivity of only about 50%. For this reason, polymerase chain reaction can be used to identify mycobacterium with a sensitivity and accuracy of 94.7% and 92%, respectively.

Imaging

Plain radiographs, CT, and MRI with contrast should be obtained in all patients. The MRI characteristics of nonpyogenic VO are similar to those of pyogenic VO, but there are features such as tuberculosis that are unique to nonpyogenic VO. Tuberculosis is often accompanied by abscess formation, a heterogenous signal, preservation of disk spaces, multiple affected vertebral bodies, and a predisposition for the thoracic spine. Radionuclide studies can be helpful.

Treatment

Medical Management

It is advantageous to include an infectious disease consultation for patients with any spinal infection. Once a culture has been obtained, empiric antibiotics should be started in the patient with sepsis or who is immunocompromised. Parenteral antibiotics tailored to the identified organism are administered for 2 to 6 weeks, and then oral therapy is administered. The length of each treatment arm will be predicated, in part, on the type of organism, host factors such as immune and nutritional status, and risk factors (for example, intravenous drug abuse, diabetes mellitus), and whether the patient has retained instrumentation. The nutritional status must be optimized. As mentioned, CRP level and ESR can be used to monitor response to medical therapy. Serial clinical examinations are also an important measure, as the resolution of pain correlates with a positive response to treatment. In the improving patient, it is not necessary to obtain serial radiographs. Infective endocarditis must be considered in patients who have spinal infections, particularly those with persistent bacteremia or fever who are not responding appropriately to medical management. An echocardiogram should be obtained to rule out endocarditis. With

tuberculosis, therapy is highly dependent on the susceptibility and immune status of the host, but is typically a prolonged multidrug regimen. With fungal infection, the appropriate regimen is delivered over a course of months.

Rigid bracing or immobilization is recommended in patients with VO, regardless of the affected region. Bracing often will help with pain relief and is effective in minimizing the development of kyphosis.

Surgical Management

There are four main indications for surgery: failure of a CT-guided biopsy or blood culture to yield an organism, thus necessitating open or percutaneous retrieval of more tissue; failure of medical therapy (persistent pain or fever); development of neurologic demise; and structural decompensation.

surgical indications

Whether the indication for surgery is neurologic or structural demise, the most appropriate surgical procedure is determined after a meticulous assessment of the structural integrity. For example, lumbar epidural abscess with neurologic impairment that occurred from direct extension of a spondylodiskitis without loss of vertebral body integrity (confirmed by CT) should be treated much differently than epidural abscess with neurologic impairment with a 50° kyphosis caused by pathologic fracture. In this example, the lumbar epidural abscess associated with spondylodiskitis can be treated with posterior decompression, evacuation of the abscess, and disk débridement. The other condition requires a more extensive débridement and reconstruction.

The algorithm for surgical treatment is actually quite simple when considering the four goals of surgical management and the pathogenesis of VO: thoroughly débriding infectious foci and necrotic material, relieving all pressure on the neural elements, restoring normal sagittal and coronal alignment, and providing rigid fixation in the presence of instability. Rigid fixation is particularly important considering the pathogenesis. As an infection progresses, thrombosis of the microvasculature limits the clearance of the infection as well as the formation of new bone. In addition, angiogenesis in the affected region is impaired with continued motion and persistent infection. Thus, rigid fixation will promote healing of the infection and ankylosis in the case of fusion.

goals of surgery

Vertebral osteomyelitis affects the ventral columns of the spine, and with loss of vertebral body integrity kyphosis often will result. It is important to thoroughly débride the disk space and body, reconstruct the cavity created, and provide adequate fixation. This can be done via a ventral approach, a combined ventral and posterior approach, or a posterior approach (costotransversectomy). The type of surgery performed will be predicated on many factors, including surgeon expertise, availability of an access surgeon, bone quality (whether osteoporosis is present), sagittal and coronal alignment, physiologic reserve of the patient, and degree of structural loss. A laminectomy is contraindi-

5: Spine

cated in patients with VO because of the kyphosis that it causes. If the appropriate surgical procedure cannot be done for whatever reason, the patient should be referred to a tertiary care center for definitive treatment. It is technically more challenging to salvage a failed first attempt at surgical management.

Although there is agreement that rigid fixation is necessary in cases of infection with loss of structural integrity (kyphosis), the optimal type of implant is controversial. Structural autograft and allograft bone and titanium and poly-ethyl-ether-ketone (PEEK) reconstruction cages are all viable options for ventral reconstruction after partial or complete corpectomy. Ventral plates and posterior pedicle fixation are added to augment the fixation when necessary. The decision to use ventral plates alone or with posterior fixation is predicated on several factors, including the degree of instability, region of the spine (thoracolumbar junction versus midthoracic spine), and surgeon experience.

Epidural Abscess

Epidemiology

Epidural abscess is a rare but serious disease that is associated with the risk of neurologic demise and even fatality. Hematogenous spread is responsible for about half of cases, direct extension from diskitis for about a third, and a source is not identified in the remaining cases. S aureus is the number one pathogen; however, methicillin-resistant S aureus is an important cause, particularly in patients with retained vascular or spinal implants. Less common etiologies include Staphylococcus epidermidis and gram-negative bacteria such as E coli (for example, urinary tract infections) and Pseudomanas aeruginosa (for example, intravenous drug abuse).[9] Anaerobic bacteria, fungi, and parasites are rare causes. Epidural abscesses are more common dorsally, and are more common in the thoracolumbar spine. Most abscesses are secondary to diskitis and osteomyelitis, and this underscores the need to treat these infections quickly. It is often difficult to obtain a thorough history and to interpret neurologic deficits (real versus secondary to cognitive deficits) in the elderly population. It is important to maintain a high index of suspicion in elderly patients to avoid a missed diagnosis of epidural abscess.

Clinical Presentation

The pathogenesis of neurologic demise may stem from direct compression and/or septic thrombophlebitis with resultant venous spinal cord infarction. The precise mechanism is not known. The clinical presentation varies and will be predicated on the degree and type of neurologic compression and region of the spine involved. Common findings include pain (three fourths of patients) in the affected region, radicular pain from root compression, or neurologic deficit (one third of patients) correlative to the compressed level of the spinal cord, cauda equina, or nerve root. Fever is pres-

ent in about 50% of patients. The reported range of symptom onset varies widely from days to months, and the period of neurologic demise ranges from hours to days.

Laboratory and Diagnostic Imaging

Although ESR, CRP level, and WBC count are typically elevated in patients with epidural abscesses, this is not a specific indication for the disease. Both MRI with gadolinium and CT myelography have a sensitivity greater than 90% for detection of an abscess, but the former is less invasive and the modality of choice to make the diagnosis. MRI with gadolinium will demonstrate the size and degree of neurologic compression. A ring-enhancing lesion is pathognomonic for abscess and distinguishes it from neoplasm. In patients who have associated diskitis or VO, then plain radiography and CT are essential to define the extent of osseous destruction.

Treatment

No randomized controlled trials have been performed to generate level I evidence on the treatment of epidural abscess. Most retrospective studies have demonstrated that the mainstay of treatment is direct surgical decompression followed by antibiotic administration tailored to the organism isolated during surgery. The type of surgery performed is predicated on the site of the abscess and degree of bony involvement. Indirect decompression (laminectomy for a ventral cervical or thoracic abscess) is typically not the procedure of choice. Antibiotic therapy alone is controversial, and results are limited to few retrospective series. It should only be attempted in patients with small abscesses and no neurologic deficits, and in patients who will have very close serial clinical follow-up. The 4% to 22% incidence of permanent paralysis in patients with epidural abscess underscores the need to promptly treat these patients and provides a strong argument for surgical management. The addition of spinal instrumentation is dependent on the type of surgery performed (such as cervical laminectomy) and the degree of bony destruction, if present. The main indicator of clinical outcome is degree of neurologic impairment preoperatively.

Postoperative Infections

Epidemiology

Infections are a relatively common acute postoperative complication.[10] The likelihood of infection varies with several factors: predisposing factors of the patient, complexity of the case, and prophylactic antibiotics. The infection rate for lumbar microdiskectomy is 0.7%, but it doubles when a microscope is used during the case. Instrumentation increases the infection rate, as does a posterior procedure. Anterior procedures are not associated with higher rates. Infection rates of 2.8% to 6.0% have been reported for elective fusion with instrumentation. Spine trauma treated surgically is associated with infection rates up to 10%, and higher rates are correlated with delay in surgery beyond 16 hours and multilevel surgery.

Risk factors include obesity (body mass index greater than 35), smoking, diabetes mellitus, alcohol abuse, malnutrition, chronic steroid use, prior infection, revision surgery, surgery longer than 3 hours, and blood loss greater than 1.0 L. Age has inconsistently been associated with an increased risk of infection. The most common pathogen is *S aureus*; however, *S epidermidis* and methicillin-resistant *S aureus* are other relatively frequent etiologies. Gram-negative and anaerobic pathogens occur less frequently, but can cause serious disease. Prevention has been extensively studied, and preoperative intravenous antibiotics are efficacious in decreasing infection rates. Cefazolin is effective against *S aureus* and *S epidermidis*, and should be given 1 hour before incision and readministered if the surgery exceeds 4 hours. Clindamycin or vancomycin should be given for patients allergic to cephalosporins.

Clinical Presentation

Postoperative infections may be classified as superficial, most commonly suprafascial, and deep. Most postoperative infections occur early within the first few weeks after the index procedure, but others occur late or latent (years after surgery). The most common presentation of an early postoperative infection is pain at the incision site. This pain usually will begin several days after the surgery and typically is progressive. Constitutional symptoms and signs such as fever, fatigue, and malaise are also common. Examination findings include drainage, which can range from serosanguinous to frankly purulent, and peri-incisional erythema, induration, warmth, and tenderness. Benign-appearing serosanguinous or serosanguinous drainage that does not cease within the first week postoperatively is worrisome for infection. In severe cases, mental status changes, high fever, and sepsis can occur, and this scenario warrants emergent surgical treatment.

Laboratory and Diagnostic Imaging

Laboratory studies should include ESR, CRP level, and complete blood cell count with differential. ESR will often remain elevated for up to 6 weeks after surgery, and this makes ESR a less useful study in the immediate postoperative period. CRP level remains elevated for up to 2 weeks postoperatively. Cultures or swabs of incision drainage often will confound the diagnosis because of skin colonization. The most reliable cultures are obtained at surgery.

Plain radiographs typically contribute much information, as the time frame between surgery and early infection is narrow. CT may show fluid collections. MRI with gadolinium should be obtained, but the results must be interpreted carefully. The normal postoperative changes can look very similar to the infection. Enhancing fluid collections are pathognomonic for infection.

Management

The treatment of postoperative infections is dependent on type of infection and the patient's immune, neurologic, and clinical status. Postdiskectomy diskitis is often an indolent infection that results in a delayed diagnosis. Patients often will present with progressive mechanical back pain and elevation of serologic markers. In the absence of a disk space abscess, a needle biopsy to obtain a pathogen can be followed by a course of appropriate antibiotics. If the infection progresses into a disk space or epidural abscess, the patient has intractable pain or develops instability or deformity, then surgery is indicated.

Postoperative wound infections generally respond poorly to antibiotic therapy alone, and surgical irrigation and débridement is indicated in most patients. Attempts to clinically treat a draining wound rarely will result in spontaneous resolution, and waiting will result in increased soft-tissue necrosis and possible progression to osteomyelitis. Hence, prompt surgical management is advantageous. The goals of surgery include evacuation of all fluid collections and a thorough mechanical débridement of all necrotic soft tissue. Instrumentation should be left in place if it remains intact, as this will aid in eradication of the infection for reasons noted earlier.[11,12] Similarly, bone graft should be left in place unless it appears grossly contaminated.

Vacuum-assisted closure has been shown to be a safe treatment of complex postoperative infections;[13] however, absolute indications have not been defined in the literature. The use of vacuum-assisted closure dressings is a reasonable approach for grossly contaminated wounds, ones with large areas of dead space, immune-incompetent patients, and patients in whom previous irrigation and débridement with attempted primary closure has failed. The VAC dressing can be used as a transition to a primary closure, or in recalcitrant cases, it can be used serially to secondary closure.

Annotated References

1. Wiley AM, Trueta J: The vascular anatomy of the spine and its relationship to pyogenic vertebral osteomyelitis. *J Bone Joint Surg Br* 1959;41:796-809.

2. Batson OV: The vertebral system of veins as a means for cancer dissemination. *Prog Clin Cancer* 1967;3:1-18.

3. Garcia A Jr, Grantham SA: Hematogenous pyogenic vertebral osteomyelitis. *J Bone Joint Surg Am* 1960;42A:429-436.

4. Eismont FJ, Bohlman HH, Soni PL, Goldberg VM, Freehafer AA: Pyogenic and fungal vertebral osteomyelitis with paralysis. *J Bone Joint Surg Am* 1983;65(1):19-29.

5. Krogsgaard MR, Wagn P, Bengtsson J: Epidemiology of acute vertebral osteomyelitis in Denmark: 137 cases in Denmark 1978-1982, compared to cases reported to the

5: Spine

National Patient Register 1991-1993. *Acta Orthop Scand* 1998;69(5):513-517.

6. Modic MT, Feiglin DH, Piraino DW, et al: Vertebral osteomyelitis: assessment using MR. *Radiology* 1985; 157(1):157-166.

7. Brodke DS, Fassett DR: Infections of the spine, in Spivak JM, Connolly PJ, eds: *Orthopaedic Knowledge Update: Spine*, ed 3. Rosemont, IL, American Academy of Orthopaedic Surgeons, 2006, pp 367-375.

8. Jain AK: Tuberculosis of the spine. A fresh look at an old disease. *J Bone Joint Surg Br* 2010;92:905-913.

   The use of antitubercular drugs, modern diagnostic aids, and advancements in surgical treatment of tuberculosis of the spine are discussed.

9. Darouiche RO: Spinal epidural abscess. *N Engl J Med* 2006;355(19):2012-2020.

10. Sasso RC, Garrido BJ: Postoperative spinal wound infections. *J Am Acad Orthop Surg* 2008;16(6):330-337.

    This article discusses spinal wound infections that occur after surgery, along with risk factors and preventive measures.

11. Mok JM, Guillaume TJ, Talu U, et al: Clinical outcome of deep wound infection after instrumented posterior spinal fusion: A matched cohort analysis. *Spine* 2009; 34(6):578-583.

    The authors determined that deep wound infection should be treated aggressively with early irrigation and débridement to allow preservation of instrumentation and successful fusion.

12. Rayes M, Colen CB, Bahgat DA, et al: Safety of instrumentation in patients with spinal infection. *J Neurosurg Spine* 2010;12(6):647-659.

    The authors concluded that instrumentation after radical débridement will not lead to an increased risk of recurrent infection. Spinal stabilization may be more beneficial and promote accelerated healing.

13. Mehbod AA, Ogilvie JW, Pinto MR, et al: Postoperative deep wound infections in adults after spinal fusion: Management with vacuum-assisted wound closure. *J Spinal Disord Tech* 2005;18(1):14-17.

Spinal Cord Injury

Brian K. Kwon, MD, PhD, FRCSC

Introduction

Each year in the United States, approximately 12,000 individuals sustain an acute spinal cord injury (SCI).[1] These individuals join a growing population of chronically paralyzed SCI patients, which recently was estimated by the Christopher Reeve Foundation to exceed 1.25 million. This figure is almost four times higher than previous estimates.[2] With the aging population, a greater number of persons older than 60 years suffer SCI. As a result, the average age at injury has risen from 29 years in the mid-1970s to almost 40 years since 2005. Irrespective of the age at which an individual has an SCI, the personal loss and societal costs are astronomical. Although personal loss cannot be quantified, recent estimates of societal costs place the lifetime medical costs of caring for a complete quadriplegic or paraplegic between $1 and $3 million.

It is hoped that the considerable research efforts currently under way will soon produce an effective treatment of SCI that will bring about a measurable and meaningful improvement in neurologic function. A greater understanding of the neurobiologic challenges imposed by SCI is emerging, and clinicians currently are witnessing a growing number of experimental treatments that are entering or have already initiated human evaluation.[3,4] The initiation of such human trials fuels the hope that an effective treatment may be imminent.

It is important that clinicians be aware of the basic principles of early management of acute SCI, and the therapies that are about to or have already begun evaluation in human clinical trials.

Early Management of Acute SCI

Emergency Assessment

Acute SCI occurs in the context of trauma, and so the initial treatment of patients with neurologic impairment is still guided by the Advanced Trauma Life Support (ATLS) protocols. The first priorities are the assessment and management of the airway, breathing,

Dr. Kwon or an immediate family member serves as a paid consultant to Medtronic Sofamor Danek and has received research or institutional support from Medtronic Sofamor Danek.

and circulation (ABCs). Although the ATLS protocols are familiar to most, there are important considerations in patients with acute SCI. First, the airway should be maintained and the cervical spine protected to minimize further displacement of cervical column injuries and additional insult to the spinal cord. Upper cervical spine injuries may impair diaphragmatic function and lead to rapid hypoxic respiratory failure (often at the injury scene). More commonly, lower cervical spine injuries and the resultant paralysis of intercostal muscles lead to poor chest wall expansion and a slower hypercarbic ventilatory failure within the first 24 to 48 hours of injury. Poor chest wall expansion and slower hypercarbic ventilator failure may require intubation and mechanical ventilation, which needs to be done with cervical spine protection. Disruption of sympathetic outflow with cervical SCI can lead to bradycardia, whereas the loss of vasomotor tone can result in profound hypotension. This combination of hypotension and bradycardia is often referred to as neurogenic shock, and requires vasopressor support with pharmacologic agents. Such interventions should be instituted only after hemorrhagic shock from other injuries is addressed with volume expansion and/or blood products. The term neurogenic shock is often confused with spinal shock, which refers to the absence of spinal reflexes that occurs after a severe SCI and is operationally defined as ending when the bulbocavernosus reflex returns.

Neurologic Assessment

The screening examination for neurologic impairment (the "D" stands for disability in the ABCs of the ATLS protocol) constitutes a quick assessment of whether the patient can voluntarily move the four extremities. The clinical characterization of the SCI, however, requires a formal neurologic assessment according to the American Spinal Injury Association (ASIA) guidelines, which have been adopted as the international standard for evaluating patients with SCI (**Figure 1**). The current ASIA examination entails a motor and sensory examination, although work is also being done to incorporate a clinical assessment of autonomic instability. The motor examination is conducted by measuring the strength of five key upper extremity myotomes (C5, elbow flexion; C6, wrist extension; C7, elbow extension, C8, long finger flexion; and T1, small finger abductors) and five lower extremity myotomes (L2, hip flexion; L3, knee extension; L4, ankle dorsiflexion; L5, great

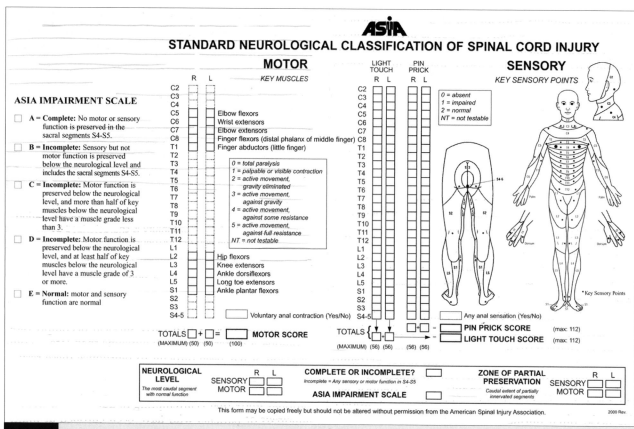

Figure 1 The American Spinal Injury Association (ASIA) Impairment Scale and Assessment Form. Acute SCI patients should be evaluated according to the ASIA standards of assessment. This involves both motor and sensory testing, and most importantly, an evaluation of function in the lowest sacral segments (S4-S5). The motor score is derived from 10 key myotomes in the upper and lower extremities. Patients are graded on the ASIA Impairment Scale based on whether or not they demonstrate function at S4-S5 (complete versus incomplete) and how much residual motor and sensory function they have maintained (to determine the extent of "incompleteness").

toe extension; and S1, ankle plantar flexion). Motor strength is documented according to the Medical Research Council (MRC) grading scheme from 0 to 5. Grade 0 represents complete paralysis, grade 1 is a palpable or visible contraction, grade 2 is full active range of motion with gravity eliminated, grade 3 is full active range of motion against gravity, grade 4 is full active range of motion against resistance, and grade 5 is normal strength. It is important during this examination not to confuse spastic or reflexive movements with voluntary motor function. For example, it is not uncommon when testing ankle plantar flexion to see reflexive extension of the great toe or ankle in response to touching the sole of the foot (akin to a Babinski reflex response). If this is witnessed by the patient or family, who are obviously desperately hopeful for some motor recovery, it can be easily misinterpreted as preserved motor function.

The sensory examination is performed by assessing light touch and pinprick sensation along 28 dermatomes (S4-S5 is one). The sensation is documented as absent, impaired, or normal and is scored 0, 1, or 2, respectively. The most common mistake in the sensory testing of individuals with SCI is misinterpreting the dermatomal distribution in the upper thorax. It is important to remember that the C4 dermatome extends down in a capelike distribution along the upper chest and shoulders, and ends just rostral to the nipple line. Because most physicians associate the nipple line with a T4 sensory distribution, it is not uncommon for the inexperienced examiner to test pinprick sensation along the upper chest, and document that there is a "T4 sensory level" because the sensation remains intact near the nipple line. This finding means that the C4 dermatome is intact.

Arguably, the most important aspect of the ASIA examination is the rectal examination. In the patient with an acute SCI, it should be determined whether he or she has pinprick and/or light touch sensation around the perianal region and voluntary anal contraction. The presence or absence of function at this S4/S5 level defines whether the patient has a complete or incomplete SCI; this distinction currently has the most significant prognostic implications for the patient. With the motor and sensory examination completed and the rectal examination completed, the severity of paralysis can be classified. The ASIA Impairment Scale is the universally accepted system for broadly categorizing the neurologic function of patients with an SCI (**Figure 1**). Patients in whom no motor or sensory function is preserved in the lowest sacral segments (S4-S5) are deemed to be ASIA A complete. Those with sensory sparing in the lowest sacral segments with no motor function are ASIA B incomplete. Those with preserved motor function below the neurologic level with the majority of myotomes having a muscle grade of two or less are ASIA C incomplete, whereas those with a muscle grade of three or more are ASIA D incomplete. Patients with normal motor and sensory function are considered to be ASIA E. The ASIA Impairment Scale highlights the importance of the rectal and perianal examination to confirm the presence or absence of sacral sparing and to determine if the SCI is complete or incomplete. A variety of "syndromes" of incomplete paralysis have been described and include central cord syndrome, Brown-Séquard syndrome, anterior or posterior cord syndrome, and cruciate paralysis. Because they all are forms of incomplete paralysis, varying degrees of neurologic improvement can be expected. The most common syndrome of incomplete paralysis is that of central cord syndrome, which is characterized by disproportionately greater deficits in the upper extremity than the lower extremity. This is most commonly observed in elderly patients with preexisting cervical spondylosis and stenosis who "kink" their spinal cord with sudden hyperextension of the neck, often during low-energy falls. Although the greater upper extremity involvement in central cord syndrome has been attributed to the arm and hand fibers of the corticospinal tract running more medially/centrally within the cord than the lower extremity fibers, this somatotopic organization of the corticospinal tract has never been anatomically demonstrated. More contemporary studies reveal that the upper extremity involvement in central cord syndrome is better explained by the dominant role that the corticospinal tract has in upper extremity function in humans (and hence, injuries to this tract are prominently manifest in the upper extremities).

Investigation

There is little argument that MRI is the most valuable imaging study for the assessment of SCI. It should be remembered that the acute SCI is an evolving biologic process, and so, the MRI appearance of the spinal cord is likely to be influenced by the timing of the imaging study. Edema and hemorrhage can be seen within the cord parenchyma, and the presence and rostrocaudal extent of these factors may be useful in predicting the eventual neurologic outcome.[5] (**Figure 2**) MRI can also help in the surgical planning to guide the decompression.

Treatment

Most acute SCIs occur with some spinal column instability, and hence, are typically treated with surgical stabilization with or without decompression. The most controversial aspect of this treatment is the timing of surgical decompression. Despite fairly convincing data

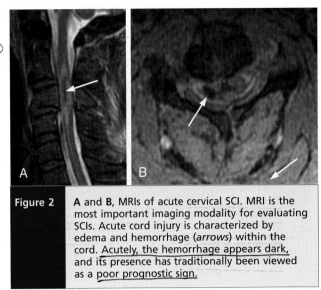

Figure 2   **A** and **B**, MRIs of acute cervical SCI. MRI is the most important imaging modality for evaluating SCIs. Acute cord injury is characterized by edema and hemorrhage (*arrows*) within the cord. Acutely, the hemorrhage appears dark, and its presence has traditionally been viewed as a poor prognostic sign.

from animal models that early surgical decompression promotes a better neurologic outcome than late decompression, it has been difficult to reproduce these results in human patients with SCI. The Surgical Treatment of Acute Spinal Cord Injury Study is a prospective observational study that is attempting to address this issue in hundreds of patients who have been enrolled at multiple North American sites. At the time of this writing, the preliminary data from this study have suggested a small benefit to early decompression. Whatever the final results of this trial, basic trauma care principles would indicate that the overall medical care of SCI patients is facilitated by expedient surgical stabilization to allow for mobilization and rehabilitation. The historical practice, therefore, of consciously delaying the surgical management of patients with spinal column injuries and spinal cord impairment with the intention of letting their spinal cords "cool down" should probably be abandoned. The one exception to this tenet is in the patient with a central cord syndrome incomplete SCI but without any spinal column instability; substantial unresolved controversy remains about whether such patients would benefit from early decompression, or a later decompression after reaching a neurologic plateau.

Biologic Challenges to Recovery

A comprehensive description of the pathophysiology and pathology of SCI is beyond the scope of this chapter. The primary injury to the spinal cord is caused by the acute traumatic forces imparted upon it by the mechanically failing spinal canal. Following the primary injury, an interrelated series of pathophysiologic processes including ischemia, excitotoxicity, inflammation, and oxidative stress contribute to further secondary damage.[6] The aim of neuroprotection strategies is to attenuate these processes and thus limit secondary damage. The recognition that ongoing ischemia may worsen secondary damage has led to the practice of aggressively avoiding hypotension and the promotion of spinal cord perfusion through an elevated mean arterial pressure (MAP).[7] Clinical practice guidelines published in 2008 by the Paralyzed Veterans of America advocate for judicious hemodynamic management, but acknowledge that the optimal MAP to maintain and for what duration remains unknown.[7] A 2009 study in which lumbar subarachnoid drains were inserted in patients with acute SCI reported that an increase in intrathecal pressure during the acute postinjury phase, and thus, the management of MAP alone may overestimate the extent to which spinal cord perfusion pressure is actually being supported.[8]

As for other relevant acute pathophysiologic mechanisms, the local and systemic inflammatory and immunologic response to SCI has garnered increasing interest in recent years. It has become evident that these are potentially important contributors not only to further neural damage and axonal retraction at the cord injury site,[9] but also for mediating the development of neuropathic pain,[10] and for increasing the vulnerability to infection.[11]

Beyond targeting the acute pathophysiologic processes that induce secondary damage during the acute stages of injury, strategies to encourage axonal sprouting and regeneration are needed to restore connectivity across the injury site. It is well recognized that such regeneration is inhibited by the nonpermissive environment of the injured central nervous system (CNS). CNS myelin contains several inhibitory molecules that block axonal growth, including Nogo, myelin-associated glycoprotein (MAG), and oligodendrocyte myelin glycoprotein (OMgp).[12] Additionally, the astrocytic response to injury elicits a glial scar, which also contains molecules that inhibit axonal growth, including chondroitin sulfate proteoglycans.[13] Overcoming these molecular inhibitors of axonal growth is the subject of intense research investigation and represents the underlying rationale for several emerging therapeutic strategies, including the anti-NOGO antibodies Cethrin, and chondroitinase ABC (ChABC).[14]

The pathology of SCI often includes some degree of cystic cavitation at the injury site,[15] and at the periphery, the demyelination of axons that have otherwise escaped disruption across the injury site.[16] The transplantation of cellular substrates into this cystic cavity has historically been done to provide a more permissive environment for axonal growth. More recently, such cell transplantation strategies have focused on the cells myelinating demyelinated axons, and thus improving signal transduction across the injury site.[17]

Experimental Therapies Currently in Human Clinical Trials

Several experimental therapies are either in the midst of human evaluation or are about to begin clinical trials. For each therapy, some of the historical and scientific background is provided to explain the biologic rationale for their evaluation in human SCI (**Table 1**).

Methylprednisolone

Although methylprednisolone is no longer in investigational human trials, its use in treating acute SCI in humans continues to be debated both in the clinical and scientific literature. Reports from the earlier half of this decade focused on the conduct and interpretation of the National Acute SCI Studies (NASCIS) 2 and 3,[18,19] which established the administration of methylprednisolone for acute SCI as a standard practice. A recent systematic review of animal studies that evaluated methylprednisolone in models of SCI revealed that beneficial effects were only reported in 34%, whereas 58% of studies reported no benefit, and 8% observed mixed results.[20] In the clinical literature, a growing number of reports have been published that describe the lack of efficacy and the increasing risk of complications such as pneumonia and sepsis with the use of methylprednisolone in humans.[21,22] A Canadian survey published in 2008 revealed that most spine surgeons (67%) no longer administer methylprednisolone for acute SCI, which is a dramatic shift in practice from 5 to 6 years prior.[23] However, in the United States, the fear of litigation will compel many surgeons to continue administering methylprednisolone despite their perspectives on its efficacy.[21,24]

Anti-Nogo Antibodies

Pioneering work in the late 1980s revealed that oligodendrocytes and their myelin membranes were inhibitory to axonal regeneration within the CNS.[25] These studies confirmed the principle that the injured spinal cord represented a nonpermissive environment to axonal growth, in contrast to the injured peripheral nerve, which was known to regenerate relatively successfully. From CNS myelin, two inhibitory fractions of 35 and 250 kDa were isolated (named NI-35 and NI-250), and then a monoclonal IgM antibody called IN-1 was developed that could block their inhibitory properties in vitro.[26] This antibody was reported to promote axonal regeneration and improve function in animal models of SCI.[27,28] The actual protein antigen that was targeted and inhibited by IN-1 was eventually characterized in 2000 and given the name "Nogo," and an IgG anti-Nogo antibody for intrathecal application after SCI was developed. The anti-Nogo antibody was subsequently shown in rat and primate models of SCI to promote axonal sprouting and functional improvements.[29,30]

This anti-Nogo IgG intrathecal approach has been commercialized by Novartis (Basel, Switzerland), which in 2006 initiated an open-label, nonrandomized human clinical trial currently being conducted as a multicenter study across Europe and in Canada (ClinicalTrials.gov Identifier: NCT00406016). Eligible patients were to be ASIA A complete thoracic paraplegics or cervical quadriplegics, with the treatment to begin between 4 and 14 days after injury. The antibody is infused intrathecally,

Table 1

Therapeutic Approaches Currently in or About to Begin Human Evaluation

Therapy	Commercial Sponsor	Therapeutic Rationale	Study Design
Anti-Nogo antibodies	Novartis (Basel, Switzerland)	Inhibit activity of Nogo-A, a protein in CNS myelin that inhibits axonal growth.	Multicenter study of ASIA A thoracic and cervical SCI began in 2006. Treatment initiated 7 to 14 days postinjury and administered intrathecally.
Cethrin	Alseres Pharmaceuticals (Hopkinton, MA)	Inhibit rho, an intracellular GTPase within the axonal growth cone that mediates the effects of inhibitory proteins (such as Nogo-A).	Multicenter study of ASIA A thoracic and cervical SCI began in 2005 and completed in 2007. Treatment applied directly to dura during surgery within 7 days of injury. Subsequent randomized trial planned.
Minocycline	None	Reduce posttraumatic inflammation and apoptotic cell death.	Single-center study of compete and incomplete SCI began in 2004 and is now analyzing data. Treatment administered intravenously within 12 h of injury.
Systemic hypothermia	None	Slow metabolic rate, reduce inflammation and oxidative stress.	Single-center study of ASIA A complete SCI began in 2006. Systemic hypothermia initiated within 12 h of injury in most patients.
Riluzole	None	A sodium channel blocker approved by the US Food and Drug Administration (FDA) for the treatment of amyotrophic lateral sclerosis.	Multicenter study of ASIA A, B, and C thoracic and cervical SCI expected to begin in 2010. Treatment to be given orally and initiated within 12 h of injury.
Magnesium (NeuroShield)	Medtronic (Memphis, TN)	A physiologic antagonist to N-methyl-D-aspartate receptors.	Multicenter study of ASIA A cervical SCI expected to begin in 2010. Treatment to be given intravenously within 12 h of injury. Phase I safety study in humans complete.
Human embryonic stem cell-derived oligodendrocyte progenitors	Geron (Menlo Park, CA)	Remyelinate demyelinated axons and restore conduction.	Multicenter study of ASIA A thoracic SCI to begin when FDA approval is granted. Transplantation of cells to occur 7 to 14 days postinjury.

initially via an indwelling catheter and more recently by repeated lumbar punctures. The clinical trial of approximately 50 patients was expected to conclude recruitment during 2010.

Cethrin

The recognition that CNS myelin prompted the cessation of axonal regeneration led researchers to question what was occurring within the tip of the axon (the axonal growth cone) that caused this response. From a therapeutic standpoint, if multiple inhibitory molecules within CNS myelin all ultimately converge upon the same intracellular signaling pathway within the axonal growth cone to halt its growth, then a single intervention targeting this pathway might counteract the effects of many inhibitors (unlike the anti-Nogo antibody, which is specific to the Nogo inhibitory protein).

Rho, a small guanosine triphosphatase, is an important intracellular signaling molecule that regulates axonal growth when exposed to inhibitory CNS myelin, and thus represents such a point of convergence for therapeutic intervention.[31] The strategy of antagonizing Rho with C3 transferase (a rho antagonist) applied directly to the cord was shown to promote recovery in an animal model of SCI.[32] Based on these preclinical findings, a cell-permeable version of C3 transferase (Cethrin) was commercialized by BioAxone Therapeutic Inc, Montreal, QC) a Canadian biotechnology firm, and a multicenter clinical trial was launched in 2005 across North America. This study included patients with cervical and thoracic SCI who were deemed to be ASIA A complete, and the treatment was administered within 7 days of injury. Cethrin was mixed within Tisseal and applied to the dura overlying the injured spinal cord at the time of spinal cord decompression. This phase IIA study was concluded in the summer of 2007 after 37 patients were enrolled. The results of this study have yet to be published. A subsequent prospective randomized clinical trial is in the planning stages.

Minocycline

Minocycline is a tetracycline antibiotic that has significant anti-inflammatory and antiapoptotic properties. Because the inflammatory response is considered to be an important contributor to secondary damage after SCI, the ability of minocycline to inhibit microglial activation and the release or activity of proinflammatory mediators (cytokines, reactive oxygen species, and matrix metalloproteinases) has made it an attractive agent to study in SCI models.[33] Numerous independent laboratories have reported on the efficacy of minocycline in various animal models of SCI.[34-36] These positive results, however, have more recently been countered by studies reporting that no functional benefit was conferred to animals treated with minocycline.[37,38]

However, the early positive data on minocycline in animal models of SCI from independent laboratories stimulated the initiation of a human clinical trial in Calgary, AB, Canada. This was a randomized controlled trial in which approximately 50 patients with acute SCI (cervical and thoracic) of both complete and incomplete injury severities were randomized to either intravenous minocycline or placebo within 12 hours of injury. At the time of this writing, the results of this study have not been published.

Systemic Hypothermia

Hypothermia has interested scientists and clinicians because it may have a neuroprotective role in traumatic and ischemic brain injury and SCI.[39] In animal models of SCI, both local and systemic hypothermia have been investigated for decades.[40] In such in vivo experiments, moderate systemic hypothermia (around 30° to 32°C) has been shown to have a wide range of histologic and biochemical effects, such as the attenuation of neutrophil invasion, reduced oxidative stress, and reduced secondary damage.

Interest in systemic hypothermia exploded in the fall of 2007 after the highly publicized case of Kevin Everett, a professional football player who suffered a cervical SCI while tackling an opposing player and was treated with systemic hypothermia (in addition to methylprednisolone and an urgent surgical decompression). Significant neurologic recovery was achieved.[41] No peer-reviewed publication describing systemic hypothermia in human SCI had been published at the time, making it difficult for scientists and clinicians to interpret the efficacy of hypothermia in general. Investigators at the Miami Project to Cure Paralysis have had a long-standing interest in hypothermia, and have conducted a pilot study on the safety and feasibility of systemic hypothermia for acute SCI. A retrospective review of 14 ASIA A acute SCI patients treated with modest systemic hypothermia (33°C) for 48 hours was performed.[42] The incidence of complications (such as atelectasis, pneumonia, acute respiratory distress syndrome) was very similar to that commonly observed in such patients.

Riluzole

Riluzole is an orally administered sodium channel blocker that is currently approved by the FDA for use in treating ALS, and hence many questions around its safety, tolerability, and pharmacokinetics in humans have been answered. Sodium channels have long been implicated in white matter damage after SCI, as the influx of sodium through voltage-gated sodium channels can ultimately lead to the loss of calcium homeostasis.[43]

Systemically administered riluzole has been evaluated by numerous investigators in acute SCI models.[44,45] These studies report a significant reduction in secondary damage around the injury site, and improved functional recovery in riluzole-treated animals.

Encouraged by these preclinical results and the established safety to human patients, a prospective multicenter clinical trial of riluzole for human patients with acute SCI is soon to be initiated through the North American Clinical Trials Network, sponsored by the Christopher and Dana Reeve Foundation. The daily dose will be that which has been previously approved by the FDA for the treatment of ALS, although it is recognized that this human oral dose is substantially less than that which has been administered via intraperitoneal injection to rats in experimental SCI studies. The investigators are currently targeting a total of 36 patients to be enrolled into this study.

Magnesium

Magnesium is a physiologic N-methyl-D-aspartate (NMDA) receptor antagonist. Glutamate levels rise rapidly after CNS injury, and glutamate's overstimulation of NMDA receptors can lead to a massive influx of calcium, leading to cell death, a process broadly referred to as excitotoxicity.[46] The widespread distribution of NMDA receptors has prompted extensive study into NMDA-receptor antagonists (including magnesium) as a neuroprotective strategy for SCI, brain injury, and other neurologic conditions.[47] The role of magnesium therapy in acute SCI models has been investigated by multiple independent laboratories. These studies have described improved biochemical, physiologic, and histologic outcomes with magnesium administration, as well as improved locomotor recovery.[48,49] However, it is important to point out that most of these studies use a magnesium dosage (approximately 300 to 600 mg/kg) that far exceeds human safety limits.

More recently, a formulation that consists of magnesium within polyethylene glycol (PEG) has been investigated as a potential neuroprotective agent for brain injury and SCI. A recent study has revealed that PEG allows for a much lower dose of magnesium to be applied effectively in SCI models.[50] This magnesium dosage is similar to that which was safely administered to patients in previous trials who had experienced stroke, cardiac arrest, and preeclampsia. This formulation of magnesium chloride within PEG (NeuroShield, Medtronic, Memphis, TN) has received FDA approval to begin human studies. A phase I study of healthy human volunteers was completed in the spring of 2009, and revealed no significant adverse events. A phase II multicenter study of human SCI patients was expected to be initiated in 2010.

Human Embryonic Stem Cell–Derived Oligodendrocyte Progenitors

As described earlier, one of the prime targets of interest for the cell transplantation field is demyelinated axons that still traverse the injury site, as the remyelination of such axons may facilitate improved signal conduction. Many different cell substrates may promote remyelination, including Schwann cells and various stem cells. Oligodendrocyte progenitor cells derived from a human embryonic stem cell (hESC) line are one such cell. As undifferentiated embryonic stem cells have the predilection to generate teratomas, the more rational approach is to control the in vitro differentiation of these multipotent cells down to an oligodendrocyte progenitor cell population, and then transplant these more "committed" cells whose fate is more certain. This strategy was demonstrated in a study that showed the implantation of hESC-derived oligodendrocyte progenitors 7 days after injury promoted remyelination and functional recovery.[51] Unfortunately, animals that received the cell transplants many months after injury (representing a chronic injury) did not experience functional recovery.

The hESC-derived oligodendrocyte progenitor technology received widespread international publicity in January 2009 when the FDA granted approval to conduct a human SCI trial with these cells, the first-ever human clinical trial using embryonic stem cell derivatives. The primary end point of this small study will be safety, as the concern for teratoma formation is of paramount importance. The trials were placed on clinical hold by the FDA in August 2009 after concerns were raised about findings from dose-escalation safety studies conducted in animal models.[52]

Emerging Concepts

There is cautious optimism that therapies for SCI will soon be emerging. The scientific community has realized that none of these therapies will represent a "cure" for SCI, and that these experimental treatments will lead to relatively small improvements in neurologic function. Such small improvements should not be dismissed, however. History will show that the widespread adoption of methylprednisolone was similarly based on very small changes in neurologic function in the NASCIS trials. Additionally, for an injury condition of such catastrophic implications, any meaningful improvement would be welcomed.

It is important to recognize that the initiation of a clinical trial is far from evidence that the therapy actually works. Although several treatments have been undergoing evaluation in human subjects, much larger, time-consuming, and expensive clinical trials to actually prove their efficacy are still necessary and will not yield an answer about the actual clinical effectiveness of these therapies for many years. The last major acute SCI intervention to be tested in a prospective randomized fashion (Sygen) took over 20 major neurotrauma institutions across North America the better part of a decade to complete.[53] There is a greater awareness of the difficulties in conducting clinical trials, with discussion in the literature.[54-57] In particular, the high rate of spontaneous neurologic recovery is highlighted, which makes it necessary to enroll large numbers of patients to have sufficient statistical power to assess neurologic

efficacy. This is particularly an issue in patients with acute/subacute SCI, where the extent of their injuries may not be so obvious, and neurologic assessment is often impaired by other factors (such as head injury or multiple trauma). All of the clinical trial initiatives discussed will enroll patients in this acute/subacute stage and all will be subject to the challenges related to high spontaneous recovery rates. Therefore, more information is needed before conclusions can be made about the efficacy of these technologies.

Annotated References

1. National Spinal Cord Injury Statistical Center: Spinal cord injury facts and figures at a glance. *J Spinal Cord Med* 2008;31(3):357-358.

   The National Spinal Cord Injury Database has been in existence since 1973 and captures data from an estimated 13% of new SCI cases in the US Since its inception, 26 federally funded Model SCI Care Systems have contributed data to the National SCI Database. As of October 2007 the database contained information on 25,415 persons who sustained traumatic SCIs.

2. *One Degree of Separation; Paralysis and Spinal Cord Injury in the United States.* Short Hills, NJ, Christopher and Dana Reeve Foundation, 2009.

   This is an extensive survey of more than 33,000 households across the United States that was conducted to capture the prevalance of SCI and paralysis across the nation. It represents one of the largest population-based samples of any disability ever conducted, and importantly, documented a far greater prevalence of paralysis than was previously estimated.

3. Hawryluk GW, Rowland J, Kwon BK, Fehlings MG: Protection and repair of the injured spinal cord: A review of completed, ongoing, and planned clinical trials for acute spinal cord injury. *Neurosurg Focus* 2008;25(5):E14.

   This is a review of past, present, and future clinical trials of therapies in acute SCI. It describes the biological rationale for a number of experimental treatments that are either in human trials currently or are about to enter clinical investigation.

4. Baptiste DC, Fehlings MG: Emerging drugs for spinal cord injury. *Expert Opin Emerg Drugs* 2008;13(1):63-80.

   This is a review of novel pharmacologic treatments that are emerging from the laboratory for the treatment of acute SCI.

5. Miyanji F, Furlan JC, Aarabi B, Arnold PM, Fehlings MG: Acute cervical traumatic spinal cord injury: MR imaging findings correlated with neurologic outcome: Prospective study with 100 consecutive patients. *Radiology* 2007;243(3):820-827.

   This study evaluated maximum spinal cord compression, maximum canal compromise, and lesion length in 100 patients with traumatic cervical SCIs. It reported

5: Spine

that maximum spinal cord compression, and the presence of hemorrhage and cord swelling were predictive of neurologic outcome.

6. Mann CM, Kwon BK: An update on the pathophysiology of acute spinal cord injury. *Semin Spine Surg* 2007; 19:272-279.

This is a review of the pathophysiologic mechanisms that are activated in acute SCI, which are thought to play a role in secondary damage. This includes such things as ischemia, oxidative stress, excitotoxicity, inflammation, and apoptosis.

7. Consortium for Spinal Cord Medicine/Paralyzed Veterans of America. *Early Acute Management in Adults with Spinal Cord Injury: A Clinical Practice Guideline for Health Care Providers*. Washington DC, Paralyzed Veterans of America, 2008.

This is an exhaustive review of the literature on the management of acute SCI. It provides guidelines for such aspects as blood pressure management, surgical decompression, and pharmacologic treatment.

8. Kwon BK, Curt A, Belanger LM, et al: Intrathecal pressure monitoring and cerebrospinal fluid drainage in acute spinal cord injury: A prospective randomized trial. *J Neurosurg Spine* 2009;10(3):181-193.

In this study, acute SCI patients had lumbar intrathecal drains inserted and CSF pressure was evaluated over 72 hours. The authors documented significant increases in CSF pressure after surgical decompression, and also during the acute postinjury period.

9. Busch SA, Horn KP, Silver DJ, Silver J: Overcoming macrophage-mediated axonal dieback following CNS injury. *J Neurosci* 2009;29(32):9967-9976.

In this study, the authors investigated the mechanisms by which the infiltration of macrophages into the injured spinal cord coincides with axonal retraction from the initial injury site. They provide interesting insights into the cellular and molecular mechanisms that are behind this macrophage-associated axonal dieback, such as the role of MMP-9.

10. Hulsebosch CE, Hains BC, Crown ED, Carlton SM: Mechanisms of chronic central neuropathic pain after spinal cord injury. *Brain Res Rev* 2009;60(1):202-213.

This is an excellent review of the genesis of neuropathic pain after SCI. In particular the role of posttraumatic inflammation and reactive oxygen species is outlined. A better understanding of the physiologic basis behind neuropathic pain would be very helpful in developing treatment strategies.

11. Popovich P, McTigue D: Damage control in the nervous system: Beware the immune system in spinal cord injury. *Nat Med* 2009;15(7):736-737.

This is an outstanding review of the role of inflammation in secondary injury after SCI. It highlights the complexity of the process, and how different elements of the inflammatory response at different time points after injury have unique effects.

12. Rowland JW, Hawryluk GW, Kwon B, Fehlings MG: Current status of acute spinal cord injury pathophysiology and emerging therapies: Promise on the horizon. *Neurosurg Focus* 2008;25(5):E2.

This is a review of the pathophysiology of acute SCI and how our understanding of this has enabled the development of a number of emerging therapies.

13. Fitch MT, Silver J: CNS injury, glial scars, and inflammation: Inhibitory extracellular matrices and regeneration failure. *Exp Neurol* 2008;209(2):294-301.

This is an in-depth review of the inflammatory response to SCI and the development of the glial scar at the site of injury. It summarizes what is understood about how the glial scar impedes axonal regeneration.

14. Rossignol S, Schwab M, Schwartz M, Fehlings MG: Spinal cord injury: Time to move? *J Neurosci* 2007;27(44): 11782-11792.

This is the summary of a symposium held at the 2006 Society for Neuroscience meeting that reviewed a number of therapeutic strategies for SCI: diminishing the repulsive barriers to axonal regeneration, cell transplants to enhance immunologic mechanisms or remyelinate axons, surgical decompression, and rehabilitative training.

15. Kakulas BA: A review of the neuropathology of human spinal cord injury with emphasis on special features. *J Spinal Cord Med* 1999;22(2):119-124.

16. Guest JD, Hiester ED, Bunge RP: Demyelination and Schwann cell responses adjacent to injury epicenter cavities following chronic human spinal cord injury. *Exp Neurol* 2005;192(2):384-393.

17. Sasaki M, Li B, Lankford KL, Radtke C, Kocsis JD: Remyelination of the injured spinal cord. *Prog Brain Res* 2007;161:419-433.

This is a review of various strategies to promote the remyelination of demyelinated axons within the injured cord. It is thought that some axons lose their myelin sheaths but are otherwise still intact across the injury site. Cells that remyelinate these axons might restore conduction and improve function.

18. Bracken MB, Shepard MJ, Collins WF, et al: A randomized, controlled trial of methylprednisolone or naloxone in the treatment of acute spinal-cord injury: Results of the Second National Acute Spinal Cord Injury Study. *N Engl J Med* 1990;322(20):1405-1411.

19. Bracken MB, Shepard MJ, Holford TR, et al: Administration of methylprednisolone for 24 or 48 hours or tirilazad mesylate for 48 hours in the treatment of acute spinal cord injury: Results of the Third National Acute Spinal Cord Injury Randomized Controlled Trial. National Acute Spinal Cord Injury Study. *JAMA* 1997; 277(20):1597-1604.

20. Akhtar AZ, Pippin JJ, Sandusky CB: Animal studies in spinal cord injury: A systematic review of methylprednisolone. *Altern Lab Anim* 2009;37(1):43-62.

This is a systematic review of all of the available studies in which methylprednisolone was administered in an animal model of acute SCI. It was concluded that in over half of the studies, methylprednisolone had no effect (or even a deleterious effect). It dispels the widely held notion that methylprednisolone was routinely effective in animal studies of SCI – a notion that biases clinicians into a more optimistic view of the benefits of the drug for human patients

21. Nicholas JS, Selassie AW, Lineberry LA, Pickelsimer EE, Haines SJ: Use and determinants of the methylprednisolone protocol for traumatic spinal cord injury in South Carolina acute care hospitals. *J Trauma* 2009;66(5): 1446-1450, discussion 1450.

    These authors sought to determine if emergency physicians in South Carolina had changed their practice of giving methylprednisolone to acute SCI patients, in light of the more recent criticisms of the NASCIS trials. They found that emergency rooms continued to have protocols for the use of steroids in acute SCI, but only one third of SCI patients who arrived at an emergency room with such a protocol ultimately received steroids.

22. Suberviola B, González-Castro A, Llorca J, Ortiz-Melón F, Miñambres E: Early complications of high-dose methylprednisolone in acute spinal cord injury patients. *Injury* 2008;39(7):748-752.

    These Spanish investigators retrospecitvely reviewed patients with SCI between 1994 and 2005 and compared those treated with or without methylprednisolone. Although no improvement in neurologic outcome was seen with methylprednisolone, those treated with the drug had a significantly higher risk of infectious and metabolic complications during their intensive care unit stay.

23. Hurlbert RJ, Hamilton MG: Methylprednisolone for acute spinal cord injury: 5-year practice reversal. *Can J Neurol Sci* 2008;35(1):41-45.

    In a survey of Canadian spine surgeons who treat acute SCI patients, approximately two thirds had abandoned the use of methylprednisolone. This was in stark contrast to a survey done by the same authors 5 years previously, in which two thirds of Canadian physicians did administer methylprednisolone for acute SCI. This highlights the fact that in the absence of a highly litigious society, Canadian physicians feel free to stop using methylprednisolone.

24. Eck JC, Nachtigall D, Humphreys SC, Hodges SD: Questionnaire survey of spine surgeons on the use of methylprednisolone for acute spinal cord injury. *Spine (Phila Pa 1976)* 2006;31(9):E250-E253.

25. Caroni P, Schwab ME: Two membrane protein fractions from rat central myelin with inhibitory properties for neurite growth and fibroblast spreading. *J Cell Biol* 1988;106(4):1281-1288.

26. Caroni P, Schwab ME: Antibody against myelin-associated inhibitor of neurite growth neutralizes nonpermissive substrate properties of CNS white matter. *Neuron* 1988;1(1):85-96.

27. Schnell L, Schwab ME: Axonal regeneration in the rat spinal cord produced by an antibody against myelin-associated neurite growth inhibitors. *Nature* 1990; 343(6255):269-272.

28. Bregman BS, Kunkel-Bagden E, Schnell L, Dai HN, Gao D, Schwab ME: Recovery from spinal cord injury mediated by antibodies to neurite growth inhibitors. *Nature* 1995;378(6556):498-501.

29. Freund P, Schmidlin E, Wannier T, et al: Anti-Nogo-A antibody treatment promotes recovery of manual dexterity after unilateral cervical lesion in adult primates: Re-examination and extension of behavioral data. *Eur J Neurosci* 2009;29(5):983-996.

    This was an important preclinical study in the development of the anti-Nogo-A antibody treatment for acute SCI. This antibody targets a protein that inhibits axonal regeneration, and here, the authors report that the intrathecal administration of this antibody in a nonhuman primate model of cervical SCI does promote recovery of hand function.

30. Wannier-Morino P, Schmidlin E, Freund P, et al: Fate of rubrospinal neurons after unilateral section of the cervical spinal cord in adult macaque monkeys: Effects of an antibody treatment neutralizing Nogo-A. *Brain Res* 2008;1217:96-109.

    This study, also in a nonhuman primate model of cervical SCI, found that the administration of the anti-Nogo antibody did not prevent rubrospinal neuron atrophy or death.

31. McKerracher L, Higuchi H: Targeting Rho to stimulate repair after spinal cord injury. *J Neurotrauma* 2006; 23(3-4):309-317.

32. Dergham P, Ellezam B, Essagian C, Avedissian H, Lubell WD, McKerracher L: Rho signaling pathway targeted to promote spinal cord repair. *J Neurosci* 2002; 22(15):6570-6577.

33. Stirling DP, Koochesfahani KM, Steeves JD, Tetzlaff W: Minocycline as a neuroprotective agent. *Neuroscientist* 2005;11(4):308-322.

34. Yune TY, Lee JY, Jung GY, et al: Minocycline alleviates death of oligodendrocytes by inhibiting pro-nerve growth factor production in microglia after spinal cord injury. *J Neurosci* 2007;27(29):7751-7761.

35. Stirling DP, Khodarahmi K, Liu J, et al: Minocycline treatment reduces delayed oligodendrocyte death, attenuates axonal dieback, and improves functional outcome after spinal cord injury. *J Neurosci* 2004;24(9):2182-2190.

36. Wells JE, Hurlbert RJ, Fehlings MG, Yong VW: Neuroprotection by minocycline facilitates significant recovery from spinal cord injury in mice. *Brain* 2003;126(Pt 7): 1628-1637.

37. Pinzon A, Marcillo A, Quintana A, et al: A reassessment of minocycline as a neuroprotective agent in a rat spinal cord contusion model. *Brain Res* 2008; 1243:146-151.

5: Spine

This is a replication of a previous study of minocycline in an animal model of SCI. In an effort to establish the "robustness" of preclinical evidence for novel therapies in animal models of SCI, the National Institutes of Health has funded a number of independent replication studies. This study was unable to replicate the effectiveness of minocycline in an animal model of SCI.

38. Saganová K, Orendáčová J, Cízková D, Vanický I: Limited minocycline neuroprotection after balloon-compression spinal cord injury in the rat. *Neurosci Lett* 2008;433(3):246-249.

This study found no benefit to using minocycline in a rodent model of compressive SCI, which stands in contrast to numerous other studies that do report a neuroprotective benefit.

39. Inamasu J, Ichikizaki K: Mild hypothermia in neurologic emergency: An update. *Ann Emerg Med* 2002; 40(2):220-230.

40. Kwon BK, Mann C, Sohn HM, et al; NASS Section on Biologics: Hypothermia for spinal cord injury. *Spine J* 2008;8(6):859-874.

This is an extensive review of the preclinical animal literature and the human literature on the use of both local and systemic hypothermia for acute SCI. At the time of this writing, there was no available human literature describing the use of systemic hypothermia in acute SCI.

41. Layden T: Kevin Everett, The Road Back. *Sports Illustrated* Dec 17, 2007;107(24):56-67.

This is the description of Kevin Everett's cervical SCI suffered while playing football for the National Football League's Buffalo Bills. Mr. Everett was treated with systemic hypothermia afterward, raising tremendous interest in the possibility that this treatment influenced his significant neurologic recovery.

42. Levi AD, Green BA, Wang MY, et al: Clinical application of modest hypothermia after spinal cord injury. *J Neurotrauma* 2009;26(3):407-415.

This is the report of a small pilot study conducted at the University of Miami to study modest systemic hypothermia in acute SCI patients. There was no significant increase in complications associated with systemic hypothermia.

43. Agrawal SK, Fehlings MG: The effect of the sodium channel blocker QX-314 on recovery after acute spinal cord injury. *J Neurotrauma* 1997;14(2):81-88.

44. Ates O, Cayli SR, Gurses I, et al: Comparative neuroprotective effect of sodium channel blockers after experimental spinal cord injury. *J Clin Neurosci* 2007;14(7): 658-665.

This study evaluated three different sodium channel blockers (phenytoin, mexiletine, and riluzole), in a model of rodent thoracic SCI. It found that mexiletine and riluzole were both more effective than phenytoin, in terms of biochemical and histologic outcomes as well as in functional recovery.

45. Schwartz G, Fehlings MG: Evaluation of the neuroprotective effects of sodium channel blockers after spinal cord injury: Improved behavioral and neuroanatomical recovery with riluzole. *J Neurosurg* 2001;94(2, Suppl): 245-256.

46. Choi DW: Excitotoxic cell death. *J Neurobiol* 1992; 23(9):1261-1276.

47. Palmer GC: Neuroprotection by NMDA receptor antagonists in a variety of neuropathologies. *Curr Drug Targets* 2001;2(3):241-271.

48. Gok B, Okutan O, Beskonakli E, Kilinc K: Effects of magnesium sulphate following spinal cord injury in rats. *Chin J Physiol* 2007;50(2):93-97.

This study evaluated magnesium sulfate as an early neuroprotective agent in thoracic SCI. It reported a reduction in posttraumatic neutrophil invasion and improved hindlimb motor function with the administration of 600 mg/kg magnesium sulfate.

49. Wiseman DB, Dailey AT, Lundin D, et al: Magnesium efficacy in a rat spinal cord injury model. *J Neurosurg Spine* 2009;10(4):308-314.

This study evaluated magnesium sulfate in a thoracic model of SCI. The authors report increased white matter sparing at the injury site and improved locomotor function in animals treated with magnesium sulfate.

50. Kwon BK, Roy J, Lee JH, et al: Magnesium chloride in a polyethylene glycol formulation as a neuroprotective therapy for acute spinal cord injury: Preclinical refinement and optimization. *J Neurotrauma* 2009;26(8): 1379-1393.

This paper reports a series of experiments conducted to refine a magnesium chloride formulation with PEG, in preparation for human translation. It describes testing different doses and time windows of intervention, and reveals a time window of 4 to 8 hours for tissue neuroprotection.

51. Keirstead HS, Nistor G, Bernal G, et al: Human embryonic stem cell-derived oligodendrocyte progenitor cell transplants remyelinate and restore locomotion after spinal cord injury. *J Neurosci* 2005;25(19):4694-4705.

52. The Medical News. FDA places Geron Corporation's IND for spinal cord injury on clinical hold. http://www.news-medical.net/news/20090819/FDA-places-Geron-Corporations-IND-for-spinal-cord-injury-on-clinical-hold.aspx. Accessed August 19, 2009.

This media report described the FDA's decision to put Geron on hold for its clinical trial. In January 2009, the approval to proceed with Geron was received. Of concern was the appearance of cystlike structures in preclinical models, prompting the need for longer term follow-up to rule out tumor formation.

53. Geisler FH, Coleman WP, Grieco G, Poonian D; Sygen Study Group: The Sygen multicenter acute spinal cord injury study. *Spine (Phila Pa 1976)* 2001;26(24, suppl): S87-S98.

5: Spine

54. Fawcett JW, Curt A, Steeves JD, et al: Guidelines for the conduct of clinical trials for spinal cord injury as developed by the ICCP panel: Spontaneous recovery after spinal cord injury and statistical power needed for therapeutic clinical trials. *Spinal Cord* 2007;45(3):190-205.

55. Lammertse D, Tuszynski MH, Steeves JD, et al; International Campaign for Cures of Spinal Cord Injury Paralysis: Guidelines for the conduct of clinical trials for spinal cord injury as developed by the ICCP panel: Clinical trial design. *Spinal Cord* 2007;45(3):232-242.

56. Steeves JD, Lammertse D, Curt A, et al; International Campaign for Cures of Spinal Cord Injury Paralysis: Guidelines for the conduct of clinical trials for spinal cord injury (SCI) as developed by the ICCP panel: Clinical trial outcome measures. *Spinal Cord* 2007;45(3):206-221.

57. Tuszynski MH, Steeves JD, Fawcett JW, et al; International Campaign for Cures of Spinal Cord Injury Paralysis: Guidelines for the conduct of clinical trials for spinal cord injury as developed by the ICCP panel: Clinical trial inclusion/exclusion criteria and ethics. *Spinal Cord* 2007;45(3):222-231.

These four papers were produced by the International Campaign to Cure Paralysis to provide guidance to the SCI community around the conduct of clinical trials for SCI. They characterize the degree of spontaneous neurologic recovery and how this influences trial design. They outline how such trials should be designed, the types of inclusion/exclusion criteria that should be applied, and the types of outcome measures that should be used. These are important guidance documents for the field of SCI.

5: Spine

Chapter 45

Adult Spinal Deformity

Michael D. Daubs, MD

Definition

Adult spinal deformity is defined by the Scoliosis Research Society as a spinal deformity with any etiology in a skeletally mature patient. Scoliosis is defined as lateral deviation of the normal vertical line of the spine of greater than 10° when measured on radiographs. This definition covers a wide range of spinal disorders, including many that begin in childhood. The key component in the definition is the requirement for skeletal maturity. The various etiologies leading to deformity may have unique clinical presentations, but the resultant spinal deformities in a skeletally mature patient are evaluated in a similar methodic manner. Regardless of whether the primary deformity is scoliosis with coronal imbalance or failed arthrodesis with fixed sagittal imbalance, the overall treatment principles remain the same.

Indications and Treatment Goals

The primary goals in treating adult spinal deformity are to gain spinal balance, halt the progression of deformity, reduce pain, and improve the patient's health-related quality of life (HRQL). Treatment should improve the patient's outcome above the natural history of the disease and avoid any deleterious long-term effects. The success of intervention is measured using validated HRQL measurement tools, which include both general health (Medical Outcomes Study 36-Item Short Form and the EuroQol-5) and disease specific (Scoliosis Research Society-30 and Oswestry Disability Index) outcome measures. To date, the treatment of adult scoliosis or adult deformity in general has not been evaluated with published randomized controlled trials with level I evidence. However, the clinical and radiologic factors that most significantly correlate with patient symptoms and functional outcomes have recently been elucidated in large case series.[1,2]

The only study of the natural history of adult scoliosis evaluated patients with untreated adolescent idiopathic scoliosis.[3] At a mean follow-up of 51 years (range, 44 to 61 years), the authors reported mean Cobb angles of 84°, 89°, and 49° for the thoracic, thoracolumbar, and lumbar spines, respectively. The study showed no difference in survival rates compared with the general population. More patients with scoliosis (77%) reported little to moderate low back pain than the control group (35%), but there was no overall difference in the ability to perform activities of daily living. Based on this study, it appears that many patients are able to tolerate high magnitudes of coronal deformity and maintain reasonable function. However, many patients with scoliosis have severe pain and functional impairment associated with curve progression and spinal imbalance. The indications for surgical treatment in adults with spinal deformity must be individualized and based on the patient's symptoms, functional impairment, evidence of curve progression, and expectations. Although previous studies have shown that curves greater than 45° can progress after maturity,[4] the results cannot be generalized. The best evidence for future curve progression is an individual patient's documented history of progression.

Patient Evaluation

Clinical Evaluation

Low back pain is the most common symptom reported by patients with adult spinal deformity. Symptoms of low back pain are also common in the general population and cannot be immediately attributed to scoliosis. A thorough history and examination is necessary to rule out other potential causes. In general, patients younger than 40 years with adult scoliosis present with symptoms similar to those of younger patients with adolescent idiopathic scoliosis. Typically, a patient's primary concerns are the probability for curve progression and the potential for long-term sequelae, poor cosmesis, and low back pain. As patients with adult idiopathic scoliosis age, their presentation is similar to those with degenerative spinal conditions. Patients older than 40 years may more often report low back pain, radicular leg pain, and neurogenic claudication. The etiology of these symptoms should be evaluated in a manner similar to that used in evaluating patients without scoliosis. Psychosocial issues can impact the treatment of all patients, including those with a spinal deformity, and should be considered in the clinical evaluation.

Dr. Daubs or an immediate family member serves as a paid consultant to or is an employee of Synthes and has received research or institutional support from Stryker.

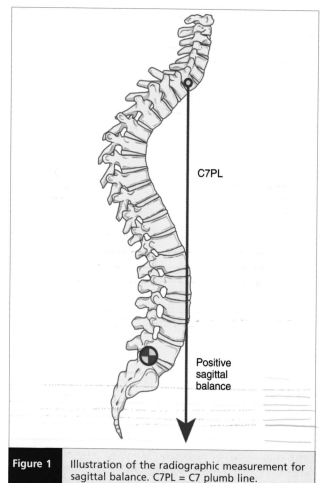

Figure 1 Illustration of the radiographic measurement for sagittal balance. C7PL = C7 plumb line.

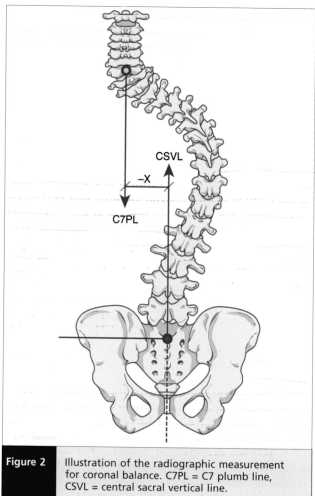

Figure 2 Illustration of the radiographic measurement for coronal balance. C7PL = C7 plumb line, CSVL = central sacral vertical line.

In addition to a thorough neurologic evaluation, a physical examination should be performed to evaluate gait and standing balance. Observing the patient's gait permits an evaluation of spinal balance while in motion. Many patients with scoliosis may stand erect in sagittal and coronal balance; however, ambulation causes fatigue, which may result in positive sagittal imbalance. Because patients with fixed sagittal imbalance often pitch forward progressively when ambulating any distance, hip and knee range of motion should be closely examined. Knees should be fully extended when evaluating standing balance. Hip range of motion should be evaluated to rule out hip flexion contractures as a contributing source of sagittal imbalance.

In general, adults with spinal deformity should be clinically evaluated in a manner similar to that used for patients presenting with a spinal disorder. The source of the patient's complaint, such as low back or leg pain, should be evaluated first. The unique dimensions of a deformity, whether it is scoliosis or fixed sagittal imbalance, should then be considered in the overall evaluation and treatment plan.

Radiographic Evaluation

Standing, 36-inch PA and lateral radiographs are needed to evaluate adult spinal deformity. The knees should be fully extended for the lateral radiograph to ensure accurate assessment of sagittal balance. The cervical, thoracic, and lumbar spines as well as the pelvis and hip joints should be visible. Cobb angles, coronal and sagittal balance, and pelvic incidence should be measured and recorded (**Figures 1** through **3**). Supine AP and lateral full-length 36-inch radiographs are helpful in determining the flexibility of coronal and sagittal plane deformities. Radiographs taken with the patient bending can be used to assess the flexibility of coronal plane deformities and may aid in surgical decision making, especially in younger adults who can be classified with the Lenke system.[5] CT with myelography may better assess spinal canal stenosis in patients with moderate to severe coronal deformity, whereas MRI may be adequate to assess patients with more minor curves.

Types of Adult Spinal Deformity

Any spinal disorder or disease that leads to scoliosis or coronal or sagittal imbalance in a skeletally mature patient is considered an adult spinal deformity. The most common categories are adult idiopathic scoliosis, adult de novo scoliosis, and fixed sagittal imbalance. Several neuromuscular disorders, such as cerebral palsy, spinal muscle atrophy, Duchenne muscular dystrophy, polio-myelitis, and posttraumatic conditions can cause spinal deformities in adulthood. Later onset adult diseases, such as Parkinson disease and multiple sclerosis, also can cause spinal deformity.

Adult Scoliosis

Adult idiopathic scoliosis is defined as scoliosis in a skeletally mature patient that existed in childhood or adolescence. Adult de novo scoliosis, or degenerative scoliosis as it is commonly termed, is a condition that did not existent before skeletal maturity and developed in adulthood. The overall prevalence of adult scoliosis increases with age.[6] Adult degenerative scoliosis pre-dominantly develops in the thoracolumbar spine;[7] how-ever, compensatory curves can also develop in the tho-racic spine. The incidence of low back pain in patients with untreated adolescent idiopathic scoliosis (mean age, 66 years) was higher than in a matched cohort (67% versus 35%). Most of the patients rated the in-tensity of pain as low or moderate.[3] There was no dif-ference in the incidence of low back pain symptoms be-tween cohorts of patients with and without adult degenerative scoliosis.[7,8] A separate cohort study evalu-ating scoliosis and nonscoliosis patients with low back pain reported that increased pain in the group with sco-liosis correlated with greater curve magnitude and rota-tion.[9] Loss of lumbar lordosis and thoracolumbar ky-phosis also has been shown to correlate with a greater incidence of reported low back pain.[10]

When evaluating HRQL outcome measures with ra-diographic parameters in adult scoliosis, curve magni-tude was not found to be a significant factor, but pa-tients with thoracolumbar and lumbar curves scored worse than patients with thoracic curves.[1] This finding agrees with the natural history of untreated adolescent idiopathic scoliosis.[3] A smaller series showed that worse patient-reported outcomes correlated with coro-nal imbalance greater than 5 cm, increased lateral lis-thesis (> 6 mm), and loss of lordosis.[11] In the largest case series to date evaluating radiographic parameters, sagittal balance was the most reliable radiographic pre-dictor of HRQL outcomes.[1,2] Patients with positive sag-ittal balance greater than 5 cm reported worse pain, physical function, and self-image.

In an attempt to better understand the factors that ultimately lead to surgical treatment for adult scoliosis, several studies[12-15] have retrospectively reviewed radio-graphic, clinical, and HRQL measures comparing sur-gically and nonsurgically treated groups. Overall, the surgically treated group reported greater frequency of leg pain, moderate to severe low back pain, and curves of greater magnitude.

As patients with adult scoliosis age, advancing de-generation leads to an increased incidence of low back pain of varying intensities. Lumbar and thoracolumbar curves are more symptomatic. HRQL measurements appear to be more influenced by the loss of lumbar lor-dosis and sagittal imbalance than by curve magnitude.

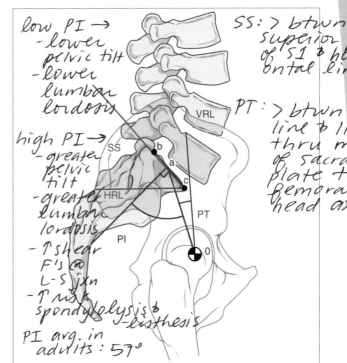

Handwritten annotations:
low PI → -lower pelvic tilt -lower lumbar lordosis
high PI → -greater pelvic tilt -greater lumbar lordosis -↑ shear F's @ L-S jxn -↑ risk spondylolysis & -listhesis
PI avg. in adults: 57°
SS: > btwn superior plate of S1 & horizontal line
PT: > btwn vert. line & line thru midpt. of sacral plate to femoral head axis

Figure 3 Illustration showing the angles and measure-ments for pelvic incidence (a), sacral slope (b), and pelvic tilt (c). SS = sacral slope, PI = pelvic incidence, PT = pelvic tilt, VRL = vertical refer-ence line, HRL = horizontal reference line.

Patients who are surgically treated for scoliosis report increased preoperative low back and leg pain and greater loss of function when compared with those who were not surgically treated.[13] In younger patients, curve magnitude is a more important factor in choosing sur-gical intervention.

Nonsurgical Treatment

There is little consensus and only weak evidence for the effectiveness of any one nonsurgical treatment method for adult scoliosis and adult deformity in general.[16] Typically, the recommended nonsurgical treatment is based on the chief symptoms reported by the patient. If low back pain is the main symptom, a structured phys-ical therapy program based on the patient's physical ca-pabilities is recommended, with emphasis on core strengthening and spinal balance. Radicular leg pain is often treated with selective nerve root injections, which can be helpful in localizing the pain generator; how-ever, lumbar epidural injections for low back pain asso-ciated with scoliosis have poor lasting effectiveness.[17] Symptoms of neurogenic claudication associated with scoliosis and stenosis are seen in older patients with adult scoliosis. Nonsurgical treatment of lumbar steno-sis is not as effective as surgical decompression.[18]

Surgical Treatment

The surgical decision-making process for adult scolio-sis is difficult. The procedures are often complex, full recovery can take up to 1 year, and complication rates as high as 20% have been reported in older patients.[19] Patients are often confused about their prognosis and fearful of the potential effects of scoliosis on their general health and appearance. Taking time to discuss the natural history of the condition and the risks for progression are helpful in alleviating the patient's fear and anxiety. Properly informing patients of the treatment options, including a thorough discussion of potential complications, is crucial for shared decision making.

The goals of surgical treatment are relief of leg and back pain, curve stabilization, and the achievement of spinal balance.

Curve Correction

Although there is evidence that coronal imbalance greater than 4 to 5 cm correlates with a reduced health status,[1,11] there is no evidence that surgical correction of coronal imbalance correlates with improved outcomes. The most important predictor of outcomes is spinal sagittal balance; however, restoring lumbar lordosis to achieve sagittal balance often requires some degree of curve correction. In adults, thoracolumbar and lumbar curves are relatively more flexible than thoracic curves. As a result, overcorrection of the lumbar curve may result in coronal imbalance. It should be stressed that spinal balance is more important than radiographic curve correction. Intraoperative PA full-length radiographs, obtained after instrumentation and any corrective maneuvers are performed, are useful in determining if spinal balance was achieved.

Selection of Fusion Levels

Selecting the appropriate cephalad and caudad levels for fusion remains an area of controversy. In a patient younger than 40 years with adult idiopathic scoliosis, the selection of fusion levels correlates more closely with recommendations for adolescent idiopathic scoliosis. The Lenke classification system can be applied and used as a general reference.[5,20] As the patient ages, curves that were once nonstructural and minor become rigid and must be treated in adulthood as true double or triple major curves.

In adults with thoracolumbar-lumbar curves, the decision-making process is more difficult. It has been commonly taught that a fusion should not end proximal to the thoracolumbar junction, but should cross the thoracolumbar junction and end in the lower thoracic spine.[21] A recent report, however, questioned this principle, and showed no difference in outcomes or the incidence of proximal junctional-related complications, regardless of whether the proximal end level of fusion was at T9, T11, or L1.[22] The authors recommended that fusions end proximally at the stable, neutral vertebrae, and that ending the fusion at the apex of the thoracic kyphosis should be avoided.

In adults, determining the distal extent of the fusion typically involves the decision whether to fuse to L5 or the sacrum, and whether pelvic fixation should be used.

In a group of patients (mean age, 45 years) with long fusions to L5, advanced disk degeneration at the L5-S1 disk developed in 69% of the patients, and 23% were subsequently treated with extension of the fusion to the sacrum. Extension to the sacrum was recommended in an additional 19% of patients, but medical morbidities prevented the procedure.[23] The high rate of disk degeneration and subsequent forward shift in sagittal alignment associated with long fusions to L5 must be weighed against the added morbidity of sacropelvic fixation and fusion to the sacrum.[24,25] Increased consensus on the indications for extending a long fusion to the sacrum include L5-S1 spondylolisthesis, L5-S1 stenosis, oblique takeoff of L5, prior L5-S1 laminectomy, and severe L5-S1 disk degeneration.[26]

The addition of iliac screws to augment lumbosacral fixation when fusing to the sacrum has shown good results at 5-year follow-up with an overall successful fusion rate of 92%.[27,28] Three of the five reported nonunions occurred in cases in which no anterior column support was used. With anterior column support, sacral and iliac screw fixation achieved a 96% fusion rate.[28] No sacral screw pull-outs, fractures, or loosening was reported; however, iliac screw loosening was reported in 43% of patients and breakage in 5%. When extending a long fusion to the sacrum, the use of illiac screw fixation and anterior column support (anterior lumbar interbody fusion, posterior lumbar interbody fusion, or transforaminal lumbar interbody fusion) decreases the rate of sacral fixation failure and pseudarthrosis.[28]

Approach

In the traditional treatment of scoliosis, anterior release combined with or without anterior fusion was believed to improve curve correction and restore alignment, especially in patients with a rigid curve. However, the anterior thoracolumbar approach can be associated with morbidity. In one study, chronic pain was associated with an anterior thoracolumbar wound in 32% of patients, and 45% reported asymmetry and abdominal bulging.[29] Recent trends have moved toward posterior-based approaches, with rigid pedicle-based instrumentation and resection osteotomies. Recently published studies reported no difference in curve correction in adult patients treated with anterior release and a posterior instrumented fusion compared with patients treated with a posterior-only approach, including resection osteotomies when indicated.[30-32] Although the added morbidity of an anterior approach has not been compared directly with the morbidity associated with posterior osteotomies in the treatment of adult scoliosis, anterior release for adult scoliosis may not be necessary to achieve comparable coronal correction and outcomes.

Decompression

Up to 64% of patients with adult scoliosis present with reports of leg pain associated with stenosis.[17] Adequate neural decompression is the first treatment priority. A wide central decompression may provide adequate treatment in many patients, but a focal radiculopathy secondary to foraminal stenosis may require further intervention. Focal radiculopathy often occurs at the apex on the concave side of a lumbar curve where there is vertebral body rotation and translation. Partially correcting the curve with distraction and in situ rod bending, along with a wide foraminal decompression through the pars interarticularis, may adequately open the foramen. If this technique is not successful, an added posterior lumbar interbody fusion or transforaminal lumbar interbody fusion may be necessary to achieve and maintain foraminal patency. An anterior lumbar interbody fusion through a standard anterior retroperitoneal or a direct lateral transpsoas approach also may be effective.

Limited Decompression and Fusion
The role for limited decompression without fusion and decompression with limited fusion in adult scoliosis is not well defined. Typically, the patient being considered for treatment with a limited approach is older, has unilateral or bilateral leg pain symptoms secondary to lumbar stenosis, and minimal or no back pain. The goal of a focused treatment is to address the primary symptomatic pathology (lumbar stenosis) without causing iatrogenic instability and rapid curve progression.

The destabilizing effect of complete unilateral or bilateral facetectomy in the lumbar spine is well reported.[33] Unilateral or bilateral limited laminotomy with partial facetectomy and preservation of the midline structures is less destabilizing;[34] however, the relevancy of these biomechanical studies to effects in the deformed spine is unknown. A partial facetectomy may be sufficient to destabilize the apex segment of a curve.

In general, a limited decompression may be considered in patients with leg pain only, lumbar curves of less than 20° minimal rotation, no radiographic instability (< 4 mm motion on dynamic radiographs and < 2 mm lateral translation), and no significant sagittal or coronal imbalance.[35,36] Indications for decompression with limited fusion are even less clear. In curves less than 20°, with an unstable segment (degenerative spondylolisthesis), decompression and fusion of the unstable segment alone may be adequate. If the unstable segment is located outside of the major curve, limited fusion also can be considered.[35,36] In general, ending a fusion adjacent to the apex of a coronal or sagittal curve is not recommended.

There are no quality randomized or cohort studies comparing outcomes of the limited approach with the standard approach for treating adult scoliosis with associated stenosis. The previous discussion presented general guidelines; all patients should be counseled on the risks of progression and the possible need for additional surgery.

Fixed Sagittal Imbalance Syndrome *"Flatback Syndrome"*
Fixed sagittal imbalance is defined as radiographic sagittal imbalance of more than 5 cm. This syndrome has multiple etiologies (**Table 1**), all of which result in pos-

Table 1
Causes of Fixed Sagittal Imbalance

Iatrogenic
   Fusion in hypolordosis
   Proximal junctional kyphosis (above a fused segment)
Ankylosing spondylitis
Congenital kyphosis
Posttraumatic conditions
Osteoporotic compression fractures *& degenerative (adult scoliosis)*
Infection, *e.g. Pott's*
Neoplasm

itive sagittal balance and the inability of the patient to stand upright. Aging is the most common cause of disk degeneration and height loss. With age, thoracic kyphosis increases and lumbar lordosis decreases. Most patients are able to maintain their sagittal balance with advancing age.[37] Patients who become symptomatic are unable to compensate for the loss of lumbar lordosis through hip extension/pelvic retroversion and knee flexion, which eventually results in positive sagittal balance (**Figure 1**). Patients typically present with chronic low back pain that worsens with prolonged standing and a pitched forward posture with knees in flexion. Extensor muscle fatigue can cause diffuse back pain that may extend to the thoracic and cervical regions.

Global sagittal balance is the result of the harmonious combination of lumbar lordosis, thoracic kyphosis, and cervical lordosis. Each anatomic region of the spine is interconnected; a change in curvature in one region causes a response in the other regions to balance the head and maintain the center of gravity over the pelvis. Because the pelvis is the foundation or base of the spine, its morphology influences the magnitude of curvature in the other regions. Pelvic incidence is a fixed, anatomic parameter of the pelvis that influences sagittal alignment. An understanding of pelvic incidence is critical in formulating the appropriate options for treating fixed sagittal imbalance. *starts @ the pelvis*

Pelvic Incidence
Pelvic incidence is defined as the angle between the line perpendicular to the middle of the sacral end plate and the line joining the middle of the sacral end plate to the center of the bicoxofemoral axis[38] (**Figure 3**). Pelvic incidence correlates strongly with sacral slope, pelvic tilt, and lumbar lordosis.[39] In simplified terms, pelvic incidence (a constant anatomic measurement determined by an individual's unique pelvic morphology) determines the sacral slope, which in turn determines the angle of take off of the lumbar spine in the sagittal plane and the resultant magnitude of lumbar lordosis. Normalized values for pelvic incidence, sacral slope, and pelvic tilt have been studied[39,40] (**Table 2**). Adult females have slightly higher angles of pelvic incidence,

Table 2

Normal Values for Pelvic Incidence, Sacral Slope, and Pelvic Tilt

Population	Radiographic Parameters (in degrees)		
	Pelvic Incidence	Sacral Slope	Pelvic Tilt
Children and adolescents (ages 3 to 18 years)			
Male	49.2 ± 11.2	41.7 ± 8.4	49.2 ± 11.2
Female	49.7 ± 10.7	41.2 ± 8.0	8.5 ± 8.3
Adults (ages 19 to 50 years)			
Male	53.2 ± 10.3	41.9 ± 8.7	11.9 ± 6.6
Female	48.2 ± 7.0	38.2 ± 7.8	10.3 ± 4.8

sacral slope, and lumbar lordosis than their male cohorts.

Several studies, have confirmed the relationship between pelvic incidence, sacral slope, pelvic tilt, and global spinal balance.[38,39,41-43] Each anatomic region of the spine and pelvis are interdependently connected to achieve spinal balance and upright posture. When a patient exhausts all compensatory mechanisms (pelvic retroversion, hip extension, knee flexion, thoracic hypokyphosis/extension) to stand upright, fixed sagittal imbalance syndrome ensues and the HRQL is negatively impacted.[2,44]

Treatment

The recommended surgical treatment of fixed sagittal imbalance is dependent on the amount of positive sagittal imbalance, the degree of flexibility of the deformity, and whether the kyphosis is focal (limited to a few spinal segments; for example, posttraumatic kyphosis) or multilevel (involving several spinal segments; for example, Scheuermann kyphosis). Pelvic incidence is also important in determining the amount of correction that is needed[45] (a patient with a higher pelvic incidence may need more lumbar lordosis to adequately correct sagittal balance). In general, fixed sagittal imbalance is surgically treated with four procedures—an interbody fusion, a Smith-Petersen osteotomy, a pedicle subtraction osteotomy, and a vertebral column resection.[46]

Interbody Fusion

Interbody fusion is limited to use in patients with minor sagittal imbalance (6 to 8 cm). Two thirds of lumbar lordosis occurs through the L4-L5 and the L5-S1 segments. Lumbar lordosis can be improved by restoring the disk height at L4-L5 and L5-S1 through the use of structural interbody allograft or cages. Because of the technical challenges and potential complications of inserting larger grafts or cages through the posterior approaches (transforaminal or posterior lumbar interbody fusions), anterior lumbar interbody fusion is pre-

ferred by many surgeons as a more effective method of regaining lordosis. For example, in a patient with a prior thoracolumbar fusion extending to L4 with disk degeneration and sagittal imbalance of 8 cm, an anterior lumbar interbody fusion at L4-L5 and L5-S1 may restore enough lordosis to obtain sagittal balance.

Smith-Petersen Osteotomy

Smith-Petersen osteotomies are usually performed at multiple levels and can restore as much as 10° of lordosis per level depending on the amount of disk mobility. A Smith-Petersen osteotomy will not be successful if there is anterior fusion, and/or will provide minimal correction if there is minimal disk height associated with large osteophytes. Less correction per level can be expected in the thoracic spine because less disk mobility is typical in this area. Smith-Petersen osteotomies can be added to the anterior lumbar interbody fusion or used in conjunction with a pedicle subtraction osteotomy to increase the magnitude of lordosis correction. Smith-Petersen osteotomies are commonly used to treat Scheuermann kyphosis, lesser degrees of thoracolumbar kyphosis, and can be used as a method of restoring lordosis and improving correction in thoracolumbar scoliosis.

Pedicle Subtraction Osteotomy

A pedicle subtraction osteotomy is indicated in patients with more severe sagittal imbalance (> 12 cm).[46] A correction of 30° to 35° can be expected in the lumbar spine and 25° in the thoracic spine.[47] These osteotomies are effective in treating focal kyphosis and can be used to treat severe scoliosis, with an asymmetric correction in the sagittal and coronal planes (Figure 4). Pedicle subtraction osteotomy can also be used when a prior circumferential fusion has been performed. A recent study (minimum 5-year follow-up) on the use of pedicle subtraction osteotomies for fixed sagittal imbalance reported no loss of regional correction in lordosis, and only a minor increase in positive sagittal balance.[48] The pseudarthrosis rate was 29%; no instances of pseudar-

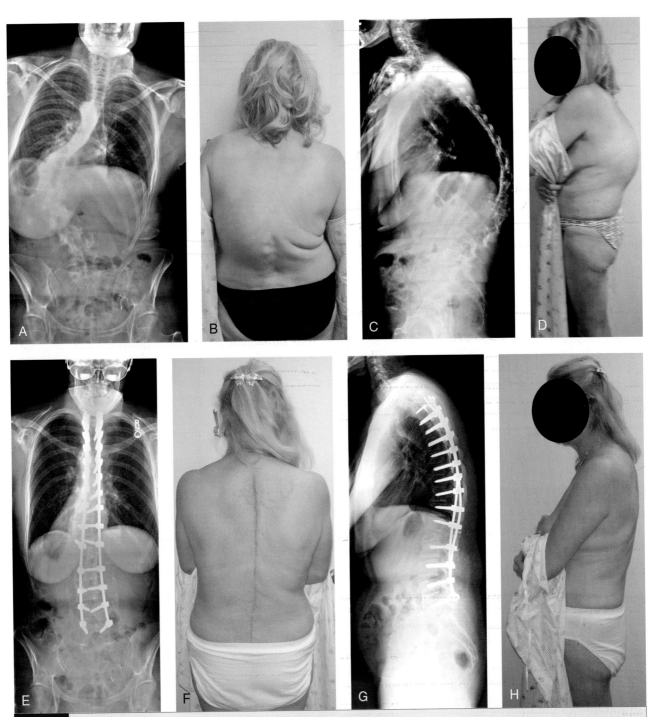

Figure 4	A 52-year-old woman with progressive adult idiopathic thoracolumbar kyphoscoliosis was treated with an asymmetric L1 pedicle subtraction osteotomy and a T3 to L5 thoracic and lumbar fusion. **A,** Preoperative AP radiograph. **B,** Preoperative AP clinical photograph. **C,** Preoperative lateral radiograph. **D,** Preoperative lateral clinical photograph. **E,** Postoperative AP radiograph. **F,** Postoperative AP clinical photograph. **G,** Postoperative lateral radiograph. **H,** Postoperative lateral clinical photograph.

throsis occurred at the osteotomy site, with most occurring at the thoracolumbar junction. The neurologic complications of pedicle subtraction osteotomies were evaluated in 108 patients with 10-year follow-ups.[49] The overall rate of neurologic deficits (defined as bowel/bladder loss, or motor loss of two or more

grades) was 11%, with permanent deficits in only 3% of patients. The mean correction in sagittal balance was 11 cm.

Vertebral Column Resection

Vertebral column resections are indicated for the correction of rigid, angular kyphosis in the thoracic spine; severe rigid scoliosis; congenital kyphosis; hemivertebrae resection in the thoracic and lumbar spines; and kyphotic deformity associated with tumor, fracture, or infection in the thoracic spine. Vertebral column resections are more commonly performed in the thoracic spine and provide more correction than pedicle subtraction osteotomies. Resections also can be performed in the lumbar spine, but are more technically difficult because of the position of the lumbar nerve root. In one report, the mean correction with a vertebral column resection was 62° in the coronal plane and 45° in the sagittal plane.[50] Vertebral column resection is an effective treatment of severe, rigid deformities. Neurologic monitoring is highly recommended. In a study of 43 patients treated with vertebral column resection (93% at the spinal cord level), 18% of patients lost motor-evoked potentials during the procedure, but all returned to normal baseline values with surgical intervention; no permanent injuries were reported.[51]

Neuromuscular Adult Scoliosis

Neuromuscular adult scoliosis covers a broad range of conditions, including cerebral palsy, spinal muscle atrophy, Duchenne muscular dystrophy, poliomyelitis, and paraplegia. Adult-onset conditions such as multiple sclerosis and Parkinson disease, which cause general weakness and balance problems, can also cause neuromuscular-type deformities. Adults typically present with pain and/or progressive deformity. The deformity can occur in any region of the spine, with the patient presenting with kyphosis, lordosis, and/or sagittal and coronal imbalance. Often, there is a long sweeping-type deformity, which may be flexible in the young adult patient. The deformities associated with multiple sclerosis and Parkinson disease may be flexible at the early onset of the disease in middle-aged and older adults but may become progressively rigid with time.

Reducing pain, halting deformity progression, and achieving spinal balance are the goals of treatment. In a patient who is confined to a wheelchair, sitting balance is key to allowing efficient use of the upper extremities and preventing skin breakdown. Because a high rate of surgical complications occurs in this group of patients, proper counseling regarding expected outcomes is important. In one of the few studies evaluating spinal surgery in patients with Parkinson disease, the rate of revision surgery was 86% and the infection rate was 14%.[52]

Intraoperative Neurophysiologic Monitoring

The evidence in support of the routine use of intraoperative neurophysiologic monitoring during the treatment of spinal deformity has strengthened. Its use aids in the early detection of impending spinal cord injury and may prevent worsening postoperative morbidity. A study of more than 1,000 patients (mean age, 14 years) surgically treated for adolescent idiopathic scoliosis

showed that changes in transcranial electric motor-evoked potentials were detected earlier than changes in somatosensory-evoked potentials.[53] Twenty-six patients had decreases in amplitude of 65% in transcranial electric motor-evoked potentials during posterior instrumentation and corrective maneuvers. Nine (35%) of these patients (0.8% of the study group) had a transient motor or sensory deficit postoperatively, all of which were detected by transcranial electric motor-evoked potentials. Changes in somatosensory-evoked potentials occurred, on average, 5 minutes after the initial changes detected by the transcranial electric motor-evoked potentials, and somatosensory-evoked potentials failed to detect a motor deficit in 4 of 7 patients. With early detection and subsequent changes in the surgical course of action, all deficits resolved by 90 days postoperatively. Although the results of this study cannot be generalized to the treatment of adult deformity, especially with regard to the rate of neurologic recovery following corrective maneuvers, it does provide excellent evidence of the potential benefits of transcranial electric motor-evoked potentials and intraoperative neurophysiologic monitoring of the spinal cord. The January 2009 position statement of the Scoliosis Research Society (www.srs.org) recommends the use of intraoperative neurophysiologic monitoring during the surgical correction of spinal deformity and considers it the preferred method for the early detection of impending or evolving spinal cord deficits.

The evidence for monitoring intraoperative nerve root function with electromyography is less clear and is controversial. The effective use of electromyography for evaluating pedicle screw placement in the thoracic[54] and lumbar[55] spine has been reported. Its role in preventing or detecting intraoperative nerve root injury is less clear.[49,56] In a large series of adult patients treated with lumbar pedicle subtraction osteotomy for adult deformity, electromyography failed to detect any of the reported nerve root injuries.[49] In many patients with adult deformity, even in surgery primarily involving the lumbar spine, the procedure involves manipulation or instrumentation of the upper lumbar or thoracolumbar region where the cord and/or conus may be affected. Intraoperative neurophysiologic monitoring is widely used and preferred in most surgical procedures for adult spinal deformity.

Challenges

The Aging Spine

The rate of complications in adult deformity surgery increase as the complexity of the surgery increases. As the population ages, there has been an increase in the number of older patients who are being surgically treated for major spinal deformities. Many complications are related to medical comorbidities and osteoporosis. The rate of major complications in patients older than 60 years was 20% in one series, with the rate of complications significantly increasing in patients older than 69 years.[19] Aggressive medical treatment and newer pharmacotherapies may reduce the risks of spinal implant failure in the osteoporotic spine. Methylmethacrylate augmentation of pedicle screw fixation improves pull-out strength and is a viable option in severe cases.[57-59] Despite the higher risk of complications, older patients have significant improvement in HRQL when compared with those treated nonsurgically.[19,60]

Corrective Osteotomies

Pedicle subtraction osteotomies and vertebral column resections allow the correction of rigid sagittal and coronal deformities, but there are increased risks with these techniques. The incidence of neurologic deficits was as high as 11% in one study, but most of the injuries were limited to the nerve root levels and eventually resolved.[49] The rate of pseudarthrosis with pedicle subtraction osteotomies was reported as high as 28% at 5-year follow-up; however, after revision surgery the HRQL measures improved and were not significantly different from those of patients without psuedoarthosis.[48] Vertebral column resections are associated with a higher rate of neurologic deficits and intraoperative neurophysiologic monitoring changes.[50,51] With monitoring, the detection of potential spinal cord deficits can be detected early and permanent deficits can be avoided.[51] Intraoperative neurophysiologic monitoring is highly recommended for these procedures.

Pseudarthrosis

Pseudarthrosis continues to be a major challenge and is one of the main complications in multilevel, adult deformity surgery. With longer term follow-up, the rate of pseudarthrosis increases. It has been reported to be 17% in one large series[61] and as high as 24% in a recent report,[62] with only 25% of the cases of pseudarthrosis detected within the 2-year follow-up period. Bone morphogenetic protein (recombinant human bone morphogenetic protein-2) mixed with tricalcium phosphate/hydroxyapatite crystals in multilevel, adult deformity surgery was found to be an adequate replacement for autogenous bone graft, with rates of fusion as high as 100% at 2-year follow-up.[63] This is an encouraging result, but longer-term follow-up is needed.

Future Directions

Over the next several years there will be a demand for better-quality scientific evidence that surgical treatment in adult spinal deformity is making a clinically significant improvement in the lives of patients. Large clinical series have shown that sagittal balance is a key predictor of improvement in HRQL. As the understanding of the role of pelvic parameters in determining sagittal balance increases, orthopaedic surgeons may become more adept at individualizing surgical interventions to restore spinal balance. Biologic proteins to improve fusion rates will continue to be discovered along with better delivery systems that may require lower doses

with fewer associated costs and complications. Drug-coated eluting devices are a future possible development. Less invasive surgical methods, such as the lateral lumbar and transpsoas interbody fusion approaches and percutaneously placed instrumentation systems, may have a role in adult deformity surgery.[64] Genetic research may allow the personalization of treatment options and early intervention to prevent the onset of severe deformity or may eradicate spinal disease through gene therapy.[65]

The treatment of adult spinal deformity is complex. The indications for surgical treatment should not be based on radiographs alone. Many patients can tolerate high magnitude curves and function well.[3] Treatment recommendations should be individualized and the impact of the deformity on the patient's daily function and quality of life should be considered.

Annotated References

1. Glassman SD, Berven S, Bridwell K, Horton W, Dimar JR: Correlation of radiographic parameters and clinical symptoms in adult scoliosis. *Spine (Phila Pa 1976)* 2005;30(6):682-688.

2. Glassman SD, Bridwell K, Dimar JR, Horton W, Berven S, Schwab F: The impact of positive sagittal balance in adult spinal deformity. *Spine (Phila Pa 1976)* 2005; 30(18):2024-2029.

3. Weinstein SL, Dolan LA, Spratt KF, Peterson KK, Spoonamore MJ, Ponseti IV: Health and function of patients with untreated idiopathic scoliosis: A 50-year natural history study. *JAMA* 2003;289(5):559-567.

4. Weinstein SL, Ponseti IV: Curve progression in idiopathic scoliosis. *J Bone Joint Surg Am* 1983;65(4): 447-455.

5. Lenke LG, Edwards CC II, Bridwell KH: The Lenke classification of adolescent idiopathic scoliosis: How it organizes curve patterns as a template to perform selective fusions of the spine. *Spine (Phila Pa 1976)* 2003; 28(20):S199-S207.

6. Schwab F, Dubey A, Gamez L, et al: Adult scoliosis: Prevalence, SF-36, and nutritional parameters in an elderly volunteer population. *Spine (Phila Pa 1976)* 2005; 30(9):1082-1085.

7. Kobayashi T, Atsuta Y, Takemitsu M, Matsuno T, Takeda N: A prospective study of de novo scoliosis in a community based cohort. *Spine (Phila Pa 1976)* 2006; 31(2):178-182.

8. Robin GC, Span Y, Steinberg R, Makin M, Menczel J: Scoliosis in the elderly: A follow-up study. *Spine (Phila Pa 1976)* 1982;7(4):355-359.

9. Gremeaux V, Casillas JM, Fabbro-Peray P, Pelissier J, Herisson C, Perennou D: Analysis of low back pain in

adults with scoliosis. *Spine (Phila Pa 1976)* 2008;33(4): 402-405.

This cohort study evaluated patients with lumbar scoliosis and chronic low back pain, and a group without scoliosis. There was no difference between the groups in regard to severity or duration of pain. Pain was increased in patients with scoliosis with a larger magnitude curve and increased rotatory olisthesis. Level of evidence: III.

10. Schwab FJ, Smith VA, Biserni M, Gamez L, Farcy JP, Pagala M: Adult scoliosis: A quantitative radiographic and clinical analysis. *Spine (Phila Pa 1976)* 2002;27(4): 387-392.

11. Ploumis A, Liu H, Mehbod AA, Transfeldt EE, Winter RB: A correlation of radiographic and functional measurements in adult degenerative scoliosis. *Spine (Phila Pa 1976)* 2009;34(15):1581-1584.

A retrospective review was performed on 58 patients with de novo scoliosis to evaluate the correlation of symptoms and radiographic findings. Coronal imbalance greater than 5 cm and loss of lordosis correlated with poorer health status. Bodily pain was higher in patients with more than 6 mm of lateral olisthesis. Level of evidence: IV.

12. Bess S, Boachie-Adjei O, Burton D, et al; International Spine Study Group: Pain and disability determine treatment modality for older patients with adult scoliosis, while deformity guides treatment for younger patients. *Spine (Phila Pa 1976)* 2009;34(20):2186-2190.

This retrospective, multicenter database review of 290 patients with adult scoliosis evaluated the determinants of surgery. Age, comorbidities, and sagittal balance did not influence the treatment modality. In younger patients, surgical treatment was determined by coronal plane deformity. Level of evidence: III.

13. Glassman SD, Schwab FJ, Bridwell KH, Ondra SL, Berven S, Lenke LG: The selection of operative versus nonoperative treatment in patients with adult scoliosis. *Spine (Phila Pa 1976)* 2007;32(1):93-97.

This retrospective case-controlled matched series compared patients treated surgically and nonsurgically to determine the factors that may have predicted one treatment over the other. Patients in the surgical group had larger curves in the thoracic and thoracolumbar/lumbar spine, greater frequency of leg pain, and a higher frequency and level of back pain compared to the patients treated nonsurgically. Level of evidence: III.

14. Pekmezci M, Berven SH, Hu SS, Deviren V: The factors that play a role in the decision-making process of adult deformity patients. *Spine (Phila Pa 1976)* 2009;34(8): 813-817.

The authors present a retrospective review evaluating the differences between patients with adult spinal deformity who underwent surgery and those who did not. There was no difference in preoperative pain levels or magnitude of back or leg pain. Patients who underwent surgery had worse scores on the Scoliosis Research Society-30 Patient Questionnaire for vitality, and on the Oswestry Disability Index for walking compared with the nonsurgical group. Level of evidence: III.

15. Smith JS, Fu KM, Urban P, Shaffrey CI: Neurological symptoms and deficits in adults with scoliosis who present to a surgical clinic: Incidence and association with the choice of operative versus nonoperative management. *J Neurosurg Spine* 2008;9(4):326-331.

Patients who underwent surgery had higher Oswestry Disability Index scores and a greater incidence of severe radiculopathy, weakness, and neurogenic claudication symptoms preoperatively compared with the nonsurgical group. Level of evidence: III.

16. Everett CR, Patel RK: A systematic literature review of nonsurgical treatment in adult scoliosis. *Spine (Phila Pa 1976)* 2007;32(19, suppl)S130-S134.

This systematic literature review concluded there was very little evidence for any type of nonsurgical care in the treatment of adult scoliosis. Level of evidence: IV.

17. Smith JS, Shaffrey CI, Berven S, et al; Spinal Deformity Study Group: Operative versus nonoperative treatment of leg pain in adults with scoliosis: A retrospective review of a prospective multicenter database with two-year follow-up. *Spine (Phila Pa 1976)* 2009;34(16): 1693-1698.

Two hundred eight patients with leg pain and adult scoliosis were evaluated. One hundred twelve were treated nonsurgically and 96 were treated with surgery. At 2-year follow-up, surgically treated patients had significantly less leg pain than the nonsurgically treated group. Level of evidence: III.

18. Weinstein JN, Tosteson TD, Lurie JD, et al; SPORT Investigators: Surgical versus nonsurgical therapy for lumbar spinal stenosis. *N Engl J Med* 2008;358(8):794-810.

A prospective, randomized study evaluating the treatment of lumbar spinal stenosis is presented. In the astreated analysis, patients who underwent surgery had significantly more improvement in all primary outcomes than did patients who were treated nonsurgically. Level of evidence: I.

19. Daubs MD, Lenke LG, Cheh G, Stobbs G, Bridwell KH: Adult spinal deformity surgery: Complications and outcomes in patients over age 60. *Spine (Phila Pa 1976)* 2007;32(20):2238-2244.

The rate of major complications was 20%, and increasing age was a significant factor in predicting the presence of a complication. Patients older than 69 years had significantly more complications. Level of evidence: IV.

20. Lenke LG: Lenke classification system of adolescent idiopathic scoliosis: Treatment recommendations. *Instr Course Lect* 2005;54:537-542.

21. Kuklo TR: Principles for selecting fusion levels in adult spinal deformity with particular attention to lumbar curves and double major curves. *Spine (Phila Pa 1976)* 2006;31(19, suppl):S132-S138.

22. Kim YJ, Bridwell KH, Lenke LG, Rhim S, Kim YW: Is

the T9, T11, or L1 the more reliable proximal level after adult lumbar or lumbosacral instrumented fusion to L5 or S1? *Spine (Phila Pa 1976)* 2007;32(24):2653-2661.

This retrospective study found no difference in revision rates, proximal junctional kyphosis, or Scoliosis Research Society outcomes when stopping the proximal fusion level at T9, T11, or L1 in a long instrumented fusion to L5 or S1. Level of evidence: IV.

23. Kuhns CA, Bridwell KH, Lenke LG, et al: Thoracolumbar deformity arthrodesis stopping at L5: Fate of the L5-S1 disc, minimum 5-year follow-up. *Spine (Phila Pa 1976)* 2007;32(24):2771-2776.

   Sixty-nine percent of patients had advanced disk degeneration at L5-S1 at 5-year follow-up following a thoracolumbar fusion that stopped at L5. Twenty-three percent had subsequent extension of their fusion to the sacrum. Level of evidence: IV.

24. Kwon BK, Elgafy H, Keynan O, et al: Progressive junctional kyphosis at the caudal end of lumbar instrumented fusion: Etiology, predictors, and treatment. *Spine (Phila Pa 1976)* 2006;31(17):1943-1951.

25. Edwards CC II, Bridwell KH, Patel A, Rinella AS, Berra A, Lenke LG: Long adult deformity fusions to L5 and the sacrum: A matched cohort analysis. *Spine (Phila Pa 1976)* 2004;29(18):1996-2005.

26. Bridwell KH: Selection of instrumentation and fusion levels for scoliosis: Where to start and where to stop. Invited submission from the Joint Section Meeting on Disorders of the Spine and Peripheral Nerves, March 2004. *J Neurosurg Spine* 2004;1(1):1-8.

27. Kuklo TR, Bridwell KH, Lewis SJ, et al: Minimum 2-year analysis of sacropelvic fixation and L5-S1 fusion using S1 and iliac screws. *Spine (Phila Pa 1976)* 2001; 26(18):1976-1983.

28. Tsuchiya K, Bridwell KH, Kuklo TR, Lenke LG, Baldus C: Minimum 5-year analysis of L5-S1 fusion using sacropelvic fixation (bilateral S1 and iliac screws) for spinal deformity. *Spine (Phila Pa 1976)* 2006;31(3): 303-308.

29. Kim YB, Lenke LG, Kim YJ, et al: The morbidity of an anterior thoracolumbar approach: Adult spinal deformity patients with greater than five-year follow-up. *Spine (Phila Pa 1976)* 2009;34(8):822-826.

   At 5-year follow-up, patients undergoing an anterior thoracolumbar approach complained of postoperative pain (32.3%), bulging (43.5%), and functional disturbance (24.2%). Level of evidence: IV.

30. Pateder DB, Kebaish KM, Cascio BM, Neubaeur P, Matusz DM, Kostuik JP: Posterior only versus combined anterior and posterior approaches to lumbar scoliosis in adults: A radiographic analysis. *Spine (Phila Pa 1976)* 2007;32(14):1551-1554.

   A retrospective, case-based comparison of posterior only versus a combined anterior and posterior approach for adult scoliosis is discussed. There were no significant differences in spinal balance or sagittal and coronal plane curve correction between the two groups.

31. Rose PS, Lenke LG, Bridwell KH, et al: Pedicle screw instrumentation for adult idiopathic scoliosis: An improvement over hook/hybrid fixation. *Spine (Phila Pa 1976)* 2009;34(8):852-857, discussion 858.

   This retrospective cohort study found significantly improved correction of the major curve, and a lower revision rate with the use of pedicle screw constructs in the treatment of adolescent idiopathic scoliosis. There were no differences in Scoliosis Research Society scores between the groups. Level of evidence: III.

32. Kim YB, Lenke LG, Kim YJ, Kim YW, Bridwell KH, Stobbs G: Surgical treatment of adult scoliosis: Is anterior apical release and fusion necessary for the lumbar curve? *Spine (Phila Pa 1976)* 2008;33(10):1125-1132.

   This is a retrospective, cohort study of 48 patients, 25 who underwent posterior instrumented fusion without an anterior apical release and 23 who underwent apical release followed by a posterior spinal fusion. There was no difference in the amount of correction, and the overall Scoliosis Research Society outcome scores were better in the group without the anterior apical relaease. Level of evidence: III.

33. Abumi K, Panjabi MM, Kramer KM, Duranceau J, Oxland T, Crisco JJ: Biomechanical evaluation of lumbar spinal stability after graded facetectomies. *Spine (Phila Pa 1976)* 1990;15(11):1142-1147.

34. Lu WW, Luk KD, Ruan DK, Fei ZQ, Leong JC: Stability of the whole lumbar spine after multilevel fenestration and discectomy. *Spine (Phila Pa 1976)* 1999; 24(13):1277-1282.

35. Weidenbaum M: Considerations for focused surgical intervention in the presence of adult spinal deformity. *Spine (Phila Pa 1976)* 2006;31(19, suppl)S139-S143.

36. Ploumis A, Transfledt EE, Denis F: Degenerative lumbar scoliosis associated with spinal stenosis. *Spine J* 2007; 7(4):428-436.

   This review paper evaluated the treatment of degenerative scoliosis with stenosis. The authors also introduce an algorithm for the treatment of degenerative scoliosis with stenosis. Level of evidence: IV.

37. Gelb DE, Lenke LG, Bridwell KH, Blanke K, McEnery KW: An analysis of sagittal spinal alignment in 100 asymptomatic middle and older aged volunteers. *Spine (Phila Pa 1976)* 1995;20(12):1351-1358.

38. Legaye J, Duval-Beaupère G, Hecquet J, Marty C: Pelvic incidence: A fundamental pelvic parameter for three-dimensional regulation of spinal sagittal curves. *Eur Spine J* 1998;7(2):99-103.

39. Vialle R, Levassor N, Rillardon L, Templier A, Skalli W, Guigui P: Radiographic analysis of the sagittal alignment and balance of the spine in asymptomatic subjects. *J Bone Joint Surg Am* 2005;87(2):260-267.

5: Spine

40. Mac-Thiong JM, Berthonnaud E, Dimar JR II, Betz RR, Labelle H: Sagittal alignment of the spine and pelvis during growth. *Spine (Phila Pa 1976)* 2004;29(15): 1642-1647.

41. Legaye J, Duval-Beaupère G: Sagittal plane alignment of the spine and gravity: A radiological and clinical evaluation. *Acta Orthop Belg* 2005;71(2):213-220.

42. Berthonnaud E, Dimnet J, Roussouly P, Labelle H: Analysis of the sagittal balance of the spine and pelvis using shape and orientation parameters. *J Spinal Disord Tech* 2005;18(1):40-47.

43. Roussouly P, Gollogly S, Berthonnaud E, Dimnet J: Classification of the normal variation in the sagittal alignment of the human lumbar spine and pelvis in the standing position. *Spine (Phila Pa 1976)* 2005;30(3): 346-353.

44. Lafage V, Schwab F, Patel A, Hawkinson N, Farcy JP: Pelvic tilt and truncal inclination: Two key radiographic parameters in the setting of adults with spinal deformity. *Spine (Phila Pa 1976)* 2009;34(17):E599-E606.

    This study evaluated 125 patients with adult deformity. Radiographic parameters were correlated with the SF-12, the Oswestry Disability Index, and the Scoliosis Research Society-30 Patient Questionnaire. Increased pelvic tilt correlated with worse outcome scores, suggesting that patients who were compensating for sagittal imbalance related worse health status. Level of evidence: III.

45. Rose PS, Bridwell KH, Lenke LG, et al: Role of pelvic incidence, thoracic kyphosis, and patient factors on sagittal plane correction following pedicle subtraction osteotomy. *Spine (Phila Pa 1976)* 2009;34(8):785-791.

    Forty patients who were treated with a pedicle subtraction osteotomy were reviewed to evaluate the role of pelvic incidence and thoracic kyphosis on the amount of lumbar lordosis needed for the restoration of sagittal balance. They arrived at a formula: PI + LL + TK < or = 45°, to help determine the amount of lumbar lordosis correction that is necessary. Level of evidence: IV.

46. Bridwell KH: Decision making regarding Smith-Petersen vs. pedicle subtraction osteotomy vs. vertebral column resection for spinal deformity. *Spine (Phila Pa 1976)* 2006;31(19, suppl):S171-S178.

47. Bridwell KH, Lewis SJ, Lenke LG, Baldus C, Blanke K: Pedicle subtraction osteotomy for the treatment of fixed sagittal imbalance. *J Bone Joint Surg Am* 2003;85(3): 454-463.

48. Kim YJ, Bridwell KH, Lenke LG, Cheh G, Baldus C: Results of lumbar pedicle subtraction osteotomies for fixed sagittal imbalance: A minimum 5-year follow-up study. *Spine (Phila Pa 1976)* 2007;32(20):2189-2197.

    Thirty-five consecutive patients with sagittal imbalance treated with lumbar pedicle subtraction osteotomies were retrospectively analyzed during an average follow-up of 5.8 years. Scoliosis Research Society outcome scores were maintained at the 5-year follow-up.

    The pseudoarthorsis rate was 29%. Level of evidence: IV.

49. Buchowski JM, Bridwell KH, Lenke LG, et al: Neurologic complications of lumbar pedicle subtraction osteotomy: A 10-year assessment. *Spine (Phila Pa 1976)* 2007;32(20):2245-2252.

    One hundred eight patients who underwent a pedicle subtraction osteotomy were reviewed to determine the incidence of neurologic complications with this procedure. The rate of neurologic complications was 11%, with only 3% resulting in a permanent deficit. Level of evidence: IV.

50. Suk SI, Kim JH, Kim WJ, Lee SM, Chung ER, Nah KH: Posterior vertebral column resection for severe spinal deformities. *Spine (Phila Pa 1976)* 2002;27(21):2374-2382.

51. Lenke LG, Sides BA, Koester LA, Hensley M, Blanke KM: Vertebral column resection for the treatment of severe spinal deformity. *Clin Orthop Relat Res* 2010; 468(3):687-699.

    This is a retrospective review of 43 patients that underwent a vertebral column resection for the treatment of severe spinal deformity. Level of evidence: IV.

52. Babat LB, McLain RF, Bingaman W, Kalfas I, Young P, Rufo-Smith C: Spinal surgery in patients with Parkinson's disease: Construct failure and progressive deformity. *Spine (Phila Pa 1976)* 2004;29(18):2006-2012.

53. Schwartz DM, Auerbach JD, Dormans JP, et al: Neurophysiological detection of impending spinal cord injury during scoliosis surgery. *J Bone Joint Surg Am* 2007; 89(11):2440-2449.

    One thousand one hundred twenty-one patients who were monitored intraoperatively with motor-evoked potentials and somatosensory-evoked potentials and who underwent surgery for adolescent idiopathic scoliosis were reviewed. A significant amplitiude change in monitoring was reported in 3.4% of the patients. Transcranial electric motor-evoked potentials were more sensitive to altered spinal cord blood flow because of hypotension or a vascular insult. Changes in motor-evoked potentials are detected earlier than changes in somatosensory-evoked potentials and result in a more rapid identification of impending spinal cord injury. Level of evidence: IV.

54. Raynor BL, Lenke LG, Kim Y, et al: Can triggered electromyograph thresholds predict safe thoracic pedicle screw placement? *Spine (Phila Pa 1976)* 2002;27(18): 2030-2035.

55. Glassman SD, Dimar JR, Puno RM, Johnson JR, Shields CB, Linden RD: A prospective analysis of intraoperative electromyographic monitoring of pedicle screw placement with computed tomographic scan confirmation. *Spine (Phila Pa 1976)* 1995;20(12):1375-1379.

56. Gunnarsson T, Krassioukov AV, Sarjeant R, Fehlings MG: Real-time continuous intraoperative electromyo-

graphic and somatosensory evoked potential recordings in spinal surgery: Correlation of clinical and electrophysiologic findings in a prospective, consecutive series of 213 cases. *Spine (Phila Pa 1976)* 2004;29(6):677-684.

57. Burval DJ, McLain RF, Milks R, Inceoglu S: Primary pedicle screw augmentation in osteoporotic lumbar vertebrae: Biomechanical analysis of pedicle fixation strength. *Spine (Phila Pa 1976)* 2007;32(10):1077-1083.

    Pedicle screw augmentation with polymethylmethacrylate in cadaver vertebrae was found to improve the initial fixation strength and fatigue strength of instrumentation in osteoporotic vertebrae. Pedicle screws augmented with polymethylmethacrylate had significantly greater pullout strength than those placed in healthy control vertebrae with no augmentation. Level of evidence: III.

58. Aydogan M, Ozturk C, Karatoprak O, Tezer M, Aksu N, Hamzaoglu A: The pedicle screw fixation with vertebroplasty augmentation in the surgical treatment of the severe osteoporotic spines. *J Spinal Disord Tech* 2009;22(6):444-447.

    Forty-nine patients who underwent pedicle screw augmentation with polymethylmethacrylate were reviewed. All patients had the T-score value of less than −2.5. There were no proximal or distal junctional segment fractures at a minimum follow-up of 24 months. Level of evidence: IV.

59. Chang MC, Liu CL, Chen TH: Polymethylmethacrylate augmentation of pedicle screw for osteoporotic spinal surgery: A novel technique. *Spine (Phila Pa 1976)* 2008;33(10):E317-E324.

    Forty-one patients with osteoporosis who underwent spinal decompression and pedicle screw instrumentation with polymethylmethacrylate augmentation were studied. There were no reported instrumentation failures or adjacent-level fractures. Level of evidence: IV.

60. Li G, Passias P, Kozanek M, et al: Adult scoliosis in patients over sixty-five years of age: Outcomes of operative versus nonoperative treatment at a minimum two-year follow-up. *Spine (Phila Pa 1976)* 2009;34(20):2165-2170.

    This is a retrospective cohort review of 83 patients older than 65 years with adult scoliosis. The study compared the Scoliosis Research Society-22 Patient Questionnaire, SF-12, EQ5D, and Oswestry Disability Index scores between those treated surgically and nonsurgically. Patients treated with surgery had significantly less pain; better health, self-image, and mental health; and were more satisfied with their treatment than patients treated nonsurgically. Level of evidence: III.

61. Kim YJ, Bridwell KH, Lenke LG, Cho KJ, Edwards CC II, Rinella AS: Pseudarthrosis in adult spinal deformity following multisegmental instrumentation and arthrodesis. *J Bone Joint Surg Am* 2006;88(4):721-728.

62. Weistroffer JK, Perra JH, Lonstein JE, et al: Complications in long fusions to the sacrum for adult scoliosis: Minimum five-year analysis of fifty patients. *Spine (Phila Pa 1976)* 2008;33(13):1478-1483.

    The authors report on a retrospective study of complications in 50 adult patients with scoliosis who were treated with long fusions to the sacrum. Pseudarthrosis was reported in 24% of the patients.

63. Mulconrey DS, Bridwell KH, Flynn J, Cronen GA, Rose PS: Bone morphogenetic protein (RhBMP-2) as a substitute for iliac crest bone graft in multilevel adult spinal deformity surgery: Minimum two-year evaluation of fusion. *Spine (Phila Pa 1976)* 2008;33(20):2153-2159.

    Ninety-eight patients who underwent adult deformity surgery supplemented with the use of bone morphogenetic protein (RhBMP-2) were prospectively followed for a minimum of 24 months. The overall fusion rate was 95%. Level of evidence: III.

64. Anand N, Baron EM, Thaiyananthan G, Khalsa K, Goldstein TB: Minimally invasive multilevel percutaneous correction and fusion for adult lumbar degenerative scoliosis: A technique and feasibility study. *J Spinal Disord Tech* 2008;21(7):459-467.

    Twelve patients were treated with a transpsoas anterior approach for an anterior fusion using a PEEK (polyether-ether ketone) cage followed by percutaneous posterior pedicle screw fixation. The mean Cobb angle preoperatively was 19° and 6° postoperatively. Level of evidence: IV.

65. Ogilvie JW, Braun J, Argyle V, Nelson L, Meade M, Ward K: The search for idiopathic scoliosis genes. *Spine (Phila Pa 1976)* 2006;31(6):679-681.

protrusion extrusion sequest

Chapter 46

Lumbar Degenerative Disease

Wellington K. Hsu, MD

Introduction

Degenerative disorders of the lumbar spine are prevalent, affect quality of life, and are a major health care concern of the general population. These conditions lead to back, buttocks, and lower extremity symptoms that result in lost work days, permanent disability, and psychological sequelae. The evolution of the orthopaedic literature has provided algorithms for surgeons to prescribe nonsurgical and surgical care in common conditions such as lumbar disk herniation, spinal stenosis, and discogenic pain. It is important to review current concepts regarding the diagnosis, management, and treatment of these conditions.

Lumbar Spinal Stenosis

Pathoanatomy/Pathophysiology

Lumbar spinal stenosis is defined as the narrowing of the spinal canal in the lumbar region that is a consequence of several pathologic conditions, the most common of which is chronic degenerative spondylosis. Narrowing of the spinal canal can occur centrally or laterally, and although either can lead to a different set of symptoms, patients often present with a combination of both. Absolute stenosis has been defined as a decrease in the midsagittal lumbar canal diameter of less than 10 mm on MRI. Furthermore, where a normal cross-sectional area of the spinal canal on an axial MRI is defined as 150 to 200 mm², measurements of less than 100 mm² have been established as central spinal stenosis. However, despite these definitions, stenosis diagnosed with radiographs often does not lead to clinically significant symptoms. Common causes of central stenosis include congenital anomalies such as short pedicle length, ligamentum flavum hypertrophy, and broad-based disk-osteophyte complexes.

Lateral stenosis can be further classified into three distinct zones: the lateral recess, foraminal zone, and extraforaminal zone (**Figure 1**). Lateral recess stenosis

Dr. Hsu or an immediate family member serves as a paid consultant to or is an employee of Stryker and has received research or institutional support from Medtronic Sofamor Danek, Baxter Northwestern Alliance, and Pioneer Surgical.

is most commonly caused by osteophyte formation and overgrowth of the superior articular facet, and foraminal stenosis usually results from a foraminal disk protrusion, posterior osteophyte formation, or loss of vertical height from degenerative collapse of the disk. The extraforaminal zone, which is defined as the area lateral to the intervertebral foramen, is most often affected by far-lateral disk and osteophyte pathology.

Mild to moderate stenosis commonly leads to symptoms related to the dynamic position of the spine. Studies have shown that during terminal extension of the lumbar spine, the central canal and foraminal diameter decreases by 20% compared to its position in terminal flexion. For this reason, patients who experience symptoms with the spine in extension (standing and walking) that are relieved with sitting should be evaluated

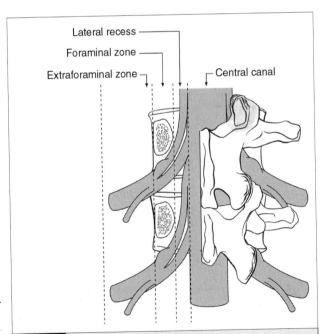

| Figure 1 | Illustration of lateral recess stenosis in which the superior articular process impinges on the traversing lumbar nerve root. The coronal section shows the relative positions of the central canal, lateral recess, foraminal zone, and extraforaminal zone. (Reproduced from Rao RD, David KS: Lumbar degenerative disorders, in Vaccaro AR, ed: *Orthopaedic Knowledge Update 8*. Rosemont, IL, American Academy of Orthopaedic Surgeons, 2005, pp 539-551.) |

5: Spine

Table 1

Distinguishing Features of Neurogenic and Vascular Claudication

Findings	Neurogenic Claudication	Vascular Claudication
Pain location	Back, buttocks, posterior thighs	Posterior calfs, heels
Radiation	Proximal to distal	Distal to proximal
Gait	Flexed posture	Upright, normal posture
Exacerbating activities	Lumbar extension, standing, walking	Any lower extremity activity
Relieving activities	Lumbar flexion, sitting	Cessation of lower extremity activity, *e.g. standing*
Lower extremity examination	Normal pulses, appearance	Diminished pulses, hair loss, diffuse edema, nail atrophy

for lumbar stenosis. These characteristics suggest that spinal stenosis is a threshold disease (having a critical spinal canal size before which patients are asymptomatic and beyond which the condition becomes apparent). Severe spinal stenosis can lead to pain that is not relieved with sitting. In these patients, the pathology may be so severe that the threshold of clinical symptoms is exceeded regardless of the position of the spine.

The symptoms associated with lumbar spinal stenosis are likely due to both mechanical and inflammatory causes. Mechanical compression results in local neural ischemia that can then lead to neuritis, reduced axonal transport, and decreased nutritional support. Because at least 50% of the vascular supply is dependent on cerebrospinal fluid diffusion, mild compression can significantly affect the local homeostasis of the involved nerve roots. Furthermore, increased neural tension can also lead to a host inflammatory response that can cause nerve irritation. Local release of inflammatory cytokines can lead to nerve root dysfunction and dorsal root ganglion irritation. There is evidence to support that a more rapid onset of canal compression leads to more severe symptoms than a chronic condition.

Clinical Presentation

Neurogenic claudication is classically described as back, buttocks, and/or posterior thigh pain that worsens with lumbar extension and is relieved by flexion. Unlike vascular claudication, pain is often more proximal in the lower extremities and is not relieved with standing (Table 1). Another common distinguishing factor between vascular and neurogenic claudication is the characteristic flexed posture on gait with lumbar stenosis that is typically not seen with peripheral vascular disease. Although central canal stenosis classically presents with bilateral lower extremity symptoms, lateral recess and foraminal stenosis can often lead to unilateral radicular pain that is worsened with extension and rotation to the affected side. Unlike radiculopathy from an acute disk herniation, pain from stenosis is not typically aggravated by sciatic tension signs such as a straight leg raise or sitting for prolonged periods of time.

Lumbar stenosis patients are also predisposed to developing concomitant pathologic changes in the cervi-

cal spine. The prevalence of tandem spinal stenosis in the lumbar stenosis patient population has been reported from 5% to 25%. A recent cadaver study reported a positive predictive value of 15.3% for the presence of cervical stenosis when lumbar stenosis was observed.[1] In cadavers with lumbar stenosis, the odds ratio for the presence of cervical stenosis was 3.58 as compared to those without lumbar findings. These studies indicate that surgeons should be keenly aware of the potential for significant and possibly asymptomatic cervical pathology during the evaluation of patients with lumbar degenerative conditions. All patients with symptomatic lumbar spinal stenosis should be questioned thoroughly on any potential symptoms of cervical myelopathy, with subsequent workup as appropriate.

Management

After the initial diagnostic evaluation with upright AP and lateral lumbar spine plain radiographs, MRI is the recommended advanced imaging modality to evaluate lumbar spinal stenosis. MRI has been shown to exhibit substantial interobserver and intraobserver reliability in the diagnosis of lumbar spinal stenosis.[2] When MRI is not possible because of the presence of ferromagnetic implants, CT myelography can be used in its place. CT is also more proficient at demonstrating bony changes, and may better demonstrate neurologic compression resulting from bony osteophytes. Although advanced imaging studies such as MRI and CT are primarily used in the diagnosis of lumbar stenosis, plain radiographs should also be carefully scrutinized to assess for degenerative instability, sagittal and coronal plane imbalance, and overall bone quality, as these conditions all are relevant in the management of this disorder.

Nonsurgical treatment with anti-inflammatory drugs, activity modification, exercise therapy, and epidural steroid injections is widely accepted as the first choice for management of lumbar spinal stenosis. Although the symptoms from lumbar stenosis often worsen with aging and the progression of spondylosis, a recent study has indicated that nonsurgical treatment can lead to maintenance of activities of daily living in most patients after 5-year follow-up.[3] Epidural steroid and/or selective nerve root injections can provide signif-

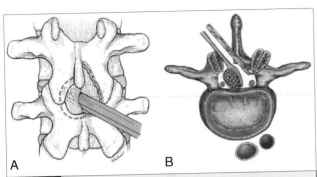

Figure 2 In a fenestration procedure, the interspinous ligament and spinous processes are preserved while the laminotomy is performed of the upper and lower lumbar segments (**A**). Through this limited approach, the undersurface of the spinous process can be resected toward the midline. Contralateral decompression after adequate dural retraction can also be performed (**B**). (Reproduced with permission from Singh K, Samartzis D, An H: Surgical techniques: Lumbar spinal stenosis. *J Am Acad Orthop Surg* 2008;16: pp 171-176.)

icant relief of the symptoms from spinal stenosis and delay the need for surgery for many patients. However, patients often experience only transient relief and require multiple injections to benefit on a long-term basis.

Surgical treatment is offered to those patients in whom initial nonsurgical therapies fail and who have significant symptoms that affect quality of life. The foundation of surgery for the treatment of lumbar spinal stenosis is an adequate decompression of the neural elements involved. Lumbar decompression usually involves resection of at least 50% of the cephalad and caudad spinous processes and associated lamina, which provides greater space for the neural elements at the level of the disk space. When advanced multilevel stenosis is diagnosed, more extensive laminectomy is required to decompress the neural elements behind the vertebral body. Care must be taken to preserve at least 50% of the facet anatomy bilaterally during decompression to avoid iatrogenic instability. Novel surgical techniques aim to preserve the midline structures such as the spinous processes and interspinous ligaments during decompression with the hope of offering long-term stability to the surgically treated lumbar segment. These techniques, often termed microdecompression, limited laminotomy, or fenestration, involve laminotomies and foraminotomies bilaterally that thoroughly decompress the nerve roots and cauda equina without resecting the superficial anatomic structures (**Figure 2**). Mild to moderate lumbar stenosis can often be treated adequately in this manner.

The results of surgical decompression were recently compared with those of nonsurgical treatment in a landmark study as part of the Spine Patient Outcomes Randomized Trial (SPORT).[4] In a clinical trial involving 654 patients, with both a randomized and observational cohort, surgical candidates with a history of at least 12 weeks of symptoms of spinal stenosis were enrolled. Patients with spondylolisthesis were excluded. Because of the high level of crossover in both patient cohorts (37% to 42%), an as-treated statistical data analysis was performed to compare clinical outcomes at various posttreatment time points from 6 weeks to 2 years. Evaluation of bodily pain and physical function scores on the Medical Outcomes Study 36-Item Short Form (SF-36) and modified Oswestry Disability Index scores demonstrated that patients who underwent surgery for lumbar spinal stenosis had a far better outcome than those treated nonsurgically as early as 6 weeks after treatment that persisted to final follow-up (2 years). The benefits from surgical treatment in spinal stenosis were significantly greater than those seen with intervertebral disk herniation from the same SPORT data because nonsurgical treatment was less effective in patients with stenosis. The significantly improved clinical outcomes from surgical treatment in comparison to nonsurgical therapies for lumbar spinal stenosis was also reported, where the effects were maintained 2 years after treatment.[5]

The indications to add a fusion procedure to surgical decompression in the treatment of lumbar spinal stenosis are the presence of degenerative spondylolisthesis, radiographic signs of instability such as scoliosis or vertebral body listhesis, or iatrogenic instability such as that created when greater than 50% of bilateral facets are removed. Recent studies in the patient population with spinal stenosis have suggested that those patients who achieve a successful lumbar fusion have superior outcomes compared to patients with pseudarthrosis.[6] Because the use of instrumentation in lumbar fusion has improved arthrodesis rates, it is thought by many authors that this leads to improved long-term clinical results. Clinical outcomes after lumbar fusion were recently stratified by diagnosis in a report of 327 patients.[7] In this study, evaluation of health-related quality of life data revealed the most substantial clinical improvement in those patients with a diagnosis of either spondylolisthesis or scoliosis. In comparison, patients with a diagnosis of adjacent segment disease with pseudarthrosis and postdiskectomy revision registered improvements in Oswestry Disability Index scores, but with smaller magnitudes of recovery.

Because lumbar spinal stenosis often affects patients older than 60 years, the associated risks and complications must be thoroughly considered before deciding on surgical treatment. As many recent studies have demonstrated the significant increase in complication risk in octogenarians, these patients must be made aware of the possible medical sequelae from surgical treatment. However, recent evidence has suggested that despite being exposed to this additional risk, patients age 60 years and older who undergo lumbar spine surgery have a reduced mortality compared to matched control subjects in the general population. In a cohort of 1,015 patients who underwent spine surgery for the diagnosis of lumbar spinal stenosis, Kaplan-Meier analyses revealed 10-year survival rates of 87.8% in patients age 60 to 70 years and 83.8% in those age 70 to 85 years,

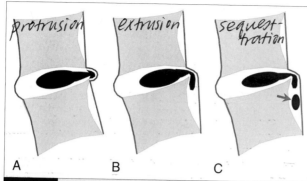

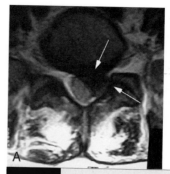

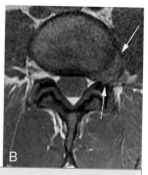

Figure 3 Schematic of different types of disk herniations. **A,** Protrusion with broad-based continuity between herniated and parent disk material. **B,** Inferior migration of disk material under the posterior longitudinal ligament. **C,** Sequestered disk fragment detached from and inferior to an extruded disk herniation. (Reproduced with permission from Fardon DF, Milette PC: Nomenclature and classification of lumbar disk pathology. *Spine* 2001;26:E93-E113.)

Figure 4 Disk herniations classified by relationship to the thecal sac. **A,** T2 axial MRI demonstrating a posterolateral disk herniation (*arrow*) typically compressing the traversing nerve root. **B,** T1 axial MRI showing a far-lateral or extraforaminal disk herniation affecting the exiting nerve root (*arrows*).

which were similar to that for joint arthroplasty surgery.[8] Furthermore, although total joint arthroplasty has been well accepted as an efficacious and cost-effective intervention, until recently, reports on the improvement in quality of life after surgical treatment of spinal stenosis have been lacking. In a study of 90 patients with a spinal decompression with or without fusion for lumbar spinal stenosis, quality-of-life measures as defined by SF-36 mental and physical component scores were compared to those after total hip and knee arthroplasty.[9] At 1- and 2-year follow-up, clinical improvement as measured by SF-36 questionnaires was comparable for patients treated surgically for spinal stenosis and joint osteoarthritis. Because total hip and knee arthroplasty patients reportedly have some of the highest self-reported quality-of-life scores in any surgical procedure, these clinical results are favorable for the surgical treatment of spinal stenosis.

Lumbar Disk Herniation

Pathoanatomy
A lumbar disk herniation is defined as a local displacement of disk contents beyond the circumferential borders of the intervertebral disk space that can lead to compression of the neural elements posteriorly.[10] A herniated disk may present as a protrusion, defined as a broad-based displacement where disk material is continuous with that of the intervertebral disk space, or extrusion, when the diameter of the disk material in the canal is greater than the distance between the edges of the base (**Figure 3**). Extrusions are termed sequestrations if no continuity exists between disk material in the spinal canal and the parent disk. Fragments can also migrate in any direction away from the site of extrusion.

Herniations are also categorized based on location of the disk fragment in relationship to the thecal sac: central, posterolateral, foraminal, or extraforaminal. Posterolateral disk herniations commonly compress the traversing nerve root at a particular level (for example, the L5 root at the L4-5 level) while the foraminal and extraforaminal (far-lateral) disk fragments affect the exiting nerve root (for example, the L4 root at the L4-5 level) (**Figure 4**). The type of disk herniation has potential implications on outcome; however, a recent study comparing lumbar disk herniation morphology on MRI between clinicians and radiologists revealed only fair agreement.[2]

Pathophysiology
The pathways by which a disk herniation can lead to radicular pain likely involve both mechanical and chemical irritation of the nerve root. Mechanical compression can lead to nerve root deformation, local ischemia, and subsequent radiating neuritis. A compounding factor with a disk herniation is the chemical effect of nucleus pulposus material directly on the nerve root that leads to the release of several inflammatory cytokines. Tumor necrosis factor-α (TNF-α), which is produced by intervertebral disk cells, has been implicated in this process. TNF-α has been demonstrated to increase localized sodium channel accretion, which predisposes nerve roots to irritation from mechanical compression. These theories are supported by animal studies that have demonstrated increased edema, fibrosis, and demyelination after exposing nerve tissue to nucleus pulposus extracts. Other cytokines have been implicated in the cause of radicular pain such as interleukin-1β, interleukin-6, prostaglandin-E2, and phospholipase-A2, which have been found in high concentrations around the nerve root and dorsal root ganglion. These factors likely act as chemical modulators of pain.[11]

[handwritten] cytokines

[handwritten] remember: nucleus pulposus is immunoprivileged → seen as foreign ... & ... elicits strong immune response

Clinical Presentation

Lumbar disk herniations usually lead to radicular complaints including pain, paresthesias, and weakness down the lower extremity in a dermatomal distribution. Referred pain, or sclerotomal pain, is characterized by pain in the low back, buttocks, or posterior thigh and originates from mesodermal tissue such as muscles, ligaments, or periosteum. Ninety-three percent of all disk herniations occur at either the L4-L5 or L5-S1 level.[12]

Patients sometimes report worsening symptoms with sitting, which places tension on the lower lumbar nerve roots. The straight leg raise test is positive when concordant, lower extremity radiculopathy is re-created with leg elevation of 35° to 70°. This test, which has demonstrated a high sensitivity but low specificity, is believed to manually stretch the L5 and S1 nerve roots on the unilateral side. The straight leg raise test on the contralateral side, which produces concordant leg symptoms with contralateral leg elevation, has a lower sensitivity but higher specificity for L4-L5 and L5-S1 disk herniations. The femoral stretch test is useful for pathology of the upper lumbar roots (L1-4), which is performed with ipsilateral hip extension and knee flexion. This test is confirmatory when it reproduces anterior thigh pain.

Severe compression of the nerve roots in the lumbosacral spine by a large disk herniation can lead to cauda equina syndrome, which is characterized by saddle anesthesia, urinary retention and overflow incontinence, impotence, bilateral leg pain, and lower extremity weakness. The severity of these symptoms increases the urgency of surgical decompression. Although clinical studies have disagreed on the exact recommendation for the timing of decompression for cauda equina syndrome, evidence suggests that longer duration and increased severity of significant symptoms lead to an increased risk of poor results. Consequently, most surgeons would advocate for decompression as soon as possible to optimize outcome. Patients with cauda equina syndrome with surgical decompression more than 48 hours after demonstrating symptoms are at greater risk for permanent urologic and sexual dysfunction, leg weakness, and chronic pain than those treated within 48 hours of symptom onset.

Management

Because most patients improve clinically within a 6-week period after the onset of back pain and radiculopathy, nonsurgical modalities are the initial mainstays of treatment. These include activity modification, physical therapy, anti-inflammatory medications, and epidural steroid injections. Although none of these treatments have been shown to alter the natural history of a lumbar disk herniation, they provide relief while the radicular symptoms can dissipate naturally. Most surgeons advocate for nonsurgical treatment of at least 6 weeks before considering other more invasive measures.

Epidural steroid injections are a low-risk alternative to surgical treatment of lumbar disk herniation. A randomized controlled trial demonstrated that 50% of patients who received an epidural steroid injection to treat a lumbar disk herniation avoided surgical intervention.[13] Although this study showed a higher satisfaction rate for patients who underwent diskectomy, the results suggest that for those who wish to avoid surgery, epidural injections can confer some pain relief and in some cases help the patient avoid a surgical procedure. Other studies of outcomes after selective nerve root injections reveal similar results in patients with lumbar radiculopathy.

The surgical treatment of a lumbar disk herniation isa diskectomy and laminotomy. Recent studies from SPORT investigators have demonstrated the improved clinical outcomes after surgery in comparison with nonsurgical treatment.[12] *SPORT Trial* Because of the inherent difficulties of randomized clinical trials in a surgical patient population, high rates of nonadherence to treatment assignment have led to several difficulties in the interpretation of the intent-to-treat statistical analyses for the SPORT studies. High crossover rates lead to a bias toward the null hypothesis in intent-to-treat analyses that inherently underestimates the true effect of surgery. However, as-treated analyses of outcome measures have suggested the advantages of surgical treatment when compared to the nonsurgical cohort. The 4-year results after continued follow-up of the randomized and observational SPORT trial revealed greater improvement in pain, function, satisfaction, and self-rated progress in the diskectomy group when compared to those treated nonsurgically. These significant improvements were seen as early as 6 weeks after surgery and reached maximum benefit by 6 months. At the 4-year time point, improvement was seen in all primary and secondary outcome measures except for work status. These authors conclude that after initial nonsurgical treatment of 6 weeks, surgery was superior to nonsurgical care in improving functional status and treating radiculopathy.[12]

Amid concerns of the surgical costs of care for spinal disorders, a follow-up study on the same patient population evaluated the cost effectiveness of surgical treatment of a lumbar disk herniation.[14] Quality-adjusted life-years (QALY), which account for both quality and length of life, have been used for the assessment of the value of interventions in health and medicine across many subspecialties. Although surgery was initially more costly than nonsurgical treatment, clinical outcomes assessed at 2-year follow-up were superior in the surgical group. The cost per QALY gained for the surgical group was estimated at $34,355 and $69,403 for the Medicare and general populations, respectively.[14] As the authors pointed out, this cost ratio compares favorably with accepted medical interventions such as that for hypertension in 60-year-old men ($59,500 per QALY).

Although diskectomy technique has changed over the past two decades, recent studies have suggested that a simple sequestrectomy, or a removal of only the disk fragments in the spinal canal and not in the disk space, can lead to excellent if not better clinical and radio-

5: Spine

graphic results than a conventional surgical protocol. In a study that compared the 2-year outcomes of patients who underwent a sequestrectomy, or a standard diskectomy in which disk tissue was removed from the intervertebral disk space, both cohorts significantly improved similarly within a 6-month period.[15] However, with measurements of parameters such as overall outcome, health-related quality-of-life scores, and analgesic use, the sequestrectomy group demonstrated significantly better outcomes. Furthermore, reherniation rates in both groups were not significantly different at 2 years. The authors postulated that more extensive removal of disk tissue can lead to pathologic changes that may manifest as increased low back pain at long-term follow-up, which can lead to significantly worse clinical outcome. A follow-up study of the same patient cohorts demonstrated significantly greater disk height loss and degeneration in the diskectomy patients at 2-year follow-up.[16] These conclusions were supported by an evidence-based review of the literature that compared conservative and aggressive approaches during a diskectomy.[17] An aggressive approach was defined as a complete removal of disk fragments with curettage of the disk space whereas a conservative diskectomy used a smaller incision with little invasion of the disk space. Similarly, these authors concluded that a more conservative approach to disk removal can lead to shorter surgical times, faster return to work, and decreased long-term back pain. However, this review did reveal a higher incidence of recurrent disk herniation in this group when compared to an "aggressive" approach.

The ability to access the neural elements through small incisions and tubular retractor systems has spawned several minimally invasive surgical techniques, with the hope that muscle-splitting approaches will result in less tissue damage and reduced postoperative morbidity compared to conventional open approaches. Earlier studies have suggested similar clinical outcomes in both of these patient groups. However, a double-blinded, randomized controlled trial in 328 patients comparing the two techniques demonstrated significantly better clinical outcomes in self-reported leg pain, back pain, and recovery rates in the conventional diskectomy cohort at 2-year follow-up.[18] The reason for these results are unclear; however, incomplete decompression of the neural elements from limited visualization in a tubular approach remains a concern for the use of this technique.

Outcomes

Although the symptoms and morphologic features of lumbar disk herniations have been studied for years, there are controversies regarding the significance of these characteristics. For example, although lumbar diskectomy has been widely thought to successfully relieve radicular pain, postoperative outcomes of low back pain are unclear. Historically, it has been thought that degenerative changes within the disk are the cause of axial symptoms that could not be relieved by nerve root decompression. However, as part of the SPORT study, a greater, more statistically significant improvement in back pain was reported as measured on a six-point scale in the diskectomy group as compared to the nonsurgical cohort.[19] Furthermore, this study demonstrated that central disk herniations were associated with more severe axial back pain than posterolateral extrusions and that after diskectomy, these patients had as successful a clinical outcome as the overall surgical cohort.

Although most lumbar disk herniations occur at the L4-L5 or L5-S1 level, significant disk pathology is also seen at the upper lumbar segments (L2-L3 and L3-L4). The greatest treatment effects from surgery were reported at these upper lumbar levels (L2-L3 and L3-L4) when compared to those seen at L4-L5 and L5-S1.[20] The authors pointed out that the primary reason for this finding was not the absolute improvement in the surgical cohort but rather the paucity of success of nonsurgical treatment in the upper lumbar level group. One possible explanation for this finding is that the cross-sectional area for the spinal canal at the upper lumbar levels is significantly smaller than the lower segments, leading to a greater intensity of symptoms. The authors also noted that upper lumbar herniations were more likely to appear in the far lateral and foraminal positions, which may be less likely to respond to nonsurgical care.

Discogenic Low Back Pain

A degenerated intervertebral disk is characterized by hydration loss, disk space narrowing, annular tears, and, ultimately, ankylosis across the lumbar segment. Discogenic pain refers to axial midline low back pain without radicular symptoms attributable to the arthritic disk pathology. However, the ubiquitous nature of degenerative disk disease and of low back pain in the general population has led to significant controversy in the diagnosis and management of this condition. Degenerative changes of the spine are prevalent in all age groups and are demonstrated in over 75% of the population older than 60 years.[21] Although 80% of the US population will experience an episode of low back pain at some point in their lifetime, only 1% of these patients will require long-term treatment. Because most individuals will not require prolonged treatment of low back pain even in the setting of lumbar degenerative spondylosis, there is difficulty in attributing back pain to degenerative disks.

Diagnostic Imaging

Plain AP and lateral radiographs are initial, inexpensive imaging tests in the assessment of discogenic pain. These images may show various signs of spondylosis, including disk space narrowing, endplate sclerosis, marginal osteophytes, instability, and facet degeneration. Flexion and extension lumbar radiographs may demonstrate further mobility across a lumbar segment; however, the tradeoff of additional irradiation for clinical

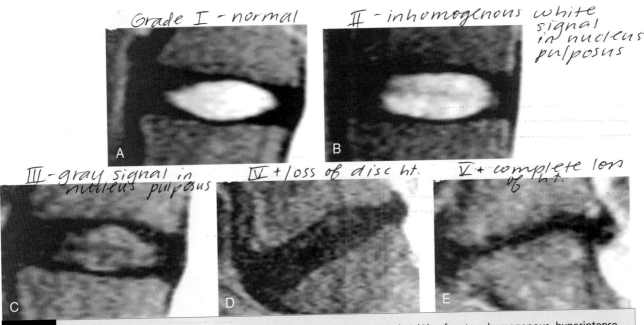

Handwritten annotations:
Grade I - normal
II - inhomogenous white signal in nucleus pulposus
III - gray signal in nucleus pulposus
IV + loss of disc ht.
V + complete loss of ht.

Figure 5 Grading system for the assessment of lumbar disk degeneration. Grade I (**A**) refers to a homogenous, hyperintense signal intensity within the disk space with normal height. Grade II (**B**) changes are defined as inhomogenous white signals with normal height. An intermediate gray signal intensity within the nucleus pulposus (**C**) is a grade III disk. Grade IV (**D**) changes are characterized by hypointense dark gray signals with mild loss of disc height. Grade V (**E**) disks have space collapse with complete loss of height. (Adapted with permission from Pfirrmann CW, Metzdorf A, Zanetti M, et al: Magnetic resonance classification of lumbar intervertebral disc degeneration. *Spine* 2001;26: 1873-1878.)

utility has led many authors to question the routine use of these images.[22]

MRI provides a much more detailed view of intervertebral disk pathology and is highly sensitive to degenerative changes. Internal disk disruption, which often cannot be seen on plain radiography, can be diagnosed on MRI with loss of signal intensity on T2-weighted images, suggesting loss of water content (**Figure 5**). Furthermore, annular tears can also be seen in the form of high-intensity zones, which is another sign of internal disk derangement. Bone marrow changes as a result of vertebral end plate changes have been associated with degenerative intervertebral disk disease. These changes have been classified into three types on the basis of chronicity of the degeneration (**Table 2**). Type I lesions are characterized by early fissuring of the cartilaginous end plate and acute vascularity within the subchondral bone (**Figure 6, A and B**). Type II changes demonstrate fatty degeneration of the adjacent bone marrow (**Figure 6, C and D**). Type III Modic findings reflect an advanced form of arthritis associated with subchondral bone sclerosis and loss of cancellous bone.

Despite the inherent value of the anatomic detail from MRI, the clinical significance of these findings is difficult to determine. Although the presence of high-intensity zones has been thought by many to correlate with chronic back pain, recent studies have suggested that this lesion does not reliably lead to a diagnosis of internal disk disruption.[23,24]

Epidemiologic studies on the relationship between lumbar spondylosis and back pain cite many confounding factors of outcome including abnormal psychomet-

Table 2

Modic Classification of Signal Changes on MRI in the Vertebral Body Marrow Adjacent to End Plates

Stage	Vertebral Body Changes
Type I	T1 – decreased signal T2 – increased signal *(acute vascularity)*
Type II	T1 – increased signal T2 – increased signal *(fatty degen.)*
Type III	T1 – decreased signal T2 – decreased signal *(sclerosis)*

ric testing, cigarette smoking, personality disorders, ongoing litigation, associated workers' compensation claims, job satisfaction, and body habitus. Furthermore, several studies have sought to correlate the presence of Modic changes with clinical symptoms; however, the results are controversial. One recent study has demonstrated that both Modic type I lesions and those changes that are seen at the L5-S1 segment are more likely to be associated with significant pain symptoms.[25] The results suggest that type I lesions may represent an early derangement phase in a pain condition that may later stabilize as disk degeneration progresses.

Provocative diskography has historically been used in confirming the diagnosis of discogenic pain. A positive result is defined as a concordant pain response elic-

Handwritten margin note: Can modic changes be correlated c pain?

Handwritten note: provocative diskography not very useful / not consistent results, many negative consequences

Type I Modic

T1   T2   *Type II Modic*   T2   T1

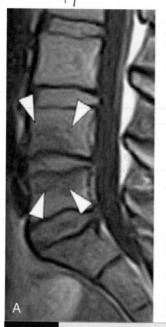
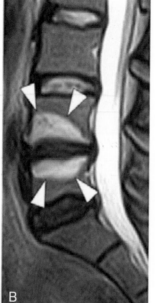
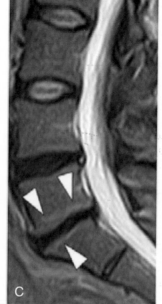
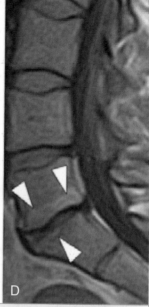

A   B   C   D

Figure 6 Typical Modic type I (**A, B**) and type II (**C, D**) changes in lumbar degenerative disk disease. Type I changes are characterized by a low intensity signal on T1-weighted (**A**) and high intensity signal on T2-weighted images (**B**). More advanced Modic type II changes are defined as high intensity signals on both T2-weighted (**C**) and T1-weighted (**D**) sagittal images. (Reproduced with permission from Albert HB, Kjaer P, Jensen TS, et al: Modic changes, possible causes, and relation to low back pain. *Med Hypothesis* 2008;70:361-368. http://www.sciencedirect.com/science/journal/03069877.)

ited from the patient with the injection of an intervertebral disk with abnormal morphology in the setting of negative control lumbar levels. It stands to reason that patients with a positive diskogram suffer from discogenic low back pain and have a higher likelihood of clinical success from a lumbar fusion. However, significant controversy in the evaluation of diskography as a diagnostic tool exists because of its operator-dependent nature, the heterogeneity of the study subjects involved, and conflicting clinical outcomes. A series of studies evaluating diskography have shown high false-positive rates (25%) in asymptomatic patients, high false-negative rates (30%) in patients with chronic low back pain, and poor positive predictive values. Furthermore, a recent study suggests that disk levels exposed to diskography result in accelerated disk degeneration, disk herniation, and end plate changes compared to matched control subjects as seen on MRI at 10-year follow-up.[26] The literature refutes diskography as a stand-alone diagnostic measure with poor predictive value, and at best, supports its use as either a confirmatory test or one piece of a complex diagnostic puzzle.

Clinical Features

Lumbar discogenic pain is classically described as a deep, aching low back pain that is mechanical in nature. Sitting, standing, bending, and axial loading are thought to exacerbate these symptoms, while rest and a supine position may provide relief. Patients often experience pain in both flexion and extension and have decreased range of motion compared to asymptomatic patients. Physical examination findings are often non-

specific and of little use in the diagnosis. Some have postulated that because instability of a lumbar motion segment is one cause of low back pain, disk degeneration may lead to micromotion that is the root cause of axial pain in these patients. However, because no diagnostic methods exist that can help elucidate this hypothesis, it remains an area for future study.

Management/Treatment

A multifaceted approach to nonsurgical care in the form of anti-inflammatory medications, fitness programs, weight loss, and functional rehabilitation remains the first-line treatment of discogenic back pain. For most patients with this condition, these measures are often effective in managing symptoms until the episode resolves. Other nonsurgical measures such as acupuncture, behavioral therapy, and exercise therapy have also demonstrated modest improvement in symptoms.[27] Although multiple different physical therapy modalities have been compared, no single program has demonstrated greater efficacy over another. Transcutaneous electrical nerve stimulation, muscle stimulation protocols, traction, and chiropractic treatment have not demonstrated long-term efficacy in the management of low back pain.[27]

When multiple modalities of nonsurgical management fail in patients diagnosed with discogenic low back pain, there are limited options for further treatment. Surgical treatment is considered a last-resort option for the patient who endures intractable symptoms for a 6-month period; however, controversy remains among experienced practitioners regarding the exact

no clear indications for surgery

surgical indications. Lumbar fusion has historically been used in the surgical treatment of degenerative disk disease; however, reported clinical outcomes are widely variable. An individual patient's response to surgery can be affected by association with workers' compensation, psychosocial comorbidities, and unrealistic expectations.

The advantages of an anterior lumbar interbody fusion (ALIF) include the avoidance of posterior muscle dissection and improved access to remove the lumbar disk resulting in increased surface area for bony healing. The potential disadvantages are the need for an access surgeon, risk of great vessel damage, and retrograde ejaculation. A recent study reported the clinical and radiographic outcomes of patients who underwent a stand-alone ALIF for the diagnosis of degenerative disk disease at the L4-L5 or L5-S1 levels with at least six-year follow-up.[28] In this study, patients were treated with recombinant human bone morphogenetic protein-2 and titanium-tapered cages at a single lumbar level. At the 6-year time point, 128 of 130 patients had a radiographically solid fusion. Clinical outcomes as determined by Oswestry Disability Index, SF-36, and back and leg pain scores demonstrated significant improvement as early as 6 weeks after surgery and sustained benefit at 6 years. The secondary surgery rate was 10% over the life of the study; however, there were no reports of vessel damage, retrograde ejaculation, or long-term complications. Lumbar total disk arthroplasty has been studied as an alternative to ALIF for the treatment of discogenic back pain; lumbar disk arthroplasty is also discussed in chapter 45.

From a posterior approach, in addition to an intertransverse fusion, either a transforaminal lumbar interbody fusion (TLIF) or a posterior lumbar interbody fusion can be performed. Both of these techniques allow for the direct decompression of the neural elements, removal of disk, and screw instrumentation through a single posterior approach. Used with posterior pedicle screw instrumentation, interbody fusions provide a 360° fusion construct that may enhance lumbar fusion rates compared to a posterolateral fusion alone. TLIF has demonstrated a lower incidence of postoperative radiculitis because of less neural retraction as compared to a posterior lumbar interbody fusion. In a retrospective analysis of 167 patients, TLIF was compared to anterior-posterior reconstructive surgery in the treatment of several degenerative conditions in the lumbar spine.[29] The authors concluded that an anterior-posterior procedure leads to significantly longer surgical and hospitalization time, increased blood loss, and twice the complication rate as does TLIF.

The outcomes of lumbar fusion for degenerative disk disease vary based upon source, patient selection criteria, outcome measures, and comorbidities. A wide spread of clinical outcomes has been reported in the literature. However, studies published in the past decade have increased understanding of the importance of patient selection and expectations from a surgical procedure. A recent systematic review compiled the literature reporting outcomes from fusion for several diagnoses.

importance of patient selection!

The authors concluded that although patients with an indication of spondylolisthesis experienced the best outcomes, fusion for the diagnosis of degenerative disk disease can lead to improved clinical outcomes.[30]

Annotated References

1. Lee MJ, Garcia R, Cassinelli EH, Furey C, Riew KD: Tandem stenosis: A cadaveric study in osseous morphology. *Spine J* 2008;8(6):1003-1006.

   The midsagittal canal diameter of cervical and lumbar spines of 440 adult skeletons from the Hamann-Todd Collection at the Cleveland Museum of Natural History was measured with digital calipers. The study demonstrated that the presence of lumbar spinal stenosis has a 15.3% positive predictive value for cervical stenosis. Level of evidence: IV.

2. Lurie JD, Doman DM, Spratt KF, Tosteson AN, Weinstein JN: Magnetic resonance imaging interpretation in patients with symptomatic lumbar spine disc herniations: Comparison of clinician and radiologist readings. *Spine (Phila Pa 1976)* 2009;34(7):701-705.

   Examination of the radiology reports from 396 patients as part of the SPORT trial demonstrated that in 42.2% of cases, the radiology reports did not clearly describe the morphology of the disk herniation. Although agreement of MRI readings between clinicians and radiologists was excellent for level and location of the disk herniation, it was only fair comparing herniation morphology. Level of evidence: IV.

3. Miyamoto H, Sumi M, Uno K, Tadokoro K, Mizuno K: Clinical outcome of nonoperative treatment for lumbar spinal stenosis, and predictive factors relating to prognosis, in a 5-year minimum follow-up. *J Spinal Disord Tech* 2008;21(8):563-568.

   A prospective study of 120 patients who received inpatient treatment of lumbar spinal stenosis in the form of anti-inflammatory medications and caudal blocks was conducted for a minimum of 5 years. In 52.5% of patients, clinical outcome was the same or better at final follow-up with patients classified as radicular type exhibiting better results than other subjects. Level of evidence: IV.

4. Weinstein JN, Tosteson TD, Lurie JD, et al; SPORT Investigators: Surgical versus nonsurgical therapy for lumbar spinal stenosis. *N Engl J Med* 2008;358(8):794-810.

   In an as-treated statistical analysis of 289 patients in a randomized cohort and 365 patients in an observational cohort with lumbar spinal stenosis, patients who underwent decompressive surgery demonstrated a significant advantage by 3 months for all primary outcome measures that remained significant at 2 years compared to nonsurgical care. Level of evidence: II.

5. Malmivaara A, Slätis P, Heliövaara M, et al; Finnish Lumbar Spinal Research Group: Surgical or nonoperative treatment for lumbar spinal stenosis? A randomized controlled trial. *Spine (Phila Pa 1976)* 2007;32(1):1-8.

5: Spine

In a randomized controlled trial of 94 patients for the surgical and nonsurgical treatment of spinal stenosis, those undergoing decompressive surgery reported greater improvement regarding leg pain, back pain, and overall disability compared with those patients who received nonsurgical care. Level of evidence: I.

6. Kornblum MB, Fischgrund JS, Herkowitz HN, Abraham DA, Berkower DL, Ditkoff JS: Degenerative lumbar spondylolisthesis with spinal stenosis: A prospective long-term study comparing fusion and pseudarthrosis. *Spine (Phila Pa 1976)* 2004;29(7):726-733, discussion 733-734.

7. Glassman SD, Carreon LY, Djurasovic M, et al: Lumbar fusion outcomes stratified by specific diagnostic indication. *Spine J* 2009;9(1):13-21.

    In a prospective study in 327 patients with a decompression and posterolateral lumbar fusion, overall clinical outcome was stratified by and correlated to initial diagnosis. The greatest improvement in Oswestry Disability Index scores were seen in patients with spondylolisthesis and scoliosis, whereas patients with disk pathology, postdiskectomy revision, instability, stenosis, and adjacent segment degeneration had a smaller magnitude of improvement. Level of evidence: II.

8. Kim HJ, Lee HM, Kim HS, et al: Life expectancy after lumbar spine surgery: One- to eleven-year follow-up of 1015 patients. *Spine (Phila Pa 1976)* 2008;33(19):2116-2121, discussion 2122-2123.

    The 10-year survival of 1,015 elderly patients older than 50 years was documented following spine surgery for lumbar spinal stenosis. The overall 10-year survival rate in patients 60 to 70 years old was 87.7%, and 83.8% in patients 70 to 85 years old. These patients had reduced mortality in comparison with the corresponding portion of the general population. Level of evidence: III.

9. Rampersaud YR, Ravi B, Lewis SJ, et al: Assessment of health-related quality of life after surgical treatment of focal symptomatic spinal stenosis compared with osteoarthritis of the hip or knee. *Spine J* 2008;8(2):296-304.

    Patients who underwent surgical treatment for spinal stenosis were compared with a matched cohort of patients who underwent total hip or total knee arthroplasty for osteoarthritis. Clinical outcomes at 1- and 2-year follow-up demonstrate that spinal stenosis surgery can lead to improvement in self-reported quality-of-life scores comparable to those of total hip and knee arthroplasty patients. Level of evidence: III.

10. Fardon DF, Milette PC; Combined Task Forces of the North American Spine Society, American Society of Spine Radiology, and American Society of Neuroradiology: Nomenclature and classification of lumbar disc pathology: Recommendations of the Combined Task Forces of the North American Spine Society, American Society of Spine Radiology, and American Society of Neuroradiology. *Spine (Phila Pa 1976)* 2001;26(5):E93-E113.

11. Doita M, Kanatani T, Harada T, Mizuno K: Immunohistologic study of the ruptured intervertebral disc of the lumbar spine. *Spine* 1996;21:235-241.

12. Weinstein JN, Lurie JD, Tosteson TD, et al: Surgical versus nonoperative treatment for lumbar disc herniation: Four-year results for the Spine Patient Outcomes Research Trial (SPORT). *Spine (Phila Pa 1976)* 2008; 33(25):2789-2800.

    Five hundred one participants enrolled in a prospective, randomized controlled trial and 743 patients in an observational cohort were treated for lumbar disk herniation with either standard open diskectomy or nonsurgical care. As-treated statistical analysis 4 years after treatment demonstrated greater improvement in all primary and secondary outcome measures after surgical treatment for lumbar disk herniation except work status. Level of evidence: II.

13. Buttermann GR: Treatment of lumbar disc herniation: Epidural steroid injection compared with discectomy. A prospective randomized study. *J Bone Joint Surg Am* 2004;86:670-679.

14. Tosteson AN, Skinner JS, Tosteson TD, et al: The cost effectiveness of surgical versus nonoperative treatment for lumbar disc herniation over two years: Evidence from the Spine Patient Outcomes Research Trial (SPORT). *Spine (Phila Pa 1976)* 2008;33(19):2108-2115.

    Using discounted cost per QALY, cost effectiveness of surgical treatment compared with nonsurgical treatment for lumbar disk herniation was evaluated. Using the patient population from the SPORT randomized and observational cohorts, at 2 years, although surgical treatment was cost effective when compared with nonsurgical treatment, the estimated economic value of surgery varied according to method of surgical cost assignment. Level of evidence: III.

15. Barth M, Weiss C, Thomé C: Two-year outcome after lumbar microdiscectomy versus microscopic sequestrectomy: Part 1. Evaluation of clinical outcome. *Spine (Phila Pa 1976)* 2008;33(3):265-272.

    Eighty-four patients with lumbar disk herniations randomized to either treatment with microdiskectomy or microscopic sequestrectomy were evaluated for clinical outcome with at least 2-year follow-up. Although both patient groups dramatically improved immediately after surgery, self-rated assessment scores continued to improve within 2 years after sequestrectomy as opposed to deterioration in the microdiskectomy group. Reherniation rates were not significantly different between the two groups. Level of evidence: I.

16. Barth M, Diepers M, Weiss C, Thomé C: Two-year outcome after lumbar microdiscectomy versus microscopic sequestrectomy: Part 2. Radiographic evaluation and correlation with clinical outcome. *Spine (Phila Pa 1976)* 2008;33(3):273-279.

    Eighty-four patients with lumbar disk herniations randomized to treatment with either microdiskectomy or simple fracture excision (sequestrectomy) underwent repeat MRI of the lumbar spine at 2-year follow-up. Modic-type end plate changes correlated with unfavorable clinical outcome after surgical treatment, and sequestrectomy demonstrated significantly less postoperative disk degeneration than standard microdiskectomy at final follow-up. Level of evidence: II.

17. Watters WC III, McGirt MJ: An evidence-based review of the literature on the consequences of conservative versus aggressive discectomy for the treatment of primary disc herniation with radiculopathy. *Spine J* 2009; 9(3):240-257.

A systematic evidence-based review of all published studies of outcomes after aggressive or conservative diskectomy was performed. Although there were no level I studies reviewed, the authors concluded that conservative diskectomy may lead to shorter surgery time, quicker return to work, and decreased incidence of long-term low back pain. However, conservative diskectomy may also lead to increased incidence of recurrent disk herniation. Level of evidence: III.

18. Arts MP, Brand R, van den Akker ME, Koes BW, Bartels RH, Peul WC; Leiden-The Hague Spine Intervention Prognostic Study Group (SIPS): Tubular diskectomy vs conventional microdiskectomy for sciatica: A randomized controlled trial. *JAMA* 2009;302(2):149-158.

A prospective controlled trial of 328 patients with radiculopathy from a lumbar disk herniation was randomized to treatment with either a tubular or conventional microdiskectomy. Using clinical outcome scores for up to 1 year after randomization, patients who underwent tubular diskectomy reported less favorable results for self-reported leg pain, back pain, and recovery. Level of evidence: I.

19. Pearson AM, Blood EA, Frymoyer JW, et al: SPORT lumbar intervertebral disk herniation and back pain: Does treatment, location, or morphology matter? *Spine (Phila Pa 1976)* 2008;33(4):428-435.

A combined analysis of 1,191 patients enrolled in the SPORT study randomized to surgical or nonsurgical treatment of lumbar disk herniations reported a significant improvement in back pain in the surgical group compared with those treated nonsurgically at 2-year follow-up. Level of evidence: III.

20. Lurie JD, Faucett SC, Hanscom B, et al: Lumbar discectomy outcomes vary by herniation level in the Spine Patient Outcomes Research Trial. *J Bone Joint Surg Am* 2008;90(9):1811-1819.

A retrospective review of 1,190 patients enrolled in the SPORT study for lumbar disk herniations correlated level of herniation to clinical outcome. At 2-year follow-up, patients with upper lumbar herniations (L3-4 and L2-3) showed a significantly greater treatment effect from surgery than did patients with L5-S1 disk herniations. This finding may have been a result of less improvement from nonsurgical treatment in the upper lumbar herniation group. Level of evidence: III.

21. Muraki S, Oka H, Akune T, et al: Prevalence of radiographic lumbar spondylosis and its association with low back pain in elderly subjects of population-based cohorts: The ROAD study. *Ann Rheum Dis* 2009;68(9):1401-1406.

The Research on Osteoarthritis Against Disability (ROAD) study evaluated 2,288 patients age 60 years or older. Clinically significant spondylosis was diagnosied in 75.8% of patients in the study, with age and body

mass index as risk factors for developing arthritic changes. Level of evidence: IV.

22. Hammouri QM, Haims AH, Simpson AK, Alqaqa A, Grauer JN: The utility of dynamic flexion-extension radiographs in the initial evaluation of the degenerative lumbar spine. *Spine (Phila Pa 1976)* 2007;32(21):2361-2364.

Of 342 plain radiographic series in the initial evaluation of the degenerative lumbar spine including flexion and extension films, only 2 had new findings not appreciated on the AP and lateral films. The authors concluded that dynamic radiographs did not significantly alter the initial course of clinical management. Level of evidence: IV.

23. Kleinstück F, Dvorak J, Mannion AF: Are "structural abnormalities" on magnetic resonance imaging a contraindication to the successful surgical treatment of chronic nonspecific low back pain? *Spine* 2006;31(19): 2250-2257.

24. Jarvik JJ, Hollingworth W, Heagerty P, Haynor DR, Deyo RA: The Longitudinal Assessment of Imaging and Disability of the Back (LAIDBack) Study: Baseline data. *Spine* 2001;26:1158-1166.

25. Kuisma M, Karppinen J, Niinimäki J, et al: Modic changes in endplates of lumbar vertebral bodies: Prevalence and association with low back and sciatic pain among middle-aged male workers. *Spine (Phila Pa 1976)* 2007;32(10):1116-1122.

In a cross-sectional study comparing self-reported low back pain symptoms and Modic changes on MRI in 228 middle-aged male workers (159 train engineers and 69 sedentary control subjects), Modic type I lesions and significant end plate changes seen at the L5-S1 level were more likely to be associated with low back pain than that seen at other lumbar levels. Level of evidence: III.

26. Carragee EJ, Don AS, Hurwitz EL, Cuellar JM, Carrino JA, Herzog R: 2009 ISSLS Prize Winner: Does discography cause accelerated progression of degeneration changes in the lumbar disc. A ten-year matched cohort study. *Spine (Phila Pa 1976)* 2009;34(21):2338-2345.

The authors concluded that modern diskography techniques resulted in accelerated disk degeneration, disk herniation, loss of disk height and signal, and the development of end plate changes.

27. Keller A, Hayden J, Bombardier C, van Tulder M: Effect sizes of non-surgical treatments of non-specific low-back pain. *Eur Spine J* 2007;16(11):1776-1788.

In a review of randomized controlled trials from systematic reviews of treatment of acute low back pain, there was a modest effect size of NSAIDs and manipulation, and for chronic low back pain, acupuncture, behavioral therapy, exercise therapy, and NSAIDs had the largest effect sizes. Level of evidence: II.

28. Burkus JK, Gornet MF, Schuler TC, Kleeman TJ, Zdeblick TA: Six-year outcomes of anterior lumbar interbody arthrodesis with use of interbody fusion cages and

5: Spine

recombinant human bone morphogenetic protein-2. *J Bone Joint Surg Am* 2009;91(5):1181-1189.

At 6-year follow-up of 130 patients treated with recombinant human bone morphogenetic protein-2 and stand-alone fusion cages, 128 patients had successful fusion. Significant improvements in Oswestry Disability Index and SF-36 scores that were seen as early as 6 weeks after surgery were maintained at 6-year follow-up. Level of evidence: IV.

29. Villavicencio AT, Burneikiene S, Bulsara KR, Thramann JJ: Perioperative complications in transforaminal lumbar interbody fusion versus anterior-posterior reconstruction for lumbar disc degeneration and instability. *J Spinal Disord Tech* 2006;19(2):92-97.

30. Carreon LY, Glassman SD, Howard J: Fusion and non-surgical treatment for symptomatic lumbar degenerative disease: A systematic review of Oswestry Disability Index and MOS Short Form-36 outcomes. *Spine J* 2008; 8(5):747-755.

A systematic review of prospective randomized controlled clinical trials in patients with low back pain of at least 12 weeks' duration was performed. In an evaluation of 25 studies, substantial improvement can be expected in patients treated with fusion when an established indication such as spondylolisthesis or degenerative disk disease is given. For patients with chronic low back pain, there is less improvement. Level of evidence: II.

Chapter 47
Cervical Degenerative Disease

John M. Rhee, MD   K. Daniel Riew, MD

Introduction

Degenerative, or spondylotic, conditions of the cervical spine constitute a spectrum of disorders. In most cases, the underlying mechanism is thought to begin with degeneration of the cervical disk, which can subsequently set off a cascade of secondary degenerative events. Depending on the presence and location of neurologic compression, the patient may present with pure axial pain, radiculopathy due to root compression, myelopathy due to cord compression, or a combination of all three conditions.

Axial Neck Pain Without Radiculopathy or Myelopathy

Clinical Evaluation

Axial neck pain is a very common problem, with an estimated lifetime prevalence of 66% in one series.[1] Most cases of axial pain arise from soft-tissue sprains and muscle strains, and are overwhelmingly benign, self-limited disorders. A smaller but still substantial population may have axial pain as a manifestation of cervical spondylosis, arising from entities such as disk degeneration, facet arthrosis, kyphosis, and less commonly,

segmental instability (**Figure 1**). Degenerative disks may lead to diffuse, poorly localized neck pain associated with other symptoms such as occipital headaches or radiation into the shoulder and scapula. Symptomatic facet arthrosis usually presents as a localized pain over the involved joint, particularly in extension. A well-described cause of axial neck pain is atlanto-axial osteoarthrosis[2] (**Figure 2**). Patients with this disorder are typically older (70 years or older) than those with subaxial arthrosis and present with pain localized to the occipitocervical junction that is typically exacerbated by rotation to the symptomatic side but not by sagittal

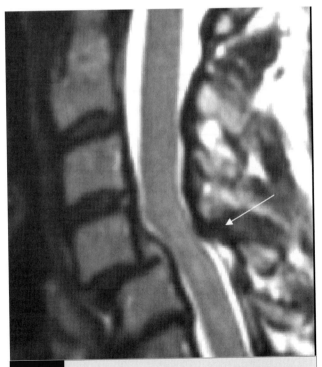

Figure 1   Cervical spondylolisthesis in a 47-year-old woman with cervical myelopathy caused by a grade II spondylolisthesis at C4-5. Associated spinal cord compression is present from the resulting narrowing of the spinal canal. Note also the buckling inward of the ligamentum flavum (*arrow*), which causes dorsal spinal cord compression. This patient also has significant disk degeneration at C5-6 and C6-7, although she has no neck pain. She was treated with anterior and posterior decompression and fusion, with complete resolution of myelopathy and solid fusion.

5: Spine

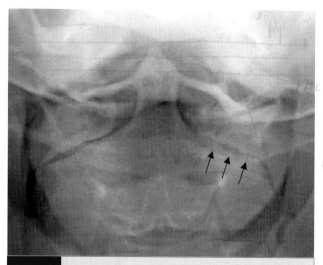

Figure 2 C1-2 facet arthrosis in a 75-year-old woman with severe left-sided neck pain occurring with rotation to the left. Open mouth odontoid view demonstrates severe facet arthrosis on the left side at C1-2 (*arrows*). Significant loss of joint space is evident on the left.

history of any injury and its mechanism should be determined. Nonspine causes of neck and shoulder pain, such as gallbladder, coronary, rotator cuff, or brachial plexus–related problems, should be investigated.

Radiographic Evaluation

Indications for obtaining radiographs include a history of trauma, prolonged duration of symptoms (longer than 1 month), presence of constitutional symptoms, suspected infection or malignancy, or known systemic disease (such as cancer or inflammatory arthritis). Plain radiographs are a reasonable initial test in the patient with axial neck pain, and perhaps are most useful in demonstrating the absence of more dangerous pathology rather than showing conditions such as degenerative disks, spurs, and other spondylotic changes that are universal during the course of normal aging.[3] If atlantoaxial arthrosis is suspected, an open mouth odontoid view may demonstrate arthritic changes in the C1-2 joints. Flexion-extension views may assist in evaluating potential instability. If tumor or infection is suspected, or if pain persists despite benign radiographs and a trial of nonsurgical treatment, MRI and/or CT may be helpful. Although imaging studies are helpful in evaluating patients with neck pain, care must be exercised in attributing symptoms to radiographic findings, as degenerative changes are more often the rule rather than the exception in the general population.

Other Diagnostic Studies

Despite clinical and radiologic studies, the exact pain generator may remain unclear in a large percentage of patients with axial pain. In such situations, more invasive tests such as diagnostic injections or diskography can be considered to further elucidate the diagnosis. However, these modalities are reserved for those in whom an initial trial of less invasive nonsurgical options has failed, which in many cases may result in resolution of symptoms despite the absence of a specific diagnosis. Facet injections may help provide both diagnostic information and therapeutic benefit in those with suspected symptomatic facet joint arthrosis. Cervical diskography can be used to identify symptomatic disk degeneration, but its true utility in predicting surgical outcomes remains controversial and is also associated with potential risks such as discitis or injury to the soft-tissue structures of the neck.

Treatment

In most patients for whom axial neck pain can be attributed to cervical spondylosis, conservative treatment is preferred because of a favorable natural history, and it is often difficult, if not sometimes impossible, to determine the exact pain generator for surgical treatment. Nonsteroidal anti-inflammatory drugs are favored over narcotic-based medications. Short-term collar immobilization may help decrease pain in those with acute symptoms. Active physical therapy, such as cervical muscle strengthening exercise, is generally preferred over passive treatment once the acute pain has im-

plane motion. Kyphosis may also be associated with neck pain. Kyphosis may occur secondary to the degenerative cascade, after multilevel cervical laminectomy, or due to myopathies that affect the cervical extensor musculature. Patients with kyphosis describe pain related to extensor muscle fatigue, as these muscles must overcome the negative biomechanical consequences of kyphosis to maintain forward gaze.

Physical examination of all patients should assess limitations in range of motion of the neck. Localized tenderness over a facet joint may be elicited in patients with symptomatic facet arthrosis, whether subaxial or atlantoaxial. In patients with atlantoaxial arthrosis, rotation to the affected side may reproduce pain, especially over the initial arc of motion when C1-2 rotation predominates over any subaxial contribution to rotation. Performing the same maneuver in the supine position with gentle traction on the cervical spine may reduce symptoms as the arthritic C1-2 facets are unloaded.

In addition to degenerative cervical spine etiologies, the differential diagnosis of isolated axial neck pain includes fractures, dislocations, inflammatory arthritides (for example, rheumatoid arthritis, ankylosing spondylitis), infections (for example, diskitis, osteomyelitis, epidural abscess), tumors (intradural, extradural), and nonspine sources. Although making a specific diagnosis can be difficult in the patient with axial neck pain, these potentially dangerous causes of neck pain should be ruled out before embarking on treatment of cervical spondylosis or neck strain/ sprain. A detailed history often provides the essential information. Constant, unremitting pain that worsens at night and is associated with constitutional symptoms such as fever, malaise, and weight loss are suggestive of tumor or infection. A

proved. Epidural injections for degenerative disks and facet joint injections for symptomatic arthrosis have been reported to provide pain relief[4,5] and may be considered if other less invasive forms of nonsurgical treatment fail. However, their true efficacy in controlled studies is lacking, and it seems doubtful that they will have any effect on the long-term natural history of these conditions.

For patients with symptomatic facet arthrosis in whom nonsurgical treatment fails, surgical fusion may yield reliable results if a specific facet joint can be implicated,[2] either in the subaxial or atlantoaxial spine. In addition, those with more readily identifiable pain generators such as kyphosis have also been shown to benefit from surgery, particularly if the kyphosis is associated with myelopathy or significant functional impairments such as loss of horizontal gaze or difficulty eating. However, considerable controversy arises in the surgical management of patients whose pain is thought to be mediated by a degenerative disk, as one of the biggest challenges in this population lies in identifying the correct pain generator because there is no unequivocal method for doing so. Furthermore, because radiographic changes of spondylosis are so prevalent, no radiographic modality alone can be relied upon to make the diagnosis. Despite these obstacles, authors have reported favorable results with anterior cervical diskectomy and fusion in patients with degenerative disks, primary reports of axial neck pain, and concordant diskograms.[6,7] However, both surgeon and patient must be aware that much more consistent results are achievable when surgically managing neural compressive pathologies, such as radiculopathy and myelopathy, instead. In the setting of radiculopathy or myelopathy, associated headaches have been shown to improve after anterior cervical diskectomy and fusion or cervical arthroplasty.[8]

Cervical Spondylotic Radiculopathy

Clinical Evaluation

Patients with cervical spondylotic radiculopathy report pain and/or neurologic dysfunction along a nerve root distribution as a result of compression of the involved root(s). The amount of weakness, numbness, or pain experienced varies. It is important to keep in mind, however, that not all patients with cervical radiculopathy have "classic" radiating arm pain symptoms. Not infrequently, radiculopathic pain is localized to one side of the neck and shoulder girdle and does not run down the arm. Trapezial and periscapular pain can be associated with radiculopathy arising from virtually any cervical level.

The two most common causes of cervical radiculopathy are soft and hard disk pathology (**Figure 3**). Soft disk pathologies represent acute ruptures with extrusion of nuclear material into the epidural space. Osteophytes in association with bulging disks may be referred to as hard disks. Disk height loss and bulging of

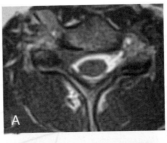
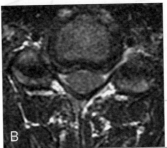
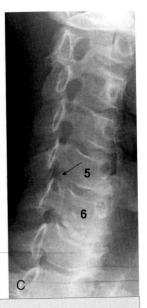

Figure 3 Soft disk herniation versus spondylotic radiculopathy and oblique radiograph. **A,** Axial MRI demonstrating a foraminal soft disk herniation. **B,** Axial MRI of a different patient demonstrating bilateral foraminal stenosis from uncinate hypertrophy, which is also demonstrated on **C,** the oblique radiograph (*arrow,* in the C5-6 foramen).

the anulus fibrosus associated with degeneration can also cause radiculopathy by decreasing the space available for the nerve root either within or as it enters the neuroforamen.

Table 1 lists typical pain and neurologic patterns associated with radiculopathies of the cervical nerve roots. The most common levels of root involvement are C6 and C7. High cervical radiculopathies (C2, C3, C4) are less common but may present with unilateral upper trapezial pain, neck pain, and headaches.

A careful physical examination should be performed to identify the nerve root involved, with the caveat that crossover within myotomes and dermatomes may be present. In contrast to the lumbar spine, posterolateral disk herniations and foraminal stenosis in the cervical spine tend to produce radiculopathy of the nerve root exiting at the same level. For example, both a C5-C6 disk herniation and C5-C6 foraminal stenosis typically produce a C6 radiculopathy. A large central to midlateral disk herniation or stenosis may, however, cause a radiculopathy of the next lower nerve root.

Several provocative tests may elicit or reproduce symptoms of radiculopathy. A Spurling maneuver may reproduce the radicular symptoms in a patient with a foraminal disk or stenosis. The neck is maximally extended and rotated to the side of the pathology. Concomitant adduction of the shoulder with extension of the elbow and wrist may accentuate the Spurling sign, as these maneuvers not only narrow the foramen but also stretch the root. Improvement of symptoms may

Table 1

Common Cervical Radiculopathy Patterns

Root	Symptoms	Motor	Reflex
C2	Posterior occipital headaches, temporal pain	-	-
C3	Occipital headache, retro-orbital or retroauricular pain	-	-
C4	Base of neck, trapezial pain	-	-
C5	Lateral arm	Deltoid	Biceps
C6	Radial forearm, thumb, and index fingers	Biceps, wrist extension	Brachioradialis
C7	Middle finger	Triceps, wrist flexion	Triceps
C8	Ring and little fingers	Finger flexors	-
T1	Ulnar forearm	Hand intrinsics	-

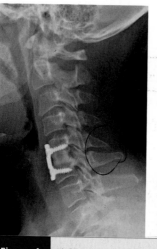
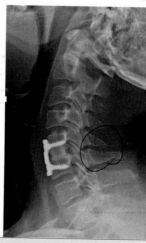

[handwritten: no motion- fusion success- ful]

Figure 4 ACDF 1 year after surgery. Flexion (**A**) and extension (**B**) radiographs 1 year after single-level ACDF with allograft and plate, demonstrating solid fusion and no motion across the spinous processes at C5-6.

occur if the patient subsequently flexes and rotates the neck to the other side and abducts the shoulder with the hand behind the neck, as these maneuvers both open up the foramen and relax the root. The presence of a Spurling sign is very helpful in determining a cervical spine origin of symptoms, as the reproduction of pain with a Spurling sign is unlikely if the cause of the pain is outside of the cervical spine.

The differential diagnosis of cervical spondylotic radiculopathy is similar to that for axial neck pain. In addition, peripheral nerve entrapment syndromes (for example, carpal or cubital tunnel syndromes) and tendinopathies of the shoulder, elbow, and wrist must be considered. Selective cervical nerve root injections can be useful in confirming the source of symptoms and may also be therapeutic, although it is uncertain whether they affect the long-term natural history of radiculopathy. Electromyography and nerve conduction

tests may help differentiate radiculopathy from peripheral entrapment neuropathies, although they are rarely needed as primary diagnostic modalities. In addition, because electrodiagnostic studies are highly operator dependent, they must be interpreted in light of the entire clinical and radiographic picture.

Radiographic Evaluation

Osteophytes causing radiculopathy can often be seen on AP, lateral, and oblique radiographs. However, definitive confirmation generally requires MRI or CT myelograms. MRI is noninvasive and may be better at identifying disk herniations (particularly those that are intraforaminal and thus lateral to the root sleeve seen on myelography) and parenchymal cord lesions, whereas CT myelography may be better at detecting bony foraminal stenosis and delineating whether root compression arises from soft disk herniations versus hard pathology such as osteophytes.

Treatment

The natural history of cervical spondylotic radiculopathy is generally favorable. Many patients with disk herniations achieve resolution of symptoms over time without surgical intervention. Furthermore, it is not common for patients with radiculopathy to progress to myelopathy.[9] Thus, in the absence of severe or progressive neurologic findings or incapacitating pain, the initial management of cervical spondylotic radiculopathy is usually nonsurgical and may include anti-inflammatory medications, physical therapy, short term immobilization, oral steroid tapers, and nerve root injections.

Surgical Treatment Options

Anterior Cervical Diskectomy and Fusion or Arthroplasty

Indications for surgery include severe or progressive neurologic deficit (weakness or numbness) or significant pain that fails to respond to nonsurgical treatment. Depending on the pathology, cervical spondylotic radiculopathy may be surgically addressed anteriorly or posteriorly. Anterior cervical diskectomy and fusion (ACDF) is currently the most common procedure in the surgical treatment of cervical radiculopathy (**Figure 4**). Although initially described with autograft and no instrumentation, many surgeons currently use allograft and a plate to avoid complications related to iliac crest autograft harvest while still achieving satisfactory arthrodesis rates and maintenance of segmental lordosis. Reported outcomes for relief of arm pain, as well as improvements in motor and sensory function are typically in the 90% range.[10] Benefits of ACDF include the direct removal of most lesions causing cervical radiculopathy (such as herniated disks or uncovertebral spurs) without requiring intraoperative neural retraction, restoration or improvement in overall cervical alignment, indirect foraminal decompression resulting from restoration of interbody height with the graft, and improvement in spondylotic neck pain with fusion. There are extremely low rates of infection or wound complications, cosmetically preferable interior scars compared to posterior incisions, and mild perioperative pain in most cases. Potential drawbacks of ACDF include pseudarthrosis (rate varies widely according to graft type and use of plate, but modern data report 5% to 10% for a single-level ACDF),[11-13] persistent speech and swallowing complications related to the anterior approach,[14,15] and the potential for accelerated adjacent segment degeneration with fusion.

Recently, cervical arthroplasty has become available for the treatment of cervical radiculopathy (**Figure 5**). Arthroplasty appears to enjoy the same set of anterior approach-related advantages as ACDF, but one major advantage over ACDF is preservation of motion and thus potentially less adjacent segment disease. Long-term studies are currently not available to determine whether arthroplasty can indeed decrease the rate of symptomatic adjacent segment disease requiring repeat surgery,[16] and debate continues as to whether adjacent segment disease is actually accelerated in those who have undergone fusion. However, The US Food and Drug Administration (FDA) Investigational Device Exemption (IDE) trial data for three different cervical arthroplasty devices have been favorable at 2-year follow-up, with at least equivalent clinical outcomes to ACDF in terms of relief of neck and arm pain. Reported device-related complications have been few, and the short-term reoperation rate may be lower than that of ACDF. Currently, the best indication for arthroplasty appears to be radiculopathy in relatively younger patients with reasonable motion at the involved segment. Potential contraindications include poor bone quality that could compromise implant stability, kyphosis, and segments that do not demonstrate significant motion preoperatively. Other contraindications include bone-forming arthropathies such as ossification of the posterior longitudinal ligament (OPLL) and diffuse idiopathic skeletal hyperostosis, instability, and neck pain due to facet arthrosis. It remains to be seen whether arthroplasty may lead to a higher rate of recurrent disease over time at the index level due to ongoing motion

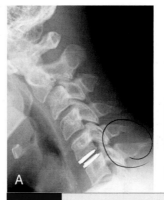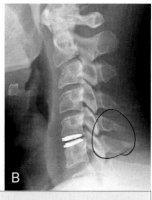

motion maintained

| **Figure 5** | Total disk replacement. Flexion (**A**) and extension (**B**) radiographs after cervical disk replacement for radiculopathy. The patient has incidental, asymptomatic upper cervical kyphosis due to an old traumatic injury. Note maintenance of motion at the level of disk replacement. |

and thus potential for osteophytic regrowth. Accordingly, a more thorough decompression is necessary when performing arthroplasty over ACDF, including bilateral foraminal decompressions and removal of all potential impinging pathology (even that which is currently asymptomatic).

Posterior Decompression

Posterior laminoforaminotomy is an alternative option in patients with radiculopathy caused by foraminal disk herniations or uncinate spurs. The ideal indication is in the patient with foraminal root compression who obtains excellent arm symptom relief by flexing the neck and rotating away from the symptomatic side (a 'reverse' Spurling sign). This position essentially mimics the neuroforaminal enlargement resulting from a foraminotomy when the medial half of the facet joint is resected. In such cases, the offending anterior osteophyte or disk herniation can but does not necessarily need to be removed to alleviate symptoms. However, poor symptom relief with the reverse Spurling maneuver may indicate the need to remove the anterior osteophyte or herniation, which may be difficult to accomplish from a posterior approach in certain cases. If so, an anterior approach may be preferable.

Major advantages of posterior foraminotomy are that it can be performed with minimal patient morbidity and it avoids both fusion and placement of an artificial disk. However, disadvantages include the possibility for incomplete decompression in the setting of anterior compressive lesions, as well as the potential for deterioration of results with time as the degenerative process continues in the absence of a fusion.[17] Despite these potential limitations, large series, including those using laminoforaminotomy through a minimally invasive approach, have reported arm pain relief in 90% to 97% of patients.[17-20]

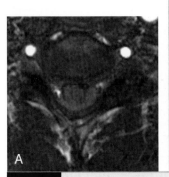
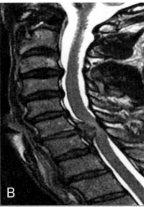

Figure 6 MRI studies demonstrating a massive herniated nucleus pulposus. Axial (**A**) and sagittal (**B**) views of the cervical spine of a 42-year-old man with severe cervical myelopathy due to a massive soft disk herniation, manifested as gait instability, bilateral hand numbness, burning dysesthesias in the arms, and hand clumsiness but minimal to no radiating neck or arm pain. Note the cord signal changes present on **B**.

Cervical Spondylotic Myelopathy

History

Cervical myelopathy describes the condition caused by compression of the spinal cord (**Figure 6**). Upper extremity symptoms include a generalized feeling of clumsiness of the arms and hands, dropping things, inability to manipulate fine objects such as coins or buttons, trouble with handwriting, and diffuse (typically nondermatomal) numbness. Lower extremity complaints include gait instability and imbalance, leading to a "drunken" gait. Patients with severe cord compression may also report symptoms of Lhermitte sign: electric shocklike sensations that radiate down the spine or into the extremities with certain offending positions of the neck.

Contrary to what the unsuspecting clinician might expect, patients with myelopathy often may not present with many of the symptoms commonly attributed to spinal column degeneration. For example, despite advanced degrees of spondylosis, many floridly myelopathic patients have no neck pain. Although radicular complaints such as radiating arm pain may coexist with myelopathy if the patient also has symptomatic nerve-root compression, many myelopathic patients have no radicular symptoms or signs despite imaging studies that clearly demonstrate root compression. It is this patient with no pain in whom myelopathy may be undiagnosed until it becomes severe. Many patients with myelopathy also deny any loss of motor strength until the condition progresses to the later stages. Subtle bowel and bladder symptoms, such as urinary urgency, can be elicited with a careful history, but frank incontinence is relatively rare and typically occurs during later stages of disease.

Physical Examination

Although a detailed neurologic and physical examination should be performed (**Table 2**), a normal neurologic examination does not exclude the diagnosis of myelopathy, just as the absence of neck or arm pain similarly does not rule out the diagnosis.[21]

Differential Diagnosis

The most common cause of cervical myelopathy in patients older than 50 years is spondylosis (degenerative changes), leading to the condition known as cervical spondylotic myelopathy (CSM). Anterior structures, such as bulging, ossified, or herniated disks, as well as osteophytic bone spurs, are the most common causes of cord compression in CSM. Degenerative spondylolisthesis of the cervical spine can also exacerbate or cause compression (**Figure 1**). Less commonly than their anterior counterparts, posterior structures, such as ligamentum flavum hypertrophy or, rarely, ossification of the ligamentum flavum, may also contribute to cord compression.

CSM commonly arises in the setting of a congenitally narrowed spinal canal. In these patients, the cord may have had sufficient space and escaped compression during the patient's relative youth until the accumulation of a threshold amount of space-occupying degenerative changes. Although CSM tends to be a disorder seen in the older patient, depending on the degree of congenital stenosis and the magnitude of the accumulated spondylotic changes, it can be seen in patients younger than 50 years.

OPLL is another major cause of cervical myelopathy (**Figure 7**). The cause of OPLL remains unclear but is most likely multifactorial, with both genetic and metabolic factors involved, including diabetes and obesity. Other causes of cervical myelopathy include various etiologies of cervical cord compression, such as tumor, epidural abscess, osteomyelitis/ diskitis, and trauma. Kyphosis, whether primary or occurring after laminectomy, can also cause cord compression and myelopathy. Whenever evaluating patients with myelopathic complaints, it is important that a broad differential diagnosis, including nonspinal conditions such as stroke, movement disorders, vitamin B_{12} deficiency, amyotrophic lateral sclerosis, and multiple sclerosis, be kept in mind.

Radiographic Evaluation

The lateral radiograph can be used to determine the degree of congenital cervical stenosis present. A Pavlov ratio (AP diameter of canal/AP diameter of vertebral body) of less than 0.8 suggests a congenitally narrow spinal canal predisposing to stenosis and cord compression. A space available for the cord of 13 mm or less also suggests a narrow sagittal diameter of the spinal canal and has been shown to correlate with neurologic injury after trauma.

To confirm spinal cord compression, advanced imaging in the form of MRI or CT myelography is necessary. MRI is noninvasive and provides adequate imag-

Table 2

Physical Findings in Cervical Myelopathy

Test	Finding	Significance
Motor examination	Weakness	Grip and intrinsic strength not uncommonly affected
Sensory examination	Alteration to touch or pinprick	Sensory levels are rarely seen, compared to thoracic myelopathy
Reflexes	Hyperreflexia	May be normal or even diminished in the presence of conditions affecting peripheral nerves (for example, diabetes, neuropathy, root compression)
Gait	Unsteady gait	May be seen with either cervical or thoracic myelopathy
Hoffman sign	Flicking the middle finger distal phalanx results in pathologic flexion of the thumb and index finger	Upper motor neuron sign
Inverted radial reflex	Diminished brachioradialis reflex with contraction of the finger flexors instead	Classically due to cord and root compression at C56, but may arise from compression at other levels
Clonus	Sustained (>3) beats	Upper motor neuron sign
Babinski	Upgoing toe	Upper motor neuron sign, may indicate poorer prognosis
Finger escape sign	Inability to maintain the ulnar digits in an extended and adducted position	Consistent with cervical myelopathy
Scapulohumeral reflex	Tapping the tip of the scapula results in brisk scapular elevation and humeral abduction	Consistent with upper cervical myelopathy
Jaw jerk	Tapping lower jaw leads to a brisk jerk	Origin of upper motor neuron findings may be in brain rather than spinal cord

ing characteristics in most patients. A closed MRI is preferred over an open study whenever possible because of its superior image quality. Signal changes within the cord may be demonstrated on MRI and are suggestive of severe compression. Signal changes seen on T1-weighted images correlate with a poorer prognosis for neurologic recovery following surgical decompression. When necessary, CT myelograms provide outstanding resolution of both bony and neural anatomy for surgical planning. Alternatively, if a high-quality MRI is present but questions remain regarding bony anatomy for the purposes of surgical planning, a noncontrast CT can be obtained to provide complementary information. OPLL and osteophytes are much easier to identify on CT than MRI.

Treatment *CSM = progressive → need surgical tx*

Unlike cervical spondylotic radiculopathy, cervical spondylotic myelopathy tends to be progressive and rarely improves in the long term without surgical management.[22] The typical progression is a stepwise clinical deterioration punctuating stable periods. Continued impingement by the spondylotic spine results in cord ischemia by compressing the anterior spinal artery and also may have a direct mechanical effect on the cord.

Vascular phenomenon

Surgical management has been shown to improve functional outcomes, pain, and neurologic status compared to nonsurgical treatment.[23] It has also been suggested that early intervention improves prognosis before permanent destructive changes occur in the spinal cord.[24] Therefore, nonsurgical treatment should be reserved for patients with mild cases or those who pose a prohibitive surgical risk. If nonsurgical treatment is elected, patients are instructed to report any progression in symptoms. An orthosis, anti-inflammatory medications, and neck strengthening exercises can be considered along with physical therapy for balance and gait training. Traction and chiropractic manipulation should probably be avoided in these patients, as they are unlikely to be of much benefit but do carry a small risk of harm.

It is not so clear, however, how best to treat patients with imaging evidence of cord compression but no clinical symptoms of myelopathy. This scenario not infrequently occurs, for example, in patients who obtained an MRI for an episode of axial neck pain that subsequently resolved. On the one hand, asymptomatic cord compression may eventually become symptomatic, particularly if the compression is severe or the patient sustains an injury. On the other hand, it is possible, espe-

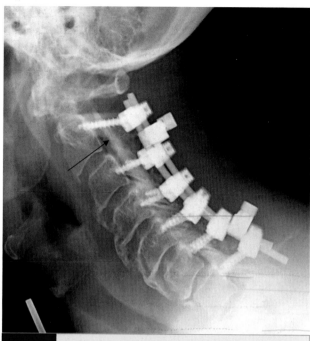

Figure 7 Radiograph of the cervical spine of a 72-year-old woman with cervical myelopathy due to massive OPLL (arrow). Note that the OPLL extends from C2-4 and is thick enough to be seen on plain radiographs. She was treated with multilevel laminectomy and fusion with excellent improvement in myelopathy and neck pain.

cially with milder degrees of stenosis, that the patient may never develop problems. Ultimately, this decision rests in the informed consent of the patient and an understanding of the risks and benefits of surgical versus nonsurgical care. Depending on the degree of cord compression or presence of spinal cord signal changes, it can be entirely reasonable to recommend surgery even in the absence of symptoms.

Surgical Treatment Options

Although there is consensus regarding the need for surgical treatment of cervical myelopathy, considerable debate exists regarding the optimal surgical approach. There are several options, including anterior decompression and fusion or arthroplasty, laminectomy, laminectomy and fusion, and laminoplasty. Each approach has its own set of advantages and disadvantages, and there is no one procedure that is clearly favorable in all circumstances. Considerations that may favor one approach over another include the number of stenotic levels present, patient factors such as comorbidities, and a desire to either limit or preserve motion.

Anterior Decompression and Fusion

The major advantage of the anterior approach for cervical myelopathy is the ability to directly decompress structures most commonly responsible for cord compression, such as herniated disks, spondylotic bars, and OPLL. Anterior decompression, in contrast to posterior

approaches, can also directly relieve neural compression resulting from kyphosis by removing the vertebral bodies over which the cord may be draped. In addition, the fusion procedure associated with anterior decompression helps to relieve spondylotic neck pain, can correct and improve kyphosis, immobilizes and therefore protects the segment of decompressed cord, and prevents recurrent disease over the fused segments. Anterior surgery also enjoys a low rate of infection and relatively mild postoperative pain. However, it is important to keep in mind that all anterior operations carry relatively small but real risks intrinsic to the anterior approach, such as persistent speech and swallowing disturbance, airway obstruction, esophageal injury, and vertebral artery injury.

Overall excellent neurologic recovery rates and outcomes have been reported with anterior surgery for myelopathy.[25] For those with myelopathy arising from one to two disk segments, the anterior approach is generally the one of choice, as it provides excellent outcomes with relatively little morbidity. The traditional approach has been ACDF. Recently, however, anterior diskectomy and total disk replacement has been reported with success in patients with single-level myelopathy, although the role of arthroplasty in myelopathy remains to be defined and currently may be best suited for those with myelopathy due to soft disk herniation rather than severe spondylosis.

The supremacy of the anterior approach is not so clear in those requiring multilevel anterior surgery. Multilevel fusions are more prone to nonunion (11% to 40% reported in the literature) and graft/plate complications.[26] In particular, long corpectomy reconstructions tend to be biomechanically unsound, even when plated, and carry a relatively high risk of graft kickout (up to 20% reported in the literature).[26] If an anterior approach is necessary in a patient with multilevel myelopathy and the pattern of cord compression allows, it may be preferable to perform multilevel ACDF. Alternatively, single-level corpectomy can be done at levels of retrovertebral compression along with diskectomy(ies) at level(s) of disk-based compression to avoid the pitfalls of long multilevel corpectomy.

[handwritten margin note: avoid multilevel corpectomy]

Laminectomy Alone or With Fusion

Although laminectomy without fusion for the treatment of cervical myelopathy is still performed, especially by neurosurgeons, there are numerous drawbacks to its use (**Figure 8**). Postlaminectomy kyphosis can occur after laminectomy and, although the true incidence in the adult population is unknown, estimates range from 11% to 47%.[27,28] Postlaminectomy kyphosis can lead to potential recurrent myelopathy if the cord becomes draped and compressed over the kyphotic area.[29] In addition to potential neurologic sequelae, the kyphosis itself can be a source of neck pain or deformity. If an aggressive facetectomy is performed along with laminectomy, spondylolisthesis can also develop and contribute to cord compression. Furthermore, if a patient requires a subsequent posterior operation, the exposed dura over the length of the laminectomy can make the revision more tedious, difficult, and risky to perform.

A posterior fusion can be added to avoid the pitfalls of laminectomy alone. Laminectomy and fusion are typically performed along with lateral mass screw instrumentation. Fusion has several potential benefits, including improvement of spondylotic neck pain, better maintenance of cervical alignment, and prevention of postlaminectomy kyphosis. In addition, mild amounts of preexisting kyphosis can be improved after laminectomy by positioning the neck in extension before securing the instrumentation. However, in those with significant or fixed kyphosis, anterior, anterior-posterior, or osteotomy based approaches may be needed to achieve satisfactory correction. For those in whom a posterior approach is desirable due to the number of levels involved but fusion is not necessary, laminoplasty may be a better choice.

Laminoplasty

Laminoplasty was designed as a procedure to achieve multilevel posterior cord decompression while avoiding postlaminectomy kyphosis, a major problem associated with laminectomy. There are many ways of performing laminoplasty, but the open door and French door techniques are the most common. The common theme in all variations of laminoplasty is the creation of a hinge at the junction of the lateral mass and lamina by thinning the dorsal cortex but not cutting completely through the ventral cortex, thereby allowing the creation of greenstick fractures. In the open door technique, the hinge is created unilaterally; in the French door version, the hinge is created bilaterally. The opening is performed on the opposite lateral mass-laminar junction in an open door procedure, or in the midline with the French door variation. Opening the laminoplasty increases the space available for the spinal cord, which drifts away from compressive lesions into the space created. The opening can then be held patent with bone (eg, autologous spinous process or rib allograft), sutures, suture-anchors, or specially designed plates[30] (**Figure 9**).

In addition to its benefits over laminectomy, laminoplasty possesses several distinct advantages over anterior surgery. First, because an indirect decompression is performed, it is in general a technically easier and quicker operation to perform than multilevel anterior corpectomy, particularly in patients with severe stenosis or OPLL. Second, laminoplasty is a motion-preserving procedure. In contrast to anterior surgery, no fusion is required with laminoplasty. The theoretical advantages of laminoplasty have been borne out in head-to-head clinical trials with multilevel anterior corpectomy. Laminoplasty and anterior surgery have similar rates of neurologic improvement, but laminoplasty has a much lower complication rate.[31,32]

Laminoplasty is clearly not a perfect operation, is not appropriate in all cases, and does have its disadvantages. Segmental root–level palsy remains a concern, with an incidence postoperatively ranging from 5% to

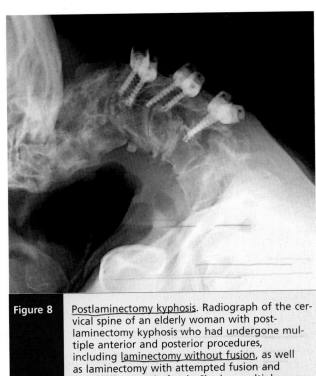

Figure 8   Postlaminectomy kyphosis. Radiograph of the cervical spine of an elderly woman with postlaminectomy kyphosis who had undergone multiple anterior and posterior procedures, including laminectomy without fusion, as well as laminectomy with attempted fusion and eventual removal of rods. She has multiple nonunions both anteriorly and posteriorly, as well as severe cervical kyphosis. It is imperative to prevent this sort of deformity from developing by avoiding cervical laminectomy alone in patients who present initially with kyphosis.

12%.[33] It most commonly affects the C5 root, resulting in deltoid and biceps weakness, although other roots can also be affected. Although typically associated with laminoplasty, root palsies appear to occur with similar frequency after all types of spinal cord decompression procedures (such as anterior surgery or laminectomy). Neck pain is often reported to be an issue in patients who have had laminoplasty. Controversy exists as to whether laminoplasty-associated neck pain is simply a persistence of the patient's preoperative spondylotic neck pain or a de novo pain arising postoperatively. However, laminoplasty is not the procedure of choice in those with significant preoperative axial neck pain. The patient with preoperative kyphosis also presents a relative contraindication to laminoplasty. Most of the compressive structures that lead to cervical myelopathy, such as disk herniations, spondylotic bars, and OPLL, arise anteriorly. Thus, laminoplasty and other posteriorly-based procedures for spinal cord decompression rely on the ability of the cord to drift away from the anterior lesions as a result of releasing the posterior tethers (laminae, ligamentum flavum). Although such drifting reliably occurs in a lordotic or neutral cervical spine, it may not occur in the setting of significant kyphosis. Laminoplasty has been shown to produce acceptable neurologic recovery rates in patients with up to 13° of kyphosis.[34] However, because some loss of lordosis occurs even with laminoplasty, laminoplasty in patients with preexisting kyphosis may

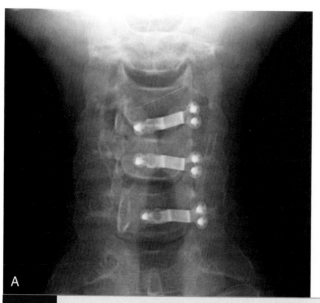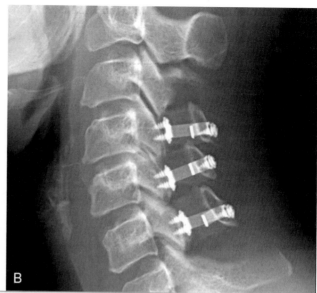

Figure 9   Laminoplasty. AP (**A**) and lateral (**B**) radiographs after open door laminoplasty with plate fixation. This 40-year-old woman had multilevel myelopathy with no axial neck pain and preserved lordosis, making her an ideal candidate for this operation. Partial inferior laminectomy of C3 and superior laminectomy of C7 were also performed to decompress the cord at the C3-4 and C6-7 disk spaces, respectively, while at the same time preserving the extensor muscular attachments as much as possible, which in turn may lessen the incidence of postoperative neck pain and loss of lordosis that can occur even with laminoplasty.

lead to acceleration of kyphosis, which in turn might cause neck pain and recurrent cord compression. In kyphotic patients with multilevel myelopathy, laminectomy with fusion may be a better alternative if the kyphosis is flexible. If the kyphosis is not flexible but instead fixed or ankylosed, the anterior approach with or without supplemental posterior surgery will likely lead to the best outcomes.

Combined Anterior and Posterior Surgery

Combined approaches are strongly recommended in patients with postlaminectomy kyphosis. In this setting, if a multilevel corpectomy is performed to decompress the cord, an extremely unstable biomechanical environment results due to the preexisting laminectomy: in essence, the right and left sides of the spine become disconnected from each other. Supplemental posterior fixation is recommended to improve construct stability.[35] Likewise, in patients needing multilevel fusion (≥ four motion segments) or those with significant kyphosis, especially in the setting of poor bone quality, supplemental posterior fixation and fusion should be considered.

Annotated References

1. Côté P, Cassidy JD, Carroll L: The Saskatchewan Health and Back Pain Survey: The prevalence of neck pain and related disability in Saskatchewan adults. *Spine (Phila Pa 1976)* 1998;23(15):1689-1698.

2. Ghanayem AJ, Leventhal M, Bohlman HH: Osteoarthrosis of the atlanto-axial joints. Long-term follow-up after treatment with arthrodesis. *J Bone Joint Surg Am* 1996;78(9):1300-1307.

3. Boden SD, McCowin PR, Davis DO, Dina TS, Mark AS, Wiesel S: Abnormal magnetic-resonance scans of the cervical spine in asymptomatic subjects. A prospective investigation. *J Bone Joint Surg Am* 1990;72(8): 1178-1184.

4. Hession WG, Stanczak JD, Davis KW, Choi JJ: Epidural steroid injections. *Semin Roentgenol* 2004;39(1):7-23.

5. Silbergleit R, Mehta BA, Sanders WP, Talati SJ: Imaging-guided injection techniques with fluoroscopy and CT for spinal pain management. *Radiographics* 2001;21(4):927-939, discussion 940-942.

6. Palit M, Schofferman J, Goldthwaite N, et al: Anterior discectomy and fusion for the management of neck pain. *Spine (Phila Pa 1976)* 1999;24(21):2224-2228.

7. Garvey TA, Transfeldt EE, Malcolm JR, Kos P: Outcome of anterior cervical discectomy and fusion as perceived by patients treated for dominant axial-mechanical cervical spine pain. *Spine (Phila Pa 1976)* 2002;27(17):1887-1895, discussion 1895.

8. Riina J, Anderson PA, Holly LT, Flint K, Davis KE, Riew KD: The effect of an anterior cervical operation for cervical radiculopathy or myelopathy on associated headaches. *J Bone Joint Surg Am* 2009;91(8):1919-1923.

Eight hundred three patients who had single-level ACDF or cervical arthroplasty in FDA IDE trials were evaluated post hoc for improvement in associated headaches. Both groups had significant improvement at 24 months after surgery. Level of evidence: I.

9. Lees F, Turner JW: Natural history and prognosis of cervical spondylosis. *Br Med J* 1963;2(5373):1607-1610.

10. Bohlman HH, Emery SE, Goodfellow DB, Jones PK: Robinson anterior cervical discectomy and arthrodesis for cervical radiculopathy: Long-term follow-up of one hundred and twenty-two patients. *J Bone Joint Surg Am* 1993;75(9):1298-1307.

11. Wang JC, McDonough PW, Endow K, Kanim LE, Delamarter RB: The effect of cervical plating on single-level anterior cervical discectomy and fusion. *J Spinal Disord* 1999;12(6):467-471.

12. Martin GJ Jr, Haid RW Jr, MacMillan M, Rodts GE Jr, Berkman R: Anterior cervical discectomy with freeze-dried fibula allograft: Overview of 317 cases and literature review. *Spine (Phila Pa 1976)* 1999;24(9):852-858, discussion 858-859.

13. Samartzis D, Shen FH, Goldberg EJ, An HS: Is autograft the gold standard in achieving radiographic fusion in one-level anterior cervical discectomy and fusion with rigid anterior plate fixation? *Spine (Phila Pa 1976)* 2005;30(15):1756-1761.

14. Bazaz R, Lee MJ, Yoo JU: Incidence of dysphagia after anterior cervical spine surgery: A prospective study. *Spine (Phila Pa 1976)* 2002;27(22):2453-2458.

15. Winslow CP, Winslow TJ, Wax MK: Dysphonia and dysphagia following the anterior approach to the cervical spine. *Arch Otolaryngol Head Neck Surg* 2001;127(1):51-55.

16. Hilibrand AS, Carlson GD, Palumbo MA, Jones PK, Bohlman HH: Radiculopathy and myelopathy at segments adjacent to the site of a previous anterior cervical arthrodesis. *J Bone Joint Surg Am* 1999;81(4):519-528.

17. Herkowitz HN, Kurz LT, Overholt DP: Surgical management of cervical soft disc herniation. A comparison between the anterior and posterior approach. *Spine (Phila Pa 1976)* 1990;15(10):1026-1030.

18. Henderson CM, Hennessy RG, Shuey HM Jr, Shackelford EG: Posterior-lateral foraminotomy as an exclusive operative technique for cervical radiculopathy: A review of 846 consecutively operated cases. *Neurosurgery* 1983;13(5):504-512.

19. Zeidman SM, Ducker TB: Posterior cervical laminoforaminotomy for radiculopathy: Review of 172 cases. *Neurosurgery* 1993;33(3):356-362.

20. Adamson TE: Microendoscopic posterior cervical laminoforaminotomy for unilateral radiculopathy: Results of a new technique in 100 cases. *J Neurosurg* 2001;95(1, suppl)51-57.

21. Rhee JM, Heflin JA, Hamasaki T, Freedman B: Prevalence of physical signs in cervical myelopathy: A prospective, controlled study. *Spine* 2009;34(9):890-895.

In a prospective evaluation of 39 patients with cervical myelopathy who were compared with 37 control subjects, myelopathic physical signs were substantially more prevalent in the myelopathy group. However, 21% of myelopathy patients (as evidenced by myelopathic symptoms, correlative spinal cord compression on imaging, and improvement in myelopathy after decompression) did not show any physical signs. Thus, the absence of myelopathic signs does not preclude the diagnosis of cervical myelopathy or its successful surgical treatment.

22. Nurick S: The pathogenesis of the spinal cord disorder associated with cervical spondylosis. *Brain* 1972;95(1):87-100.

23. Sampath P, Bendebba M, Davis JD, Ducker TB: Outcome of patients treated for cervical myelopathy: A prospective, multicenter study with independent clinical review. *Spine (Phila Pa 1976)* 2000;25(6):670-676.

24. Emery SE, Smith MD, Bohlman HH: Upper-airway obstruction after multilevel cervical corpectomy for myelopathy. *J Bone Joint Surg Am* 1991;73(4):544-551.

25. Emery SE, Bohlman HH, Bolesta MJ, Jones PK: Anterior cervical decompression and arthrodesis for the treatment of cervical spondylotic myelopathy: Two to seventeen-year follow-up. *J Bone Joint Surg Am* 1998;80(7):941-951.

26. Rhee JM: Posterior surgery for cervical spondylotic myelopathy. *Semin Spine Surg* 2004;16:255-263.

27. Kato Y, Iwasaki M, Fuji T, Yonenobu K, Ochi T: Long-term follow-up results of laminectomy for cervical myelopathy caused by ossification of the posterior longitudinal ligament. *J Neurosurg* 1998;89(2):217-223.

28. Mikawa Y, Shikata J, Yamamuro T: Spinal deformity and instability after multilevel cervical laminectomy. *Spine (Phila Pa 1976)* 1987;12(1):6-11.

29. Guigui P, Benoist M, Deburge A: Spinal deformity and instability after multilevel cervical laminectomy for spondylotic myelopathy. *Spine (Phila Pa 1976)* 1998;23(4):440-447.

30. Park AE, Heller JG: Cervical laminoplasty: Use of a novel titanium plate to maintain canal expansion—surgical technique. *J Spinal Disord Tech* 2004;17(4):265-271.

31. Yonenobu K, Hosono N, Iwasaki M, Asano M, Ono K: Laminoplasty versus subtotal corpectomy: A comparative study of results in multisegmental cervical spondy-

5: Spine

lotic myelopathy. *Spine (Phila Pa 1976)* 1992;17(11): 1281-1284.

32. Edwards CC II, Heller JG, Murakami H: Corpectomy versus laminoplasty for multilevel cervical myelopathy: An independent matched-cohort analysis. *Spine (Phila Pa 1976)* 2002;27(11):1168-1175.

33. Uematsu Y, Tokuhashi Y, Matsuzaki H: Radiculopathy after laminoplasty of the cervical spine. *Spine (Phila Pa 1976)* 1998;23(19):2057-2062.

34. Suda K, Abumi K, Ito M, Shono Y, Kaneda K, Fujiya M: Local kyphosis reduces surgical outcomes of expansive open-door laminoplasty for cervical spondylotic myelopathy. *Spine (Phila Pa 1976)* 2003;28(12):1258-1262.

35. Riew KD, Hilibrand AS, Palumbo MA, Bohlman HH: Anterior cervical corpectomy in patients previously managed with a laminectomy: Short-term complications. *J Bone Joint Surg Am* 1999;81(7):950-957.

Chapter 48

Cervical Spine Trauma

Jens R. Chapman, MD   Richard J. Bransford, MD

Epidemiologic Factors

Cervical spine injuries are particularly challenging to treat despite dramatic improvements in diagnostic and treatment capabilities. The cervical spine allows considerable head motion while it protects the spinal cord, the exiting nerve roots, and the accompanying vascular structures. The exposed position, high carrying load, expansive range of motion, and limited intrinsic bony stability of the spine in the neck region mean that it is exposed to a wide range of injuries, from soft-tissue sprains to severe fracture-dislocations with associated neurovascular injury. Cervical spine trauma is estimated to lead to 25,000 new fractures per year in the United States, affecting 2% to 3% of all patients with blunt trauma.[1] The estimated incidence is 10 to 50 fractures per 1 million population. The leading injury mechanisms are motor vehicle crashes, falls from a height, and sports-related incidents.

Important dynamic changes are occurring in the prevalent types of injuries and the affected populations.

Dr. Chapman or an immediate family member serves as a board member, owner, officer, or committee member of the North American Spine Society, AO Spine International, AO Spine North America, and the Cervical Spine Research Society; is a member of a speakers' bureau or has made paid presentations on behalf of Medtronic Sofamor Danek and Synthes USA; serves as a paid consultant to Synthes USA; serves as an unpaid consultant to DePuy (a Johnson & Johnson Company), Stryker, Alseres Pharmaceuticals, and Paradigm Spine; has received research or institutional support from DePuy (a Johnson & Johnson Company), Medtronic Sofamor Danek, Synthes, Stryker, HansJoerg and the Wyss Foundation; and has received nonincome support (such as equipment or services), commercially derived honoraria, or other non-research–related funding (such as paid travel) from Synthes, Stryker, and Medtronic Sofamor Danek. Dr. Bransford or an immediate family member is a member of a speakers' bureau or has made paid presentations on behalf of AO and Synthes; serves as a paid consultant to Synthes; and has received research or institutional support from AO, Biomet, Pfizer, Wright Medical Technology, DePuy (a Johnson & Johnson Company), Spinevision, Stryker, and Synthes.

Historically, the focus of cervical spine trauma care has been on high–kinetic energy injuries affecting relatively young and healthy individuals. Decreasing rates of cervical spine trauma have been reported in this demographic group, along with increasing rates of survival. The cause may be improvements in automobile safety features, such as airbags. However, in patients older than 65 years, injuries resulting from low-energy mechanisms or preexisting spine or systemic comorbidities are of increasing concern because of the risk of morbidity and mortality. More than 20% of all cervical spine trauma is estimated to occur in patients older than 65 years. The population older than 85 years is projected to double by 2025.[2] Unstable injuries, such as odontoid fractures, are the most common injury variant in patients older than 65 years.[3]

Injury Assessment Strategies and Clearance

Clinicians treating trauma patients must effectively assess and predict the structural integrity of the entire spine, and especially the cervical spine because of its exposed position. Spine assessment and clearance are best accomplished with a systematic clinical evaluation and appropriate imaging studies. Knowledge of the injury mechanism, the patient's preinjury functional status, and injury-related changes in neurologic function are important in a spine injury assessment. Posterior neck tenderness, ecchymosis, and interspinous crepitus or gapping are key examination findings. A formal neurologic evaluation, including mental status and extremity assessment, using the American Spinal Injury Association (ASIA) template (http://www.asia-spinalinjury.org/publications/2006_Classif_worksheet.pdf) should be part of a routine examination. It is very important to formally document these neurologic assessments in an ongoing fashion to provide a timeline of neurologic status. Chapter 44 provides specific information on neurologic status assessment.

The greatest impact on outcome is prevention of secondary neurologic deterioration in a patient who is initially neurologically intact. It is important to optimize the chances for recovery in a patient with an established spinal cord injury. The risk of secondary neurologic injury and long-term patient morbidity is largely correlated with the presence of a spine injury that was overlooked because of inadequate imaging studies. Therefore, an effective spine clearance algorithm and

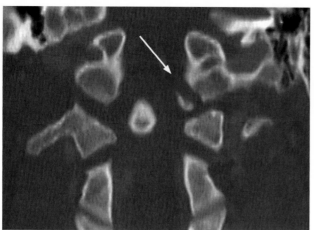

Figure 1 Coronal CT reformat of a 24-year-old man with type III occipital condyle fracture in the setting of a highly unstable occipitocervical dissociation with occiput-C1 widening and C1-C2 widening (*arrow*).

implementation of spinal column protection are integral to the overall trauma care pathway.

Triage of patients who may need spine imaging and immobilization can follow several suggested pathways. The widely accepted, relatively simple National Emergency X-Radiology Utilization Study (NEXUS) criteria for clinical cervical spine clearance includes five points: the patient (1) is cognitively unimpaired; (2) does not have neck pain; (3) has a nonfocal neurologic examination; (4) does not have tenderness, swelling, ecchymosis, or major lacerations in the head-neck area; and (5) has a pain-free neck range of motion. Patients who meet these criteria do not need further cervical spine imaging.[4] Spine injury is suspected in any patient who has been involved in a traumatic event and does not meet all of these criteria. A formal, methodical clinical evaluation is required, including documentation of the injury history, neck inspection and palpation, and a neurologic assessment using the ASIA standards. The role of routine cervical screening radiographs has been reevaluated based on several large-scale studies, and the increasingly common availability of rapid-acquisition CT technology in emergency departments has made CT the preferred imaging modality.[5] The inherent limitations of conventional radiographs include limited visualization of the transition zones, especially in the craniocervical and cervicothoracic region. Helical cervical spine CT increasingly is being validated as the preferred diagnostic modality for at-risk patients. More specifically, routine screening CT of the cervical spine has been recommended for patients with craniofacial, long bone, or pelvic trauma; impaired cognitive status; focal neurologic findings on examination; a history of an ankylosing spine disorder; a history of high-energy trauma (such as a fall of ≥ 10 feet or a motor vehicle crash at a speed of ≥ 30 miles per hour); or if there was an associated death at the scene of the traumatic

event.[4-6] The disadvantage of this imaging approach is the considerable radiation dose to the thyroid and other soft tissues. Neck clearance continues to be challenging in patients with a persistent severe cognitive impairment, although recent studies suggest that these patients can be cleared of a clinically unstable injury if CT reveals no abnormality.[4] Most centers use a three-phase protocol for spine clearance for at-risk patients. In the first phase, a helical CT of the entire cervical spine, with sagittal and coronal reformatted views, is reviewed and presumably cleared. The second phase involves a secondary review of all spine imaging studies after an attempt at clinical reevaluation. If the absence of any radiographic sign of injury is confirmed, the third phase is initiated, in which upright lateral spine radiographs are used to assess for the presence of new-onset deformity. Another approach is the use of MRI as a screening tool for these patients in the third phase. The considerable cost and logistic factors related to MRI use have continued to limit its popularity.

For patients with questionable ligamentous instability, a traction test can be helpful in demonstrating relevant disruption. This test is done under fluoroscopy by an experienced examiner (preferably a surgeon) and uses low in-line weight application of no more than 10 lb. Flexion-extension radiographs remain a mainstay of cervical spine instability evaluation for awake patients without known neurologic or major musculoskeletal injury but not for patients with severe head injury. For now, plain CT with a secondary review protocol remains a reasonable clearance system for patients with a protracted lack of interactive cognitive skills.

Routine MRI has been recommended for any patient with cervical spinal cord injury and for screening a patient with an ankylosing disorder or a possible occult spine injury.[7] In addition to revealing acute hemorrhage and cord signal changes, some imaging sequences, such as T2-weighted fat suppression views, also can show acute ligament injuries of the cervical spine. There is a strong relationship between mechanism of injury, cord signal changes, and severity of spinal cord injury as seen on MRI.

Injury Classification

Upper Cervical Spine
Occipital condyle fractures have received increased attention as detection rates have increased with the routine use of CT in trauma applications. The simple Anderson-Montesano three-part system has remained largely unchallenged and provides helpful guidance for management.[8]

This system differentiates impaction injuries (type I) from shear injuries that extend into the skull base (type II). Both of these injury types usually are inherently stable, but little is known about their long-term clinical outcomes. A type III injury is an avulsion injury of the alar ligaments, and it has the potential to be a highly unstable craniocervical disruption (**Figure 1**).

The Traynelis classification of atlanto-occipital dissociations depends on the direction of displacement.[9] This system is limited by absence of a severity component and is likely to disproportionately show anterior cranial displacement relative to the cervical spine because of the size of the head. As with a true ligamentous disruption of any joint in the body, an injury description using the direction of displacement can be somewhat misleading if the two adjoining bony ends can be manipulated in any direction.

The Harborview craniocervical injury classification attempts to identify the severity of the traumatic disruption in a three-tier system analogous to that of basic ligamentous extremity injury.[10] Type I injuries are isolated and can be treated nonsurgically; these include stable, unilateral type III occipital condyle injuries or isolated alar ligament tears. A type III injury is an obvious complete disruption of all interconnecting ligaments; patients are subclassified on the basis of whether they survive to reach the emergency department. The limitation of this system lies in the ambiguous definition of a type II injury, which is a craniocervical disruption with borderline radiographic screening values. These injuries are inherently unstable but may be missed on cursory evaluation. This injury category points out the potential for incomplete and occult craniocervical disruption, which remains a challenge to timely recognition. Studies have suggested at least a 30% delay in diagnosis with potential for serious secondary neurologic deterioration in patients with these potentially life-threatening injuries.[10] The advent of a systematic head-and-neck CT protocol and increased awareness of this injury has reduced the incidence of missed craniocervical injuries.

There have been few concerted efforts to revise the existing classification systems for atlas fractures.[11] The basic questions pertain to stability prediction and the fate of displaced intra-articular fractures. The Levine classification differentiates problematic fractures from injuries with an anticipated uncomplicated course.[12] The less concerning fractures include posterior arch fractures, transverse process injuries, and some lateral mass fractures. Segmental anterior arch fractures and displaced intra-articular injuries, as well as comminuted three- or four-part bursting injuries, are of concern because of their instability and complex management course. One of the key factors in determining the stability of atlas fractures is the integrity of the transverse atlantal ligament (TAL), which is not specifically addressed in the Levine classification system. Previously it was believed that a combined overhang of the C1 lateral masses by more than 6.9 mm, as measured on open-mouth odontoid radiographs, was indicative of a TAL disruption. However, this long-held belief was challenged by study of advanced imaging modalities, which found that only 39% of atlas fractures with a disrupted TAL were detected if radiographs alone were used.[13] The 7-mm overhang criterion for determining a TAL disruption is no longer believed to be relevant as a screening tool; scrutiny of relevant CT and MRI is recommended instead. A simple categorization of TAL injuries into bony avulsion injury (type I) or ligamentous injury (type II) has been suggested because of the inherently different likelihood of healing with nonsurgical care.[12] Purely ligamentous TAL disruption has almost no chance of healing, but most bony avulsion injuries can be expected to heal with appropriate nonsurgical management.

Odontoid fractures are represented by the well-known Anderson-d'Alonzo spine injury classification.[14] Although simple and intuitively clear, this system includes an exceedingly rare injury in its type I category, and it does not differentiate type II injuries by the severity-related factors that distinguish their prognosis or treatment. Some subtypes of type II fractures are useful for avoiding management pitfalls, but they are not part of a systematic, integrated odontoid classification system.[15]

Fractures of the axis have been divided into the broad categories of vertebral body fractures and hangman's fractures. The four-tiered classification of hangman's fracture separates type II fractures into type II and type IIA.[16] Type II fractures are intrinsically more stable from a discoligamentous standpoint; they can usually be managed in traction and converted to external immobilization. Type IIA fractures feature flexion-distraction through the C2-3 disk with posterior ligamentous disruption. An additional subtype, the Eismont-Starr atypical hangman variant, is associated with a much higher neurologic injury rate (**Figure 2**). The Francis fracture severity scale is a relatively simple and reproducible means of describing angulation and translational displacement. In general, the upper cervical spine injury classifications are highly specific and very detailed, but a systematic regional classification has proved elusive.[11]

It is important to remember that a specific injury entity must be seen in the context of its possible association with other upper cervical spine injuries. For instance, an odontoid fracture may be associated with a TAL disruption, and this injury is dramatically less likely to heal nonsurgically. Similarly, an isolated atlantoaxial rotatory subluxation may be eminently treatable with nonsurgical means. However, this injury may be associated with a contralateral atlantoaxial joint disruption that renders the entire upper cervical spine unstable in the form of a craniocervical disruption. These combination injuries are not uncommon in the upper cervical spine. A detailed assessment of the entire functional unit is required, with subsequent comprehensive treatment to optimize the result.

Lower Cervical Spine and Cervicothoracic Junction

Classifications of lower cervical spine injuries have been formulated around anatomic, biomechanical, or combined concepts and features. A lack of basic characteristics such as simplicity and interobserver-intraobserver reliability, as well as a lack of relevance to treatment and outcomes, has limited the general acceptance of lower cervical spine classification systems.[17]

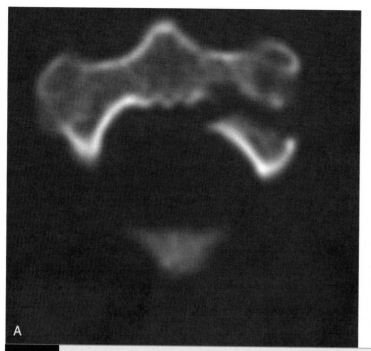

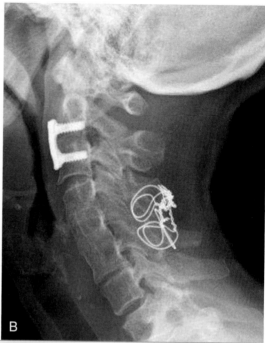

Figure 2 **A,** Preoperative axial CT scan of an atypical hangman's fracture in a 73-year-old woman with a history of C4-C6 fusion presenting with ASIA D spinal cord injury. **B,** Postoperative lateral radiograph after C2-C3 anterior cervical diskectomy and instrumented fusion.

Conceptually, the AO-ASIF system accepted by the Orthopaedic Trauma Association has the merit of combining widely accepted injury types with some correlation to treatment algorithms. The three basic injury categories consist of a simple type A injury, including inherently stable fractures that usually result from an axial loading mechanism; a type B injury, including bending injuries such as a unilateral or bilateral dislocation with or without fractures; and a type C injury, including circumferentially destabilized fracture-dislocations. Unfortunately, a tiered system of subcategories has greatly increased the complexity of this system at the cost of reproducibility. This system has limited relevance for management. The most detailed system that incorporates an injury severity gradient is the mechanistic Allen-Ferguson model.[18] This system is based on the assumption of a unidirectional force of varying grades of energy applied in a highly predictable manner. However, this system is hampered by a lack of discrete differentiators and insufficient interobserver reliability; it has had limited use for research purposes.

Recently, attempts to simplify pleomorphic lower cervical spine injuries into the simple injury categories typical of conventional classification systems have been expanded by the concept of severity scores, which attempt to quantify injuries by attaching a numeric score to key elements of the cervical spinal column. The Cervical Spine Injury Severity Scale (CSISS) measures displacement of injury in the anterior, posterior, and two lateral columns and assigns a total score.[19] The alternative Spine Trauma Study Group system is referred to as the subaxial injury classification. This system derives an injury score from a combination of three components: injury morphology, integrity of the diskoligamentous complex, and neurologic injury.[20] Neurologic injury status, as determined from the physical examination, is incorporated into the overall injury description. There is general agreement that neither severity scale will serve as the sole tool for stability assessment or treatment decision making. However, by providing a checklist of the important components of cervical spine stability, these classifications help clinicians create a more reproducible decision-making process and invite researchers to compare treatment results based on injury severity calculations. The intraobserver and interobserver evaluations have been encouraging.

No single system or concept has emerged as clearly preferable to the other systems. However, recent studies have found that the interobserver and intraobserver reliability of both severity scales is better than that of the more traditional classification systems. These severity scales have the potential to improve understanding of injuries by providing a checklist for complete evaluation, and they may improve understanding of treatment outcomes relative to injury severity.

Management

Emergency Management in the Field

The emergency management of patients with a spine trauma is important for limiting the potential of further injury to a destabilized spinal column and for minimizing further bleeding and pain. The basic concepts of first responder care include avoidance of neck and back manipulation. Supine immobilization on a rigid backboard is used with full spine precautions and a rigid neck collar. The resuscitation phase consists of maintaining normal or near-normal blood pressures to maximize cord perfusion while seeking to normalize tissue oxygenation and striving for a hematocrit level above 30%. Manual inline traction, awake, fiberoptic intubation, and transnasal intubation are recommended as adjuvant techniques to establish formal airway access for patients with a potential cervical spine injury while minimizing the potential for secondary injury displacement.[21]

Reduction

Traction-induced realignment is a very important emergent intervention option for a displaced cervical spine injury, with the potential to achieve indirect neural canal decompression. The timing and technique of reduction of a cervical spine fracture-dislocation remains controversial, however, with respect to neuroimaging.[22] Secondary neurologic deterioration may occur as a result of disk or bone fragments being dislodged into the spinal canal during a reduction maneuver. The additional diagnostic insight afforded by MRI must be balanced against the potential for damage from leaving a cervical spine fracture-dislocation unreduced and the need to subject a patient with a dislocated neck to additional transfers. Even in an efficient and well-equipped trauma center, MRI is time consuming. The actual incidence of clinically threatening mass effects in patients with a subaxial fracture-dislocation was found to be much lower than originally feared, however.[23] Prospective studies found that it is safe for an awake, alert, examinable patient with spinal cord injury to undergo closed reduction with sequential skeletal traction and avoidance of neck manipulation before MRI is performed.[24] Early reduction of cervical fracture-dislocations may improve the prospects for neural injury recovery, although the incidence and specific circumstances leading to improvement remain unclear. The current general recommendation is that patients with a confirmed spinal cord injury should receive an attempt at formal closed reduction with skeletal cranial traction aided by serial neurologic checks and followed by a postreduction neuroimaging study to assess for ongoing cord compression.[22] If the patient has ongoing cord compression, emergent surgical intervention with removal of impinging structures and stabilization is encouraged. For a patient who is neurologically intact, closed reduction before MRI remains an option if MRI is not immediately available. Closed reduction of a dislocated cervical spine in an unresponsive or otherwise unexaminable patient usually is discouraged until neuroimaging has been obtained and has confirmed the absence of ongoing cord compression from a disk or bone fragment. As the use of open anterior or posterior cervical spine decompression and instrumentation techniques has increased, there has been a recent trend toward bypassing closed reduction and taking patients directly to the operating room for definitive surgical decompression and instrumentation (**Figure 3**).

Any form of neck traction is generally contraindicated in the presence of distraction trauma in the cervical spine because of the danger of increasing neural trauma and compromising arterial flow to the brain and spinal cord. The application of cranial tongs may be contraindicated in some types of skull fractures for fear of causing a fracture propagation and secondary brain injury. Therefore, application of skull tongs in the presence of fractures is not advisable unless approved by a surgeon familiar with neurotrauma.

Closed reduction of a dislocated lower cervical spine should be performed in a controlled setting. The principles include patient monitoring (cardiovascular, respiratory, and neurologic), incrementally increased skeletal traction using fluoroscopy or serial radiographs, intravenous analgesia, and muscle relaxation. As traction is applied to the cervical spine, periodic radiographs assess for overdistraction in any of its segments. Manual reduction attempts are generally discouraged because they can exert uncontrollable forces on the neck and may cause a disk or bone fragment to shear off into the canal. Cervical reduction efforts should be abandoned and an urgent MRI should be obtained if the patient's neurologic status deteriorates during reduction efforts. Reduction also is usually abandoned if realignment fails with traction weight amounting to two thirds of the patient's body weight. This weight recommendation is not absolute, however, and it depends on individual clamp specifications. For most graphite-based tongs, a fixed limitation of 80 lb has been suggested because of the risk of clamp deformation at higher loads, with subsequent clamp pullout. In patients with a persistent impinging spinal cord lesion, emergency surgical intervention aimed at neural element decompression and stabilization of the affected injury segment may have to be considered (**Figure 3**).

Acute Steroid Administration

This topic is discussed in greater detail in chapter 44. The pharmacologic care options for patients with a suspected spinal cord injury generally are limited to intravenous administration of methylprednisolone. Blood pressure and cardiac output support are provided through intravenous administration of vasopressors to patients with neurogenic shock.[21] The popularity of aggressive steroid management has tapered off considerably because of the absence of a demonstrable major clinical impact on cord recovery since completion of the North American Spinal Cord Injury (NASCIS) studies.[25] There have been persistent questions about the methodology used in these studies, however. The general recommendation is that intravenous steroid administration is only a treatment option and not a recommendation or a standard of care. Steroid use has not been formally studied in patients with a nerve root injury or gunshot injury and, therefore, is not recommended for these indications.

5: Spine

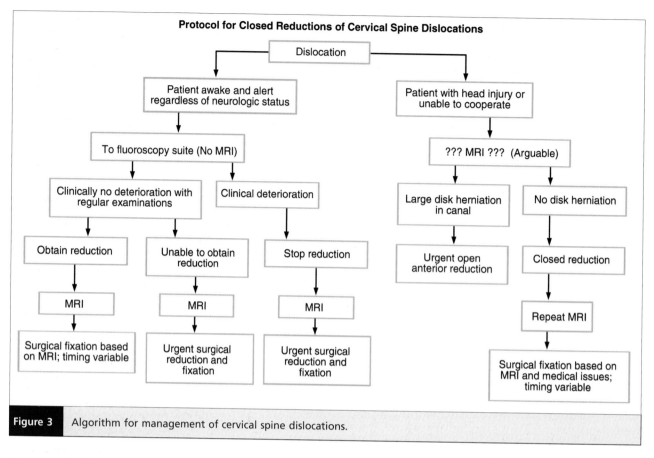

Protocol for Closed Reductions of Cervical Spine Dislocations

Figure 3   Algorithm for management of cervical spine dislocations.

Nonsurgical Care

Sound decision making for treatment of any spine trauma is based on a comprehensive multifactorial assessment that defies the use of a simple binary algorithm. The scientific literature does not provide decisive guidance on preferred treatments. There is a prevalence of type III and IV evidence based on small patient cohorts and personal observations. Treatment preferences strongly differ based on the clinician's training background, type of practice, and practice location.[26] In addition to the considerations for the thoracolumbar spine, the neck has complexities related to its exposed location and delicate bony structures in close proximity to vital arteries, neural elements, and pharyngeal structures. Craniocervical injuries and penetrating trauma can pose an immediate vital threat from airway compromise and anoxia. Usually decisive emergency surgical intervention is required. Vertebral artery injuries may considerably alter the usual diagnostic and treatment algorithm for trauma patients. For instance, anterior neck procedures, although they are less invasive than thoracolumbar procedures, have difficulties related to biomechanical limitations and potential postoperative aspiration and dysphagia, especially in patients older than 65 years. The important decision-making factors include the presence of neurologic injury, structural damage to key supporting structures, differentiation of osseous and ligamentous trauma, and specific injury mechanisms.[19,20] Other patient factors also heavily influence treatment decision making, in-

cluding patient age and size, quality of bone structure, preoperative alignment, presence of ankylosing spine disorders, overall injury load, and other preexistent comorbidities. General factors that favor a successful outcome of nonsurgical care include an absence of neurologic injury, predominantly bony injuries with intact key supporting ligaments, preservation of a satisfactory alignment, and a single-system injury. The choices of nonsurgical care range from activity restriction for a patient with an inherently stable injury to external immobilization with a brace or halo vest or prolonged recumbent skeletal traction for a patient with a very unstable injury. Soft collars have no inherent biomechanical stabilizing effects on the lower cervical spine and usually are reserved for symptom reduction in patients with neck muscle sprains. Rigid neck collars are suitable for external immobilization after surgery and can be considered for patients with a minimally deformed compression fracture or an apophyseal injury. However, conventional neck collars offer little stabilization to the transition zones, such as the cervicothoracic region. Some additional stability can be provided by thoracic and cranial attachments to a rigid neck collar. Nevertheless, injuries treated with such combination devices need to have some inherent stability because in actual use there often is a fair amount of subaxial motion.

Halo vests continue to provide the most rigid form of cervical spine external immobilization. However, a halo vest assembly cannot fully immobilize the midcervical spine. In a phenomenon known as snaking, focal kyphosis in the midcervical spine can be seen on a recumbent lateral radiograph, but an upright lateral radiograph shows maintained lordosis. For this reason a halo vest assembly is primarily used in patients with an upper cervical spine injury. In general, halo vest treatment is unsuitable for patients who have extreme obesity, polytrauma, or chest deformity or injury. Halo vests also are unsuitable for patients who are frail and elderly, primarily because the pulmonary constraint increases the risk of aspiration. Halo ring applications usually are contraindicated for patients with a skull fracture or another cranial defect. Several studies described the limitations of these devices and emphasized the high complication rates from infection, pin site loosening, or failure of stabilization.[27,28] Complications occurred in as many as 35% of patients. Most of the complications were minor, however, and 84% of patients had satisfactory healing without surgery.[27] Properly applied halo vest immobilization remains the most useful nonsurgical treatment for a select group of mainly osseous cervical spine injuries.

Surgical Principles: Timing and General Concepts

The timing of surgical intervention for cervical spine trauma is somewhat controversial, in part because of the vague nature of definitions regarding emergent care. The most commonly used timeline to differentiate early and late surgery in spine trauma is 72 hours, although 48 and 24 hours also have been suggested. Interventions taking place after 24 hours are not considered acute in many other specialties, however. A feasibility study found that surgical intervention within 8 hours was possible for no more than 10% of patients.[29] Important considerations in the timing of surgery for spine injury include the overall injury burden (injury severity) and the presence of comorbidities, ankylosis of the spinal column, vertebral artery injury, ability to reduce dislocations, persistent cord compression, or neurologic injury. The five basic categories of neurologic injury are applicable to the cervical spine: neurologically intact status, incomplete spinal cord injury, complete spinal cord injury, root injury, and status unknown because of persistent cognitive impairment. The presence of neurologic injury, especially with persistent cord compression, is commonly regarded as an indication for emergent decompression. Early surgical spine intervention for trauma has been overwhelmingly described as safe in studies mostly of patients with thoracolumbar injury.[30] In general, early surgical intervention for spine trauma results in reduced overall length of stay and decreased intensive care stay as well as pulmonary deterioration. Treatment at a trauma center decreases the likelihood of paralysis by 33%, compared with treatment at a nontrauma center.[31] A more aggressive approach toward spinal column trauma management and more effective integrated care were identified as possible causes for this finding, which was based on the study of large administrative databases. If early surgical intervention for cervical spine trauma is chosen, adherence to trauma management principles is recommended, such as maintenance of spine immobilization, physiologic blood pressure (mean arterial pressure > 85 mm Hg), hematocrit level (> 30), and oxygenation as well as atraumatic airway management. Maintenance of physiologic blood pressure has been increasingly emphasized to avoid a second-shock trauma to the neural elements. Secondary postresuscitation hypotension is particularly damaging in patients with central nervous system injuries and should be avoided if possible. If available, electrophysiologic neuromonitoring may be useful in acute surgical spine trauma management.

Despite absence of specific pertinent studies, the important factors in recommending early surgical care for patients with a confirmed complete spinal cord injury are expedited mobilization, improved skin care, simplified chemical deep venous thrombosis–pulmonary embolism prophylaxis, and early rehabilitation care. There are no clear guidelines as to the timing of surgery for patients with a cervical spine fracture and concurrent neurologic injury. Despite animal studies with findings favoring early surgical intervention,[32-36] this practice has not been fully validated in clinical studies. Emerging studies have found neurologic improvement with early decompression and stabilization, however. The unpublished Surgical Treatment for Acute Spinal Cord Injury Study, which retrospectively assessed the timing of intervention in more than 200 patients with incomplete spinal cord injury, found an improved motor score and ASIA status for patients treated early.

The goals of surgical treatment of cervical spine injuries are to restore physiologic alignment, protect and decompress the compromised neural elements, and provide effective stabilization to incapacitated segments. Ideally, these goals are achieved by using the least invasive and atraumatic technique possible and involving the fewest possible motion segments in any arthrodesis construct. Most spine trauma can be treated from either an anterior or posterior approach, with combined anterior-posterior procedures reserved for the most complex injuries or for patients with preexisting concurrent multifocal stenosis or deformity. Insights gained from advanced neuroimaging and refinements in surgical implants for the cervical spine are expanding the treatment options. Ultimately, cervical spine surgery will allow rapid mobilization of a patient with minimal reliance on external immobilization devices.

Craniocervical Injuries

Recognition of potentially unstable craniocervical dissociation can be lifesaving in some patients, and it represents the most important step in preventing further damage to patients with a nondisrupted spinal cord. An injury affecting any component of the upper cervical spine should be scrutinized for a more complex injury because the upper cervical spine forms an integrated anatomic and functional unit.[10] Occasionally, a surgeon may need to differentiate a truly unstable injury from a

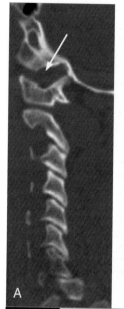
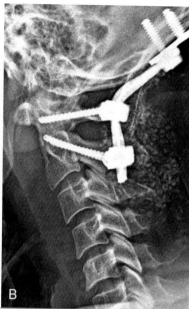

Figure 4 **A,** Parasagittal CT reformat in a 23-year-old man involved in a high-speed motor vehicle collision with obvious occiput – C1 distraction and occipital-cervical dissociation (*arrow*). **B,** Postoperative lateral radiograph demonstrating occiput to C2 posterior instrumented fusion with structural iliac crest allograft and morcellized autograft and bone graft extenders.

partially disrupted injury by using a traction test if there is still uncertainty after a dedicated CT and MRI of the craniocervical junction. Traction is generally undesirable for craniocervical dissociations because it can subject the upper cervical spinal cord to undue tension and aggravate any underlying neurologic injury. Even a halo ring and vest offer only marginal immobilization of a truly unstable craniocervical dissociation, while tending to distract the head from the neck. Temporary immobilization using sandbags around the head and crossover tape may afford better immobilization to the injured region until definitive surgery is performed. Surgical stabilization should be done as early as is medically safe. Preoperative baseline electrophysiologic assessment with motor- and somatosensory-evoked potentials can aid in safely positioning a patient with an unstable injury. The preferred surgical management consists of an occipitocervical arthrodesis to C2 or C3, using rigid segmental fixation and posterior decompression as necessary (**Figure 4**). More limited fixation, as from the occiput to the C1 ring, does not treat the more global instability of a disrupted craniocervical junction.

Atlas and Transverse Atlantal Ligament Injury

In general, most atlas fractures can be treated nonsurgically with suitable immobilization. The subtypes with a high likelihood of unsatisfactory nonsurgical outcome include disruption of the TAL or a displaced fracture of the lateral mass such as a sagittal split injury.[37] Atlantoaxial instability with eventual cord compression, a

painful cock-robin position of the head, and suboccipital headache can be the result of lack of congruous healing of the C1 lateral masses between the occipital condyles and the C2 superior articular processes. An atlantal fracture malunion or nonunion usually requires a challenging late craniocervical reconstruction. In contrast, early recognition of an unstable atlantal fracture may allow atlantoaxial motion-preserving C1 primary internal fixation with posterior lateral mass screws and direct internal reduction without fusion.

Most patients with a confirmed TAL disruption require atlantoaxial instrumented arthrodesis. This procedure is most commonly done through posterior surgery with rigid segmental fixation, although anterior techniques have been used. Cable or wire fixation of C1 and C2 has a secondary role of securing bone graft because of its inherent biomechanical limitations. The segmental fixation options include C1-C2 transarticular screws, C1 lateral mass screws, and C2 fixation achieved with pedicle, pars, or translaminar screws.[38] These instrumentation options offer an unprecedented ability to adapt to the patient's individual anatomic and biomechanical needs, with reliable fracture healing.

Odontoid Injuries

Most odontoid fractures are amenable to successful nonsurgical management. Type I injury is rare and requires close evaluation for a potential craniocervical dissociation. Similarly, most type III fractures, in which the typical fracture pattern reaches into the cancellous body of the axis, can be expected to heal well with appropriate nonsurgical realignment and immobilizations. Type II odontoid fractures continue to be the subject of considerable debate and uncertainty. For well-selected patients, nonsurgical treatment is likely to lead to union. The prognostically favorable factors include minimal fracture translation, angulation, and absence of comminution. Patient-related factors, including good general health, no nicotine use, and no other cervical spine abnormalities, are another key to successful treatment. For a patient with good bone quality who has an unstable odontoid fracture of a suitable pattern, anterior odontoid screws placed by an experienced surgeon in atraumatic fashion offer the potential for primary fracture healing with preservation of some atlantoaxial motion[15] (**Figure 5**). Typically, a single well-placed screw offers sufficient biomechanical fracture fixation, with healing rates similar to those of dual screws.

There remains significant controversy as to the preferred management of type II odontoid fractures, which are encountered with increasing frequency in geriatric patients.[39] The treatment recommendations range from surgery with an attempt at anterior odontoid screw fixation or primary posterior arthrodesis and fixation to palliative soft neck collar placement, which can be expected to result in nonunion. Posterior atlantoaxial segmental arthrodesis offers the advantage of immediate stability and mobilization, with minimal reliance on external immobilization. Regardless of the treatment,

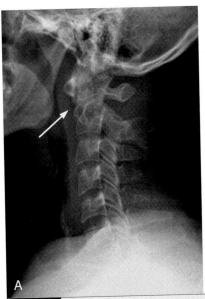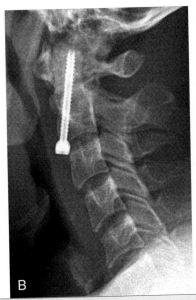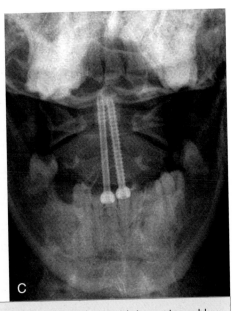

Figure 5 **A,** Preoperative lateral radiograph of a 24-year-old man initially managed in a halo vest but with increasing subluxation of his type II dens fracture (*arrow*). **B,** Postoperative lateral radiograph after placement of two cannulated odontoid screws. **C,** Postoperative open-mouth radiograph of two cannulated odontoid screws.

there is a high risk of swallowing difficulty or aspiration. The 1-year mortality rate is as high as 40% for these patients.[39]

Because of disagreement as to the treatment algorithm for unstable type II odontoid fractures, its management depends on the surgeon's preference and the perceived patient needs. In general, posterior atlantoaxial arthrodesis using segmental fixation offers the greatest likelihood of successful healing of an unstable type II odontoid injury, with the least reliance on external mobilization. Treatment recommendations for an impaired elderly patient remain to be clarified. Palliative management using a soft neck collar is acceptable for a medically compromised elderly patient with a short expected life span.

Hangman's Fracture

Most type I and most type II hangman's fractures can be treated nonsurgically with immobilization. However, a type IIA fracture, with a typical C2-3 disk disruption and accompanying kyphosis and translation, can be treated with more predictable results using surgical stabilization. Either posterior C1-C3 posterior instrumented fusion or anterior C2-C3 cervical decompression and instrumented fusion can be used. Despite the biomechanical advantages of posterior instrumentation, the necessary incorporation of the C1 segment limits its appeal, unless direct pars fracture with internal fixation screws is feasible. Anterior C2-C3 fixation offers preservation of atlantoaxial motion, but it is less than straightforward because of the approach and several technical challenges.

In a type III injury, there is a bilateral pars fracture and subluxation of the C2 facet joint on C3. It is difficult to achieve closed reduction of the dislocation and common concurrent spinal cord injury, and closed reduction may be impossible because the C2 posterior pars and lamina are dissociated from both the proximal and caudal spine elements. Early open reduction followed by C1-C3 or C2-C3 instrumented fusion using segmental fixation is recommended.

Lower Cervical Spine Injuries

With the advent of modern rigid fixation systems, surgeons frequently are able to reliably achieve stability using anterior or posterior fixation only. Posterior instrumentation offers better biomechanical fixation stiffness in flexion, the ability to reduce dislocated facet joints directly, the ability to perform stable multilevel fixation extending into the transition zones, higher union rates with segmental fixation, and the opportunity to perform a multilevel neural element decompression of cord and individual roots. However, anterior neck surgery performed in a simple supine position is less painful and prone to complications than posterior surgery. The potential for a more meaningful neurologic recovery is afforded by decompression of the anterolateral corticospinal tracts, with better biomechanics in extension loading. In a prospective comparison of anterior-posterior cervical surgery, 70% of patients treated with anterior surgery improved at least one Frankel grade, compared with 57% of patients treated with posterior surgery.[40] Posterior cervical spine surgery has been associated with increased bleeding, more wound-healing complications, and prolonged myofascial incisional pain. This constellation has led to a trend toward anterior neck surgery for most types of unstable lower cervical spine trauma.

As a general strategy, the approach to an injured lower cervical spine should be chosen based on the lo-

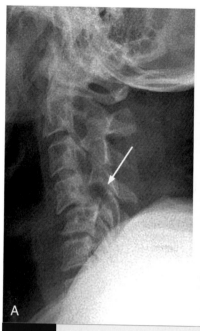
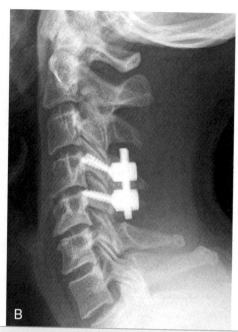
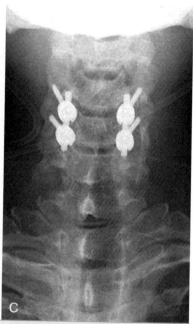

Figure 6 A, Trauma lateral radiograph showing C4-C5 bilateral jumped facets (*arrow*) in a 52-year-old man after a 20-foot fall. Postoperative lateral **(B)** and AP **(C)** radiographs after closed reduction in a fluoroscopy suite and then surgical fixation with lateral mass screws into C4 and C5.

cation of the most severe structural damage. This principle implies, for example, that burst fractures should be treated via an anterior approach, and facet dislocations, with or without fracture, should be treated via a posterior approach. Similarly, depressed lamina fractures are treated through a posterior approach. As in any trauma surgery, a neural decompression should be accompanied by rigid internal fixation and arthrodesis to maintain lasting physiologic alignment.

The posterior implant options primarily consist of rod-and-screw systems, with lateral mass screw placement being the standard of care for the C3 through C6 segments (**Figure 6**). Over the past decade, these techniques have been established as safe and effective for posterior cervical stabilization. In contrast, pedicle screw fixation of the C3 through C6 segments has been used only for stabilization of certain degenerative conditions and has not become a primary form of posterior cervical spine fixation. Because of the absence of suitable lateral masses at the axis and in the cervicothoracic junction, pedicle screw fixation has emerged as the posterior fixation technique of choice for instrumentation of the C2, C7, and upper thoracic segments.

Common trauma indications for anterior subaxial cervical spine surgery include unstable burst fracture in a metabolically healthy patient or a patient with a previously reduced lower cervical spine fracture-dislocation. The limitations of anterior subaxial trauma surgery, compared to posterior neck procedures, include the usual exposure restriction to two or three motion segments, poor access to the cervical transition zones, and increased exposure-related morbidity such as dysphagia. Anterior cervical plating offers less stiffness in

flexion, torsion, and axial loading than segmental posterior stabilization techniques. Higher rates of nonunion and hardware failure are reported than with posterior procedures in patients who undergo multilevel anterior arthrodesis and in patients with osteopenia.

Anterior subaxial neck procedures can be divided into three phases: decompression, anterior column reconstruction, and anterior stabilization. Several treatment variables apply to each phase. Depending on the indication, anterior cervical decompression surgery can be accomplished with either diskectomy or corpectomy. In an acute trauma setting, multilevel anterior corpectomies are rarely if ever indicated. A corpectomy has a significantly more destabilizing effect on the neck than a diskectomy. Thus, a patient's need for decompression must be weighed against the patient's biomechanical needs and physiologic circumstances. If supplemental posterior surgery is not needed, anterior stabilization can be achieved with a low-profile plate and unicortical vertebral body screws that are rigidly locked into the plate. Although bicortical fixation has been recommended to increase biomechanical stability in the presence of trauma, this factor must be weighed against the risk of dural or neurologic injury. Rigid anterior plate fixation has minimized the need for supplemental external immobilization with a halo vest, and it improves the ability to maintain physiologic neck alignment until bony healing has been achieved. Dynamic locking plates have been introduced with the goal of improving graft healing by load sharing in patients with degenerative indications. However, these devices have little or no place in the treatment of a traumatically disrupted spinal column. The results of anterior surgery in pa-

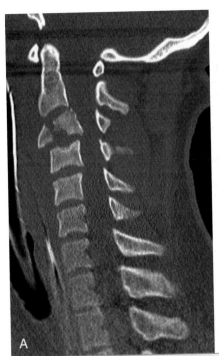
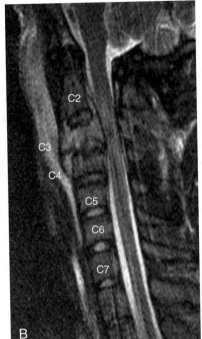
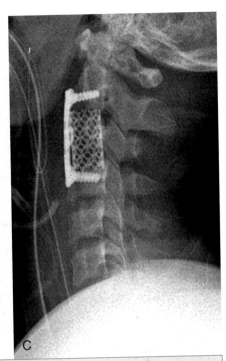

Figure 7 A, Preoperative sagittal CT scan in a 17-year-old boy who jumped over a fence and landed on his head, sustaining a C3 axial load, burst-type injury with ASIA type A spinal cord injury. B, Preoperative T2 sagittal MRI scan demonstrating high signal in the patient's spinal cord. C, Postoperative lateral radiograph after a C3 corpectomy and reconstruction with a titanium cage and anterior plating.

tients with subaxial spine trauma in general have been favorable, even in patients with a flexion-type injury and despite the inherently more limited biomechanical stiffness of these constructs compared with posterior devices.[41]

Combined anterior-posterior surgery for patients with subaxial trauma has been superseded by third-generation anterior-posterior instrumentation systems, which offer rigid fixation options. The exception is in patients with an unusually severe fracture-dislocation, fracture malunion, displaced fracture-dislocation in conjunction with an ankylosing disorder or other deformity, or severe multilevel posttraumatic myelopathy combined with cervical stenosis. For some of these patients, staging procedures on separate days can achieve the treatment goals while lessening the physiologic impact of a same-day combined procedure. The specific approach is chosen largely on the basis of the individual patient's injury and comorbidities. For instance, an initial posterior approach is more effective for reduction and stabilization in most patients with a fracture-dislocation or ankylosing spine disease. A supplemental anterior approach can be used at a later date. In contrast, patients with kyphotic fracture malunion or a severe burst fracture first usually require an anterior approach, followed by a secondary posterior stabilization and decompression of neural elements, as needed.

Burst–Axial Load Injuries

High-grade burst fractures are most commonly treated with a corpectomy, anterior strut grafting, and rigid an-

terior plate fixation (**Figure 7**). Supplemental posterior fixation may be considered if the patient is osteopenic or if there are other concerns about stability.[42] Reconstruction of an anterior column defect can be achieved with a tricortical structural iliac crest graft, structural fibular allograft, or a structural cage with autologous local bone graft core. Anterior column reconstruction options have emerged from concerns about morbidity associated with autologous iliac crest bone graft. No major study has compared the healing rates of patients who received autologous iliac crest graft for a traumatic injury and those who underwent anterior column corpectomy reconstruction using fibula allograft or a titanium cage.

Unilateral Facet Fracture-Dislocations

Unilateral facet fracture-dislocations are relatively uncommon and have been reported in less than 6% of cervical spine fractures.[43,44] These injuries are believed to occur as a result of flexion and rotatory forces acting on the spine during the injury sequence. The typical radiographic features include modest kyphosis and translation of as much as 25% of vertebral body width. The reported incidence of traumatic disk herniations is 23%.[14] The fracture may involve the superior or inferior articular processes or a comminuted lateral mass. A floating lateral mass is a separation from the vertebral body with a varying amount of facet joint disruption. There have been several attempts to classify unilateral facet fracture-dislocation, but the great injury variability has precluded any widely accepted standard interpretation. A recent categorization consists of three types with three subcategories each.[45] Type A injuries have a facet fracture, type B injuries have a dislocation without fracture, and type C injuries feature a combination. This classification system has not yet undergone validation studies.

Patients with these injuries usually are treated with closed reduction and postreduction neuroimaging to assess for neural element compression. Nerve root injury is the prevalent form of neurologic injury in these patients, usually on the side of the dislocation. Nonsurgical treatment has been suggested for patients with normal or near-normal alignment and minimal or improving neurologic symptoms. This treatment usually consists of closed reduction for a period of time, followed by external immobilization with a cervicothoracic brace or halo vest. Follow-up radiographs are reviewed for maintenance of alignment. The surgical options include anterior diskectomy and bone grafting with locking-plate fixation, posterior foraminotomy and arthrodesis using bone graft, and segmental stabilization with a screw-and-rod construct. Posterior fixation usually necessitates sacrificing an additional motion segment because of compromised fixation on the side with the fractured lateral mass. Other factors to be considered include the need for a foraminotomy, which is best accomplished from the posterior approach; and the quality of bone, with posterior segmental instrumentation offering better fixation than anterior surgery. In a study of 90 patients with isolated facet injuries, surgical care was associated with better outcomes in terms of pain and functional scores than nonsurgical care, although the length of stay was nearly twice as long in the surgically treated patients.[45] Persistent instability and further settling in the injury zone were possible causes.

Bilateral Facet Fracture-Dislocations

Bilateral facet fracture-dislocation from a bending mechanism is a serious injury because of its potential impact on the spinal cord. Although the incidence of traumatic disk herniation in bilateral facet fracture-dislocation is as low as 13%, its propensity to induce potential secondary neurologic deterioration after closed reduction is a cause for concern. Closed reduction under controlled circumstances, followed by neuroimaging, is a well-supported treatment for a communicative patient or a patient with severe spinal cord injury. Definitive segmental surgical stabilization and decompression, as needed, have been widely recommended. These goals can be accomplished with posterior segmental fixation using a screw-based system or with anterior stabilization in a patient with good bone quality. The posterior technique is preferred if the patient has poor bone quality or if posterior decompression of displaced laminar and facet fragments is necessary (**Figure 6**).

Flexion-Teardrop Injuries

A flexion-teardrop injury occurs when there is a combined loss of anterior column integrity in flexion and tensile failure of the posterior ligamentous complex. A teardrop-shaped triangular fragment typically is avulsed from the inferior edge of the rostral vertebral body while the vertebral body is pushed back into the spinal canal. The presence of neurologic injury is variable. The treatment recommendations range from nonsurgical care to anterior, posterior, or combined anterior-posterior surgery. A comparison of treatment with a halo vest to surgical care with anterior corpectomy, strut grafting, and plating found that the surgical procedure had superior radiographic and health-related quality-of-life outcomes.[40] Although this study reported no complications of surgical treatment and found that outcomes were correlated with an absence of kyphosis, other studies reported complications after anterior-only fixation in the presence of osteopenia, incomplete reduction, or major disengagement of facet joints. Overall, anterior treatment alone appears to offer a reasonably good outcome under the correct circumstances. A combination of anterior decompression and strut grafting with posterior instrumentation remains an option for patients with impaired bone quality.

Extension Injuries

Hyperextension fractures are commonly associated with an ankylosing spine condition such as disseminated idiopathic skeletal hyperostosis or ankylosing spondylitis. In patients with a pretraumatic spinal column kyphosis, fractures in an ankylosing spine often appear as a hyperextension injury. The frequently irregular fracture planes typically indicate the presence of a fracture-dislocation with inherent structural compromise.[7] Closed reduction should be attempted with the greatest of care in a patient with this type of injury because secondary spinal cord injury can occur with uncontrolled neck manipulation. If medically feasible, early surgical intervention is frequently desirable because closed reduction is difficult if not impossible to maintain, and epidural hematoma formation can further compromise the spinal cord. Typically, definitive care consists of a multilevel posterior segmental stabilization in association with posterior spinal canal decompression (**Figure 8**). In patients with an anterior column gap, secondary anterior stabilization can be achieved with a structural bone graft and plate fixation. Given the long lever arms of the spinal column and the presence of vertebral osteopenia in patients with an ankylosing spine disorder, fixation failure is somewhat likely after isolated anterior fracture stabilization.[7]

Fracture-Dislocations

Fracture-dislocation is commonly associated with spinal cord injury. Patients with cervical fracture-dislocation often have significant translational displacement, and they may need to be evaluated for a potential vertebral artery injury if the transverse foramina have fracture involvement. Closed reduction can be difficult

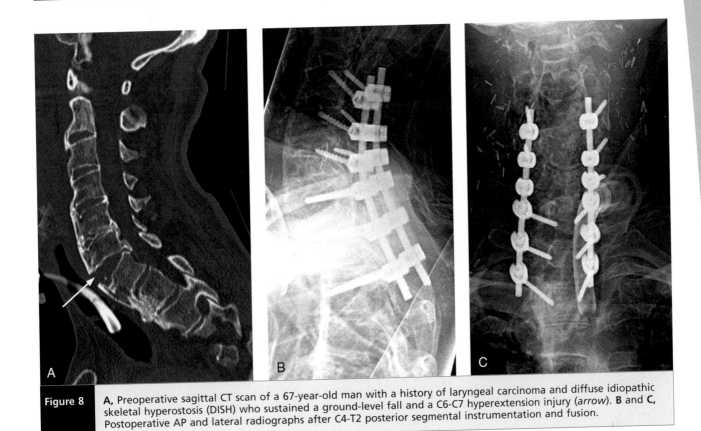

Figure 8 **A,** Preoperative sagittal CT scan of a 67-year-old man with a history of laryngeal carcinoma and diffuse idiopathic skeletal hyperostosis (DISH) who sustained a ground-level fall and a C6-C7 hyperextension injury (*arrow*). **B** and **C,** Postoperative AP and lateral radiographs after C4-T2 posterior segmental instrumentation and fusion.

to maintain because of loss of key structural elements such as facet joints and soft-tissue attachments. After the best possible closed reduction is achieved and neuroimaging is performed, the early surgical care usually involves posterior multilevel segmental instrumentation and arthrodesis. Secondary anterior column reconstruction may be necessary, depending on whether the anterior column is restored through indirect posterior reduction.

Cervicothoracic Junction Injuries

Injuries to the cervicothoracic junction (C7-T2) are only sporadically reported, but they may amount to as high as 9% of all blunt neck trauma.[46] The high rate of missed or delayed diagnosis probably results from the difficulty of imaging in this region. The increasing use of CT with reformatting as a primary screening tool may decrease the incidence of missed injuries. The most common cervicothoracic junction injuries are of the flexion type. These injuries are difficult to reduce closed because of the steep inclination angle of the facet joints of C7 and T1 and the other upper thoracic segments. In nonsurgical treatment, there is an inability to compensate for the bending forces typically exerted on the cervicothoracic junction. Posterior segmental instrumented fusion generally is the primary treatment for an unstable cervicothoracic injury. Anterior treatment is not preferred in this transition zone because of limited access, approach-related morbidity, and poor biomechanical fixation strength in the vertebral bodies of the upper thoracic spine.

Special Circumstances

Ankylosing Spine Conditions

The incidence of fractures in patients with ankylosing spondylitis, disseminated idiopathic skeletal hyperostosis, and end-stage spondylosis appears to be increasing. Injuries in an ankylosing spine may be the result of a high–kinetic energy impact mechanism or a low-impact event such as a ground-level fall. Patients with an ankylosing spine condition require an increased index of suspicion; the onus is on the clinician to prove the absence rather than the presence of a fracture. Even the slightest crack may indicate an unstable injury. Radiographic identification may be difficult because of the presence of other radiographic abnormalities. Other medical comorbidities are frequently encountered and may demand urgent medical attention, thus distracting from the spine care needs. Preinjury spine deformities are common, and frequently they pose serious immobilization and transfer problems. Most injuries in patients with an ankylosing spine condition are of the extension type and are around C5-C7, although injuries such as an odontoid fracture also can occur. The possibility of noncontiguous injuries in more than 10% of patients is a reason to perform advanced neuroimaging of the entire spinal column for detection. Other management concerns revolve around impaired bone quality from the underlying musculoskeletal disease, the potential for epidural hematoma formation in hyperemic inflammatory tissues disrupted by trauma, and the possibility of occult esophageal or aortic injuries. For all but non-displaced injuries, the preferred management usually is multisegmental posterior instrumentation and neural element decompression, as clinically indicated (**Figure 8**). Anterior surgery has a supplemental role because of the inherent biomechanical limitations and limited surgical access. Positioning of the patient for prone surgery can be daunting. A neurologically intact patient with a kyphotic deformity in the presence of an ankylosing spine disorder is in danger of secondary neurologic deterioration during any transfer or unguided realignment attempt. Realignment can be undertaken under certain conditions, but usually the spinal column is left close to its normal preinjury position to minimize the chance of uncontrolled displacement of the spinal canal. Intraoperative imaging can be difficult, and posterior bony landmarks may be severely distorted from the underlying inflammatory disease process and multilevel autofusions. Despite comprehensive multispecialty care, the survival rates in patients older than 80 years have been poor.[7]

Spine Injuries in Elderly Patients
The prevalence of cervical spine fractures is 2.4% to 4.7% in elderly patients, generally categorized as those older than 65 years.[47,48] The injury is caused by a ground-level fall in 62% of these patients. A spine fracture in elderly patients generally is more difficult to diagnose than in younger individuals because baseline, widespread spondylosis and deformity are often present. Like a fracture in a patient with an ankylosing spine condition, a fracture in these patients may be overlooked because of the low-impact injury mechanism, such as a ground-level fall, and the paucity of focal examination findings. Unstable type II odontoid fractures pose a particular treatment dilemma in this population.

Certain types of short-segment fixation that are suitable for a similar injury in younger patients are far more likely to fail in patients with age-related osteopenia and loss of physiologic mobility of the spinal column. There are greater perioperative risks such as aspiration, intolerance of external immobilization devices, and a need for anticoagulation for concurrent comorbidities. Much work remains to be done to identify optimal integrated treatment pathways for the elderly patient with cervical spine fracture.[49]

Vertebral Artery Injuries
Approximately 11% of patients with a significant cervical spine injury such as an unstable burst fracture or fracture-dislocation have disruption of physiologic vertebral artery flow.[50] If imaging reveals a displaced fracture involving the foramen transversarium, further assessment with CT angiography or magnetic resonance angiography is recommended. When aggressive screening and an individualized treatment protocol are used for blunt vertebral artery injuries, potentially preventable stroke or death is rare. No high-quality comparative studies have convincingly demonstrated improvements in overall outcomes with screening or treatment programs.[51] Transcranial Doppler screening may help identify clinically relevant flow disruption. Long-term follow-up studies have revealed persistent vertebral artery occlusion beyond 26 months following an initial injury.[52,53] A confirmed vertebral artery injury may considerably affect surgical planning because of the need to provide antiembolic coverage and ensure preservation of the artery during surgery. The management options consist of endovascular stenting or embolization and expedient surgical instrumentation of the injured segments. As with extremity injuries and concurrent arterial injuries, early decisive surgical stabilization usually is preferable to prolonged recumbence in traction. Any surgery must minimize the risk of perioperative injury to the remaining intact vertebral artery.

Emerging Concepts
With the availability of advanced spine imaging on an unprecedented scale, the increasing implementation of proven trauma recovery and resuscitation algorithms, and sophisticated and safe instrumentation systems, several advances are overdue related to relatively straightforward issues in cervical spine trauma care. The assessment and treatment of cervical spine fractures remains highly variable and inconsistent, despite many areas of improvement. There is a lack of implementation of a universal systematic evaluation and classification system for cervical spine trauma, despite their increasingly well-proven efficacy. The ongoing state of diversity and personal preferences has been detrimental to education and has diminished attempts at scientific comparison. Despite an absence of absolute scientific proof of intervention variables such as timing to neural decompression, the implementation of certain standardized treatment algorithms appears to be desirable and preferable to individualized care. Emerging data on the care of patients with severe spine injury in tertiary care centers may underscore the advantages of systematic care for this at-risk population.

Annotated References

1. Irwin ZN, Arthur M, Mullins RJ, Hart RA: Variations in injury patterns, treatment, and outcome for spinal fracture and paralysis in adult versus geriatric patients. *Spine (Phila Pa 1976)* 2004;29(7):796-802.

2. US Census Bureau: *Population Projections of the United States by Age, Sex, Race, and Hispanic Origin: 1995-2050.* Washington, DC, US Department of Commerce (Publication No P25-1130), 1995.

3. Sokolowski MJ, Jackson AP, Haak MH, Meyer PR Jr, Szewczyk Sokolowski M: Acute outcomes of cervical spine injuries in the elderly: Atlantaxial vs subaxial injuries. *J Spinal Cord Med* 2007;30(3):238-242.

This retrospective database review of 193 consecutive patients older than 65 years over a 12-year period concluded that surgical treatment of subaxial injuries was associated with an improved survival rate versus non-surgical management.

4. Harris TJ, Blackmore CC, Mirza SK, Jurkovich GJ: Clearing the cervical spine in obtunded patients. *Spine (Phila Pa 1976)* 2008;33(14):1547-1553.

 A retrospective cohort study of 367 obtunded trauma patients showed that initial CT imaging identified all unstable cervical spine injuries, and subsequent upright radiographs did not identify any additional injuries but significantly delayed spine clearance.

5. Blackmore CC, Mann FA, Wilson AJ: Helical CT in the primary trauma evaluation of the cervical spine: An evidence-based approach. *Skeletal Radiol* 2000;29(11): 632-639.

6. Bailitz J, Starr F, Beecroft M, et al: CT should replace three-view radiographs as the initial screening test in patients at high, moderate, and low risk for blunt cervical spine injury: A prospective comparison. *J Trauma* 2009; 66(6):1605-1609.

 This prospective study of 1,583 consecutive patients comparing cervical spine radiographs to CT concluded that CT should replace plain radiographs for the initial evaluation of blunt cervical spine injury in patients at any risk for injury.

7. Caron T, Bransford R, Nguyen Q, Agel J, Chapman J, Bellabarba C: Spine fractures in patients with ankylosing spinal disorders. *Spine (Phila Pa 1976)* 2010;35(11): E458-E464.

 This retrospective review of 122 spine fractures in 112 patients with ankylosing spinal disorders concludes that these patients are at high risk for complications and death and should be counseled accordingly. Multilevel posterior segmental instrumentation allows effective fracture healing.

8. Anderson PA, Montesano PX. Morphology and treatment of occipital condyle fractures. *Spine (Phila Pa 1976)*. 1988;13(7):731-736.

9. Traynelis VC, Marano GD, Dunker RO, et al. Traumatic atlanto-occipital dislocation: Case report. *J Neurosurg* 1986;65:863-870.

10. Bellabarba C, Mirza SK, West GA, et al: Diagnosis and treatment of craniocervical dislocation in a series of 17 consecutive survivors during an 8-year period. *J Neurosurg Spine* 2006;4(6):429-440.

11. Bono CM, Vaccaro AR, Fehlings M, et al; Spine Trauma Study Group: Measurement techniques for upper cervical spine injuries: Consensus statement of the Spine Trauma Study Group. *Spine (Phila Pa 1976)* 2007; 32(5):593-600.

 This review article from the Spine Trauma Study Group discusses the various imaging measurements available and how these measurements are documented.

12. Levine AM, Edwards CC: Traumatic lesions of the occipitoatlantoaxial complex. *Clin Orthop Relat Res* 1989;239:53-68.

13. Dickman CA, Greene KA, Sonntag VK: Injuries involving the transverse atlantal ligament: Classification and treatment guidelines based upon experience with 39 injuries. *Neurosurgery* 1996;38(1):44-50.

14. Anderson LD, D'Alonzo RT: Fractures of the odontoid process of the axis. *J Bone Joint Surg Am* 1974;56(8): 1663-1674.

15. Levine AM, Edwards CC: The management of traumatic spondylolisthesis of the axis. *J Bone Joint Surg Am* 1985;67(2):217-226.

16. Maak TG, Grauer JN: The contemporary treatment of odontoid injuries. *Spine (Phila Pa 1976)* 2006;31(11, suppl):S53-S60, discussion S61.

17. Kwon BK, Vaccaro AR, Grauer JN, Fisher CG, Dvorak MF: Subaxial cervical spine trauma. *J Am Acad Orthop Surg* 2006;14(2):78-89.

18. Allen BL Jr, Ferguson RL, Lehmann TR, O'Brien RP. A mechanical classification of closed, indirect fractures and dislocations of the lower cervical spine. *Spine (Phila Pa 1976)* 1982;7(1):1-27.

19. Moore TA, Vaccaro AR, Anderson PA: Classification of lower cervical spine injuries. *Spine (Phila Pa 1976)* 2006;31(11, suppl):S37-S43, discussion S61.

20. Vaccaro AR, Hulbert RJ, Patel AA, et al; Spine Trauma Study Group: The subaxial cervical spine injury classification system: A novel approach to recognize the importance of morphology, neurology, and integrity of the disco-ligamentous complex. *Spine (Phila Pa 1976)* 2007;32(21):2365-2374.

 The authors compared the subaxial cervical spine injury classification system (SLIC) to the Harris and Ferguson and Allen systems by 20 spine surgeons to 11 cervical trauma cases. They concluded that the SLIC provides a comprehensive classification system for subaxial cervical trauma.

21. Baptiste DC, Fehlings MG: Update on the treatment of spinal cord injury. *Prog Brain Res* 2007;161:217-233.

 The authors present an overview of the pathobiology of spinal cord injury and current treatment choices before focusing the rest of the discussion on the variety of promising neuroprotective and cell-based approaches that have recently moved or are very close to clinical testing.

22. Grauer JN, Vaccaro AR, Lee JY, et al: The timing and influence of MRI on the management of patients with cervical facet dislocations remains highly variable: A survey of members of the Spine Trauma Study Group. *J Spinal Disord Tech* 2009;22(2):96-99.

 In this questionnaire study sent to 25 fellowship-trained spine surgeons, the authors conclude that the timing and utilization of MRI for patients with traumatic cervical facet dislocations remain variable.

23. Grant GA, Mirza SK, Chapman JR, et al: Risk of early closed reduction in cervical spine subluxation injuries. *J Neurosurg* 1999;90(1, suppl)13-18.

24. Vaccaro AR, Falatyn SP, Flanders AE, et al: Magnetic resonance evaluation of the intervertebral disc, spinal ligaments, and spinal cord before and after closed traction reduction of cervical spine dislocations. *Spine* 1999;24(12):1210-1217.

25. Suberviola B, González-Castro A, Llorca J, Ortiz-Melón F, Miñambres E: Early complications of high-dose methylprednisolone in acute spinal cord injury patients. *Injury* 2008;39(7):748-752.

This retrospective review of 82 patients with acute spinal cord injuries concludes that the use of methylprednisolone is not associated with an improvement in neurologic function and is associated with an increased risk of infectious and metabolic complications.

26. Grauer JN, Vaccaro AR, Beiner JM, et al: Similarities and differences in the treatment of spine trauma between surgical specialties and location of practice. *Spine (Phila Pa 1976)* 2004;29(6):685-696.

27. Bransford RJ, Stevens DW, Uyeji S, Bellabarba C, Chapman JR: Halo vest treatment of cervical spine injuries: A success and survivorship analysis. *Spine (Phila Pa 1976)* 2009;34(15):1561-1566.

This retrospective review of 342 patients with cervical spine fractures treated with halo vest immobilization found treatment was successful in 85% of patients, and 74% of survivors completed their intended treatment period. Complications, though common, were mostly not severe.

28. Glaser JA, Whitehall R, Stamp WG, et al: Complications associated with the halo-vest: A review of 245 cases. *J Neurosurg* 1986;65(6):762-769.

29. Levi AD, Hurlbert RJ, Anderson P, et al: Neurologic deterioration secondary to unrecognized spinal instability following trauma: A multicenter study. *Spine (Phila Pa 1976)* 2006;31(4):451-458.

30. Bellabarba C, Fisher C, Chapman JR, Dettori JR, Norvell DC: Does early fracture fixation of thoracolumbar spine fractures decrease morbidity or mortality? *Spine (Phila Pa 1976)* 2010;35(9, suppl):S138-S145.

In this systematic review of articles between January 1990 and December 2008, 68 articles were screened and 9 met criteria. The authors conclude that patients with unstable thoracic fractures should undergo early (< 72 hours) stabilization of their injury to reduce morbidity and, possibly, mortality.

31. Macias CA, Rosengart MR, Puyana JC, et al: The effects of trauma center care, admission volume, and surgical volume on paralysis after traumatic spinal cord injury. *Ann Surg* 2009;249(1):10-17.

The authors studied 4,121 patients diagnosed with traumatic spinal cord injuries and concluded that trauma center care is associated with reduced paralysis. National guidelines to triage all such patients to trauma centers are followed little more than half the time.

32. Carlson GD, Gordon CD, Oliff HS, Pillai JJ, LaManna JC: Sustained spinal cord compression. *J Bone Joint Surg Am* 2003;85:86-94.

33. Dimar JR, Glassman SD, Raque GH, Zhang YP, Shields CB: The influence of spinal canal narrowing and timing of decompression on neurologic recovery after spinal cord contusion in a rat model. *Spine* 1999;24:1623-1633.

34. Fehlings MG, Sekhon LH, Tator C: The role and timing of decompression in acute spinal cord injury. *Spine* 2001;26:s101-s110.

35. Fehlings MG, Tator CH: An evidence-based review of decompressive surgery in acute spinal cord injury: Rationale, indications, and timing based on experimental and clinical studies. *J Neurosurg Spine* 1999;91:1-11.

36. Shields CB, Zhang YP, Shields LB, Han Y, Burke DA, Mayer NW: The therapeutic window for spinal cord decompression in a rat spinal cord injury model. *J Neurosurg Spine* 2005;3:302-307.

37. Bransford RJ, Falicov A, Nguyen QT, Chapman JR: The C1 lateral mass sagittal split fracture: An unstable Jefferson fracture variant. *J Neurosurg Spine* 2009; 10(5):466-473.

In this retrospective review of all C1 ring fractures, the authors review three surviving patients with C1 unilateral sagittal splits treated nonsurgically who went on to develop cock-robin deformities and eventually required occiput to C2 fusions.

38. Wright NM: Posterior C2 fixation using bilateral, crossing C2 laminar screws: Case series and technical note. *J Spinal Disord Tech* 2004;17(2):158-162.

39. Smith HE, Kerr SM, Fehlings MG, et al: Trends in epidemiology and management of type II odontoid fractures: 20-Year experience at a model system spine injury tertiary referral center. *J Spinal Disord Tech* 2010; October. Epub ahead of print.

The authors retrospectively reviewed 263 consecutive type II odontoid fractures and found a statistically significant increase in the rate of presentation of type II odontoid fractures with time.

40. Brodke DS, Anderson PA, Newell DW, Grady MS, Chapman JR: Comparison of anterior and posterior approaches in cervical spinal cord injuries. *J Spinal Disord Tech* 2003;16(3):229-235.

41. Fisher CG, Dvorak MF, Leith J, Wing PC: Comparison of outcomes for unstable lower cervical flexion teardrop fractures managed with halo thoracic vest versus anterior corpectomy and plating. *Spine (Phila Pa 1976)* 2002;27(2):160-166.

42. Johnson MG, Fisher CG, Boyd M, Pitzen T, Oxland TR, Dvorak MF: The radiographic failure of single segment anterior cervical plate fixation in traumatic cervical flexion distraction injuries. *Spine (Phila Pa 1976)* 2004;29(24):2815-2820.

43. Lowery DW, Wald MM, Browne BJ, et al: Epidemiology of cervical spine injury victims. *Ann Emerg Med* 2001;38:12-16.

44. Hadley MN, Fitzpatrick BC, Sonntag VK, et al: Facet fracture-dislocation injuries of the cervical spine. *Neurosurgery* 1992;30:661-666.

45. Dvorak MF, Fisher CG, Aarabi B, et al: Clinical outcomes of 90 isolated unilateral facet fractures, subluxations, and dislocations treated surgically and nonoperatively. *Spine (Phila Pa 1976)* 2007;32(26):3007-3013.

    This retrospective outcomes study looked at 90 isolated unilateral facet fractures, subluxations, and dislocations and concluded that nonsurgically treated patients report worse outcomes than surgically treated patients, particularly at longer follow-up.

46. Nichols CG, Young DH, Schiller WR: Evaluation of cervicothoracic junction injury. *Ann Emerg Med* 1987;16: 640-642.

47. Ngo B, Hoffman JR, Mower WR: Cervical spine injury in the very elderly. *Emerg Radiol* 2000;7:287-291.

48. Schrag SP, Toedter LJ, McQuay N Jr: Cervical spine fractures in geriatric blunt trauma patients with low-energy mechanism: Are clinical predictors adequate? *Am J Surg* 2008;195(2):170-173.

    This retrospective case-control study of 99 patients examined clinical predictors in geriatric patients with blunt trauma and concluded that predictors are inade-quate for the evaluation of the cervical spine in geriatric trauma patients with a low-energy injury mechanism.

49. Sokolowski MJ, Jackson AP, Haak MH, Meyer PR Jr, Sokolowski MS: Acute mortality and complications of cervical spine injuries in the elderly at a single tertiary care center. *J Spinal Disord Tech* 2007;20(5):352-356.

    The authors carried out a retrospective database review of 979 patients older than 65 years with cervical spine injuries and concluded that statistically comparable survival rates were achieved in both surgically treated and nonsurgically treated patient populations.

50. Anonymous: Management of vertebral artery injuries after nonpenetrating cervical trauma. *Neurosurgery* 2002;50(3, suppl):S173-S178.

51. Fassett DR, Dailey AT, Vaccaro AR: Vertebral artery injuries associated with cervical spine injuries: A review of the literature. *J Spinal Disord Tech* 2008;21(4):252-258.

    A literature review was performed assessing vertebral artery injuries associated with cervical spine injuries and concluded that screening for and treatment of asymptomatic vertebral artery injuries may be considered, but it is unclear based on the current literature whether these strategies improve outcomes.

52. Biffl WL, Ray CE Jr, Moore EE, et al: Treatment-related outcomes from blunt cerebrovascular injuries: The importance of routine follow-up arteriography. *Ann Surg* 2002;235:699-707.

53. Miller PR, Fabian TC, Croce MA, et al: Prospective screening for blunt cerebrovascular injuries: Analysis of diagnostic modalities and outcomes. *Ann Surg* 2002; 236:386-395.

5: Spine

Chapter 49

Thoracolumbar Trauma

Normal Chutkan, MD   Jonathan Tuttle, MD

Introduction

Traumatic spinal fractures occur in approximately 150,000 patients in North America annually.[1] The thoracolumbar region is one of the most commonly affected areas and can result in significant disability. There is a bimodal distribution that tends to differ by age and mechanism. In the younger patient population, high-energy mechanisms such as a fall from a height or a high-speed motor vehicle collision predominate. In elderly patients, a fall from standing height can be significant enough to cause an osteoporotic compression fracture. The management of these two types of fracture mechanisms may differ significantly. Controversy exists with regard to the best management approach because both surgical and nonsurgical treatment have been reported to be successful in the literature. This is confounded by the heterogeneous nature of trauma patients and the many variables that need to be considered such as body habitus, presence or absence of closed head injury, polytrauma, osteoporosis, spondyloarthropathy, and medical comorbidities.

Anatomy

The thoracolumbar junction is defined as T11–L2. In this region the relatively rigid thoracic spine transitions into a more mobile lumbar spine. A change in the facet orientation also affects motion when transitioning from the thoracic into the lumbar spine. The thoracic facets have a more coronal orientation that resists flexion and extension while allowing more torsional and lateral bending movements. The lumbar facets have a more sagittal orientation to allow for significant flexion and extension. The thoracic spine is additionally stabilized by the rib cage and costovertebral articulations. In the sagittal plane the thoracic spine normally has an average of 35° of kyphosis (range, 20° to 50°) whereas the lumbar spine averages 40° of lordosis (range, 30° to 50°).

The posterior ligamentous complex (PLC) is an important component when determining the stability of a fracture. The PLC is composed of the facet capsules, ligamentum flavum, and interspinous and supraspinous ligaments and is sometimes referred to as the posterior tension band. The PLC makes up one of the three categories in the most recently devised fracture classification system.

The normal adult spinal cord terminates in the conus medullaris at the L1 level, which means the spinal cord is at risk for injury throughout much of the thoracolumbar junction. The spinal canal diameter in the thoracic spine is relatively narrow and therefore not able to tolerate significant canal intrusion. The blood supply to the spinal cord is via a single anterior spinal artery and two posterior spinal arteries. Both the anterior and posterior spinal arteries are perfused in a segmental fashion from radicular arteries arising from the posterior intercostal arteries. The artery of Adamkiewicz is thought to be a dominant anterior radicular artery originating from a left intercostal vessel between T8-L2 and is seen in 10% to 16% of patients. In these patients it may provide a major portion of the blood supply to the anterior thoracolumbar spinal cord.

Assessment

Initial Assessment

Initial treatment of thoracolumbar injuries begins in the field with adherence to the Basic Life Support and Advanced Trauma Life Support guidelines and attention to airway, breathing, and circulation. Hypotension with bradycardia may be caused by loss of central sympathetic regulation after a spinal cord injury at or above T6, which is termed spinal or neurogenic shock. Precautionary cervical spine immobilization and use of a rigid backboard are essential. Information on the mechanism of injury, gross neurologic status, and associated injuries is helpful in initiating appropriate treatment. Transportation to the nearest facility with the resources to manage acute trauma is warranted.

Dr. Chutkan or an immediate family member serves as a board member, owner, officer, or committee member of Walton Rehabilitation Hospital, Medical College of Georgia, and AO North America; has received royalties from Globus Medical; serves as a paid consultant to or is an employee of Globus Medical; and has received research or institutional support from Synthes. Dr. Tuttle or an immediate family member is a member of a speakers' bureau or has made paid presentations on behalf of AO and has received research or institutional support from Synthes.

5: Spine

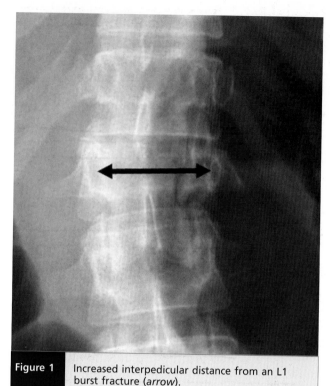

Figure 1 Increased interpedicular distance from an L1 burst fracture (*arrow*).

Physical Examination

A detailed examination is necessary and should include major muscle groups, light touch and pinprick sensation, deep tendon and bulbocavernosus reflexes, rectal tone, and perianal sensation. The sensory examination may be more useful for determining the level of injury, especially in the thoracic spine. The umbilicus is innervated by T10, whereas T12 innervates the lower abdomen. The first lumbar nerve root innervates the inguinal region. Voluntary anal sphincter tone and perianal sensation may signify an incomplete spinal cord injury. Useful scales to guide evaluation of the patient with spinal injury are the American Spinal Injury Association form and the Frankel Impairment Scale.[2,3]

Physical examination should include a thorough evaluation of the entire spine. Careful log rolling will allow for inspection and palpation of the back. Any wounds, palpable step-offs, or areas of tenderness are to be noted. Because there is an 8% to 11% chance of cervical injury associated with thoracolumbar trauma, radiographic evaluation of the entire spine is indicated.

Imaging

Initial imaging of the trauma patient includes either plain radiographs, CT, or both.[4] Traditionally AP and lateral plain radiographs were used to screen patients at risk for fracture based on mechanism of injury or clinical suspicion of fracture, and advanced imaging modalities such as CT and MRI were reserved for more detailed evaluation once an injury had been identified. There is now literature to support a move from plain radiographs to CT for initial fracture evaluation as

rapid screening with helical CT of the head, thorax, abdomen, and pelvis is often a routine part of the trauma evaluation.[5]

CT allows axial images as well as sagittal and coronal reformats that are superior to plain films when evaluating fractures or dislocations. Both plain radiographs and CT show spinal alignment and bony morphology; however, CT shows greater detail and helps prevent missing smaller fractures or underestimating fracture severity. CT can be particularly helpful in obese patients in whom fine detail may be lost on plain films and for visualization of transition zones except when the patient weighs too much for the CT table. Another issue with CT in patients with spine trauma is the amount of radiation exposure.

Plain Radiographs

Plain radiographs can still provide useful information. The lateral view allows for evaluation of the sagittal alignment and measurement of any kyphotic deformity. Screening lateral films are usually taken in the supine position. Alignment may worsen on weight bearing, alerting the clinician to the possibility of a more serious injury and/or disruption of the PLC. Upright conventional radiography continues to allow unequaled insight into postural alignment and segmental stability. Vertebral body height can also be evaluated; a loss of height of more than 50% may be indicative of a posterior ligamentous injury. The AP view is helpful in evaluating coronal alignment. Malalignment of the spinous processes is suggestive of a rotational injury, whereas widening of the interpedicular distance (**Figure 1**) may indicate a burst fracture. An increase in the interspinous distance may indicate a flexion injury. Focal scoliosis may be present in lateral compressive injuries.

Computed Tomography

CT is becoming the screening tool of choice at many institutions. Although reformatted sagittal and coronal images can be obtained, the quality of the reformatted images is dependent on the slice thickness of the screening studies. Once an injury is detected, if there is any question as to the quality of the screening studies, it is recommended that a more detailed thin-cut (2-mm) study be obtained at that level. CT is considered the gold standard for evaluating the osseous structures and is particularly helpful in assessing canal encroachment. Facet fractures and dislocations are easily evaluated with CT, and any asymmetry or malalignment should be noted. The "naked" or "empty" facet sign may signify a subluxation or dislocation (**Figure 2**). Careful evaluation of combined axial and reformatted images can help delineate osseous injury morphology and often leads to an appreciation of possible concomitant ligamentous or soft-tissue injuries.

Magnetic Resonance Imaging

MRI is helpful in evaluating nonosseous structures, the neural elements, and the PLC.[6-8] Disk herniations, epidural hematomas, occult injuries, and other possible

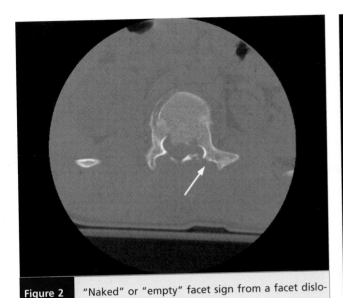

Figure 2 | "Naked" or "empty" facet sign from a facet dislocation (*arrow*).

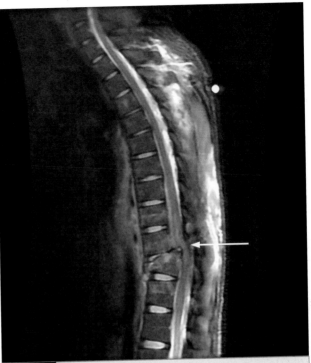

Figure 3 | Increased signal within the spinal cord on a T2-weighted MRI after a fracture-dislocation injury (*arrow*).

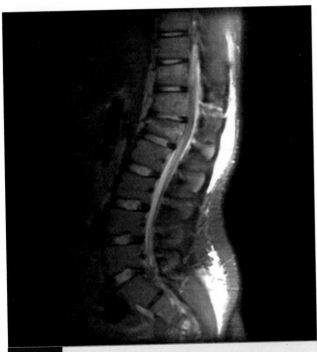

Figure 4 | Ligamentum flavum, interspinous, and supraspinous ligament injury after facet dislocation.

soft-tissue neural compressive lesions are best demonstrated with MRI. The sensitivity for detecting PLC injury on physical examination alone is relatively low. T2-weighted and fat-suppressed T2-weighted images are helpful in evaluating the PLC. Increased signal is indicative of edema or frank disruption and may signal a more severe or unstable injury. The anulus fibrosus, anterior longitudinal ligament, posterior longitudinal ligament, and spinal cord will also show increased signal on T2-weighted MRI when injured (**Figures 3** and **4**). Increased signal within the spinal cord is seen with

hemorrhage and/or edema and is a poor prognostic sign. T2-weighted MRI or short tau inversion recovery MRI is also useful to identify occult fractures that may be missed on plain films and CT. MRI can be particularly helpful in patients with multiple osteoporotic compression fractures with acute fractures showing increased T2 signal compared to normal signal in chronic fractures.

Spinal Stability

Instability has been defined as the loss of the ability of the spine under physiologic loads to maintain its pattern of displacement so that there is no initial or additional neurologic deficit, no major deformity, and no incapacitating pain.[9] A scoring system was developed to aid in determining stability; however, many of these data were based on in vitro data, and a true objective clinical definition remains elusive.

Fracture Classification

The goal of any fracture classification system includes ease of application, ability to guide treatment, and excellent interobserver and intraobserver reliability. An initial thoracolumbar classification described the fracture by anatomic deformation and mechanism of injury.[10] This work was later revised; one concept that was added was the integrity of the PLC and its importance in stability. A later classification system used a

5: Spine

Table 1

Thoracolumbar Injury Classification Scale

Category	Points
Injury morphology	
Compression	1
Burst	+1
Translational/rotational	3
Distraction	4
Neurologic status	
Intact	0
Nerve root	2
Cord, conus medullaris	
Incomplete	3
Complete	2
Cauda equina	3
PLC	
Intact	0
Injury suspected/indeterminate	2
Injured	3

(Adapted with permission from Vaccaro AR, Lehman RA Jr, Hurlbert RJ, et al: A new classification of thoracolumbar injuries: The importance of injury morphology, the integrity of the posterior ligamentous complex, and neurologic status. *Spine (Phila Pa 1976)* 2005;30:2325-2333.)

two-column model.[11] Yet another fracture morphology classification system separated degrees of instability in an effort to devise a treatment strategy.[12] A middle column was added to the two-column model. The load-sharing classification system warned of the dangers of short-segment posterior fixation for highly comminuted, kyphotic, and poorly apposed burst-type fractures due to the likelihood of construct failure.[13]

The AO Spine classification system was much more comprehensive and categorized fractures into three main types (A, B, and C), which were then further subclassified into three subtypes that were also broken into three subgroups.[14] Type A fractures were caused by compression injuries. Type B fractures resulted from distraction, and type C injuries were rotational. One drawback to this system, like the Denis system, is the further into the classification subtypes an observer reported, the less reliable the results. However, the interobserver and intraobserver reliability are on par or slightly better than the Denis system.[15]

The Spine Study Trauma Group devised a thoracolumbar injury classification system based on expert opinion from multiple level I trauma centers.[16-18] The system was first published containing a mechanistic injury model called the Thoracolumbar Injury Severity Score (TLISS) and was later revised to a fracture morphology system. The fracture morphology version was referred to as the Thoracolumbar Injury Classification System (TLICS) and it defined three main areas to evaluate: fracture morphology, PLC injury, and neurologic status (**Table 1**).

Fracture morphology was divided into four main categories that are progressively more severe: compression, burst, translation/rotational, and distraction. Compression fractures are the least severe and are characterized by loss of vertebral body height without retropulsion of bone into the spinal canal. Burst fractures are defined by a portion of the fractured vertebral body retropulsed into the spinal canal and may be an axial, lateral, or flexion type. When combined with rotation or translation, a burst fracture is classified as the more severe translation or rotational fracture morphology, which also includes unilateral or bilateral facet dislocations and translation/rotational fractures not associated with a compression or burst fracture. The final category is distraction and includes both flexion-distraction and extension-distraction injuries; flexion-distraction injuries are more common. A Chance fracture can be considered a flexion-distraction injury where the anterior and posterior elements all fail in tension. The Chance fracture can be entirely within osseous structures or can be a combination of osseous and ligamentous tissues. A true bony Chance fracture can be treated with extension bracing or a cast, whereas an osteoligamentous Chance fracture usually requires surgical stabilization.

The goal of the TLICS was to guide treatment with reliability and reproducibility. Evaluation has shown improved reliability compared to previously published data from the AO or Denis classification systems and among different spine specialties. The interobserver and intraobserver reliability showed slightly better kappa values than published results for the Denis and the AO Spine classification systems, indicating better reliability.[19-22] Another study indicated there was moderate reliability when comparing a set of cases between fellowship-trained orthopaedic spine surgeons and neurosurgeons.[23]

Treatment Options

The treatment options for managing thoracolumbar fractures are based on stability. Determining stability is sometimes more difficult than would initially be expected, and controversy exists in the literature as to the most effective treatment.[24-29] Conservative treatment such as bracing with activity modification, pain medication, and serial imaging is adequate for less severe fractures and avoids the potential complications of surgery. With more severe fractures, such as a fracture-dislocation with translation or rotation, surgical intervention is frequently warranted. A classification system may be useful to help the clinician determine the relative stability of the spine. It is also important to design an instrumentation construct that is unlikely to fail, and the load-sharing classification of thoracolumbar fractures may be helpful.[30-32]

Surgical stabilization may be more advantageous when it occurs early after trauma and for factors other

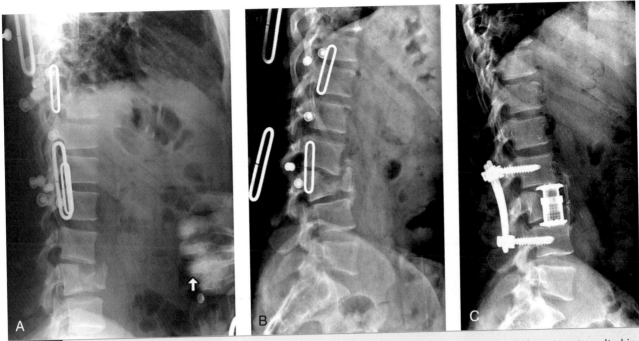

Figure 5   A, Initial standing film showing a TLSO after lumbar pincer-type fracture. **B**, Failed nonsurgical treatment resulted in increased kyphosis and increasing back pain 3 months after injury and treatment in TLSO. **C**, Radiograph 1 year after anterior approach for corpectomy and posterior approach for short-segment pedicle screw instrumentation.

than neurologic deficit.[33-35] Data from retrospective studies suggest that patients with thoracolumbar trauma may have fewer days in intensive care and on a ventilator, a shorter hospital stay, and fewer respiratory infections when surgery is completed within 3 days of hospitalization. Large prospective studies would be helpful to delineate the effect on outcome related to the timing of stabilization. One difficulty encountered when trying to devise a study related to trauma patients is the lack of patient uniformity (patients may or may not have single or multisystem injuries, traumatic brain injury, spinal-related neurologic deficit, and underlying ankylosing disorder, or may be thin or obese).

Conservative treatment is used for neurologically intact patients with stable fractures such as compression fractures, one-column and minor injuries using the Denis classification, type A injuries using the AO system, and TLICS scores lower than 4. Pain medication, bracing or casting in extension, activity modification, and serial imaging are usually effective. A removable thoracolumbosacral orthosis (TLSO) is the most commonly used form of immobilization; however, hyperextension casting with a Risser-type body cast may also be used but is less well tolerated by patients. Immobilization has been recommended for a minimum of 10 to 12 weeks; however, new data suggest stable AO type A3 fractures may not need bracing in certain patient populations.[25] Serial imaging and follow-up are necessary to detect any evidence of progressive spinal deformity and to monitor fracture healing. Progressive improvement in pain and return to function can be expected for most patients. Nonsurgical management has been associated with equivalent functional outcomes with less

pain, fewer complications, and lower cost when compared with surgical management in neurologically intact patients with stable burst fractures. A recent study of interim results found AO type A3 fractures to have similar outcomes when treated with a custom TLSO compared to no orthosis.[36] Failure of nonsurgical management may be manifested by patient inability to tolerate brace or cast immobilization, incapacitating pain, progressive deformity, or progressive neurologic impairment.

Surgery is often warranted in patients with unstable spine injuries. These patients frequently have a major spine injury causing mechanical instability, neurologic instability, or both, according to the Denis classification. When the AO classification or TLICS is applied, these patients tend to have type B or C injuries or a TLICS greater than 4, respectively. Decompression in addition to spinal stabilization may be required if a neurologic injury is present, particularly if the injury is incomplete.

Surgical intervention may be needed for the patient in whom nonsurgical treatment has failed (**Figure 5**). Early standing films may show significantly increased segmental kyphosis and increasing neurologic deficit; continued pain or failure of immobilization may occur later. After 3 to 4 weeks, a reconstructive procedure may be necessary and can be much more involved than surgical intervention immediately after injury. The patient discussed in **Figure 5** required anterior corpectomy with release of the anterior longitudinal ligament and posterior osteotomies to correct sagittal malalignment because of a 3-month delay in surgical treatment after initial injury.

Table 2

TLICS Surgical Approach Algorithm

Neurologic Status	Posterior Ligamentous Complex	
	Intact	**Disrupted**
Intact	Posterior approach	Posterior approach
Root injury	Posterior approach	Posterior approach
Incomplete spinal cord or cauda equina injury		Combined approach
Complete spinal cord or cauda equina injury	Posterior (anterior) approach	Posterior (combined) approach

(Adapted with permission from Vaccaro AR, Lehman RA Jr, Hurlbert RJ, et al: A new classification of thoracolumbar injuries: The importance of injury morphology, the integrity of the posterior ligamentous complex, and neurologic status. *Spine (Phila Pa 1976)* 2005;30:2325-2333.)

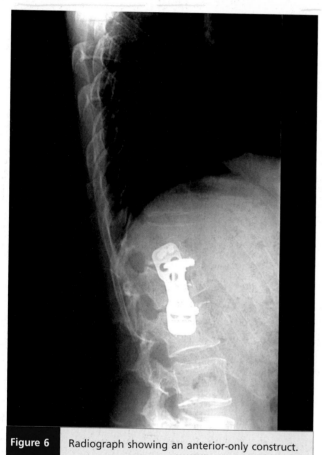

Figure 6 Radiograph showing an anterior-only construct.

Surgical intervention can be anterior, posterior, or circumferential. The TLICS system suggested a surgical approach based on the neurologic status of the patient and the integrity of the PLC. A posterior approach alone was recommended for patients with intact neurologic status or root injury, whereas an anterior approach alone was recommended for an incomplete spinal cord injury with an intact PLC. Patients presenting with a cauda equina syndrome may be treated with an anterior, posterior, or combined approach depending upon where decompression and stabilization are needed. Complete spinal cord injury patients are treated in a manner similar to cauda equina patients,

with a preference for the posterior approach. One study noted that many institutions would consider decompression of the spinal cord or cauda equina with associated PLC injury to maintain cerebrospinal fluid dynamics and prevent the formation of syringomyelia,[16] despite the patient having a complete spinal cord injury. (**Table 2**). Combined or circumferential approaches are usually reserved for patients who require anterior column decompression and/or reconstruction following posterior realignment and stabilization.

Anterior surgery is frequently indicated for an incomplete spinal cord injury or cauda equina syndrome resulting from retropulsed bone due to a burst-type fracture. A subtotal corpectomy with removal of retropulsed bone is often required to decompress the canal. A structural cadaver allograft or a cage may be used to reconstruct the anterior column and maintain alignment following decompression. In two studies reviewing neurologic improvement, the Frankel grade was noted to improve by one grade; in one study, the average kyphosis was improved from 22.7° to 7.4° with loss of sagittal alignment averaging 2.1° after treatment. For most patients with an intact PLC, the use of anterior instrumentation allows for an anterior-only construct (**Figure 6**). In patients with evidence of PLC disruption (AO type B), the use of anterior-only constructs is controversial. Although there are limited reports of successful use of this technique in the literature, it should be considered with caution. Anterior surgery is also an option for pincer-type fractures due to the high risk of nonunion and persistent pain. In stable burst fractures there is often the option of anterior or posterior procedures. One study showed better outcomes among patients treated with anterior-only surgery compared with posterior-only surgery.[29]

Posterior surgery can be useful for direct and indirect decompression and stabilization. Direct decompression can be achieved by removing the facet/lamina/pedicle ipsilateral to the retropulsed bone within the spinal canal and removing the fracture fragment or tapping it anterior. This procedure is particularly useful in patients with an incomplete neurologic injury and canal encroachment from retropulsed bone. In neurologically intact patients, decompression may not be necessary because it further destabilizes the spine and may increase the possibility of dural tear or neural injury. The spinal canal has the potential to remodel as it heals with increased spinal canal diameter over time.

Indirect decompression can be achieved in a patient with an intact posterior longitudinal ligament using posterior instrumentation. Postural reduction and distraction in the sagittal plane allows for fracture reduction via ligamentotaxis. The most popular way to provide stabilization is via pedicle screws and rods (**Figure 7**), although a hook-and-rod construct may be used. Pedicle screw constructs spanning at least two levels above and two levels below the fracture have been found to decrease the occurrence of progressive kyphosis and hardware failure. Progressive kyphosis without hardware failure is not necessarily a clinical problem but should be monitored with radiographs. Short segment instrumentation (one level above to one level below) is usually sufficient for Chance-type fractures, compression fractures, and some burst fractures but has been associated with increased hardware failure and progressive kyphosis, especially when the anterior column is incompetent and unable to provide stability. One study showed that increased vertebral body comminution, poor bony fragment apposition, and increased kyphosis can help predict short segment instrumentation failure.[13] Rotational injuries and fracture-dislocations are usually best managed by a posterior approach, which allows for realignment and multilevel fixation.

Combined anterior-posterior procedures are generally reserved for severe injuries with significant posterior column disruption and loss of anterior column integrity. These injuries usually are treated with initial stabilization and realignment via a posterior approach followed by anterior column reconstruction either at the same setting or as a staged procedure. A disadvantage of the combined procedure is the added morbidity of both an anterior and posterior approach. Another indication for combined procedures is in the setting of significant osteoporosis, where a combined approach may reduce the risk of hardware failure.

Osteoporotic Vertebral Compression Fractures

With an aging baby boomer generation, the incidence of osteoporotic vertebral compression fracture (VCF) is likely to increase. Currently, approximately 700,000 VCFs occur per year in the United States. VCF is the most common osteoporotic fracture, occurring twice as often as hip fractures.[37] The literature suggests approximately 20% to 25% of patients older than 70 years will experience a VCF; this percentage increases to about 50% for patients older than 80 years.[37] Other studies have found that a patient with one VCF is five times as likely to experience a second VCF within 1 year. Two VCFs result in an even higher risk of the occurrence of a third VCF.[37]

VCFs may be treated nonsurgically or surgically. Most patients respond to nonsurgical treatment, which

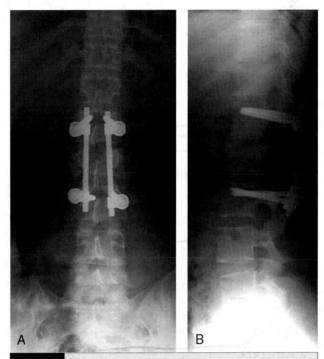

Figure 7   AP (**A**) and lateral (**B**) radiographs of a patient who underwent short-segment pedicle screw fixation for a burst fracture.

involves medical management of the underlying osteoporosis, pain medication, bracing, and activity modification. Surgical treatment includes percutaneous options such as vertebroplasty or kyphoplasty, or open surgery. Open surgical treatment may be indicated for patients with a neurologic deficit from a significant kyphotic deformity or retropulsed bone, or for reconstruction of significant spinal malalignment as a salvage procedure. When open surgery is necessary, serious consideration should be given to long constructs with multiple fixation points and/or combined anterior-posterior procedures to reduce the risk of hardware failure because of osteoporotic bone.

Most patients with VCFs do not have a neurologic deficit; the primary indication for surgical intervention tends to be intractable pain. These patients often have significant medical comorbidities that may limit surgical options. Minimally invasive techniques have been developed that allow surgical treatment of painful VCFs with minimal surgical morbidity. Percutaneous vertebroplasty and kyphoplasty involve injection of polymethylmethacrylate cement into the fractured body. In contrast to vertebroplasty, cavity creation in kyphoplasty is with a balloon tamp with injection of a more viscous cement. Both procedures result in significant pain reduction in the immediate postoperative period (60% to 100%); however, kyphoplasty reportedly has less chance of cement extravasation. Kyphoplasty also is advantageous because it can partially restore vertebral body height and correct kyphosis, although the clinical significance of this benefit remains controversial. To date there are no long-term studies showing

5: Spine

a clinical benefit of kyphoplasty over vertebroplasty. However, kyphoplasty is more expensive than vertebroplasty. One randomized controlled study found that pain related outcomes were similar when comparing patients treated with kyphoplasty and those treated nonsurgically at the 1-year follow-up visit.[38] The study also noted at the 1-year follow-up that the kyphoplasty patients were more likely to require less activity restriction and narcotic use than control subjects treated nonsurgically. The kyphoplasty results are in contrast to a recently published study where the role of vertebroplasty was called into question when compared to a sham surgery.[39] This study had methodological errors that made it difficult to compare its results to those of other kyphoplasty studies or to studies retrospectively comparing vertebroplasty to routine nonsurgical treatment.

Emerging Concepts

Minimally invasive surgery is gaining ground in the treatment of thoracolumbar trauma. Most of the literature is from case series and retrospective studies, and these techniques have not been accepted as the standard of care for treating trauma patients. A 2008 study documented the treatment of AO A2- and A3-type fractures in 18 patients with combined short-segment minimally invasive pedicle screw instrumentation and kyphoplasty using calcium phosphate cement in the fractured vertebral body.[40] The patients did not have progressive kyphosis beyond 1° to 5°, and no additional compression fractures were noted during the average 22-month follow-up period.

Another review of currently available technology discussed anterior endoscopic approaches as well as percutaneous pedicle screw placement.[1] The authors noted that technology is still evolving for these approaches and that there is a learning curve associated more with anterior endoscopic approaches than posterior percutaneous pedicle screw placement. With improved three-dimensional imaging and navigation systems, the role of minimally invasive surgery may continue to increase in popularity.

Annotated References

1. Rampersaud YR, Annand N, Dekutoski MB: Use of minimally invasive surgical techniques in the management of thoracolumbar trauma: Current concepts. *Spine (Phila Pa 1976)* 2006;31(11, suppl):S96-S102, discussion S104.

2. Maynard FM Jr, Bracken MB, Creasey G, et al; American Spinal Injury Association: International standards for neurological and functional classification of spinal cord injury. *Spinal Cord* 1997;35(5):266-274.

3. Frankel HL, Hancock DO, Hyslop G, et al: The value of postural reduction in the initial management of closed

injuries of the spine with paraplegia and tetraplegia: I. *Paraplegia* 1969;7(3):179-192.

4. Dai LY, Wang XY, Jiang LS, Jiang SD, Xu HZ: Plain radiography versus computed tomography scans in the diagnosis and management of thoracolumbar burst fractures. *Spine (Phila Pa 1976)* 2008;33(16):E548-E552.

This study reviewed the difference between compression and burst fractures based on plain radiography diagnosis compared with CT diagnosis. The authors found that vertebral body comminution was often underestimated with plain radiographs, which was not the case when evaluating fractures with CT. They concluded treatment is better directed from CT than plain radiography.

5. Hauser CJ, Visvikis G, Hinrichs C, et al: Prospective validation of computed tomographic screening of the thoracolumbar spine in trauma. *J Trauma* 2003;55:228-235.

6. Lee HM, Kim HS, Kim DJ, Suk KS, Park JO, Kim NH: Reliability of magnetic resonance imaging in detecting posterior ligament complex injury in thoracolumbar spinal fractures. *Spine (Phila Pa 1976)* 2000;25(16):2079-2084.

7. Dai LY, Ding WG, Wang XY, Jiang LS, Jiang SD, Xu HZ: Assessment of ligamentous injury in patients with thoracolumbar burst fractures using MRI. *J Trauma* 2009;66(6):1610-1615.

A retrospective study validating the use of MRI as an imaging modality to determine PLC injury is presented. The authors noted that the PLC injury did not correlate with neurologic injury or fracture severity.

8. Oner FC, van Gils AP, Faber JA, Dhert WJ, Verbout AJ: Some complications of common treatment schemes of thoracolumbar spine fractures can be predicted with magnetic resonance imaging: Prospective study of 53 patients with 71 fractures. *Spine (Phila Pa 1976)* 2002;27(6):629-636.

9. White A, Panjabi M: The problem of clinical instability in the human spine: A systematic approach, in *Clinical Biomechanics of the Spine*, ed 2. Philadelphia, PA, JB Lippincott, 1990, pp 277-378.

10. Sethi MK, Schoenfeld AJ, Bono CM, Harris MB: The evolution of thoracolumbar injury classification systems. *Spine J* 2009;9(9):780-788.

The authors document the challenges and evolution of the thoracolumbar classification systems.

11. Holdsworth FW: Fractures, dislocations, and fracture-dislocations of the spine. *J Bone Joint Surg Am* 1970;52(8):1534-1551.

12. Denis F: The three column spine and its significance in the classification of acute thoracolumbar spinal injuries. *Spine (Phila Pa 1976)* 1983;8(8):817-831.

13. McCormack T, Karaikovic E, Gaines RW: The load sharing classification of spine fractures. *Spine (Phila Pa 1976)* 1994;19(15):1741-1744.

14. Magerl F, Aebi M, Gertzbein SD, Harms J, Nazarian S: A comprehensive classification of thoracic and lumbar injuries. *Eur Spine J* 1994;3(4):184-201.

15. Wood KB, Khanna G, Vaccaro AR, Arnold PM, Harris MB, Mehbod AA: Assessment of two thoracolumbar fracture classification systems as used by multiple surgeons. *J Bone Joint Surg Am* 2005;87(7):1423-1429.

16. Vaccaro AR, Lehman RA Jr, Hurlbert RJ, et al: A new classification of thoracolumbar injuries: The importance of injury morphology, the integrity of the posterior ligamentous complex, and neurologic status. *Spine (Phila Pa 1976)* 2005;30(20):2325-2333.

17. Vaccaro AR, Zeiller SC, Hulbert RJ, et al: The thoracolumbar injury severity score: A proposed treatment algorithm. *J Spinal Disord Tech* 2005;18(3):209-215.

18. Patel AA, Dailey A, Brodke DS, et al; Spine Trauma Study Group: Thoracolumbar spine trauma classification: The Thoracolumbar Injury Classification and Severity Score system and case examples. *J Neurosurg Spine* 2009;10(3):201-206.

    A description of the TLICS scheme and its application to three clinical case vignettes are discussed.

19. Patel AA, Vaccaro AR, Albert TJ, et al: The adoption of a new classification system: Time-dependent variation in interobserver reliability of the thoracolumbar injury severity score classification system. *Spine (Phila Pa 1976)* 2007;32(3):E105-E110.

    A review of the interobserver reliability when using the mechanistic TLISS classification system, the precursor to the TLICS, is presented. This study reviewed the TLISS system and showed how it compared favorably to prior thoracolumbar classification systems, such as the AO and Denis classifications.

20. Harrop JS, Vaccaro AR, Hurlbert RJ, et al; Spine Trauma Study Group: Intrarater and interrater reliability and validity in the assessment of the mechanism of injury and integrity of the posterior ligamentous complex: A novel injury severity scoring system for thoracolumbar injuries. Invited submission from the Joint Section Meeting On Disorders of the Spine and Peripheral Nerves, March 2005. *J Neurosurg Spine* 2006;4(2):118-122.

21. Vaccaro AR, Baron EM, Sanfilippo J, et al: Reliability of a novel classification system for thoracolumbar injuries: The Thoracolumbar Injury Severity Score. *Spine (Phila Pa 1976)* 2006;31(11, Suppl)S62-S69, discussion S104.

22. Whang PG, Vaccaro AR, Poelstra KA, et al: The influence of fracture mechanism and morphology on the reliability and validity of two novel thoracolumbar injury classification systems. *Spine (Phila Pa 1976)* 2007; 32(7):791-795.

    The interrater reliability of the TLICS is on par or better than that of the AO or the Denis classification systems.

23. Raja Rampersaud Y, Fisher C, Wilsey J, et al: Agreement between orthopedic surgeons and neurosurgeons regarding a new algorithm for the treatment of thoracolumbar injuries: A multicenter reliability study. *J Spinal Disord Tech* 2006;19:477-482.

24. Wood K, Buttermann G, Mehbod A, et al: Operative compared with nonoperative treatment of a thoracolumbar burst fracture without neurological deficit: A prospective, randomized study. *J Bone Joint Surg Am* 2003;85(5):773-781.

25. Bailey CS, Dvorak MF, Thomas KC, et al: Comparison of thoracolumbosacral orthosis and no orthosis for the treatment of thoracolumbar burst fractures: Interim analysis of a multicenter randomized clinical equivalence trial. *J Neurosurg Spine* 2009;11(3):295-303.

    This study is ongoing but interim results show comparable outcomes in treating AO type A3 burst fractures with or without a custom TLSO. Participants could not have greater than 35° of kyphosis or a neurologic deficit. No statistically significant outcome has been identified between the two groups.

26. Shen WJ, Shen YS: Nonsurgical treatment of three-column thoracolumbar junction burst fractures without neurologic deficit. *Spine (Phila Pa 1976)* 1999;24(4):412-415.

27. Siebenga J, Leferink VJ, Segers MJ, et al: Treatment of traumatic thoracolumbar spine fractures: A multicenter prospective randomized study of operative versus nonsurgical treatment. *Spine (Phila Pa 1976)* 2006;31(25):2881-2890.

28. Thomas KC, Bailey CS, Dvorak MF, Kwon B, Fisher C: Comparison of operative and nonoperative treatment for thoracolumbar burst fractures in patients without neurological deficit: A systematic review. *J Neurosurg Spine* 2006;4(5):351-358.

29. Wood KB, Bohn D, Mehbod A: Anterior versus posterior treatment of stable thoracolumbar burst fractures without neurologic deficit: A prospective, randomized study. *J Spinal Disord Tech* 2005;18(suppl, Suppl)S15-S23.

30. Wang XY, Dai LY, Xu HZ, Chi YL: The load-sharing classification of thoracolumbar fractures: An in vitro biomechanical validation. *Spine (Phila Pa 1976)* 2007; 32(11):1214-1219.

    This study used previously established in vitro biomechanical approaches and concluded that the load-sharing classification system was valid for determining stability.

31. Dai LY, Jin WJ: Interobserver and intraobserver reliability in the load sharing classification of the assessment of thoracolumbar burst fractures. *Spine (Phila Pa 1976)* 2005;30(3):354-358.

32. Dai LY, Jiang LS, Jiang SD: Conservative treatment of thoracolumbar burst fractures: A long-term follow-up

5: Spine

[Handwritten note at top of page: note: sacralization of L5 — congenital anomaly; incidence ~35% — TP of L5 fuses to sacrum or ilium, b/l > unilateral — L5-S1 disk may be thin & narrow — asymptomatic v. symptomatic (usually 2/2 altered biomechanics)]

results with special reference to the load sharing classification. *Spine (Phila Pa 1976)* 2008;33(23):2536-2544.

A retrospective review of 127 patients treated conservatively and followed for a minimum of 3 years concluded that the load-sharing classification system can help predict failure of conservative management. This study is unique because it included patients with neurologic deficit as well as those without deficit. Thirty-seven patients included in the study had refused surgical intervention and underwent nonsurgical treatment.

33. McHenry TP, Mirza SK, Wang J, et al: Risk factors for respiratory failure following operative stabilization of thoracic and lumbar spine fractures. *J Bone Joint Surg Am* 2006;88(5):997-1005.

34. Croce MA, Bee TK, Pritchard E, Miller PR, Fabian TC: Does optimal timing for spine fracture fixation exist? *Ann Surg* 2001;233(6):851-858.

35. Kerwin AJ, Frykberg ER, Schinco MA, Griffen MM, Murphy T, Tepas JJ: The effect of early spine fixation on non-neurologic outcome. *J Trauma* 2005;58(1):15-21.

36. Bailey CS, Dvorak MF, Thomas KC, et al: Comparison of thoracolumbosacral orthosis and no orthosis for the treatment of thoracolumbar burst fractures: Interim analysis of a multicenter randomized clinical equivalence trial. *J Neurosurg Spine* 2009;11:295-303.

The authors found equivalence between treatment with a TLSO and no orthosis for thoracolumbar burst fractures. No significant difference was found between treatment groups.

37. Cauley JA, Hochberg MC, Lui LY, et al: Long-term risk of incident vertebral fractures. *JAMA* 2007;298(23):2761-2767.

The authors present a population-based cohort study that followed 2,680 white women for up to 15 years to evaluate their risk of developing an osteoporotic compression fracture based on the presence of vertebral compression fractures and bone mineral density.

38. Wardlaw D, Cummings SR, Van Meirhaeghe J, et al: Efficacy and safety of balloon kyphoplasty compared with non-surgical care for vertebral compression fracture (FREE): A randomised controlled trial. *Lancet* 2009;373(9668):1016-1024.

This randomized study compared patients undergoing kyphoplasty for an osteoporotic compression fracture with conservative management. The patients treated with kyphoplasty required less narcotic and had increased activity in comparison with the nonsurgically treated patients.

39. Kallmes DF, Comstock BA, Heagerty PJ, et al: A randomized trial of vertebroplasty for osteoporotic spinal fractures. *N Engl J Med* 2009;361(6):569-579.

A randomized controlled study comparing sham surgery to vertebroplasty found similar outcomes at 1 month after the procedure.

40. Korovessis P, Hadjipavlou A, Repantis T: Minimal invasive short posterior instrumentation plus balloon kyphoplasty with calcium phosphate for burst and severe compression lumbar fractures. *Spine (Phila Pa 1976)* 2008;33(6):658-667.

A case series review is presented of 18 patients treated with balloon kyphoplasty and short-segment percutaneous pedicle screw instrumentation for L1-L4 compression or burst-type fractures.

[Vertical text in left margin: 5: Spine]

Chapter 50
Lumbar Spondylolisthesis

Toshinori Sakai, MD, PhD   Koichi Sairyo, MD, PhD   Nitin N. Bhatia, MD

Introduction

Spondylolisthesis is the displacement of one vertebra over the subjacent vertebra. This slippage, which can occur at anytime from infancy through adulthood, has several different causes. Based on the underlying cause of the slippage, spondylolisthesis is subdivided into five types: isthmic, degenerative, dysplastic, congenital (pathologic), and traumatic (**Table 1**). Although the radiographic translation seen in a spondylolisthesis is independent of the underlying cause, it is important to identify the cause because the natural history, symptoms, and treatment of the disorder differ based on the etiology.

Epidemiology

The various types of spondylolisthesis have different fundamental causes. Isthmic spondylolisthesis is caused by a defect in the pars interarticularis, which is called a spondylolysis, pars defect, or pars fracture (**Figure 1**). Along with the degenerative type, the isthmic type is one of the two most common forms of spondylolisthesis. Lumbar spondylolysis and isthmic spondylolisthesis occur in approximately 6% of the general population, and occur most commonly at the L5-S1 level. This in-

cidence varies considerably among different ethnic groups. The incidence of lumbar spondylolysis is 6.4% in Caucasian males, 2.8% in African-American males, 2.3% in Caucasian females, and 1.1% in African-American females.[1] The highest incidence reported is 54% in native residents of Greenland.[2] These results suggest that a genetic or hereditary factor may play a role in the development of spondylolysis.

The incidence of spondylolysis and isthmic spondylolisthesis varies depending on the method of analysis. Studies using plain radiographs have shown a 4.6% incidence of spondylolysis, whereas studies using CT have shown rates between 5.7% and 5.9%.[3,4] The fifth lumbar vertebra (L5) accounts for approximately 90% of spondylolysis cases, and unilateral spondylolysis is found in approximately 22% of cases. Multiple-level spondylolysis is rare and seen in less than 0.5% of cases.

Degenerative spondylolisthesis has a 3:1 prevalence in women, with African-American women affected three times more frequently than Caucasian women. The most commonly involved level is L4-L5, followed by L3-L4. Unlike isthmic spondylolisthesis, the L5-S1 level is rarely affected by degenerative spondylolisthesis. As the name implies, degenerative spondylolisthesis is caused by degenerative changes in the disk and facet complex, which lead to instability at the affected level. Because this type of spondylolisthesis is a degenerative

Dr. Sairyo or an immediate family member has received royalties from Japan MDM; is a member of a speakers' bureau or has made paid presentations on behalf of Japan MCM; serves as an unpaid consultant to Japan Kyphoon; and has received research or institutional support from Alphatec Spine, Medtronic Sofamor Danek, Senko, and Stryker. Dr. Bhatia or an immediate family member has received royalties from Alphatec Spine; is a member of a speakers' bureau or has made paid presentations on behalf of Biomet, Stryker, Alphatec Spine, Seaspine, and Globus Medical; serves as a paid consultant to Alphatec Spine, Biomet, and Seaspine; and has received research or institutional support from Alphatec Spine, Biomet, Arthrex, National Institutes of Health (NIAMS & NICHD), and Spinewave. Neither Dr. Sakai nor any immediate family member has received anything of value from or owns stock in a commercial company or institution related directly or indirectly to the subject of this chapter.

Table 1

Wiltse Classification of Spondylolisthesis

Type	Description
I	Dysplastic: congenital abnormality of the upper sacrum or the arch of L5
II	Isthmic: lesion in the pars interarticularis A. Lytic: fatigue fracture of the pars B. Elongated but intact pars C. Acute fracture
III	Degenerative: resulting from long-standing intersegmental disease
IV	Traumatic: fracture in region other than the pars
V	Pathologic: generalized or local bone disease

(Reproduced from Jones TR, Rao RD: Adult isthmic spondylolisthesis. *J Am Acad Orthop Surg* 2009;17(10):609-617.)

[Handwritten annotations: deficiency of facet jts. or sagittal align.; L5-S1; #1 L5-S1; restability (can be traumatic); #2 L4-5, L3-4 @ disk & facet; acute fractures; VI Post-surgical/iatrogenic; lamina in btwn superior facets; inferior sup; jxn btwn superior facet & lamina; facet, pedicle across sacrum causing dislocate or sublux L spine]

5: Spine

note: Sacralization of L5
- congenital anomaly; incidence ~3.5%
- TP of L5 fuses to sacrum or ilium; b/l > unilateral
- L5-S1 disk may be thin & narrow
- asymptomatic v. symptomatic (usually 2/2 altered biomechanics)

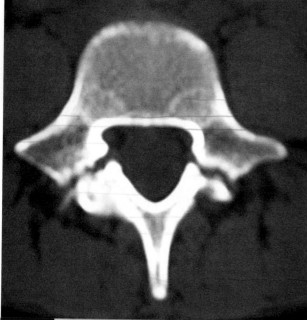

Figure 1   Axial CT image of L5 spondylolysis (also known as a pars fracture or pars defect). (Reproduced with permission from Cavalier R, Herman MY, Cheung EV, Pizzutillo PD: Spondylolysis and Spondylolisthesis in children and adolescents: I. Diagnosis, natural history, and nonsurgical mamagement. *J Bone Joint Surg Am* 2006;14:417-424.)

crum. This lesion is caused by high-energy trauma and is rarely isolated. Most instances of traumatic spondylolisthesis are accompanied by multiple traumatic injuries and visceral, vascular, and neurologic symptoms. Because many patients die soon after the initial traumatic event, many cases of traumatic spondylolisthesis are not identified. A review of the literature reported approximately 30 cases of traumatic lumbosacral dislocation;[8] however, it is likely that this number underrepresents the actual incidence of this type of injury.

Pathogenesis

Various theories have been put forth regarding the possible cause of lumbar spondylolysis. Many authors believe that lumbar spondylolysis is a stress fracture of the pars interarticularis because spondylolysis frequently occurs in athletes in sports requiring repetitive trunk movements, especially extension;[9-12] it frequently occurs in athetoid palsy patients with involuntary trunk movements.[13] Spondylolysis has not been reported in fetuses, infants, or nonambulatory patients.[14,15] The radiologic course is similar to that of a stress fracture of a long bone. The pars defects can heal with nonsurgical management.[16-18]

The pathogenesis of isthmic spondylolisthesis following spondylolysis also has been extensively studied. By definition, isthmic spondylolisthesis is slippage associated with a spondylolysis of the cephalad involved vertebra; however, spondylolysis does not develop in all patients with this type of anterior slippage. In a study describing the natural history of spondylolysis and isthmic spondylolisthesis in 30 patients, the greatest slip progression occurred early in life.[19] During the first decade of follow-up evaluation, the average slip progression was 7% for those that progressed. Progression in the second and third decades averaged 4%. In the fourth decade of follow-up, the average progression was only 2%. Therefore, the progression of isthmic spondylolisthesis occurs in younger patients; this type of spondylolisthesis may gradually stabilize as the patient ages.

Degenerative spondylolisthesis is a disorder that affects older patients. Chronic degenerative changes that occur in the facet joint and disk space result in the loss of normal segmental stability. Certain anatomic variants, including hyperlordosis, sagittal orientation of the facet joints, and sacralization of the L5 vertebral body can predispose a patient to the development of degenerative spondylolisthesis. Chronic, low-level instability leads to further degenerative changes, including facet joint subluxation with capsular laxity, osteophyte formation, and disk-space narrowing. These changes lead to compression of the traversing nerve root of the involved level. In the most common expressions of L4-L5 degenerative spondylolisthesis, the L5 nerve root is often symptomatic, with resultant lower lateral leg radiculopathy and possible foot and toe dorsiflexion weakness. The amount of displacement in degenerative spondylolisthesis tends to be limited to less than 40%

(margin note, right) predisposing risks

condition, it most commonly occurs in older patients. The records and radiographs of 949 women and 120 men age 50 years and older who had been treated by a spinal surgeon for low back pain were reviewed.[5] Women who had borne children had a significantly higher incidence of degenerative spondylolisthesis than nulliparous women (28% versus 16.7%, respectively). The incidence of degenerative spondylolisthesis was 7.5% in the men, which was significantly less than in the women (P = 0.031).

In congenital and dysplastic spondylolisthesis, the pars interarticularis is intact but the L5-S1 facet joints are abnormally developed. This deficiency in the facet joints leads to instability and the resultant anterior translation of the L5 vertebral body. Because the posterior arch is not fractured, as in isthmic spondylolisthesis, the L5 lamina translates anteriorly with the vertebral body and can cause central spinal canal stenosis, with symptoms of stenosis occurring with slippages of more than 35% (**Figure 2**). The exact incidences of these types of spondylolisthesis are unknown, but an incidence of 14% to 21% has been reported in relatively large series of patients treated for spondylolithesis.[6,7]

Traumatic spondylolisthesis is characterized by a dislocated or subluxated lumbar spine, which has moved anterior to the sacrum because of bilateral dislocations or fractures of the L5-S1 facet joints, pedicles, pars interarticularis, or a fracture line crossing the sa-

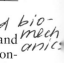

5: Spine

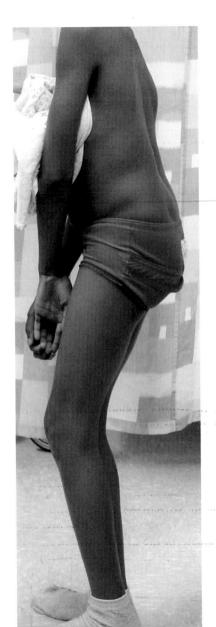

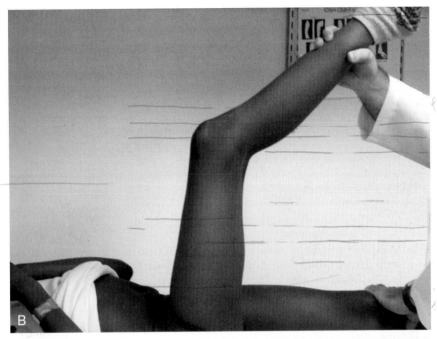

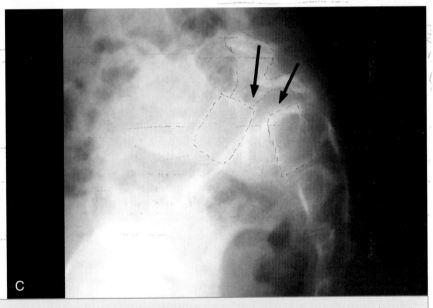

Figure 2   **A,** Photograph of a 9-year-old girl with grade IV dysplastic (Wiltse type I) spondylolisthesis of L5-S1. Note the position of flexion of her hips and knees. **B,** Popliteal angle measurement of 55° secondary to contracture of hamstring muscles. **C,** Standing lateral radiograph of the lumbosacral spine of the same patient, illustrating high-grade spondylolisthesis with lumbosacral kyphosis (*arrows*). (Reproduced with permission from Cavalier R, Herman MY, Cheung EV, Pizzutillo PD: Spondylolysis and Spondylolisthesis in children and adolescents: I. Diagnosis, natural history, and nonsurgical management. *J Bone Joint Surg Am* 2006;14:417-424.)

because of the eventual contact between the superior articular facet of the inferior level and the pars interarticularis of the superior level. Central spinal stenosis can occur as a result of facet joint hypertrophy, ligamentum flavum redundancy, and disk-space bulging.

In congenital and dysplastic spondylolisthesis, abnormalities of the vertebral arch or facet joints lead to spondylolisthesis at the lumbosacral junction. Abnormalities include failure of formation of the facet joint or sagittal alignment of the L5-S1 facet complex. Spon-

dylolysis, by definition, does not occur with dysplastic or congenital spondylolisthesis; therefore, the intact L5 lamina may translate anteriorly with the vertebral body and can cause severe central spinal stenosis. This disorder usually becomes symptomatic in early adolescence, and it affects females approximately twice as frequently as males.

Traumatic spondylolisthesis involves a bony or ligamentous injury that results in acute instability of the involved level. This type of injury can include high-energy trauma resulting in ligamentous rupture, facet complex fracture, and possible facet subluxation and dislocation. Acute pars fractures secondary to high-energy fractures also can be classified as traumatic injuries. Although the traumatic pars fracture is seemingly similar to the spondylolytic pars fracture seen in isthmic spondylolisthesis, the traumatic pars fracture occurs when the pars fails under abnormal and excessive stress, whereas the spondylolytic defect occurs under normal physiologic stress.

Clinical Presentation

Chronic isthmic spondylolisthesis frequently causes low back pain in adult patients. Radiculopathy may eventually develop in the lower extremities because of the fibrocartilaginous proliferation around the pars defect. This radiculopathy involves the exiting nerve root, which is the L5 nerve root in the most common type of L5 spondylolysis. The typical symptoms of chronic isthmic spondylolisthesis are low back pain caused by spinal instability and radiating leg pain caused by compression of the exiting nerve root.

In degenerative spondylolisthesis, lateral recess and foraminal stenosis result in radiculopathy caused by compression of the traversing nerve root. Hypertrophy and subluxation of the involved facet complex, combined with the common degenerative changes of disk bulging and ligamentum flavum redundancy, cause compression on the exiting nerve root at that level. Central stenosis can occur in more advanced cases. Because the L4-L5 level is most commonly affected by degenerative spondylolisthesis, L5 radiculopathy from compression of the traversing L5 nerve root is the most common neural finding in these patients.

The clinical presentations of congenital, dysplastic, and traumatic spondylolisthesis were discussed previously in this chapter.

Treatment

Isthmic Spondylolisthesis and Spondylolysis
Nonsurgical Treatment
Spondylolysis is relatively common in children and adolescents. A prospective study reported a diagnosis of spondylolysis, with or without spondylolisthesis, in 9 of 73 pediatric patients (12.3%) with a chief report of low back pain.[20] Most adolescents with isthmic spondylolisthesis or spondylolysis can be successfully managed with nonsurgical treatment. In one recent meta-analysis study, 83.9% of adolescent patients who were nonsurgically treated for lumbar spondylolysis had a successful clinical outcome after at least 1 year, and bracing did not influence this outcome.[21]

Bony union of the pars defect can be achieved in adolescents if they refrain from participation in sports activities and wear a trunk brace, although fracture healing is variable. Early diagnosis may be extremely

important in attaining bony healing of the pars. Based on a retrospective review of CT of 239 pars defects in 134 young patients treated nonsurgically, an early stage of the defects at first presentation was an important prognostic indicator in attaining osseous healing with nonsurgical treatment.[17] Nonsurgical treatments include nonsteroidal anti-inflammatory drugs, brace therapy, sports activity restrictions, and, occasionally, short-term bed rest. Regardless of whether the pars defect heals, most symptoms resolve over time with conservative treatment.

It is likely that an adult patient with a long-standing lumbar spondylolysis and isthmic spondylolisthesis would also benefit from a nonsurgical treatment protocol. Physical therapy, home-based strengthening programs, weight reduction, activity modification, and possible injection therapy, including epidural injections, facet blocks, and pars injections, may be beneficial in certain patients. The associated degenerative changes that occur in the adult patient with a chronic lumbar isthmic spondylolisthesis, however, may require surgical decompression of the compressed nerve root or stabilization of the degenerative motion segment.

Direct Repair of Spondylolysis
Various techniques to directly repair a pars defect have been described. These techniques include bone grafting with the placement of wires, screws, or hook-screw constructs to stabilize the fractured pars. Minimally invasive repair techniques also have been described (Figure 3). The goal of these procedures is to restore the normal anatomy and save a spinal motion segment to retain the associated spinal mobility. For these procedures to be successful, the pain source must be the pars defect itself. The pain generator can be preoperatively verified by injecting the defect with a local anesthetic. In patients who do not respond to the local anesthetic injection, direct repair of the pars defect is not recommended; other causes of low back pain should be evaluated. If significant displacement has occurred at the site of the spondylolysis, direct repair of the defect may not be highly successful because of difficulty in achieving solid bony healing.

Decompression of Lumbar Nerve Roots Affected by Spondylolysis
Radiculopathy can develop in an adult patient with spondylolysis as the condition becomes more chronic. The radiculopathy affects the exiting nerve root associated with the cephalad vertebra of the involved spinal segment because this nerve root is compressed by scar formation around the spondylolysis site. In the most common L5 spondylolysis with an L5-S1 spondylolisthesis, the L5 nerve root is involved. Decompressive laminectomy (the Gill procedure) has been described for patients with lumbar spondylolysis and associated radiculopathy. Subsequently, some authors reported that the Gill procedure can result in further vertebral slippage postoperatively and recommended spinal fusion in addition to laminectomy.[22,23]

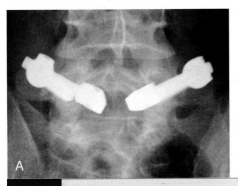
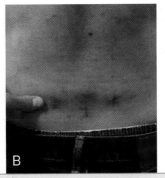
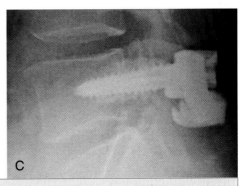

Figure 3 Minimally invasive technique for the direct repair of a pars defect. **A,** AP radiograph showing instrumentation placement. **B,** Postoperative photograph demonstrating incision size and location. **C,** Lateral radiograph showing instrumentation construct. (Reproduced with permission from Sairyo K, Sakai T, Yasui N: Minimally invasive technique for direct repair of the pars defects in young adults using a percutaneous pedicle screw and hook-rod system: A technical note. *J Neurosurg Spine* 2009;10:492-495.)

Less invasive techniques to decompress the involved nerve root in patients with spondylolysis have been developed.[24] These decompression-only procedures are indicated in patients older than 40 years and in those with radiculopathy without low back pain and no evidence of spinal instability on dynamic radiographs. Good clinical outcomes with a mean follow-up period of 11.7 months have been reported. The advantage of these minimally invasive techniques is the feasibility of excising the edge of the spondylolysis site and associated scar tissue, with possibly less damage to the posterior elements, paravertebral muscles, and posterior ligamentous structures. Patients treated with a decompression-only procedure for spondylolysis should be counseled that their instability may continue to progress and that further surgery, including surgical fusion, may ultimately be necessary.

Low-Grade Isthmic Spondylolisthesis
Noninstrumented Fusion
Because of the risk of increased spondylolisthesis following posterior decompression alone, spinal stabilization in addition to decompression has been recommended in adult patients with symptomatic isthmic spondylolisthesis.[25] In one prospective randomized study comparing instrumented and noninstrumented lumbar posterolateral fusion for adult isthmic spondylolisthesis, posterolateral fusion performed without instrumentation relieved pain and improved function; the use of supplementary transpedicular instrumentation did not improve the fusion rate or the clinical outcomes.[25]

The authors of a recent study retrospectively reviewed the long-term follow-up (mean, 19.7 years) outcomes of uninstrumented posterolateral spinal arthrodesis in adolescents with low-grade (grade I or II) lumbar isthmic spondylolisthesis.[26] The outcome of spinal fusion was good, with 43 of 49 patients (87.7%) attaining solid fusion; 6 patients (12.3%) had a pseudarthrosis. The satisfactory results obtained in 94% of patients were closely associated with the rate of successful fusion.

Instrumented Fusion
Numerous surgical procedures have been described for isthmic spondylolisthesis, including decompression with or without posterolateral lumbar fusion and (possibly) with instrumentation and the addition of an interbody fusion. In a systematic review of the radiographic and clinical outcomes of adult patients who were surgically treated for low-grade isthmic spondylolisthesis, the authors concluded that a combined anterior and posterior procedure most reliably achieves fusion and a successful clinical outcome.[27] However, a recent study reported that circumferential fusion achieved significantly better results than posterolateral fusion at 6 months and 1 year, although the difference diminished with time and was not significant at 2 years postoperatively.[28]

In a prospective study to compare the outcomes of posterior lumbar interbody fusion and posterolateral fusion in patients with adult isthmic spondylolisthesis, the type of fusion did not affect the 2-year outcome.[29] In another prospective study, 164 adult patients with isthmic spondylolisthesis were evaluated to determine predicative factors for outcomes of spinal fusion.[30] Patients who worked prior to surgery, males, and those who exercised regularly had better outcomes after fusion. The results of a systematic review of 29 selected high-quality studies on lumbar fusion showed no difference in outcomes between different fusion techniques.[31] Overall, the optimal type of surgery for low-grade adult isthmic spondylolisthesis remains controversial.

High-Grade Spondylolisthesis
Although high-grade isthmic spondylolisthesis (grade III, IV, or V) accounts for a distinct minority of all patients with spondylolisthesis, the treatment of high-grade spondylolisthesis can be complex and difficult. The optimal treatment of this pathology remains controversial. The clinical indications for the surgical treatment of a high-grade spondylolisthesis include continued pain despite conservative treatments, the progression of spinal deformity, and the presence of neurologic symptoms.

5: Spine

Most patients with high-grade spondylolisthesis or spondyloptosis (complete subluxation of the cephalad vertebra off the lower vertebra; grade V spondylolisthesis) become symptomatic during adolescence. A recent literature review evaluated the surgical treatment of high-grade spondylolisthesis in the pediatric population.[32] The authors concluded that it was impossible to formulate clear guidelines for treating high-grade spondylolisthesis based on the best evidence available in the published literature because of the paucity of high-level studies on the topic. Various surgical techniques have been described, each with advantages and disadvantages.[33-40] A study evaluating the long-term results of anterior, posterior, and circumferential in situ fusion for high-grade isthmic spondylolisthesis reported the superiority of circumferential fusion over the other methods studied.[41]

Degenerative Spondylolisthesis
Nonsurgical Treatment
As in many spinal disorders, the preferred initial treatment of patients with degenerative spondylolisthesis is nonsurgical. Nonsurgical treatment includes anti-inflammatory medications, physical therapy, activity modification, and home-based exercise programs. Exercise programs frequently focus on core strengthening and aerobic conditioning, although no prospective randomized trials have been performed to identify the optimal nonsurgical modality. Other techniques used in conjunction with physical therapy include electrical stimulation, massage, heat packs, cold packs, ultrasound, and acupuncture; however, there are few high quality data supporting the use of these modalities.

Epidural steroid injections are often used in the treatment of degenerative spinal conditions, including spinal stenosis and spondylolisthesis. The theoretic benefit of an epidural corticosteroid is its potent local anti-inflammatory effect, which decreases the radicular and local pain caused by the degenerative joint changes and nerve compression. Although epidural steroid injections are frequently used and may temporarily improve symptoms, there have been no prospective randomized studies evaluating the efficacy of epidural injections for the long-term relief of symptoms in patients with degenerative spondylolisthesis. Two high-quality studies evaluating surgical treatment for symptomatic degenerative spondylolisthesis have shown that patients treated with conservative methods have inferior outcomes after at least 2 years of treatment compared with those treated surgically.[42,43]

Surgical Treatment
The primary surgical treatments for degenerative spondylolisthesis are decompression alone, decompression with noninstrumented fusion, and decompression with instrumented fusion. Surgical indications include back pain or leg symptoms that are recalcitrant to nonsurgical treatment, lead to a significant impairment in quality of life, and have associated significant or progressive neurologic deficits or neurogenic bowel or bladder symptoms. The results of surgical treatments for radiculopathy and neurogenic claudication are believed to be better than results after surgical treatment for isolated axial back pain in patients with degenerative disease.

Decompression Alone
The goal of surgical decompression is the relief of symptomatic neurologic compression. The treatment of degenerative spondylolisthesis frequently includes central and lateral recess decompression because of the combined central spinal stenosis and facet joint changes that lead to lateral recess stenosis. Laminectomy is commonly performed in this setting. Several studies evaluated decompression alone in this patient population.[44-46] The effectiveness of laminectomy alone has been described, with more than 80% of patients having good or excellent outcomes. Care must be taken, however, to prevent iatrogenic stability or worsen underlying instability. In one study, only 33% of patients treated with total facetectomy as part of the decompression procedure had good or excellent results versus 80% in those whose treatment included facet preservation.[46] Most of these studies have limited value because of the small number of patients, retrospective analyses, and suboptimal follow-up periods. Overall, decompression alone can be used to treat selected patients with stable spondylolisthesis, but further instability may result and require additional surgical treatment.

Decompression With Noninstrumented Fusion
Because of the risk of worsening instability and vertebral body translation following decompression of a lumbar spondylolisthesis, a fusion has been advocated in conjunction with the decompressive procedure. Noninstrumented posterolateral lumbar fusion was among the first types of lumbar fusions advocated for this use. Several studies evaluated the success of noninstrumented fusion in patients with degenerative lumbar spondylolisthesis.[46-48] In one study, 33% of the patients with degenerative spondylolisthesis had good or excellent results following laminectomy with total facetectomy, and 80% of the patients achieved good or excellent results following laminectomy with preservation of the facet joints.[46] When a noninstrumented posterolateral fusion was added, the rate of good and excellent results increased to 90%, suggesting that the added stability provided by the fusion may improve results in this patient population.

In a prospective, randomized study evaluating 50 consecutive patients with degenerative lumbar spondylolisthesis,[47] the patients were treated with either decompression alone or decompression with posterolateral fusion. The fusion group had significantly improved outcomes compared with the nonfusion group. These results were confirmed by other authors.[48]

Decompression With Instrumented Fusion
With the widespread acceptance of lumbar pedicle screws, instrumented lumbar fusions have become both

technically feasible and commonplace. The success rates of instrumented posterolateral lumbar fusions in association with decompression for degenerative spondylolisthesis have been evaluated. In a study comparing the results of decompression with instrumented fusion versus decompression with noninstrumented fusion for degenerative spondylolisthesis, the addition of instrumentation lead to a higher fusion rate (82% versus 45%, P = 0.0015), but the clinical difference between patients treated with instrumented and noninstrumented fusion was not statistically significant at 2-year follow-up (P = 0.435).[49] In a longer term study of this same patient group (evaluated at least 5 years postoperatively), the achievement of solid fusion resulted in better clinical outcomes than in instances when solid fusion was not accomplished.[50] The authors suggested that because the addition of instrumentation led to higher fusion rates, which resulted in improved long-term clinical outcomes, instrumented fusion should be considered in the surgical treatment of lumbar degenerative spondylolisthesis.

The most comprehensive prospective study evaluating the surgical treatments of degenerative spondylolisthesis was an arm of the Spine Patient Outcome Research Trial.[43] At 4-year follow-up in randomized and observational cohorts, patients with degenerative spondylolisthesis who were treated surgically had greater pain relief and improvement in function throughout that time frame when compared with patients treated nonsurgically. Because various surgical treatments were used in the study, conclusions regarding the optimal surgical approach require further data analysis.

Congenital and Dysplastic Spondylolisthesis

Patients with congenital or dysplastic spondylolisthesis often become symptomatic in early adolescence as the slippage increases. Back pain, hamstring tightness, and spinal canal stenosis are caused by the intact posterior elements. After these symptoms develop, conservative treatment is rarely useful. Surgical treatment consists of stabilizing the motion segment with neural decompression if necessary. Various techniques have been used, but no high-quality studies comparing these techniques have been performed.

Traumatic Spondylolisthesis

Traumatic spondylolisthesis injuries are high-energy, unstable injuries that are frequently accompanied by other multisystem trauma. The initial treatment of these patients includes stabilization of the associated traumatic injuries and appropriate evaluation and diagnosis of the spondylolisthesis. Clinical and radiographic workups for possible bony or soft-tissue pelvic injuries and other noncontiguous spinal injuries should be included in the workup.

The treatment of the traumatic spondylolisthesis requires stabilization of the subluxation or dislocation, usually with an instrumented fusion. Instrumentation to the pelvis or proximal to the involved motion segment may be needed to provide appropriate fixation. Pelvic fixation may be required if there is an associated pelvic fracture or ligamentous injury. Significant neurologic injury can occur because of the rapid neurologic compression that occurs with these injuries, and decompression of compressed nerve roots or the central canal may be required.

Annotated References

1. Roche MB, Rowe GG: The incidence of separate neural arch and coincident bone variations: A survey of 4,200 skeletons. *Anat Rec* 1951;109(2):233-252.

2. Simper LB: Spondylolysis in Eskimo skeletons. *Acta Orthop Scand* 1986;57(1):78-80.

3. Sonne-Holm S, Jacobsen S, Rovsing HC, Monrad H, Gebuhr P: Lumbar spondylolysis: A life long dynamic condition? A cross sectional survey of 4,151 adults. *Eur Spine J* 2007;16(6):821-828.

   A survey of 4,151 individuals was used to identify the distribution and risk factors for lumbar spondylolysis. Men were significantly more at risk for L5 spondylolysis. In women, increased lumbar lordosis had a significant association with L5 spondylolysis. Increased pelvic inclination was associated with L5 spondylolysis in both men and women.

4. Belfi LM, Ortiz AO, Katz DS: Computed tomography evaluation of spondylolysis and spondylolisthesis in asymptomatic patients. *Spine (Phila Pa 1976)* 2006;31(24):E907-E910.

5. Sanderson PL, Fraser RD: The influence of pregnancy on the development of degenerative spondylolisthesis. *J Bone Joint Surg Br* 1996;78(6):951-954.

6. Newman PH: Stenosis of the lumbar spine in spondylolisthesis. *Clin Orthop Relat Res* 1976;115(115):116-121.

7. Boxall D, Bradford DS, Winter RB, Moe JH: Management of severe spondylolisthesis in children and adolescents. *J Bone Joint Surg Am* 1979;61(4):479-495.

8. Vialle R, Wolff S, Pauthier F, et al: Traumatic lumbosacral dislocation: Four cases and review of literature. *Clin Orthop Relat Res* 2004;419(419):91-97.

9. Jackson DW, Wiltse LL, Cirincoine RJ: Spondylolysis in the female gymnast. *Clin Orthop Relat Res* 1976;117(117):68-73.

10. Seitsalo S, Antila H, Karrinaho T, et al: Spondylolysis in ballet dancers. *J Dance Med Sci* 1997;1:51-54.

11. Soler T, Calderón C: The prevalence of spondylolysis in the Spanish elite athlete. *Am J Sports Med* 2000;28(1):57-62.

12. Teitz CC: Sports medicine concerns in dance and gymnastics. *Pediatr Clin North Am* 1982;29(6):1399-1421.

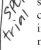

5: Spine

13. Sakai T, Yamada H, Nakamura T, et al: Lumbar spinal disorders in patients with athetoid cerebral palsy: A clinical and biomechanical study. *Spine (Phila Pa 1976)* 2006;31(3):E66-E70.

14. Rowe GG, Roche MB: The etiology of separate neural arch. *J Bone Joint Surg Am* 1953;35(1):102-110.

15. Rosenberg NJ, Bargar WL, Friedman B: The incidence of spondylolysis and spondylolisthesis in nonambulatory patients. *Spine (Phila Pa 1976)* 1981;6(1):35-38.

16. Morita T, Ikata T, Katoh S, Miyake R: Lumbar spondylolysis in children and adolescents. *J Bone Joint Surg Br* 1995;77(4):620-625.

17. Fujii K, Katoh S, Sairyo K, Ikata T, Yasui N: Union of defects in the pars interarticularis of the lumbar spine in children and adolescents: The radiological outcome after conservative treatment. *J Bone Joint Surg Br* 2004; 86(2):225-231.

18. Sairyo K, Sakai T, Yasui N: Conservative treatment of lumbar spondylolysis in childhood and adolescence: The radiological signs which predict healing. *J Bone Joint Surg Br* 2009;91(2):206-209.

    The stage of the spondylolysis defect on CT and the presence or absence of high-signal change in the adjacent pedicle on T2-weighted MRI were evaluated to determine their relationship to bony healing in nonsurgically treated children. The authors reported that 87% of the early defects healed, 32% of progressive defects healed, and no terminal defects healed. In the defects with positive high-signal change, 77% healed after conservative treatment.

19. Beutler WJ, Fredrickson BE, Murtland A, Sweeney CA, Grant WD, Baker D: The natural history of spondylolysis and spondylolisthesis: 45-year follow-up evaluation. *Spine (Phila Pa 1976)* 2003;28(10):1027-1035, discussion 1035.

20. Bhatia NN, Chow G, Timon SJ, Watts HG: Diagnostic modalities for the evaluation of pediatric back pain: A prospective study. *J Pediatr Orthop* 2008;28(2):230-233.

    A prospective study was performed to examine the diagnosis rate in pediatric patients with back pain. Of 73 patients presenting with back pain, no diagnosis was made in 57 patients (78.1%). These results suggest that pediatric back pain frequently does not carry a definitive diagnosis.

21. Klein G, Mehlman CT, McCarty M: Nonoperative treatment of spondylolysis and grade I spondylolisthesis in children and young adults: A meta-analysis of observational studies. *J Pediatr Orthop* 2009;29(2):146-156.

    Meta-analysis suggested that 83.9% of patients with spondylolysis and grade I spondylolisthesis who were treated nonsurgically had a successful clinical outcome after at least 1 year. Bracing did not seem to influence outcomes. In contrast to the high rate of success with clinical parameters, most defects did not heal with nonsurgical treatment.

22. Osterman K, Lindholm TS, Laurent LE: Late results of removal of the loose posterior element (Gills operation) in the treatment of lytic lumbar spondylolisthesis. *Clin Orthop Relat Res* 1976;117(117):121-128.

23. Sairyo K, Goel VK, Masuda A, et al: Biomechanical rationale of endoscopic decompression for lumbar spondylolysis as an effective minimally invasive procedure: A study based on the finite element analysis. *Minim Invasive Neurosurg* 2005;48(2):119-122.

24. Sairyo K, Katoh S, Sakamaki T, Komatsubara S, Yasui N: A new endoscopic technique to decompress lumbar nerve roots affected by spondylolysis: Technical note. *J Neurosurg* 2003;98(3, suppl):290-293.

25. Möller H, Hedlund R: Instrumented and noninstrumented posterolateral fusion in adult spondylolisthesis: A prospective randomized study. Part 2. *Spine (Phila Pa 1976)* 2000;25(13):1716-1721.

26. Girardo M, Bettini N, Dema E, Cervellati S: Uninstrumented posterolateral spinal arthrodesis: Is it the gold standard technique for I degrees and II degrees grade spondylolisthesis in adolescence? *Eur Spine J* 2009; 18(Suppl 1):126-132.

    A retrospective review of the outcome of uninstrumented posterolateral spinal arthrodesis in adolescents with low-grade isthmic spondylolisthesis is presented. Good outcomes were reported, with 87.7% of patients attaining solid fusion. Pseudarthrosis was reported in 12.3% of patients. The satisfactory results obtained in 94% of patients were closely associated with the rate of successful fusion.

27. Kwon BK, Hilibrand AS, Malloy K, et al: A critical analysis of the literature regarding surgical approach and outcome for adult low-grade isthmic spondylolisthesis. *J Spinal Disord Tech* 2005;18(suppl):S30-S40.

28. Swan J, Hurwitz E, Malek F, et al: Surgical treatment for unstable low-grade isthmic spondylolisthesis in adults: A prospective controlled study of posterior instrumented fusion compared with combined anterior-posterior fusion. *Spine J* 2006;6(6):606-614.

29. Ekman P, Möller H, Tullberg T, Neumann P, Hedlund R: Posterior lumbar interbody fusion versus posterolateral fusion in adult isthmic spondylolisthesis. *Spine (Phila Pa 1976)* 2007;32(20):2178-2183.

    The authors report on a prospective study to compare the outcome of posterior lumber interbody fusion and posterolateral fusion in patients with adult isthmic spondylolisthesis. The type of fusion did not affect the 2-year outcomes. Despite the theoretic advantages of posterior lumber interbody fusion, no improvements in patient outcomes over posterolateral fusion were demonstrated.

30. Ekman P, Möller H, Hedlund R: Predictive factors for the outcome of fusion in adult isthmic spondylolisthesis. *Spine (Phila Pa 1976)* 2009;34(11):1204-1210.

    The authors conducted a prospective study to determine predictive factors in the outcomes of 164 adult patients with isthmic spondylolisthesis who were surgically treated with fusion. The results showed that patients working prior to surgery had more favorable outcomes. Male gender and participation in regular exercise also were indicators of a better outcome after fusion.

31. Jacobs WC, Vreeling A, De Kleuver M: Fusion for low-grade adult isthmic spondylolisthesis: A systematic review of the literature. *Eur Spine J* 2006;15(4):391-402.

32. Transfeldt EE, Mehbod AA: Evidence-based medicine analysis of isthmic spondylolisthesis treatment including reduction versus fusion in situ for high-grade slips. *Spine (Phila Pa 1976)* 2007;32(19, suppl):S126-S129.

The authors reviewed the available literature in an attempt to formulate evidence-based recommendations for the surgical treatment of high-grade spondylolisthesis in the pediatric population. Pseudarthrosis rates were decreased by performing an instrumented reduction with a fusion; however, there was no significant difference in clinical outcomes in patients treated with fusion in situ and reduction and fusion.

33. Sasso RC, Shively KD, Reilly TM: Transvertebral Transsacral strut grafting for high-grade isthmic spondylolisthesis L5-S1 with fibular allograft. *J Spinal Disord Tech* 2008;21(5):328-333.

A retrospective study was conducted to evaluate the clinical and radiographic outcomes of 25 patients with high-grade isthmic spondylolisthesis treated with decompression and transvertebral, transsacral, strut grafting with a fibular allograft. Although there was no reduction in translational deformity, this technique offered excellent fusion results and good clinical outcomes, and it prevented the progression of sagittal translation and lumbosacral kyphosis.

34. Smith MD, Bohlman HH: Spondylolisthesis treated by a single-stage operation combining decompression with in situ posterolateral and anterior fusion: An analysis of eleven patients who had long-term follow-up. *J Bone Joint Surg Am* 1990;72(3):415-421.

35. Minamide A, Akamaru T, Yoon ST, Tamaki T, Rhee JM, Hutton WC: Transdiscal L5-S1 screws for the fixation of isthmic spondylolisthesis: A biomechanical evaluation. *J Spinal Disord Tech* 2003;16(2):144-149.

36. Gaines RW: L5 vertebrectomy for the surgical treatment of spondyloptosis: Thirty cases in 25 years. *Spine (Phila Pa 1976)* 2005;30(6, suppl):S66-S70.

37. Hu SS, Bradford DS, Transfeldt EE, Cohen M: Reduction of high-grade spondylolisthesis using Edwards instrumentation. *Spine (Phila Pa 1976)* 1996;21(3):367-371.

38. Floman Y, Millgram MA, Ashkenazi E, Smorgick Y, Rand N: Instrumented slip reduction and fusion for painful unstable isthmic spondylolisthesis in adults. *J Spinal Disord Tech* 2008;21(7):477-483.

The safety and clinical outcomes of surgically instrumented slip reduction in 12 adults with isthmic spondylolisthesis was evaluated. The slip was anatomically reduced by 100% in five patients and between 90% and 95% in seven patients. Minimal loss of correction (5%) was observed in two patients. No neurologic complications were reported.

39. Goyal N, Wimberley DW, Hyatt A, et al: Radiographic and clinical outcomes after instrumented reduction and transforaminal lumbar interbody fusion of mid and high-grade isthmic spondylolisthesis. *J Spinal Disord Tech* 2009;22(5):321-327.

The authors report on a retrospective cohort study of instrumented reduction and transforaminal lumbar interbody fusion in mid- and high-grade cases of adult isthmic spondylolisthesis. The average anterolisthesis was 51.0% preoperatively, 13.2% in the immediate postoperative period, and 17.0% at final follow-up.

40. Doita M, Uno K, Maeno K, et al: Two-stage decompression, reduction, and interbody fusion for lumbosacral spondyloptosis through a posterior approach using Ilizarov external fixation. *J Neurosurg Spine* 2008;8(2):186-192.

A 33-year-old woman with spondyloptosis was treated with a two-stage surgical procedure involving decompression, reduction, and posterior fusion using an Ilizarov external fixator and transpedicular fixation system. The spondylolisthesis was partially reduced without neurologic alterations and without complications.

41. Helenius I, Lamberg T, Osterman K, et al: Posterolateral, anterior, or circumferential fusion in situ for high-grade spondylolisthesis in young patients: A long-term evaluation using the Scoliosis Research Society questionnaire. *Spine (Phila Pa 1976)* 2006;31(2):190-196.

42. Anderson PA, Tribus CB, Kitchel SH: Treatment of neurogenic claudication by interspinous decompression: Application of the X STOP device in patients with lumbar degenerative spondylolisthesis. *J Neurosurg Spine* 2006;4(6):463-471.

43. Weinstein JN, Lurie JD, Tosteson TD, et al: Surgical versus nonsurgical treatment for lumbar degenerative spondylolisthesis. *N Engl J Med* 2007;356(22):2257-2270.

In a comparison of surgical and nonsurgical treatment for lumbar degenerative spondylolisthesis, patients with degenerative spondylolisthesis and spinal stenosis who were treated surgically had substantially greater improvement in pain relief and function over a 2-year period than patients treated nonsurgically.

44. Fitzgerald JA, Newman PH: Degenerative spondylolisthesis. *J Bone Joint Surg Br* 1976;58(2):184-192.

45. Epstein NE: Decompression in the surgical management of degenerative spondylolisthesis: Advantages of a conservative approach in 290 patients. *J Spinal Disord* 1998;11(2):116-122.

46. Lombardi JS, Wiltse LL, Reynolds J, Widell EH, Spencer C III: Treatment of degenerative spondylolisthesis. *Spine (Phila Pa 1976)* 1985;10(9):821-827.

5: Spine

47. Herkowitz HN, Kurz LT: Degenerative lumbar spondylolisthesis with spinal stenosis: A prospective study comparing decompression with decompression and intertransverse process arthrodesis. *J Bone Joint Surg Am* 1991;73(6):802-808.

48. Ghogawala Z, Benzel EC, Amin-Hanjani S, et al: Prospective outcomes evaluation after decompression with or without instrumented fusion for lumbar stenosis and degenerative Grade I spondylolisthesis. *J Neurosurg Spine* 2004;1(3):267-272.

49. Fischgrund JS, Mackay M, Herkowitz HN, Brower R, Montgomery DM, Kurz LT: Degenerative lumbar spondylolisthesis with spinal stenosis: A prospective, randomized study comparing decompressive laminectomy and arthrodesis with and without spinal instrumentation. *Spine (Phila Pa 1976)* 1997;22(24):2807-2812.

50. Kornblum MB, Fischgrund JS, Herkowitz HN, Abraham DA, Berkower DL, Ditkoff JS: Degenerative lumbar spondylolisthesis with spinal stenosis: A prospective long-term study comparing fusion and pseudarthrosis. *Spine (Phila Pa 1976)* 2004;29(7):726-733, discussion 733-734.

Chapter 51

Thoracic Disk Herniation

Mark B. Dekutoski, MD

Incidence

Thoracic disk herniation detected by MRI is present in 20% to 40% of asymptomatic control subjects.[1,2] Thoracic diskectomy for clinically symptomatic patients accounts for less than 1% of all diskectomies performed in North America.[3,4]

Classification

Disk herniations of the thoracic spine are classified based on their segmental level, canal location, size, imaging characteristics, and clinical presentation. Symptomatic thoracic disks tend to occur with greater prevalence in the junctional segments than in the rigid segments and are often classified as cervical and/or upper lumbar disk herniations. Central and large disks (greater than 40% of canal diameter) are associated with a greater incidence of myelopathy and worse functional outcomes.[5] Calcific changes to the disk and dural interface noted on CT can predict a greater likelihood of cerebrospinal fluid complications with intervention. Classification based on clinical presentation is common and follows the spectrum of asymptomatic axial pain syndromes provoked by rotation to radicular syndromes and/or myelopathy.

Etiology

The thoracic spine includes mobile areas of transition at the junctions and areas of relative stiffness in flexion

Dr. Dekutoski or an immediate family member serves as a board member, owner, officer, or committee member of AOSpine North America and AOSpine North America Education Committee; has received royalties from Medtronic Sofamor Danek; is a member of a speakers' bureau or has made paid presentations on behalf of Medtronic Sofamor Danek; serves as a paid consultant to Medtronic Sofamor Danek; has received research or institutional support from Mayo Clinic Practice and Mayo Clinic Foundation; and has received nonincome support (such as equipment or services), commercially derived honoraria, or other non–research-related funding (such as paid travel) from Medtronic Sofamor Danek.

secondary to the ribs. Costovertebral articulations, however, allow the coupled motions of lateral bending and rotation. Annular disruption, disk and plate fissuring, and the cascade of disk repair and degeneration are associated with repetitive rotation. Although trauma has been documented to cause defects in the end plate (Schmorl nodes), disk herniation is generally associated with the apoptotic changes that occur with aging and stiffening of the spine. Thoracic disk herniation also occurs with the spectrum of conditions marked by diskopathy of the thoracic disks and is hallmarked by the condition of diffuse idiopathic skeletal hyperostosis and the enthesopathic condition of ankylosing spondylitis. Intradiskal calcification and calcification of the extruded thoracic disk occur more commonly in the thoracic spine.

Clinical Presentation

Patients present with a spectrum of symptoms that can vary from thoracic pain, which is typically aggravated by rotation, to radicular complaints, to presentation of long track signs as evidence of myelopathy. Onset typically occurs during the fourth through sixth decades of life. Symptoms commonly occur in the cervical thoracic junction, usually marked by interscapular pain. Midthoracic pathology can cause pain with radicular or myelopathic features, and lower thoracic disk herniations can cause groin pain or even lower root symptoms because the thoracic disk can have a mass effect on the concomitant anatomic motor cells of the ventral cord. This condition manifests as a lower motor neuropathy. The typical motor neuron presentation may include bladder dysfunction and gait disturbance. The slow, insidious onset can make diagnosis more difficult.

Delayed diagnosis is common because of the nonspecific nature of the symptoms. The differential diagnosis should include rare neurologic conditions that present with imbalance and/or central radicular features, including amyotrophic lateral sclerosis, multiple sclerosis, transverse myelitis, and more common syndromes such as those seen with shingles/herpes zoster, rib fractures, cholecystitis, kidney stones, pleuritic syndromes, and scapulothoracic bursal syndromes.

5: Spine

Physical Examination

The physical examination should evaluate for thoracic tenderness and pain with rotation. A detailed neurologic examination should assess the sensory dermatome level, long track signs, evidence of spasticity or hyperreflexia, gait disturbance, and sphincter tone. Clinical findings can present as radicular symptoms, incomplete cord syndrome, and/or more unilateral cord symptoms.

Imaging

MRI should follow the clinical history and the development of a differential diagnosis. Decisions regarding imaging require clinical validation because population-based control studies have demonstrated image findings consistent with thoracic disk herniation in 37% of asymptomatic individuals.[1,2] The differential diagnoses should include retroperitoneal neoplasm and other intra-abdominal and/or intrathoracic pathology. Syndromes that create intrinsic cord pathology, such as arteriovenous malformation, and demyelinating conditions such as amyotrophic lateral sclerosis, transverse myelitis, and cord tumors also should be considered. Concomitant CT is of value in assessing the calcific character of the disk and dural interface.

Natural History

The natural history of thoracic disk injury has been studied in small case series.[3,5-10] Most patients with intermittent mechanical and/or radicular pain have a period of inflammatory symptoms marked by back and/or chest wall pain that gradually subsides over 6 to 18 months. This condition is typically commensurate with a reduction in rotational activities that aggravate symptoms such as shoveling, golf, or hitting a slap shot in hockey. Imaging studies of patients with symptomatic thoracic disk herniations have revealed associated symptom reduction with a reduction in the extruded disk volume on follow-up MRI studies.

Nonsurgical treatments include analgesic support, core stabilization, and radicular anesthetic blocks. Immobilization with corsets and/or braces can be considered. There are few quality data to support these treatment methods.

Surgical intervention is stratified by neurologic status. In patients with myelopathy and/or progression of neurologic deficit, cord decompression affords the potential to stabilize or improve symptoms. For patients with radicular symptoms, persistent, unremitting pain, and disability that is refractory to pain management and therapeutic injections, surgical decompression may be of significant benefit. Patients who are not neurologically compromised and have pain that interferes substantially with their quality of life after an active period (longer than 6 months) of nonsurgical management may be considered to have a limited indication for surgery. The patient with axial pain syndromes must be well informed about the significant surgical and neurologic risks and the limited functional benefit described in several large clinical series.

MRI should be part of the preoperative evaluation and surgical planning, and can be supplemented with CT to assess calcification. The presence of calcification can predict the surgical finding of significant resorption and adherence of the dura to the disk and the potential need for dural reconstruction at the time of resection. Because disk herniations tend to be more chronic and more adherent to the dura, dural repair is commonly needed and should be planned for when calcification is present.

Surgical Approach

Thoracic disk herniations are more commonly located anteromedial rather than lateral to the dural contents. Traditional posterior laminectomy often requires medial retraction and manipulation of the cord, which can provoke neurologic defects. A spectrum of approaches and techniques, globally described as anterolateral or posterolateral techniques, have been used to effect decompression of the thoracic spinal cord (**Figure 1**). All approaches other than laminotomy destabilize the facet, costotransverse joint, and posterolateral disk complex. Several recent case series have highlighted and illustrated these techniques.[11,12]

Anterior or anterolateral techniques comprise transthoracic and/or a variance of transpleural and retropleural techniques that involve resection of the rib head and a lateral approach to the vertebral body and foramen. During these procedures, the posterior portion of the disk and/or body is excised to access the midline and ventral disk herniation. Fusion is commonly necessary to avoid iatrogenic instability, further disk collapse, further segmental instability symptoms, and progression of the local inflammatory cascade and/or neural compression. Video-assisted thoracic techniques in noncalcified and smaller-volume compressive lesions have equivalent outcomes to thoracotomy when performed by experienced surgeons.

Posterolateral procedures are variants of a costotransversectomy and transpedicular and oblique approaches to the anterolateral dura that limit cord retraction. These posterolateral techniques involve resection of the lateral lamina, facet, pedicle, and costovertebral joint to create an oblique window to access the anterolateral and lateral aspects of the spinal canal. These approaches have a more limited window, require significant bony resection, and are also associated with significant postlaminectomy and postfacetectomy instability unless they are combined with a posterolateral fusion.

Most authors vary their approach based on the disk level and characteristics. For calcified disks, large disks, and those with a more midline location, an anterolateral approach provides the greatest access for dural repair with the least amount of neural retraction. Compressive lesions located in upper thoracic levels may

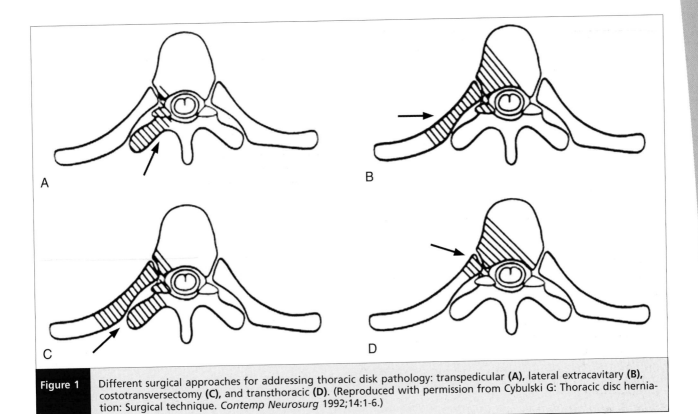

Figure 1 Different surgical approaches for addressing thoracic disk pathology: transpedicular **(A)**, lateral extracavitary **(B)**, costotransversectomy **(C)**, and transthoracic **(D)**. (Reproduced with permission from Cybulski G: Thoracic disc herniation: Surgical technique. *Contemp Neurosurg* 1992;14:1-6.)

require sternotomy and/or use of the venacaval window to access the levels. Most posterolateral disks and upper thoracic–level disks (T3 through T5) are readily accessed via posterolateral approaches. Midthoracic and posterolateral disks are accessible via either approach. Communication of the relative risks, approach-related complications, outcomes, and surgeon experience are part of the surgical choice of an informed patient.

One of the greatest risks in performing a thoracic disk herniation is wrong-level surgery. It is important to have a direct comparison of the axial imaging and the intraoperative radiographic technique by counting ribs. The ability to accurately identify a level for thoracic disk herniation also can be supplemented by placing a percutaneous fiducial into the pedicle or posterior elements and confirming this in the preoperative setting with CT and fluoroscopic imaging.[13]

Outcomes for procedures for thoracic disk herniations have been limited to several small series.[14-16] There is no evidence other than case series to guide therapy, and the limited volume of these cases precludes randomization. In larger series from referral centers, large disk size, midline location, and the presence of a calcific disk-dural interface were associated with more complications and worse functional outcomes.

Annotated References

1. Wood KB, Garvey TA, Gundry C, Heithoff KB: Magnetic resonance imaging of the thoracic spine: Evaluation of asymptomatic individuals. *J Bone Joint Surg Am* 1995;77(11):1631-1638.

2. Wood KB, Blair JM, Aepple DM, et al: The natural history of asymptomatic thoracic disc herniations. *Spine (Phila Pa 1976)* 1997;22(5):525-529, discussion 529-530.

3. Brown CW, Deffer PA Jr, Akmakjian J, Donaldson DH, Brugman JL: The natural history of thoracic disc herniation. *Spine (Phila Pa 1976)* 1992;17(6, suppl): S97-S102.

4. Regan JJ: Percutaneous endoscopic thoracic discectomy. *Neurosurg Clin N Am* 1996;7(1):87-98.

5. Hott JS, Feiz-Erfan I, Kenny K, Dickman CA: Surgical management of giant herniated thoracic discs: Analysis of 20 cases. *J Neurosurg Spine* 2005;3(3):191-197.

6. Bozzao A, Gallucci M, Masciocchi C, Aprile I, Barile A, Passariello R: Lumbar disk herniation: MR imaging assessment of natural history in patients treated without surgery. *Radiology* 1992;185(1):135-141.

7. Delauche-Cavallier MC, Budet C, Laredo JD, et al: Lumbar disc herniation: Computed tomography scan changes after conservative treatment of nerve root compression. *Spine (Phila Pa 1976)* 1992;17(8):927-933.

8. Ellenberg MR, Ross ML, Honet JC, Schwartz M, Chodoroff G, Enochs S: Prospective evaluation of the course of disc herniations in patients with proven radiculopathy. *Arch Phys Med Rehabil* 1993;74(1):3-8.

5: Spine

9. Maigne J-Y, Rime B, Deligne B: Computed tomographic follow-up study of forty-eight cases of nonoperatively treated lumbar intervertebral disc herniation. *Spine (Phila Pa 1976)* 1992;17(9):1071-1074.

10. Saal JA, Saal JS, Herzog RJ: The natural history of lumbar intervertebral disc extrusions treated nonoperatively. *Spine (Phila Pa 1976)* 1990;15(7):683-686.

11. Ayhan S, Nelson C, Gok B, et al: Transthoracic surgical treatment for centrally located thoracic disc herniations presenting with myelopathy: A 5-year institutional experience. *J Spinal Disord Tech* 2010;23(2):79-88.

    A well-illustrated, select case series is presented by a highly experienced, reputable, referral spine practice. Level of evidence: IV.

12. Bransford R: Early experience treating thoracic disc herniations using a modified transfacet pedicle-sparing decompression and fusion. *J Neurosurg Spine* 2010;12(2):221-231.

    A well-illustrated and described surgical technique in a small case series is presented by an experienced, self-critical, referral spine practice. Level of evidence: IV.

13. Hsu W, Sciubba DM, Sasson AD, et al: Intraoperative localization of thoracic spine level with preoperative percutaneous placement of intravertebral polymethylmethacrylate. *J Spinal Disord Tech* 2008;21(1):72-75.

    This article is an important technical reference to help with level localization and avoid wrong-level surgery. Level of evidence: IV.

14. Ohnishi K, Miyamoto K, Kanamori Y, Kodama H, Hosoe H, Shimizu K: Anterior decompression and fusion for multiple thoracic disc herniation. *J Bone Joint Surg Br* 2005;87(3):356-360.

15. Sheikh H, Samartzis D, Perez-Cruet MJ: Techniques for the operative management of thoracic disc herniation: Minimally invasive thoracic microdiscectomy. *Orthop Clin North Am* 2007;38(3):351-361, abstract vi.

    A technique paper with case illustration is presented. Level of evidence: IV.

16. Bartels RH, Peul WC: Mini-thoracotomy or thoracoscopic treatment for medially located thoracic herniated disc? *Spine (Phila Pa 1976)* 2007;32(20):E581-E584.

    A small case series with technical notes is presented. Level of evidence: IV.

Chapter 52

New Technologies in Spine Surgery

Lauren M. Burke, MD, MPH   Joseph R. O'Brien, MD, MPH   Michael T. Benke, MD
Warren D. Yu, MD

Introduction

New technologies in spine surgery are rapidly evolving, with the current focus on motion conservation and nonfusion options. Development of these technologies aims at reducing arthodesis-related morbidities, such as bone graft donor site pain, pseudarthrosis, approach-related morbidity, and adjacent-level degeneration. Cervical disk replacement shows promise with new data becoming available, yet the role for lumbar disk replacement is yet to be fully defined. Prospective controlled studies are currently under way for dynamic stabilization and facet replacement. Conclusions about efficacy and safety should be withheld until these data are available. Early results of interspinous spacers are promising as a minimally invasive alternative to decompression and fusion, and indications may continue to expand. More recently, novel tissue engineering strategies are being explored as potential treatment of degenerative disk disease.

Disk Arthroplasty

Cervical disk arthroplasty (CDA) has the potential to be superior to anterior diskectomy and fusion (ACDF). As the gold standard, ACDF has remarkable success, with

excellent long-term results reported above the 90th percentile. Fusion rates follow the same trend. The most compelling argument for a motion-preserving alternative to fusion is the incidence of symptomatic adjacent-level disease, believed to be approximately 3% annually. Approximately 25% of these patients may require reoperation for symptomatic adjacent-segment degeneration at 10 years. Some authors hypothesize that stiffening the spine through fusion accelerates degeneration at the adjacent segments. Disk arthroplasty aims to decrease adjacent-segment degeneration through motion preservation.

CDA is a motion-preserving procedure with limited indications, which currently include primarily radiculopathy caused by the compressive effect of a herniated cervical disk or osseous foraminal stenosis limited to one- and two-level disease (**Figure 1**). Treatment of myelopathy with CDA is still controversial, but is possible if the symptoms are mild and anterior compression is present. Although axial neck pain is currently not an indication for arthroplasty, it is being studied. Spondylolysis, deformity, instability, and subluxation are contraindications.[1] Other relative contraindications include osteopenia, osteoporosis, autoimmune disorders including rheumatoid arthritis, prior infection, and congenital stenosis.

One limitation of recent literature on CDA is the lack of long-term results. This is a fairly new procedure, still undergoing several Food and Drug Administration (FDA) Investigational Device Exemption (IDE) clinical trials; however, the early 2- and 3-year follow-up results are promising. The recent literature shows better clinical outcomes in the CDA groups compared to those receiving ACDF, although both treatment arms show statistically significant excellent outcomes when compared to preoperative scores. Some authors attribute patient enthusiasm for being selected for the disk replacement group as an etiology for improved outcomes in the CDA group as compared to the ACDF group.

A group of authors reported their experience with the Bryan CDA (Medtronic Sofamor Danek, Memphis, TN) at 2-year follow-up in 2003.[2] This study included 103 single-level patients and 44 bilevel patients followed for 1 to 2 years. Success rates for single-level CDA and bilevel CDA were 90% and 94%, respectively. Another study reported 93% success rates at 3-year follow-up in 2007.[1] Yet another study demonstrated success rates in

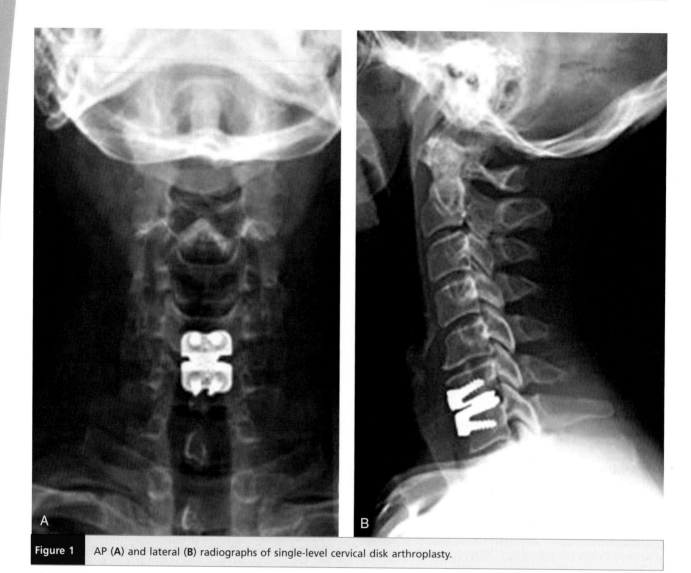

Figure 1 AP (**A**) and lateral (**B**) radiographs of single-level cervical disk arthroplasty.

single-level and bilevel CDA of 90% and 96%, respectively.[3] These success rates are comparable to those of ACDF. The literature also supports a complication rate equal to or less than that of ACDF.

Although CDA holds promise, few long-term data are available and the long-term durability of these implants remains to be seen. Wear debris may be an issue. Like all surgical procedures, patients must be carefully chosen for the appropriate procedure.

Comparison of CDA to lumbar replacement surgery is inevitable, but they are two highly different procedures. Lumbar disk arthroplasty has been used for the treatment of axial back pain; surgical treatment generally has lower clinical success rates. Axial back pain may be treated surgically if a 6- to 12-month course of nonsurgical treatment was unsuccessful. Preoperative disability should be significant and gauged with standardized outcome measures such as the Oswestry Disability Index (ODI). Most studies on surgery for axial back pain define success as improvement (but not elimination) of disability. Most patients will continue postoperative narcotic use, and only 10% on average return to work. Additionally, isolation of a pain-generating segment is a crucial part of the algorithm for back pain surgery. Some authors advocate diskography or MRI for this purpose, but others think that facet blocks and localizing injections can help determine the pain generator. However the pain generator is identified, it is important to note that outcomes decline for multilevel procedures. For axial back pain surgery, one-level surgical outcomes are the best.

Treatment of discogenic back pain may involve fusion or arthroplasty (**Figure 2**). Theoretically, lumbar arthroplasty should reduce or eliminate pain from a degenerated disk and restore or maintain normal motion at the index level, theoretically decreasing adjacent-segment disease. Indications for lumbar disk arthroplasty are similar to those of fusion. Patients should have intractable back pain due to discogenic disk disease. Accompanying radicular pain should be less prevalent than back pain. All patients should have at least 6 months of unsuccessful nonsurgical treatment. Contraindications include previous laminectomy, pars defect, facet disease, deformity, and instability.

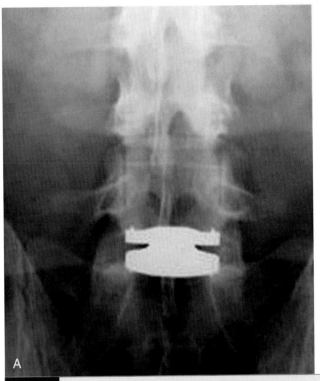
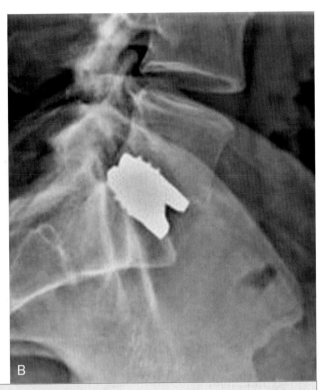

Figure 2   AP (**A**) and lateral (**B**) radiographs of single-level lumbar disk arthroplasty. (Courtesy of Khaled Kebaish, MD.)

Variable results have been reported in the literature. A 2007 study reported a mean 13.2-year follow-up on 106 patients treated with lumbar disk arthroplasty, with 82% good or excellent outcome at final follow-up. In addition, 7.5% of patients required additional surgery and posterior instrumentation for fusion and of those, 2.8% because of adjacent-level disease. Ninety percent of implants retained at least 4° of motion at 10 years.[4] More recent reported results are not as promising. A retrospective review compared one-level and two-level disk arthroplasty groups.[5] There was no statistical significance between the two groups and no control group in the study. Overall satisfaction was 70% at 2 years. An important issue addressed in a prospective study is the difference in results at particular levels.[6] Most arthroplasty procedures are performed at L4-5 or L5-S1 levels, or are bilevel procedures. The reported results showed a decline in overall outcomes when the lumbosacral junction is included, as well as increased complication rates.[6]

Lumbar disk arthroplasty is a relatively new procedure with variable evidence. Choosing the right patient for this surgery is most challenging, as the absence of improvement in back pain is common after surgery for discogenic disk disease. Revisions are exceedingly difficult, with injury to the great vessels sometimes an unforgiving complication. Future studies and long-term results are in progress.

Dynamic Stabilization

Several pedicle-based dynamic stabilization systems have been developed and are in various stages of biomechanical and clinical evaluation. These systems stabilize a spinal segment without rigid arthrodesis to theoretically decrease the incidence of adjacent-level degeneration. These implants are pedicle based and control motion at the index level. Variation occurs at the interpedicular spacer. Graf Artificial Ligament System (SEM Co, Montrouge, France) and Dynesys Dynamic Stabilization System (Zimmer Spine, Minneapolis, MN) (**Figure 3**) are two with the longest clinical experience.

Potential indications for dynamic stabilization are grade I spondylolisthesis, spinal stenosis with instability, recurring disk herniation, and degenerative disk disease with mechanical back pain. All patients undergoing dynamic stabilization should have had an unsuccessful course of nonsurgical treatment. Contraindications to this surgery are similar to those of other spine surgery with instrumentation, as these implants use pedicle screws. Poor bone stock, metabolic bone disease, and active infection, as well as scoliosis, severe spondylolisthesis, and postlaminectomy destabilization are all contraindications.

The limited data available for dynamic stabilization are contradictory and inconclusive. Some report positive clinical outcomes at 10-year follow-up in patients with degenerative spondylolisthesis and flexion insta-

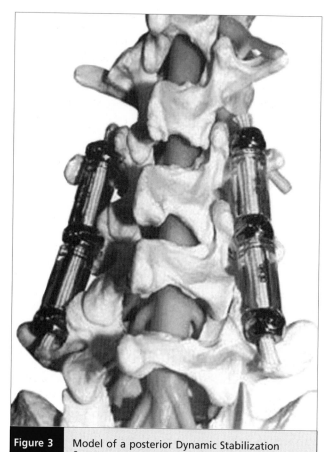

Figure 3 | Model of a posterior Dynamic Stabilization System.

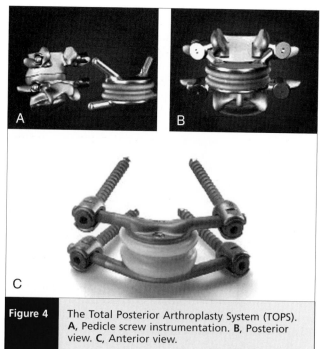

Figure 4 | The Total Posterior Arthroplasty System (TOPS). **A,** Pedicle screw instrumentation. **B,** Posterior view. **C,** Anterior view.

bility, but results are less favorable in this time period in patients with degenerative scoliosis.[7] Prospective data reports vary on clinical outcomes. Results on single-level dynamic stabilization for spondylolisthesis suggest that clinical outcomes are favorable and remain that way for a minimum 4-year follow-up.[8] According to one study, 21% of patients had evidence of screw loosening or breakage at 2-year follow-up; however, no reoperations occurred for this hardware failure.[8] A reported 47% of patients in this study showed adjacent-segment degeneration, which was statistically significant. Another prospective study of microdecompression and the Dynesys system reported only 50% favorable outcome, with 30% of patients reporting persistent lumbar pain at 12-month follow-up.[9] Reoperation rates reached 19% due to hardware complications.[9] Current data suggest dynamic stabilization may be an acceptable alternative to fusion in selected cases of one- and two-level degenerative lumbar pathologies.

The discussed implants are nonfusion devices. Other constructs are being developed that are hybrids, allowing fusion at one level and dynamic stabilization at the adjacent segment in hopes of slowing or preventing degeneration at levels adjacent to a fusion. Although some early clinical outcomes have been positive, published data remain limited. Further studies are imperative to establish efficacy and potential risks.

Facet Replacement

Facet arthroplasty is the newest form of posterior dynamic or nonfusion stabilization. The spinal unit is composed of the disk and two facet joints. Each of these three joints has the potential for degeneration and pain generation. Facet arthroplasty, following standard decompression of the neural elements, allows for the replacement of the diseased facets with preservation of motion as an alternative to traditional spinal fusion. Although several designs are in various stages of development, only two have published literature. The first is an anatomic reconstruction where each facet joint is replaced with unlinked articulating metal-on-metal components (Total Facet Arthroplasty System [TFAS], Archus Orthopedics, Redmond, WA). The second design is a nonanatomic reconstruction of the posterior articulating elements. Both facet joints are replaced with a single nonanatomic linked articulating core composed of polycarbonate urethane (Total Posterior Arthroplasty System [TOPS], Impliant, Ramat Poleg, Israel) (**Figure 4**).

Potential indications for facet arthroplasty have focused on spinal stenosis patients with or without grade I spondylolisthesis. Facet removal allows for wide decompression whereas facet arthroplasty confers stability with motion and precludes the need for fusion. IDE trials are currently under way for both the anatomic design (TFAS) and the nonanatomic design (TOPS). Each randomized, controlled, prospective IDE trial is comparing the facet replacement device with instrumented fusion. To date, there are no published data from these trials.

Recent biomechanical data are available for each of the facet arthroplasty designs. In a cadaver study, three-dimensional kinematics of TFAS-implanted spines were compared to those of intact spines and spines with posterior pedicle screw stabilization at the L4-5 level. Range of motion of the TFAS was 81% of the intact spine in flexion, 68% in extension, 88% in lateral bending, and 128% in axial rotation.[10] A similar cadaver study was done comparing multidirectional mobility of the TOPS implanted spine to the intact spine at the L4-5 level. Range of motion was almost ideally restored in lateral bending and axial rotation, and allowed 85% of the intact range of motion in flexion and extension.[11]

Authors of a 2007 study reported on 29 patients who underwent decompression and implantation of TOPS as part of a prospective, multicenter, pilot study performed outside the United States.[12] All patients had spinal stenosis and/or spondylolisthesis at L3-4 or L4-5 due to facet arthropathy. Visual analog score for leg pain improved from 88 to 12, ODI score dropped from 57% to 16%, and the Zurich Claudication Questionnaire score decreased from 57% to 26% at 1-year follow-up. No cases of slip progression and no signs of screw loosening were found.

Other potential indications for facet replacement may be for axial low back pain generated from facet arthropathy. This small subset of patients is difficult to define. Another possible indication for facet arthroplasty may be in conjunction with lumbar disk arthroplasty. In theory, this technology would replace all three degenerated joints of the functional spinal unit. Cost and implant failure may limit the combined use of these two technologies.

The goal of facet replacement is to attain posterior stabilization without fusion while allowing wide posterior decompression. As in total disk replacement, motion segment wear is inherent to arthroplasty systems in general and may be problematic in facet replacements. Like posterior dynamic stabilization systems, current facet arthroplasty systems are pedicle based and subject to hardware loosening and failure. Further research is required before the widespread use of facet arthroplasty can be advocated and before conclusions can be made on efficacy and safety.

Interspinous Spacer Technology

Neurogenic claudication is a common spinal pathology that historically was treated nonsurgically with activity modification, nonsteroidal anti-inflammatory medications, and epidural steroid injections. Open surgical decompression is indicated in recalcitrant cases. The common reports of neurogenic claudication are pain with ambulation that is exacerbated by standing upright and lumbar extension, but symptomatic relief with lumbar flexion. The shopping cart sign is commonly seen in stenotic patients with neurogenic claudication. These patients have improved walking endurance when leaning forward on a shopping cart, which provides relative flexion in the lumbar spine, opens the canal, and stretches the redundant ligamentum flavum that causes

neural compression. Nonsurgical treatment has limited effects, and symptoms may deteriorate over time.

Interspinous spacer technology has been developed for treatment of mild to moderate intermittent neurogenic claudication. Implants are placed between the spinous processes through a small posterior incision, as far anterior as allowed, sacrificing the interspinous ligaments. They produce relative kyphosis at the index level without disrupting overall sagittal balance. Biomechanical studies showed an increase in canal area by 18%, foraminal area by 25%, and foraminal width by 41% with the X-STOP device (Medtronic, Minneapolis, MN)[13] (**Figure 5**).

Since 2005, when the FDA approved the first and only implant (X-STOP) for neurogenic claudication, other devices have been developed, with clinical trials under way for many. Based on a multicenter, prospective, randomized IDE trial, early clinical data for the X-STOP demonstrate good to excellent results at 2 years compared to nonsurgical treatment. Outcomes were assessed using the Zurich Claudication Questionnaire, ODI and Medical Outcomes Study Short Form-36, and all demonstrated statistically significant improvement in the X-STOP group at all time points relative to the control group.[14] Patient satisfaction in the X-STOP group was 73% compared to 36% of control patients. In a smaller prospective study, 24 patients showed a 71% satisfaction rate at 1-year follow-up; however, 29% of this group required epidural steroid injections for recurrence of symptoms.[15] A subsequent study of intermediate follow-up (average, 4.2 years) found that outcomes of X-STOP surgery are stable over time as measured by ODI.[16]

Implantation of these devices is not without risk. Fracture of the spinous processes can occur intraoperatively or postoperatively. Depending on symptoms, fracture may necessitate surgical decompression and fusion. One case of bilateral posterior facet stress fractures after insertion of an interspinous implant has been reported in the literature.[17]

With many of these devices in clinical trials, more data will become available on their efficacy and safety. Currently long-term data are limited; however, interspinous devices are an attractive option for elderly or medically frail patients with neurogenic claudication who may not be able to tolerate a more extensive procedure.

Disk Regeneration

A separate, more novel approach to the treatment of degenerative disk disease is through the regeneration of intervertebral disk tissue via tissue engineering strategies. Degeneration is characterized by the loss of water content from the nucleus pulposus, the loss of macromolecules such as aggrecan, the loss of blood supply from the capillary beds, and increased enzymatic activity such as that from the matrix metalloproteinase (MMP) family. Through the modulation of intervertebral disk biology with the administration of cells or

5: Spine

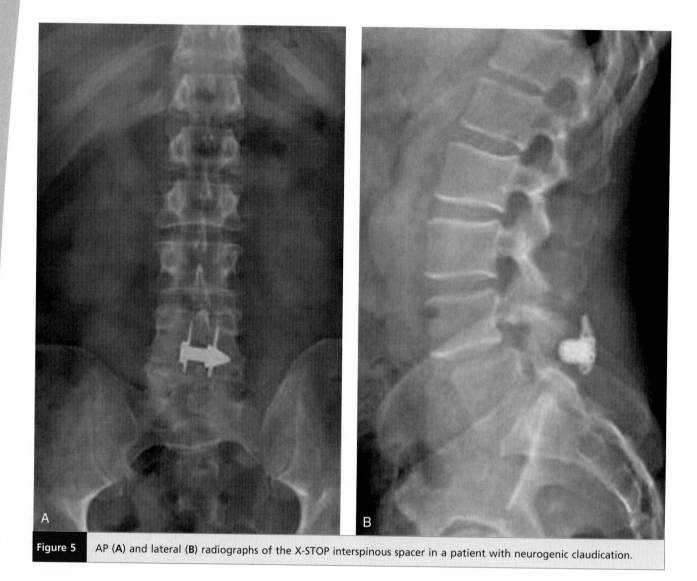

Figure 5 AP (**A**) and lateral (**B**) radiographs of the X-STOP interspinous spacer in a patient with neurogenic claudication.

growth factors, many researchers are investigating methods to alter the biologic imbalance of catabolism and anabolism that leads to loss of disk height, annular tears, and disk herniation.

Gene therapy represents one approach in this research arena. In recent studies, cells have been induced to produce factors such as transforming growth factor–β1; tissue inhibitors of metalloproteinases (TIMPs); and Lin-11, Isl-1, Mec-3) mineralization protein (LMP-1). Significant in vitro work has been done to modulate the expression of these factors to potentially reverse the molecular processes that occur during disk degeneration. Both viral and nonviral vectors have been studied in the delivery of the transgenes to cells. Although many vectors have exhibited high transfection rates with minimal immunogenicity such as adeno-associated virus, significant safety precautions remain in the translation of gene therapy to humans. Nonviral delivery methods such as DNA liposomes and plasmid DNA accompanied by an ultrasonography contrast agent ("microbubbles") have been studied in hopes of bypassing the safety issues with viral transduction.

Autologous cell–based therapy has shown promise because of its avoidance of viral vectors, multipotent differentiation, and proliferation potential. Exposing mesenchymal stem cells to various media conditions can initiate differentiation down different pathways, including that of the chondrogenic lineage, which shows similarities to that of intervertebral disk tissue. Researchers have demonstrated that rabbit mesenchymal stem cells transplanted into healthy rabbit disks can survive for up to 24 weeks,[18] suggesting that long-term survival is realistic. Studies characterizing the strategies of disk regeneration currently are still in the early stages as more data are required to progress to clinical trials.

Future Directions

Interest is growing in the development of minimally invasive surgery, motion-preserving surgical procedures, and regenerative technologies. Spine surgery is an evolving field with pronounced interest in preventing adjacent-segment degeneration and disease as well as avoiding revision surgeries. With many new technologies in clinical trials, future data regarding the safety and efficacy of these devices and techniques can be anticipated.

Annotated References

1. Pimenta L, McAfee PC, Cappuccino A, Cunningham BW, Diaz R, Coutinho E: Superiority of multilevel cervical arthroplasty outcomes versus single-level outcomes: 229 consecutive PCM prostheses. *Spine (Phila Pa 1976)* 2007;32(12):1337-1344.

   In a prospective series, multilevel cervical arthroplasty demonstrated significantly improved clinical outcomes in comparison with single-level outcomes, while reoperation rates leveled at 3-year follow-up. Level of evidence: II.

2. Goffin J, Van Calenbergh F, van Loon J, et al: Intermediate follow-up after treatment of degenerative disc disease with the Bryan Cervical Disc Prosthesis: Single-level and bi-level. *Spine (Phila Pa 1976)* 2003;28(24):2673-2678.

3. Sasso RC, Smucker JD, Hacker RJ, Heller JG: Artificial disc versus fusion: A prospective, randomized study with 2-year follow-up on 99 patients. *Spine (Phila Pa 1976)* 2007;32(26):2933-2940, discussion 2941-2942.

   In this prospective study, the authors demonstrated that single-level cervical arthroplasty was comparable to the "gold standard" ACDF in clinical outcomes and reoperation rates, while preserving motion at the index level.

4. David T: Long-term results of one-level lumbar arthroplasty: Minimum 10-year follow-up of the CHARITE artificial disc in 106 patients. *Spine (Phila Pa 1976)* 2007;32(6):661-666.

   A retrospective chart review of 106 patients who underwent one-level arthroplasty at either L4-5 or L5-S1 is presented. This study revealed durability at minimum 10-year follow-up and a low reoperation rate for adjacent-level disease.

5. Siepe CJ, Mayer HM, Heinz-Leisenheimer M, Korge A: Total lumbar disc replacement: Different results for different levels. *Spine (Phila Pa 1976)* 2007;32(7):782-790.

   This article presents midterm clinical results from a prospective study of lumbar total disk replacement at different segments (L4-5, L5-S1, and bilevel L4-5 and L5-S1). The results note significant differences between single-level and bilevel arthroplasty. Outcomes were reported to be significantly lower in bilevel total disk replacement with higher complication rates.

6. Hannibal M, Thomas DJ, Low J, Hsu KY, Zucherman J: ProDisc-L total disc replacement: A comparison of 1-level versus 2-level arthroplasty patients with a minimum 2-year follow-up. *Spine (Phila Pa 1976)* 2007;32(21):2322-2326.

   This article presents early results for patients enrolled in two concurrent FDA IDE lumbar arthroplasty clinical trials at a single institution. The authors found no statistical significance between the two groups at 2-year follow-up, although the two-level arthroplasty group scored marginally lower on evaluations.

7. Kanayama M, Hashimoto T, Shigenobu K, Togawa D, Oha F: A minimum 10-year follow-up of posterior dynamic stabilization using Graf artificial ligament. *Spine (Phila Pa 1976)* 2007;32(18):1992-1996, discussion 1997.

   The authors present a retrospective review of 56 patients showing improvement in outcomes for patients with degenerative spondylolisthesis and flexion instability. Results for those with laterolisthesis and degenerative scoliosis were poor.

8. Schaeren S, Broger I, Jeanneret B: Minimum four-year follow-up of spinal stenosis with degenerative spondylolisthesis treated with decompression and dynamic stabilization. *Spine (Phila Pa 1976)* 2008;33(18):E636-E642.

   This prospective study reported a minimum 4-year follow-up of single-level spondylolisthesis. Good clinical outcomes that hold up after 4 years were reported, but a 21% rate of screw loosening and breakage and a 47% rate of adjacent-level degeneration were seen.

9. Würgler-Hauri CC, Kalbarczyk A, Wiesli M, Landolt H, Fandino J: Dynamic neutralization of the lumbar spine after microsurgical decompression in acquired lumbar spinal stenosis and segmental instability. *Spine (Phila Pa 1976)* 2008;33(3):E66-E72.

   The authors report a high incidence of hardware failure and improved clinical outcomes mainly due to microscopic decompression in this prospective study. Thirty percent of patients had continued reports of lumbar pain at 1-year follow-up.

10. Zhu Q, Larson CR, Sjovold SG, et al: Biomechanical evaluation of the Total Facet Arthroplasty System: 3-dimensional kinematics. *Spine (Phila Pa 1976)* 2007;32(1):55-62.

    A biomechanical evaluation of the TFAS is presented. Range of motion was 81% of the intact spine in flexion, 68% in extension, 88% in lateral bending, and 128% in axial rotation.

11. Wilke HJ, Schmidt H, Werner K, Schmölz W, Drumm J: Biomechanical evaluation of a new total posterior-element replacement system. *Spine (Phila Pa 1976)* 2006;31(24):2790-2796, discussion 2797.

12. McAfee P, Khoo LT, Pimenta L, et al: Treatment of lumbar spinal stenosis with a total posterior arthroplasty prosthesis: Implant description, surgical technique, and a prospective report on 29 patients. *Neurosurg Focus* 2007;22(1):E13.

    A prospective, multicenter, pilot study performed outside the United States assessed 29 patients who underwent TOPS implantation. Visual analog scale for leg pain improved from 88 to 12 points, ODI dropped from

5: Spine

57% to 16%, and the Zurich Claudication Questionnaire dropped from 57% to 26% at 1-year follow-up. No cases of slip progression and no signs of screw loosening were found.

13. Richards JC, Majumdar S, Lindsey DP, Beaupré GS, Yerby SA: The treatment mechanism of an interspinous process implant for lumbar neurogenic intermittent claudication. *Spine (Phila Pa 1976)* 2005;30(7):744-749.

14. Zucherman JF, Hsu KY, Hartjen CA, et al: A multicenter, prospective, randomized trial evaluating the X STOP interspinous process decompression system for the treatment of neurogenic intermittent claudication: Two-year follow-up results. *Spine (Phila Pa 1976)* 2005; 30(12):1351-1358.

15. Siddiqui M, Smith FW, Wardlaw D: One-year results of X Stop interspinous implant for the treatment of lumbar spinal stenosis. *Spine (Phila Pa 1976)* 2007;32(12): 1345-1348.

This prospective study looks at a small group of patients with lumbar stenosis treated with the X-STOP device. Results are from 12-month follow-up. The data reported showed 71% clinical improvement, but 7 of 24 patients (29%) had recurrence of symptoms at 1 year.

16. Kondrashov DG, Hannibal M, Hsu KY, Zucherman JF: Interspinous process decompression with the X-STOP device for lumbar spinal stenosis: A 4-year follow-up study. *J Spinal Disord Tech* 2006;19(5):323-327.

17. Chung KJ, Hwang YS, Koh SH: Stress fracture of bilateral posterior facet after insertion of interspinous implant. *Spine (Phila Pa 1976)* 2009;34(10):E380-E383.

The authors present a case report of stress fractures of bilateral inferior articular processes of L4 6 years after insertion of an interspinous spacer at L4-5.

18. Sobajima S, Vadala G, Shimer A, Kim JS, Gilbertson LG, Kang JD: Feasibility of a stem cell therapy for intervertebral disc degeneration. *Spine J* 2008;8(6):888-896.

This two-part in vitro and in vivo study looked at the feasibility of stem cell therapy for disk disease. Results showed extracellular matrix production in vitro by human stem cells, and incorporation of transplanted stem cells in rabbit intervertebral disks at 24 weeks. It was concluded that stem cells may have multiple mechanisms to confer therapeutic effect in disc degeneration.

Section 6

Pediatrics

SECTION EDITOR:

KENNETH J. NOONAN, MD

Chapter 53

Shoulder, Upper Arm, and Elbow Trauma: Pediatrics

J. Michael Wattenbarger, MD   Steven L. Frick, MD

Injuries to the Sternoclavicular Joint and Clavicle

The sternoclavicular joint connects the upper extremity to the axial skeleton. This joint is susceptible to injury from a direct blow or other force applied laterally to the clavicle, acromion, or shoulder. The medial clavicle ossification center appears during the late teenage years, and the physis closes between age 20 and 25 years. As a result, sternoclavicular injuries in teenagers and young adults often are physeal injuries that mimic dislocations. A delay in diagnosis is common because physical examination and plain radiography can be unreliable for assessing displacement. For a patient with pain and swelling near the sternoclavicular joint, axial CT is recommended to assess for dislocation or physeal injury and to clarify the direction and magnitude of any displacement. An injury with anterior instability usually is treated nonsurgically. A posteriorly displaced fracture or dislocation can cause injury or compression to the great vessels, trachea, and esophagus, and usually it is treated with closed or open reduction to restore anatomic alignment (**Figure 1**). Although some authors believe that medial physeal injuries have remodeling potential and can be treated nonsurgically, others have noted a high frequency of persistent instability after reduction and recommend open reduction and stabilization with suture or wires.[1-3] Pin fixation in this region is not recommended because of the risk of pin migration and injury to nearby vital structures. It is recommended that a vascular or cardiothoracic surgeon be notified and available during the reduction because of the potential for catastrophic hemorrhage. Closed

reduction probably should not be attempted for a chronic injury (an injury of more than 2 weeks' duration) because the clavicle may be adhering to mediastinal vascular structures. Instead, open reduction should be performed with careful circumferential dissection around the medial clavicle.

Clavicle Fractures

Diaphyseal clavicle fractures occur in patients of any age, including newborn infants. Clavicle fracture in a newborn is treated with immobilization that can be as simple as pinning the sleeve covering the affected arm into the desired position. Brachial plexus injury may occur in conjunction with clavicle fracture in a newborn. A child with a clavicle fracture may have pseudoparalysis of the upper extremity from pain, however. If the clinician is unable to assess the neurovascular sta-

Dr. Wattenbarger or an immediate family member serves as a board member, owner, officer, or committee member of the Pediatric Orthopaedic Society of North America and has received research or institutional support from Biomet. Dr. Frick or an immediate family member serves as a board member, owner, officer, or committee member of the American Orthopaedic Association, the J. Robert Gladden Society, the Pediatric Orthopaedic Society of North America, and the American Academy of Orthopaedic Surgeons; and has received research or institutional support from Biomet.

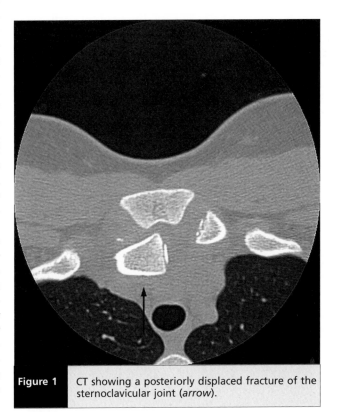

Figure 1   CT showing a posteriorly displaced fracture of the sternoclavicular joint (*arrow*).

6: Pediatrics

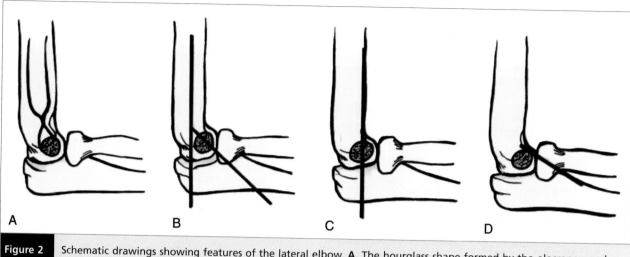

Figure 2	Schematic drawings showing features of the lateral elbow. **A,** The hourglass shape formed by the olecranon and coronoid fossa. **B,** The humeral-capitellar angle, which is 40° in children of all ages. **C,** The anterior humeral line, which in most children should bisect the capitellum; in young children, the anterior humeral line should intersect the anterior third of the capitellum. **D,** A smooth arc from the anterior humerus capitellum and coronoid process should be present. (Adapted from Herring JA, Tachdjian MO, eds: *Tachdjian's Pediatric Orthopedics,* ed 4. Philadelphia, PA, Saunders, 2008, p 2461.)

tus of the upper extremity at the time of injury, the child should be examined several weeks later to rule out a brachial plexus injury.

More than 80% of clavicle fractures in children are diaphyseal, and almost all of them will heal with non-surgical treatment. A review of pediatric clavicle fractures over a 20-year period in a busy trauma center found that only 15 children were surgically treated.[4] The indications for surgical treatment of a pediatric clavicle fracture included tenting of the skin, an open fracture, severe shortening of the shoulder girdle, and risk to the neurologic or vascular structures.

A distal clavicle fracture also can usually be treated nonsurgically in children. The strong periosteal sleeve typically is not displaced with the fracture. Therefore, a distal fracture often heals with what appears to be two clavicles in bayonet apposition, and this so-called double clavicle usually remodels.

Proximal Humerus Fractures

The growth potential of the proximal humeral physis (which contributes 80% of the humerus length) and the range of motion of the shoulder joint mean that most proximal humerus fractures in children and adolescents can be treated nonsurgically with excellent functional results. Most fractures of the proximal humerus are in the Salter-Harris type II pattern, with the distal shaft fragment displaced through the thinner anterior periosteal sleeve. In the Neer-Horowitz classification, which is most commonly used, type I is a minimally displaced fracture, type II is displaced less than one third of the width of the shaft, type III is displaced one third to two thirds of the width of the shaft, and type IV is displaced more than two thirds of the width of shaft.[5]

The treatment of proximal humerus fractures in children age 6 years or younger is not controversial. Even a type III or IV fracture can be treated nonsurgically with a good functional outcome. Concern about the lack of remodeling potential in adolescents has led some to recommend surgical treatment of these fractures. According to an early report, surgically treated patients had a higher rate of complications than patients treated with closed reduction.[6] However, a later study found that proximal humerus fractures in adolescents can be treated safely with open reduction and fixation with either pins or screws.[7] Because of complications related to wires, the use of retrograde flexible nails has been recommended for the surgical treatment of these fractures.[8] It should be noted that most studies have reported good functional results even after closed treatment of severely displaced and angulated proximal humerus fractures in adolescents.[9]

Nerve and vascular injuries are uncommon in association with proximal humerus fractures. One study found associated nerve injuries in only 4 of 578 patients with proximal humerus fracture (0.7%), all of them with valgus displacement (shaft is displaced medially).[10] These nerve deficits resolved within 9 months without treatment.

Elbow Injuries

Elbow injuries are common in children. The radiographic evaluation should include AP and lateral radiographs. An internal oblique radiograph is helpful for evaluating a minimally displaced lateral condyle fracture.[11] An understanding of the normal radiographic appearance of a child's elbow anatomy is necessary for the initial evaluation and may help in determining the treatment. A true lateral radiograph should show the hourglass appearance of the olecranon fossa and supracondylar area (**Figure 2**), but the medial epicondyle should not be seen, and there should be no widening of the metaphyseal area. The humeral condylar angle, formed by a line along the shaft of the humerus and a line perpendicular to the capitellar physis, is 40° in children of all ages.[12] The anterior humeral line is drawn down the anterior shaft of the humerus and should bisect the capitellum; however, in children younger than 4 years it should intersect the anterior third of the capitellum.[12] In all radiographic views, the radius should be aligned with the capitellum, as shown by the radiocapitellar line (a line drawn down the radial shaft should intersect the capitellum). On an AP radiograph, the Baumann angle is formed by a line drawn through the long axis of the humerus and a line drawn along the flat metaphyseal region adjacent to the capitellar physis. The Baumann angle averages 72° in children, but it can range from 64° to 81°[13] (**Figure 3**). This angle can be useful in assessing the coronal alignment of the elbow after reduction of a supracondylar humerus fracture.[14]

The presence of the posterior fat pad sign was associated with an occult fracture in 76% of children whose radiographs were otherwise negative.[15] Thus, most children with a posterior fat pad sign are assumed to have a nondisplaced elbow fracture. Typically these children receive cast treatment for 3 weeks.

Supracondylar fracture accounts for as many as 60% of elbow fractures in children; it is the most common type of elbow fracture in children. The lateral condyle fracture represents approximately half of the remaining 40% of elbow fractures in children. Medial epicondyle, medial condyle, olecranon, and transphyseal fractures occur much less frequently.

Supracondylar Humerus Fractures

A supracondylar humerus fracture can occur in extension or flexion. An extension injury to the humerus represents 97% of supracondylar humerus fractures. The Gartland classification of extension-type fractures has been modified to include flexion-type fractures.[16] A Gartland type I fracture is minimally displaced. A type II fracture is incomplete; one cortex is intact, there is either posterior (extension) or anterior (flexion) angulation, and fracture displacement is more than 3 mm. A type III fracture is completely displaced. A recently proposed type IV fracture has multidirectional instability, often diagnosed when the flexion reduction maneuver for an extension-type fracture causes the distal fragment to move anterior to the proximal fragment.[17]

There is little disagreement on the treatment of a type I fracture, which is with casting, usually for 3 weeks. The initial evaluation of these fractures should include a careful evaluation of the medial distal humerus, with consideration of the need for contralateral comparison radiographs. Subtle comminution of the medial distal humerus in an otherwise minimally displaced fracture can lead to cubitus varus. Fractures with medial comminution and varus malalignment should be treated surgically[18] (**Figure 4**). Physical examination and radiographs of the contralateral elbow can help determine whether a minimally displaced supracondylar fracture is in varus.

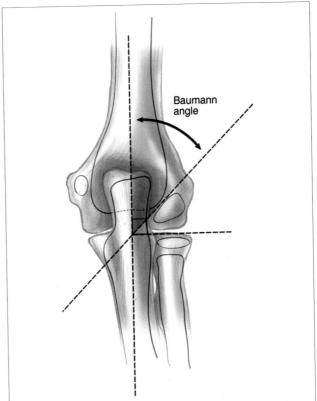

| Figure 3 | Schematic drawing showing the Baumann angle, which is formed by a line parallel to the humeral shaft and a line parallel to the lateral condyle physis. (Reproduced with permission from Yen YM, Kocher MS: Lateral entry compared with medial and lateral entry pin fixation for completely displaced supracondylar humeral fractures in children: Surgical technique. *J Bone Joint Surg Am* 2008;90[suppl 2, pt 1]:20-30.) |

The techniques for the treatment of displaced supracondylar humerus fracture include skeletal traction, closed reduction, and casting. With the advent of intraoperative fluoroscopy, closed reduction and pinning have become the treatment of choice for a type II or III supracondylar humerus fracture.[16,19,20] In the past, type II fractures were often treated with closed reduction and casting, but concern about loss of reduction and malunion have led to recommendations for surgical treatment of these fractures. A study of displaced type II fractures after closed reduction found that a third of the fractures lost position and 17% ultimately needed secondary reduction and pinning.[21] There also are concerns that deformities in the sagittal plane of a child's elbow will not remodel well. A study of the long-term effects of elbow malreduction found that 50% had radiographic abnormalities and 50% had limited elbow motion.[22] The practice of flexing the elbow to 120° during treatment to avoid loss of reduction has been questioned by recent studies; these studies found an increase in forearm compartment pressure and a loss of the radial pulse when the elbow was flexed past 90°.[23,24]

6: Pediatrics

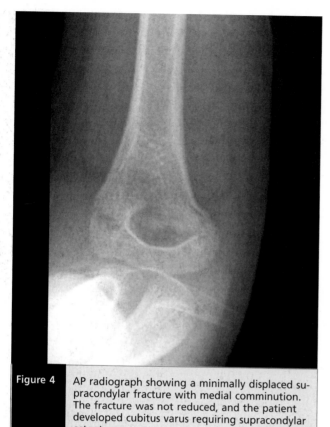

Figure 4 AP radiograph showing a minimally displaced supracondylar fracture with medial comminution. The fracture was not reduced, and the patient developed cubitus varus requiring supracondylar osteotomy.

Closed reduction and percutaneous pinning of type II fractures had a low complication rate in 189 patients treated at one institution.[19] There were no malunions, no surgical complications, and no anesthesia complications. Four patients (2.1%) had an infection; three of the infections were superficial and were treated with oral antibiotics. The patient with a deep infection was the only one requiring reoperation. The authors concluded that surgical treatment of type II supracondylar fractures is safe. Other authors also stressed the low complication rate associated with closed reduction and pinning, and they recommend this treatment of angulated type II fractures.[16,20]

Type III fractures are treated surgically with closed reduction under fluoroscopic guidance and pin fixation. Modern pinning techniques have been well studied and found to have low complication rates.[19,20,25-27] Volkmann ischemia is rarely seen with fracture pinning and postoperative elbow immobilization at less than 90° of flexion. Malunion also rarely occurs. Only 1 malunion was reported in a study of 622 surgically treated supracondylar fractures.[20] No malunions occurred in 189 surgically treated type II fractures,[19] and only 1 malunion occurred in 203 surgically treated fractures.[28] In a good-quality reduction, the anterior humeral line should bisect the capitellum, and the humerocondylar and Baumann angles should be close to normal. Mild rotational malalignment is well tolerated because of shoulder motion, and translational deformi-

ties have good remodeling potential. Intraoperative internal and external oblique radiographs are helpful for judging the reduction.

The most common complications in most large studies are pin migration (approximately 2% of patients) and infection (1% to 2.4%).[19,20,27] The infections associated with closed reduction and pinning usually are superficial and can be treated with oral antibiotics. Rarely, the infection is deep and requires surgical débridement. A comparison of semisterile technique and full surgical preparation found no difference in infection rates; the infection rate remained low even if preoperative antibiotics were not used.[20,27] Three weeks of pin fixation is sufficient for almost all supracondylar humerus fractures in children. A longer period of pin fixation provides bacteria and foreign material with an entry portal for a longer period of time and thereby fosters infection. In an adolescent with supracondylar humerus fracture, the duration of pin fixation is 4 to 6 weeks, and the rate of deep infection is correspondingly higher. In these patients, burying the pins beneath the skin may decrease the infection risk.

Studies of the pin configuration for supracondylar fractures have compared the use of medial- and lateral-entry crossed pins with the use of lateral-entry pins alone. Biomechanical studies found that crossed pins are stronger in torsion than a lateral-entry construct. Proponents of lateral-only pins cite a lower incidence of iatrogenic nerve injury with these pins. A systematic review of 35 studies that included 2,054 children found that an iatrogenic nerve injury was 1.84 times more likely when medial- and lateral-entry pins were used, compared with lateral-entry pins alone.[29] The probability of loss of reduction was 0.58 times lower when medial- and lateral- entry crossed pins were used than with lateral-entry-only pins. Recent prospective studies found no difference in loss of reduction or iatrogenic nerve injury based on pin configuration.[30,31]

The incidence of iatrogenic ulnar nerve injury may be lower in more recent studies because of a better understanding of its cause and the use of safer techniques for medial pinning. For instance, it is known that the ulnar nerve will subluxate anteriorly when the elbow is hyperflexed in some children.[32,33] Therefore, most surgeons who use medial- and lateral-entry pins reduce an extension-type fracture in flexion before placing one or two lateral pins, and they extend the elbow before placing the medial pin[30,31,34,35] (**Figure 5**). If palpating the cubital tunnel is difficult because of swelling, a small medial incision is recommended to make sure the ulnar nerve is out of the way before the medial pin is placed.[20] The medial pin should be removed if the patient's hand moves as it is being placed.

More recent studies have described the technique of using lateral entry pins to decrease the risk of loss of reduction. Loss of reduction in 9 of 322 fractures (2.9%) was caused by failure to engage both fragments with two or more pins, failure to achieve bicortical fixation with two or more pins, or failure to achieve adequate pin separation (more than 2 mm) at the fracture site.[36] The researchers now use three lateral pins for a type III

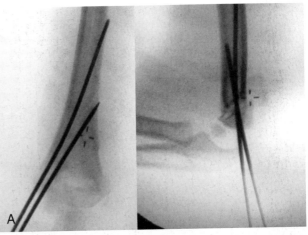

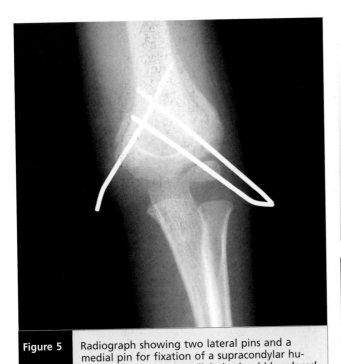

Figure 5 Radiograph showing two lateral pins and a medial pin for fixation of a supracondylar humerus fracture. The medial pin should be placed with the elbow extended to avoid entrapment of the ulnar nerve.

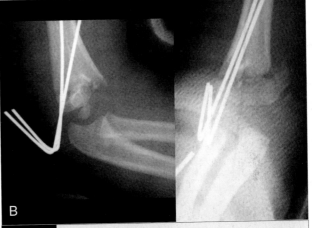

Figure 6 A, Fluoroscopic images showing improper placement of lateral entry pins for fixation of a supracondylar fracture. There is very little spread between the pins. B, Radiographs showing loss of reduction 2 weeks after pinning.

fracture (**Figures 6** and **7**). Other researchers state that one lateral pin must engage the lateral column and the other pin must engage the central column.[34] A prospective study of intraoperative internal and external oblique fluoroscopy used to assess rotational stability after pinning found that only 26% of type III fractures were stable after two lateral-only pins were used.[37] A third pin was added to the unstable fractures, with resulting stability in an additional 50%. In the fractures that remained unstable, a medial pin was added.

Flexion-type fractures are rare and are more difficult to treat than extension-type fractures. Open reduction is more often required, and preoperative ulnar nerve symptoms are more common.[38,39] A type IV fracture has multidirectional instability, with no intact periosteum to help with the reduction. These fractures can often be treated closed by using pins as a joystick in the distal fragment and by rotating the C-arm rather than the patient's arm to obtain orthogonal views during pinning.[17,19]

It has been established that closed supracondylar humerus fractures without vascular injury or severe soft-tissue swelling can be managed as surgical "urgencies," requiring prompt but not immediate treatment.[40-43] According to many protocols, the fracture should be splinted in 30° to 40° of elbow flexion; the patient should be admitted for observation, with closed reduction and pinning as soon as the patient's stomach is empty and an expert surgical team is available. There is concern that swelling may lead to vascular compromise or a compartment syndrome if treatment is delayed, or that an acceptable closed reduction may become more

difficult to achieve. The argument that a delay in treatment can lead to a need for open reduction is difficult to assess because the indications for open reduction have not been defined. Although nonemergent treatment is often implemented, one study found that compartment syndrome developed in 11 patients with a low-energy fracture although they had no initial sign of vascular compromise; there was an average delay to surgery of 22 hours.[44] The authors recommended early surgical treatment of patients with a red-flag warning sign such as severe elbow swelling, ecchymosis, neurologic deficit, or diminished or absent radial pulse. Patients with an ipsilateral forearm or wrist fracture also are at increased risk for developing a compartment syndrome and should be carefully monitored.[45]

In a patient with a supracondylar fracture and absent radial and ulnar pulses, distal perfusion is determined to be adequate (a pink hand) or inadequate (a white hand). A patient with a white hand often has a ruptured or entrapped brachial artery with inadequate collateral circulation, and the surgical team should be

6: Pediatrics

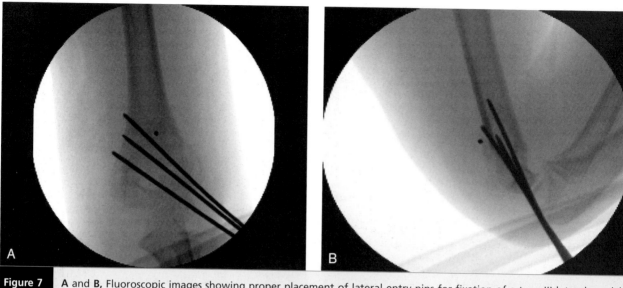

Figure 7 **A** and **B,** Fluoroscopic images showing proper placement of lateral entry pins for fixation of a type III lateral condyle fracture. The spread between the pins at the fracture site is adequate, and the pins engage both cortices.

prepared to explore and repair or reconstruct the brachial artery after reducing and pinning the fracture. Arteriography is not indicated for an isolated injury. A patient with a pink hand should undergo closed reduction and pinning. A near-anatomic reduction with no gapping should be obtained to avoid artery entrapment or tethering by soft tissues pulled into the fracture. If an acceptable closed reduction cannot be obtained, an anterior approach should be used for open reduction to allow visualization of the artery. If the pulse returns after closed reduction, the patient is admitted for observation. If the pulse does not return but there is a Doppler signal at the wrist and the hand remains well perfused, the recommendation is to admit the patient and carefully monitor perfusion and active finger motion over the next 48 hours. Some authors recommend a more aggressive approach, with earlier exploration of the brachial artery if the pulse does not return after reduction. If the pulse is lost after closed reduction and pinning in a patient with an intact preoperative pulse, open reduction usually is indicated to assess the artery. The elbow should not be flexed more than 90° for postoperative cast immobilization.

Lateral Condyle Fractures

Treatment of a lateral condyle fracture is based on the amount of displacement seen on radiographs and whether there is an intact articular cartilage hinge. Internal oblique radiographs are useful in assessing the amount of displacement in a lateral condyle fracture[11] (**Figure 8**). An intact articular surface can be expected if there is less than 2 mm of displacement in any radiographic view. An incomplete fracture should have an intact articular cartilage surface, which suggests a relatively stable fracture.

Lateral condyle fractures traditionally are classified using the Milch system; however, it is not useful for guiding modern treatments. A new classification system

for lateral condyle fractures has been proposed based on the amount of displacement of the fracture and whether the articular cartilage is intact on arthrogram.[46] A type I fracture has less than 2 mm of displacement, a type II fracture has more than 2 mm of displacement and intact articular cartilage, and a type III fracture has more than 2 mm of displacement and incongruent articular cartilage. Intraoperative arthrography is recommended for fractures with more than 2 mm of displacement if it is unclear whether the articular surface is intact. With an intact articular surface, closed reduction and pinning are recommended. An open reduction and pinning are performed if the articular surface is not intact.[46] There were three times as many complications among type III fractures as among type II fractures; all type III fractures had displacement of at least 4 mm.

In a study of treatment for lateral condyle fractures, closed reduction was attempted for all fractures. If the fracture could be reduced to less than 2 mm of displacement, closed pinning was performed. Fractures that could not be reduced to less then 2 mm of displacement were treated with open reduction and internal fixation. Although severely displaced fractures were most likely to require open reduction and internal fixation, many of these fractures could be treated closed. There was no osteonecrosis, nonunion, or physeal arrest.[47]

Lateral overgrowth or a lateral bump sometimes appears, regardless of whether a lateral condyle fracture was treated surgically or with casting alone. A 10% incidence of lateral overgrowth was reported in surgically treated lateral condyle fractures. The possibility of lateral overgrowth should be discussed with the family before surgery.

Fractures that are minimally displaced (less than 2 mm) can be treated with a cast and close follow-up. Only a small percentage of minimally displaced frac-

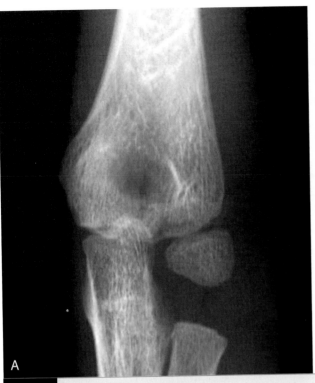
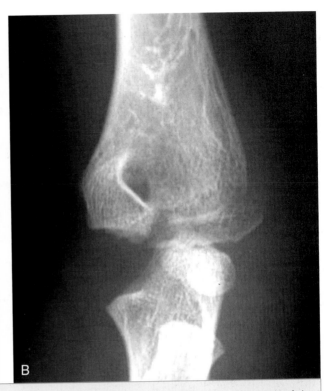

Figure 8 **A,** AP radiograph of a lateral condyle fracture showing minimal displacement. **B,** Internal oblique radiograph of the same elbow, clearly showing a displaced lateral condyle fracture. (Reproduced with permission from Song KS, Kang CH, Min BW, Bae KC, Cho CH: Internal oblique radiographs for diagnosis of nondisplaced or minimally displaced lateral condylar fractures of the humerus in children. *J Bone Joint Surg Am* 2007;89[1]:58-63.)

tures go on to nonunion. If a minimally displaced fracture does not heal, pinning is recommended.

Nonunion of lateral condyle fractures can lead to cubitus valgus and tardy ulnar nerve palsy. There have been historically high rates of osteonecrosis in fractures treated with late open reduction and internal fixation (more than 3 weeks after initial injury). Open reduction and internal fixation has been recommended for late-identified fractures, with a goal of union of the fragment rather than anatomic reduction.[48] Such a fracture should be fixed in the position that provides the best range of motion and carrying angle. Soft-tissue stripping should be avoided.

Transphyseal Fractures

Transphyseal fractures are relatively uncommon, usually occurring in children younger than 2 years. Half of these fractures are associated with child abuse. The differential diagnosis includes lateral condyle fracture and elbow dislocation. In a transphyseal fracture, the relationship of the radial head and capitellum is intact. The fracture usually is treated with closed reduction and pinning. Casting alone has a higher rate of cubitus varus.

Medial Epicondyle Fractures

Fifty percent of medial epicondyle fractures are associated with a dislocated elbow. Postreduction radiographs of an elbow dislocation always should be eval-

uated for the presence of an entrapped medial epicondyle. There is agreement that fractures with less than 5 mm of displacement can be treated with 1 to 2 weeks of immobilization, followed by resumption of activities. The treatment of fractures with more than 5 mm of displacement is more controversial. For a high-demand athlete, surgical treatment may be recommended to avoid the possibility of instability. A study with long-term follow-up of medial epicondyle fractures displaced 5 to 15 mm found that patients had similar results regardless of whether they were treated with casting or with open reduction and internal fixation.[49]

Monteggia Fracture-Dislocations

Late recognition of Monteggia fracture-dislocations still occurs and necessitates difficult reconstructive procedures. Closed treatment after early recognition usually is successful and typically leads to healing in an anatomic position, with good function. To prevent missing the diagnosis, the radiocapitellar line should be assessed on every lateral radiograph of the elbow; a line down the radial shaft should pass through the center of the capitellar ossification center (**Figure 9**). Closed reduction of the ulnar shaft deformity usually results in reduction of the dislocated radial head. If closed reduction is not possible, open reduction through a lateral approach is indicated, with preservation or repair of the annular ligament. In patients age 8 years and older

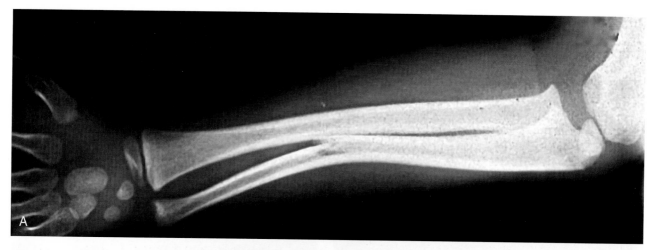

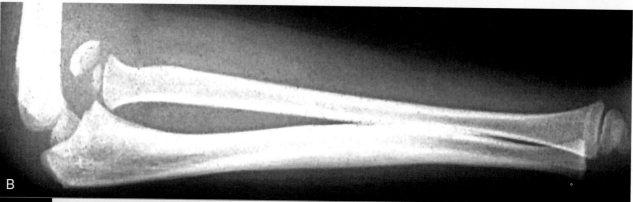

Figure 9   **A,** Radiograph showing a greenstick ulna fracture. The radial head is dislocated (a line drawn through the proximal radius does not line up with the capitellum). This Monteggia fracture was initially missed. **B,** Lateral radiograph of the same fracture 3 months later, clearly showing the dislocated radial head. The ulna is not straight; this characteristic suggests the possibility of a dislocated radial head.

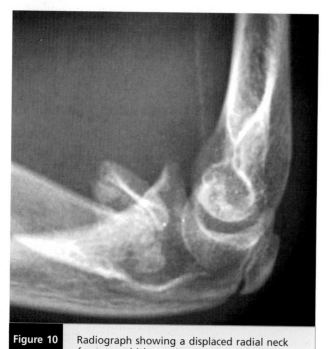

Figure 10   Radiograph showing a displaced radial neck fracture, which requires surgical treatment. The fracture has almost 90° of angulation.

with a length-unstable ulna fracture, plate fixation may be indicated to maintain the length and reduction of the radiocapitellar joint. Late reconstruction of a missed Monteggia injury is considered if the radial head retains its concave structure; typically it involves osteotomy of the ulna to correct the angular and length deformity, with or without annular ligament reconstruction.

Completely Displaced Radial Neck Fractures

A radial neck fracture with less than 30° of angulation and less than 3 to 5 mm of translation is managed with 2 to 3 weeks of immobilization followed by a gradual return to function (**Figure 10**). Healing with greater angulation or translation can result in a cam effect that disrupts the rotational arc of the radius around the ulna, limiting forearm supination and pronation. Open reduction of a displaced radial neck fracture is associated with several complications, including stiffness and osteonecrosis. Because of these risks, there should be an attempt at closed reduction with percutaneous pin reduction, intramedullary pin reduction, or manipulation of the radial neck with a curved elevator, while avoiding opening the fracture or radiocapitellar joint. Multiple methods of closed manipulation can be attempted before a more invasive method is used. A stout pin placed distal and posterior to the fracture can be used to lever the radial head back onto the neck, or the pin can be used to directly push on the radial head. If such a reduction method is successful, stability is tested with supination and pronation under fluoroscopy. If necessary, the fracture is stabilized with obliquely directed wires. Excellent success and functional results have been reported with the use of a retrograde intramedullary rod, which is driven up to the fracture, rotated, and driven into the radial neck-head fragment.[50] Rotation of the rod reduces the fracture and provides internal fixation.

If these techniques are not successful, a formal open reduction is done with a lateral approach to the radiocapitellar joint. Usually the radial head fragment is displaced laterally and distally, and care is taken during exposure to preserve any intact soft-tissue attachments, which may provide vascularity to the fragment. The annular ligament should be evaluated; it may need to be divided and repaired later to reposition the radial head in anatomic position in the joint. Fixation is done using obliquely placed wires, small screws, or an intramedullary rod.

Annotated References

1. Wirth MA, Rockwood CA Jr: Acute and chronic traumatic injuries of the sternoclavicular joint. *J Am Acad Orthop Surg* 1996;4(5):268-278.

2. Lewonowski K, Bassett GS: Complete posterior sternoclavicular epiphyseal separation: A case report and review of the literature. *Clin Orthop Relat Res* 1992;281:84-88.

3. Waters PM, Bae DS, Kadiyala RK: Short-term outcomes after surgical treatment of traumatic posterior sternoclavicular fracture-dislocations in children and adolescents. *J Pediatr Orthop* 2003;23(4):464-469.

4. Kubiak R, Slongo T: Operative treatment of clavicle fractures in children: A review of 21 years. *J Pediatr Orthop* 2002;22(6):736-739.

5. Neer CS II, Horwitz BS: Fractures of the proximal humeral epiphysial plate. *Clin Orthop Relat Res* 1965;41:24-31.

6. Beringer DC, Weiner DS, Noble JS, Bell RH: Severely displaced proximal humeral epiphyseal fractures: A follow-up study. *J Pediatr Orthop* 1998;18(1):31-37.

7. Dobbs MB, Luhmann SL, Gordon JE, Strecker WB, Schoenecker PL: Severely displaced proximal humeral epiphyseal fractures. *J Pediatr Orthop* 2003;23(2):208-215.

8. Rajan RA, Hawkins KJ, Metcalfe J, Konstantoulakis C, Jones S, Fernandes J: Elastic stable intramedullary nailing for displaced proximal humeral fractures in older children. *J Child Orthop* 2008;2(1):15-19.

Fourteen older patients with displaced proximal humerus fractures were treated with open or closed reduction and stabilization with elastic nails. The procedure was safe and resulted in good outcomes as measured by outcomes scores and patient satisfaction.

9. Bahrs C, Zipplies S, Ochs BG, et al: Proximal humeral fractures in children and adolescents. *J Pediatr Orthop* 2009;29(3):238-242.

Of 43 proximal humerus fractures in patients age 6 to 16 years, 33 were treated surgically. An anatomic closed reduction was obtained in 16 of the 33 patients after reduction under general anesthesia. Open reduction was then performed in 17 patients. Soft tissue including periosteum (two patients) and biceps tendon with periosteum (seven patients) was found in the fracture site. All patients had an excellent result. Level of evidence: IV.

10. Hwang RW, Bae DS, Waters PM: Brachial plexus palsy following proximal humerus fracture in patients who are skeletally immature. *J Orthop Trauma* 2008;22(4):286-290.

Neurologic injury is extremely uncommon in patients with proximal humerus fractures. In this series, 0.4% of patients had a neurologic deficit, and all resolved with observation. Level of evidence: IV.

11. Song KS, Kang CH, Min BW, Bae KC, Cho CH: Internal oblique radiographs for diagnosis of nondisplaced or minimally displaced lateral condylar fractures of the humerus in children. *J Bone Joint Surg Am* 2007;89(1):58-63.

In a prospective study of 54 minimally displaced lateral condyle fractures, the efficacy of internal oblique views for determining the amount of displacement and, therefore, instability in lateral condyle fractures was assessed. Different displacement was seen on the AP and internal oblique radiographs in 70% of the fractures. Level of evidence: I.

12. Simanovsky N, Lamdan R, Hiller N, Simanovsky N: The measurements and standardization of humerocondylar angle in children. *J Pediatr Orthop* 2008;28(4):463-465.

A study of humerocondylar angle in normal children divided the children by age group as younger than 5 years, 5 to 10 years, and 10 to 15 years. In all age groups the humerocondylar angle was found to be 40°.

13. Herman MJ, Boardman MJ, Hoover JR, Chafetz RS: Relationship of the anterior humeral line to the capitellar ossific nucleus: Variability with age. *J Bone Joint Surg Am* 2009;91(9):2188-2193.

The anterior humeral line passes through the middle third of the capitellum in most children. However, the location of this line is more variable in children who are younger than 4 years, passing almost equally through either the middle third or the anterior third of the capitellum.

6: Pediatrics

14. Williamson DM, Coates CJ, Miller RK, Cole WG: Normal characteristics of the Baumann (humerocapitellar) angle: An aid in assessment of supracondylar fractures. *J Pediatr Orthop* 1992;12(5):636-639.

15. Skaggs DL, Mirzayan R: The posterior fat pad sign in association with occult fracture of the elbow in children. *J Bone Joint Surg Am* 1999;81(10):1429-1433.

16. Omid R, Choi PD, Skaggs DL: Supracondylar humeral fractures in children. *J Bone Joint Surg Am* 2008;90(5): 1121-1132.

    This is an excellent review of the literature on the evaluation, treatment, and complications of supracondylar humerus fractures.

17. Leitch KK, Kay RM, Femino JD, Tolo VT, Storer SK, Skaggs DL: Treatment of multidirectionally unstable supracondylar humeral fractures in children: A modified Gartland type-IV fracture. *J Bone Joint Surg Am* 2006; 88(5):980-985.

18. De Boeck H, De Smet P, Penders W, De Rydt D: Supracondylar elbow fractures with impaction of the medial condyle in children. *J Pediatr Orthop* 1995;15(4):444-448.

19. Skaggs DL, Sankar WN, Albrektson J, Vaishnav S, Choi PD, Kay RM: How safe is the operative treatment of Gartland type 2 supracondylar humerus fractures in children? *J Pediatr Orthop* 2008;28(2):139-141.

    This is a retrospective review of 189 type II supracondylar fractures treated at one institution with closed reduction and pinning. Three superficial infections were treated with oral antibiotics. One patient had a deep infection. The authors recommend surgical treatment of type II fractures based on the complication rate in other studies of similar fractures.

20. Bashyal RK, Chu JY, Schoenecker PL, Dobbs MB, Luhmann SJ, Gordon JE: Complications after pinning of supracondylar distal humerus fractures. *J Pediatr Orthop* 2009;29(7):704-708.

    This review of complications associated with pinning of 622 supracondylar humerus fractures at one institution specifically compared the infection rate with various types of preparations. A minimal preparation without preoperative antibiotics did not lead to a higher infection rate. The authors describe a technique for placing a medial pin, if needed. Only one iatrogenic ulnar nerve injury was found in 311 patients treated with a medial pin (0.3%). Preoperative nerve deficit was most common in flexion and type III fractures. Level of evidence: III.

21. Parikh SN, Wall EJ, Foad S, Wiersema B, Nolte B: Displaced type II extension supracondylar humerus fractures: Do they all need pinning? *J Pediatr Orthop* 2004; 24(4):380-384.

    A study of 24 type II fractures treated with closed reduction and casting found that 7 fractures lost position, and 4 of the 7 required secondary reduction and pinning. Two fractures had an unsatisfactory outcome.

22. Simanovsky N, Lamdan R, Mosheiff R, Simanovsky N: Underreduced supracondylar fracture of the humerus in children: Clinical significance at skeletal maturity. *J Pediatr Orthop* 2007;27(7):733-738.

    At final follow-up, 50% of 22 patients with a supracondylar humerus fracture that was initially underreduced in the sagittal plane had radiographic abnormality of the humerocondylar angle, 50% had limited elbow flexion, and 31% were aware of their limited elbow flexion at skeletal maturity. Only three patients felt minor functional disability. Ten patients had an unsatisfactory result. The authors recommend surgical treatment with pinning for a moderately displaced fracture to avoid late deformity and loss of motion.

23. Battaglia TC, Armstrong DG, Schwend RM: Factors affecting forearm compartment pressures in children with supracondylar fractures of the humerus. *J Pediatr Orthop* 2002;22(4):431-439.

24. Mapes RC, Hennrikus WL: The effect of elbow position on the radial pulse measured by Doppler ultrasonography after surgical treatment of supracondylar elbow fractures in children. *J Pediatr Orthop* 1998;18(4):441-444.

25. Skaggs DL, Cluck MW, Mostofi A, Flynn JM, Kay RM: Lateral-entry pin fixation in the management of supracondylar fractures in children. *J Bone Joint Surg Am* 2004;86(4):702-707.

26. Skaggs DL, Hale JM, Bassett J, Kaminsky C, Kay RM, Tolo VT: Operative treatment of supracondylar fractures of the humerus in children: The consequences of pin placement. *J Bone Joint Surg Am* 2001;83(5):735-740.

27. Iobst CA, Spurdle C, King WF, Lopez M: Percutaneous pinning of pediatric supracondylar humerus fractures with the semisterile technique: The Miami experience. *J Pediatr Orthop* 2007;27(1):17-22.

    A review of 304 supracondylar humerus fractures treated with a semisterile technique found an overall infection rate of 2.34%, with a deep infection rate of 0.47%. Perioperative antibiotics were not used in 68% of the patients. Level of evidence: IV.

28. Bahk MS, Srikumaran U, Ain MC, et al: Patterns of pediatric supracondylar humerus fractures. *J Pediatr Orthop* 2008;28(5):493-499.

    The coronal and sagittal angle of supracondylar humerus fractures was studied in 203 fractures. Fractures with a coronal obliquity of more than 10° had greater comminution and rotational malunion. Similarly, fractures with a sagittal obliquity of more than 20° were associated with a higher incidence of additional injuries and malunion in extension than fractures with less than 20° of sagittal obliquity.

29. Brauer CA, Lee BM, Bae DS, Waters PM, Kocher MS: A systematic review of medial and lateral entry pinning versus lateral entry pinning for supracondylar fractures of the humerus. *J Pediatr Orthop* 2007;27(2):181-186.

Medial-lateral pin configuration and lateral pin configuration were systematically reviewed using data from 35 studies including 2,054 children. Iatrogenic nerve injury was 1.84 times more common with medial- and lateral-entry pins than with lateral-entry pins alone. The probability of loss of reduction was 0.58 times lower with medial- and lateral-entry pinning. In recent prospective studies there was no difference in loss of reduction and iatrogenic nerve injury between medial- and lateral-entry pins and lateral-entry pins alone. Medial- and lateral-entry pinning was found to be more stable.

30. Kocher MS, Kasser JR, Waters PM, et al: Lateral entry compared with medial and lateral entry pin fixation for completely displaced supracondylar humeral fractures in children: A randomized clinical trial. *J Bone Joint Surg Am* 2007;89(4):706-712.

    A prospective study compared the use of crossed pins (*n* = 24) and lateral-entry pins (*n* = 28) in type III extension-type supracondylar fractures. There was no significant difference in mild loss of reduction (one in the crossed-pins patient group and six in the lateral pin patient group) or radiographic parameters. There were no iatrogenic ulnar nerve injuries in either group. Both lateral-entry and crossed-pin fixation are effective in the treatment of type III supracondylar humerus fractures. Level of evidence: I.

31. Tripuraneni KR, Bosch PP, Schwend RM, Yaste JJ: Prospective, surgeon-randomized evaluation of crossed pins versus lateral pins for unstable supracondylar humerus fractures in children. *J Pediatr Orthop B* 2009;18(2):93-98.

    In a prospective review of supracondylar fractures treated with crossed pins (*n* = 20) and those treated with lateral pins only (*n* = 20), patients were randomized based on surgeon preference. There was no between-group difference in outcome with regard to final range of motion or radiographic parameters. One patient in each group had a change in treatment plan: in the lateral pin only group, the surgeon chose to use a medial pin because of medial comminution, and in the crossed-pin group the surgeon used only lateral pins because of a subluxating ulnar nerve.

32. Zaltz I, Waters PM, Kasser JR: Ulnar nerve instability in children. *J Pediatr Orthop* 1996;16(5):567-569.

33. Belhan O, Karakurt L, Ozdemir H, et al: Dynamics of the ulnar nerve after percutaneous pinning of supracondylar humeral fractures in children. *J Pediatr Orthop B* 2009;18(1):29-33.

    The authors prospectively studied ulnar nerve morphology and dynamics using ultrasound in patients treated with either cross-pinning or lateral-entry-only pinning. They recommend lateral-entry pinning as the safer procedure.

34. Yen YM, Kocher MS: Lateral entry compared with medial and lateral entry pin fixation for completely displaced supracondylar humeral fractures in children: Surgical technique. *J Bone Joint Surg Am* 2008;90(suppl 2, pt 1):20-30.

    The technique for pinning supracondylar humerus fractures is reviewed.

35. Eidelman M, Hos N, Katzman A, Bialik V: Prevention of ulnar nerve injury during fixation of supracondylar fractures in children by 'flexion-extension cross-pinning' technique. *J Pediatr Orthop B* 2007;16(3):221-224.

    Sixty-seven supracondylar fractures were treated with two lateral pins and one medial pin. The lateral pins were placed with the patient's arm flexed, and the medial pin was placed with the arm extended. There were no iatrogenic ulnar nerve injuries.

36. Sankar WN, Hebela NM, Skaggs DL, Flynn JM: Loss of pin fixation in displaced supracondylar humeral fractures in children: Causes and prevention. *J Bone Joint Surg Am* 2007;89(4):713-717.

    A study of 322 supracondylar humerus fractures examined the incidence and causes of postoperative displacement. All of the eight fractures that lost reduction (2.9%) were Gartland type III; seven were treated with two lateral pins, and one was treated with crossed pins. Loss of reduction was more often avoided when three lateral pins were used. Three types of pin fixation errors were identified.

37. Zenios M, Ramachandran M, Milne B, Little D, Smith N: Intraoperative stability testing of lateral-entry pin fixation of pediatric supracondylar humeral fractures. *J Pediatr Orthop* 2007;27(6):695-702.

    A prospective study of 21 patients with a type III supracondylar humerus fracture found that only 26% of the fractures were stable after two lateral pins were used, based on a comparison of lateral intraoperative fluoroscopic views in internal and external rotation. Stability was achieved with a third lateral pin in 48% of patients. An additional medial pin and medial-entry wire were placed and if the fracture was not stable after three lateral wires were used. Twenty-four percent of the fractures needed a medial pin to achieve stability. After the stability testing protocol was instituted, no patient had a return to the operating room for loss of reduction.

38. Mahan ST, May CD, Kocher MS: Operative management of displaced flexion supracondylar humerus fractures in children. *J Pediatr Orthop* 2007;27(5):551-556.

    A retrospective review found that type III flexion-type supracondylar humerus fractures were more likely to require open reduction (31%) than type III extension-type fractures (10%). Patients with a flexion-type fracture had more preoperative ulnar nerve symptoms (19%) than those with an extension-type fracture (3%). Flexion-type fractures are more difficult to treat than extension-type fractures and should be recognized preoperatively.

39. Steinman S, Bastrom TP, Newton PO, Mubarak SJ: Beware of ulnar nerve entrapment in flexion-type supracondylar humerus fractures. *J Child Orthop* 2007;1(3):177-180.

    A retrospective study of supracondylar fractures requiring open reduction found that, although flexion-type fractures accounted for only 2% to 3% of the supracondylar fractures, 20% of the fractures requiring open reduction were of the flexion type; in half of those, the ulnar nerve was entrapped in the fracture.

40. Iyengar SR, Hoffinger SA, Townsend DR: Early versus delayed reduction and pinning of type III displaced supracondylar fractures of the humerus in children: A comparative study. *J Orthop Trauma* 1999;13(1):51-55.

41. Mehlman CT, Strub WM, Roy DR, Wall EJ, Crawford AH: The effect of surgical timing on the perioperative complications of treatment of supracondylar humeral fractures in children. *J Bone Joint Surg Am* 2001;83(3): 323-327.

42. Gupta N, Kay RM, Leitch K, Femino JD, Tolo VT, Skaggs DL: Effect of surgical delay on perioperative complications and need for open reduction in supracondylar humerus fractures in children. *J Pediatr Orthop* 2004; 24(3):245-248.

43. Leet AI, Frisancho J, Ebramzadeh E: Delayed treatment of type 3 supracondylar humerus fractures in children. *J Pediatr Orthop* 2002;22(2):203-207.

44. Ramachandran M, Skaggs DL, Crawford HA, et al: Delaying treatment of supracondylar fractures in children: Has the pendulum swung too far? *J Bone Joint Surg Br* 2008;90(9):1228-1233.

    In a multicenter retrospective study, 11 pediatric patients with an isolated supracondylar humerus fracture and no vascular initial compromise later developed a compartment syndrome. Significant swelling at presentation and delay in fracture reduction may be important warning signs for the development of a compartment syndrome in children with a supracondylar humerus fracture.

45. Blakemore LC, Cooperman DR, Thompson GH, Wathey C, Ballock RT: Compartment syndrome in ipsilateral humerus and forearm fractures in children. *Clin Orthop Relat Res* 2000;376:32-38.

46. Weiss JM, Graves S, Yang S, Mendelsohn E, Kay RM, Skaggs DL: A new classification system predictive of complications in surgically treated pediatric humeral lateral condyle fractures. *J Pediatr Orthop* 2009;29(6): 602-605.

    A proposed classification of lateral condyle fractures was based on a retrospective review of children treated at one institution over a 7-year period. The overall complication rate was 25%.

47. Song KS, Kang CH, Min BW, Bae KC, Cho CH, Lee JH: Closed reduction and internal fixation of displaced unstable lateral condylar fractures of the humerus in children. *J Bone Joint Surg Am* 2008;90(12):2673-2681.

    A prospective study reviewed the results of closed reduction with percutaneous Kirschner wire fixation in unstable fractures of the lateral condyle. Fractures were classified into five types based on AP and internal oblique radiographs. Fractures were pinned closed if the fracture gap after reduction was less than 2 mm. There were no major complications after 63 fractures. Level of evidence: IV.

48. Wattenbarger JM, Gerardi J, Johnston CE: Late open reduction internal fixation of lateral condyle fractures. *J Pediatr Orthop* 2002;22(3):394-398.

49. Farsetti P, Potenza V, Caterini R, Ippolito E: Long-term results of treatment of fractures of the medial humeral epicondyle in children. *J Bone Joint Surg Am* 2001; 83-A:1299-1305.

50. Schmittenbecher PP, Haevernick B, Herold A, Knorr P, Schmid E: Treatment decision, method of osteosynthesis, and outcome in radial neck fractures in children: A multicenter study. *J Pediatr Orthop* 2005;25(1):45-50.

Forearm, Wrist, and Hand Trauma: Pediatrics

Howard R. Epps, MD   Michelle S. Caird, MD

Introduction

Trauma of the forearm and hand are among the most common injuries sustained in children, representing over 40% of all fractures. Injuries are slightly more common in boys and usually result from falls, sports participation, or the use of playground equipment.[1] Most injuries occur in isolation. In the multitrauma setting, management becomes prioritized by the primary and secondary survey.

Management of fractures depends on the fracture pattern (torus, greenstick, complete, or plastic deformation), the fracture location, and the age of the patient. Historically, it was widely believed that practically all forearm and hand fractures could be managed primarily with closed techniques. It is currently recognized that certain fractures are best managed with surgical intervention, yet the bulk of these fractures are managed closed.

The age of the patient and the amount of displacement still guide the treatment plan, but other factors also play a prominent role. The surgeon must consider the remodeling potential of the fracture,[2,3] the cost to the family of surgical care, patient and family expectations, and the family's personal beliefs. Guidelines for acceptable alignment provide some direction but are not evidence based. These other factors must be considered during shared decision making for each patient. Counseling from the outset and careful monitoring of unstable fractures should lead to a final result that meets the expectations of all parties.

When fractures require reduction, multiple options exist for anesthesia in the emergency department. Options include conscious sedation with nitrous oxide, ketamine, or short-acting benzodiazepines with possi-

ble hematoma block supplementation.[4,5] Intravenous regional anesthesia has the advantage of avoiding the systemic effects of conscious sedation.[6]

Forearm Diaphyseal Fractures

Forearm fractures are very common in children. These injuries can be plastic deformation of the forearm, greenstick fractures, or complete fractures of both bones. As with other pediatric fractures, treatment depends on fracture type and location, adequacy of reduction, associated soft-tissue injuries, and the age of the patient.[7] A thorough evaluation includes assessment for associated injuries, especially to the wrist or elbow.

Most fractures in the diaphysis of the forearm in children can be treated with closed reduction and immobilization in a cast.[8,9] Plastic deformation is a deforming injury to the bone without frank fracture and results in painful, visibly bent bones. If reduction is required (greater than 20° of angulation), steady three-point bend pressure sustained over minutes may be needed. Cast immobilization provides protection and pain reduction. Greenstick fractures are well treated with closed reduction and well-molded casting (**Figure 1**).

Patient age and fracture location help define acceptable alignment with more remodeling potential in younger children and in those with more distal fractures. Ten degrees of angulation, bayonet apposition, and 30° of malrotation are well tolerated in complete diaphyseal fractures in children age 10 years or younger.[10] Children younger than 8 years can tolerate up to 20° of angulation, full translation, and up to 45° of malrotation.[11] Except for obvious malrotation, the assessment of rotation is challenging and may be detected on forearm radiographs as a mismatch of cortical thickness at the fracture site or in the relationship between the bicipital tuberosity and the radial styloid on an AP radiograph, which should be 180° from each other. Close monitoring in the cast with weekly radiographs for the first 3 to 4 weeks following reduction allows identification and treatment of unstable fractures. A full treatment course is often 6 to 12 weeks of immobilization. Complications can occur with these injuries. Malunion may decrease forearm rotation and, if insuf-

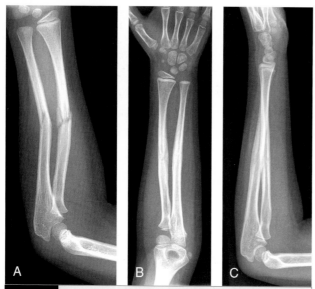

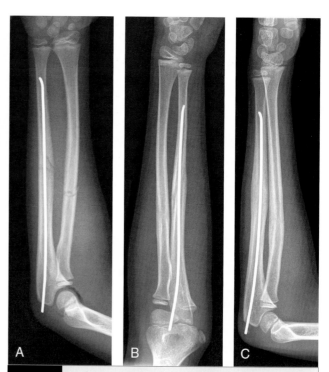

Figure 1 Radiographic studies of a 6-year-old girl with a greenstick fracture of the diaphysis of the radius and ulna with approximately 15° of angulation. **A,** The fracture was treated with closed reduction and casting. This resulted in return of full forearm motion and good alignment on AP **(B)** and lateral **(C)** radiographs.

Figure 2 Radiographic studies of an 8-year-old boy with a midshaft forearm fracture of the radius and ulna. The ulna fracture, which was open, was treated with irrigation and débridement and intramedullary nailing of the ulna combined with cast immobilization. **A,** Radiograph at operation. AP **(B)** and lateral **(C)** radiographs after healing.

ficient growth and remodeling potential remains, corrective osteotomies may be required.[12] Refractures occur in 8% of children and often require open reduction with internal fixation.

Indications for surgical intervention include open fractures, fractures with significant soft-tissue injury or swelling, unstable fractures, and fractures with unacceptable alignment after reduction attempts. Surgical techniques include reduction with intramedullary stabilization of both bones, fixation with plating of both bones, a hybrid construct with plating of one bone and intramedullary fixation of the other, or single-bone fixation combined with long arm casting until union is achieved[13,14] (**Figure 2**). When properly executed each method provides similar results.

Compartment syndrome can occur in association with forearm fractures treated operatively[15] and nonsurgically. Multiple passes with flexible intramedullary nails in attempted reduction increases the risk for compartment syndrome.[15] A high index of suspicion in high-energy injury patterns and early recognition of signs including increasing requirement for pain medication can lead to prompt treatment with forearm fasciotomies.[16] All open forearm fractures require thorough irrigation and débridement at the time of injury and may be stabilized safely at the same time if deemed necessary.[17] Healing time may be delayed in 4% to 5% of open fractures, but nonunion is rare.

Galeazzi fractures are fractures of the distal third of the radial diaphysis with dislocation at the distal radioulnar joint (DRUJ). The injury occurs infrequently in the pediatric population and is most often seen in adolescents. Many of these injuries go unrecognized. Good results are achieved with anatomic reduction of the radius fracture (either closed or with open reduction and internal fixation) and immobilization of the DRUJ in a reduced position. This often requires supination of the forearm, or in very rare instances, pinning of the DRUJ in a reduced position.[18]

Distal Radius and Ulna Metaphyseal Fractures

Fractures of the distal radius metaphysis occur in all age groups, but the peak incidence occurs during the adolescent growth spurt.[1,19] High-resolution peripheral quantitative CT has shown transient changes in the bone architecture during the latter half of puberty. The proportion of load borne by cortical bone decreases and the porosity of the cortex increases, which may explain this phenomenon.[20]

Torus fractures of the metaphysis are inherently stable. They heal uneventfully in 3 weeks with treatment in a below-elbow cast or a removable splint. Previous studies reported comparable outcomes but superior patient and parent satisfaction when patients were treated with a removable device that could be discontinued at home.[21-23] More recent work, however, showed that patients treated with a removable splint experienced pain for a longer period of time and required more time to

Table 1

Acceptable Angulation for Distal Radius Fractures in Degrees

Age (Years)	Sagittal Plane, Boys	Sagittal Plane, Girls	Frontal Plane
4-9	20	15	15
9-11	15	10	5
11-13	10	10	0
>13	5	0	0

(Data from Waters PM, Mih AD: Fractures of the distal radius and ulna, in Beaty JH, Kasser JR, eds: *Rockwood and Wilkins' Fractures in Children*, ed 6. Philadephia, PA, Lippincott Williams & Wilkins, 2006, p 370.)

resume their normal activity level.[24] Parents can thus choose between the convenience of a removable splint with the possibility of some increased discomfort early in the healing process, or better control of pain but potentially more difficulties related to a cast. Careful interpretation of radiographs is mandatory to differentiate between a true torus fracture that is amenable to this treatment protocol and a subtle nondisplaced greenstick fracture that has a higher risk of displacement.

Greenstick fractures and complete fractures of the metaphyseal region may be unstable and require close monitoring. Acceptable alignment for metaphyseal fractures with displacement depends on age (**Table 1**). Greenstick fractures of the metaphysis are potentially unstable and should be monitored closely. The proximity to the physis gives the surgeon some leeway in the amount of acceptable displacement. Recent work suggests that fractures with minimal displacement (15° or less of angulation on the sagittal view and 0.5 cm of displacement) have low risk of displacement when monitored closely and managed in an appropriately molded cast.[3] With this protocol more than 85% of patients' fractures healed with less than 20° of angulation, and all patients had normal function at 6 weeks. The potential for displacement, however, is well established. Close observation with weekly radiographs can help prevent the unpleasant surprise of a deformed arm when the cast is removed after several weeks (**Figure 3**).

Complete metaphyseal fractures requiring reduction have a high risk of redisplacement, particularly in children older than 10 years. Loss of reduction remains problematic and exceeds 30% in some series. Short arm casts and long arm casts are equally effective provided they are appropriately applied with careful molding.[9,25] A prospective study of 75 distal radial fractures requiring reduction showed that initial complete displacement, the degree of obliquity of the fracture line, and the quality of casting technique are correlated with loss of reduction.[26] Defined as the ratio of the width of the cast in the sagittal view to the width of the cast in the coronal view at the fracture, a cast index of less than 0.7 was associated with a low rate of remanipulation.[27]

Closed reduction with percutaneous fixation has been shown to reduce the rate of redisplacement of fractures requiring reduction.[28] This approach has been recommended for older children because their risk of redisplacement is higher and the potential for remodeling is lower. Percutaneous fixation also provides stability when excessive swelling, soft-tissue concerns, or neurologic symptoms preclude immobilization with a snug cast.[7] Pin configurations include metaphyseal pins, smooth transphyseal pins, and transradioulnar pin fixation.[29,30] Rare considerations with these methods include early physeal arrest with transphyseal pinning[31] and formation of a radioulnar synostosis with transradioulnar pin fixation.

Distal Radius and Ulna Physeal Fractures

Physeal fractures of the distal radius and ulna are 20% of the physeal fractures sustained by children.[7] This area has the largest remodeling potential of all forearm fractures, but growth disturbance remains a concern. The fractures occur most commonly in adolescents, so the proximity to skeletal maturity becomes an important factor in guidelines for acceptable alignment.

Fractures requiring reduction should be reduced as gently as possible with adequate sedation and muscle relaxation to minimize injury to the physis. Fractures present longer than 1 week should not be reduced because of the risk of iatrogenic injury to the physis.[32] In children with significant growth remaining at the time of injury, fractures can be followed after healing to detect growth arrest, which occurs in approximately 1% to 7% of these injuries. If growth potential is preserved, the patient can still benefit from fracture remodeling, and a corrective osteotomy can be performed at skeletal maturity if the deformity remains excessive. Fractures determined to be markedly unstable at reduction can be supplemented with smooth wire fixation to enhance stability. Though rare, displaced intra-articular fractures of the distal radial epiphysis require anatomic reduction and stabilization.

Ulnar styloid fractures have a low rate of union. A review of 46 ulnar styloid fractures associated with distal radius fractures revealed a nonunion rate of 80% (**Figure 3**). Seven patients developed symptomatic nonunions, and all were found to have pathology involving the triangular fibrocartilage complex (TFCC).[33] Persistent symptoms on the ulnar side of the wrist warrant investigation of the integrity of the TFCC. Physeal frac-

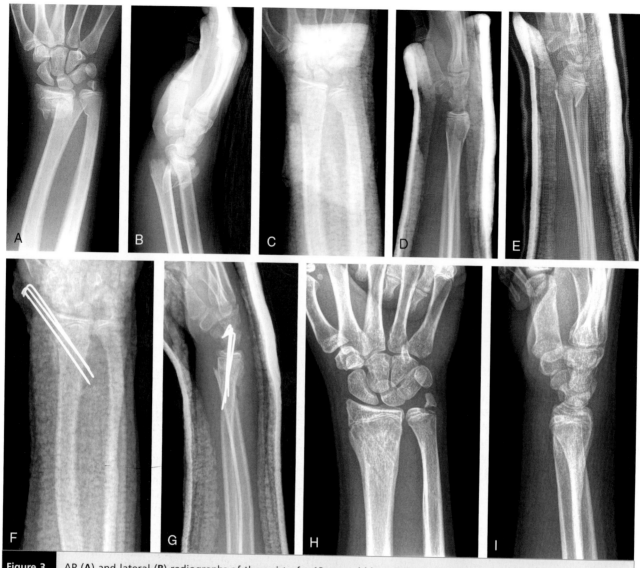

Figure 3 AP (**A**) and lateral (**B**) radiographs of the wrist of a 13-year-old boy with distal metaphyseal fractures of the radius and ulna with an associated ulnar styloid fracture. Good reduction was achieved on AP (**C**) and lateral (**D**) radiographs, but reduction was lost over the first 2 weeks of sugar tong splint treatment as shown on the lateral radiograph (**E**). The patient underwent closed reduction and percutaneous pin fixation as seen on AP (**F**) and lateral (**G**) radiographs. he fracture healed and the patient returned to full activities without pain despite ulnar styloid nonunion (**H** and **I**).

tures of the distal ulna have a significantly higher risk of growth arrest (50%) than fractures of the distal radius.[34] This fact should be conveyed to families of children with this injury, and the patients should be followed after healing to detect growth disturbance.

Carpal Injuries

Scaphoid Fractures

Injuries to the carpal bones are rare in children. Most carpal injuries in children are scaphoid fractures and occur after age 11 years. Wrist and snuffbox tenderness are suggestive of fracture. Early plain radiographs may not reveal the fracture, and inadequate treatment can

lead to nonunion. Therefore, children with suspected injury should be immobilized in a thumb spica cast with repeat radiographs at 10 to 14 days after injury, and cast wear should be continued if there is evidence of fracture. Authors of a 2009 study found that 30% of pediatric patients with suspected injury treated in this manner went on to have radiographic evidence of scaphoid fracture at follow-up.[35] According to results from a 2007 study, 94% of pediatric patients with scaphoid fractures had good or excellent results by objective and self-assessment scores.[36] Treatment of documented fractures follows the general recommendations of immobilization for nondisplaced fractures, closed or open reduction with compression screw fixation for displaced fractures, and surgical treatment of nonunions.[37]

Table 2

Hand Fractures Requiring Surgical Treatment in Children

Fracture	Treatment	Potential Complications of Missed Injury
Phalangeal neck fracture	Reduction of the extension at the fracture and pin fixation	Loss of flexion
Phalangeal condyle fracture	Reduction of intra-articular fracture with pin fixation	Malunion and loss of motion
Seymour fracture (open Salter-Harris type I or II fracture of distal phalanx with interposition of germinal matrix into physis)	Nail plate removal, irrigation and débridement, reduction of open fracture, nail bed repair	Osteomyelitis and nail abnormalities
Metacarpal and phalangeal shaft fractures	Reduction of malrotation and pin fixation	Malrotation
Bennett fracture (intra-articular fracture of the thumb metacarpal base)	Reduction of the shortening, angulation, and malrotation at the fracture and pin fixation	Malunion and arthritis
Gamekeeper's fracture (Salter-Harris type III intra-articular fracture at thumb proximal phalanx)	Open reduction of intra-articular fracture with pin fixation	Nonunion and instability

Fractures of Other Carpal Bones

Fractures and injuries to other carpal bones are rare, and mainly case reports exist. These include transscaphoid perilunate dislocations, pisiform fracture-dislocations associated with distal radius fractures,[38] and trapezial fractures associated with first carpal metacarpal dislocations.[39] Many of these fractures are associated with other wrist injuries, and treatment is individualized.

Hand Injuries

The hand is the most frequently injured part of the body in children. The patterns and mechanisms of injury differ between age groups, with more soft-tissue crush injuries in toddlers and primarily bony sports injuries in older children.[40] The small finger and its metacarpal are most commonly fractured followed by the thumb. Phalangeal fractures are slightly more common than metacarpal fractures. Most of these injuries are best treated nonsurgically.[41]

Hand Fractures and Dislocations

Most phalangeal fractures occur at the base or the proximal metaphysis, are minimally displaced, and require nonsurgical treatment with buddy taping or splinting. Metacarpal fractures most commonly are diaphyseal and should be scrutinized for malrotation.

Some pediatric hand fractures require surgical intervention, and these are detailed in **Table 2**. Phalangeal neck fractures frequently have a rotation and extension deformity that requires closed reduction and pin fixation to prevent loss of flexion.[41-43] Phalangeal condyle fractures are intra-articular, and most require reduction and pinning (**Figure 4**). Seymour fractures are open

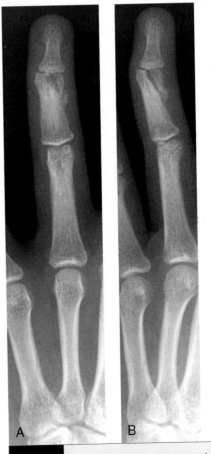

Figure 4	A 15-year-old boy presented for treatment 6 weeks after sustaining a unicondylar fracture of the middle phalanx. AP (**A**) and oblique (**B**) radiographs show intra-articular displacement and moderate healing. When unrecognized, this fracture will heal with limited motion at the distal interphalangeal joint.

6: Pediatrics

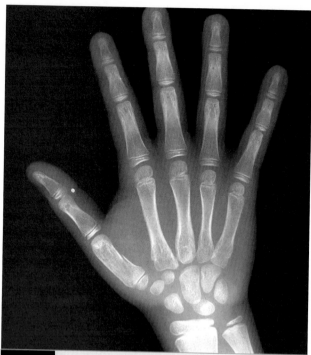

Figure 5 A nondisplaced fracture of the base of the thumb metacarpal in a 9-year-old boy healed with closed treatment and weekly monitoring with radiographs. These fractures may displace and then require reduction and percutaneous pin fixation until union.

Salter-Harris type I or II fractures of the distal phalanx with a tear of the germinal matrix and interposition of soft tissue into the physis. These fractures should be treated with nail plate removal; irrigation and débridement; reduction of the open fracture; nail bed repair; and replacement of the nail plate into the eponychial fold. Phalangeal and metacarpal fractures associated with malrotation should be reduced and stabilized until healed. Intra-articular fractures of the first metacarpal base (Bennett fractures) may displace due to the pull of the abductor pollicus longus on the distal radial fragment. Displaced fractures here require reduction of the shortened, angled, and rotated fragments with percutaneous pins until fracture union (**Figure 5**). Although older children and teens may sustain an ulnar collateral ligament injury at the thumb metacarpophalangeal joint, more commonly the same mechanism results in a Salter-Harris type III intra-articular fracture at the thumb proximal phalanx. If the fracture is displaced, open reduction and pinning are necessary.

Extensor Tendon Injuries

Extensor tendon injuries are much less common than flexor tendon injuries in children. They can be detected with loss of tenodesis of the fingers with flexion and extension of the wrist. In a retrospective study of primary repair and outcome, 98% of patients had good or excellent total active motion.[44] Twenty-two percent had some extension lag or loss of flexion (more likely with patients younger than 5 years, complete laceration, or zone I, II, or III injury). Mallet finger injuries occur more commonly in adolescents and are treated in the same manner as in adults.

Flexor Tendon Injuries

Flexor tendon injuries in children most often occur as a result of a cut by glass. These injuries may be difficult to diagnose depending on patient age and cooperation. Complete laceration can alter the resting posture of the hand. Early diagnosis and repair with techniques used in adults leads to good results in children.[45-47] There is controversy surrounding postoperative protocols, with both full immobilization and early mobilization methods showing good results.[48]

Annotated References

1. Beaty J, Kasser J, eds: *Rockwood and Wilkins' Fractures in Children*, ed 6. Philadelphia, PA, Lippincott Williams & Wilkins, 2006.

2. Do TT, Strub WM, Foad SL, Mehlman CT, Crawford AH: Reduction versus remodeling in pediatric distal forearm fractures: A preliminary cost analysis. *J Pediatr Orthop B* 2003;12(2):109-115.

3. Al-Ansari K, Howard A, Seeto B, Yoo S, Zaki S, Boutis K: Minimally angulated pediatric wrist fractures: Is immobilization without manipulation enough? *CJEM* 2007;9(1):9-15.

   This retrospective cohort study examined bicortical distal radius fractures with minimal angulation (≤15° of sagittal plane angulation and ≤0.5 cm of displacement). Most patients (89%) healed with less than 20° of angulation. Level of evidence: IV.

4. Marcus RJ, Thompson JP: Anaesthesia for manipulation of forearm fractures in children: A survey of current practice. *Paediatr Anaesth* 2000;10(3):273-277.

5. Cimpello LB, Khine H, Avner JR: Practice patterns of pediatric versus general emergency physicians for pain management of fractures in pediatric patients. *Pediatr Emerg Care* 2004;20(4):228-232.

6. Werk LN, Lewis M, Armatti-Wiltrout S, Loveless EA: Comparing the effectiveness of modified forearm and conventional minidose intravenous regional anesthesia for reduction of distal forearm fractures in children. *J Pediatr Orthop* 2008;28(4):410-416.

   Sixty-two patients with acute forearm fractures requiring reduction in the emergency department were randomized to conventional minidose or modified forearm intravenous regional anesthesia. Outcomes were similar. Level of evidence: I.

7. Bae DS: Pediatric distal radius and forearm fractures. *J Hand Surg Am* 2008;33(10):1911-1923.

   A comprehensive review of the literature is presented.

8. Zionts LE, Zalavras CG, Gerhardt MB: Closed treatment of displaced diaphyseal both-bone forearm fractures in older children and adolescents. *J Pediatr Orthop* 2005;25(4):507-512.

9. Webb GR, Galpin RD, Armstrong DG: Comparison of short and long arm plaster casts for displaced fractures in the distal third of the forearm in children. *J Bone Joint Surg Am* 2006;88(1):9-17.

10. Price CT, Scott DS, Kurzner ME, Flynn JC: Malunited forearm fractures in children. *J Pediatr Orthop* 1990; 10(6):705-712.

11. Ploegmakers JJ, Verheyen CC: Acceptance of angulation in the non-operative treatment of paediatric forearm fractures. *J Pediatr Orthop B* 2006;15(6):428-432.

12. Price CT, Knapp DR: Osteotomy for malunited forearm shaft fractures in children. *J Pediatr Orthop* 2006;26(2): 193-196.

    The authors performed radius and ulna osteotomies for nine malunited forearm fractures in this retrospective case series. The average improvement in forearm rotation was 102° after correction. Level of evidence: IV.

13. Garg NK, Ballal MS, Malek IA, Webster RA, Bruce CE: Use of elastic stable intramedullary nailing for treating unstable forearm fractures in children. *J Trauma* 2008; 65(1):109-115.

    In this retrospective study of children with unstable forearm fractures that were treated with flexible intramedullary nails, the authors found a delayed union and a nonunion. Overall, complications were considered few, and functional outcome was good. Level of evidence: IV.

14. Reinhardt KR, Feldman DS, Green DW, Sala DA, Widmann RF, Scher DM: Comparison of intramedullary nailing to plating for both-bone forearm fractures in older children. *J Pediatr Orthop* 2008;28(4):403-409.

    This study retrospectively compared functional and radiographic outcomes of length-stable both-bone forearm fractures that were treated with intramedullary fixation or compression plating in children 10 to 16 years of age, Outcomes and rates of complications were comparable. Level of evidence: III.

15. Yuan PS, Pring ME, Gaynor TP, Mubarak SJ, Newton PO: Compartment syndrome following intramedullary fixation of pediatric forearm fractures. *J Pediatr Orthop* 2004;24(4):370-375.

16. Bae DS, Kadiyala RK, Waters PM: Acute compartment syndrome in children: Contemporary diagnosis, treatment, and outcome. *J Pediatr Orthop* 2001;21(5):680-688.

17. Luhmann SJ, Schootman M, Schoenecker PL, Dobbs MB, Gordon JE: Complications and outcomes of open pediatric forearm fractures. *J Pediatr Orthop* 2004; 24(1):1-6.

18. Eberl R, Singer G, Schalamon J, Petnehazy T, Hoellwarth ME: Galeazzi lesions in children and adolescents: Treatment and outcome. *Clin Orthop Relat Res* 2008; 466(7):1705-1709.

    In this retrospective study of Galeazzi fractures in children, 31% were initially recognized. Twenty-two of 26 patients were treated with reduction and a long or short arm cast, and 4 of 26 were treated surgically. Outcomes were good (3 patients) or excellent (23 patients) in all cases. Level of evidence: IV.

19. Hove LM, Brudvik C: Displaced paediatric fractures of the distal radius. *Arch Orthop Trauma Surg* 2008; 128(1):55-60.

    The authors examined incidence, fracture pattern, treatment, and radiologic outcome of all pediatric distal radius fractures treated in a single city in 1 year.

20. Kirmani S, Christen D, van Lenthe GH, et al: Bone structure at the distal radius during adolescent growth. *J Bone Miner Res* 2009;24(6):1033-1042.

    The authors performed high-resolution peripheral quantitative CT on healthy children 6 to 21 years of age. Bone strength increased with age, but the porosity of cortical bone peaked transiently during puberty.

21. Abraham A, Handoll HH, Khan T: Interventions for treating wrist fractures in children. *Cochrane Database Syst Rev* 2008;2:CD004576.

    The authors performed a systematic review of 10 randomized controlled trials treating pediatric distal radius fractures to determine risks and benefits of various methods of treatment. Level of evidence: II.

22. Plint AC, Perry JJ, Correll R, Gaboury I, Lawton L: A randomized, controlled trial of removable splinting versus casting for wrist buckle fractures in children. *Pediatrics* 2006;117(3):691-697.

23. Symons S, Rowsell M, Bhowal B, Dias JJ: Hospital versus home management of children with buckle fractures of the distal radius: A prospective, randomised trial. *J Bone Joint Surg Br* 2001;83(4):556-560.

24. Oakley EA, Ooi KS, Barnett PL: A randomized controlled trial of 2 methods of immobilizing torus fractures of the distal forearm. *Pediatr Emerg Care* 2008; 24(2):65-70.

    Children with distal radius torus fractures were randomized to a volar fiberglass splint or a short arm plaster cast. Patients treated with a splint had increased duration of pain ($P = 0.009$) and took more time to resume normal activities ($P = 0.001$). Patients wearing a cast had significantly more problems with the appliance ($P = 0.004$). Level of evidence: II.

25. Bohm ER, Bubbar V, Yong Hing K, Dzus A: Above and below-the-elbow plaster casts for distal forearm fractures in children: A randomized controlled trial. *J Bone Joint Surg Am* 2006;88(1):1-8.

26. Alemdaroglu KB, Iltar S, Cimen O, Uysal M, Alagöz E, Atlihan D: Risk factors in redisplacement of distal ra-

6: Pediatrics

dial fractures in children. *J Bone Joint Surg Am* 2008; 90(6):1224-1230.

The authors prospectively analyzed 75 displaced or severely angulated pediatric wrist fractures. Completely displaced fractures were 11.7 times more likely to redisplace after reduction than angulated fractures. The degree of obliquity of the fracture line was also strongly correlated with redisplacement. Level of evidence: I.

27. Chess DG, Hyndman JC, Leahey JL, Brown DC, Sinclair AM: Short arm plaster cast for distal pediatric forearm fractures. *J Pediatr Orthop* 1994;14(2):211-213.

28. McLauchlan GJ, Cowan B, Annan IH, Robb JE: Management of completely displaced metaphyseal fractures of the distal radius in children: A prospective, randomised controlled trial. *J Bone Joint Surg Br* 2002; 84(3):413-417.

29. Jung HJ, Jung YB, Jang EC, et al: Transradioulnar single Kirschner-wire fixation versus conventional Kirschner-wire fixation for unstable fractures of both of the distal forearm bones in children. *J Pediatr Orthop* 2007;27(8):867-872.

The authors describe a technique to treat unstable distal both-bone forearm fractures with a single Kirschner wire traversing the radius and the ulna without violating the physis. Cases were compared with a historical group treated with conventional pinning techniques. Outcomes were similar. Level of evidence: III.

30. Choi KY, Chan WS, Lam TP, Cheng JC: Percutaneous Kirschner-wire pinning for severely displaced distal radial fractures in children: A report of 157 cases. *J Bone Joint Surg Br* 1995;77(5):797-801.

31. Boyden EM, Peterson HA: Partial premature closure of the distal radial physis associated with Kirschner wire fixation. *Orthopedics* 1991;14(5):585-588.

32. Waters PM, Bae DS, Montgomery KD: Surgical management of posttraumatic distal radial growth arrest in adolescents. *J Pediatr Orthop* 2002;22(6):717-724.

33. Abid A, Accadbled F, Kany J, de Gauzy JS, Darodes P, Cahuzac JP: Ulnar styloid fracture in children: A retrospective study of 46 cases. *J Pediatr Orthop B* 2008; 17(1):15-19.

Forty-six ulnar styloid fractures associated with distal radius fractures were reviewed retrospectively. Eighty percent failed to unite. All patients with chronic symptoms had pathology involving the TFCC. Level of evidence: IV.

34. Golz RJ, Grogan DP, Greene TL, Belsole RJ, Ogden JA: Distal ulnar physeal injury. *J Pediatr Orthop* 1991; 11(3):318-326.

35. Evenski AJ, Adamczyk MJ, Steiner RP, Morscher MA, Riley PM: Clinically suspected scaphoid fractures in children. *J Pediatr Orthop* 2009;29(4):352-355.

In this retrospective study, 30% of pediatric patients with suspected but radiographically negative scaphoid fractures went on to show radiographic evidence of fracture at 1.5 to 2-week follow-up. The authors recommend thumb spica immobilization of suspected scaphoid fractures until follow-up radiographs are normal. Level of evidence: IV.

36. Huckstadt T, Klitscher D, Weltzien A, Müller LP, Rommens PM, Schier F: Pediatric fractures of the carpal scaphoid: A retrospective clinical and radiological study. *J Pediatr Orthop* 2007;27(4):447-450.

In this retrospective study, 22 pediatric patients with scaphoid fractures were reviewed, with 17 receiving cast immobilization and 5 requiring open reduction and screw fixation for displacement or nonunion. A total of 94% were scored good or excellent by the Cooney score and by patient self-assessment. Level of evidence: IV.

37. Henderson B, Letts M: Operative management of pediatric scaphoid fracture nonunion. *J Pediatr Orthop* 2003;23(3):402-406.

38. Mancini F, De Maio F, Ippolito E: Pisiform bone fracture-dislocation and distal radius physeal fracture in two children. *J Pediatr Orthop B* 2005;14(4):303-306.

39. Parker WL, Czerwinski M, Lee C: First carpal-metacarpal joint dislocation and trapezial fracture treated with external fixation in an adolescent. *Ann Plast Surg* 2008;61(5):506-510.

This case report describes this extremely rare injury in a teenager who had a good outcome and recommends external fixation as a possible treatment in the pediatric population. Level of evidence: V.

40. Vadivelu R, Dias JJ, Burke FD, Stanton J: Hand injuries in children: A prospective study. *J Pediatr Orthop* 2006; 26(1):29-35.

41. Valencia J, Leyva F, Gomez-Bajo GJ: Pediatric hand trauma. *Clin Orthop Relat Res* 2005;432(432):77-86.

42. Cornwall R, Ricchetti ET: Pediatric phalanx fractures: Unique challenges and pitfalls. *Clin Orthop Relat Res* 2006;445:146-156.

43. Waters PM: Operative carpal and hand injuries in children. *J Bone Joint Surg Am* 2007;89(9):2064-2074.

The authors present a review of surgically treated injuries in children. Level of evidence: V.

44. Fitoussi F, Badina A, Ilhareborde B, Morel E, Ear R, Pennecot GF: Extensor tendon injuries in children. *J Pediatr Orthop* 2007;27(8):863-866.

This retrospective study of extensor tendon repairs in children showed 98% good or excellent total active motion. Twenty-two percent had extension lag or flexion loss that was more likely in patients younger than 5 years, complete laceration, or zone I, II, or III injury. Level of evidence: IV.

45. Nietosvaara Y, Lindfors NC, Palmu S, Rautakorpi S, Ristaniemi N: Flexor tendon injuries in pediatric patients. *J Hand Surg Am* 2007;32(10):1549-1557.

    This retrospective study of children who underwent flexor tendon repair showed good subjective and objective outcomes with multistrand repair at all levels with an active-motion rehabilitation program. Level of evidence: IV.

46. Darlis NA, Beris AE, Korompilias AV, Vekris MD, Mitsionis GI, Soucacos PN: Two-stage flexor tendon reconstruction in zone 2 of the hand in children. *J Pediatr Orthop* 2005;25(3):382-386.

47. Kato H, Minami A, Suenaga N, Iwasaki N, Kimura T: Long-term results after primary repairs of zone 2 flexor tendon lacerations in children younger than age 6 years. *J Pediatr Orthop* 2002;22(6):732-735.

48. Moehrlen U, Mazzone L, Bieli C, Weber DM: Early mobilization after flexor tendon repair in children. *Eur J Pediatr Surg* 2009;19(2):83-86.

    This retrospective study of children who underwent flexor tendon repair and an age-adapted early motion rehabilitation protocol showed 93% total active motion and 93% good or excellent results. Level of evidence: IV.

6: Pediatrics

Chapter 55

Upper Extremity Disorders: Pediatrics

Dan A. Zlotolow, MD   Scott H. Kozin, MD

Introduction

Upper limb deformities make up a full 10% of all congenital anomalies, second only in incidence to cardiac anomalies.[1] Although teratogens often are blamed for such congenital differences, most occur spontaneously or are genetically determined. Many deformities, such as thrombocytopenia-absent radius, follow a set pattern, and others, such as central deficiencies and symbrachydactyly, have a spectrum of phenotypic variants that make them difficult to classify.

Recent advances in cell-signaling research have enriched our understanding of anomalous limb development. The limb bud begins to develop 26 days after fertilization, when the embryo is smaller than a grain of rice. By the eighth week, the embryo is approximately 1 inch in length, and the upper limb is fully formed (**Figure 1**). Congenital deformities that affect limb formation occur during this period. Further differentiation and growth of the limbs occurs during the subsequent fetal period. Longitudinal growth of the limb is coordinated by the apical ectodermal ridge (AER), an ectodermal condensation that forms a cap over the lengthening limb. Lateral plate mesoderm (destined to become bone, cartilage, and tendon) and somatic mesoderm (muscle, nerve, and vasculature) grow out from the embryo under the AER.[2] Anteroposterior radioulnar differentiation is determined by the zone of polarizing activity (ZPA) through the sonic hedgehog pathway. Duplication of the ZPA results in mirror-image duplication of the limb. Dorsoventral development is coordinated by the wingless-type signaling pathway in the dorsal non-AER ectoderm. Removal of the AER results in a truncated limb, but its influence on the underlying mesoderm can be overcome by the addition of fibroblast growth factors to the apex of the limb bud.[3] The

ZPA also is necessary for longitudinal growth via induction of the gremlin protein. Both gremlin and bone morphogenetic proteins are produced in the growing limb mesoderm. The antagonistic effects of gremlin on bone morphogenetic proteins prevent premature limb maturation and cessation of longitudinal development.[4] The wingless-type signaling pathway also is necessary for longitudinal growth because it influences the establishment and maintenance of the AER.[5]

The most commonly used classification scheme is based on the understanding of embryogenesis, but it is limited because of its reliance on clinical judgment as well as the overlap of deformities (**Table 1**). Great variations in the clinical appearance of the same embryologic malformation can challenge the clinician who is trying to identify an anomaly. Often, the pattern of deformity (one or all limbs affected) and its associations (for example, Poland syndrome in symbrachydactyly) offer clues to accurate diagnosis and classification. At initial diagnosis, the primary goal of the surgeon is to

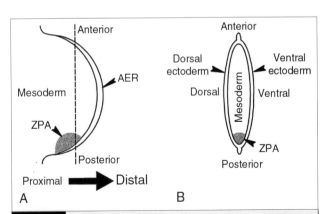

Figure 1 Schematic drawings showing the development of the limb bud in a proximal-to-distal direction coordinated by the apical ectodermal ridge (AER). The zone of polarizing activity (ZPA) signals the differentiation of radius- and ulna-side structures. **A,** The limb bud in the frontal plane. **B,** A cross section of the limb bud at the dashed line shown in A. (Adapted with permission from Daluiski A, YiS E, Lyons KM: The molecular control of upper extremity development: Implications for congenital hand anomalies. *J Hand Surg Am* 2001;26[1]:8-22.)

Dr. Zlotolow or an immediate family member is an unpaid consultant to Arthrex and serves as a board member, owner, officer, or committee member of the American Society for Surgery of the Hand. Dr. Kozin or an immediate family member serves as a board member, owner, officer, or committee member of the American Society for Surgery of the Hand.

6: Pediatrics

assist the family in understanding and coping with the child's condition.

Failure of Formation

Radial Longitudinal Deficiencies

Two thirds of all radial longitudinal deficiencies are diagnosed as part of a syndrome, often involving the heart, kidney, bone marrow, or gastrointestinal tract. The more severe the deficiency, the more likely it is to be associated with a syndrome.[6] Half of these deficiencies are bilateral. Boys are more often affected than girls, by a ratio of 3 to 2. The occurrence usually is sporadic, with minimal influence of family history. Radial longitudinal deficiency may be the only observable sign of a syndrome, and its presence should trigger a full workup of the heart, kidney, bone marrow, and gastrointestinal tract, as well as a general pediatric orthopaedic examination. A chromosomal challenge test should be performed to detect Fanconi anemia before bone marrow failure can occur.[7]

The classification is based upon the extent of deficiency, from thumb hypoplasia to complete absence of the radius (**Table 2**). Complete absence of the radius is most common, accompanied by a shortened forearm segment and a radial deviation of the wrist. The ulna is typically 60% shorter on the affected side than on the contralateral side, and often it is bowed and thickened[8] (**Figure 2**).

Thrombocytopenia-Absent Radius Syndrome

Thrombocytopenia-absent radius syndrome is characterized by complete bilateral absence of the radii and preservation of the thumbs (**Figure 2**). Its incidence is 1 to 2 per 1 million live births.[9] Although the phenotype is well understood, the predominantly autosomal recessive genotype is only beginning to be determined. Transient hypomegakaryotic thrombocytopenia is present at birth and tends to improve if the child survives the first year of life.

Fanconi Anemia

Fanconi anemia is a pancytopenia associated with radial longitudinal deficiency. Unlike thrombocytopenia-absent radius syndrome, this hematologic disorder appears when the child is age 3 to 12 years. The diagnosis

Table 1

The Embryologic Classification of Congenital Anomalies

Primary Classification	Secondary Classification
I. Failure of formation	A. Transverse arrest B. Longitudinal arrest
II. Failure of differentiation	A. Soft tissue B. Skeletal C. Tumorous
III. Duplication	A. Whole limb B. Humeral C. Radial D. Ulnar E. Digit
IV. Overgrowth	A. Whole limb B. Partial limb C. Digit
V. Undergrowth	A. Whole limb B. Whole hand C. Metacarpal D. Digit
VI. Constriction band syndrome	
VII. Generalized skeletal abnormality	

Table 2

The Global Classification of Radial Longitudinal Deficiencies

Type	Thumb	Carpus[a]	Distal Radius	Proximal Radius
N	Absence or hypoplasia	Normal	Normal	Normal
O	Absence or hypoplasia	Absence, hypoplasia, or coalition	Normal	Normal, radioulnar synostosis, or radial head dislocation
1	Absence or hypoplasia	Absence, hypoplasia, or coalition	>2 mm shorter than ulna	Normal, radioulnar synostosis, or radial head dislocation
2	Absence or hypoplasia	Absence, hypoplasia, or coalition	Hypoplasia	Hypoplasia
3	Absence or hypoplasia	Absence, hypoplasia, or coalition	Physis absence	Variable hypoplasia
4	Absence or hypoplasia	Absence, hypoplasia, or coalition	Absence	Absence

[a]A carpal anomaly implies hypoplasia, coalition, absence, or bipartite carpal bones. Hypoplasia and absence are more common on the radial side of the carpus, and coalitions are more frequent on the ulnar side. Radiographic findings are valid only if the child is older than 8 years, to allow for ossification of the carpal bones.

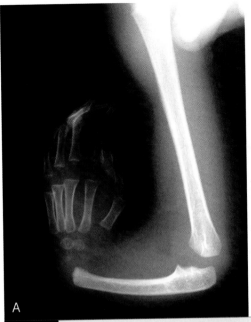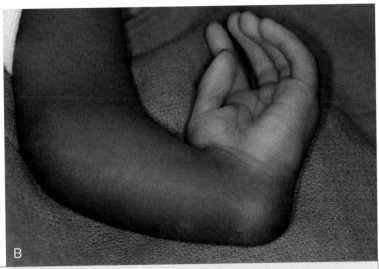

Figure 2 A child with thrombocytopenia-absent radius syndrome. Ulnar bowing at the forearm and preservation of the thumb can be seen in the AP radiograph of the hand and lateral forearm (**A**) and a photograph (**B**). (Courtesy of Shriners Hospital for Children, Philadelphia, PA.)

can easily be missed, with tragic consequences. Every child with any radial longitudinal deficiency should undergo a chromosomal challenge test to rule out Fanconi anemia. Unless bone marrow transplantation is successful, the pancytopenia is progressive and lethal. Children with Fanconi anemia are susceptible to acute myelogenous leukemia as well as solid tumors of the head, neck, breast, liver, esophagus, and vulva. The pancytopenia may be accompanied by anomalies in other organ systems, including the skin and kidneys.[10]

VACTERL Association
The term VACTERL association is commonly used to include cardiac malformations and limb anomalies in association with vertebral defects, anal atresia, tracheoesophageal fistula with esophageal atresia, renal anomalies, and radial dysplasia. At least three systems must be affected for the diagnosis of VACTERL association to be made. The limb deformities include the spectrum of radial longitudinal deficiencies as well as syndactyly and polydactyly. No reliable inheritance pattern or teratogenic exposure has been identified for the VACTERL association, possibly because it represents a common but highly variable phenotypic terminus for various chromosomal or environmental insults.

Holt-Oram Syndrome
With an incidence of 1 per 100,000 live births, Holt-Oram syndrome is the most common of all heart-limb syndromes.[10] The severity of the limb deformity is not predictive of the extent of cardiac involvement and can vary greatly across generations. Most deformities are limited to thumb hypoplasia, but more severe radial de-

ficiencies and even ulna-side deficiencies can occur. More than 70 mutations in the *TBX5* transcription factor gene have been associated with Holt-Oram syndrome. Not all people with a *TBX5* mutation have the disease, however, and only 35% of patients with the syndrome have a *TBX5* mutation.[11] The inheritance pattern is autosomal dominant with variable expression.

Thumb Hypoplasia
Radial longitudinal deficiencies may occur without affecting the thumb, as in thrombocytopenia-absent radius syndrome, or may affect only the thumb. As with any radius-side deficiency, the presence of an associated syndrome or anomaly should be suspected and ruled out. Evaluation of a hypoplastic thumb primarily hinges on the status of the basal joint. A thumb with a stable basal joint usually can be salvaged with a combination of skin flaps, ligament reconstructions, and tendon transfers. An unstable thumb will not function well, and the best treatment is ablation and pollicization. The Manske modification of the Blauth classification differentiates types IIIA and IIIB based on basal joint stability (**Table 3**).

Treatment
As soon as the diagnosis of radial longitudinal deficiency is made, a passive stretching protocol should be instituted under the supervision of a therapist. Tight radius-side structures should be stretched every time the child's diaper is changed and at bedtime. Progressive splinting can begin as soon as the limb is long enough to accommodate it. A severely affected patient

6: Pediatrics

Table 3

The Classification of Thumb Deficiency

Type	Clinical Findings	Treatment
I	Minor generalized hypoplasia	Augmentation
II	Absence of intrinsic thenar muscles Narrowing of first web space Ulnar collateral ligament insufficiency	Opponensplasty First web release Ulnar collateral ligament reconstruction
III	Absence of intrinsic thenar muscles Narrowing of first web space Ulnar collateral ligament insufficiency Extrinsic muscle and tendon abnormalities Skeletal deficiency IIIA: Stable carpometacarpal joint IIIB: Unstable carpometacarpal joint	IIIA: Reconstruction IIIB: Pollicization
IV	Floating thumb	Pollicization
V	Absence of thumb	Pollicization

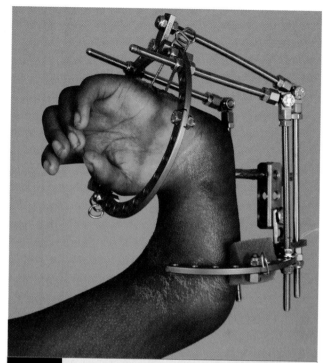

Figure 3 Photograph showing the use of a hybrid fixator to slowly correct soft-tissue balance before surgical centralization in a child with radial dysplasia. (Courtesy of Shriners Hospital for Children, Philadelphia, PA.)

or a patient who has undergone unsuccessful nonsurgical management may benefit from centralization procedures to correct the radial deviation of the wrist. An older patient who has functionally compensated for the deformity, a patient with a proximate terminal condition, or a patient with an extension contracture of the elbow who relies on the radial deviation to reach the mouth is a poor candidate for any surgical procedure. A supposedly successful operation may make such a patient's condition worse. The results of centralization remain unpredictable despite recent technical advances. Even when an excellent correction is achieved, recurrence of the deformity is common. An alternative may be gradual distraction lengthening of the tight radius-side structures using an Ilizarov-type ring fixator (**Figure 3**). When correction of the wrist position is achieved, a centralization procedure can be performed with little to no tension on the radius side. The results of this technique have been promising, although recurrence remains a concern.[12,13] Ulna lengthening via distraction osteogenesis may need to be performed several times to achieve adequate length at maturity. Despite high complication rates, ulna lengthening remains appealing because it can improve the use of the hand if near-normal length is achieved.[14]

The treatment of thumb hypoplasia hinges on the stability of the carpometacarpal joint. The child typically does not use the thumb if the basal joint is unstable because insufficient power is available for pinching and grasping. As the child grows, he or she will learn to bypass the thumb in favor of scissor grasping between the index and long fingers. Cortical representation will not develop in an unused thumb, and heroic measures

to salvage such a thumb will not lead to its use. Pollicization is the preferred option because it effectively takes advantage of the child's developing index–long finger pinch pattern.

A type I thumb requires no treatment. A type II thumb has deficient intrinsic musculature and can be reconstructed with an opponensplasty and a four-flap Z-plasty for web space deepening. Ulnar collateral ligament reconstruction and, if necessary, radial collateral ligament reconstruction may be accomplished at the same time. Pollex abductus (an interconnection between the flexor and extensor systems along the radial aspect of the thumb) can occur with a type II or IIIA thumb. These thumbs require a pulley reconstruction and recentralization of the flexor tendon. A type IIIA thumb is missing extrinsic motors and requires tendon transfers to provide extensor pollicis longus and/or flexor pollicis longus function. A type IIIB, IV, or V thumb is best treated with ablation and pollicization (**Figure 4**). The results of pollicization are correlated with the condition of the index finger and its associated musculature before pollicization.[15-17] Children who develop a good grip-and-pinch pattern after pollicization are likely to maintain the pattern into adulthood.[16]

Ulnar Deficiencies

Unlike a radius-side deficiency, the loss of ulna-side structures in the upper limb rarely is accompanied by abnormalities in other organ systems. Concomitant

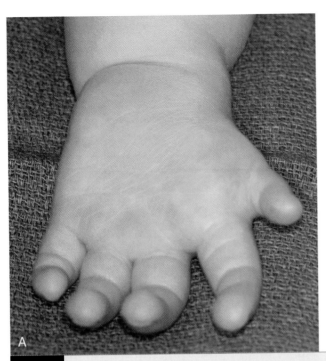
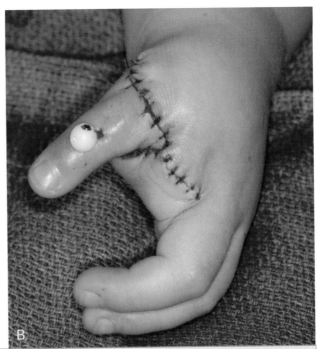

Figure 4	Type IIIB thumb hypoplasia before **(A)** and after **(B)** thumb ablation and index pollicization. It can be difficult for parents to understand the need for surgery, particularly if the thumb is of adequate size. However, the function and appearance of the hand can be dramatically improved through a well-done pollicization. (Courtesy of Shriners Hospital for Children, Philadelphia, PA.)

skeletal abnormality can exist, however, including pre-axial abnormality, fibular hemimelia, or proximal focal femoral deficiency (**Figure 5**). Bilaterality occurs only in approximately one quarter of patients.

The classification is based on the severity of elbow and forearm involvement, as well as the condition of the thumb and thumb–index finger web space[18] (**Table 4**). Hand involvement varies greatly, with almost all children having absent ulna-side digits, and some children having absent or anomalous radius-side digits. The wrist is in mild to moderate ulnar deviation, and the forearm segment may be markedly shortened. Elbow range of motion can be limited or absent.

As with a radial deficiency, the progression of deformity can be limited by early stretching and splinting. Corrective procedures can be considered when the child is at least 6 months of age. Syndactyly releases and deepening of the thumb–index finger web space can improve the appearance and function of the hand. Creation of a one-bone forearm occasionally is necessary to stabilize the forearm, but it results in the loss of any forearm rotation. Correction of the ulnar deviation posture is rarely necessary. No predictable procedures exist for restoring elbow motion in these children.

Central Deficiencies

A cleft hand results from a failure of formation of the center of the limb. The inherited forms typically become more severe with each generation, and affected families should undergo genetic counseling. Sporadic incidences may represent a spontaneous mutation. Bi-

lateral foot and hand involvement (split hand–split foot syndrome) has been located on chromosome 7[19] (**Figure 6**). The clinical deformity ranges from a slightly shortened third ray to only one ulnar digit (in the monodactylous type). Bizarre combinations and orientations of the carpals, metacarpals, and phalanges can occur, as well as syndactyly and synostoses. The presence of nubbins suggests the diagnosis of an atypical cleft hand (symbrachydactyly).

The cleft hand has been called "a functional triumph, yet a social disaster."[20] The cleft in a mildly affected hand can be closed to optimize its appearance and help the child use the hand to carry small objects and liquids. A two-digit hand is cosmetically challenging for most children, but its function is excellent if the length of the digits is adequate. Length augmentation of the thumb or short finger may be of benefit. Syndactyly releases may be indicated as well. The reconstructive options are limited for a monodactylous hand.

Symbrachydactyly

The diagnosis of symbrachydactyly includes a wide range from transverse deficiency above the elbow to mild hypoplasia of the hand. Unlike cleft hand, symbrachydactyly predominantly affects only one limb. The monodactylous form preserves the thumb (**Figure 7**). The etiology is believed to be an interruption of the vascular supply to the end of the limb, resulting in loss of the mesodermal cells destined to become terminal limb structures. Transverse deficiencies with nubbin formation may indicate that, although the AER contin-

6: Pediatrics

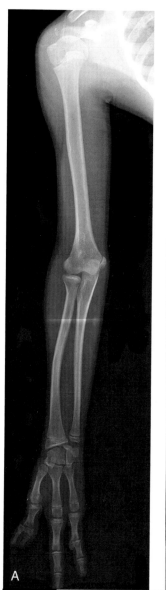
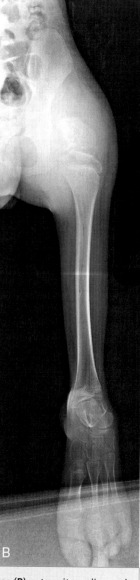

Figure 5 AP upper (**A**) and lower (**B**) extremity radiographs of a child with ulnar dysplasia with thumb duplication, as well as associated fibular hemimelia and proximal focal femoral deficiency. (Courtesy of Shriners Hospital for Children, Philadelphia, PA.)

Table 4

The Classification of Ulnar Deficiencies (0-IV) and Subgroup Classification by Abnormality of the First Web Space (A-D)

Type	Grade	Characteristics
0		Normal forearm Deficiencies in hand and carpus
I	Hypoplasia	Hypoplasia of the ulna with presence of distal and proximal ulnar epiphysis Minimal shortening
II	Partial aplasia	Partial aplasia with absence of the distal or middle third of the ulna
III	Complete aplasia	Total agenesis of the ulna
IV	Synostosis	Fusion of the radius to the humerus

Subtype	Grade	Characteristics
A	Normal	Normal first web space and normal thumb
B	Mild	Mild first web space deficiency and mild thumb hypoplasia with intact opposition and extrinsic tendon function
C	Moderate to severe	Moderate to severe first web space deficiency and similar thumb hypoplasia with malrotation into the plane of the digits Loss of opposition Dysfunction of the extrinsic tendons
D	Absence	Absence of the thumb

ued to signal the limb to grow, only the ectoderm was available for forming terminal structures. A transverse deficiency without nubbins is believed to result from a loss of the AER with truncation of limb growth.[21]

In the short-finger type of symbrachydactyly, the triad of syndactyly, brachydactyly, and symphalangism is most common (**Figure 8**). A severely affected hand can resemble a cleft hand, but the presence of nubbins and the involvement of only one limb differentiates the two diagnoses. Poland syndrome may be present, with absence of the sternal head of the pectoralis major, and the patient also may have a loss of breast tissue and a chest wall deficiency (**Figure 9**). The monodactylous

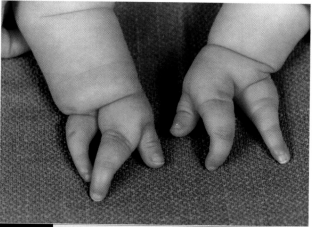

Figure 6 Photograph showing a child's split hands (central deficiency). The child's feet had a similar deformity. (Courtesy of Shriners Hospital for Children, Philadelphia, PA.)

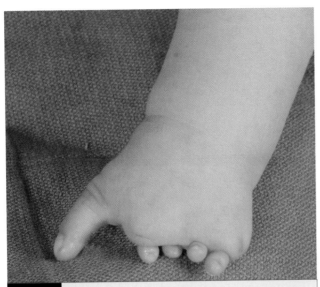

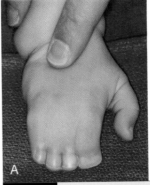

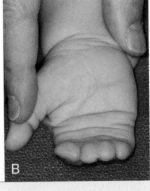

Figure 8 Photographs showing the dorsal (**A**) and volar (**B**) aspects of a hand with short-finger symbrachydactyly, which is characterized by the triad of syndactyly, brachydactyly, and symphalangism. (Courtesy of Shriners Hospital for Children, Philadelphia, PA.)

Figure 7 Photograph showing a child's hand with monodactylous symbrachydactyly, with the thumb preserved. (Courtesy of Shriners Hospital for Children, Philadelphia, PA.)

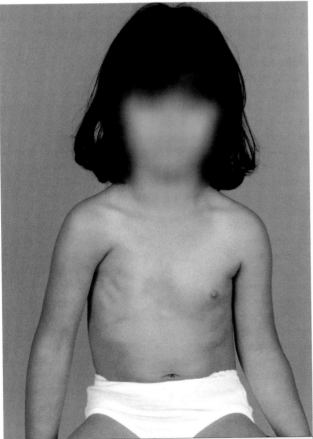

Figure 9 Photograph of a girl with severe Poland syndrome. The absence of the pectoralis muscles and a nipple can be seen. More commonly, only the sternal head of the pectoralis major is absent. (Courtesy of Shriners Hospital for Children, Philadelphia, PA.)

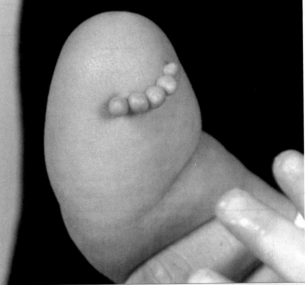

Figure 10 Photograph showing a transverse deficiency just below the elbow with terminal nubbins (peromelic symbrachydactyly). (Courtesy of Shriners Hospital for Children, Philadelphia, PA.)

form can be differentiated from a cleft hand by preservation of the thumb. Nubbins may be absent. The peromelic form is a transverse deficiency with loss of all digits (**Figure 10**). Nubbins can be seen at the terminus of the limb.

Syndactyly releases are indicated for a child with the short-finger type. Redundant soft tissue at the end of the limb allows nonvascularized toe proximal phalanges to be transferred to gain digital length. The growth of these transferred phalanges has been variable, although preservation of the periosteum and collateral ligaments appears to improve the results.[22] Vascularized toe transfers are technically more challenging than nonvascularized phalangeal transfers, but they can add greater length and provide more mobile joints. Vascu-

of radius, ulna, and combined deficiencies.[25] Severe forms of Holt-Oram syndrome are similar in appearance, and associated cardiac anomalies therefore should be ruled out. The truncated limb length means that a prosthesis can provide substantial functional improvement. Early fitting is indicated to optimize acceptance of the prosthesis.

Failure of Differentiation

Syndactyly

Failure of separation of the digits occurs in 3 per 10,000 live births. Although an autosomal dominant inheritance pattern is common, the expression is variable and penetrance is incomplete. The genetic defect has been localized to chromosome 2 (2q34-q36).[26] Syndromic associations are relatively uncommon, although Apert syndrome (**Figure 12**), Poland syndrome, symbrachydactyly, amnionic disruption sequence, cleft hand, and ulnar longitudinal deficiency can occur. Amnionic bands cause a fenestrated type of syndactyly known as acrosyndactyly, with retention of a narrow remnant of the proximal web space.

The classification of syndactyly is straightforward. The presence or absence of a synostosis determines whether the syndactyly is simple or complex. The term synonychia refers to a joint nail plate and indicates a synostosis of the distal phalanges. A complete syndactyly extends to the fingertip, and an incomplete syndactyly does not. Apert syndrome is classified as a complete or complicated syndactyly.

Reconstruction to obtain an adequate web space usually is indicated for functional and aesthetic reasons. The timing of surgery is controversial, but most surgeons agree that early separation of a complete syndactyly is warranted for border digits, particularly the thumb and index finger. Because of the disparity in length between the ring and small fingers and the thumb and index finger, the shorter digit will tether the longer digit, creating joint contractures and rotational deformities. Release of the thumb–index finger web should be performed by age 6 months to allow development of prehensile grasp-and-pinch patterns. Separation of the long and ring fingers can be delayed until the hand is larger and easier to reconstruct. At least 3 months should be allowed between procedures to separate adjacent digits.

The commissure and the lateral nail fold are the most challenging areas to reconstruct in simple syndactyly. The commissure should be free of any suture lines and grafts to prevent later scarring and contracture (web creep). A full-thickness skin graft is almost always necessary to cover any remaining defects, and harvesting can be easily done from the wrist crease, with virtually no harvest site morbidity (**Figure 13**). A complex syndactyly may require soft-tissue transfers. The digital neurovascular bundles may be abnormal or absent if a synostosis is present.

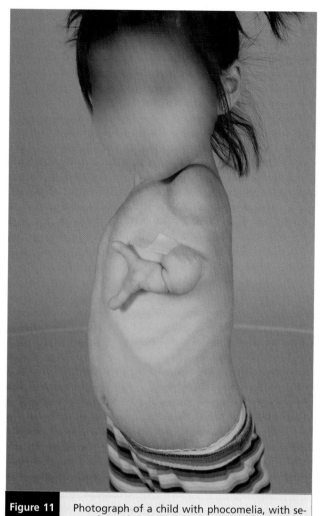

larized toe transfers can be used for some monodactylous and peromelic-type hands.[23] Distraction osteogenesis is another option; a 30% to 100% increase in phalangeal length has been reported, with no donor site morbidity.[24] Prosthesis fitting at age 6 months was considered mandatory for a child with the peromelic type of syndactyly, particularly at the midforearm or above-elbow level. However, the children rarely rely on the prosthesis for functioning unless the deficiencies are bilateral, and the adage "fit when they sit" may no longer apply.

Phocomelia

Phocomelia became famous as a consequence of maternal thalidomide use to treat pregnancy-related nausea, but otherwise it is quite rare. The syndrome is characterized by short or absent long bones and a flipperlike appearance of the hands and/or feet. Intercalary aplasia results in the loss of forearm segments or the entire arm. The hands and feet sometimes arise directly from the trunk (**Figure 11**). Phocomelia may be the most severe form of longitudinal deficiency along the spectrum

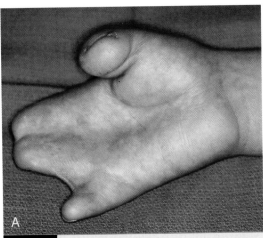
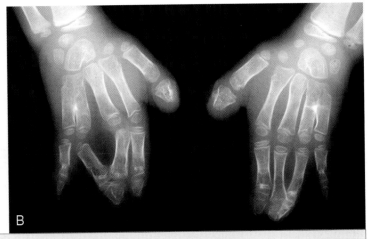

Figure 12 Photograph **(A)** and AP radiograph **(B)** showing a complicated syndactyly in a child with Apert syndrome. (Courtesy of Shriners Hospital for Children, Philadelphia, PA.)

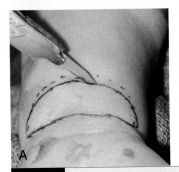
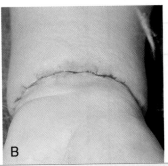
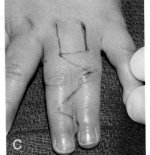
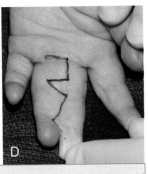

Figure 13 Photographs showing the location of full-thickness skin graft harvesting and flaps used for the release of a syndactyly. The wrist crease is an excellent source of skin graft **(A)**, with minimal postoperative morbidity **(B)**. Dorsal **(C)** and volar **(D)** flaps should be designed to minimize suturing at the commissure. (Courtesy of Shriners Hospital for Children, Philadelphia, PA.)

Camptodactyly

Proximal interphalangeal joint contractures can result from a fracture or a tendon laceration or avulsion, or they may occur spontaneously or as part of a syndrome. It may be difficult to differentiate camptodactyly from posttraumatic proximal interphalangeal joint contractures or boutonniere deformities, particularly in young children. True camptodactyly occurs in as many as 1% of the population. When familial, it has an autosomal dominant inheritance pattern.[27] The congenital type has no sex predilection, but the adolescent type occurs more often in girls. The small finger is most commonly affected.

Clinodactyly

Partial damage to the physis as a result of trauma, a thermal injury, or a physeal abnormality inherited as an autosomal dominant trait can lead to progressive radioulnar angular deformity. The middle phalanx of the small finger is most commonly affected, with a typical bend toward the ring finger. Radiographs may reveal a C-shaped physis that results in a triangular delta phalanx (**Figure 14**). The curvature begins to interfere with daily activities when the deformity reaches 30° to 40°.[28]

Kirner Deformity

Kirner deformity is a combined flexion and radial deviation deformity of the small finger that occurs spontaneously or may have a genetic component. The finger has an angulated distal interphalangeal joint with a curved, beak-shaped nail similar to that found in nail clubbing. However, the deformity itself is at the distal phalanx and not at the joint. Treatment is rarely necessary.

Congenital Synostoses

Synostosis Across the Elbow

Humeroradial synostosis can occur with ulnar hypoplasia (type I), or with a normal ulna (type II). Although type II is more commonly familial than type I, both types occur in a variety of genetic syndromes or with other skeletal or extraskeletal anomalies.[29] The child should be referred to a geneticist as well as to appropriate pediatric subspecialists. In type I humeroradial synostosis, the elbow usually is fused in extension, making some daily tasks difficult. When the elbow is fused in a flexed position, as is more common in type II, patients are better able to perform bimanual tasks and to feed and groom themselves. Severe hyperexten-

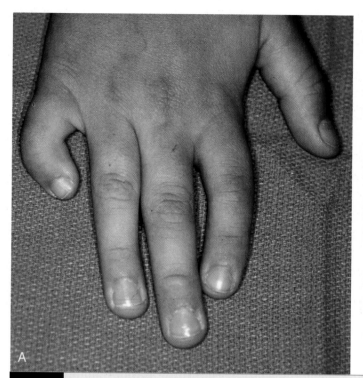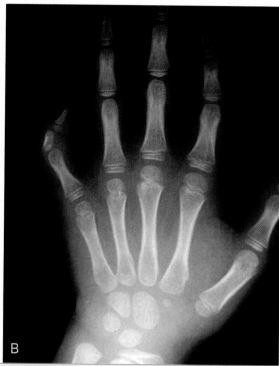

Figure 14 Photograph **(A)** and PA radiograph **(B)** showing the hand of a child with bilateral clinodactyly. (Courtesy of Shriners Hospital for Children, Philadelphia, PA.)

sion may warrant a corrective osteotomy to improve function.

Radioulnar Synostosis

The most common upper extremity synostosis is found between the radius and ulna. The diagnosis is often missed because function is maintained through compensatory hyperrotation at the wrist (sometimes of more than 100°) as well as and rotation at the shoulder.[30] Although there is an autosomal dominant transmission pattern, penetrance is variable and the synostosis can occur sporadically. Radiographs show a well-formed fusion mass across the proximal radius and ulna, often with a radial head dislocation (**Figure 15**). Most synostoses are in a near-neutral position and are well tolerated, requiring no treatment unless the child is limited in specific daily activities. Takedown of the synostosis to achieve forearm motion is almost always unsuccessful.[31] Rotational osteotomies can position the arm in a more favorable position. The optimal position for function is controversial, although slight pronation of both arms may be most useful for computer use. Supination of the nondominant side may facilitate perineal care.

Sprengel Deformity

Failure of the scapula to descend during embryogenesis results in a congenital elevation of the scapula. The deformity is sporadic and typically unilateral. An omovertebral band almost always is present. The treatment remains controversial. If functional or cosmetic consid-

erations warrant surgical intervention, procedures ranging from soft-tissue releases to scapular osteotomies can be considered.

Duplication

Thumb (Preaxial) Polydactyly

Thumb duplication most commonly occurs in white children and typically is unilateral and sporadic. The etiology is a split rather than a true duplication. Both thumbs are smaller than the thumb on the unaffected contralateral side. The ulnar-sided thumb tends to be larger and better formed than the radial-sided thumb (**Figure 16**). A simple count of the abnormal bones yields the Wassel stage. In a Wassel type IV thumb (the most common duplication), there are four abnormal bones including two distal and two proximal phalanges.[32]

Surgical reconstruction is indicated for most patients. Because the thumb to be preserved is usually smaller than the unaffected contralateral thumb, bulk from the thumb to be ablated should be preserved to augment the final reconstruction. The collateral ligaments should be preserved or repaired and reconstructed.

Ulnar Polydactyly

Postaxial polydactyly is most common in children of African descent; it has an autosomal dominant transmission pattern with high penetrance.[33] Often one of

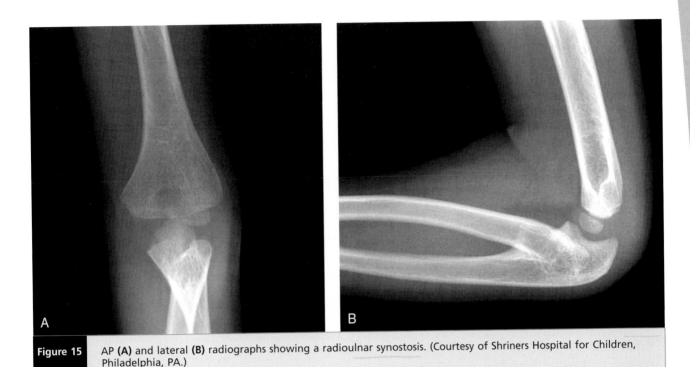

Figure 15 AP **(A)** and lateral **(B)** radiographs showing a radioulnar synostosis. (Courtesy of Shriners Hospital for Children, Philadelphia, PA.)

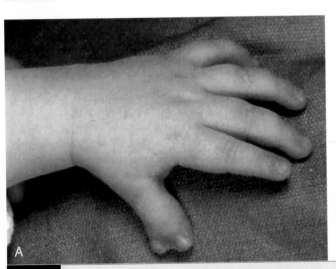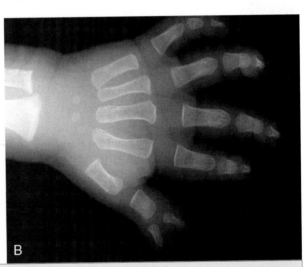

Figure 16 Photograph **(A)** and PA radiograph **(B)** showing a type II thumb duplication. Note that two phalanges are affected. (Courtesy of Shriners Hospital for Children, Philadelphia, PA.)

the child's parents will have bilateral bumps on the ulnar side of the hand because a polydactylous digit was tied off at a young age. The child should receive a routine physical examination to detect any other skeletal system abnormalities. An extra digit on the ulnar side of the hand of a child of European descent should trigger an evaluation to detect a possible cardiac septal defect, thoracic dystrophy, hypogenitalism or ambiguous genitalia, ocular disorder, cleft lip or palate, mental retardation, cutaneous and nail dysplasia, or renal anomaly. Ellis–van Creveld syndrome should be suspected in a child from a genetically isolated population such as the Amish. Genetic counseling is recommended if the polydactyly is associated with other findings.

In type A, the extra digit is well formed; in type B, it is little more than a skin tag (**Figure 17**). A type A digit requires surgical excision; in-office ablation should not be attempted. A type B digit traditionally has been tied off with clips or suture ligature. Surgical ablation may be preferred to obtain a better long-term cosmetic result and avoid the necessity of the parents' observing the digit necrosis and eventual autoamputation.[33] A type B ablation can be performed in the office with a portable electrocautery device, under local anesthesia.

Ulnar Dimelia
Mirror hand is a rare duplication centered about the index finger. The hand has as many as eight fingers but

6: Pediatrics

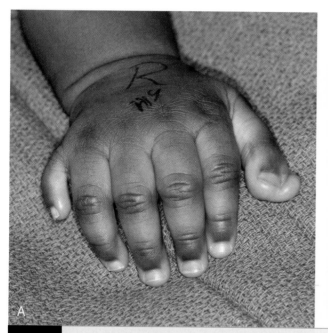

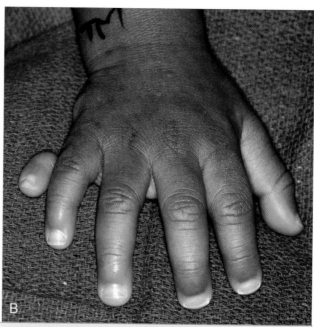

Figure 17 Photographs showing a type A **(A)** and a type B **(B)** postaxial duplication. A well-formed digit should be excised in the operating room, but a vestigial digit with a small skin and vascular pedicle can be excised in the office. (Courtesy of Shriners Hospital for Children, Philadelphia, PA.)

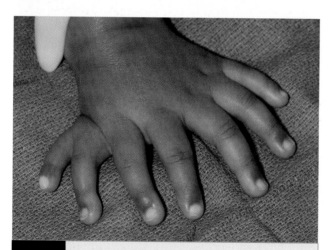

Figure 18 Photograph showing the classic appearance of ulnar dimelia (mirror hand). The ulna-side structures are duplicated, and the thumb is absent. (Courtesy of Shriners Hospital for Children, Philadelphia, PA.)

no thumb (**Figure 18**). The radius is absent, and two ulnae are present instead. Duplication of the ZPA is thought to lead to the formation of two ulnar halves of the limb. The treatment involves pollicization of the best radial digit and ablation of the rest to create a thumb and four fingers. The supranumerary digits often yield viable tendons for transfer, which may be needed particularly if wrist extensors are absent. The elbow, forearm, and wrist motion is limited because of the double ulnae.

Overgrowth

Macrodactyly

Overgrowth of one or more digits occurs sporadically or as part of neurofibromatosis or Klippel-Trenaunay-Weber, Ollier-Maffucci, or Proteus syndrome. All components of the digit are enlarged, commonly with angular deformity and joint contracture (**Figure 19**). In static macrodactyly, a congenital finger enlargement grows proportionally to the other digits. Progressive macrodactyly is more common. The finger is of normal size at birth but exhibits disproportionate growth that leads to worsening joint stiffness. Type I is the most common, with fatty infiltration of the median nerve within the carpal tunnel extending distally to the digital nerves. Type II is associated with neurofibromatosis and skeletal enlargement with osteochondromas. Type II is characterized by digital hyperostosis, periarticular osteochondromas, stiff joints, and no nerve hypertrophy. Type IV is macrodactyly in the setting of hemihypertrophy of the entire limb.[34] Debulking procedures can lead to further joint stiffness and may need to be repeated. Closing-wedge osteotomies through the physis can halt longitudinal growth and correct angulation of the digit, but they do not arrest appositional growth and may result in further joint stiffness. Ray amputation may be the most viable option for a stiff finger that interferes with functioning.

Constriction Band Syndrome

Strands of the amnionic membrane can detach from the innermost layer of the placenta and entrap the develop-

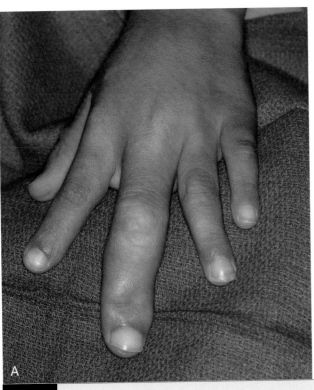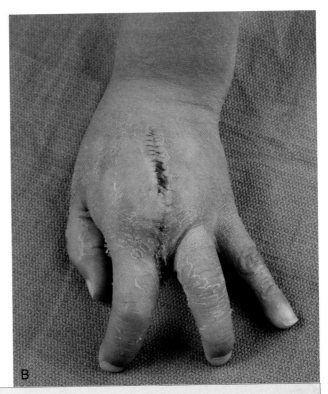

Figure 19 Photographs showing macrodactyly of the long finger. **A**, The typical angulation and joint contractures can be seen. **B**, Ray amputation and index transposition yielded a more functional hand. (Courtesy of Shriners Hospital for Children, Philadelphia, PA.)

ing fetus. The result is constricting rings that can lead to amputations and syndactyly. Facial or cranial clefts can result if the fetus swallows these bands. There is no consensus as to the nomenclature, and the phenomenon has been called constriction ring syndrome, amnionic band syndrome, Streeter dysplasia, or annular constriction rings. Differentiating amnionic disruption sequence from symbrachydactyly or a central deficiency can be difficult. Constriction bands and acrosyndactyly are pathognomonic (**Figure 20**). Inclusion cysts sometimes are seen at the level of an amputation. An impending amputation in a neonate is a surgical emergency. The constriction should be released with Z-plasties as soon as possible. In contrast, a minor band that does not place the limb at risk can be observed, and typically it requires no treatment.

Brachial Plexus Injury

The incidence of neonatal brachial plexus palsy is approximately 1 to 2 per 1,000 live births, although it may be declining despite an overall increase in fetal weight at term delivery. In addition to fetal macrosomia, the risk factors include prolonged or difficult labor, shoulder dystocia, breech presentation, forceful extraction with the aid of vacuum or forceps, a uterine anomaly, and a previous child with a brachial plexus injury. A caesarian delivery decreases but does not eliminate the risk of a brachial plexus injury.

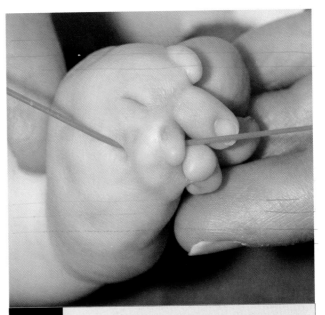

Figure 20 Photograph showing vessel loops through the remnant of the web space in a child with acrosyndactyly from constriction band syndrome. (Courtesy of Shriners Hospital for Children, Philadelphia, PA.)

The right side is most often injured. An upper trunk injury at C5-C6 is most common (Erb palsy). An extended upper plexus lesion involves C7, and a global

6: Pediatrics

Table 5

Patterns of Brachial Plexus Injuries

Pattern	Involved Nerve Roots	Primary Deficiency
Erb-Duchenne lesion Upper brachial plexus	C5-C6	Shoulder abduction and external rotation Elbow flexion
Extended Erb lesion Upper and middle plexus	C5-C7	Shoulder abduction and external rotation Elbow flexion Elbow and finger extension
Dejerine-Klumpke lesion Lower brachial plexus	C8-T1	Hand intrinsic muscles Finger flexors
Total or global lesion Entire brachial plexus	C5-T1	Entire extremity

plexus injury continues to C8-T1 (**Table 5**). An isolated lower plexus injury (Klumpke palsy) is rare. Involvement of the lower plexus can result in a Horner syndrome, characterized by ptosis, miosis, enophthalmos, and anhidrosis. Most neonatal palsies are neurapraxic injuries that improve within 2 months. Axonometric injuries undergo Wallerian degeneration and require nerve regeneration within an intact nerve sheath. Functional recovery of elbow flexion by age 4 to 6 months indicates that at least a portion of the nerve is in continuity. Limited or absent elbow flexion at age 6 months suggests a neurotmetic injury. Because the nerves have been disrupted, spontaneous recovery in the long term is unlikely.

Patients with a neurotmetic rupture require excision of the neuroma and cable grafting of the defect with autograft nerve (most commonly the sural nerve). Direct repair usually is not possible. Nerve root avulsion from the spinal cord is a preganglionic injury and is not repairable by any means. Nerve grafting from viable roots and/or delayed tendon transfers are required to improve function. An avulsion injury should be suspected if the child has phrenic nerve dysfunction with an elevated hemidiaphragm on inspiratory imaging, Horner syndrome, or scapular winging.

Incomplete recovery in the shoulder typically favors the C6-C7 innervated internal rotators and adductors over the C5-C6 innervated external rotators and abductors. Untreated, a posterior moment is placed across the glenohumeral joint, resulting in anterior capsular and muscular tightness, posterior glenohumeral subluxation, posterior glenoid version, and eventually formation of a pseudoglenoid on the posterior surface of the scapula. The process is similar to that of developmental dysplasia of the hip joint.

The treatment begins during the neonatal period with passive abduction and external rotation stretching by the caretaker at every diaper change. If the shoulder contracture persists after stretching, botulinum toxin injections can be used. Late-appearing or resistant contractures require an open or arthroscopic glenohumeral reduction, with or without tendon transfers. A humeral rotational osteotomy can be considered to orient the forearm into a better position for feeding and grooming.

Developmental Conditions

Pediatric Trigger Thumb

Trigger thumb in children is no longer believed to be congenital, but its etiology is unknown.[35-37] At age 1 year, the prevalence is 3 per 1,000 children.[36] Although the rate of spontaneous resolution is undefined, surgical release remains the mainstay of treatment.[37-40]

Trigger Finger

Trigger finger in adults and trigger thumb in children and adults respond predictably to A1 pulley release, but trigger finger in children does not. Unlike pediatric trigger thumb, in pediatric trigger finger there is often an anatomic variance that leads to the triggering effect. Abnormal interconnections between the superficialis and profundus tendons have been implicated. Surgical release requires a more extensive exposure than for an adult trigger finger and may require exposure of the entire flexor system in the hand and finger. Release of the A1 pulley with resection of one slip of the flexor digitorum superficialis tendon has been recommended.[41]

Madelung Deformity

The cause of Madelung deformity is controversial. The characteristic feature is undergrowth of the volar-ulnar corner of the distal radius (**Figure 21**). Tension from a restraining Vickers ligament may limit growth at that portion of the distal radius.[42] Most incidences are sporadic, but mutations in the *SHOX* gene can lead to Leri-Weill dyschondrosteosis, in which the patient has short stature, mesomelic upper and lower limb shortening, and Madelung deformity. Mutations can occur spontaneously or be inherited via autosomal dominant transmission. Girls are more often affected than boys.[43] A similar deformity can result from repetitive ballistic loading of the wrist and is common in young female gymnasts.

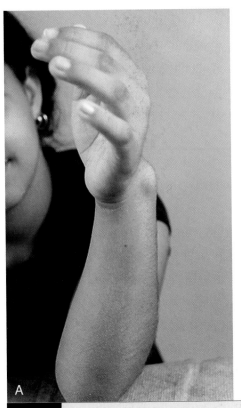
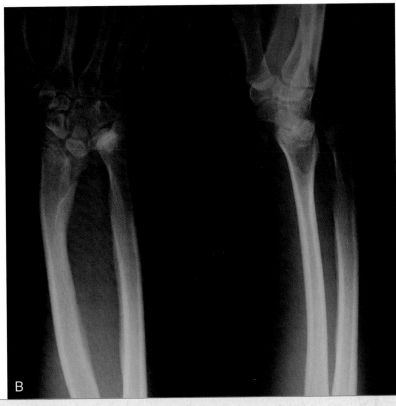

| Figure 21 | Photograph (A) and AP and lateral radiographs (B) showing Madelung deformity. (Courtesy of Shriners Hospital for Children, Philadelphia, PA.) |

Madelung deformity usually requires no treatment, and even a gross deformity is well tolerated. Early release of the Vickers ligament and physiolysis has been recommended to prevent worsening of the deformity and allow some spontaneous correction.[44] Gymnasts should cease weight-bearing activities until the pain resolves. The indications for surgical correction include pain and aesthetic concerns. A dome osteotomy can correct the increased tilt and inclination and can restore a more neutral ulnar variance.[45] If the child's symptoms are primarily from ulnocarpal impaction, ulnar shortening may be added to a radial osteotomy or used primarily.[46,47]

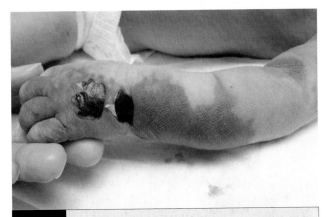

| Figure 22 | Photograph showing neonatal compartment syndrome, with the pathognomonic skin lesion and peripheral ischemia. (Courtesy of Shriners Hospital for Children, Philadelphia, PA.) |

Vasculocutaneous Catastrophe of the Newborn (Intrauterine Compartment Syndrome)

A neonatal compartment syndrome always is accompanied by a skin lesion over the affected limb (**Figure 22**).[48] The telltale signs usually are visible at birth, although they often are missed. The limb is edematous with tip necrosis or ischemia. If the compartments are not released, the limb progresses to necrosis and digital contractures. The late appearance of this syndrome is typical of a Volkmann ischemic contracture. The differential diagnosis includes amnionic disruption sequence (identified by the presence of a band proximal to the level of the ischemia or necrosis), cord strangulation, arterial thrombosis, and cellulitis. Emergency compartment release is the only treatment in the acute setting. A child with a late-appearing syndrome may benefit from release of the entire flexor-pronator origin, neurolysis, and débridement of necrotic tissue.

6: Pediatrics

Annotated References

1. Bamshad M, Watkins WS, Dixon ME, et al: Reconstructing the history of human limb development: Lessons from birth defects. *Pediatr Res* 1999;45(3):291-299.

2. Daluiski A, Yi SE, Lyons KM: The molecular control of upper extremity development: Implications for congenital hand anomalies. *J Hand Surg Am* 2001;26(1):8-22.

3. Riddle RD, Tabin C: How limbs develop. *Sci Am* 1999;280(2):74-79.

4. Lyons K, Ezaki M: Molecular regulation of limb growth. *J Bone Joint Surg Am* 2009;91(suppl 4):47-52.

   The known molecular regulators of limb development are concisely and clearly reviewed. The clinical sequelae of breakdowns in the regulatory pathways are considered.

5. Barrow JR, Thomas KR, Boussadia-Zahui O, et al: Ectodermal Wnt3/beta-catenin signaling is required for the establishment and maintenance of the apical ectodermal ridge. *Genes Dev* 2003;17(3):394-409.

6. Goldfarb CA, Wall L, Manske PR: Radial longitudinal deficiency: The incidence of associated medical and musculoskeletal conditions. *J Hand Surg Am* 2006;31(7):1176-1182.

7. Auerbach AD, Rogatko A, Schroeder-Kurth TM: International Fanconi Anemia Registry: Relation of clinical symptoms to diepoxybutane sensitivity. *Blood* 1989;73(2):391-396.

8. Lourie GM, Lins RE: Radial longitudinal deficiency: A review and update. *Hand Clin* 1998;14(1):85-99.

9. Hall JG: Thrombocytopenia and absent radius (TAR) syndrome. *J Med Genet* 1987;24(2):79-83.

10. Klopocki E, Schulze H, Strauss G, et al: Complex inheritance pattern resembling autosomal recessive inheritance involving a microdeletion in thrombocytopenia-absent radius syndrome. *Am J Hum Genet* 2007;80(2):232-240.

    A microdeletion of chromosome 1q21.1 was consistently found in 30 patients with TAR syndrome. The deletion occurred de novo in 25% of cases.

11. Brassington AM, Sung SS, Toydemir RM, et al: Expressivity of Holt-Oram syndrome is not predicted by TBX5 genotype. *Am J Hum Genet* 2003;73(1):74-85.

12. Goldfarb CA, Murtha YM, Gordon JE, Manske PR: Soft-tissue distraction with a ring external fixator before centralization for radial longitudinal deficiency. *J Hand Surg Am* 2006;31(6):952-959.

13. Sabharwal S, Finuoli AL, Ghobadi F: Pre-centralization soft tissue distraction for Bayne type IV congenital radial deficiency in children. *J Pediatr Orthop* 2005;25(3):377-381.

14. Pickford MA, Scheker LR: Distraction lengthening of the ulna in radial club hand using the Ilizarov technique. *J Hand Surg Br* 1998;23(2):186-191.

15. Kozin SH, Weiss AA, Webber JB, Betz RR, Clancy M, Steel HH: Index finger pollicization for congenital aplasia or hypoplasia of the thumb. *J Hand Surg Am* 1992;17(5):880-884.

16. Clark DI, Chell J, Davis TR: Pollicisation of the index finger: A 27-year follow-up study. *J Bone Joint Surg Br* 1998;80(4):631-635.

17. Manske PR, McCaroll HR Jr: Index finger pollicization for a congenitally absent or nonfunctioning thumb. *J Hand Surg Am* 1985;10(5):606-613.

18. Cole RJ, Manske PR: Classification of ulnar deficiency according to the thumb and first web. *J Hand Surg Am* 1997;22(3):479-488.

19. Buss PW: Cleft hand/foot: Clinical and developmental aspects. *J Med Genet* 1994;31(9):726-730.

20. Flatt AE: Cleft hand and central defects, in Flatt AE, ed: *The Care of Congenital Hand Anomalies*, ed 2. St. Louis, MO, Quality Medical Publishing, 1994, pp 337-365.

21. Summerbell D: A quantitative analysis of the effect of excision of the AER from the chick limb-bud. *J Embryol Exp Morphol* 1974;32(3):651-660.

22. Radocha RF, Netscher D, Kleinert HE: Toe phalangeal grafts in congenital hand anomalies. *J Hand Surg Am* 1993;18(5):833-841.

23. Kay SP, Wiberg M: Toe to hand transfer in children: Part 1. Technical aspects. *J Hand Surg Br* 1996;21(6):723-734.

24. Dhalla R, Strecker W, Manske PR: A comparison of two techniques for digital distraction lengthening in skeletally immature patients. *J Hand Surg Am* 2001;26(4):603-610.

25. Goldfarb CA, Manske PR, Busa R, Mills J, Carter P, Ezaki M: Upper-extremity phocomelia reexamined: A longitudinal dysplasia. *J Bone Joint Surg Am* 2005;87(12):2639-2648.

26. Kozin SH: Syndactyly. *J Am Soc Surg Hand* 2001;1:1-13.

27. Engber WD, Flatt AE: Camptodactyly: An analysis of sixty-six patients and twenty-four operations. *J Hand Surg Am* 1977;2(3):216-224.

28. Burke F, Flatt A: Clinodactyly: A review of a series of cases. *Hand* 1979;11(3):269-280.

29. McIntyre JD, Benson MK: An aetiological classification for developmental synostoses at the elbow. *J Pediatr Orthop B* 2002;11(4):313-319.

30. Ogino T, Hikino K: Congenital radio-ulnar synostosis: Compensatory rotation around the wrist and rotation osteotomy. *J Hand Surg Br* 1987;12(2):173-178.

31. Kanaya F, Ibaraki K: Mobilization of a congenital proximal radioulnar synostosis with use of a free vascularized fascio-fat graft. *J Bone Joint Surg Am* 1998;80(8): 1186-1192.

32. Wassel HD: The results of surgery for polydactyly of the thumb: A review. *Clin Orthop Relat Res* 1969;64:175-193.

33. Watson BT, Hennrikus WL: Postaxial type-B polydactyly: Prevalence and treatment. *J Bone Joint Surg Am* 1997;79(1):65-68.

34. O'Rahilly R: Morphological patterns in limb deficiencies and duplications. *Am J Anat* 1951;89(2):135-193.

35. Slakey JB, Hennrikus WL: Acquired thumb flexion contracture in children: Congenital trigger thumb. *J Bone Joint Surg Br* 1996;78(3):481-483.

36. Kikuchi N, Ogino T: Incidence and development of trigger thumb in children. *J Hand Surg Am* 2006;31(4): 541-543.

37. Rodgers WB, Waters PM: Incidence of trigger digits in newborns. *J Hand Surg Am* 1994;19(3):364-368.

38. Dinham JM, Meggitt BF: Trigger thumbs in children: A review of the natural history and indications for treatment in 105 patients. *J Bone Joint Surg Br* 1974;56(1): 153-155.

39. McAdams TR, Moneim MS, Omer GE Jr: Long-term follow-up of surgical release of the A(1) pulley in childhood trigger thumb. *J Pediatr Orthop* 2002;22(1): 41-43.

40. Skov O, Bach A, Hammer A: Trigger thumbs in children: A follow-up study of 37 children below 15 years of age. *J Hand Surg Br* 1990;15(4):466-467.

41. Bae DS, Sodha S, Waters PM: Surgical treatment of the pediatric trigger finger. *J Hand Surg Am* 2007;32(7): 1043-1047.

   A retrospective study of 18 consecutive patients found a 91% resolution of trigger fingers in children treated with A1 pulley release and partial flexor digitorum superficialis resection. Level of evidence: IV.

42. Stehling C, Langer M, Nassenstein I, Bachmann R, Heindel W, Vieth V: High resolution 3.0 Tesla MR imaging findings in patients with bilateral Madelung's deformity. *Surg Radiol Anat* 2009;31(7):551-557.

   MRI of three patients with Madelung deformity revealed a stout Vickers ligament and pyramidization of the proximal carpal row, along with an anomalous hypertrophied and elongated volar radiotriquetral ligament.

43. Huber C, Rosilio M, Munnich A, Cormier-Daire V; French SHOX GeNeSIS Module: High incidence of SHOX anomalies in individuals with short stature. *J Med Genet* 2006;43(9):735-739.

44. Vickers D, Nielsen G: Madelung deformity: Surgical prophylaxis (physiolysis) during the late growth period by resection of the dyschondrosteosis lesion. *J Hand Surg Br* 1992;17(4):401-407.

45. Harley BJ, Brown C, Cummings K, Carter PR, Ezaki M: Volar ligament release and distal radius dome osteotomy for correction of Madelung's deformity. *J Hand Surg Am* 2006;31(9):1499-1506.

46. Salon A, Serra M, Pouliquen JC: Long-term follow-up of surgical correction of Madelung's deformity with conservation of the distal radioulnar joint in teenagers. *J Hand Surg Br* 2000;25(1):22-25.

47. Bruno RJ, Blank JE, Ruby LK, Cassidy C, Cohen G, Bergfield TG: Treatment of Madelung's deformity in adults by ulna reduction osteotomy. *J Hand Surg Am* 2003;28(3):421-426.

48. Ragland R III, Moukoko D, Ezaki M, Carter PR, Mills J: Forearm compartment syndrome in the newborn: Report of 24 cases. *J Hand Surg Am* 2005;30(5):997-1003.

6: Pediatrics

Chapter 56

Spine Trauma and Disorders: Pediatrics

Anthony Scaduto, MD   Daniel Hedequist, MD

Congenital Anomalies

Congenital abnormalities of the spine are caused by an embryologic insult that occurs between the 8th and 12th weeks of gestation. These anomalies traditionally are classified as a failure of formation, a failure of segmentation, or mixed. In clinical practice, defining the anomaly and trying to predict growth potential and potential curve progression have useful treatment implications. Plain radiographs remain the simplest means of classifying congenital spine deformities. Three-dimensional CT provides greater clarity when defining specific anomalies (**Figure 1**). In a patient undergoing surgery, the anomaly is best studied and classified using three-dimensional CT.[1] Routine use of CT is not warranted in patients with a nonprogressive deformity that does not require treatment.

The spinal column develops at the same embryologic stage as the spinal cord and organ systems, including the genitourinary and cardiac systems. A spinal cord abnormality (tethered cord, diastematomyelia, or Chiari malformation) is present in as many as 30% of patients with congenital scoliosis. Patients who have associated cutaneous signs of dysraphism, a neurologic abnormality, or curve progression requiring surgery should undergo screening of the spinal axis. The genitourinary system should be evaluated with screening ultrasonography of the kidneys, ureters, and bladder; the cardiac system should be evaluated with a thorough cardiac examination, with imaging if necessary.

The prognosis depends on the anomaly and its potential for progression. A wedge vertebra, unsegmented hemivertebra, or block vertebra has little potential for progression and requires only minimal observation. A simple deformity such as a hemivertebra (with healthy disks above and below) has a greater potential for progression and should be carefully observed. A tether to growth (a failure of segmentation) has a significant tendency to cause rapid and severe growth abnormalities including unilateral bars and bars associated with multiple concave rib fusions.

The surgical treatment of congenital scoliosis or kyphosis revolves around early diagnosis and treatment, before the development of spinal decompensation. In order of importance, the goals of surgery are to prevent progression, safely correct the deformity, and maintain flexibility and balance. The surgical treatment ranges from in situ fusion to convex epiphysiodesis to hemivertebra resection. Fusion and instrumentation can be effectively done with spine instrumentation and allograft, even in very young patients.[2] The use of neurologic monitoring through somatosensory- and motor-evoked potentials is paramount because of the great risk of neurologic injury during surgery for a congenital spine deformity.

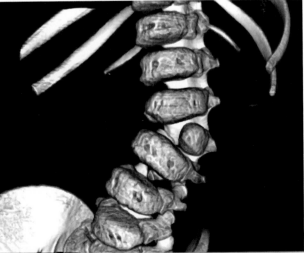

Figure 1   Three-dimensional CT of an isolated hemivertebra. The disk spaces above and below the hemivertebra can be clearly seen. A fully segmented hemivertebra is associated with a high risk of progressive scoliosis.

Dr. Scaduto or an immediate family member is a member of a speakers' bureau or has made paid presentations on behalf of Abbott and Zimmer; serves as a paid consultant to or is an employee of Abbott and Zimmer; and has received research or institutional support from DePuy, a Johnson & Johnson Company. Dr. Hedequist or an immediate family member is a member of a speakers' bureau or has made paid presentations on behalf of Medtronic Sofamor Danek.

6: Pediatrics

Congenital spine deformities occasionally are seen in concert with congenital rib fusions. The disorder can lead to a hypoplastic chest on one side, with resultant respiratory decompensation (called thoracic insufficiency). The interrelationship between the congenital deformed spine and the deformed chest is well recognized, and it has treatment ramifications. The development of the vertical expandable prosthetic titanium rib (VEPTR) has allowed improvement in spine growth, curve control, and expansion of the hypoplastic chest in some patients with congenital spine deformities. The management of severe deformities continues to evolve, and long-term follow-up is needed to determine the efficacy of the VEPTR.

Klippel-Feil Syndrome

A patient with Klippel-Feil syndrome has congenital cervical fusions as well as a low posterior hairline and a short neck secondary to the cervical fusions. Klippel-Feil syndrome sometimes is erroneously diagnosed as congenital muscular torticollis because of the head tilt and limited motion that characterizes both conditions. As many as a third of patients with Klippel-Feil syndrome also have an elevated scapula (Sprengel deformity) or partial hearing loss. In general, patients require little orthopaedic intervention beyond counseling to avoid activities that place the neck at high risk, such as football, gymnastics, and trampoline use. Some pediatric patients develop instability or degeneration of adjacent normal, unfused cervical spine segments because of increased biomechanical stress. These patients can be treated with an instrumented cervical arthrodesis of the affected spine area.[3]

Os Odontoideum

Os odontoideum is an anomaly of the axis that frequently appears during childhood with neck pain, transient paresthesias, or myelopathy. This disorder is believed to result from an unrecognized fracture of C2 in early childhood, with subsequent instability caused by nonunion. An os odontoideum is best recognized on CT; it is characterized by an ossicle at the top of the dens above the C1-C2 articulation, with sclerotic borders. Plain radiographs in flexion and extension are used to document the associated C1-C2 instability. Half of patients with an os odontoideum have myelopathy, and MRI frequently shows signal changes in the spinal cord (**Figure 2**). The treatment of os odontoideum is surgical. Patients treated nonsurgically may develop neurologic signs. The surgery entails a C1-C2 posterior arthrodesis using autograft wires, transarticular screws, or a C1-C2 screw rod construct.[4]

Idiopathic Scoliosis

Idiopathic scoliosis is a curvature of the spine of unknown etiology. The three categories, based on the patient's age at diagnosis, are infantile (before age 3 years), juvenile (age 3 to 10 years), and adolescent (age 11 years or older). Infantile scoliosis more commonly affects boys than girls. Most infantile curves are left thoracic, with little rotation in the spine, and most resolve spontaneously over time with no treatment. The incidence of a neural axis abnormality is higher in infantile scoliosis than in adolescent scoliosis, and therefore the physical examination should focus on detecting any neurologic signs and any signs of spinal dysraphism. Analysis of the coronal radiographs allows measurement of the Cobb angle, the rib-vertebral angle difference of Mehta, and rib overlap of the apical vertebral body. These measurements reveal the presence of spinal rotation and determine whether the child has structural scoliosis, which is most likely to progress. Untreated progressive infantile scoliosis can lead to restrictive lung disease, cor pulmonale, and early death.

Treatment usually is reserved for a progressive infantile curve of more than 25°. A thoracolumbosacral orthosis or derotation casting can be used. The curve can be completely resolved with casting in children younger than 20 months who have a Cobb angle of less than 60°.[5] Derotation casting often is unsuccessful if the curve is more than 60° or the child is older than 20 months. These patients are best treated surgically with a growing rod spine construct. The growing-rod or VEPTR method allows spine and lung growth until definitive fusion can be performed.[6]

Juvenile scoliosis is more common in girls than in boys and tends to appear as a right-side thoracic curvature. The incidence of spinal dysraphism in these patients is higher than that of adolescent scoliosis. Large curves require MRI screening of the spinal axis. A progressive curve with a Cobb angle of more than 25° is best treated with bracing either for 18 hours a day or at nighttime. Surgical intervention is reserved for patients with a Cobb angle of more than 50° (**Figure 3**). Depending on the size and age of the patient, the surgical treatment may be definitive instrumented fusion, or fusion may be delayed in favor of initial treatment with growing rods.

Adolescent idiopathic scoliosis is the most common type of scoliosis. Most patients are healthy girls. The likelihood of curve progression depends on the size of the Cobb angle and the amount of remaining growth. The amount of remaining growth can be correlated with a left hand-and-wrist radiograph to determine bone age. The stages of the adolescent growth spurt were recently correlated with the bone age.[7] These findings are used to determine whether the best treatment is observation, bracing, or surgery. Observation is appropriate for a skeletally immature patient with a Cobb angle of less than 25° or for a skeletally mature patient with a Cobb angle of more than 25° and a curve of less than 50° in the thoracic spine and less than 35° to 40° in the thoracolumbar or lumbar spine.

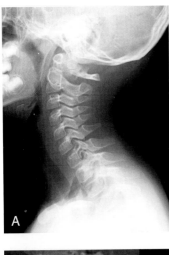

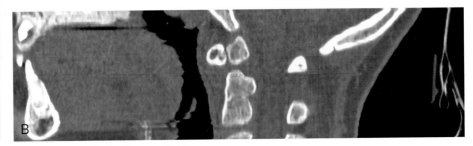

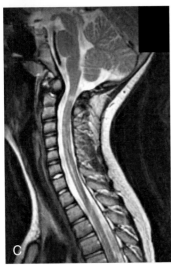

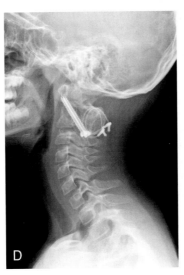

Figure 2   Os odontoideum in an 11-year-old gymnast who reported arm weakness after a fall. **A,** Lateral radiograph of the cervical spine. Note the position of the anterior ring of the atlas and its relation to the body of the axis. **B,** CT showing a well-demarcated os odontoideum and its anatomic location. **C,** MRI showing cord signal changes at the level of the os odontoideum. **D,** Lateral radiograph 1 year after fusion with transarticular screws and iliac crest bone graft and cable grafting.

Brace treatment to prevent curve progression is generally warranted in a child with significant remaining growth and a curve of 25° to 40°. Brace use is recommended for 18 to 22 hours a day, although some braces are designed for nighttime use only. Ideally, brace use should lead to a 50% correction of the curve. Brace use is less likely to be successful if the in-brace correction is poor; there is hypokyphosis; or the patient is male, obese, or noncompliant. A multicenter randomized brace study (the BrAIST study [www.clinicaltrials.gov]) is under way to determine the efficacy of brace use. Idiopathic curves larger than 50° are at risk for progression even after skeletal maturity is achieved. Instrumented fusion can improve the cosmetic deformity and stabilize pulmonary function. The Lenke classification is used to identify the major structural curve and any minor curves.[8] The major curve must be included in the instrumented fusion. The decision to include a minor curve depends on curve flexibility, as determined from side-bending radiographs, and the sagittal alignment of the spine on a lateral radiograph. The fusion should extend sufficiently distal to ensure sagittal and coronal balance, but otherwise it should be limited as much as possible to preserve motion.

The surgical options include an open anterior fusion with instrumentation, a thoracoscopic fusion with instrumentation, a posterior fusion with instrumentation, and a circumferential fusion with instrumentation. An open anterior procedure with instrumentation is best performed for a thoracolumbar curve with a normal sagittal profile. This procedure is ideal if levels can be spared by performing an anterior instrumented fusion. Thoracoscopic instrumentation and fusion is efficacious and associated with improved subjective patient outcomes.[9] The instrumentation choices for posterior segmental fixation include hooks, wires, cables, and pedicle screws. The off-label use of segmental pedicle screw fixation has improved coronal plane correction in posterior instrumented fusion, but it has not yet been established whether the additional coronal correction will improve the long-term outcome. Segmental screw fixation has allowed many large curves to be managed effectively without an anterior release[10] (**Figure 3**).

Neurologic monitoring is paramount during every procedure for spine deformity. Standard monitoring should include detection of changes in somatosensory- and motor-evoked potentials. Motor-evoked potentials in particular can provide an excellent warning of im-

6: Pediatrics

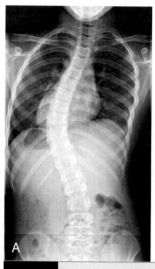
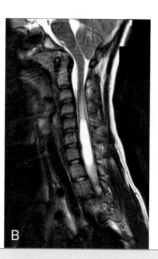
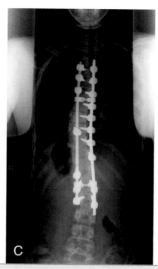
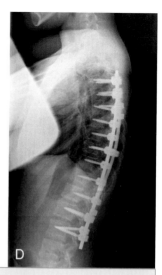

Figure 3 An atypical left-side thoracic curve in an 8-year-old girl who reported headaches. **A,** AP radiograph. Spinal dysraphism is more common in juvenile scoliosis than it is in adolescent scoliosis. MRI screening of the spinal axis is required for a curve requiring intervention. **B,** MRI showing the presence of a Chiari malformation and spinal cord syrinx. The curve progressed despite Chiari decompression and bracing. AP **(C)** and lateral **(D)** radiographs showing definitive fusion with segmental screw fixation.

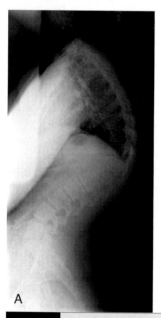
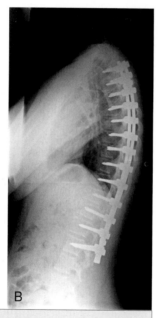

Figure 4 A 14-year-old girl with Scheuermann kyphosis. Lateral radiographs before **(A)** and after **(B)** posterior Ponte osteotomies and segmental pedicle screw fixation and fusion.

pending spinal cord dysfunction.[11] Triggered electromyography can aid the surgeon in determining the safety of placement for thoracic pedicle screws.

Scheuermann Kyphosis

The most common type of structural kyphosis in adolescents is Scheuermann kyphosis, which can have different effects in the thoracic, thoracolumbar, and lumbar spine. Although the exact etiology is unknown, the result is an abnormality of the end plate apophysis that leads to vertebral wedging, Schmorl nodes, and sagittal plane kyphosis. In the thoracic spine, Scheuermann kyphosis is radiographically defined as three consecutive vertebral bodies with wedging of more than 5° each. Thoracic Scheuermann kyphosis appears in adolescents as pain, deformity, or both. An affected individual has back pain during daily life and a tendency toward jobs that require less physical labor. A significant curve in early adolescence tends to progress during peak height velocity, leading to fixed thoracic kyphosis, increased lumbar lordosis with resultant sagittal imbalance, and cervical lordosis.

Brace treatment for Scheuermann kyphosis can be considered in a growing child who has 50° or more of thoracic kyphosis. A Milwaukee brace or a Boston brace is used, the latter with a superstructure to allow overall control of sagittal alignment. Surgical treatment is indicated if the patient has progressive deformity, back pain, and cosmetic deformity. The radiographic criterion usually is 75° of thoracic kyphosis or 40° of thoracolumbar kyphosis. The surgical treatment usually is posterior only, even for a severe deformity. Segmental pedicle screw fixation with foramen-to-foramen osteotomies is required to obtain correction[12] (**Figure 4**). Overcorrection of the deformity in the thoracic spine should be avoided because it can lead to proximal or distal junctional kyphosis. Neurologic deficits are more common with correction of kyphosis than correction of scoliosis, and monitoring with somatosensory- and motor-evoked potentials is necessary.

The term atypical Scheuermann kyphosis usually refers to end plate irregularities, vertebral wedging, and loss of alignment in the lumbar spine. Atypical Scheuermann kyphosis can cause back pain and discomfort during adolescence, especially in active patients. The resultant spasms and hamstring tightness can be treated with physical therapy, nonsteroidal anti-inflammatory drugs (NSAIDs), and occasionally bracing. The disorder is self-limiting; usually the symptoms resolve after growth is complete, with no long-term consequences.

Spondylolysis and Spondylolisthesis

The term spondylolysis refers to a fracture or defect of the pars interarticularis. This injury is a common cause of low back pain in children and especially in adolescent athletes. Spondylolysis is common among gymnasts, who are subjected to many hyperextension forces. The symptoms include activity-related back pain without a true radicular component. Usually the pain is nonradiating and increases with hyperextension because of impingement by the facet joint immediately above the fracture region. The diagnosis can be made using plain radiographs, although subsequent single-photon emission CT bone scanning or CT may be required. The pars fracture can be acute, but a chronic defect should be suspected if CT reveals wide fracture lines and sclerosis of the fracture edges. In general, the goal of treatment is to resolve the symptoms. Nonsurgical treatment focuses on physical therapy to strengthen the core and relieve any associated hamstring or hip flexor tightness. NSAIDs are useful for reducing any acute inflammation, and bracing can minimize repetitive hyperextension forces that can aggravate the condition. Although the rate of defect healing with nonsurgical treatment is only 28%, 83% of patients were found to have symptom improvement.[13] A patient who has no symptom relief after significant nonsurgical treatment may be a candidate for a localized fusion (if the pars fracture is at the last lumbar vertebra), or for a surgical repair of the pars (if the fracture involves a more cephalad lumbar vertebra).

Spondylolisthesis is the anterior displacement of a vertebral segment relative to the next adjacent vertebral level. Spondylolisthesis develops from a pars defect or a congenital anomaly of the posterior elements. This condition sometimes is mild and self-limiting (low-grade spondylolisthesis), but it can cause significant back pain, neurologic symptoms, and cosmetic deformity (high-grade spondylolisthesis). The prognosis depends on the patient's age and the extent of vertebral subluxation at presentation. The slippage can be measured by calculating the slip angle or measuring the percentage of subluxation. Patients with low-grade spondylolisthesis can be treated nonsurgically, with plain radiographic follow-up every 6 to 12 months.

The surgical treatment of spondylolisthesis varies widely, depending on the overall deformity, the amount of slip, and the presence of neurologic symptoms. Patients with significant slippage usually develop neurologic symptoms similar to those of spinal stenosis. These patients require a posterior decompression, in which the posterior elements in the area of the slip are removed and the nerve roots are decompressed out to the foramina. Further progression of the slip is prevented by a fusion. Modern instrumentation techniques generally are used to provide stability to the arthrodesis bed and avoid casting. Partial surgical realignment may be indicated to improve the overall sagittal balance of the patient. Usually a realignment procedure entails anterior column support, sometimes in concert with a decompression, through a posterior interbody fusion with transpedicular segmental instrumentation. Spondylolisthesis also is discussed in chapter 50.

Back Pain

Back pain is uncommon in children younger than 12 years, but almost half of children have experienced an episode of low back pain by age 18 years.[14] A thorough patient history and examination are essential for identifying pathologic back pain, which is continuous, limits walking, or interferes with sleep. Pathologic back pain differs from benign, mechanical back pain, which usually is activity related and improves with rest. An exhaustive evaluation is not required for all children with back pain, and the diagnosis usually is made from plain radiographs only.[15] Spondylolysis and Scheuermann kyphosis are the common causes of pathologic back pain in children. Less common conditions include infection, neoplastic disorders, and juvenile arthritis. Laboratory studies (complete blood count, erythrocyte sedimentation rate, and C-reactive protein level), CT, MRI, or bone scanning may be necessary. MRI is best used if there is disk pathology or a neurologic finding. CT allows bony changes to be seen, as in spondylolysis or an osteoid osteoma. A technetium Tc 99m bone scan can allow detection of a tumor, infection, or fracture. Most patients with benign mechanical back pain respond to rest, NSAIDs, and a home training program or supervised physical therapy.[16] School-age children should be counseled on proper backpack use.

Pediatric Spine Trauma

Spine injuries are rare in children; only 1% of all pediatric injuries involve the spine. The most common causes of spine injury in children are motor vehicle crashes, falls, sports injuries, and child abuse. Injury patterns in young children differ from those of adults, in part because of the child's greater spine elasticity, head size, and horizontal facet orientation. The cervical spine is the most frequently injured region, but thoracic or lumbar spine injury becomes more common with increasing age.[17] In comparison to spine injuries in adolescents and adults, cord injury is more common and more lethal in children younger than 8 years, but the prognosis for recovery is better.[18] Upper cervical spine injury (occiput to C3) is more common than lower cervical spine injury in children younger than 8 years.[19]

A thorough examination is essential for any child with a spine injury because of the high incidence of associated injuries and noncontiguous spine trauma. In

6: Pediatrics

an unconscious child, the only sign of injury may be a palpable defect between spinous processes, facial bruising, or passenger restraint contusions. The examination can be challenging even if the child is conscious. As many as 20% of children with a spine fracture from blunt trauma have a normal initial examination, and therefore repeated examination is warranted.[20]

Anatomy and Radiographic Evaluation

The cervical, thoracic, and lumbar vertebral bodies develop from three primary ossification centers; the lateral ossification centers form each side of the neural arch, and the vertebral body arises from a central ossification center (**Figure 5**). The posterior arches fuse to each other by age 3 years, and the neural arch fuses to the body by age 7 years. Radiographic findings suggestive of injury in an adult may be within normal limits in a child. These findings include prevertebral soft-tissue thickening, an increased atlantodens interval, pseudosubluxation of C2-C3 or C3-C4, wedging of cervical vertebral bodies, and loss of cervical lordosis (**Table 1**).

The radiographic evaluation of a child suspected of having a spine injury begins with AP and lateral radiographs; if the child is older than 5 years, an open-mouth odontoid radiograph is added. Although CT of the entire cervical spine is routinely used to rule out injury in an adult, the use of CT as the primary imaging modality for cervical spine injury in children remains controversial.[21,22] On CT or a plain radiograph, a radiolucent synchondrosis can be mistaken for a fracture line. Conversely, a fracture through the physis may be overlooked. If the initial radiographic findings are equivocal, CT with three-dimensional reconstruction can accurately detect upper osseous cervical injuries. MRI is superior to CT for delineating the soft-tissue anatomy, and it alters the initial diagnosis based on plain radiography or CT in as many as two thirds of patients.[23,24] MRI is best reserved for patients who are unconscious, have neurologic findings or a suspicious mechanism of injury; or if a standard clinical and radiographic evaluation cannot be performed.

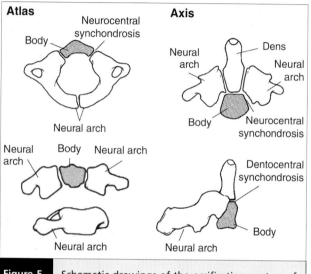

Figure 5 Schematic drawings of the ossification centers of the atlas and axis. (Adapted from Copley LA, Dormans JP: Cervical spine disorders in infants and children. *J Am Acad Orthop Surg* 1998; 6:205.)

Spinal Cord Injury Without Radiographic Abnormality

In as many as 34% of spinal cord injuries in children younger than 8 years, no abnormalities can be seen on the initial plain radiographs. Evidence of injury usually

---

Table 1

Pediatric Cervical Spine Characteristics That May Be Mistaken for a Sign of Injury

Radiographic Finding	Patient Age (Range, in Years)	Physiologic Limits
Wide atlantodens interval	0-8	≤5 mm Space available for cord ≥ 13 mm
Dentrocentral synchondrosis	0-7	Fusion line may be visible until age 11 years
Secondary ossification center at tip of dens	6-12	Appears around age 6 years Fuses with dens by age 12 years
C2-C3 or C3-C4 pseudosubluxation	0-8	<4 mm Smooth, contiguous posterior laminar line (Swischuk line)
Prevertebral soft-tissue swelling	0-8	<2/3 of adjacent vertebral width on lateral film Prevertebral tissue is enlarged in a crying child
Interspace angulation	0-8	Occurs in 16% of healthy children
Wedging of vertebral body	0-12	Vertebral bodies are ovoid at birth 7% of healthy children have a wedged C3 body
Absence of cervical lordosis	0-12	Occurs in 14% of healthy children

---

is apparent on MRI during the immediate postinjury period, but the MRI evidence is more specific after 48 hours. The soft-tissue abnormalities can be intraneural, as in cord edema or hematoma, or extraneural, as in longitudinal or interspinous ligament edema. Approximately 40% of children who have a spinal cord injury without radiographic abnormality (SCIWORA) completely recover, but 40% do not recover neurologic function and 20% have partial recovery. The rigidity of immobilization influences recovery. If stabilization is unachievable through external means (a collar or halo), surgical stabilization should be undertaken. Recurrence of injury was reported in 17% of patients with SCIWORA who had external immobilization lasting no more than 8 weeks, but it did not recur with immobilization for 12 weeks.[25]

Spine Fracture Management

Initial and Nonsurgical Management

The management of a cervical spine fracture begins with immobilization in a pediatric-size collar. The disproportionate head-to-torso ratio of young children can cause as much as 15° of cervical flexion in the supine position, even with a well-fitting cervical collar. Thus, transportation of children younger than 8 years requires a spine board with an occipital depression or sufficient thoracic elevation to align the cervical and thoracic spines.

The National Acute Spinal Cord Injury Study protocol recommends administering methylprednisolone sodium succinate for 23 hours within 3 hours of a spinal cord injury.[26] The drug is administered for 48 hours if it is started 3 to 8 hours after the injury. The initial bolus dose of 30 mg/kg over 15 minutes is followed by a maintenance infusion of 5.4 mg/kg/h. Few data exist on the use of methylprednisolone for pediatric patients, and its use as a standard treatment for spinal cord injury has recently been questioned.[27,28]

Spine fractures in children often can be managed nonsurgically because of the child's bone quality and excellent potential for remodeling. Depending on the level of injury, halo vest immobilization and a thoracic lumbosacral orthosis may maintain spine alignment and prevent instability during healing.

Pediatric Spine Instrumentation

Brace management may be insufficient to impart stability after a severe pediatric spine injury. Ideally, surgery with instrumentation should restore stability, enhance fusion, and lead to as little loss in mobility as possible. Pediatric cervical spine instrumentation in the past consisted of wire constructs augmented with halo vest immobilization. There is growing interest in applying the rigid fixation techniques developed for adults to pediatric patients. In the cervical spine, the options include occipital plates, transarticular screws (C1-C2), pedicle screws, lateral mass screws, pars screws, and intralaminar screws (**Figure 6**). Several recent studies found that these techniques can be safely applied in children as young as 3 years. Proper surgical planning is essential, including CT to confirm favorable bone size and rule out atypical anatomy.[4,29,30] Pedicle screw fixation is a powerful means of reducing and stabilizing fractures of the thoracic and lumbar spine in children. Its advantages include the possibility of limiting fusion to one or two levels above and below the fracture and reducing or eliminating the need for a brace. Additional study is needed to determine whether the use of pedicle screws that cross an open neurocentral synchondrosis in a young child can lead to iatrogenic spinal stenosis or scoliosis.[31,32]

Cervical Spine Fractures

Occipitoatlantal Dislocation

Occipitoatlantal injuries often are fatal. If the child survives the initial injury, complete tetraplegia is likely, with ventilator dependence. Identifying this injury can be difficult. A Powers ratio higher than 1 or lower than 0.55 is indicative, respectively, of anterior or posterior displacement of the occiput on the atlas. Immobilization without traction (in a halo or Minerva cast) is essential to initial treatment. Definitive stabilization requires fusion of the occiput to C1 or C2.

Atlas Fracture

A burst fracture of C1 (the Jefferson fracture) is rare but may be underappreciated in children.[33] An atlas fracture occurs when an axial load of the head is transmitted through the occipital condyles to the lateral masses at C1. This injury is difficult to appreciate on radiographs. CT can be useful for assessing the injury or confirming healing. Neurologic injury is unlikely. The treatment usually is simple immobilization with a halo vest or cast for 2 to 3 months.

Odontoid Fracture

An odontoid fracture in a child younger than 7 years occurs through the synchondrosis at the base of the dens. In older children, odontoid fractures are similar to those in adults. The common symptoms are neck and occipital pain or a limited cervical range of motion. Neurologic deficits are rare. Plain radiographs may show an anterior angulation and translation of the odontoid, but spontaneous reduction is possible and may lead to a missed diagnosis. CT or MRI should be used if the diagnosis is questionable.

The injury heals well with adequate immobilization for 8 to 10 weeks. The choice of a rigid collar or a halo vest depends on the stability of the fracture and the size of the patient. Anterior displacement is reduced with mild extension and posterior translation when the halo is applied. Halo pin insertion into the thin calvaria of a young child is most safely accomplished by using 8 to 12 pins and limiting the insertional torque of each pin. In general, the insertional torque of each halo pin should equal the age of the child (for example, 4 ft-lb of torque are used for a 4-year-old child); the upper limit is 8 ft-lb. A thermoplastic Minerva body jacket can be used as an alternative to halo immobilization in a very young child.[34] This device avoids the possibility

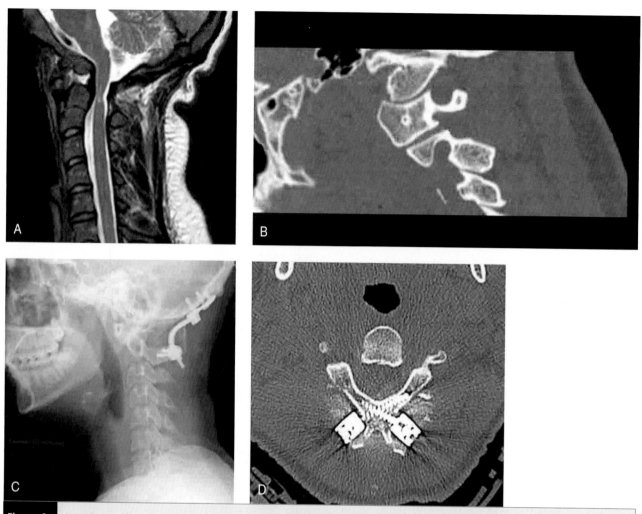

Figure 6 Imaging studies of a 17-year-old girl. **A,** MRI showing an injury to the upper cervical spine resulting from a motor vehicle crash and complicated by the presence of congenital stenosis at C1. **B,** CT showing a high-riding vertebral artery at C2, which precluded the use of transarticular C1-C2 screws. CT is essential in planning cervical instrumentation in children. Lateral radiograph (**C**) and CT (**D**) showing occiput-to-C2 fusion with an occipital plate and intralaminar C2 screws.

of pin complications and pin artifact on MRI or CT, but it allows slightly more motion.[35]

Atlantoaxial Instability and Rotatory Subluxation
Isolated rupture of the transverse ligament of the atlas is an uncommon injury in children. The resultant C1-C2 instability is suggested by an atlantodens interval greater than 5 mm on a lateral radiograph. Treatment of an acute rupture is possible with halo cast immobilization for 8 to 12 weeks. Marked instability is best managed with C1-C2 fusion.[36]

Atlantoaxial rotatory subluxation is an acquired alteration of the articulation between the atlas and axis. It can result from minor trauma but more commonly occurs after an upper respiratory infection (Grisel syndrome) or a nasopharyngeal procedure. Head movement causes pain, and C1-C2 rotation is significantly limited or completely fixed. The child has torticollis, in which the chin is rotated to one side and the head is tilted to the opposite side. Unlike congenital muscular torticollis, which is caused by a tight sternocleidomastoid, this condition is characterized by tenseness in the muscle that opposes the head position on the long side.

Rotatory subluxation is suggested by asymmetry of the C1 lateral masses on an open-mouth odontoid radiograph or overlapping of C1 onto C2 on a lateral radiograph. Dynamic CT can confirm the diagnosis by revealing a loss of the normal atlantoaxial rotation with attempted maximal head rotation. Many atlantoaxial rotatory displacements resolve spontaneously. The treatment depends on the duration of symptoms.[37] During the first week, the treatment consists of immobilization with a soft collar, NSAIDs, and range-of-motion exercises. If symptoms persist, inpatient cervical halter traction, muscle relaxants, and analgesics are used. A halo cast sometimes is applied for 4 to 6 weeks after reduction is achieved. If painful rotatory subluxation persists or recurs, fusion of C1-C2, with or without reduction, is indicated.

Hangman's Fracture

Spondylolisthesis secondary to a bilateral pedicle fracture at C2 results from forced hyperextension and is called a hangman's fracture. Anterior displacement of the posterior arch of C2 more than 2 mm from the spinolaminar line (the Swischuk line) suggests injury. This fracture heals with immobilization for 12 weeks and rarely requires C1-C3 fusion.

Subaxial Fracture

Subaxial injury (C3-C7) is most common in children age 9 years or older, and usually occurs between C5 and C7.[38] The most common injury patterns involve compression fracture of the vertebral body or facet dislocation. These injuries often are managed with initial traction to realign the kyphosis and reduce any dislocated facet. Approximately two thirds of children with a subaxial injury can be treated with a rigid collar or halo vest only. Excessive cervical flexion or extension in children can also lead to the separation of the cartilaginous end plate from the vertebral body. This injury is extremely unstable and may require surgical fixation.

Thoracolumbar Spine Injuries

Injury to the thoracic or lumbar spine in children is less common than cervical spine injury. The injury tends to occur at the thoracolumbar junction, usually as the result of a motor vehicle crash or sports injury.[39] The three-column classification of spine injuries in adults also is applicable to children. The mechanism of injury and its stability are determined by the extent of injury to the anterior, middle, and posterior columns. The injury is classified as a compression fracture, burst fracture, flexion-distraction injury, or fracture-dislocation.

Compression fractures involve a failure of the anterior column without injury to the middle or posterior column. A compression fracture can occur at multiple levels as the result of a flexion mechanism of injury. A compression fracture with a less than 50% loss of height is considered stable and unlikely to have any associated neurologic injury. The injury will heal with 4 to 6 weeks of brace immobilization. Vertebral body height can partially reconstitute itself if significant growth remains. Posterior surgical stabilization may be needed if there is significant kyphosis from multiple compression fractures.

Burst fractures involve a failure of the anterior and middle columns. A burst fracture is most common in adolescents and young adults who sustain an axial load, as with a fall from a height. An associated neurologic injury is likely to be caused by the retropulsed fragments into the canal or neuroforamina. The evaluation should include an MRI before reduction to rule out a dural tear or nerve root entrapment. Stabilization with posterior instrumentation is preferred in children with significant remaining anterior growth. A pedicle screw construct that includes one or two levels above and below the fracture site sometimes can restore sufficient sagittal alignment. Anterior column reconstruction may be needed if the vertebral body height is less than 60% or for anterior decompression of the canal.

A flexion-distraction injury, also known as a Chance fracture, is a compression fracture of the anterior column with a distraction injury to the middle and posterior columns. In children, the posterior and middle column injury can be osseous or ligamentous. The ligamentous injury propagates between the spinous processes, and the end plate separates from the vertebral body. This fracture is best appreciated on MRI.[40] Nearly all of these fractures are seat belt injuries, usually in children younger than 10 years. They may be accompanied by major abdominal injuries including aortic dissection.[20] Injuries involving bony elements with less than 15° of segmental kyphosis can be treated with an extension cast or a brace, if adequate reduction is achieved. Surgical stabilization with pedicle screws or wires is preferable if significant kyphosis or ligamentous injury exists.

A fracture-dislocation is a rare injury that involves a failure of all three columns. The thoracolumbar junction is the most common site of injury. These highly unstable fractures almost always require surgical reduction, decompression, and internal fixation. Neurologic injury is likely.

Annotated References

1. Kawakami N, Tsuji T, Imagama S, Lenke LG, Puno RM, Kuklo TR; Spinal Deformity Study Group: Classification of congenital scoliosis and kyphosis: A new approach to the three-dimensional classification for progressive vertebral anomalies requiring operative treatment. *Spine (Phila Pa 1976)* 2009;34(17):1756-1765.

   Three-dimensional CT led to a more comprehensive understanding of anomalies than the classic classification scheme.

2. Hedequist DJ: Instrumentation and fusion for congenital spine deformities. *Spine (Phila Pa 1976)* 2009;34(17):1783-1790.

   Modern instrumentation and fusion techniques for congenital scoliosis are reviewed.

3. Hedequist D, Hresko T, Proctor M: Modern cervical spine instrumentation in children. *Spine (Phila Pa 1976)* 2008;33(4):379-383.

   Twenty-five patients were treated surgically with modern implants for a cervical spine disorder. The authors conclude this is a safe and efficacious technique, even in young children.

4. Klimo P Jr, Kan P, Rao G, Apfelbaum R, Brockmeyer D: Os odontoideum: Presentation, diagnosis, and treatment in a series of 78 patients. *J Neurosurg Spine* 2008; 9(4):332-342.

   A retrospective review of 78 patients with os odontoideum included three patients who were asymptomatic at the time of diagnosis and were observed. All three patients developed neurologic symptoms, leading the authors to conclude that this disorder requires posterior

6. Pediatrics

cervical arthrodesis. Transarticular screws can be successfully used in the pediatric population.

5. Sanders JO, D'Astous J, Fitzgerald M, Khoury JG, Kishan S, Sturm PF: Derotational casting for progressive infantile scoliosis. *J Pediatr Orthop* 2009;29(6):581-587.

    The authors' experience with derotation casting for infantile scoliosis is reviewed. This prospective study found that casting is best for patients younger than 20 months with a Cobb angle of less than 60°. Older patients with a larger Cobb angle tended to have a poorer outcome with serial casting.

6. Thompson GH, Akbarnia BA, Campbell RM Jr: Growing rod techniques in early-onset scoliosis. *J Pediatr Orthop* 2007;27(3):354-361.

    The use of growing-rod techniques for early-onset scoliosis is reviewed. This technique allows continued growth of the spine while controlling curvature. The complication rate, while moderate, is acceptable and relates to hook disengagement or rod breakage.

7. Sanders JO, Khoury JG, Kishan S, et al: Predicting scoliosis progression from skeletal maturity: A simplified classification during adolescence. *J Bone Joint Surg Am* 2008;90(3):540-553.

    The radiographic appearance of the epiphyses of the phalanges, metacarpals, and distal radius are correlated with the adolescent growth phases. A useful classification system is presented for determining the timing of growth in relation to a bone age radiograph. The information is useful for determining the potential for successful bracing in patients with idiopathic scoliosis.

8. Lenke LG, Betz RR, Harms J, et al: Adolescent idiopathic scoliosis: A new classification to determine extent of spinal arthrodesis. *J Bone Joint Surg Am* 2001;83(8):1169-1181.

9. Newton PO, Upasani VV, Lhamby J, Ugrinow VL, Pawelek JB, Bastrom TP: Surgical treatment of main thoracic scoliosis with thoracoscopic anterior instrumentation: A five-year follow-up study. *J Bone Joint Surg Am* 2008;90(10):2077-2089.

    Forty-one patients were treated with anterior thoracoscopic fusion and instrumentation for adolescent idiopathic scoliosis, with 5-year follow-up. The advantages of limited scar and muscle dissection must be weighed against the increased risk of pseudarthrosis and implant failure, compared with posterior instrumentation techniques.

10. Suk SI, Kim JH, Cho KJ, Kim SS, Lee JJ, Han YT: Is anterior release necessary in severe scoliosis treated by posterior segmental pedicle screw fixation? *Eur Spine J* 2007;16(9):1359-1365.

    Thirty-five patients with curves greater than 70° treated with posterior surgery alone were retrospectively reviewed. Satisfactory coronal and sagital correction was achieved with segmental pedicle screw fixation.

11. Schwartz DM, Auerbach JD, Dormans JP, et al: Neurophysiological detection of impending spinal cord injury during scoliosis surgery. *J Bone Joint Surg Am* 2007;89(11):2440-2449.

    A clinical study of 1,121 patients who underwent instrumented spine fusion for adolescent idiopathic scoliosis found that transcranial monitoring of motor-evoked potentials is more specific than monitoring of somatosensory-evoked potentials with regard to spinal cord insult. Both motor- and somatosensory-evoked potentials should be used for spine deformity surgery.

12. Geck MJ, Macagno A, Ponte A, Shufflebarger HL: The Ponte procedure: Posterior only treatment of Scheuermann's kyphosis using segmental posterior shortening and pedicle screw instrumentation. *J Spinal Disord Tech* 2007;20(8):586-593.

    A prospective study of 17 patients treated with Ponte osteotomies and posterior instrumentation for Scheuermann kyphosis found that even for larger degrees of kyphosis, correction is possible with apical osteotomies and pedicle screw fixation from a posterior-only approach.

13. Klein G, Mehlman CT, McCarty M: Nonoperative treatment of spondylolysis and grade I spondylolisthesis in children and young adults: A meta-analysis of observational studies. *J Pediatr Orthop* 2009;29(2):146-156.

    A meta-analysis of 15 observational studies found 83.9% of patients treated nonsurgically for spondylolysis had a successful clinical outcome after at least 1 year.

14. Leboeuf-Yde C, Kyvik KO: At what age does low back pain become a common problem? A study of 29,424 individuals aged 12-41 years. *Spine (Phila Pa 1976)* 1998;23(2):228-234.

15. Bhatia NN, Chow G, Timon SJ, Watts HG: Diagnostic modalities for the evaluation of pediatric back pain: A prospective study. *J Pediatr Orthop* 2008;28(2):230-233.

    The authors present level II evidence that exhaustive diagnostic testing for pediatric back pain infrequently leads to a definitive diagnosis.

16. Ahlqwist A, Hagman M, Kjellby-Wendt G, Beckung E: Physical therapy treatment of back complaints on children and adolescents. *Spine (Phila Pa 1976)* 2008;33(20):E721-E727.

    In a randomized study, 45 children with back complaints demonstrated improvement with both individualized and nonindividualized physical therapy but shorter duration of pain with an individualized therapy program.

17. Bilston LE, Brown J: Pediatric spinal injury type and severity are age and mechanism dependent. *Spine (Phila Pa 1976)* 2007;32(21):2339-2347.

    A retrospective review of 340 patients with pediatric spine trauma found that in older children spine injuries are likely to result from sports and recreation, and they become more evenly distributed between the cervical and thoracolumbar spine.

18. Carreon LY, Glassman SD, Campbell MJ: Pediatric spine fractures: A review of 137 hospital admissions. *J Spinal Disord Tech* 2004;17(6):477-482.

19. Polk-Williams A, Carr BG, Blinman TA, Masiakos PT, Wiebe DJ, Nance ML: Cervical spine injury in young children: A National Trauma Data Bank review. *J Pediatr Surg* 2008;43(9):1718-1721.

    The study reviewed 95,654 blunt traumas in children younger than 3 years. The rate and type of spinal column injuries in this population are detailed.

20. Junkins EP Jr, Stotts A, Santiago R, Guenther E: The clinical presentation of pediatric thoracolumbar fractures: A prospective study. *J Trauma* 2008;65(5):1066-1071.

    This prospective study of children at a level I trauma center during a 1-year period found that examination was only 81% sensitive and 68% specific for diagnosing a thoracolumbar fracture.

21. Jimenez RR, Deguzman MA, Shiran S, Karrellas A, Lorenzo RL: CT versus plain radiographs for evaluation of c-spine injury in young children: Do benefits outweigh risks? *Pediatr Radiol* 2008;38(6):635-644.

    CT and conventional radiography are compared as a primary screening tool for pediatric spine injury. Radiation exposure is as much as 90 times greater with CT, but CT often was used as a screening tool regardless of injury severity.

22. Rana AR, Drongowski R, Breckner G, Ehrlich PF: Traumatic cervical spine injuries: Characteristics of missed injuries. *J Pediatr Surg* 2009;44(1):151-155, discussion 155.

    This study of 1,307 patients suggested that CT is the optimal primary means of detecting cervical spine injuries.

23. Flynn JM, Closkey RF, Mahboubi S, Dormans JP: Role of magnetic resonance imaging in the assessment of pediatric cervical spine injuries. *J Pediatr Orthop* 2002;22(5):573-577.

24. Junewick JJ, Meesa IR, Luttenton CR, Hinman JM: Occult injury of the pediatric craniocervical junction. *Emerg Radiol* 2009;16(6):483-488.

25. Launay F, Leet AI, Sponseller PD: Pediatric spinal cord injury without radiographic abnormality: A meta-analysis. *Clin Orthop Relat Res* 2005;433:166-170.

26. Bracken MB, Shepard MJ, Collins WF, et al: A randomized controlled trial of methylprednisolone or naloxone in the treatment of acute spinal cord injury: Results of the second national acute spinal cord injury study. *N Engl J Med* 1990;322:1405-1411.

27. Ito Y, Sugimoto Y, Tomioka M, Kai N, Tanaka M: Does high dose methylprednisolone sodium succinate really improve neurological status in patient with acute cervical cord injury? A prospective study about neurological recovery and early complications. *Spine (Phila Pa 1976)* 2009;34(20):2121-2124.

    This retrospective comparison of adults treated with or without steroids at the time of spinal cord injury failed to find any neurologic benefit to steroids while noting a higher rate of pulmonary complications in patients who received steroids.

28. Pereira JE, Costa LM, Cabrita AM, et al: Methylprednisolone fails to improve functional and histological outcome following spinal cord injury in rats. *Exp Neurol* 2009;220(1):71-81.

    The effects of methylprednisolone were compared with saline solution in the treatment of rats with a T10 contusion injury. Results indicate that methylprednisolone does not lead to improved functional outcome.

29. Hedequist D, Proctor M: Screw fixation to C2 in children: A case series and technical report. *J Pediatr Orthop* 2009;29(1):21-25.

    This is one of the first reports on the safety and efficacy of various screw fixation techniques to C2, even in young children.

30. Reilly CW, Choit RL: Transarticular screws in the management of C1-C2 instability in children. *J Pediatr Orthop* 2006;26(5):582-588.

31. Cil A, Yazici M, Daglioglu K, et al: The effect of pedicle screw placement with or without application of compression across the neurocentral cartilage on the morphology of the spinal canal and pedicle in immature pigs. *Spine (Phila Pa 1976)* 2005;30(11):1287-1293.

32. Zhang H, Sucato DJ: Unilateral pedicle screw epiphysiodesis of the neurocentral synchondrosis: Production of idiopathic-like scoliosis in an immature animal model. *J Bone Joint Surg Am* 2008;90(11):2460-2469.

    The authors induced scoliosis in young pigs by placing unilateral pedicle screws across the neurocentral synchondrosis.

33. AuYong N, Piatt J Jr: Jefferson fractures of the immature spine: Report of 3 cases. *J Neurosurg Pediatr* 2009;3(1):15-19.

    This article describes common findings and possible sources for missing Jefferson fractures in young children.

34. Skaggs DL, Lerman LD, Albrektson J, Lerman M, Stewart DG, Tolo VT: Use of a noninvasive halo in children. *Spine (Phila Pa 1976)* 2008;33(15):1650-1654.

    Twenty-nine of 30 children were successfully immobilized with a new pinless halo, including seven with cervical fusion and five with atlantoaxial rotatory instability.

35. Mandabach M, Ruge JR, Hahn YS, McLone DG: Pediatric axis fractures: Early halo immobilization, management and outcome. *Pediatr Neurosurg* 1993;19(5):225-232.

36. Reilly CW: Pediatric spine trauma. *J Bone Joint Surg Am* 2007;89(suppl 1):98-107.

6: Pediatrics

The authors present a review article on pediatric spine trauma.

37. Pang D, Li V: Atlantoaxial rotatory fixation: Part III. A prospective study of the clinical manifestation, diagnosis, management, and outcome of children with atlanto-axial rotatory fixation. *Neurosurgery* 2005;57(5):954-972, discussion 954-972.

38. Dogan S, Safavi-Abbasi S, Theodore N, Horn E, Rekate HL, Sonntag VK: Pediatric subaxial cervical spine injuries: Origins, management, and outcome in 51 patients. *Neurosurg Focus* 2006;20(2):E1.

39. Dogan S, Safavi-Abbasi S, Theodore N, et al: Thoracolumbar and sacral spinal injuries in children and adolescents: A review of 89 cases. *J Neurosurg* 2007;106(6, suppl):426-433.

This large retrospective study of children with thoracolumbar injuries describes the common location, associated injuries, and rates of recovery.

40. de Gauzy JS, Jouve JL, Violas P, et al: Classification of Chance fracture in children using magnetic resonance imaging. *Spine (Phila Pa 1976)* 2007;32(2):E89-E92.

Three types of Chance fracture lesions in children are all well visualized on MRI.

Chapter 57

Pelvis, Hip, and Femur Trauma: Pediatrics

Amy L. McIntosh, MD   Karl E. Rathjen, MD

Introduction

Injury to the pelvis, hip, or femur in a child usually is the result of high-energy trauma. The possibility of nonaccidental trauma must be remembered if the child is younger than 2 years. It is important that the assessment of every child with an injury to the pelvis, hip, or femur begins with basic trauma care. When it has been determined the patient is stable and all injuries have been identified, a treatment plan can be developed that takes into consideration the unique characteristics of the immature skeleton as well as the patient's specific injuries.

Pelvic Fracture

Characteristics

Pelvic fractures include pelvic ring injuries, acetabular fractures, and apophyseal avulsion fractures (also discussed in chapter 61). Pelvic ring and acetabular fractures in children most commonly result from a pedestrian–motor vehicle collision or a motor vehicle crash. Pelvic ring injuries are more common than acetabular fractures, which were found to account for only 13% of pelvic injuries.[1,2] Although two studies attempted to identify risk factors for pelvic fracture,[3,4] it is important to remember that 30% of patients had a normal physical examination.[2] With all traumatic injuries, the treating personnel must maintain a high degree of suspicion as well as a low threshold for obtaining appropriate radiographs. Children can sustain an open pelvic injury, although this injury is uncommon. It is important that a child with a pelvic fracture receive a thorough rectal and genitourinary examination.[5,6]

Neither Dr. McIntosh nor any immediate family member has received anything of value from or owns stock in a commercial company or institution related directly or indirectly to the subject of this chapter. Dr. Rathjen or an immediate family member serves as an unpaid consultant to Orthopediatrics.

Treatment

Most pelvic fractures in children are stable and can be treated nonsurgically with spica casting or protected weight bearing. Adolescents are more likely to have an unstable injury requiring surgical stabilization. In a review of 166 pediatric patients with a pelvic fracture, all patients requiring open reduction and internal fixation were found to have a closed triradiate cartilage.[7] However, a review of 148 pediatric patients with a pelvic fracture found that a third of the 18 patients requiring open reduction had an open triradiate cartilage.[8] The indications for surgical management in children are similar to those for adults; they include pelvic ring disruption with more than 2 cm of displacement, acetabular fracture, and triradiate cartilage injury with more than 2 mm of displacement.[9]

Complications

Death is uncommon in children with a pelvic fracture, and it almost always is the result of a head or visceral injury. Pelvic fracture–associated hemorrhage is less common in children than in adults. A solid visceral injury is more likely than a pelvic vascular disruption to cause massive blood loss in children with a pelvic fracture.[10-12]

Pelvic ring disruption is unlikely to remodel, and healing with more than 1 cm of pelvic asymmetry may increase the risk of nonstructural scoliosis, lumbar pain, the Trendelenburg sign, or sacroiliac joint tenderness and pain.[13] Patients with acetabular fractures generally do well with treatment, but those with triradiate cartilage injury may not and conditions can deteriorate over time.[14] Injury to the triradiate cartilage may produce physeal arrest and subsequent hip dysplasia.[15,16] If a triradiate physeal bar is identified early, it may be possible to excise it and prevent or limit subsequent dysplasia.[17]

Hip Dislocation

Characteristics

Most traumatic hip dislocations are posterior, although anterior dislocations do occur. A careful examination should be performed to delineate all associated injuries.

6: Pediatrics

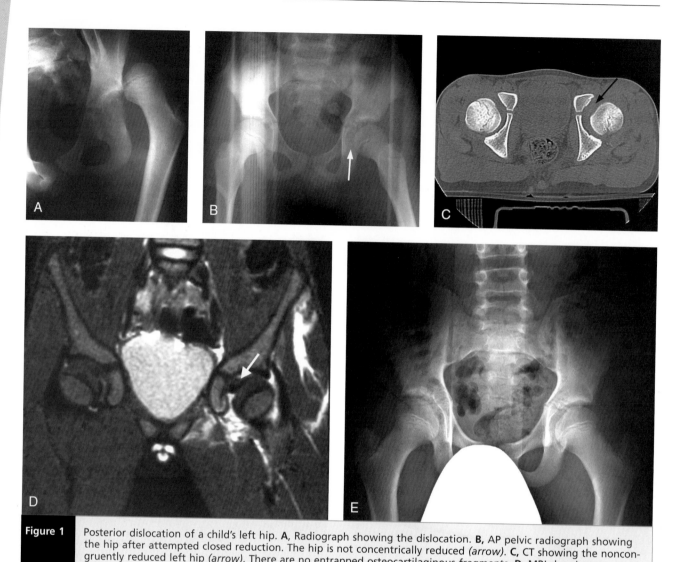

Figure 1 Posterior dislocation of a child's left hip. **A,** Radiograph showing the dislocation. **B,** AP pelvic radiograph showing the hip after attempted closed reduction. The hip is not concentrically reduced *(arrow)*. **C,** CT showing the noncongruently reduced left hip *(arrow)*. There are no entrapped osteocartilaginous fragments. **D,** MRI showing an enfolded ligamentum teres or capsule *(arrow)* causing the nonconcentric hip reduction. **E,** AP pelvic radiograph showing mild coxa magna and subtle femoral neck deformity 4 years after open reduction and removal of entrapped capsule and ligamentum.

An associated fracture (particularly fracture of the proximal femoral epiphysis), a nerve injury (most commonly to the peroneal branch of the sciatic nerve), or an ipsilateral knee injury is reported in 5% to 30% of patients.[18-21]

Treatment

A timely attempt at closed reduction is the first treatment for all traumatic hip dislocations. Closed reduction is successful for most dislocated hips. Because of the possibility of displacing the proximal femoral epiphysis, it is imperative that closed reduction be done with appropriate sedation or anesthesia. To prevent proximal femoral physeal separation, the use of fluoroscopy during the reduction has been recommended.[22] Postreduction radiographs should be carefully assessed. In children, a nonconcentric reduction may be caused by interposed capsule or labrum. Unlike osteocartilagi-

nous fragments in adults, the interposed soft tissue is not evident on postreduction CT. It is important to remember that subtle asymmetry on postreduction radiographs may be the only indication that an open reduction is necessary[19,23-26] (**Figure 1**). If open reduction is required, the traditional surgical approach is in the direction of the dislocation (most commonly posteriorly). However, the Ganz surgical dislocation technique can be used to provide excellent circumferential exposure of the labrum.[27,28]

Traumatic hip dislocation in children generally has a good long-term outcome. In 42 children with a traumatic hip dislocation, 95% had mild pain (usually weather related) or no pain, and 78% continued to participate in high-demand activities such as football, soccer, and basketball.[20] Traumatic hip dislocations still may be neglected in the developing world; these patients may benefit from open reduction.[29,30]

Complications

The complications of traumatic hip dislocation in children include nerve injury, redislocation, coxa magna, and osteonecrosis. Osteonecrosis in children who have traumatic hip dislocation without femoral neck fracture is less common than in adults, and it may be related to a delay in reduction.[20] Coxa magna is a common radiographic finding that is not associated with functional limitation. Redislocation is rare and can be treated with prolonged immobilization or capsulorrhaphy, depending on the age of the patient and the time elapsed since injury.[31] In adults, 60% to 70% of nerve injuries associated with hip dislocation spontaneously improve.[21]

Femoral Neck Fracture

Characteristics

Femoral neck fractures in children are classified using the Delbet system. Type I is a transphyseal separation, type II is transcervical, type III is basicervical, and type IV is intertrochanteric. A femoral neck fracture in the absence of a history of high-energy trauma should raise suspicion of nonaccidental trauma or pathologic bone.[32,33]

Treatment

Displaced physeal separation in an infant sometimes occurs as a result of obstetric or nonaccidental trauma. Because of an infant's tremendous remodeling potential, this injury can be successfully treated with immobilization in a Pavlik harness or spica cast. In these children, a nondisplaced, incomplete femoral neck fracture resulting from low-energy trauma can be managed with spica casting and close follow-up to ensure displacement and deformity do not develop. Because of a child's propensity to develop progressive deformity, protected weight bearing should be undertaken with extreme caution.[34]

Almost all other displaced femoral neck fractures in children should be managed with urgent anatomic reduction, stable fixation, and external immobilization. No conclusive evidence has established the superiority of a closed reduction or an open reduction. However, the time to reduction and the quality of the reduction influence the risk of osteonecrosis.[35,36] Thus, it is imperative that the reduction be timely and anatomic, regardless of whether the surgeon chooses closed reduction and percutaneous fixation, an anterior approach with percutaneous fixation, or an anterolateral approach for reduction and fixation. Recent studies suggested that decompression of the hip capsule may decrease the incidence of osteonecrosis[37,38]

Because of the relatively frequent occurrence of delayed union or nonunion, fracture stability should take precedence over physeal viability. Surgeons should cross the physis with implants whenever necessary; the implants can be removed after the fracture has healed[36] (**Figure 2**). Adequate fixation is important, and supplemental immobilization with a hip spica cast is effective

at decreasing the rotational forces produced by the distal fragment. It is wise to recognize that the leg is an exceptionally long moment arm that can produce tremendous rotational forces at the fracture site even when it is not bearing weight. Avoidance of weight bearing is not always achievable in children, and therefore it is not surprising that supplemental spica casting is associated with low rates of delayed union or nonunion.[39]

Complications

Osteonecrosis is the most common and significant complication of femoral neck fracture in children. A review of 25 femoral neck fractures with a meta-analysis of an additional 335 fractures found that the development of osteonecrosis was correlated with the age of the patient and the type of fracture. For each year of increasing age, patients were 1.14 times more likely to develop osteonecrosis. The rate of osteonecrosis was 38% for Delbet type I fractures, 28% for type II fractures, 18% for type III fractures, and 5% for type IV fractures.[40]

Delayed union or nonunion has been reported to occur after 3% to 67% of femoral neck fractures in children.[41,42] Delayed union and nonunion can be successfully managed with proximal femoral valgus osteotomy[43] (**Figure 2**). Other reported complications include coxa vara, coxa valga, coxa magna, premature physeal closure, limb-length difference, and infection.[41,42,44]

Subtrochanteric Femur Fracture

Characteristics

In adults, a subtrochanteric femur fracture is defined as a fracture no more than 5 cm below the lesser trochanter. As modified for children, the definition is a fracture within 10% of the total femoral length of the lesser trochanter.[45] A subtrochanteric fracture resulting from low-energy trauma should raise suspicion of a preexisting pathologic lesion.[46]

Treatment and Complications

Subtrochanteric femur fractures can be treated with spica casting, traction followed by spica casting, or surgical stabilization using external fixation or a plate-and-screw or intramedullary device.[47] These fractures tend to develop unacceptable varus and shortening, and therefore displaced fractures should be managed with some form of stabilization.[45,48,49] An incomplete and nondisplaced fracture can be managed in an immediate spica cast, but it should be followed closely during the first 2 to 3 weeks to ensure that deformity does not develop.[47] Limb-length discrepancy and angular malalignment are the most commonly reported complications of subtrochanteric femur fracture. Careful attention to detail during treatment may limit the risk of these complications. Osteonecrosis of the femoral head, heterotopic ossification, and infection also can occur.

6: Pediatrics

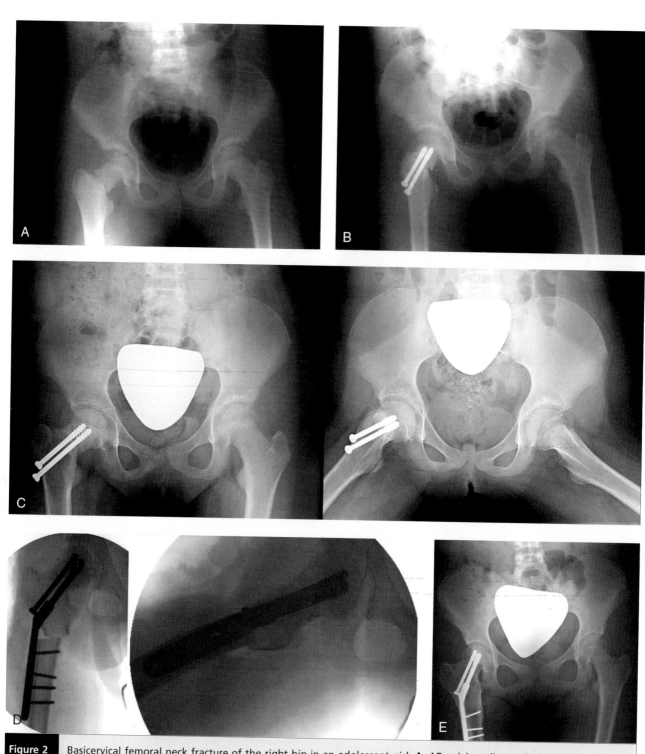

Figure 2   Basicervical femoral neck fracture of the right hip in an adolescent girl. **A,** AP pelvic radiograph showing the fracture. **B,** AP pelvic radiograph taken immediately after attempted percutaneous reduction. The reduction is not anatomic. To avoid crossing the physis, relatively short screws were used. **C,** AP *(left)* and frog-lateral *(right)* pelvic radiographs taken 4 months after injury, showing slight varus collapse, backing out of the screws, and delayed fracture union. **D,** AP *(left)* and lateral *(right)* fluoroscopic views showing valgus osteotomy, revision fixation, and bone grafting of the femoral neck site through the compression hip screw tract. **E,** AP pelvic radiograph taken 2 years after valgus osteotomy, showing the slightly shortened femoral neck.

Femoral Shaft Fracture

Fractures of the femoral shaft are common, and most orthopaedic surgeons treat them on a regular basis. Cortical thickness increases throughout childhood; the mechanism of injury in femoral shaft fractures therefore is correlated with age. A fall is the most common mechanism of injury in toddlers and children younger than 10 years. The most common mechanism among older children and adolescents is a pedestrian–motor vehicle collision or a motor vehicle crash.[50]

Repeated fractures or a fracture after minor trauma should alert the clinician to the possibility of an underlying pathologic condition. Osteogenesis imperfecta is diagnosed based on the presence of multiple fractures and other typical signs including dentinogenesis imperfecta, blue sclerae, and hearing loss. The diagnosis can be confirmed by analysis of collagen produced by cultured dermal fibroblasts. Generalized osteopenia from cerebral palsy, myelomeningocele, and other neuromuscular conditions also leads to a predisposition to fracture.[51] Radiographs always should be carefully evaluated for localized pathologic conditions that could predispose the patient to fracture. The most common benign conditions include a unicameral bone cyst, nonossifying fibroma, eosinophilic granuloma, or aneurysmal bone cyst. Malignant conditions are far less common; they include osteogenic sarcoma, Ewing sarcoma, and lymphoma.

Nonaccidental trauma accounts for 50% to 69% of all fractures in children younger than 1 year.[52] Such fractures are the second most common symptom of child abuse, after soft-tissue injury such as bruising or burn injury. Among child abuse–related long bone injuries, humerus fractures are the most common and femur fractures are the second most common. The age of the patient is important in identifying injury patterns that may be related to abuse. A rib, tibia-fibula, humerus, or femur fracture is more likely to be the result of nonaccidental trauma in a patient younger than 18 months than in an older patient.[53]

Characteristics

The classification of femoral shaft fractures, like that of most diaphyseal fractures, is based on the radiographic examination and the condition of the soft-tissue envelope (that is, whether the fracture is closed or open). Radiographs are evaluated for fracture location (proximal, middle, or distal third), configuration (transverse, oblique, or spiral), angulation, the extent of comminution, and the amount of displacement, translation, and shortening. Spiral and oblique fractures are differentiated based on the length of the fracture. A fracture is classified as spiral if its length is more than twice the femoral diameter at the level of the fracture. A fracture that is shorter than twice the femoral diameter at the level of the fracture is considered oblique.[54,55] Femur fractures are designated as length stable or unstable. Stable fractures are transverse or oblique, and unstable fractures are spiral or comminuted.[54] Shortening also

---

Table 1

Age-Based Treatment Recommendations for Femoral Diaphyseal Fractures

Age: 0-6 months
Pavlik harness or spica casting

Age: 7 months-5 years
Early spica cast if ≤ 2cm of initial shortening
If > 2 cm of shortening or polytrauma/open fracture:
  Flexible Intramedullary fixation
  Bridge versus open plating
  Skeletal traction for 2-3 weeks, followed by spica cast
  External fixator

Age: 6-11 years
Flexible intramedullary nails if the fracture pattern is length stable
Length stable fracture patterns are either transverse or oblique. An oblique fracture is < 2 times the femoral diameter at the level of the fracture.
Submuscular bridge plating if the fracture pattern is length unstable or is a very proximal/distal fracture.
Length unstable fractures patterns are comminuted and/or spiral. A spiral fracture is ≥ 2 times the femoral diameter at the level of the fracture.

Age: > 11 years
Flexible intramedullary nails if length stable, and patient weighs ≤ 100 lb
Rigid trochanteric entry nail if length unstable, or patient weighs > 100 lb
Submuscular bridge plate if length unstable or very proximal/distal fracture

---

helps define stability and is best classified at the time of initial evaluation as unacceptable (more than 3 cm of shortening) or acceptable (less than 3 cm of shortening).

Treatment and Complications

The American Academy of Orthopaedic Surgeons has published a guideline on the treatment of pediatric diaphyseal femur fractures[56] (**Table 1**). Several methods can be used to treat femoral shaft fractures in children. The age and size of the child are the most important factors in deciding which treatment modality is most appropriate. In general, infants and children younger than 5 years are treated nonsurgically in a Pavlik harness or hip spica cast. Children older than 5 years may be treated with some form of skeletal fixation. Additional factors to consider include the mechanism of injury, the presence of multiple injuries, the condition of the soft tissue, the family support environment, and the available economic resources. As with any form of orthopaedic treatment, the experience, skill, and preference of the treating physician may be significant in determining the treatment. Guidelines based on the age of the patient can be used.

6: Pediatrics

Birth to Age 6 Months

The Pavlik harness can be used for treatment of a femur fracture in infants younger than 6 months. The advantages of the Pavlik harness include ease of application without sedation or general anesthesia, ability to adjust the harness if fracture manipulation is necessary, ease of diapering, and absence of the skin irritation commonly associated with casting.[57] Excessive hip flexion in the presence of a swollen thigh may compress the femoral nerve, and the surgeon should monitor quadriceps function during treatment to detect such an injury.

Age 7 Months to 5 Years

In children age 7 months to 5 years without extenuating circumstances such as polytrauma, neurovascular injury, or open injury, nonsurgical treatment is with closed reduction and immediate spica cast application. Preschool-age children tolerate a spica cast much better than school-age children because they can be transported more easily and have shorter healing times. An unstable fracture with more than 2 to 3 cm of initial shortening may be difficult to manage in a spica cast.

After conscious sedation or general anesthesia has been administered, an appropriately sized protective liner is applied. The child should be placed on the spica table. Towels are folded and placed under the liner in the chest and abdominal areas to create room for breathing and abdominal distention after eating. The surgeon holds the legs with the child's hips in approximately 60° to 90° of flexion and 30° of abduction. The more proximal the fracture, the more the hips should be flexed. The knees should be flexed to 90°. Some external rotation will correct the rotational deformity of the distal fragment. An experienced assistant applies the cast, and a good condylar and buttock mold is placed into the cast to maintain the reduction. Care must be taken to avoid excessive compression or traction through the region of the popliteal fossa.

Compartment syndrome of the leg is a recognized complication of early spica casting.[58,59] The risk of this serious complication can be minimized by avoiding excessive traction while placing the cast, avoiding knee flexion of more than 90°, and creating a smoothly contoured popliteal fossa. The patient's level of comfort as well as neurologic and vascular status should be checked and documented before discharge.

Fluoroscopy is used while the cast hardens to allow mild manipulation, and cast wedging also can be used as needed in the hardened cast. The acceptable alignment depends on the age of the patient, but in general no more than 10° of deformity in the coronal plane and 20° of deformity in the sagittal plane are considered acceptable. Shortening should not exceed 2.0 cm. Radiographs should be obtained weekly during the first 2 to 3 weeks to allow any loss of the initial reduction to be corrected. The time to healing ranges from 4 to 8 weeks, depending on the age of the child. Physical therapy is not routinely necessary after cast removal. A special child seat is needed for safe transport in an automobile.

Children who are age 7 months to 5 years should be treated surgically if there are extenuating circumstances such as polytrauma, open fracture, or a length-unstable fracture pattern. The surgical options include external fixation, flexible intramedullary fixation, bridge plating, and skeletal traction. Skeletal traction can be applied after placement of a distal femoral traction pin. After early callus has formed in 2 to 3 weeks, a spica cast can be placed.

Age 6 to 11 Years

Flexible (elastic) intramedullary nails are the preferred treatment of a length-stable (transverse or short oblique) femoral shaft fracture in children age 6 to 11 years. The elastic nail provides three-point intramedullary contact and load sharing, thus allowing more rapid mobilization (Figure 3). The rate of complications is greater in children older than 11 to 12 years and/or heavier than 100 lb.[60,61] The most common minor complication of flexible intramedullary nail fixation is pain at the insertion site in the distal femur, which occurs in 40% of patients.[62] Because the pain is associated with the amount of distal nail protrusion, it is recommended that no more than 25 mm of the nail should be left protruding from the cortex, with a minimal bend of the nail. A patient with a very proximal or distal fracture or a length-unstable fracture is at relatively high risk of a complication. These patients may be best treated with a more rigid surgical device such as a bridge plate or rigid intramedullary nails.

Preoperative planning for the use of flexible intramedullary nails includes measuring the narrowest diameter of the femoral canal and multiplying it by 0.4 to determine the nail size that will produce the desired 80% canal fill. The patient is placed on a radiolucent table or fracture table, with the unaffected leg abducted out of the way. The nails are inserted retrograde; they should enter the femur 2 to 2.5 cm proximal to the distal femoral physis. Care is taken to avoid dissection about the distal femoral physis and to avoid entering the knee joint. The time to union is 10 to 12 weeks. Most surgeons remove the nails within 1 year of insertion.

Age 12 Years or Older

Treatment options in children age 12 years or older include flexible intramedullary rodding, bridge plating, and rigid locked intramedullary nailing using a lateral trochanteric entry site. The preferred option depends on the fracture stability and the weight of the patient. An adolescent who weighs less than 100 lb and has a length-stable (transverse or short oblique) fracture can usually be treated using flexible nails. Submuscular bridge plating for the treatment of a length-unstable, very proximal, or distal femur fracture offers several advantages, including stability, early mobility, avoidance of growth plates, preservation of the proximal femoral blood supply, and limited surgical exposure and soft-tissue dissection. The disadvantages of submuscular bridge plating include the technical demand-

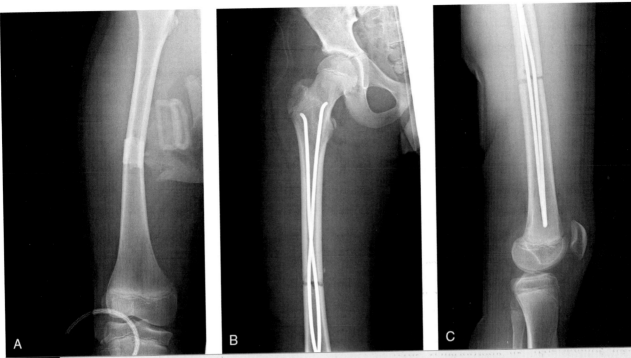

Figure 3 Radiographs of a transverse diaphyseal femur fracture (a length-stable fracture) in an 11-year-old boy weighing less than 100 lb. **A,** AP radiograph showing the fracture. AP (**B**) and lateral (**C**) radiographs showing treatment with flexible intramedullary nails.

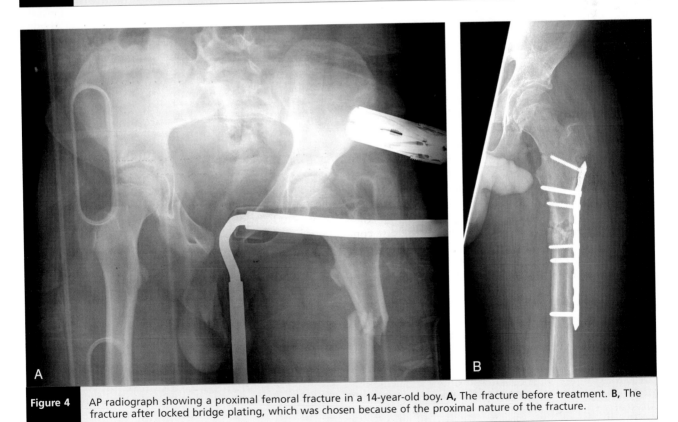

Figure 4 AP radiograph showing a proximal femoral fracture in a 14-year-old boy. **A,** The fracture before treatment. **B,** The fracture after locked bridge plating, which was chosen because of the proximal nature of the fracture.

ing application and the time-consuming removal procedure (**Figure 4**). Before application of the plate, the fracture must be provisionally reduced with the aid of traction or a pillow. A 4.5-mm narrow, low-contact dynamic compression plate can be used for most patients. Locking plates can be used if the patient has osteopenia or a proximal or distal fracture with limited room for screw placement. Self-tapping screws facilitate insertion, and absorbable suture can be tied around the head to avoid loss of the screw in the soft tissues. The plate offers 12 to 16 holes over its length and should allow placement of three screws above and three screws below the fracture. A tabletop bender is used to bend the plate to accommodate the proximal femur and distal metaphysis. A small incision is made distally to allow for insertion. The plate is tunneled between the femoral periosteum and the vastus lateralis, and it is provisionally fixed with Kirschner wires or Steinmann pins in the most proximal and distal holes. A third wire can be placed in the middle portion of the plate to prevent recurvatum. The patient must not bear weight until callus formation is visible radiographically, at an average of 5 weeks after surgery.[63]

Rigid interlocking intramedullary nails have been successfully used to treat femoral shaft fractures in adolescents. The rigid fixation imparted by the nail, along with the rotational control from the interlocking screws, allows this device to be used in highly unstable fractures, permits weight bearing immediately after surgery, limits the risk of angular deformity, and can be dynamized to promote fracture healing.

Osteonecrosis of the femoral head is the most severe complication of intramedullary nailing of a femoral shaft fracture in an adolescent, although it is relatively rare. It is believed that injury to the medial circumflex artery occurs during insertion of the nail medial to the tip of the greater trochanter. Osteonecrosis has occurred in at least 18 children and adolescents after intramedullary nailing with large, adult-sized nails placed through the piriformis fossa. At least one incident of osteonecrosis was associated with a rigid nail placed through the tip of the greater trochanter. Nails placed through the tip of the greater trochanter also have been associated with premature greater trochanteric epiphysiodesis, coxa valga, and hip subluxation.[64] However, more recent studies did not find these changes in the proximal femur after lateral trochanteric entry.[65] When using rigid nailing, the surgeon should take great care to avoid drifting into the region medial to the tip of the trochanter and should consider nail removal only after closure of the physis. Osteonecrosis can occur from nail placement or from damage of the vessels at nail removal.

External Fixation

The primary current indications for external fixation are an open fracture; severe disruption of the soft-tissue envelope, including severe burn injury; multiple trauma; an extremity with an arterial injury requiring immediate revascularization of the extremity; an unstable fracture pattern; and unsuccessful nonsurgical management. The fixators generally are applied for 10 to 16 weeks, until solid union has been achieved. Weight bearing is permitted as early as tolerated, with consideration of the stability of the fracture and the external fixator.

Pin tract infection accounts for approximately 50% of complications of treatment with an external fixator. In general, pin tract infection responds to good pin care and antibiotics. Rates of nonunion, delayed union, and angular deformity are generally reported to be slightly higher than with more rigid fixation techniques. Delayed union and refracture also are more common, with a reported incidence of 1.5% to 21%.[66] These complications are most common in short oblique fractures because the use of a rigid external fixator means that secondary callus is less likely to form.[66] When refracture occurs at the previous fracture site as a consequence of incomplete union, the fixator should be left in place until solid union is seen radiographically. To avoid this complication, the surgeon may consider leaving the pins for a few days after the fixator is removed, so as to allow fixator replacement if a fracture occurs. Complete apposition of the fracture fragments should be achieved at the time of initial reduction.[66]

Annotated References

1. Banerjee S, Barry MJ, Paterson JM: Paediatric pelvic fractures: 10 years experience in a trauma centre. *Injury* 2009;40(4):410-413.

   In a retrospective review, the authors found that pelvic fractures in children have a good long-term outcome when treated nonsurgically but are an indicator of other serious injuries with a high rate of mortality.

2. Junkins EP Jr, Nelson DS, Carroll KL, Hansen K, Furnival RA: A prospective evaluation of the clinical presentation of pediatric pelvic fractures. *J Trauma* 2001; 51(1):64-68.

3. Ramirez DW, Schuette JJ, Knight V, Johnson E, Denise J, Walker AR: Necessity of routine pelvic radiograph in the pediatric blunt trauma patient. *Clin Pediatr (Phila)* 2008;47(9):935-940.

   The authors determined that clinical indicators may be needed to determine the necessity of pelvic radiographs in awake and alert pediatric patients who have experienced blunt trauma.

4. Nabaweesi R, Arnold MA, Chang DC, et al: Prehospital predictors of risk for pelvic fractures in pediatric trauma patients. *Pediatr Surg Int* 2008;24(9):1053-1056.

   The authors found that identification of risk factors in pediatric trauma patients may help determine which are at highest risk of pelvic fracture and may most benefit from pelvic radiography.

5. Mosheiff R, Suchar A, Porat S, Shmushkevich A, Segal D, Liebergall M: The "crushed open pelvis" in children. *Injury* 1999;30(suppl 2):B14-B18.

6. Davidson BS, Simmons GT, Williamson PR, Buerk CA: Pelvic fractures associated with open perineal wounds: A survivable injury. *J Trauma* 1993;35(1):36-39.

7. Silber JS, Flynn JM: Changing patterns of pediatric pel-

vic fractures with skeletal maturation: Implications for classification and management. *J Pediatr Orthop* 2002; 22(1):22-26.

8. Karunakar MA, Goulet JA, Mueller KL, Bedi A, Le TT: Operative treatment of unstable pediatric pelvis and acetabular fractures. *J Pediatr Orthop* 2004;25(1):34-38.

9. Holden CP, Holman J, Herman MJ: Pediatric pelvic fractures. *J Am Acad Orthop Surg* 2007;15(3):172-177.

   The authors discuss treatment and complications associated with pelvic fractures in children.

10. Demetriades D, Karaiskakis M, Velmahos GC, Alo K, Murray J, Chan L: Pelvic fractures in pediatric and adult trauma patients: Are they different injuries? *J Trauma* 2003;54(6):1146-1151, discussion 1151.

11. Grisoni N, Connor S, Marsh E, Thompson GH, Cooperman DR, Blakemore LC: Pelvic fractures in a pediatric level I trauma center. *J Orthop Trauma* 2002;16(7):458-463.

12. Ismail N, Bellemare JF, Mollitt DL, DiScala C, Koeppel B, Tepas JJ III: Death from pelvic fracture: Children are different. *J Pediatr Surg* 1996;31(1):82-85.

13. Smith W, Shurnas P, Morgan S, et al: Clinical outcomes of unstable pelvic fractures in skeletally immature patients. *J Bone Joint Surg Am* 2005;87(11):2423-2431.

14. Heeg M, de Ridder VA, Tornetta P III, de Lange S, Klasen HJ: Acetabular fractures in children and adolescents. *Clin Orthop Relat Res* 2000;376:80-86.

15. Trousdale RT, Ganz R: Posttraumatic acetabular dysplasia. *Clin Orthop Relat Res* 1994;305:124-132.

16. Bucholz RW, Ezaki M, Ogden JA: Injury to the acetabular triradiate physeal cartilage. *J Bone Joint Surg Am* 1982;64(4):600-609.

17. Peterson HA, Robertson RC: Premature partial closure of the triradiate cartilage treated with excision of a physical osseous bar: Case report with a fourteen-year follow-up. *J Bone Joint Surg Am* 1997;79(5):767-770.

18. Schmidt GL, Sciulli R, Altman GT: Knee injury in patients experiencing a high-energy traumatic ipsilateral hip dislocation. *J Bone Joint Surg Am* 2005;87(6):1200-1204.

19. Vialle R, Pannier S, Odent T, Schmit P, Pauthier F, Glorion C: Imaging of traumatic dislocation of the hip in childhood. *Pediatr Radiol* 2004;34(12):970-979.

20. Mehlman CT, Hubbard GW, Crawford AH, Roy DR, Wall EJ: Traumatic hip dislocation in children: Long-term followup of 42 patients. *Clin Orthop Relat Res* 2000;376:68-79.

21. Cornwall R, Radomisli TE: Nerve injury in traumatic dislocation of the hip. *Clin Orthop Relat Res* 2000;377:84-91.

22. Herrera-Soto JA, Price CT, Reuss BL, Riley P, Kasser JR, Beaty JH: Proximal femoral epiphysiolysis during reduction of hip dislocation in adolescents. *J Pediatr Orthop* 2006;26(3):371-374.

23. Herrera-Soto JA, Price CT: Traumatic hip dislocations in children and adolescents: Pitfalls and complications. *J Am Acad Orthop Surg* 2009;17(1):15-21.

   The authors discuss the treatment of traumatic hip dislocations in children and late complications such as osteonecrosis, coxa magna, and osteoarthritis.

24. Chun KA, Morcuende J, El-Khoury GY: Entrapment of the acetabular labrum following reduction of traumatic hip dislocation in a child. *Skeletal Radiol* 2004;33(12):728-731.

25. Price CT, Pyevich MT, Knapp DR, Phillips JH, Hawker JJ: Traumatic hip dislocation with spontaneous incomplete reduction: A diagnostic trap. *J Orthop Trauma* 2002;16(10):730-735.

26. Shea KP, Kalamchi A, Thompson GH: Acetabular epiphysis-labrum entrapment following traumatic anterior dislocation of the hip in children. *J Pediatr Orthop* 1986;6(2):215-219.

27. Ganz R, Huff TW, Leunig M: Extended retinacular soft-tissue flap for intra-articular hip surgery: Surgical technique, indications, and results of application. *Instr Course Lect* 2009;58:241-255.

   The authors discuss the implications of using the extended retinacular soft-tissue flap as an intra-articular procedure.

28. Ganz R, Gill TJ, Gautier E, Ganz K, Krügel N, Berlemann U: Surgical dislocation of the adult hip: A technique with full access to the femoral head and acetabulum without the risk of avascular necrosis. *J Bone Joint Surg Br* 2001;83(8):1119-1124.

29. Banskota AK, Spiegel DA, Shrestha S, Shrestha OP, Rajbhandary T: Open reduction for neglected traumatic hip dislocation in children and adolescents. *J Pediatr Orthop* 2007;27(2):187-191.

   In a retrospective case series, the authors found that surgical reduction may be preferable to other methods of treating neglected traumatic hip dislocation in children and adolescents.

30. Kumar S, Jain AK: Open reduction of late unreduced traumatic posterior hip dislocation in 12 children. *Acta Orthop Scand* 1999;70(6):599-602.

31. Nirmal Kumar J, Hazra S, Yun HH: Redislocation after treatment of traumatic dislocation of hip in children: A report of two cases and literature review. *Arch Orthop Trauma Surg* 2009;129(6):823-826.

   The authors treated five patients with traumatic dislocation of the hip; two patients, age 2 and 3 years, had redislocation. Closed reduction was found to be an effective treatment, but adequate immobilization and protected weight bearing are necessary in children younger than 10 years to avoid redislocation.

32. Gholve P, Arkader A, Gaugler R, Wells L: Femoral neck fracture as an atypical presentation of child abuse. *Orthopedics* 2008;31(3):271.

The authors discuss an atypical presentation of nonaccidental injury in a 3-year-old child with femoral neck fracture. The diagnostic rationale for the nonaccidental injury is discussed.

33. Shrader MW, Schwab JH, Shaughnessy WJ, Jacofsky DJ: Pathologic femoral neck fractures in children. *Am J Orthop (Belle Mead NJ)* 2009;38(2):83-86, discussion 86.

The authors discuss a large series of pathologic femoral neck fractures in a pediatric population and review treatment methods and complication rates.

34. Forster NA, Ramseier LE, Exner GU: Undisplaced femoral neck fractures in children have a high risk of secondary displacement. *J Pediatr Orthop B* 2006;15(2):131-133.

35. Shrader MW, Jacofsky DJ, Stans AA, Shaughnessy WJ, Haidukewych GJ: Femoral neck fractures in pediatric patients: 30 years experience at a level 1 trauma center. *Clin Orthop Relat Res* 2007;454:169-173.

The authors discuss the factors that contribute to the occurrence of femoral head osteonecrosis in skeletally immature patients with femoral neck fractures. In 20 patients studied, 18 had fracture healing with no complications.

36. Boardman MJ, Herman MJ, Buck B, Pizzutillo PD: Hip fractures in children. *J Am Acad Orthop Surg* 2009;17(3):162-173.

The authors discuss hip fractures and review complications and surgical options.

37. Cheng JC, Tang N: Decompression and stable internal fixation of femoral neck fractures in children can affect the outcome. *J Pediatr Orthop* 1999;19(3):338-343.

38. Ng GP, Cole WG: Effect of early hip decompression on the frequency of avascular necrosis in children with fractures of the neck of the femur. *Injury* 1996;27(6):419-421.

39. Flynn JM, Wong KL, Yeh GL, Meyer JS, Davidson RS: Displaced fractures of the hip in children: Management by early operation and immobilisation in a hip spica cast. *J Bone Joint Surg Br* 2002;84(1):108-112.

40. Moon ES, Mehlman CT: Risk factors for avascular necrosis after femoral neck fractures in children: 25 Cincinnati cases and meta-analysis of 360 cases. *J Orthop Trauma* 2006;20(5):323-329.

41. Canale ST, Bourland WL: Fracture of the neck and intertrochanteric region of the femur in children. *J Bone Joint Surg Am* 1977;59(4):431-443.

42. Morsy HA: Complications of fracture of the neck of the femur in children: A long-term follow-up study. *Injury* 2001;32(1):45-51.

43. Magu NK, Singh R, Sharma AK, Ummat V: Modified Pauwels' intertrochanteric osteotomy in neglected femoral neck fractures in children: A report of 10 cases followed for a minimum of 5 years. *J Orthop Trauma* 2007;21(4):237-243.

The authors studied the role of a modified Pauwels intertrochanteric osteotomy in treating neglected femoral fractures in children and determined that this procedure creates a biomechanical environment conducive to healing while simultaneously correcting associated coxa vara.

44. Togrul E, Bayram H, Gulsen M, Kalaci A, Ozbarlas S: Fractures of the femoral neck in children: Long-term follow-up in 62 hip fractures. *Injury* 2005;36(1):123-130.

45. Pombo MW, Shilt JS: The definition and treatment of pediatric subtrochanteric femur fractures with titanium elastic nails. *J Pediatr Orthop* 2006;26(3):364-370.

46. Vigler M, Weigl D, Schwarz M, Ben-Itzhak I, Salai M, Bar-On E: Subtrochanteric femoral fractures due to simple bone cysts in children. *J Pediatr Orthop B* 2006;15(6):439-442.

47. Jeng C, Sponseller PD, Yates A, Paletta G: Subtrochanteric femoral fractures in children: Alignment after 90 degrees-90 degrees traction and cast application. *Clin Orthop Relat Res* 1997;341:170-174.

48. Jarvis J, Davidson D, Letts M: Management of subtrochanteric fractures in skeletally immature adolescents. *J Trauma* 2006;60(3):613-619.

49. Segal LS: Custom 95 degree condylar blade plate for pediatric subtrochanteric femur fractures. *Orthopedics* 2000;23(2):103-107.

50. Loder RT, O'Donnell PW, Feinberg JR: Epidemiology and mechanisms of femur fractures in children. *J Pediatr Orthop* 2006;26(5):561-566.

51. Fry K, Hoffer MM, Brink J: Femoral shaft fractures in brain-injured children. *J Trauma* 1976;16(5):371-373.

52. Banaszkiewicz PA, Scotland TR, Myerscough EJ: Fractures in children younger than age 1 year: Importance of collaboration with child protection services. *J Pediatr Orthop* 2002;22(6):740-744.

53. Pandya NK, Baldwin K, Wolfgruber H, Christian CW, Drummond DS, Hosalkar HS: Child abuse and orthopaedic injury patterns: Analysis at a level I pediatric trauma center. *J Pediatr Orthop* 2009;29(6):618-625.

A retrospective review of prospectively collected information from an urban level I pediatric trauma center found 500 patients with child abuse (age birth to 48 months) and compared them with 985 accidental trauma control patients from 2000 to 2003. Victims of abuse were generally younger. There was no difference when comparing the sex of the children. Patients younger than 18 months with rib, tibia/fibula, humerus, or femur fractures are more likely to be victims of non-accidental trauma. Long bone fractures (humerus and femur) in patients older than 18 months were more likely due to accidental trauma than to child abuse. Level of evidence: III.

54. Rathjen KE, Riccio AI, De La Garza D: Stainless steel flexible intramedullary fixation of unstable femoral shaft fractures in children. *J Pediatr Orthop* 2007;27(4):432-441.

    Stainless steel flexible intramedullary fixation of 40 unstable femur fractures (spiral and/or comminuted) were compared to 41 stable (transverse or oblique) femur fractures treated with stainless steel flexible intramedullary fixation. Stainless steel intramedullary fixation was effective treatment for unstable femur fractures if cortical abutment was present. Level of evidence: III.

55. Winquist RA, Hansen ST Jr, Clawson DK: Closed intramedullary nailing of femoral fractures: A report of five hundred and twenty cases. *J Bone Joint Surg Am* 1984;66(4):529-539.

56. Kocher MS, Sink EL, Blasier RD, et al: Treatment of pediatric diaphyseal femur fractures. *J Am Acad Orthop Surg* 2009;17(11):718-725.

    This article discusses an AAOS-approved clinical practice guideline that reviews the evidence published from 1966 through October 1, 2008. It reviews the good evidence, shows where evidence is lacking, and pinpoints topics that future research must target to improve the treatment of children with isolated diaphyseal femur fractures.

57. Podeszwa DA, Mooney JF III, Cramer KE, Mendelow MJ: Comparison of Pavlik harness application and immediate spica casting for femur fractures in infants. *J Pediatr Orthop* 2004;24(5):460-462.

58. Halanski M, Noonan KJ: Cast and splint immobilization: Complications. *J Am Acad Orthop Surg* 2008;16(1):30-40.

    This review article discusses materials and techniques to avoid casting and splinting complications.

59. Mubarak SJ, Frick S, Sink E, Rathjen K, Noonan KJ: Volkmann contracture and compartment syndromes after femur fractures in children treated with 90/90 spica casts. *J Pediatr Orthop* 2006;26(5):567-572.

60. Ho CA, Skaggs DL, Tang CW, Kay RM: Use of flexible intramedullary nails in pediatric femur fractures. *J Pediatr Orthop* 2006;26(4):497-504.

61. Moroz LA, Launay F, Kocher MS, et al: Titanium elastic nailing of fractures of the femur in children: Predictors of complications and poor outcome. *J Bone Joint Surg Br* 2006;88(10):1361-1366.

62. Luhmann SJ, Schootman M, Schoenecker PL, Dobbs MB, Gordon JE: Complications of titanium elastic nails for pediatric femoral shaft fractures. *J Pediatr Orthop* 2003;23(4):443-447.

63. Sink EL, Hedequist D, Morgan SJ, Hresko T: Results and technique of unstable pediatric femoral fractures treated with submuscular bridge plating. *J Pediatr Orthop* 2006;26(2):177-181.

64. Gordon JE, Swenning TA, Burd TA, Szymanski DA, Schoenecker PL: Proximal femoral radiographic changes after lateral transtrochanteric intramedullary nail placement in children. *J Bone Joint Surg Am* 2003;85(7):1295-1301.

65. Keeler KA, Dart B, Luhmann SJ, et al: Antegrade intramedullary nailing of pediatric femoral fractures using an interlocking pediatric femoral nail and a lateral trochanteric entry point. *J Pediatr Orthop* 2009;29(4):345-351.

    In a retrospective review, 78 femoral shaft fractures in children and adolescents age 8 to 18 years were treated with lateral trochanteric entry rigid intramedullary nail fixation. All patients progressed to union at an average of 7 weeks, with less than 10° of malalignment in all planes. No patient developed osteonecrosis or significant differences in their neck-shaft angle or articulotrochanteric distance. Level of evidence: III.

66. Carmichael KD, Bynum J, Goucher N: Rates of refracture associated with external fixation in pediatric femur fractures. *Am J Orthop (Belle Mead NJ)* 2005;34(9):439-444, discussion 444.

Developmental Dysplasia of the Hip

Developmental dysplasia of the hip (DDH) is the most common orthopaedic defect in newborns. DDH encompasses the spectrum of abnormalities involving the growing hip, including radiographic differences of the proximal femur or acetabulum and subluxation or dislocation of the hip joint. The incidence of DDH is estimated to range from 1 to more than 35 per 1,000 live births, based on the age at diagnosis or the method used for detection. For all newborn infants, a physical examination using the Ortolani and Barlow maneuvers is the most useful procedure to detect instability.

A discussion of treatment for adolescents and young adults with DDH from the perspective of adult reconstruction surgeons is presented in chapter 32.

Etiology and Pathogenesis

All components of the hip develop from the same primitive mesenchymal cells. Around the seventh week of intrauterine life, a cleft develops, defining the future femoral head and acetabulum. By the 11th intrauterine week, the hip joint is fully formed; this is the first time a dislocation can occur. The abnormalities resulting from an early dislocation are so severe that these dislocations are termed teratologic. Many teratologic dislocations are associated with certain neuromuscular conditions and genetic syndromes, especially those in which there is decreased or abnormal fetal movement, such as arthrogryposis or spina bifida.

There is a genetic component to DDH. The risk is increased twelvefold if a first-degree relative has DDH.[1]

Dr. Zaltz or an immediate family member serves as a board member, owner, officer, or committee member of the Michigan Orthopaedic Society and has received non-income support (such as equipment or services), commercially derived honoraria, or other non-research–related funding (such as paid travel) from DePuy, a Johnson & Johnson Company. Neither Dr. Castaneda nor any immediate family member has received anything of value from or owns stock in a commercial company or institution related directly or indirectly to the subject of this chapter.

The condition is most prevalent among Native Americans and Laplanders and is rarely seen in infants of African descent. Cultural traditions, such as swaddling infants with the hips held in extension, also have been implicated as important causative factors. Approximately 80% of affected infants are girls; this pattern is believed to be related to the perinatal ligamentous laxity caused by infant and maternal hormones. The left hip is affected in 60% of children, the right hip in 20%, and both hips in 20%. It is believed that the left side is more frequently involved because the left femur is adducted against the mother's lumbosacral spine in the most common intrauterine position (left occiput anterior), and instability is likely to develop as less femoral epiphysis is contained by the acetabulum. Infants in the breech position during the third trimester also are at increased risk for DDH.

Diagnosis
Physical Examination

In the newborn, the palpable sensation of the hip sliding into or out of the acetabulum is the mainstay of a positive diagnosis. The Ortolani test is a gentle maneuver in which the examiner feels the dislocated hip reducing as the flexed hip is abducted while the greater trochanter is anteriorly lifted. In the Barlow test, the examiner gently presses posterior on the flexed, adducted thigh to detect instability of a located hip that subluxates or dislocates (**Figure 1**). A palpable reduction or dislocation constitutes a positive test. Many infants are referred to an orthopaedic surgeon because the referring provider has detected soft-tissue clicks. Often the referring provider has ordered an ultrasonogram because of these clicks. An ultrasonogram performed before 6 weeks of age may spuriously indicate acetabular dysplasia, however. Infants with normal ultrasonographic findings in the presence of a soft-tissue click have normal hip development.[2]

The Ortolani and Barlow signs are rarely present after 3 months of age because of soft-tissue contracture. A dislocation can become fixed, and limited hip abduction in flexion will be present on the affected side. Detection is relatively easy in unilateral dislocation but more difficult in bilateral dislocation, where both hips are symmetrically limited. In unilateral dislocation, apparent shortening of the thigh (the Galeazzi sign) is

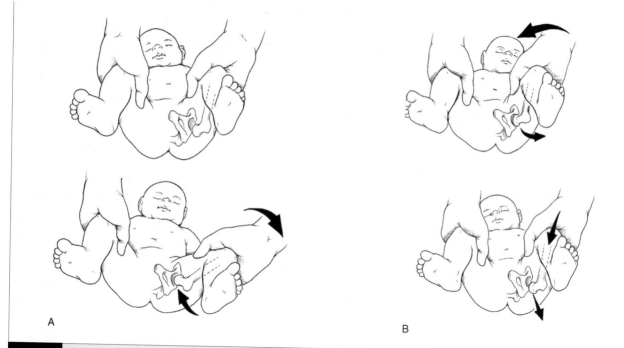

Figure 1 Drawings showing the clinical tests for detecting developmental dysplasia of the hip. **A,** The Ortolani test. **B,** The Barlow test. (Reproduced from Guille JT, Pizzutillo PD, MacEwen GD: Developmental dysplasia of the hip from birth to six months. *J Am Acad Orthop Surg* 2000;8:232-224.)

detected when the infant is positioned supine with both hips and knees flexed and the ankles level on the examination table. A walking child with unilateral dislocation may toe walk to compensate for the relative shortening. After a child reaches walking age, bilateral dislocation can cause a hip flexion contracture that is compensated for with increased lumbar lordosis. These patients may walk with a waddle because of bilateral gluteus medius functional insufficiency. Dysplasia without dislocation can be clinically silent in a child but may appear with hip pain or degenerative disease in adolescence or adulthood.

Imaging

In the normal newborn with clinical evidence of DDH, routine radiography of the hips and pelvis may be confirmatory. A normal radiograph does not exclude the presence of instability, however. The most common method of imaging the neonatal hip is ultrasonography, which offers distinct advantages compared with other imaging techniques. Unlike plain radiography, it can distinguish the cartilaginous components of the acetabulum and the femoral head, and there is no ionizing radiation. Real-time ultrasonography permits multiplanar examination that can clearly determine the position of the femoral head with respect to the acetabulum and permits observation of changes in hip position with movement. Unlike other techniques such as MRI, ultrasonography does not require sedation.

The pioneering work on ultrasonographic examination emphasized a morphologic approach and was

based on a static coronal image obtained through a lateral approach, with the infant in the lateral decubitus position. A subsequent approach was based on a dynamic multiplanar examination that assessed the hip in positions produced by the Ortolani and Barlow maneuvers.[3-5]

These two approaches complement each other. Most clinicians now use the so-called dynamic standard minimum examination, which includes assessment in the coronal plane with the hip at rest and assessment in the transverse plane with the hip under stress. At rest, two angles are measured in the coronal plane. A reference line is drawn above the acetabulum along the lateral wall of the ilium. The α angle is formed between the reference line and a line drawn tangential to the bony roof of the acetabulum; the β angle is formed between the reference line and a line drawn tangential to the cartilaginous labrum. In general, a normal mature infant hip should have an α angle of more than 60° and a β angle of less than 55°. The dynamic assessment monitors the position of the head in relation to the posterior bony wall of the acetabulum while a modified Barlow test is being performed (**Figure 2**).

Universal screening of newborns is neither cost effective nor practical, and it can lead to overdiagnosis, especially if performed before age 6 weeks. The current recommendation is that infants with a risk factor or an equivocal physical finding be referred for ultrasonographic screening. Recent data suggest that physical examination of all neonates for hip dysplasia and selective ultrasonography for infants at high risk are the

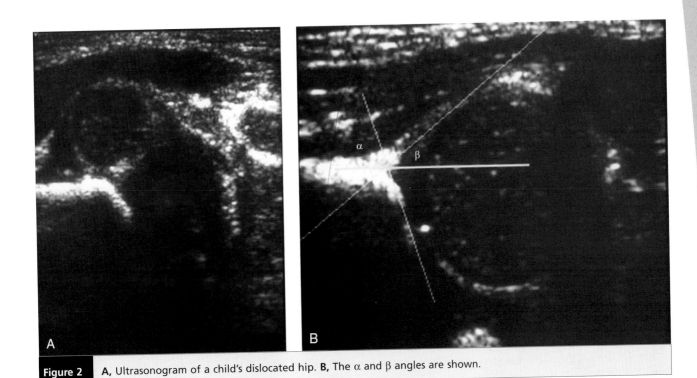

Figure 2   A, Ultrasonogram of a child's dislocated hip. **B,** The α and β angles are shown.

best means of decreasing the incidence of arthritic hips at age 60 years.[6] The ossific nucleus of the femoral head usually appears on ultrasonographic images at approximately 12 weeks of age, and it becomes apparent on plain radiographs by approximately 4 to 6 months. At that time, plain radiography becomes the primary imaging modality for DDH. Several lines can be projected on the AP radiograph of the pelvis (**Figure 3**). The acetabular index typically has been used to objectively assess the contour of the acetabulum; the normal value is less than 25° in children older than 6 months.

Arthrography, CT, and MRI have narrow indications and are not used in the primary diagnosis of DDH. Although arthrography provides information about soft-tissue impediments during closed reduction, it is an invasive study that requires anesthesia, and the interpretation is partially subjective. CT is the method of choice for evaluating the position of the femoral head after a closed or open reduction. Sedation is seldom required, as the patient is immobilized in a cast. Some centers use MRI after reduction to confirm the hip position and define the soft-tissue structures about the hip.

Treatment

The fundamental goal of treatment for DDH is to obtain a concentric and stable reduction with a minimal risk of aseptic necrosis. The complexity, risk, and rate of complications after treatment increase with a delay in diagnosis.

Splinting

Most affected infants who are younger than 6 months have hips that are dysplastic, subluxatable (Barlow pos-

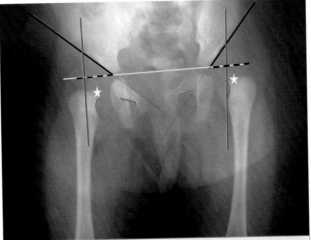

Figure 3   Radiograph of a hip with DDH, showing the Hilgenreiner line (yellow), the Perkin line (red), the Shenton line (green), and the acetabular index (black and yellow angle). The proximal medial metaphysis (star) of a located hip should be in the inferior medial quadrant of the grid formed by the Hilgenreiner and Perkins lines. The right is located and the left is dislocated with a break in the Shenton line, with displaced metaphysic and a higher acetabular index.

itive), or reducible (Ortolani positive). These children can be successfully treated with splinting in flexion and abduction. The Pavlik harness is the most commonly used splint in the United States (**Figure 4**). This device is a dynamic splint that requires normal muscle function; it is not used in children who have spina bifida or spasticity. Success with the Pavlik harness depends on the

6: Pediatrics

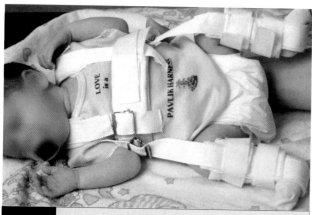

Figure 4 Photograph of a child wearing a Pavlik harness.

age at which it is applied and the time spent in the harness. Although an older child sometimes can be treated with the harness, most babies who are older than 6 months and are crawling should be treated with a different method.

The infant is placed in the harness with the anterior straps holding the hips in flexion and the posterior straps gradually stretching the hips out into abduction. The harness is typically applied with the hips in 90° to 100° of flexion. Hyperflexion should be avoided to prevent femoral nerve palsy or inferior hip dislocation, and wide abduction (more than 60°) should not be forced because of the risk of necrosis. The harness is worn continuously until the hip is stable. Harness use is suspended if the hip is found to be displaced in a posterior position, which can cause a failure of development of the posterior wall of the acetabulum, resulting in a severe form of acetabular dysplasia (Pavlik harness disease). Ultrasonography is used to help identify hips that are not developing adequately and may require another form of treatment.[7] Use of the harness should be continued until normal hip anatomy develops, typically between 6 and 8 weeks after stability is achieved. Other abduction splints, such as the Von Rosen and Hoffmann-Daimler splints, also have been used successfully. Regardless of the orthosis, extreme abduction should be avoided. If concentric reduction is not obtained within 2 to 4 weeks, another method of treatment should be selected.

Closed Reduction

In infants who are older than 6 months or who have had unsuccessful abduction splinting, closed reduction under general anesthesia with an arthrogram should be attempted. Excessive force should be avoided because it can cause ischemic necrosis. An arthrogram can provide useful information on the quality of the reduction and anatomic elements that could impede the hip reduction (the ligamentum teres, pulvinar, and transverse ligament). In the presence of a soft-tissue contracture, an adductor and/or psoas tenotomy can be considered to minimize force. After reduction has been obtained, the safe zone of abduction should be assessed. The safe zone is an arc of stable positioning between redislocation (adduction) and the limit of comfortable abduction. The patient is placed in a spica cast in the so-called human position, with 100° of flexion, 45° of abduction, and neutral rotation, for at least 6 weeks. The patient should then be placed in a second cast or an orthosis to maintain abduction until acetabular remodeling is complete. Even after a successful reduction, the hip must be followed to detect late acetabular dysplasia requiring a secondary procedure.

Open Reduction

Failure to obtain a concentric or stable closed reduction is an indication for open reduction in a patient of any age. Most children older than 18 months require open reduction. The anteromedial and medial surgical approaches have been used in children younger than 2 years. These approaches involve dividing the adductor longus and psoas tendons to allow direct access to the anteromedial hip capsule, which is opened to reach the intra-articular obstacles to reduction. The opportunity to perform a capsulorrhaphy is limited, but the ligamentum teres can be shortened and transferred to the medial capsule in an effort to increase hip stability. The risks of the medial approach include osteonecrosis and upper femoral growth disturbance.

The most commonly used method for open hip reduction is the anterior Smith-Petersen approach. The anterior approach is suitable for a patient of any age because the dissection preserves the medial femoral circumflex vessels and allows for a capsulorrhaphy and, if needed, a pelvic osteotomy. A separate groin incision allows tenotomy of the adductor longus and facilitates hip abduction. The dissection is deepened between the tensor fascia lata and the rectus femoris through a bikini incision parallel to the groin flexion crease. The direct origin of the rectus femoris is divided to expose the superior and lateral hip capsule. The psoas is found in the inferior wound and cut. Once the hip capsule is opened, the intra-articular structures obstructing reduction including the pulvinar, ligamentum teres, and transverse ligaments should be removed or transected as necessary. The labrum often is found to be tight before division of the transverse ligament. Radial cuts in the labrum should be avoided because they are a significant risk factor for early osteoarthritis.[8] Postoperative immobilization should be in a functional position, with the hip in 15° of flexion, 15° of abduction, and neutral rotation.

Femoral shortening during the open reduction has replaced preoperative traction for reducing the soft-tissue tension around the hip. The procedure is routinely performed in children older than 3 or 4 years, and it is considered necessary for any child if a gentle reduction is not obtained. The femur is shortened in the subtrochanteric region. With the hip reduced, the amount of femoral overlap is assessed and resected, and the femur is internally fixed with a plate and screws. Varus and rotation can be treated through this osteotomy as needed, but excessive retroversion of the femur should be avoided.

6: Pediatrics

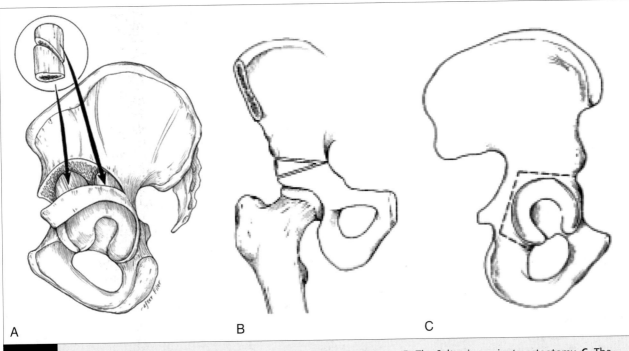

Figure 5 Drawings showing three pelvic osteotomies. **A,** The Dega osteotomy. **B,** The Salter innominate osteotomy. **C,** The Ganz periacetabular osteotomy. (Reproduced from Gillingham BL, Sanchez AA, Wenger DR: Pelvic osteotomies for the treatment of hip dysplasia in children and young adults. *J Am Acad Orthop Surg* 1999;7:325-337.)

Pelvic Osteotomy

In an older child, the acetabulum may be severely dysplastic with anterolateral insufficiency. If this condition is found, a pelvic osteotomy should be considered during the open reduction to maximize stability. The Salter innominate osteotomy is a redirectional osteotomy that hinges through the pubic symphysis and restores approximately 25° of lateral coverage and 10° of anterior coverage. The Pemberton and Dega osteotomies have been extensively used, with similar results[9] (**Figure 5**).

Age Limits for Reduction

The long-term results are best if a patient with DDH is diagnosed and treated at a young age. The rate of complications increases proportionally with age, and diminished results can be expected with increasing age. Beyond a certain age, surgical treatment is unlikely to produce a stable, mobile, and pain-free joint for the long term.[10] Despite the obvious gait abnormalities, pain-free bilateral dislocations probably should not be reduced after the child reaches age 4 to 5 years. Unilateral dislocations can be more problematic because of limb-length inequality and pelvic obliquity, but even these generally fare better without treatment beyond age 6 years.[11] An appropriately performed epiphysiodesis can treat the limb-length discrepancy in these patients.

Redislocation

Redislocation after a closed reduction usually is treated with a repeat closed reduction or an open reduction, without deleterious effects on the long-term outcome.

Redislocation after open reduction often is attributable to actions taken during the initial procedure, such as insufficient capsular release, inadequate capsulorrhaphy, or combined femoral and pelvic osteotomies resulting in posterior instability. These actions almost always necessitate repeat surgery, and the results may deteriorate depending on the duration of the redislocation.

Ischemic Necrosis

Ischemic necrosis can result from extrinsic compression of the vasculature supplying the capital femoral epiphysis and excessive direct pressure on the cartilaginous head; these can be provoked by excessive or forceful abduction, multiple attempts at closed reduction, or repeat surgery. The radiographic appearance of ischemic necrosis may include failure of the ossific nucleus to develop within 1 year after reduction, broadening of the femoral neck, increased density or fragmentation of the capital femoral epiphysis, or residual deformity of the femoral head and neck after ossification. The most common classification of ischemic necrosis distinguishes between epiphyseal and metaphyseal involvement. Treatment depends on the degree of severity as well as the presence of symptoms related to deformity of the femoral neck or upper femur.

Late Dysplasia

Children who are diagnosed with DDH should be followed until skeletal maturity, even after a successful closed or open reduction. Serial radiographs should be obtained. The acetabulum continues to develop until approximately age 6 years, and failure of the acetabulum to develop normally may be an indication for intervention.

The presence of asymptomatic dysplasia in an adolescent warrants further follow-up. CT or MRI can provide important information in symptomatic patients. Radiographic dysplasia such as a decreased lateral center-edge angle (the angle of Wiberg) or an anterior center-edge angle (the angle of Lequesne) is associated with early osteoarthritis, especially in the presence of a labral tear. This dysplasia is an indication for surgery in a symptomatic patient. In experienced hands, the Ganz periacetabular osteotomy is the procedure of choice for the correction of the bony dysplasia (**Figure 5, C**). The labral tear should be repaired through an open or arthroscopic approach.[12]

Developmental Coxa Vara

Developmental coxa vara is relatively uncommon, with an incidence of 1 in 25,000 live births. There is bilateral involvement in 30% to 50% of patients. Although the etiology is unknown, developmental coxa vara has been considered an unusual localized dysplasia that occurs if an unspecified primary ossification defect in the inferior femoral neck undergoes fatigue failure when bearing weight, resulting in progressive varus displacement. Radiographically, a decreased femoral neck-shaft angle is noted with an associated decrease in the articulotrochanteric distance and increased femoral retroversion. The classic radiographic changes include an inverted Y-shaped radiolucency in the inferior femoral neck. The position of the physeal plate should be measured using the Hilgenreiner physeal angle, which is determined from an AP radiograph as the angle between the Hilgenreiner line and the plane of the proximal femoral physis. A normal Hilgenreiner angle should be less than 25°. With an increasing Hilgenreiner angle, there is a greater chance of progression of the coxa vara, stress fracture, nonunion of the femoral neck, and early degenerative arthritis of the hip.

Patients typically have a progressive but painless limp during early childhood, with the coxa vara creating a high-riding position of the greater trochanter and subsequent functional weakening of the abductors. Children with bilateral involvement walk with a waddling gait and may have increased lumbar lordosis. Unilateral involvement causes a Trendelenburg gait, and the limb-length inequality can accentuate the limping.

Nonsurgical treatment has not proved effective. Surgical correction should address the deformity in both the sagittal and coronal planes. A valgus and derotational osteotomy is indicated if the femoral neck-shaft angle is less than 90°, the Hilgenreiner angle is greater than 60°, or the physeal angle is greater than 45°. Surgical treatment should aim for overcorrection of the neck-shaft angle to approximately 160°, restoration of the Hilgenreiner angle to approximately 25°, and normalization of femoral rotation. Supplemental bone grafting is generally not necessary. Internal fixation

with plates allows early mobilization. Percutaneous techniques with external fixation have also been used successfully.[13]

If adequate correction is achieved, the defect in the neck closes within approximately 6 months after surgery. The physis closes approximately 24 months after surgery, even if it has not been violated. The patient must be monitored for limb-length inequality. Recurrence of the varus is unusual if adequate valgus has been achieved.

Legg-Calvé-Perthes Disease

Legg-Calvé-Perthes (LCP) disease is widely believed to result from an initial interruption of the blood supply to a variable portion of the proximal femoral epiphysis, possibly extending to the adjacent femoral growth plate and metaphysis. The condition is not simply ischemic; the consequences of epiphyseal bone resorption, collapse, and repair affect the course of the disease. LCP disease has a variable course to final healing of the femoral epiphysis. The symptoms can extend over 2 to 5 years. Most patients recover satisfactory, minimally symptomatic function. There are rare incidences of minimal disease with little or no permanent change in the contour of the femoral head, but most patients have moderately severe disease that results in an aspherical femoral head at maturity. Approximately half of patients develop premature osteoarthritis.

Epidemiology and Etiology

The disease most commonly occurs in boys age 4 and 10 years, although it can occur in children as young as 2 years and occasionally occurs in teenagers. The male-to-female ratio is approximately 5 to 1. LCP disease is distinguished from adult osteonecrosis because of the greater potential for healing and remodeling. The disease is bilateral in approximately 10% of children, but it does not appear at the same stage in both hips. Simultaneous bilateral involvement should alert the clinician to the possibility of a different diagnosis. Conditions that should be ruled out include multiple epiphyseal dysplasia, spondyloepiphyseal dysplasia, sickle cell disease, Gaucher disease, and hypothyroidism.

Despite some causal associations, including parental smoking, thrombophilic disorders, and cartilage gene mutations, no conclusive cause has been identified. Children with LCP disease tend to be of short stature and have delayed bone maturation compared with normally developing children. There is a significant rate of attention deficit disorder among affected children.

Pathogenesis

There are numerous experiments in which Perthes-like changes are produced without injuring the arterial supply.[14,15] There is growing experimental evidence of recurrent injury to the circumflex arteries in animals that mimics the appearance of LCP disease, suggesting that

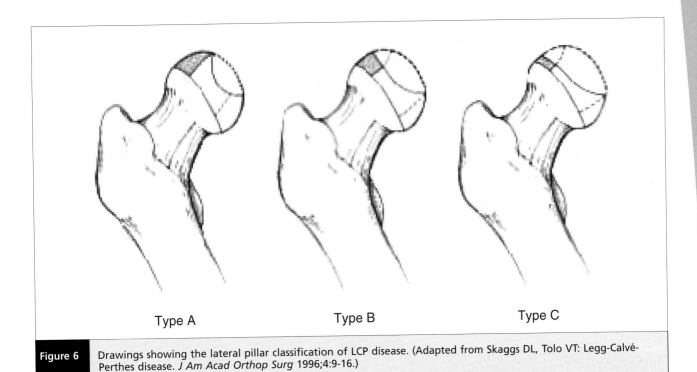

Type A   Type B   Type C

Figure 6 Drawings showing the lateral pillar classification of LCP disease. (Adapted from Skaggs DL, Tolo VT: Legg-Calvé-Perthes disease. *J Am Acad Orthop Surg* 1996;4:9-16.)

the bone necrosis and repair develop over time after repetitive ischemic insults. A porcine model of LCP disease suggests that the physeal tissue is most often spared.[16] Iliac crest biopsy specimens from patients with LCP disease suggested the presence of cytoplasmic granules containing lipid and fibrillar material, but the clinical significance is unknown.[17] Linkage studies of a family with a history of LCP disease and precocious arthritis revealed a mutation in *COL2A1* gene that decreases collagen helical mechanical properties.[18]

Clinical Evaluation, Imaging, and Classification

A child with LCP disease typically has a Trendelenburg gait or antalgic limp that is intermittently painful. Discomfort may be referred to the thigh, knee, or groin. The clinical examination reveals variable hip irritability and stiffness; limitation in abduction and internal rotation are most common. In severe LCP disease, a limb-length discrepancy may be present later in the course of the disease. The differential diagnosis includes septic arthritis, transient synovitis, proximal femoral osteomyelitis, and pyomyositis. Infectious processes are differentiated by the clinical setting and laboratory analysis.

MRI, CT, and bone scanning have been investigated for imaging hips with LCP disease, but their clinical value has not yet been clearly established. MRI is well established for the diagnosis of labral and articular cartilage anomalies, particularly in skeletally mature patients with healed LCP. Standard radiographs are the basis for classification and treatment. The radiographic course of LCP is divided into four stages. The initial stage, characterized by apparent widening of the joint and mild symptoms, is presumed to occur after infarc-

tion and can extend as long as 6 months. The fragmentation stage can last from 6 months to 2 years. Hip-related symptoms are most prevalent during this period. Fragmentation is thought to begin when a subchondral lucent line (the crescent sign) appears and there is progressive radiographic dissolution of the epiphysis. A crescent sign may be present, involving less or more than half of the epiphysis (Salter-Thompson type A or B, respectively). The Catterall classification is based on the extent of epiphyseal fragmentation; it has poor interobserver and intraobserver reliability and is of historical importance only. Currently, the most widely used system for the fragmentation stage is the lateral pillar classification[19] (**Figure 6**). This system is based on the first AP hip radiograph obtained during the fragmentation stage. The lateral third of the epiphysis, usually located lateral to the central sequestrum, is compared to that of the contralateral hip and is measured for grading. The epiphysis is considered type A if its height is equal to that of the contralateral epiphysis, type B if there is collapse and the height of the epiphysis is greater than 50%, and type C if there is greater collapse and the height is less than 50% of that of the contralateral epiphysis. A fourth type, called type B/C borderline, was recently added to categorize hips with a thin or poorly ossified lateral pillar and loss of exactly 50% of the original height of the lateral pillar. This classification system has good intraobserver and interobserver reliability and is well correlated with the prognosis.[20] The lateral pillar classification progresses during fragmentation in approximately 30% of hips, and changes are more common in extensively involved hips.[21] Lateral subluxation and hinge abduction are definitively related to a poor prognosis.[22] Hinge abduc-

6: Pediatrics

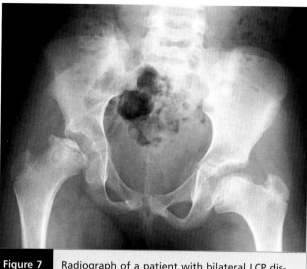

| Figure 7 | Radiograph of a patient with bilateral LCP disease. The left hip is almost completely healed while the right hip is in the early reossification stage. Lateral subluxation and deformity of the right epiphysis suggests hinge abduction. |

tion, in which a deformity of the lateral epiphysis prevents abduction and causes hinging on the lateral acetabulum, is diagnosed using an AP pelvic radiograph with the hips abducted (**Figure 7**).

Reossification, the third radiographic phase of LCP disease, occurs when new bone formation is clearly recognizable on radiographs. This phase may last as long as 18 months. Healing or remodeling, the fourth stage, begins when the epiphyseal bone density normalizes and trabecular patterns appear. The common residual deformities may be more recognizable at this stage, including femoral neck shortening (coxa breva), head widening (coxa magna), and flattening (coxa plana). With involvement of the capital femoral growth plate, there can be tilting of the femoral neck (coxa valga) and relative overgrowth of the greater trochanter. Secondary changes in acetabulum depth and orientation occur throughout the course of LCP disease and partially determine joint congruence, hip motion, and the long-term durability of the hip.[23] The Stulberg classification is used to assess joint congruity at skeletal maturity. Type I is defined as a completely normal hip. A type II hip (spherically congruent) has a spherical femoral head that may be larger than normal and has a short neck or an abnormal acetabulum. A type III hip (aspherically congruent) is nonspherical, with an ovoid, mushroom, or umbrella shape that is not flat. A type IV hip (also aspherically congruent) is flat and articulates with a correspondingly flat acetabulum. A type V hip (incongruent) has a flat or deformed femoral head that articulates with a differently shaped acetabulum. The accuracy of the Stulberg classification system has been questioned.[24] The interobserver and intraobserver reliability of this system is moderate. Only type I and some type II hips seem to function well over the course of a lifetime. By the fifth or sixth decade of life, most patients with Stulberg types develop degenerative arthritis.[20,25]

Natural History and Prognosis

Patients with LCP disease with significant femoral head deformity function relatively well into the fourth and fifth decades of life. The long-term prognosis is best with a young age at onset; approximately 80% of children with onset before age 6 years have a favorable prognosis. Poor results can be predicted for patients with type B/C or C hips whose age at onset was 4 or 5 years.[26,27] In an older patient, less residual joint deformity is associated with an improved prognosis.

Treatment

Treatment during the initial symptomatic phase includes rest, activity modification, the use of nonsteroidal anti-inflammatory drugs, and physical therapy to maintain hip motion and muscle strength. Bracing and casting have no significant benefit. Surgical treatment is controversial; a recent landmark study determined that patients who are older than 8 years at onset and have a hip in the lateral pillar B group or the B/C border group have a better outcome with surgical treatment than with nonsurgical treatment.[25]

Children who are younger than 8 years at onset and have a group A or B hip have a very favorable outcome unrelated to treatment. Children of any age with a group C hip frequently have a poor outcome; the hip is unaffected by treatment. The timing of surgery has a significant impact on the result; no positive effect has been found from containment surgery performed after the initial or early fragmentation stage. Surgical options to improve containment include femoral varus osteotomy, acetabular enhancement procedures such as periacetabular osteotomy, or shelf arthroplasty. Successful treatment of established hinge abduction has been reported using a valgus or abduction-type procedure, intertrochanteric osteotomy, or shelf arthroplasty.[28]

Occasionally, a patient with LCP disease develops mechanical symptoms related to loose fragments of cartilage or labral pathology. The diagnosis of internal derangement has been facilitated by magnetic resonance arthrography. Management of hip abnormalities related to LCP disease is evolving with the increasing understanding of femoroacetabular impingement and patterns of labral and chondral injury. Surgical treatment using hip arthroscopy and surgical dislocation is emerging for the management of disorders related to LCP disease.

Slipped Capital Femoral Epiphysis

Slipped capital femoral epiphysis (SCFE) is a disorder characterized by posterior and interior displacement of the epiphysis on the femoral neck. It is the most common disorder affecting adolescent hips, although younger children with hormonal or systemic disorders can also be affected. Patients with SCFE may have acute or chronic symptoms as a result of varying de-

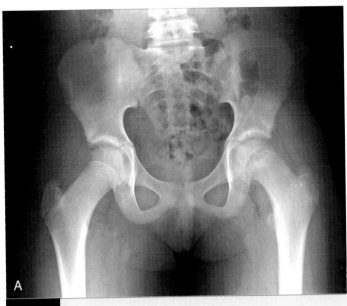
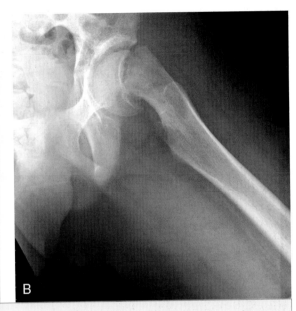

Figure 8   A and B, Radiographs showing an unstable SCFE.

grees of epiphyseal stability that may affect the ability of the child to ambulate.

Etiology

Mechanical forces acting through a susceptible physis are thought to be responsible for the observed translation. Children affected by a hormonal abnormality or imbalance may be more susceptible to SCFE at an earlier age. Disorders of vitamin D metabolism, thyroid hormone production, renal osteodystrophy, pelvic radiation therapy, and parenteral administration of growth hormone are associated with SCFE. Other factors associated with SCFE include femoral retroversion and obesity. A recent study using laser capture techniques to examine chondrocytes from the physeal plates of patients with SCFE found downregulation of gene expression for type II collagen and aggrecan.[29] It is not known whether this finding is a cause of or a response to SCFE.

Incidence

SCFE is more prevalent in boys than in girls and, in decreasing frequency, affects children of African, Hispanic, Native American, and Caucasian descent. Recent multistate data from the United States suggest an incidence of 10 per 100,000.[30] Obesity is the single greatest risk factor for the development of SCFE; approximately 75% of affected children have a weight above the 90th percentile. SCFE has not been shown to be linked to other obesity-related disorders such as tibia vara or type II diabetes.[31] Although the historically reported incidence of SCFE is variable, recent reports suggest that the overall rate of disease may be increasing, probably as a result of the increased prevalence of pediatric obesity.[30,32] The severity of SCFE has been shown to be proportionate to both body mass index and duration of symptoms.[33]

Clinical Evaluation and Classification

The mean age at presentation is 13.4 years for boys and 12.2 years for girls. The classification of SCFE is based on epiphyseal stability.[34] A stable slip is defined by the ability of the patient to walk or bear weight on the extremity. An unstable slip is defined by the inability to bear weight. A patient with unstable SCFE is more likely to develop osteonecrosis of the epiphysis; the reported rate of osteonecrosis in unstable SCFE ranges from 0 to 54.5%, with an average of 22%.[35,36]

In general, patients with an unstable slip show guarding on attempted passive examination as well as an inability to walk. The slip in these patients is likely to be quite unstable, with an externally rotated, shortened limb that is akin to an acute fracture. Most patients have a stable slip. Their symptoms are more indolent and have an average duration of 5.7 months.[37] These patients have pain in the groin, thigh, knee, buttock, or peritrochanteric region. An external rotation limp usually is present and is correlated with both the severity of the proximal femoral deformity and the stability of the physeal plate. Passive flexion of the involved hip produces obligatory external rotation, and attempted passive internal rotation often produces discomfort.

Imaging

Traditional plain radiographs, including pelvic AP and true lateral views, are used to establish the diagnosis of SCFE (**Figure 8**). SCFE is most readily seen on lateral radiographs. The reliability of the Klein line, a traditional diagnostic sign, has recently been questioned.[38] Depending on the chronicity of the symptoms, a variable amount of femoral metaphyseal remodeling is radiographically visible.

Two methods are used to estimate the anatomic severity of SCFE. On the lateral radiograph, the slip an-

6: Pediatrics

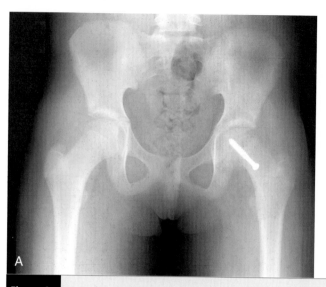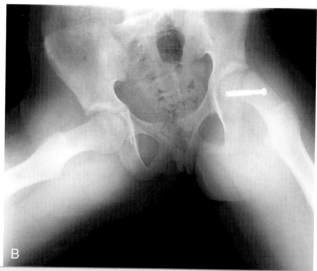

| **Figure 9** | **A** and **B**, Radiographs after initial treatment with in situ pinning in the patient whose radiographs are shown in Figure 8. The patient continued to have symptoms related to impingement. |

gle measures angulation between the femoral epiphysis and the femoral neck as mild (less than 30°), moderate (30° to 60°), or severe (more than 60°). The slip percentage measures translation between the epiphysis and femoral neck on AP or lateral views as mild (less than 25%), moderate (25% to 50%), or severe (more than 50%). Recent CT data suggest that a plain radiographic assessment of SCFE may underestimate the anatomic SCFE deformity and, thus, its long-term consequences.[39]

Treatment

A stable SCFE is treated with stabilization of the epiphysis to prevent further displacement and to promote stability and healing of the physis (**Figure 9**). For this purpose, percutaneous in situ fixation is used with a cannulated screw inserted into the center of the epiphysis and a minimum of four threads crossing the physis. The outcome of the procedure is predictable in most patients. The few complications of in situ pinning include insertion site femoral fracture, acetabular screw impingement, progressive slip after pin insertion, and chondrolysis.[40] Patients with stable SCFE are permitted to bear full weight with crutches after the first 4 to 6 weeks after screw insertion.

The traditional treatment of unstable SCFE is in situ fixation using one central cannulated screw; a second screw is added if necessary for stability. Forceful closed manipulative reduction is not recommended because it increases the risk of osteonecrosis. The use of emergency anterior capsulotomy with hematoma or fluid evacuation, followed by controlled epiphyseal reduction to the preslip position and smooth Kirschner wire fixation, also has been reported for managing unstable SCFE.[41] The long-term anatomic consequences of a slipped epiphysis, the association between femoroacetabular impingement and the development of osteoarthritis, and applied understanding of the vascular anat-

omy of the upper femoral epiphysis are changing the traditional approaches to unstable and some high-grade stable SCFEs. Two techniques permit controlled reduction of the epiphysis. Epiphyseal reorientation using a surgical dislocation approach and a modified Dunn procedure are reported to permit full correction at the site of deformity and stabilization of the epiphysis while protecting the epiphyseal vascular flap.[42]

Recent midterm data on 105 patients with severe SCFE treated with in situ fixation found that 49% had an excellent result, 26% a good result, and 24% a fair or poor result. The mean Iowa hip score was 84.7.[43] A study of symptomatic femoroacetabular impingement after SCFE treatment found that 31% of patients had symptomatic hips and 32% had clinical evidence of impingement at a mean 6.1 years after treatment.[44]

The presence of symptomatic impingement was not correlated with slip severity but with the α angle (head-neck junction morphology) after healing. The natural history of an individual patient with SCFE and the ideal hip for acute operative reduction remain undetermined.

The role of prophylactic contralateral in situ fixation remains controversial in both stable and unstable SCFE. It is difficult to predict the occurrence of a contralateral slip in patients with a unilateral SCFE, and prediction accuracy may vary considerably depending on the population. A high percentage of patients who develop a contralateral SCFE are not symptomatic.[45] The prevalence of contralateral SCFE ranges from 20% to 60% and is higher in patients younger than 10 years.[46,47] The prevalence of simultaneous bilateral SCFE is approximately 20%.[48] Data accumulated over a 10-year period revealed contralateral SCFE in 36% of patients. Of these patients, 22% had a severe slip, and 6% developed osteonecrosis or chondrolysis. Contralateral pinning was determined to be safer than observation until symptoms develop.[49] Contralateral pinning is

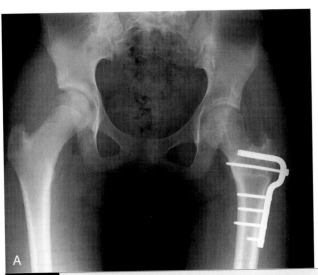
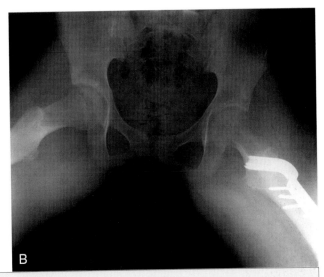

| Figure 10 | **A** and **B**, Radiographs after a surgical hip dislocation, head and neck osteochondroplasty, and intertrochanteric flexion derotational osteotomy in the patient discussed in Figures 8 and 9. |

commonly recommended for patients who have unstable SCFE, are younger than 10 years, or have a systemic metabolic disorder.

Complications

Complications resulting from the treatment of SCFE include osteonecrosis, chondrolysis, slip progression, pinning-associated femur fracture, screw impingement, and painful or function-limiting upper femoral deformity. The reported incidence of osteonecrosis in stable SCFE is approximately 4%, and the incidence in unstable SCFE averages 22%.[35,50]

The treatment of established osteonecrosis depends on the location of the necrotic segment, healing of the physeal plate, extent of epiphyseal involvement, and any associated deformity. The evaluation should include plain radiographs, CT with sagittal and coronal reformatting, and MRI. Screw removal is often necessary after physeal healing to prevent intra-articular penetration and facilitate imaging. Small, non–weight-bearing zone lesions are observed. Reconstructive procedures include realignment osteotomies, distraction, and vascularized fibular transfers.[44] Salvage procedures include arthrodesis and total hip arthroplasty. The role of bisphosphonates for treating post-SCFE osteonecrosis is under investigation.[51]

The indications for treatment and the surgical techniques for reconstructing painful or function-limiting upper femoral deformities are evolving. The patients most at risk include those with an increased α angle and/or an associated acetabular retroversion or anterior overcoverage.[44] If feasible, the preoperative evaluation of these patients should include magnetic resonance arthrography to assess labral damage and chondral injury. The traditional treatments include flexion-valgus-derotational osteotomies of the femur at the intertrochanteric or subtrochanteric level. The use of surgical dislocation to reach the labrum, acetabulum,

and head-neck junction may improve the efficacy of traditional realignment procedures. The role of head-neck junction osteoplasty and subcapital osteotomy remains to be determined[52-54] (**Figure 10**).

Annotated References

1. Stevenson DA, Mineau G, Kerber RA, Viskochil DH, Schaefer C, Roach JW: Familial predisposition to developmental dysplasia of the hip. *J Pediatr Orthop* 2009; 29(5):463-466.

    A large database was reviewed to determine the incidence of DDH as well as the relative risk associated with a familial history. The finding that there is a significantly increased risk if a first-degree relative is affected should lead to future research into the phenotypic characterization of patients with DDH, as well as genetic analysis.

2. Kane TP, Harvey JR, Richards RH, Burby NG, Clarke NM: Radiological outcome of innocent infant hip clicks. *J Pediatr Orthop B* 2003;12(4):259-263.

3. Grissom LE, Harke HT: Developmental dysplasia of the pediatric hip with emphasis on sonographic evaluation. *Semin Musculoskelet Radiol* 1999;3(4):359-370.

4. Graf R: Fundamentals of sonographic diagnosis of infant hip dysplasia. *J Pediatr Orthop* 1984;4(6):735-740.

5. Harcke HT, Kumar SJ: Current concepts review: The role of ultrasound in the diagnosis and management of congenital dislocation and dysplasia of the hip. *J Bone Joint Surg Am* 1991;73:622-628.

6. Mahan ST, Katz JN, Kim YJ: To screen or not to screen? A decision analysis of the utility of screening for developmental dysplasia of the hip. *J Bone Joint Surg Am* 2009;91(7):1705-1719.

6: Pediatrics

Decision analysis was applied to reach a concise and clinically relevant conclusion: the highest probability of having a nonarthritic hip at age 60 years results from screening all neonates clinically for hip dysplasia and using imaging modalities in selected infants.

7. Lerman JA, Emans JB, Millis MB, Share J, Zurakowski D, Kasser JR: Early failure of Pavlik harness treatment for developmental hip dysplasia: Clinical and ultrasound predictors. *J Pediatr Orthop* 2001;21(3):348-353.

8. Jessel RH, Zurakowski D, Zilkens C, Burstein D, Gray ML, Kim YJ: Radiographic and patient factors associated with pre-radiographic osteoarthritis in hip dysplasia. *J Bone Joint Surg Am* 2009;91(5):1120-1129.

An unequivocal relationship is established among DDH, osteoarthritis with increasing age, and the severity of the dysplasia, as shown by decreased center-edge angles as well as the presence of labral tears.

9. López-Carreño E, Carillo H, Gutiérrez M: Dega versus Salter osteotomy for the treatment of developmental dysplasia of the hip. *J Pediatr Orthop B* 2008;17(5): 213-221.

Patients treated with Dega and Salter osteotomies had similar results at midterm follow-up.

10. Vallamshetla VR, Mughal E, O'Hara JN: Congenital dislocation of the hip: A re-appraisal of the upper age limit for treatment. *J Bone Joint Surg Br* 2006;88(8): 1076-1081.

11. Crawford AH, Mehlman CT, Slovek RW: The fate of untreated developmental dislocation of the hip: Long-term follow-up of eleven patients. *J Pediatr Orthop* 1999;19(5):641-644.

12. Trousdale RT: Acetabular osteotomy: Indications and results. *Clin Orthop Relat Res* 2004;429:182-187.

13. Sabharwal S, Mittal R, Cox G: Percutaneous triplanar femoral osteotomy correction for developmental coxa vara: A new technique. *J Pediatr Orthop* 2005;25(1): 28-33.

14. Liu SL, Ho TC: The role of venous hypertension in the pathogenesis of Legg-Perthes disease: A clinical and experimental study. *J Bone Joint Surg Am* 1991;73(2): 194-200.

15. Boss JH, Misselevich I: Osteonecrosis of the femoral head of laboratory animals: The lessons learned from a comparative study of osteonecrosis in man and experimental animals. *Vet Pathol* 2003;40(4):345-354.

16. Kim HK, Stephenson N, Garces A, Aya-ay J, Bian H: Effects of disruption of epiphyseal vasculature on the proximal femoral growth plate. *J Bone Joint Surg Am* 2009;91(5):1149-1158.

The authors evaluated the viability of physeal chondrocytes and the architecture of the proximal femoral physis after suture ligature–induced epiphyseal osteonecrosis in a porcine model. Most animals with surgically induced necrosis had no visible physeal abnormality.

17. Kitoh H, Kitakoji T, Kawasumi M, Ishiguro N: A histological and ultrastructural study of the iliac crest apophysis in Legg-Calve-Perthes disease. *J Pediatr Orthop* 2008;28(4):435-439.

Eleven iliac crest biopsies from patients with LCP disease were compared with 10 iliac crest biopsies from patients with hip dysplasia. Resting zone chondrocytes were found to have cytoplasmic granules thought to be lipid material and fibrillar inclusions.

18. Su P, Li R, Liu S, et al: Age at onset-dependent presentations of premature hip osteoarthritis, avascular necrosis of the femoral head, or Legg-Calvé-Perthes disease in a single family, consequent upon a p.Gly1170Ser mutation of COL2A1. *Arthritis Rheum* 2008;58(6):1701-1706.

A review of 42 members of a five-generation family with a history of premature osteoarthritis found that a serine-to-glycine mutation of *COL2A1* may loosen the helical structure of collagen segregated in patients with LCP disease.

19. Herring JA, Kim HT, Browne R: Legg-Calve-Perthes disease: Part I. Classification of radiographs with use of the modified lateral pillar and Stulberg classifications. *J Bone Joint Surg Am* 2004;86(10):2103-2120.

20. Akgun R, Yazici M, Aksoy MC, Cil A, Alpaslan AM, Tumer Y: The accuracy and reliability of estimation of lateral pillar height in determining the herring grade in Legg-CalvePerthes disease. *J Pediatr Orthop* 2004; 24(6):651-653.

21. Kuroda T, Mitani S, Sugimoto Y, et al: Changes in the lateral pillar classification in Perthes' disease. *J Pediatr Orthop B* 2009;18(3):116-119.

A retrospective review of 102 patients with LCP disease found changes in lateral pillar morphology and classification after initial classification. Change was observed in 31%, and this finding was more prevalent in patients with extensive disease.

22. Gigante C, Frizziero P, Turra S: Prognostic value of Catterall and Herring classification in Legg-Calve-Perthes disease: Follow-up to skeletal maturity of 32 patients. *J Pediatr Orthop* 2002;22(3):345-349.

23. Sankar WN, Flynn JM: The development of acetabular retroversion in children with Legg-Calvé-Perthes disease. *J Pediatr Orthop* 2008;28(4):440-443.

In 53 patients with axial imaging obtained early in the course of LCP disease, there was a 1.8% incidence of retroversion. Following skeletal maturation, 5 of 16 hips had plain radiographic evidence of retroversion, suggesting adaptive development during the disease course.

24. Neyt JG, Weinstein SL, Spratt KF, et al: Stulberg classification system for evaluation of Legg-Calve-Perthes disease: Intra-rater and inter-rater reliability. *J Bone Joint Surg Am* 1999;81(9):1209-1216.

25. Herring JA, Kim HT, Browne R: Legg-Calve-Perthes disease: Part II. Prospective multicenter study of the effect of treatment on outcome. *J Bone Joint Surg Am* 2004;86(10):2121-2134.

26. Canavese F, Dimeglio A: Perthes' disease: Prognosis in children under six years of age. *J Bone Joint Surg Br* 2008;90(7):940-945.

    A retrospective review of 166 patients younger than 6 years when LCP disease appeared found that mild LCP disease had a generally good radiographic outcome and that severe disease did not benefit from containment treatment using the Salter innominate osteotomy, compared with nonsurgical treatment.

27. Rosenfeld SB, Herring JA, Chao JC: Legg-calve-perthes disease: A review of cases with onset before six years of age. *J Bone Joint Surg Am* 2007;89(12):2712-2722.

    A retrospective review of 188 patients with LCP disease appearing before age 6 years found that all had a Stulberg type I or II radiographic outcome, except for those classified into the lateral column B/C or C group and those age 5 years or older.

28. Freeman RT, Wainwright AM, Theologis TN, Benson MK: The outcome of patients with hinge abduction in severe Perthes disease treated by shelf acetabuloplasty. *J Pediatr Orthop* 2008;28(6):619-625.

    In a retrospective review of the outcomes of arthrographically proved hinge abduction and subsequent treatment with the Staheli shelf arthroplasty, 52% of the patients had Stulberg type I or II disease. Decreased medial joint space and improved acetabular coverage were reported.

29. Scharschmidt T, Jacquet R, Weiner D, Lowder E, Schrickel T, Landis WJ: Gene expression in slipped capital femoral epiphysis: Evaluation with laser capture microdissection and quantitative reverse transcription-polymerase chain reaction. *J Bone Joint Surg Am* 2009; 91(2):366-377.

    The authors evaluated expression of mRNA for key structural molecules in growth plate chondrocytes of patients with SCFE.

30. Benson EC, Miller M, Bosch P, Szalay EA: A new look at the incidence of slipped capital femoral epiphysis in New Mexico. *J Pediatr Orthop* 2008;28(5):529-533.

    The current and past reported incidences of SCFE were compared to identify factors related to the fivefold increased incidence of SCFE since the 1960s.

31. Bowen JR, Assis M, Sinha K, Hassink S, Littleton A: Associations among slipped capital femoral epiphysis, tibia vara, and type 2 juvenile diabetes. *J Pediatr Orthop* 2009;29(4):341-344.

    A retrospective review investigated multiple disease occurrence in adolescents with obesity. No disease coexistence was established among tibia vara, SCFE, and type II diabetes.

32. Murray AW, Wilson NI: Changing incidence of slipped capital femoral epiphysis: A relationship with obesity? *J Bone Joint Surg Br* 2008;90(1):92-94.

    Increasing rates of childhood obesity and SCFE are investigated in the Scottish population.

33. Loder RT: Correlation of radiographic changes with disease severity and demographic variables in children with stable slipped capital femoral epiphysis. *J Pediatr Orthop* 2008;28(3):284-290.

    A retrospective review of 97 patients treated for stable SCFE correlated slip severity, symptom severity, and metaphyseal deformity with the duration of symptoms.

34. Loder RT, Richards BS, Shapiro PS, Reznick LR, Aronson DD: Acute slipped capital femoral epiphysis: The importance of physeal stability. *J Bone Joint Surg Am* 1993;75(8):1134-1140.

35. Phillips SA, Griffiths WE, Clarke NM: The timing of reduction and stabilisation of the acute, unstable, slipped upper femoral epiphysis. *J Bone Joint Surg Br* 2001; 83(7):1046-1049.

36. Tokmakova KP, Stanton RP, Mason DE: Factors influencing the development of osteonecrosis in patients treated for slipped capital femoral epiphysis. *J Bone Joint Surg Am* 2003;85(5):798-801.

37. Green DW, Reynolds RA, Khan SN, Tolo V: The delay in diagnosis of slipped capital femoral epiphysis: A review of 102 patients. *HSS J* 2005;1(1):103-106.

38. Loder RT: Correlation of radiographic changes with disease severity and demographic variables in children with stable slipped capital femoral epiphysis. *J Pediatr Orthop* 2008;28(3):284-290.

39. Mamisch TC, Kim YJ, Richolt JA, Millis MB, Kordelle J: Femoral morphology due to impingement influences the range of motion in slipped capital femoral epiphysis. *Clin Orthop Relat Res* 2009;467(3):692-698.

    Computer reconstruction was used to evaluate the effect of metaphyseal morphology on post-SCFE femoral acetabular impingement. The presence of metaphyseal deformity and decreased head-neck offset increases the likelihood of impingement with relatively mild slip severity.

40. Goodwin RC, Mahar AT, Oswald TS, Wenger DR: Screw head impingement after in situ fixation in moderate and severe slipped capital femoral epiphysis. *J Pediatr Orthop* 2007;27(3):319-325.

    An in vitro study evaluated arc of motion and screw-head acetabular impingement in a cadaver model. Using perpendicular technique, the authors found flexion-related impingement at 70° in moderate SCFE and 50° in severe SCFE.

41. Parsch K, Weller S, Parsch D: Open reduction and smooth Kirschner wire fixation for unstable slipped capital femoral epiphysis. *J Pediatr Orthop* 2009;29(1): 1-8.

    At 5-year follow-up after urgent anterior capsulotomy with controlled epiphyseal reduction and fixation using smooth Kirschner wires, the overall rate of osteonecrosis was 4.7% and the average Iowa hip score was 94.5.

42. Ziebarth K, Zilkens C, Spencer S, Leunig M, Ganz R, Kim YJ: Capital realignment for moderate and severe SCFE using a modified Dunn procedure. *Clin Orthop Relat Res* 2009;467(3):704-716.

No osteonecrosis was reported in 40 patients at two institutions after moderate or severe SCFE was reduced with surgical dislocation and modified Dunn osteotomy. Significant intra-articular pathology was reported at the time of open reduction.

43. Castañeda P, Macías C, Rocha A, Harfush A, Cassis N: Functional outcome of stable grade III slipped capital femoral epiphysis treated with in situ pinning. *J Pediatr Orthop* 2009;29(5):454-458.

In 129 severe slips retrospectively analyzed at an average of 5 years after in situ fixation, the lowest Iowa hip scores and the highest complication rate were noted in patients in whom pin placement was inadequate.

44. Dodds MK, McCormack D, Mulhall KJ: Femoroacetabular impingement after slipped capital femoral epiphysis: Does slip severity predict clinical symptoms? *J Pediatr Orthop* 2009;29(6):535-539.

Retrospective evaluation of 49 patients at a mean 6 years after in situ pinning for SCFE found that femoroacetabular impingement is correlated with the α angle and not with slip severity.

45. Koenig KM, Thomson JD, Anderson KL, Carney BT: Does skeletal maturity predict sequential contralateral involvement after fixation of slipped capital femoral epiphysis? *J Pediatr Orthop* 2007;27(7):796-800.

In a retrospective review of 71 patients with unilateral SCFE, 23% of patients with open triradiate cartilage developed mild contralateral SCFE. No single factor predicted sequential slip.

46. Jerre R, Billing L, Hansson G, Karlsson J, Wallin J: Bilaterality in slipped capital femoral epiphysis: Importance of a reliable radiographic method. *J Pediatr Orthop B* 1996;5(2):80-84.

47. Azzopardi T, Sharma S, Bennet GC: Slipped capital femoral epiphysis in children aged less than 10 years. *J Pediatr Orthop B* 2010;19(1):13-18.

The authors studied 10 children younger than 10 years with SCFE and found that obesity is closely related to the development of the condition in younger children.

48. Kamarulzaman MA, Abdul Halim AR, Ibrahim S: Slipped capital femoral epiphysis (SCFE): A 12-year review. *Med J Malaysia* 2006;61(suppl A):71-87.

49. Yildirim Y, Bautista S, Davidson RS: Chondrolysis, osteonecrosis, and slip severity in patients with subsequent contralateral slipped capital femoral epiphysis. *J Bone Joint Surg Am* 2008;90(3):485-492.

Retrospective evaluation of 227 patients treated for unilateral SCFE from 1993 to 2003 found that 36% developed contralateral SCFE within 6.5 months. Based on severity and complications related to SCFE, prophylactic pinning was determined to be warranted.

50. Palocaren T, Holmes L, Rogers K, Kumar SJ: Outcome of in situ pinning in patients with unstable slipped capital femoral epiphysis: Assessment of risk factors associated with avascular necrosis. *J Pediatr Orthop* 2010; 30(1):31-36.

The authors determined that female sex and slip magnitude are potential predisposing factors for the development of osteonecrosis.

51. Ramachandran M, Ward K, Brown RR, Munns CF, Cowell CT, Little DG: Intravenous bisphosphonate therapy for traumatic osteonecrosis of the femoral head in adolescents. *J Bone Joint Surg Am* 2007;89(8):1727-1734.

A prospective, nonrandomized study of bisphosphonate use in patients at risk for developing osteonecrosis was based on posttreatment bone scans. At a mean 38-month follow-up, all hips were rated good or excellent.

52. Gomez JA, Matsumoto H, Roye DP Jr, et al: Articulated hip distraction: A treatment option for femoral head avascular necrosis in adolescence. *J Pediatr Orthop* 2009;29(2):163-169.

A retrospective review of arthrodiastasis in the treatment of osteonecrosis found that patients with SCFE-associated osteonecrosis were least likely to benefit from the procedure.

53. Rebello G, Spencer S, Millis MB, Kim YJ: Surgical dislocation in the management of pediatric and adolescent hip deformity. *Clin Orthop Relat Res* 2009;467(3):724-731.

A surgical dislocation approach was used in the management of a variety of pediatric hip disorders. Four of 58 patients developed osteonecrosis.

54. Mamisch TC, Kim YJ, Richolt J, et al: Range of motion after computed tomography-based simulation of intertrochanteric corrective osteotomy in cases of slipped capital femoral epiphysis: Comparison of uniplanar flexion osteotomy and multiplanar flexion, valgisation, and rotational osteotomies. *J Pediatr Orthop* 2009;29:336-340.

Computer simulation was used to compare corrective uniplanar flexion with corrective mulitplanar osteotomies in the management of post-SCFE deformity. Similar improvement was noted in flexion and internal rotation regardless of the procedure. Multiplanar osteotomies offered superior restoration of abduction.

Chapter 59

Knee, Leg, Ankle, and Foot Trauma: Pediatrics

Matthew A. Halanski, MD   José A. Herrera-Soto, MD

Introduction

Injuries in the lower extremity occur frequently in children and vary in their complexity, treatment, and outcomes. Because most lower extremity growth occurs at the physes about the knee, posttraumatic growth arrest can lead to significant malalignment or limb-length discrepancies. Injuries such as corner fractures, Salter-Harris type I fractures of the distal femur, patellar sleeve fractures, and Tillaux fractures may be subtle on radiographs, yet significant long-term consequences exist if they are not managed appropriately. Pediatric polytrauma patients may present with multiple lower extremity injuries and the clinician must be vigilant in looking for all injuries even in the face of obvious fractures (**Figure 1**). Thus "satisfaction of search"[1,2] has the potential to miss other injuries and complications such as compartment syndrome as seen in some tibia fractures.

Distal Femoral Metaphyseal Fractures

Distal metaphyseal fractures occur proximal to the growth plate, and most are unstable after reduction unless fixation is obtained with a construct such as crossed smooth Kirschner wires (K-wires). The physis should be avoided with these wires, but those fractures in close proximity to the growth plate mandate crossing the physis to achieve fracture stability. With the use of crossed K-wires, the surgeon must recognize the risk of joint sepsis from pin tract infection. To avoid this, burying the wires or using a retrograde fixation method is recommended. In this manner a wire is introduced in a distal-to-proximal direction. Once the wire has crossed the fracture and the far cortex, it is gently advanced proximally until out of the skin, where it is bent over. In the older patient with limited growth, plating may be valuable,[3] especially in more proximal fractures where there is a lower risk to the physis.

When a small peripheral metaphyseal fragment of bone (corner fracture) is found in the young child, nonaccidental trauma should be suspected. This very subtle radiologic finding is the result of violent force and is often seen in the distal femur and the proximal and distal tibia (**Figure 2**). Nonaccidental trauma should always be expected when the history is discordant or when long bone fractures occur in nonambulatory children. A complete skeletal survey and child protective services consultation should be obtained in these cases.

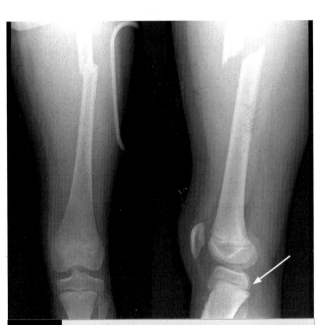

Figure 1 AP and lateral radiographs of a 13-year-old boy with an obvious femoral shaft fracture from an motor vehicle accident. One day later, after femoral fixation, the patient kept reporting knee pain that led to late diagnosis of a proximal tibia physeal fracture (*arrow*) that required fixation.

Dr. Herrera-Soto or an immediate family member has received royalties from Biomet; is a member of a speakers' bureau or has made paid presentations on behalf of Bonutti Technologies and Biomet; serves as a paid consultant to Biomet; and has received research or institutional support from Biomet. Neither Dr. Halanski nor any immediate family member has received anything of value from or owns stock in a commercial company or institution related directly or indirectly to the subject of this chapter.

6: Pediatrics

Distal Femur Physeal Injuries

The distal femoral growth plate accounts for 70% of the growth from the femur and contributes to 40% of the whole lower extremity. When a fracture occurs, multiple zones of the growth plate can be damaged and result in partial or complete premature physeal closure. Thus, the younger the patient at the time of injury, the worse the angular deformity or limb-length inequality will be. Fortunately, distal femoral physeal injuries are relatively uncommon, as they account for less than 2% of all injuries to the physes. A varus or valgus mechanism of injury and associated injuries around the knee should alert the physician to the possibility of this injury.

Nondisplaced injuries (≤2 mm) are amenable to long leg casting. Typically these patients present with pain and swelling in the affected extremity and normal radiographs, making confirmation of the presence of injury difficult. The best tool for evaluation is still the physical examination, which will alert the examiner to tenderness along the physis with an associated effusion. In the past, stress radiographs were used to confirm this injury; however, MRI or ultrasound is now the diagnostic modality of choice. If MRI is not available, the surgeon may place the extremity in a cast and watch for callus formation within 2 to 3 weeks after injury. Although most authors agree that casting alone is sufficient for these injuries, they may displace even after well-molded casting and should be monitored closely. If any signs of displacement are present, fixation is warranted. Also, any patients not amenable to casting (obese patients or those with a closed head injury) may benefit from fixation to avoid loss of reduction.

Fracture fragments displaced over 50% of the bone diameter have a high potential for growth plate arrest (**Figure 3**). Hence, anatomic physeal alignment is of utmost importance. Salter-Harris I injuries and Salter-Harris II injuries with a small metaphyseal fragment are best managed with crossed K-wires (**Figure 4**). Smooth K-wires that do not cross at the fracture site should be used for maximal stability. If these wires are placed in a retrograde manner (from the epiphysis into the metaphysis), they will traverse the knee joint and

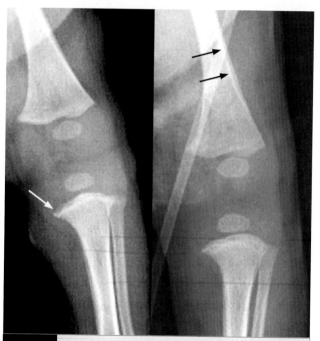

Figure 2 | Radiographs of the knee in a 9-month-old patient demonstrates a corner fracture of the proximal tibia (*white arrow*). Corner fractures and multiple fractures at different stages of healing are pathognomonic for nonaccidental fractures. Fractures at different stages of healing (*black arrows*) can be seen in this example, with periosteal healing of the femur indicating a likely older occult injury to the femur as well as a corner fracture of the tibia.

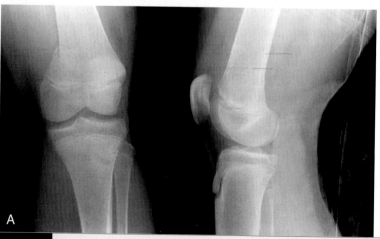
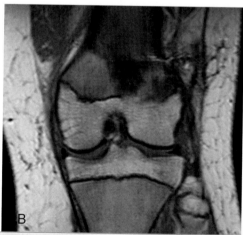

Figure 3 | **A,** AP and lateral radiographs of the knee of a 14-year-old girl who was hit by a car and sustained a Salter-Harris type II fracture. **B,** Coronal MRI of the femur 9 months after open reduction and internal fixation. The patient has asymmetric growth plate closure from the trauma. Yet due to relative skeletal maturity, little effect on limb length is expected.

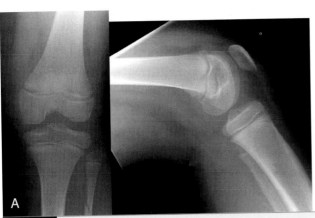
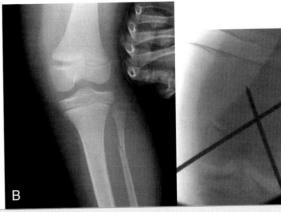

Figure 4   **A,** Radiographs showing a proximal fibula greenstick fracture in a patient who injured the lateral aspect of her knee when she was hit by a car. On physical examination she presented with swelling and severe pain to manipulation. The femoral growth plate appears wide. **B,** The patient was obese; therefore, percutaneous fixation was recommended. Intraoperative stress films show fracture gap with valgus stress. MRI would be the current modality of choice to diagnose this injury. These pins traverse the knee joint and should be buried or pulled through to decrease the risk of joint infection.

should be buried to prevent pin tract–induced septic arthritis. Placing these wires in an antegrade fashion or pulling them through the skin proximally after retrograde placement is an alternative that reduces the risk of septic arthritis from pin tract infection. In type II injuries with a large metaphyseal fragment, screw fixation may be used. The screws are usually placed from the side of the metaphyseal fragment (Thurston Holland), thus fixing the distal fragment to the intact metaphysis.

Displaced intra-articular injuries or Salter-Harris type III and IV injuries (>2 mm) must be reduced to prevent articular step-off and early arthrosis. Open reduction and fixation of intra-articular injuries with screws parallel to the growth plate is the recommended method. Recently, arthroscopic assessment of reduction after fixation has been suggested as an alternative.[4]

The most common complications are partial growth disturbance with residual angular deformity or shortening. The likelihood of physeal growth disturbance is greater when initial displacement is segmented. The need for additional surgery can occur in about 40% to 60% of the cases, and has been reported in up to 50% of patients regardless of an anatomic reduction. The treating physician should avoid performing multiple attempts at closed manipulation because the risk of growth disturbance may increase. Ligament injuries have been associated with these injuries.[5]

Patella Fractures

Patella fractures are less common in children than in adults. Most patella fractures in children occur from either a direct blow or a sudden contraction of the extensor mechanism. Avulsion fractures of the patella, on the other hand, are more common in children and may be difficult to diagnose.[6] The sleeve fracture is unique to children and consists of a large articular chondral frag-

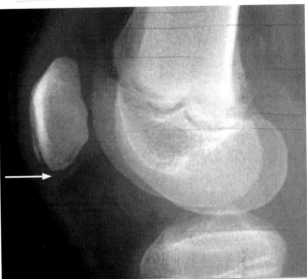

Figure 5   Lateral radiograph of the knee demonstrates a small fleck of bone at the inferior pole of the patella (*arrow*). Inability to perform a straight leg raise indicates extensor mechanism disruption and requires surgical fixation. The treating surgeon should be aware of possible articular flap consistent with a sleeve fracture.

ment with a small bone fragment pulled from the ossification center. Radiographic examination reveals a small fleck of bone inferiorly and an associated patella alta (**Figure 5**). A high index of suspicion is needed to prevent this pitfall. Physical examination will demonstrate knee effusion and inability to fully extend the knee.

In general, patella fractures in children can be treated similarly to those in adults. Nondisplaced fractures with an intact extensor mechanism can be treated with long leg or cylinder casting. Progressive weight

6: Pediatrics

bearing as tolerated can be started once pain control is adequate. In patients with displaced fractures the restoration of knee extension function and articular congruity are the goals of treatment. This requires an anatomic reduction and stabilization of the fracture fragments.[7] Internal fixation is performed using a figure-of-8 tension band of either wire or nonabsorbable sutures or tape, which are tied around either smooth K-wires or cannulated screws. A recent study concluded that a horizontal figure-of-8 band with two twists of wire at contiguous corners provides the greatest compression and stability.[8] Sleeve fractures require open reduction and internal fixation of the patellar tendon to the distal patella.

Proximal Tibial Physeal Fractures

Proximal tibial fractures are common in the pediatric population. Several anatomic regions and fracture patterns correlate with the child's age and the mechanism of injury.[9] Intra-articular injuries are rare and correlate with adultlike injury patterns, whereas metaphyseal fractures are seen in the younger patient. Physeal injuries account for less than 1% of all physeal injuries. This growth plate has added stability because of the anterior epiphyseal extension of the tibial tubercle. There are also significant contributions to fragment stability from the collateral ligaments and the fibula. As a result, it requires a high-energy injury to incite a fracture of the proximal tibia epiphysis.

Nondisplaced fractures are treated by long leg casting and can be followed closely to assess maintenance of reduction. A bivalved long leg cast allows fracture stabilization while allowing swelling to occur. Displaced fractures also can be treated by closed manipulation and casting. These patients should be admitted for observation in light of the potential development of compartment syndrome. When intra-articular injuries are treated closed, CT after casting can help in the evaluation of joint congruity. Should internal fixation be needed, epiphyseal screws that are parallel to the growth plate are the most desirable. This is especially true in skeletally immature children with over 2 years of growth remaining. However, as in distal femoral injuries, stability must never be sacrificed to avoid a potential growth plate arrest and, if necessary, smooth wires across the physis may be needed.

A feared complication is the potential development of vascular injury and/or compartment syndrome as a result of the tethering effect of the popliteal artery. It is important to recognize that spontaneous reduction may occur and all proximal tibial physeal fractures may have vascular compromise. In displaced fractures, many of these vascular occlusions resolve once reduction is achieved. Nevertheless, careful observation is warranted during and after the treatment. Other possible complications are partial or premature growth arrest leading to angular deformity and limb-length inequality.

Tibial Tubercle Fractures

Avulsion fractures of the tibial tubercle occur mostly in adolescents during a sporting (jumping) activity and represent less than 1% of all physeal injuries. The patient often presents with a knee effusion, inability to extend the knee, and an anterior knee mass. Minimally displaced fractures can be treated with long leg or cylinder casting. Intra-articular fractures and those with more than 2 mm of displacement require anatomic reduction; many can be percutaneously stabilized with screw fixation after closed manipulation. Open reduction and fixation is warranted if the fracture is displaced despite closed reduction attempts. Anterior compartment syndrome may result from bleeding of the recurrent anterior tibial artery after tibial tubercle fractures. For open treatment, a prophylactic fasciotomy of the anterior compartment may reduce the risk of compartment syndrome in patients with marked swelling and pain in the anterior compartment. Screw prominence is a common complication; once the fracture has healed, removal will alleviate the symptoms. Growth arrest and recurvatum is possible; however, most patients are adolescents with less risk of progressive deformity.

Metaphyseal Fractures

Proximal metaphyseal fractures in young children may provoke overgrowth of the medial aspect of the proximal tibia leading to genu valgum (Cozen fracture); this deformity peaks around 1 year after injury. Families are instructed to watch for progressive deformity. Some studies have shown that the associated valgus deformity will resolve spontaneously.[10] In a long-term study with an average 15-year follow-up, almost 50% of the patients with posttraumatic tibial valgus had reports of knee and/or ankle pain on the affected side with 6° more in valgus than the contralateral side.[11] The mechanical axis eventually improved in all, giving them an S-shape tibia or increase in ankle varus. Careful follow-up and little tolerance to valgus progression is warranted. Hemiepiphysiodesis with guided growth is the recommended treatment of this relatively rare residual deformity.[12]

Tibial Shaft Fractures

Tibial shaft fractures are among the most common pediatric fractures. Treatment is tailored according patient age and type of injury. Most can be treated by closed methods. Nondisplaced or minimally displaced tibia fractures are best managed by long leg casting. The most common method of managing displaced tibial shaft fractures is closed reduction and long leg casting. Close follow-up is needed to ensure maintenance of alignment. Alignment is based on the age of the patient: the younger the patient, the more angulation that can be accepted.

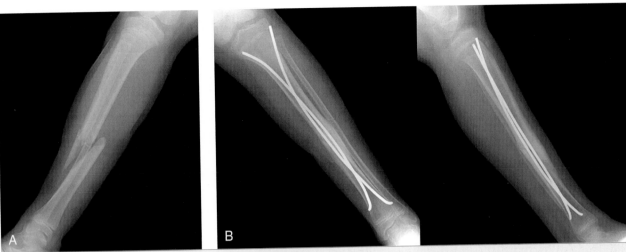

Figure 6 Radiographs showing a comminuted tibial shaft fracture in a 10-year-old girl. **A,** This unstable fracture is amenable to internal fixation. **B,** Three months after flexible nailing, the patient presented with no pain and a united fracture. Nail removal was performed 6 months after surgery.

Recent reports reviewed the efficacy of elastic intramedullary nailing for comminuted shaft fractures[13,14] (Figure 6). The average time to healing was longer in comparison to the expected 10 weeks in patients with casts for less significant fractures. Several complications were reported to each group including infection, malunion, nonunion (10%), skin irritation, and limb-length inequality. Another method of treatment is external fixation, which is primarily reserved for open injuries with severe soft-tissue damage.[15] Malunion is the most common complication, and nonunion occurs in about 2% of the cases.

Although compartment syndrome is less common in children than adults, it may occur with almost any injury to the lower extremity. It has to be suspected in both closed and open injuries when a patient presents with pain out of proportion to his or her injury. Evaluation of compartment syndrome in children can be difficult. Increased anxiety, agitation, and an increasing need for narcotics for pain relief, especially after reduction and immobilization, should alert the clinician to this possibility. Immediate evaluation and fasciotomies can prevent permanent sequelae.

Ankle Sprains

Ankle injuries are common in the pediatric patient. As the ligamentous structures about the ankle are often stronger than the distal tibial and fibular physis, occult physeal injuries may be misdiagnosed as ankle sprains. However, isolated soft-tissue injuries do occur in the pediatric population and have been seen on postinjury MRI.[16] High-resolution ultrasound has also helped differentiate ankle sprains and occult fractures.[17] Overweight children may be at more risk for ankle injury.[18] There does not appear to be a clear advantage to casting versus symptomatic treatment of children with true ankle sprains or occult ankle fractures.[19]

Distal Tibial Physeal Fractures

Distal tibial physeal injuries or separations (Salter Harris type I and II) tend to occur most often in children age 11 to 13 years.[20] Many of these injuries are treated with closed reduction and long leg casting. Occasionally open reduction with or without fixation is required to improve reduction and remove interposed periosteum. Despite the fracture's overall benign appearance, up to 25% of patients with type II injuries may show signs of premature growth plate closure.[20,21] In addition, symptoms resembling those of compartment syndrome have been reported due to impingement of the extensor hallucis longus and deep peroneal nerve in displaced fractures (extensor retinacular syndrome).[22,23]

Salter-Harris type III and IV fractures of the distal tibial epiphysis are both physeal and intra-articular. Nondisplaced fractures can be treated with casting; however, intra-articular displacement greater than 2 mm should be treated with open reduction and internal fixation to anatomically align the joint space and the physis. It is generally thought that diastasis at the fracture site may be better tolerated than articular step-off; however, there is no pediatric literature to support this theory. CT to evaluate the amount of displacement can guide treatment in borderline cases. Screw fixation of these fractures is often used; the screws are placed within the epiphyseal fragment and often parallel the physis and joint surface. If crossing the physis is necessary, smooth wires are typically used. Recently, transepiphyseal bioabsorbable implants have been shown to offer equivalent clinical results without requiring later implant removal.[24]

Transitional fractures of the adolescent distal tibia occur as the distal tibial physis begins to close in a predictable fashion, from anteromedial to posterior to lateral and finally to anterolateral. As the distal tibial physis closes, the remaining open portions of the physis are susceptible to injury. Because the physis closes in a

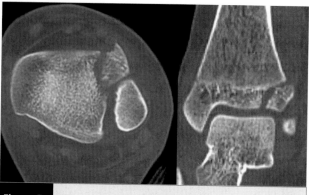

Figure 7 CT in an almost skeletally mature individual with a displaced juvenile Tillaux fracture.

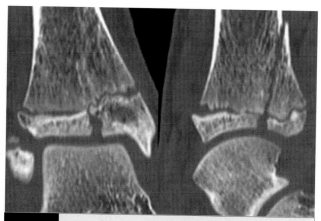

Figure 8 Coronal and sagittal CT demonstrates a triplane fracture with a sagittal split of the epiphysis, an axial separation of the physis, and a coronal splint extending from the metaphysis and through the epiphysis. The lateral image demonstrates both anterior displacement of the Tillaux fracture and posterior displacement of the metaphyseal portion. This would imply that the Tillaux fragment is separated and is a three-part fracture.

sequential manner two main types of transitional fractures occur: the Tillaux fracture and the triplane fracture.

The Tillaux fracture is only seen during adolescence as an intra-articular Salter-Harris type III fracture. It occurs when the medial physis has closed and the anterior lateral physis remains open in children age 11 to 16 years. When the ankle is subjected to an external rotation force, the anterolateral portion of the physis is avulsed with the anterior tibiofibular ligament (**Figure 7**). Although the potential for premature growth arrest is low (the physis has already begun to close), intra-articular displacement greater than 2 mm may lead to early joint arthritis and tibiofibular instability. CT should be used to assess fracture displacement after casting. Clearly displaced fractures or those found to be displaced (>2 mm) after reduction on CT should be treated with open or closed reduction and internal fixation.[25] Arthroscopically assisted reduction and percutaneous fixation have also been described.[26,27]

Salter-Harris type IV fractures involving the distal tibial epiphysis, the physis, and the tibial metaphysis are called triplane fractures. This fracture most often occurs in patients age 12 to 15 years. Different variants (medial and lateral, intra-malleolar, and three- and four-part fractures) exist,[28] but most commonly the epiphysis is fractured in the sagittal plane, the physis is separated in the axial plane, and the metaphysis is fractured posteriorly in the coronal plane (**Figure 8**). The lateral portion of the epiphysis is essentially fractured from the medial portion, which has already fused with the distal tibia. As with other Salter-Harris type III and IV injuries, cast immobilization can be used for nondisplaced fractures, and a closed reduction should be attempted on displaced intra-articular fractures (>2 mm). CT should be performed in patients in whom reduction was attempted to accurately assess fracture displacement. Any fractures not satisfactorily reduced should undergo open reduction and internal fixation. CT can help with preoperative planning of such surgery and can aid in the detection of occult talar dome injuries.[29] Recently, arthroscopically aided reduction and percutaneous fixation has been used with success in treating these fractures.[30]

Fractures of the Distal Fibula

Factures of the distal fibula are relatively common, and most are Salter-Harris type I or type II fractures. When the fibular physis is at the level of the tibiotalar joint, the physis is more likely to fracture; when the fibular physis is below the tibiotalar joint, a metaphyseal injury is more likely.[31] Isolated nondisplaced fractures may be treated with immobilization. Functional bracing has been shown to be superior to casting for nondisplaced fractures.[32] These injuries may occur in isolation or may be associated with distal tibial fractures; in these cases the tibia fracture guides treatment and the fibula rarely requires fixation. Pinning or plating of fibular fractures is occasionally necessary, especially when an unstable ankle injury exists secondary to an additional medial-sided injury. Complications of these fractures are rare, but nonunions[33] and growth arrests leading to fibular shortening[34] have been described.

Talus Fractures

Fractures of the talar neck are rare in children and are a result of forced dorsiflexion. The medial malleolus may be involved if supination was a component of the injury. Nondisplaced fractures of the talar neck can be managed with immobilization and no weight bearing. Displaced fractures (>5 mm of displacement or 5° of malalignment) should undergo attempted closed reduction, and, if stable, a cast can be worn. If the reduction is unacceptable or cannot be maintained, open reduction is necessary. A limited anterior approach can be made to aid in reduction while pin or screw fixation can be placed posterior laterally.[35] As in adults, osteonecrosis is a complication with these fractures. Although most other talus fractures are rare, there has been an increase in the number of lateral process fractures seen in snowboarders.[36] Nondisplaced fractures may be immobilized, whereas small symptomatic fragments may require excision.

Calcaneal Fractures

Closed calcaneal fractures are rare injuries in children and typically are a result of a fall. Extra-articular fractures can be managed with immobilization and restricted weight bearing. In the past, intra-articular fractures have been treated closed with good results. The ability of the talus and calcaneus to remodel at the subtalar joint in the growing child has been thought to lead to these results. Recently, surgical treatment of displaced (>2 mm) intra-articular fractures, using a lateral buttress plate, has been shown to be safer in children than in adults and to provide generally good to excellent outcomes.[37]

Fractures of the Midfoot

Midfoot fractures are relatively benign and may involve compression-type fractures or avulsions that require a period of immobilization. The "nutcracker," cuboid fracture is a burst-type fracture that occurs when the foot is forcefully abducted and sustains an axial load,[38] a condition that can lead to significant lateral column shortening that should be surgically restored. This type of injury and other midfoot injuries have been associated with equestrian sports.[39]

Metatarsal Fractures

Stress fractures in adolescent athletes involving the second metatarsal respond to decreased activity and either casting or a rigid-soled shoe.[40] In children younger than 5 years the first metatarsal is most likely to be fractured, often as a result of a fall from a height, whereas in the older patient the fifth metatarsal is more likely to be injured during athletics.[41] Most of these fractures may be treated symptomatically in a walking cast. Multiple or severely angulated metatarsal fractures may require surgical fixation. For displaced or intra-articular fractures of the fifth metatarsal, a non–weight-bearing cast should be implemented.[42] Surgical treatment of proximal fractures of the fifth metatarsal (Jones fracture) may allow a quicker return to activities.[42]

Toe Injuries

Toe injuries in children result from direct trauma to the toe or from kicking an inanimate object. Similar to the Seymour fracture of distal phalanx in the hand, open Salter-Harris fractures of the distal phalanx in the toes

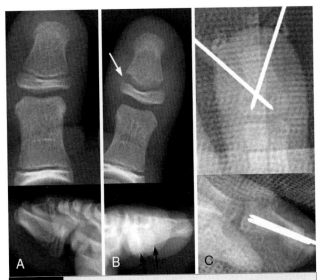

Figure 9 Radiographs of the great toe of a 10-year-old child who presented late with pain and purulence after "stubbing" her toe and who had bleeding from her nail fold. Radiographs of the contralateral toe (**A**), and injured toe (**B**) demonstrate physeal widening and step-off (*arrows*). The treatment included nail plate removal, débridement, reduction, and fixation (**C**). This patient had an unrecognized open physeal fracture, which became secondarily infected.

can occur. These innocuous and initially innocent-appearing "stubbed toes" are actually open injuries associated with nail bed lacerations and require a formal débridement with or without fixation and treatment with antibiotics (**Figure 9**). In most patients with simple toe fracture, buddy taping and a stiff-soled shoe is all that is required. Fractures with significant deformity may require closed reduction and/or pinning to maintain their position. Open dislocations of the great toe interphalangeal joint have been described in children participating in martial arts activities. These injuries are typically treated with irrigation, reduction, closure, and immobilization.[43]

Lawn Mower Injuries and Traumatic Amputations

Lawn mower injuries continue to be a source of significant morbidity, with an incidence of 11 in 100,00 US children,[44] and result in amputations or significant impairments of the limb. These injuries require early antibiotics, irrigation, and débridement.[45] Early primary closure after adequate débridement and treatment of vascular injury and osseous stabilization has been described.[46] Frequently however, repetitive débridements, soft-tissue flaps, and skin grafting are necessary to treat these injuries. Another source of severe foot injuries has been seen with the use of all-terrain vehicles. Often the child's limb gets caught in the vehicle's chain mechanism, causing either a crushing or degloving injury that can result in a midfoot amputation.[47]

Annotated References

1. Ashman CJ, Yu JS, Wolfman D: Satisfaction of search in osteoradiology. *AJR Am J Roentgenol* 2000;175(2): 541-544.

2. Berbaum KS, Franken EA Jr, Dorfman DD, et al: Satisfaction of search in diagnostic radiology. *Invest Radiol* 1990;25(2):133-140.

3. Vander Have K, Herrera J, Kohen R, Karunakar M: The use of locked plating in skeletally immature patients. *J Am Acad Orthop Surg* 2008;16(8):436-441.

   The authors review the current use of locked plates in the pediatric population. Level of evidence: IV.

4. Lee YS, Jung YB, Ahn JH, Shim JS, Nam DC: Arthroscopic assisted reduction and internal fixation of lateral femoral epiphyseal injury in adolescent soccer player: A report of one case. *Knee Surg Sports Traumatol Arthrosc* 2007;15(6):744-746.

   A case report using arthroscopic-assisted reduction and fixation of distal femoral fracture is discussed. Level of evidence: IV.

5. Bertin KC, Goble EM: Ligament injuries associated with physeal fractures about the knee. *Clin Orthop Relat Res* 1983;177 :188-195.

6. Hunt DM, Somashekar N: A review of sleeve fractures of the patella in children. *Knee* 2005;12(1):3-7.

7. Dai LY, Zhang WM: Fractures of the patella in children. *Knee Surg Sports Traumatol Arthrosc* 1999;7(4): 243-245.

8. Rabalais RD, Burger E, Lu Y, Mansour A, Baratta RV: Comparison of two tension-band fixation materials and techniques in transverse patella fractures: A biomechanical study. *Orthopedics* 2008;31(2):128.

   The authors of a biomechanical cadaver study looked at the use of figure-of-8 versus parallel wire arrangement and stainless steel wire versus ultra-high–molecular-weight polyethylene tape in transverse patellar fractures. Type of material made little difference in results; however, the parallel arrangement demonstrated less fracture distraction.

9. Mubarak SJ, Kim JR, Edmonds EW, Pring ME, Bastrom TP: Classification of proximal tibial fractures in children. *J Child Orthop* 2009;3(3):191-197.

   The authors evaluated 135 pediatric proximal tibia fractures and propose a new classification scheme that reflects both the direction of force and a fracture pattern that appears to be age dependent. Level of evidence: IV.

10. Zionts LE, MacEwen GD: Spontaneous improvement of post-traumatic tibia valga. *J Bone Joint Surg Am* 1986; 68(5):680-687.

11. Tuten HR, Keeler KA, Gabos PG, Zionts LE, MacKenzie WG: Posttraumatic tibia valga in children: A long-term follow-up note. *J Bone Joint Surg Am* 1999;81(6): 799-810.

12. Stevens PM, Pease F: Hemiepiphysiodesis for posttraumatic tibial valgus. *J Pediatr Orthop* 2006;26(3):385-392.

13. Gordon JE, Gregush RV, Schoenecker PL, Dobbs MB, Luhmann SJ: Complications after titanium elastic nailing of pediatric tibial fractures. *J Pediatr Orthop* 2007; 27(4):442-446.

   Fifty children with 51 diaphyseal tibial shaft fractures were followed until union; five patients had delayed healing. Patients with delayed healing were older (mean age, 14.1 years) versus the study population as a whole (mean age, 11.7 years). Other complications included malunion, osteomyelitis at the fracture site, and nail migration through the skin. Level of evidence: IV.

14. Srivastava AK, Mehlman CT, Wall EJ, Do TT: Elastic stable intramedullary nailing of tibial shaft fractures in children. *J Pediatr Orthop* 2008;28(2):152-158.

   The authors reviewed 24 tibial shaft fractures in 24 patients treated surgically by elastic-stable intramedullary nailing. The average union time for all tibia fractures was 20.4 weeks. Complications include two neurovascular (8%), two infections (8%), two malunions (8%), and one limb-length discrepancy (4%).

15. Myers SH, Spiegel D, Flynn JM: External fixation of high-energy tibia fractures. *J Pediatr Orthop* 2007; 27(5):537-539.

   The authors discuss a retrospective review of 31 children treated with external fixation for high-energy tibial shaft fractures. The authors show a long union time (6 months) in those older than 12 years and increased risk of limb-length discrepancy in those younger than 11 years.

16. Launay F, Barrau K, Petit P, Jouve JL, Auquier P, Bollini G: [Ankle injuries without fracture in children: Prospective study with magnetic resonance in 116 patients]. *Rev Chir Orthop Reparatrice Appar Mot* 2008;94(5): 427-433.

   One hundred two MRIs were examined in children with ankle injuries without fractures on plain films. Minor ligament injury was noted in 20 patients and ligament tear in 5; minor bone injury was noted in 42 patients and fracture in 7. None of these fractures were visible on the plain radiographs. Level of evidence: IV.

17. Simanovsky N, Lamdan R, Hiller N, Simanovsky N: Sonographic detection of radiographically occult fractures in pediatric ankle and wrist injuries. *J Pediatr Orthop* 2009;29(2):142-145.

   Fifty-eight children age 2 to 16 years who sustained an acute ankle and wrist injury suggestive of fracture on clinical examination, but with negative radiograph, were referred for high-resolution ultrasound. All patients with negative ultrasound studies had negative follow-up radiographs. In 13 patients with positive ultrasound, the follow-up radiographs demonstrated a periosteal reaction. Level of evidence: I.

18. Zonfrillo MR, Seiden JA, House EM, et al: The association of overweight and ankle injuries in children. *Ambul Pediatr* 2008;8(1):66-69.

    The authors used 180 patients and 180 control subjects to look for an increased risk of ankle injury in the overweight population and observed a significant association between children being overweight and ankle injury. Level of evidence: III.

19. Launay F, Barrau K, Simeoni MC, Jouve JL, Bollini G, Auquier P: [Ankle injury without fracture in children: Cast immobilization versus symptomatic treatment. Impact on absenteeism and quality of life]. *Arch Pediatr* 2008;15(12):1749-1755.

    The authors discuss a prospective, randomized study of treating ankle injuries without fracture with either symptomatic care or cast immobilization. No differences in clinical progression were found; however, parental and child absenteeism was higher in the casted group. Level of evidence: II.

20. Kraus R, Kaiser M: Growth disturbances of the distal tibia after physeal separation: What do we know, what do we believe we know? A review of current literature. *Eur J Pediatr Surg* 2008;18(5):295-299.

    An in-depth review of the current literature on distal tibial epiphyseal injuries is presented.

21. Leary JT, Handling M, Talerico M, Yong L, Bowe JA: Physeal fractures of the distal tibia: Predictive factors of premature physeal closure and growth arrest. *J Pediatr Orthop* 2009;29(4):356-361.

    Chart review of 124 pediatric patients with distal tibia physeal fractures demonstrates a significant correlation between premature physeal closure and both the mechanism of injury and the amount of initial fracture displacement. Level of evidence: III.

22. Cox G, Thambapillay S, Templeton PA: Compartment syndrome with an isolated Salter Harris II fracture of the distal tibia. *J Orthop Trauma* 2008;22(2):148-150.

    The authors present a case report demonstrating a compartment syndrome after a Salter-Harris type II fracture of the distal tibia.

23. Haumont T, Gauchard GC, Zabee L, Arnoux JM, Journeau P, Lascombes P: Extensor retinaculum syndrome after distal tibial fractures: Anatomical basis. *Surg Radiol Anat* 2007;29(4):303-311.

    An anatomic study is presented that provides an anatomic explanation for the clinically described extensor retinaculum syndrome. Level of evidence: IV.

24. Podeszwa DA, Wilson PL, Holland AR, Copley LA: Comparison of bioabsorbable versus metallic implant fixation for physeal and epiphyseal fractures of the distal tibia. *J Pediatr Orthop* 2008;28(8):859-863.

    Comparison between metallic (n = 26) and bioabsorbable (n = 24) implants used in treating distal tibial epiphyseal fractures found no significant difference between implants. Level of evidence: III.

25. Kaya A, Altay T, Ozturk H, Karapinar L: Open reduction and internal fixation in displaced juvenile Tillaux fractures. *Injury* 2007;38(2):201-205.

    Ten patients with juvenile Tillaux fractures were treated by open reduction and internal fixation and had an average 99.3/100 American Orthopaedic Foot and Ankle Society score at follow-up. Level of evidence: IV.

26. Panagopoulos A, van Niekerk L: Arthroscopic assisted reduction and fixation of a juvenile Tillaux fracture. *Knee Surg Sports Traumatol Arthrosc* 2007;15(4):415-417.

    A case report demonstrating the usefulness of ankle arthroscopy in treating a juvenile Tillaux fracture is presented.

27. Thaunat M, Billot N, Bauer T, Hardy P: Arthroscopic treatment of a juvenile tillaux fracture. *Knee Surg Sports Traumatol Arthrosc* 2007;15(3):286-288.

    A case report demonstrating the usefulness of ankle arthroscopy in treating a juvenile Tillaux fracture is presented.

28. Schnetzler KA, Hoernschemeyer D: The pediatric triplane ankle fracture. *J Am Acad Orthop Surg* 2007; 15(12):738-747.

    The authors present a thorough review of pediatric triplane fractures.

29. Heusch WL, Albers HW: Intramalleolar triplane fracture with osteochondral talar defect. *Am J Orthop (Belle Mead NJ)* 2008;37(5):262-266.

    A case report of a concomitant medial talar osteochondral injury and triplane fracture is presented.

30. Jennings MM, Lagaay P, Schuberth JM: Arthroscopic assisted fixation of juvenile intra-articular epiphyseal ankle fractures. *J Foot Ankle Surg* 2007;46(5):376-386.

    The authors present long-term follow-up on six patients with arthroscopic-assisted, percutaneous fixation of intra-articular juvenile epiphyseal ankle fracture. All of the patients returned to full activity within 14 weeks of surgery. Level of evidence: IV.

31. Pesl T, Havranek P, Nanka O: Mutual position of the distal fibular physis and the tibiotalar joint space: Radiological typology and clinical significance. *Eur J Pediatr Surg* 2007;17(5):348-353.

    The authors found a correlation between the location of the fibular physis in relation to the tibiotalar joint and the level of fibular fracture in pediatric ankle injuries. Level of evidence: III.

32. Boutis K, Willan AR, Babyn P, Narayanan UG, Alman B, Schuh S: A randomized, controlled trial of a removable brace versus casting in children with low-risk ankle fractures. *Pediatrics* 2007;119(6):e1256-e1263.

    Children with low-risk ankle fractures were randomized to receive a removable ankle brace or a below-knee walking cast. The removable ankle brace was found to be more effective than the cast with respect to recovery of physical function, was associated with a faster return to baseline activities, was superior with respect to pa-

6: Pediatrics

tient preferences, and was also cost-effective. Level of evidence: II.

33. Mirmiran R, Schuberth JM: Non union of an epiphyseal fibular fracture in a pediatric patient. *J Foot Ankle Surg* 2006;45(6):410-412.

34. Lui TH, Chan KB, Ngai WK: Premature closure of distal fibular growth plate: A case of longitudinal syndesmosis instability. *Arch Orthop Trauma Surg* 2008; 128(1):45-48.

    A case report describing fibular physeal closure, which resulted in a shortened fibula and syndesmotic instability, is presented.

35. Beaty JH, Kasser JR: *Rockwood and Green's Fractures in Children*, ed 5. Philadelphia, PA, Lippincott Williams & Wilkins, 2009, pp 1172-1175.

36. von Knoch F, Reckord U, von Knoch M, Sommer C: Fracture of the lateral process of the talus in snowboarders. *J Bone Joint Surg Br* 2007;89(6):772-777.

    Twenty-three snowboarders with lateral process fractures of the talus were followed. An average American Orthopaedic Foot and Ankle Society hindfoot score of 94 was found, including nonsurgically and surgically treated fractures. Level of evidence: IV.

37. Petit CJ, Lee BM, Kasser JR, Kocher MS: Operative treatment of intraarticular calcaneal fractures in the pediatric population. *J Pediatr Orthop* 2007;27(8):856-862.

    The authors present 14 closed calcaneal fractures treated with open reduction and internal fixation. The authors found most children with displaced intra-articular calcaneal fractures treated with open reduction and internal fixation had a good clinical outcome with few complications. Level of evidence: IV.

38. Ceroni D, De Rosa V, De Coulon G, Kaelin A: Cuboid nutcracker fracture due to horseback riding in children: Case series and review of the literature. *J Pediatr Orthop* 2007;27(5):557-561.

    The authors discuss a case series of four children with cuboid injuries sustained during equestrian accidents. Level of evidence: IV.

39. Ceroni D, De Rosa V, De Coulon G, Kaelin A: The importance of proper shoe gear and safety stirrups in the prevention of equestrian foot injuries. *J Foot Ankle Surg* 2007;46(1):32-39.

    This is a case series of foot injuries which occurred during equestrian accidents and stresses the importance of proper safety equipment for young riders. Level of evidence: IV.

40. Niemeyer P, Weinberg A, Schmitt H, Kreuz PC, Ewerbeck V, Kasten P: Stress fractures in adolescent competitive athletes with open physis. *Knee Surg Sports Traumatol Arthrosc* 2006;14(8):771-777.

41. Singer G, Cichocki M, Schalamon J, Eberl R, Höllwarth ME: A study of metatarsal fractures in children. *J Bone Joint Surg Am* 2008;90(4):772-776.

    One hundred sixty-six metatarsal fractures in children were reviewed. In patients who were 5 years old or younger, the primary mechanism was a fall from a height and the first metatarsal was most commonly injured. In patients who were older than 5 years, most accidents occurred at sports facilities, were caused by a fall on a level surface, and most commonly affected the fifth metatarsal. Level of evidence: IV.

42. Herrera-Soto JA, Scherb M, Duffy MF, Albright JC: Fractures of the fifth metatarsal in children and adolescents. *J Pediatr Orthop* 2007;27(4):427-431.

    A total of 103 patients with fifth metatarsal fractures were reviewed. Most fractures of the fifth metatarsal did well after a course of walking cast, unless the fracture was an intra-articular displaced fracture type or the fracture occured in the proximal diaphyseal area. The authors recommend non–weight-bearing casts for all angulated or displaced intra-articular injuries to avoid delays in healing and angulation. Level of evidence: IV.

43. Shin YW, Choi IH, Rhee NK: Open lateral collateral ligament injury of the interphalangeal joint of the great toe in adolescents during Taekwondo. *Am J Sports Med* 2008;36(1):158-161.

    Seven study subjects all had an open wound on the dorsolateral aspect of the interphalangeal joint of the hallux. All seven patients regained full great toe function after surgical repair. Level of evidence: IV.

44. Vollman D, Smith GA: Epidemiology of lawn-mower-related injuries to children in the United States, 1990-2004. *Pediatrics* 2006;118(2):e273-e278.

45. Nguyen A, Raymond S, Morgan V, Peters J, Macgill K, Johnstone B: Lawn mower injuries in children: A 30-year experience. *ANZ J Surg* 2008;78(9):759-763.

    This is a 30-year retrospective review of lawn mower injuries. Admissions for lawn mower injury decreased over time but the frequency of admission for ride-on lawn mower injuries increased over time. Ride-on lawn mowers caused significantly more severe injuries requiring longer periods of recovery in comparison with standard mowers. Level of evidence: IV.

46. Goldsmith JR, Massa EG: Primary closure of lawn mower injuries to the foot: A case series. *J Foot Ankle Surg* 2007;46(5):366-371.

    The authors discuss a case series of nine lawn mower injuries in which primary closure was performed. The hospital courses for this patient population were remarkably lower than those previously reported in the literature. Level of evidence: IV.

47. Thompson TM, Latch R, Parnell D, Dick R, Aitken ME, Graham J: Foot injuries associated with all-terrain vehicle use in children and adolescents. *Pediatr Emerg Care* 2008;24(7):466-467.

    Ten cases of foot injury were identified in patients with a median age of 3 years. Eight had forefoot injuries, including six who had amputation of the great toe, and all but one patient had multiple open foot fractures. Level of evidence: IV.

Chapter 60

Lower Extremity and Foot Disorders: Pediatrics

J. Eric Gordon, MD   Matthew B. Dobbs, MD

Lower Extremity Alignment

Axial Development and Alignment

At birth, nearly all infants have physiologic hip and knee flexion contractures combined with an external rotation contracture of the hips, making the assessment of axial alignment difficult. When examined carefully, infants are noted to have significant genu varum. The hip and knee flexion contractures resolve as children approach walking age; this varus becomes more apparent leading to parental concern about this physiologic deformity. The genu varum begins to improve toward neutral alignment in most children at approximately age 8 months, with neutral alignment normally achieved between the ages of 18 to 24 months. Beyond this age, alignment continues to change toward increasing genu valgum, which peaks at approximately age 5 years. This physiologic valgus spontaneously corrects by approximately age 7 years to neutral adult alignment.[1] Whenever children are seen for reports of lower extremity malalignment, a detailed family history and the age at which the malalignment was first noted is important. A careful physical examination noting the presence of rotational alignment and abnormalities in gait is crucial.

Rotational Development and Alignment

At birth, significant femoral anteversion and internal tibial torsion are present in almost all infants. Internal tibial torsion progressively remodels spontaneously until approximately age 5 to 6 years. After this age, minimal change in tibial torsion occurs. The typical toddler's gait pattern arises when children have some

Dr. Gordon or an immediate family member has received royalties from Orthopediatrics and serves as a paid consultant to Orthopediatrics. Dr. Dobbs or an immediate family member serves as a board member, owner, officer, or committee member of the Association of Bone and Joint Surgeons, the Orthopaedic Research and Education Foundation, the Pediatric Orthopaedic Society of North America, and Scoliosis Research; has received royalties from D-Bar Enterprises; and serves as a paid consultant to D-Bar Enterprises.

persistence of the external rotation hip contracture as they begin walking, and outtoeing occurs as a physiologic mechanism to aid in balance. As the child continues to grow, the external hip contractures decrease and the femoral anteversion becomes more obvious with an intoed gait pattern that can be exacerbated by persistent tibial torsion. Nearly all children correct the excessive femoral anteversion that is often present at age 5 years by age 8 to 9 years. Avoiding W-sitting (the child's bottom is planted between the feet), walking with the feet turned outward, heel wedges, and twister cables have all been recommended to promote remodeling and improvement, but there is no evidence that any of these interventions changes the natural history of femoral anteversion. Symmetric intoeing or outtoeing is not a pathologic condition, but hip dysplasia should be suspected in children with asymmetric excessive femoral anteversion. Children with excessive unilateral external femoral rotation and a positive Galeazzi sign should also be evaluated carefully for evidence of congenital coxa vara.

Radiographic Analysis and Planning

The primary tool for evaluating children and adolescents with suspected lower extremity coronal plane deformities is the standing long cassette radiograph,[2,3] obtained with the child or adolescent standing with the knee facing directly anteriorly; the patella is centered over the femoral condyles and the distal femur should be symmetric with a true anteroposterior appearance. The position of the foot should be ignored, as rotational abnormalities of the tibia can lead to malpositioning of the radiograph and greatly lower its diagnostic value. Ideally, the patient should be able to bear weight on both extremities, and both extremities from the hip to the ankle should be seen on the same radiograph. Severe genu varum or valgum deformities may prohibit both extremities from being seen on the same radiograph; if so, the extremities may be imaged separately.

Once the radiograph is inspected for adequacy, the malalignment test is performed by drawing the mechanical axis, a line from the center of the femoral head to the center of the ankle. The distance from the center of the knee to the line is measured and the direction noted. Normal values and ranges for the mechanical

6: Pediatrics

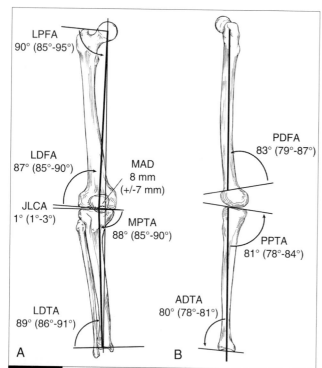

| Figure 1 | **A,** Illustration showing the measurement of the mechanical axis deviation (MAD), lateral proximal femoral angle (LPFA), lateral distal femoral angle (LDFA), medial proximal tibial angle (MPTA), and lateral distal tibial angle (LDTA) and their normal values and ranges. JLCA = joint line congruity angle. **B,** The measurement of the posterior distal femoral angle (PDFA), posterior proximal tibial angle (PPTA), and anterior distal tibial angle (ADTA) and their normal values. |

axis deviation (MAD) and other measurements are noted in **Figure 1**. If the MAD is outside the normal range, further analysis must be performed to determine the source of the malalignment.

The source of the malalignment may be due to bony deformity in the femur, tibia, or joint or due to ligamentous laxity within the knee joint or some combination of these conditions. To determine the source of the malalignment, either mechanical axis planning or anatomic axis planning may be performed. With either method, comparison to the normal side allows one to determine the amount of deformity present. Should both sides be affected, population-based averages can be used.

In mechanical axis planning, a line is drawn from the center of the femoral head to the center of the knee representing the mechanical axis of the femur. A second line is then constructed across the distal femoral condyles. The lateral angle measured by the intersection of these lines is the lateral distal femoral angle (normal average is 87°). A third line is then drawn from the tip of the greater trochanter to the center of the femoral head and the lateral angle formed with the femoral mechanical axis is measured as the lateral proximal femoral angle (normal average spine is 90°). Next, a line is

drawn from the center of the knee to the center of the ankle representing the mechanical axis of the tibia. A line is then drawn across the proximal tibial condyles and the intersection with the mechanical axis of the tibia is measured medially as the medial proximal tibial angle (normal average is 87°). Distally, a line is drawn along the distal tibial articular surface and the lateral intersection with the tibial mechanical axis is measured as the lateral distal tibial angle (normal average is 90°). Finally, the intersection of the lines created across the distal femoral condyles and the proximal tibial condyles can be measured as the joint line congruity angle (normal average is 0°) to assess intrarticular pathology (**Figure 1,** *A*).

The site of bony malalignment can be identified in simple or uniapical deformities by reconstructing normal proximal and distal axes of the involved bone and resolving these axes into a center of rotation angulation (CORA). The CORA identifies the site within the bone where the deformity resides. Correction of the deformity should be around the CORA (**Figure 2**). Lateral axes at the distal femur, proximal tibia, and distal tibia also exist and should be taken into account when correcting lower extremity deformities (**Figure 1,** *B*).

Principles of Deformity Correction: Osteotomy and Physeal Modification

Axial lower extremity deformities can be corrected by osteotomy combined with either internal or external fixation. Skeletally immature individuals can also be treated by physeal modification using either permanent or temporary hemiepiphysiodesis. When an osteotomy is selected, the correction should be about the previously measured CORA. The position of the osteotomy should be chosen based on the CORA as well as physiologic and biologic factors.

Conditions Causing Malalignment
Metabolic Bone Disease

Metabolic bone disease often results in deformity by causing weakness within the physis, allowing worsening of existing deformity, or preventing the normal progression of alignment changes as outlined in the previous section. The deformity that is produced can be predicted based on the age of onset of the metabolic bone disease. Rickets, either from dietary causes or as X-linked hypophosphatemic rickets, produces very early changes in the physis that lead to an inability to remodel early physiologic genu varum with a persistent and worsening varus deformity, with characteristic physeal widening, and trumpeting of the metaphysis (**Figure 3**). Chronic renal failure produces a somewhat later onset metabolic bone disease with similar physeal widening but a characteristic valgus deformity due to failure to remodel the later physiologic genu valgum deformity (**Figure 4**). Deformities caused by metabolic bone disease can be successfully corrected by either hemiepiphysiodesis or osteotomy. If the deformity is corrected using temporary hemiepiphysiodesis, improvement in the radiographic appearance of the physis

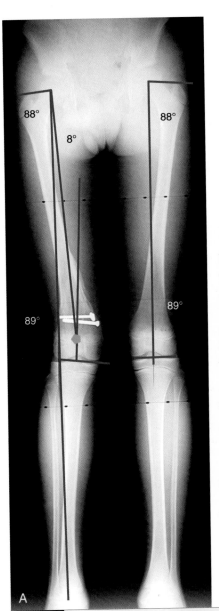
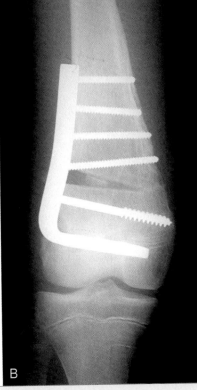
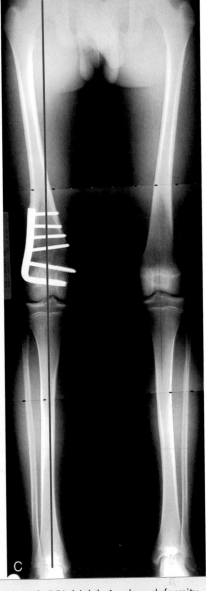

Figure 2   **A,** Standing AP radiograph of both lower extremities showing the normal LPFA and LDFA (*right*). A valgus deformity is demonstrated by lateral deviation of the MAD due to a lateral physeal arrest of the distal femur after a physeal fracture (*left*). The normal LPFA and LDFA have been reconstructed to identify the CORA (*green dot*) with an 8° deformity. **B,** An AP view of the right knee 2 weeks after an 8° varus distal femoral opening wedge osteotomy stabilized with a blade plate. **C,** Standing AP radiograph of both lower extremities showing a normal MAD 1 year after osteotomy.

is noted as alignment improves.[4] Alternatively, correction can be performed successfully using circular external fixation.[5]

Tibia Vara

Tibia vara or Blount disease is a complex deformity of the lower extremity characterized by progressive varus of the lower extremity centered at the tibia. Secondary deformities include femoral deformity, internal tibial torsion, procurvatum of the proximal tibia, and distal tibial valgus. Tibia vara can occur as early-onset or infantile disease, in which bowing is first noted between birth and 3 years of age, and late-onset disease, in which bowing is first noted at age 4 years or older. The late-onset group can be subdivided into a juvenile form, with bowing noted at age 4 to 10 years, and an adolescent form, in which bowing is noted at age 11 years or older.[6]

Infantile tibia vara can often be difficult to differentiate from physiologic bowing of the lower extremity. Most commonly, the metaphyseal-diaphyseal angle is used to diagnose tibia vara in the population younger than 3 years. Metaphyseal-diaphyseal angles less than 9° almost universally indicate the presence of physio-

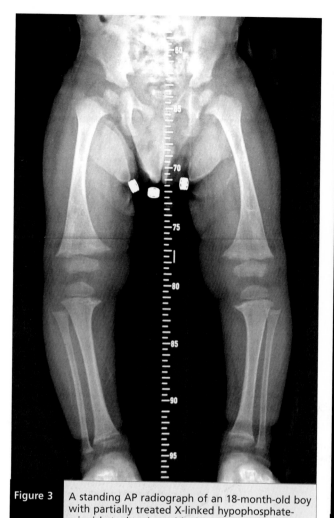

Figure 3 A standing AP radiograph of an 18-month-old boy with partially treated X-linked hypophosphatemic rickets showing widening of all of the physes and mild trumpeting of the distal femoral metaphyses.

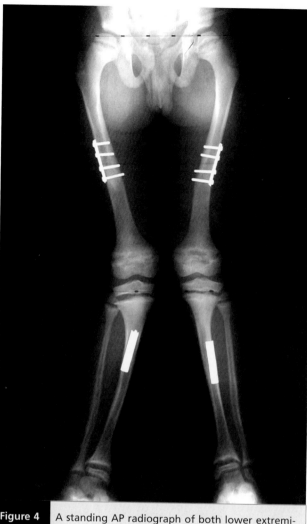

Figure 4 A standing AP radiograph of both lower extremities in a 10-year-old boy with chronic renal failure showing a valgus deformity with severe widening of the physes.

logic bowing. Angles of 9° to 15° are intermediate, and angles of 16° or more nearly always indicate the presence of tibia vara.[7,8] The reliability of this measurement was recently confirmed on digital radiographs.[9] Early-onset tibia vara can be classified according to the classification system developed by Langenskiöld as stages I through VI.[10] Physeal bar formation is present in stages V and VI (**Figure 5**). Older patients with early-onset tibia vara frequently develop severe varus deformities that can be associated with medial joint depression. In severe neglected cases, mild compensatory distal femoral valgus can infrequently occur. After the initial diagnosis in children 21 months to 4 years, it is believed that early-onset tibia vara can be successfully treated with daytime bracing. Instrumented hemiepiphysiodesis may also be an option in this younger age group. If varus is present after age 4 years, proximal tibial osteotomy is indicated to correct the deformity. If a physeal bar has formed medially, epiphyseolysis should be considered in conjunction with the tibial osteotomy to allow growth. When diagnosis is delayed and the patient has developed joint line depression, plateau eleva-

tion can also be performed either as an initial procedure in a staged reconstruction or as a single-stage procedure with tibial osteotomy (**Figure 6**).

Late-Onset Tibia Vara

Late-onset tibia vara does not have classic Langenskiöld changes and is characterized by more mild deformities than are found in early-onset disease. Although the name would suggest that the deformity is solely in the tibia, varus deformity in the femur is commonly present and can account for half of the deformity in many patients.[11] Approximately 60% of patients with growth remaining can be treated with hemiepiphysiodesis.[12] Authors of a 2009 study suggested younger patients with less deformity were somewhat more likely to correct after epiphysiodesis but were unable to identify strong prognostic factors.[13] Patients in whom full correction fails with hemiepiphysiodesis, who are skeletally mature, or who have significant pain with ambulation can be treated with definitive correction in a

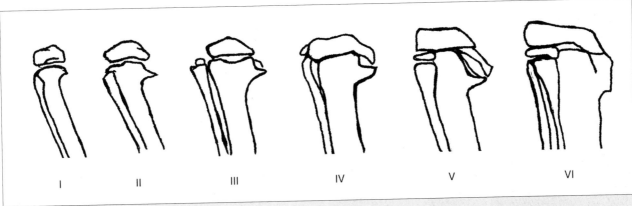

Figure 5 The Langenskiöld classification of early-onset tibia vara, showing stages I through VI. (Adapted from Langenskiöld, A: Tibia vara. *J Pediatr Orthop* 1994;14[2]:141-142.)

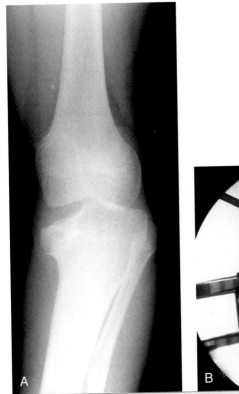
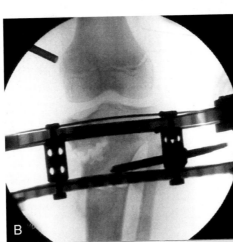
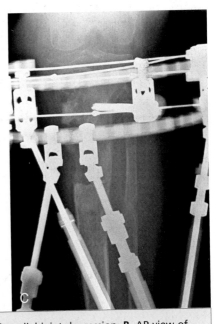

Figure 6 **A,** AP view of the knee in a 10-year-old girl with early-onset tibia vara and medial joint depression. **B,** AP view of the knee after medial plateau elevation and simultaneous proximal tibial metaphyseal osteotomy with fixation by a circular external fixator. **C,** AP radiograph of the proximal tibia 2 months after surgery showing progressive healing of the plateau elevation and regenerate bone after gradual correction and lengthening of the metaphyseal osteotomy.

single-stage procedure with distal femoral and proximal tibial osteotomies, if needed.[14-18] The proximal tibial osteotomy can be performed with either acute or gradual correction using a variety of different plates or monolateral, circular, or computer-driven external fixation systems. Fibular osteotomy does not seem to be necessary when a computer-driven external fixation system is used with gradual correction.[18] Gradual correction can also allow distal transport of the proximal

fibula to tighten the lateral collateral ligament in patients who have developed joint laxity.[17]

Genu Valgum
Idiopathic genu valgum can occur in patients with incomplete remodeling after physiologic valgus. Minimal correction of frontal plane alignment occurs after age 10 years. After this age, when the deformity is significant and the patient is symptomatic with either knee

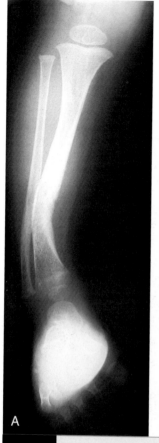
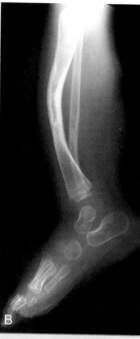

Figure 7   AP (**A**) and lateral (**B**) radiographs of the tibia in a 2-year-old girl with anterolateral bowing without a fracture.

pain or difficulty performing athletic activities, hemi-epiphysiodesis is the preferred technique to correct the deformity while growth remains. After skeletal maturity, in severe cases, corrective osteotomy can be performed to correct the deformity in the involved bone.

Congenital Pseudarthrosis of the Tibia

Congenital pseudarthrosis of the tibia is associated with anterolateral bowing of the tibia, which can lead to dysplastic changes in the tibia and fibula and in most cases to fracture with persistent pseudarthrosis of the tibia. The initial fracture can occur at any time from the neonatal period into late childhood. Neurofibromatosis type I is found in approximately 50% of patients with congenital pseudarthrosis of the tibia. Prior to fracture (**Figure 7**), protective bracing with a clamshell-type brace is indicated and should be maintained until the end of growth or beyond. After fracture, long leg casting can sometimes result in bony union but should be attempted. When the fragments are extremely dystrophic or if nonsurgical treatment leads to no evidence of healing after 3 to 4 months, surgical treatment is indicated. Treatment with open reduction, iliac crest bone grafting, and circular external fixation with or without proximal lengthening has been successful in

obtaining healing of the pseudarthrosis.[19] Unfortunately, without intramedullary fixation, a high rate of refracture with pseudarthrosis development has been observed.[20] This has led some to recommend placement of intramedullary stabilization at the time of external fixator removal. Others have recommended vascularized fibula transfer from the contralateral limb. Although it leads to a high rate of healing, vascularized fibula transfer has been associated with donor-site morbidity including ankle valgus and ipsilateral fracture with pseudarthrosis reformation at either the proximal or distal end of the vascularized graft. Finally, several authors have advocated open reduction with resection of the pseudarthrosis, iliac crest bone grafting, and intramedullary fixation using a Williams rod.[20] This treatment has been complicated by persistence of the pseudarthrosis and problems with late calcaneus foot deformities and long-term weakness of the gastrocnemius-soleus complex. Other approaches have included creation of a one-bone lower leg by synostosis to the fibula and the use of an allograft fibula to bypass a dysplastic tibia and prevent fracture.[21,22] Most recently, success has been reported with the use of bone morphogenetic protein to increase the healing rate.[23-25]

Rotational Malalignment

Increased Femoral Anteversion

After age 8 years, minimal changes in femoral anteversion occur, and some children have persistent intoeing due to the residual excessive femoral anteversion. Several studies have failed to show any association of persistent anteversion into adulthood with degenerative changes of the hip or knee. Although this intoeing is usually asymptomatic, children older than 8 years with external hip rotation less than 20° in extension can have functional limitations in sports and activities of daily living (such as tripping during walking or running) that in selected cases make treatment indicated. Nonsurgical treatment of femoral anteversion in both older and younger children is not effective. Derotational osteotomies can be performed proximally, or distally with an open technique and Kirschner wire fixation with a cast or plate fixation. Derotational osteotomies can also be performed percutaneously in the diaphysis and stabilized with a transtrochanteric femoral nail.[26,27]

Tibial Torsion

Although less common than increased femoral anteversion, persistent internal tibial torsion can be a cause of persistent intoeing that can produce functional problems during sports or activities of daily living. Children older than 6 years with more than 10° of internal rotation that produces functional problems can be treated by derotational osteotomy.

External tibial torsion can occasionally produce knee or ankle pain when a thigh-foot angle over 20° exists in conjunction with hindfoot valgus. Most commonly this condition is seen in patients older than 8 years in conjunction with a tight Achilles tendon. Surgical correction is indicated when pain persists despite an adequate physical therapy program emphasizing Achilles tendon stretching. Surgical correction of either internal or external tibial torsion is most commonly performed in the distal metaphysis and can be stabilized by Kirschner wires or staples and a cast or a small plate with or without fibular osteotomy.[28,29]

Miserable or Malignant Malalignment

Combined excessive or increased femoral anteversion with external tibial torsion often produces knee pain through shear at the joint surface during ambulation or by producing anterior knee pain leading to a condition identified as miserable or malignant malalignment. Patients will ambulate with the foot facing forward but with the anterior knee pointing medially. Patients with mild amounts of femoral anteversion and tibial torsion can sometimes be treated successfully by a physical therapy program emphasizing vastus medialis obliquus strengthening and hamstring stretching. Significant combined increased femoral anteversion and external tibial torsion can be effectively treated surgically with combined femoral and tibial derotational osteotomies in a single or staged fashion.

Limb-Length Discrepancy

Epiphysiodesis, Closed Femoral Shortening, Limb Lengthening

Limb-length discrepancy can occur because of either traumatic or congenital etiologies. Mild discrepancies less than 2 cm are common and require no treatment. A lift is almost always an option to help equalize limb lengths and should be used by children with discrepancies more than 2 cm.

Evaluation of patients with limb-length discrepancy who are still growing should include a projection of the discrepancy at maturity. The growth-remaining method, Mosley straight-line graph method, or multiplier method can all lead to accurate predictions when combined with accurate bone ages. For patients with a projected discrepancy of 2 to 4 cm, contralateral epiphysiodesis is most commonly used. Larger discrepancies can be addressed in individual patients using this technique. Percutaneous epiphysiodesis, after careful planning and evaluation, has proved safe and has a low complication rate.[30] Skeletally mature patients who have discrepancies of 2 to 5 cm can also be treated by open shortening with blade plate fixation or closed femoral shortening using an intramedullary saw and intramedullary fixation.

Discrepancies greater than 4 cm are amenable to limb lengthening using distraction osteogenesis as described by Ilizarov. This can be accomplished using several available circular, computer-driven, or monolateral devices with typical lengthening rates of 1 mm per day. Very long discrepancies of up to 15 to 20 cm can be addressed using a combination of multiple lengthenings and epiphyseodeses. Larger discrepancies can be treated with amputation and prosthetic fitting to equalize limb lengths.

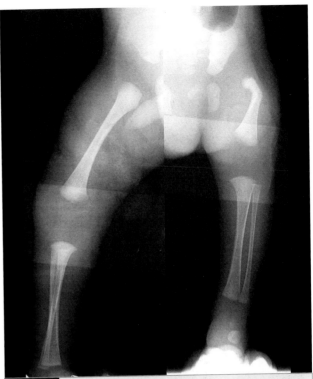

| Figure 8 | AP radiograph of both lower extremities in a patient with left proximal femoral focal deficiency, showing proximal femoral varus and significant shortening of the femur. |

Congenital Femoral Deficiency

Congenital femoral deficiency includes congenital short femur, proximal femoral focal deficiency, and femoral hypoplasia. Shortening of the femur is associated with varying degrees of proximal femoral varus, distal femoral valgus, femoral retroversion, acetabular dysplasia, and congenital absence or incompetence of the cruciate ligaments of the knee (**Figure 8**). Approximately half of these patients will have associated fibular hemimelia. Several different classification schemes have been developed to guide treatment. These classification systems focus on stability of the hip and the amount of shortening noted in the femur.

The projected limb-length discrepancy and the stability of the associated joints as well as the severity of the associated deformities determine treatment options. Patients with a projected limb-length discrepancy of less than 15 to 20 cm with relatively stable or surgically stable joints and a functional, plantigrade foot are often candidates for limb lengthening. The presence of projected limb-length discrepancies of more than 20 cm, very unstable joints, or a nonfunctional foot are relative indications for ablation. This most often takes the form of a Syme amputation with or without a knee arthrodesis. Selected patients with severe femoral deficiency and a functional ankle and foot can be treated by knee arthrodesis combined with Van Ness rotationplasty. This allows the rotated foot to serve as a knee joint allowing active flexion of the knee.

6: Pediatrics

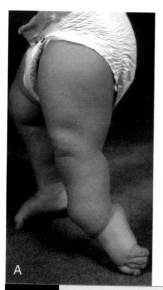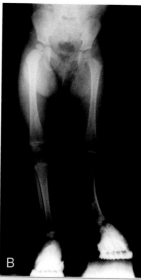

Figure 9 **A,** Photograph of the left lower extremity of a 14-month-old patient with fibular hemimelia showing significant anterior bowing with an apical dimple, shortening of the limb, a foot with four toes, and an equinus contracture. **B,** A standing AP radiograph of a 2-year-old girl with fibular hemimelia showing an absent fibula and significant limb-length discrepancy as a result of a shortened tibia.

Fibular Hemimelia

Fibular hemimelia is the most common of the congenital long bone deficiencies and is characterized by shortening or complete absence of the fibula, genu valgum, mild femoral shortening, and absence of one to three rays in the foot. Half of children with fibular hemimelia have tarsal coalitions, often severe coalitions involving the talus and calcaneus that may not be noted on initial radiographs due to the cartilaginous nature of the bones in early development. This severe coalition can lead to ball-and-socket changes in the ankle. Fibular hemimelia is often associated with anterior bowing of the tibia with a skin dimple noted anteriorly and an equinovalgus contracture of the ankle (**Figure 9**). Classification depends on the amount of fibular shortening or complete absence of the fibula. Treatment of fibular hemimelia is determined primarily by the stability and function of the foot and ankle and to a lesser extent by the projected limb-length discrepancy. Patients with mild projected limb-length discrepancy (less than 5 cm) and a stable foot can be managed with contralateral epiphysiodesis. Limb lengthening should be considered for patients with a stable plantigrade foot regardless of the number of rays present. Even patients with a three-toe foot, when associated with a stable ankle and a plantigrade functional foot, may be good candidates for limb lengthening. Patients with unstable valgus foot deformities often function better with Syme amputation at approximately 1 year of age with subsequent prosthetic fitting.

Tibial Hemimelia

Tibial hemimelia is a very rare condition associated with absence of part or the entire tibia. Deficiency of either the proximal or distal tibia can occur. This is a genetically linked syndrome[31,32] that is associated with ulnar aplasia and other musculoskeletal conditions and can be passed down to descendents. Patients often present with shortening of the lower leg and severe clubfoot deformities. Treatment is primarily based on the stability of the knee joint. Patients with an ossified proximal tibia can be treated by synostosis of the tibia and proximal fibula and a modified Syme amputation, leaving a stump ending in the fibula. Patients without a proximal tibia have been historically treated by the Brown procedure, with centralization of the proximal tibia beneath the femur to reconstruct the knee. This has been universally unsuccessful, leading to flexion contracture of the knee and very limited function. These patients are best treated with knee disarticulation and prosthetic fitting. Patients with distal tibial deficiency can be treated with limb lengthening after stabilization of the foot.

Posteromedial Bowing

Posteromedial bowing of the tibia is differentiated from anterolateral bowing seen in patients with congenital pseudarthrosis of the tibia. Posteromedial bowing of the tibia is associated frequently with a calcaneovalgus foot deformity (**Figure 10**). Although the etiology is unknown, a mechanism of mechanical trauma associated with in utero rupture of the amnion has been suggested.[33] Most frequently the bowing deformity will gradually improve with age, with some children having persistent bowing after age 4 years.[8] Some children will be left with mild ankle and knee valgus in spite of remodeling. Most children will have mild shortening of the limb at birth of approximately 1 to 2 cm. This will progress to an average shortening of 4 cm at maturity with occasional children developing more severe length discrepancies. Treatment of the limb-length discrepancy can be accomplished by wearing a lift, or surgically via limb lengthening or contralateral epiphysiodesis.

Hemiatrophy

Anisomelia with the shorter limb appearing to be abnormally small is known as hemiatrophy. Children with this condition are usually otherwise normal and the limb-length discrepancy between the two limbs is usually small. Most often this condition is treated with shoe lifts in younger children with subsequent definitive contralateral epiphysiodesis or limb lengthening in patients with greater ultimate limb-length discrepancy.

Hemihypertrophy

Anisomelia with the larger limb appearing to be abnormally large is known as hemihypertrophy. The difference in limb diameter often has little relationship to the projected or existing limb-length discrepancy. Hemihypertrophy is sometimes associated with the development of abdominal or retroperitoneal tumors such as hepatoblastoma, Wilms tumor, or neuroblastoma. The

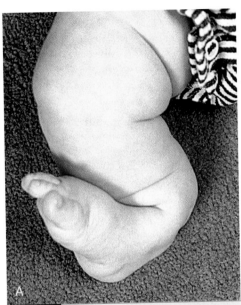
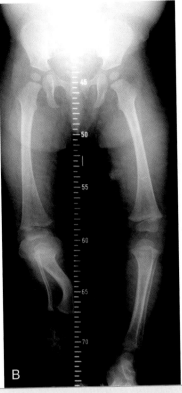
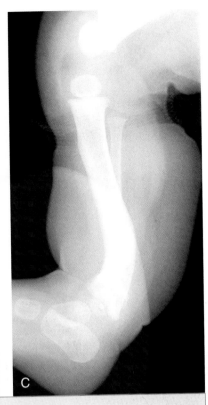

Figure 10   **A,** Photograph of posteromedial bowing in a 3-month old girl showing a calcaneovalgus foot and a tibia with an obvious bowing deformity. **B,** An AP radiograph of both lower extremities in a 1-year-old girl with posteromedial bowing, showing a significant limb-length discrepancy and tibial deformity. **C,** Lateral radiograph of the tibia in the patient in **B,** showing significant unresolved tibial bowing.

hemihypertrophy is not caused by the tumor, which is often identified years after the diagnosis of hemihypertrophy. Because of the risk of malignant tumor development, some recommendations include serum α-fetoprotein levels every 6 weeks from the time of diagnosis until age 4 years and abdominal ultrasound examinations every 3 months until age 6 to 9 years. Orthopaedic management includes appropriate lifts under the normal limb and following the patient for serial determinations of limb-length discrepancy until definitive epiphysiodesis at an appropriate age. Limb lengthening should rarely be considered, as the normal limb is the short limb.

Other Conditions
Congenital Dislocation of the Patella
Children with congenital dislocation of the patella are frequently diagnosed with an irreducible laterally dislocated patella before age 5 years. This condition should be differentiated from the much more common situation in which the patella is unstable or dislocates with activity in teens or young adults. Congenital dislocation of the patella is frequently associated with genu valgum flexion contracture of the knee and external tibial torsion. Although most often asymptomatic in younger children, the knee frequently becomes symptomatic with reports of pain and difficulty running as children

approach adolescence. Surgical correction involves a comprehensive approach with proximal and distal realignment and careful balancing of the soft tissues to avoid redislocation because of the shallow trochlear groove. Surgery can be successful even in very young children by transfer of the entire distal insertion of the patellar tendon from its pathologic lateral position to a more normal anteromedial position.[20]

Congenital Knee Dislocation
Congenital knee dislocation encompasses a spectrum of disorders ranging from simple hyperextension of the knee in which the tibia dislocates anterior to the femur but can be reduced by simple flexion of the knee, to rigid disorders in which the dislocation is fixed with the tibia translated anteriorly and proximally. Approximately 50% of patients with congenital dislocation of the knee will have hip dysplasia affecting either or both hips. Flexing the knee and applying a long leg splint with the knee in a flexed position can treat simple hyperextension. Patients with both hip dysplasia and congenital knee dislocation can frequently be treated for both disorders with a Pavlik harness. Rigid dislocations often require initial serial casting or splinting and either percutaneous quadriceps tendon lengthening or open quadricepsplasty.

6: Pediatrics

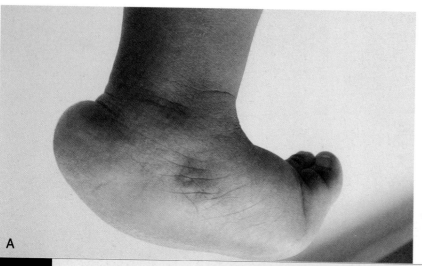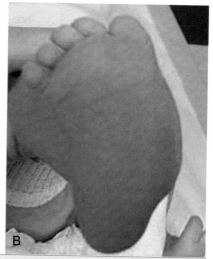

Figure 11 Clinical photographs demonstrating the features of congenital vertical talus. **A,** Unilateral congenital vertical talus deformity in a 6-week-old infant demonstrating the convex plantar surface of the foot. **B,** Plantar aspect of the foot showing forefoot abduction deformity.

Foot Disorders

Congenital Vertical Talus

Congenital vertical talus is a rare foot deformity that is present at birth and has an estimated incidence of 1 in 10,000. The hallmark of the deformity is a fixed dorsal dislocation of the navicular on the head of the talus resulting in a rigid flatfoot deformity. It occurs as an isolated deformity (idiopathic) in approximately half of all cases and is associated with neuromuscular and genetic disorders in the remaining cases. A careful neurologic examination should be performed in all vertical talus patients, and MRI evaluation of the neural axis should be considered to rule out spinal cord anomalies. Half of the children have bilateral involvement and there is male predominance over females by a ratio of 2:1. The etiology of idiopathic vertical talus has a genetic basis. This is supported by a positive family history in up to 20% of patients and the recent findings that mutations in the *HOXD10* gene, a member of a large family of highly conserved transcription factors that regulate limb development, are responsible for vertical talus in several familial cases.[34]

Congenital vertical talus is characterized by hindfoot equinus and valgus due to contractures of the Achilles and peroneal tendons and forefoot abduction and dorsiflexion due to contractures of the extensor digitorum longus, extensor hallucis longus, and anterior tibialis tendons (**Figure 11**). It is usually recognizable in the newborn by the rigidity of the deformities, but it must be differentiated from the more common calcaneovalgus foot, posterior medial bowing of the tibia, flexible flatfoot, and the oblique talus. Forced plantar flexion and dorsiflexion lateral radiographs can confirm the diagnosis of vertical talus. The forced plantar flexion lateral radiograph in a true vertical talus demonstrates persistent dorsal dislocation of the first metatarsal axis

to the longitudinal axis of the talus, while the forced dorsiflexion lateral radiograph demonstrates a persistently decreased tibiocalcaneal angle indicating fixed hindfoot equinus (**Figure 12**).

The goals of treatment are to restore the normal anatomic relationship between the talus, the navicular, and the calcaneus to provide a normal weight distribution through the foot. Many short- and long-term complications associated with extensive soft-tissue release surgeries for vertical talus have been noted. As such, efforts have been made recently to identify a less invasive approach for correcting this deformity.[34,35] This new approach uses serial casting to stretch the contracted dorsal and lateral soft tissues and gradually reduce the talonavicular joint. The principles used for casting are similar to those used in the Ponseti method of clubfoot correction. Once reduction is achieved with casting, the talonavicular joint is reduced (open or closed) and pinned in the operating room. Percutaneous tenotomy of the Achilles tendon is performed to correct the residual equinus contracture. Excellent early results have been reported from multiple centers.[34-36] Longer follow-up will be necessary to ensure maintenance of correction.

Clubfoot

Clubfoot is one of the most common birth defects involving the musculoskeletal system, with a worldwide incidence of about 1 in 1,000 live births. Approximately 80% of clubfeet are isolated birth defects and are considered idiopathic. The remaining 20% of clubfeet are associated with neuromuscular conditions and genetic syndromes. Although the exact etiology of idiopathic clubfoot is not known, a genetic component is suggested by the 33% concordance of identical twins and familial occurrence in 25% of cases. Additional evidence for a genetic etiology is provided by differences in clubfoot prevalence across ethnic populations, with

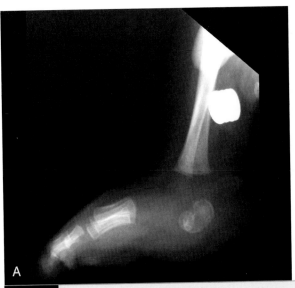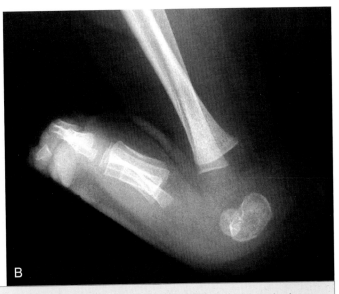

Figure 12	**A,** Plantar flexion lateral radiograph of the right foot of the patient in **Figure 11** with congenital vertical talus, showing persistent dorsal translation of the forefoot on the hindfoot. **B,** Lateral dorsiflexion radiograph of the same foot, showing persistent plantar flexion of the talus and calcaneus.

the lowest prevalence in the Chinese population and the highest in Hawaiians and Maoris. Idiopathic clubfoot is not a single gene disorder. Instead, clubfoot is heterogeneous and likely due to multiple genes and epigenetic factors most of which are not yet understood.[37] A recent study has identified *PITX1*, a transcription factor critical for limb development, as the gene responsible for clubfoot in a five-generation family.[31] This is the first gene identified to date for idiopathic clubfoot. A common genetic pathway for vertical talus and clubfoot is likely because many families have been reported in which both disorders are seen, as well as individuals with clubfoot on one side and vertical talus on the other.

Clubfoot is a complex congenital foot deformity that can be difficult to treat. It is recognizable at birth and is characterized by hindfoot equinus, hindfoot varus, midfoot adduction, and midfoot cavus (**Figure 13**). Clubfoot can be differentiated from the more common positional foot anomalies on the basis of the rigid equinus deformity seen in clubfoot and its resistance to gentle passive correction. Several classification systems exist but their clinical utility is questionable. In the future a genetic classification for clubfoot may be available that would allow patients to be categorized in a manner that would help physicians predict response to treatment.

Historically, treatment of clubfoot has consisted of serial casting followed by extensive soft-tissue release surgery. In addition to the many reported short-term complications associated with this procedure, long-term studies have shown many patients treated with extensive soft-tissue releases for clubfoot develop pain, arthritis, and difficulty ambulating as adults. The Ponseti method of serial casting, a percutaneous tenotomy of the Achilles tendon, and foot abduction bracing avoids

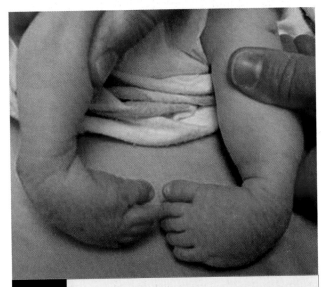

Figure 13	Photograph showing bilateral clubfoot in a 2-week-old boy, demonstrating hindfoot varus, hindfoot equinus, midfoot adduction, and midfoot cavus.

the need for extensive surgery in most patients with idiopathic clubfeet and has become the gold standard of treatment in North American and many parts of the world. The upper age limit of a child with clubfoot who can be treated with the Ponseti method is yet to be defined, with reports of correction obtained in children as old as 10 years at the initiation of treatment. In addition, there are recent reports of success using the Ponseti method to treat nonidiopathic clubfeet, including clubfeet in patients with distal arthrogryposis, myelomeningocele, and a variety of genetic syndromes.[38-40] The Ponseti method has also been applied successfully

6: Pediatrics

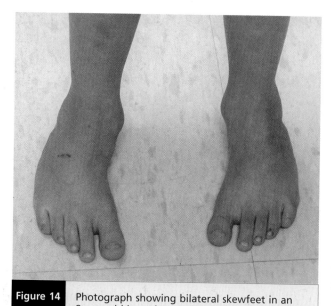

Figure 14 Photograph showing bilateral skewfeet in an 8-year-old boy, characterized by forefoot adduction, midfoot abduction, and hindfoot valgus.

in children previously treated with extensive soft-tissue release who later suffered a relapse.[41] As a result, there is no type of clubfoot or situation for which the Ponseti method should not be initially applied. Even in the most difficult feet, the method allows partial correction that then limits the amount of surgery needed. The goal in treatment of all clubfeet should be to obtain plantigrade, mobile feet with the least invasive method possible.

Metatarsus Adductus

Metatarsus adductus is a common foot deformity characterized by adduction of the forefoot with respect to the hindfoot. The lateral border of the foot has a convex contour, with the actual curvature occurring at the tarsometatarsal joints. There is no deformity in the hindfoot, with full range of motion present in the ankle and subtalar joints. The incidence is approximately 1 in 1,000 births with equal frequency in boys and girls and bilaterality occurring 50% of the time. Metatarsus adductus is a molding deformity that occurs due to fetal crowding as seen in late pregnancy, first pregnancies, twin pregnancies, and oligohydramnios.

Most cases (90%) of metatarsus adductus are mild and spontaneously resolve in the first year of life or with gentle stretching exercises. An additional 5% of cases resolve in the early walking years (1 to 4 years of age). In the remaining 5% of cases, the foot is stiffer at the outset and the deformity is likely to persist. However, long-term studies have shown that residual metatarsus adductus causes no problems in terms of pain or foot function. Given the benign natural history of metatarsus adductus, aggressive treatment is generally not warranted. Those parents distressed about the position of the foot can be taught stretching exercises to perform at diaper changes several times a day. The par-

ents must be taught how to perform the exercises correctly by abducting the forefoot using a thumb on the cuboid as a fulcrum. The stretch is held for a few seconds and repeated 20 times per session. If the forefoot is abducted without applying pressure on the cuboid, heel valgus may result without correction of the adductus, possibly leading to a skewfoot.

If the parents are still bothered by the appearance of the child's foot at 7 months of age, serial casting can be performed with two to three casts changed at 2-week intervals. The foot is manipulated as just described followed by application of a long leg plaster cast with the knee bent 90° and the plaster well molded with the forefoot in abduction. Most feet that are stiff enough to warrant casting should be placed into a nighttime foot abduction brace for up to 1 year to maintain correction. In the rare 4- to 5-year-old child with severe deformity, midfoot osteotomies can be considered.

Positional Calcaneovalgus

This common foot deformity is recognizable at birth due to the characteristic appearance of the forefoot resting on the anterior surface of the lower leg. The deformity is thought to be positional in nature, is more common in firstborn children, and has a predilection for females. It is important to differentiate this condition from more serious disorders that can have similar presentations, such as congenital vertical talus, posteromedial bow of the tiba, and paralytic calcaneus foot deformity. When there is confusion between a calcaneovalgus foot deformity and a true vertical talus, a plantar-flexion lateral radiograph is indicated. Treatment of a positional calcaneovalgus foot is not necessary, as spontaneous improvement is the norm.

Skewfoot

Skewfoot (also termed Z-foot and serpentine foot) is a rare, complex deformity characterized by forefoot adduction, midfoot abduction, and hindfoot valgus (**Figure 14**). The pathogenesis and natural history of this deformity remain unknown. Some cases may result from improper casting of metatarsus adductus and/or clubfoot. It is difficult to differentiate skewfoot from metatarsus adductus radiographically in the infant because of a lack of ossification of the navicular and medial cuneiform. The diagnosis can often be made clinically based on the presence of significant hindfoot valgus in combination with the forefoot adduction. In the older child and adolescent, radiographs demonstrate the deformities in the hindfoot, midfoot, and forefoot (**Figure 15**). Nonsurgical management in childhood consists of stretching a tight Achilles tendon as well as custom soft orthotics to support the talar head with weight bearing. Surgery is rarely indicated if nonsurgical treatment fails to relieve pain, and usually involves osteotomies to correct both hindfoot and forefoot deformities as well as lengthening of the heel cord and medial reefing of the talonavicular joint.

Flexible Flatfoot

The incidence of flatfoot is unknown, but the condition is most common in infants and decreases with age. Approximately 20% of adults have flatfoot. All flatfeet are characterized by a decrease in the medial longitudinal arch with sagging of the midfoot combined with hindfoot valgus, and abduction of the forefoot. There are three main types of flatfoot: hypermobile flexible flatfoot, flexible flatfoot with a short Achilles tendon, and rigid flatfoot. The hypermobile flexible flatfoot accounts for most types of flatfeet in children and is rarely a clinical problem. This type of flatfoot has excellent mobility of the subtalar joint demonstrated by the heel correcting to a varus position with the patient standing on toes. The loss of arch is only seen with weight bearing. A rigid flatfoot does not correct into hindfoot varus with toe rise, indicating limitation of motion in the subtalar joint. This is the least common type of flatfoot in children, and tarsal coalitions should be ruled out in these cases, as they often require surgical treatment. Those patients with a flexible flatfoot and tight heel cord should be treated with heel cord stretching because this deformity has the potential to cause pain. Surgery is indicated when heel cord stretching fails to relieve symptoms. If the flatfoot is mild, a lengthening of the gastrocnemius fascia or the heel cord (if the soleus is also tight) may be all that is necessary. For a more severe deformity, heel cord lengthening should be combined with osteotomies to correct the deformity. Patients with hypermobile flatfeet, if symptomatic, can be treated with soft orthotics to change the shoe wear pattern and decrease symptoms. Surgery is rarely indicated for the flexible flatfoot.

Tarsal Coalition

A tarsal coalition refers to a fibrous, cartilaginous, or bony union between two or more bones of the midfoot or hindfoot. The incidence is not well known but is thought to be between 3% to 6% of the general population, with a 2:1 male-to-female distribution. The most common coalitions are the calcaneonavicular and the talocalcaneal (middle facet). Together these account for 90% of all coalitions. Bilaterality occurs in 50% to 60% of cases, and there is a genetic predisposition evidenced by positive family histories and an autosomal dominant pattern of inheritance.[42]

Symptoms of activity-related pain may develop as a coalition changes from a cartilaginous to a bony union. This change occurs commonly between age 8 and 12 years for calcaneonavicular coalitions and between age 12 and 16 years for talocalcaneal coalitions. The pain in the talocalcaneal coalitions is often poorly localized in the hindfoot, whereas a calcaneonavicular coalition usually causes pain dorsolaterally in the area of the coalition. A common presentation with a coalition is a history of repeated ankle sprains due to limitation of subtalar motion. On physical examination there is a rigid flatfoot deformity with minimal subtalar motion, such that the hindfoot does not invert into varus with toe standing.

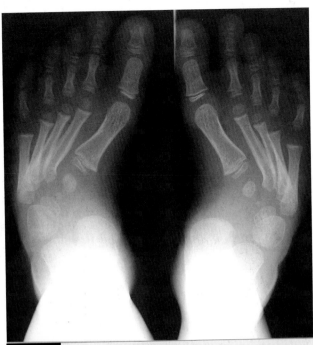

Figure 15   AP radiographs of the patient in Figure 14 with bilateral skewfeet, demonstrating lateral translation of the midfoot on the hindfoot.

The calcaneonavicular coalition can be diagnosed with an internal oblique radiograph of the foot, which demonstrates the bony bridge. A standing lateral radiograph may demonstrate a long anterior process of the calcaneus, called the anteater sign. Talocalcaneal coalitions are more difficult to diagnose on plain radiographs, and a CT or MRI is usually necessary. Only symptomatic coalitions should be treated because up to 75% of coalitions do not cause pain or disability. The initial treatment of a symptomatic coalition includes a below-the-knee walking cast for 4 weeks. If the pain is not relieved immediately during cast wear, then the coalition may be only an incidental finding. A soft insert is used after cast removal, and approximately one third of patients will remain symptom free. If symptoms recur, surgery is warranted. Resection of the coalition and interposition of fat or the extensor digitorum brevis muscle is successful in most cases of calcaneonavicular coalitions. Overall, the results of talocalcaneal coalition resections and fat interposition are less favorable. In particular, if more than 50% of the subtalar joint is affected by the coalition, then resection alone is less likely to relieve symptoms. In addition, if there is excessive hindfoot valgus, a valgus-correcting osteotomy should be considered at the time of resection. Arthrodesis of the subtalar joint is reserved for patients with subtalar arthritis.

Juvenile Hallux Valgus

Hallux valgus or bunion deformity is an abnormal prominence on the medial side of the first metatarsal head with its accompanying bursa (**Figure 16**). A juve-

6: Pediatrics

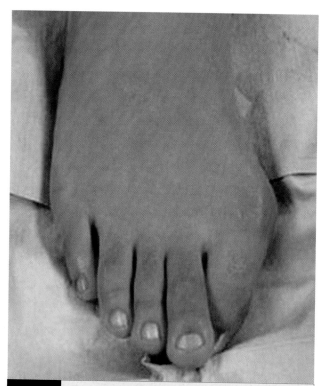

Figure 16 Photograph of the foot of an adolescent boy with significant hallux valgus deformity. The first toe is laterally deviated at the metatarsophalangeal joint causing overlap of the second toe onto the first.

nile bunion has its onset in the preteen or teenage years, when the growth plates of the metatarsals and phalanges are still open. The incidence is unknown but there is a female predilection with 80% of surgically treated cases. Although the cause is unknown, there is a strong genetic component with reports of X-linked, autosomal dominant, and polygenic modes of transmission. Standing AP and lateral radiographs of the foot can help determine the site of the deformities. Typical measurements recorded are the first-second intermetatarsal angle, the first metatarsal–proximal phalanx angle, the distal metatarsal articular angle, and metatarsophalangeal (MTP) joint congruity. The natural history of juvenile hallux valgus is not known. Most experts concur that a congruous MTP joint is stable and less likely to progress than those with subluxation.

Most adolescents with hallux valgus are asymptomatic and should not undergo any form of treatment. Children with pain related to their bunion should first have nonsurgical management, including the use of shoes with an adequate toe box and a low heel. Splinting can relieve pressure over the deformity but does not provide correction long term. Surgery is indicated only when prolonged attempts at nonsurgical management have failed. The ideal time for surgery is when the physes are closed because open physes contribute to an increased incidence of recurrent deformity. The exact procedure chosen is based on the type of deformity

present but usually consists of a combination of bony osteotomies and/or soft-tissue rebalancing.[43] One of the most important considerations to make preoperatively is whether the MTP joint is subluxated. If so, treatment must include a distal soft-tissue realignment. Lateral hemiepiphysiodesis of the great toe metatarsal has been recently proposed as an alternative treatment in the juvenile patient that allows correction to be achieved slowly with continued growth of the child.[44] Additional studies are needed to confirm the efficacy of the procedure and establish treatment guidelines.

Cavus Foot Deformity

A cavus foot is characterized by a rigid plantar flexion of the forefoot in relation to the hindfoot, resulting in an abnormally high arch. The high arch may be due to plantar flexion of the first ray alone or may involve plantar flexion of all of the metatarsals. The heel in the cavus foot may be in neutral, valgus, varus (cavovarus foot) (**Figure 17,** *A*), calcaneus (calcaneocavus foot), or equinus position. A careful physical examination is required in all patients with a cavus foot deformity because most cases are due to an underlying neuromuscular disorder. Unilateral deformities can be associated with syringomyelia, lipomeningocele, spinal cord tumor, diastematomyelia, or tethered cord diagnosed on MRI of the spine. Genetic testing and a consultation with a pediatric neurologist are appropriate; an electromyogram and nerve conduction velocity studies may be ordered. Bilateral cases are often due to hereditary sensorimotor neuropathies such as Charcot-Marie-Tooth disease and Friedreich ataxia. Because of the familial nature of these conditions, examining the feet of the parents and other family members should be done if possible.

Patients typically present to the orthopaedic surgeon because of difficulty with shoe fitting, pain under the metatarsal heads, clawing of the toes, and a history of repeated ankle sprains. The deformities seen in the foot are caused by muscle imbalance. Relative weakness of the anterior tibialis compared to the peroneus longus results in plantar flexion of the first ray and the cavus deformity. Atrophy of the intrinsic muscles of the foot leads to hyperextension of the MTP joints and resulting tightening of the plantar fascia. The hindfoot deformities seen with the cavus foot develop last. In the most common examples of the cavovarus foot, the hindfoot varus develops as a direct result of the plantar-flexed first ray. If the first ray is in plantar flexion, the only way to maintain the tripod of the foot and get the heel on the ground is for the heel to go into varus. This position is reinforced by the relative strength of the posterior tibialis compared to the peroneus brevis.

Radiographic evaluation of the patient with pes cavus should include AP and lateral radiographs of the spine to look for interpedicular distance widening, congenital malformations, or atypical pattern scoliosis. Foot radiographs should include standing AP and lateral views. A cavus foot is characterized by plantar flexion of the axis of the first metatarsal in relation to

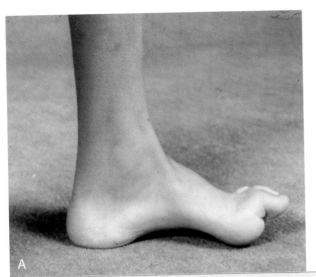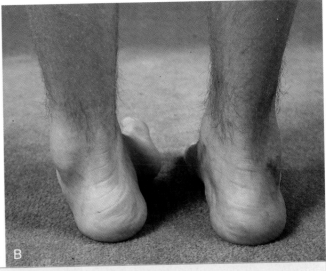

Figure 17 **A,** Photograph of a cavus foot deformity in a 14-year-old girl with a peripheral neuropathy. **B,** Unilateral cavovarus foot deformity due to Charcot-Marie-Tooth disease is shown in a 16-year-old boy. Although patients with hereditary sensory motor neuropathy typically have bilateral deformity, unilateral deformity can still occur.

the axis of the talus on the lateral view. The hindfoot can be in varus, valgus, or equinus, although varus is most common (**Figure 17, B**).

Arch supports and stretching may be appropriate in the earliest stages of a developing cavus foot deformity. Surgery is indicated for patients with painful calluses under the metatarsal heads or on the dorsum of the MTP joints, difficulty with shoe wear, and progressive deformity with ankle instability. The principles of surgery are to correct the deformities and to balance the soft tissues to maintain correction and prevent recurrences. Correction of the deformities involves release of the soft-tissue contractures combined with appropriate osteotomies.[45] The Coleman block test can be used to assess the flexibility of the hindfoot varus and help predict whether hindfoot correction can be maintained with forefoot procedures alone, or whether additional osteotomies of the hindfoot may be necessary. The block test is performed by placing a block under the lateral border of the foot while the patient is bearing weight. The block allows the forefoot to pronate; if the hindfoot is flexible, the subtalar joint will correct to neutral. Correction of the rigid subtalar joint will not occur with this maneuver, indicating that osteotomy of the hindfoot will be necessary.

Osteochondroses of the Foot

Kohler disease is an osteochondrosis that affects the tarsal navicular. It is a self-limited condition characterized by pain or swelling in the area of the tarsal navicular in association with distinct radiographic findings. It occurs in patients 4 to 7 years of age, with 80% of cases occurring in boys. The cause is unknown, but it is thought to be related to repetitive trauma. On physical examination there is typically soft-tissue swelling, erythema, and tenderness to palpation over the tarsal navicular. Active and passive range of motion is normal.

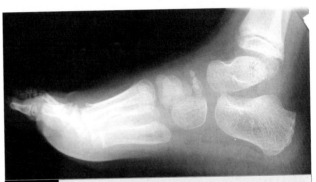

Figure 18 Lateral radiograph of the foot in a patient with Kohler disease, demonstrating the sclerotic and flattened appearance of the navicular.

The classic radiographic findings include flattening and patchy ossification of the navicular bone with preservation of its joint surfaces (**Figure 18**). The goal of treatment should be relief of symptoms, which can usually be accomplished with a short leg weight-bearing cast worn for 3 to 4 weeks. Without treatment, most patients have intermittent activity-related symptoms for 1 to 3 years. Radiographic improvement is noted over a 1-year period from onset of symptoms, and no long-term disabilities have been reported.

Freiberg infraction is an osteochondrosis characterized by osteonecrosis of the metatarsal head, the second metatarsal being most often affected. This condition is most commonly seen in patients age 13 to 18 years and is more common in girls than boys. Patients present with pain and tenderness around the second MTP joint. The second metatarsal head has a flattened appearance on radiographs, with areas of increased sclerosis and fragmentation. The natural history is variable. Many cases are self-limited, with revascularization of the

6: Pediatrics

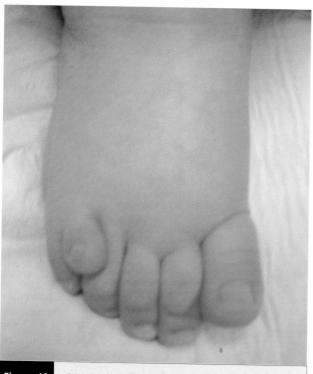

Figure 19 Postaxial polydactyly in a 6-month-old child.

metatarsal head. Some cases, however, result in significant deformity and secondary degenerative changes at the MTP joint. Initial treatment should be nonsurgical and includes activity modification and the use of metatarsal pads in the shoes. In some acute cases, casting may be beneficial. Surgery is rarely indicated and should be reserved for chronic cases unresponsive to nonsurgical treatment. Surgery can range from metatarsal neck osteotomy and joint débridement to resection of the metatarsal head.

Accessory Navicular

Approximately 10% of the population older than 5 years of age has an accessory navicular, with symptoms more commonly developing in girls. Pain and tenderness are localized to the prominent accessory navicular on the plantar medial aspect of the foot at the insertion of the posterior tibialis tendon. Accessory navicular can be classified as type I, a small sesamoid bone in the substance of the posterior tibialis tendon; type II, a large wedge-shaped bone fragment that appears to be congruous with the navicular through a synchondrosis; or type III, a large horn-shaped navicular, likely resulting from an earlier fusion of a type II deformity. Evaluation of the symptomatic patient should include an external oblique radiograph of the foot to better visualize the accessory ossification center.

Nonsurgical management includes activity modifications, foot orthotics, or a short leg walking cast for 3 to 4 weeks. The goal with nonsurgical management is to decrease pressure over the bony prominence and reduce strain on the posterior tibialis tendon. If pain persists,

surgical resection of the bony prominence is warranted, with reattachment of any posterior tibialis tendon that was removed during the bone resection. It is important to remove enough bone so the navicular is flush with the medial cuneiform on an AP radiograph of the foot. Most surgical failures are the result of inadequate removal of bone.

Lesser Toe Deformities

A curly toe is a common deformity in which the proximal interphalangeal joint is flexed and medially deviated so it underlaps the adjacent toe. The third and fourth toes are most commonly involved and the deformities are often bilateral and familial. The etiology is congenital tightness and shortening of the toe flexors. Most patients are asymptomatic, and approximately 25% of cases will resolve spontaneously. Treatment with stretching and taping can be used but has not been shown to provide long-term correction. Surgery is indicated for patients with pain and difficulty with shoe wear. Release of the long toe flexor at the level of the distal interphalangeal joint is effective in most cases.

Congenital overriding fifth toe is a familial disorder in which the fifth toe is dorsiflexed, adducted, and overrides the fourth toe. It is often bilateral and there is no sex predilection. Unlike the curly toe, which is flexible, the overriding fifth toe is a rigid deformity that often requires treatment in half of all patients. Treatment is indicated for persistent symptoms despite shoe wear modifications. Nonsurgical measures such as taping, stretching, and splinting are ineffective. Surgical treatment involves releasing the contracted MTP joint capsule, lengthening the extensor tendon, and pinning the toe in the corrected position. A dorsal incision is usually avoided because contracture of the scar can lead to recurrent deformity.

Polydactyly is the duplication of a digit and is the most common congenital toe deformity. It is often familial and is bilateral in 50% of cases. The fifth toe is the most commonly duplicated digit; this condition is called postaxial polydactyly (**Figure 19**). Duplication of the great toe is called preaxial polydactyly and occurs frequently with tibial hemimelia. *PITX1* is the first gene identified for the combination of preaxial polydactyly, clubfoot, and tibial hemimelia.[31] Treatment is generally surgical because of difficulties with shoe wear due to the widened forefoot. The procedure is usually performed between 9 and 12 months of age. Radiographs are required to assess the extent of the duplication and decide which digit to excise.

Bunionette deformity is a painful osseous prominence on the lateral aspect of the head of the fifth metatarsal (**Figure 20**) that is less common than hallux valgus deformity. It is more common in females and the exact prevalence of the deformity is unknown. Patients usually present because of a painful bursa that develops over the prominent fifth metatarsal head. Initial treatment, as with hallux valgus deformities, is shoe wear modification, to which most patients respond favorably. For persistent symptoms, surgery may be indi-

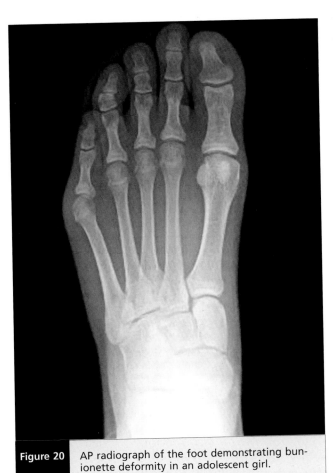

Figure 20 | AP radiograph of the foot demonstrating bunionette deformity in an adolescent girl.

cated. The most common procedure is a fifth metatarsal sliding osteotomy, which has been shown to be safe and effective.

Idiopathic Toe Walking

Idiopathic toe walking is usually easy to recognize, but it is a diagnosis of exclusion. Patients walk on their toes and the condition is usually bilateral. It is more common in males and there is a genetic etiology seen with many patients having a positive family history. Patients typically present for evaluation at age 3 or 4 years. Toe walking is normal and is often seen in children who are beginning to walk. However, by the age of 3 years, children should walk with a heel strike gait. Persistent toe walking beyond this age is abnormal and should be further evaluated. It is important in early-onset toe walking to rule out neuromuscular etiologies such as spastic diplegia. If toe walking develops in a child with a previously normal gait then it is necessary to rule out primary muscle diseases such as muscular dystrophy, myotonic dystrophy, dystonia, tethered cord, and central nervous system disorders. Unilateral toe walking should also be a red flag for an underlying neurologic etiology.

Physical examination of the child with idiopathic toe walking demonstrates a loss of passive ankle dorsiflexion. Neurologic examination will be normal. Treatment begins with instructions to parents on stretching exercises and dorsiflexion strengthening exercises. This treatment is most effective in the young patient, age 3 or 4 years. If improvement is not seen with several months of aggressive therapy done by parents and/or outside physical therapy, then serial casting can be used. A series of two or three short leg casts changed every 2 weeks is recommended. At each cast change further stretching of the Achilles tendon is attempted. For those patients who do not respond to casting or those who are older than 7 years, Vulpius lengthening of the gastrocnemius or heel cord lengthening (if both the soleus and gastrocnemius are tight) should be considered. The heel cord can be lengthened percutaneously in a stepwise manner by starting 1 cm proximal to the heel cord and releasing the medial half of the tendon. The lateral half is released 1 cm proximal to the first cut, and the medial half is released 1 cm proximal to the last cut. This allows the tendon to be lengthened but still maintain fiber continuity. The patient is placed in a short leg walking cast for 4 weeks followed by a walking boot for another 2 weeks. Physical therapy is initiated when the patient gets out of the cast. The emphasis is on maintaining ankle dorsiflexion and improving strength in the gastrocnemius. Results are very satisfactory with this procedure.

Annotated References

1. Sabharwal S, Zhao C, Edgar M: Lower limb alignment in children: Reference values based on a full-length standing radiograph. *J Pediatr Orthop* 2008;28(7):740-746.

   The authors analyzed 354 normal lower extremity long cassette radiographs in children of various ages. Initial varus alignment corrected to valgus by age 3 years. After age 7 years, the mechanical axis deviation, lateral distal tibial angle, and medial proximal tibial angle had normalized to values considered normal for adults.

2. Inan M, Jeong C, Chan G, Mackenzie WG, Glutting J: Analysis of lower extremity alignment in achondroplasia: Interobserver reliability and intraobserver reproducibility. *J Pediatr Orthop* 2006;26(1):75-78.

3. Gordon JE, Chen RC, Dobbs MB, Luhmann SJ, Rich MM, Schoenecker PL: Interobserver and intraobserver reliability in the evaluation of mechanical axis deviation. *J Pediatr Orthop* 2009;29(3):281-284.

   The authors evaluated interobserver and intraobserver reliabilities for mechanical axis deviation, lateral distal femoral angle, and medial proximal tibial angle in 35 pediatric radiographs with a variety of deformities. Measurements demonstrated excellent intraobserver and interobserver reliabilities regardless of the experience of the observer.

4. Stevens PM, Klatt JB: Guided growth for pathological physes: Radiographic improvement during realignment. *J Pediatr Orthop* 2008;28(6):632-639.

6: Pediatrics

The authors treated 14 patients with rickets using guided growth with either staples or 8-plates. When using staples, migration was common and rebound occurred in 41% of physes. No 8-plate migration occurred. As the deformities corrected, the appearance and width of the physis improved.

5. Bar-On E, Horesh Z, Katz K, et al: Correction of lower limb deformities in children with renal osteodystrophy by the Ilizarov method. *J Pediatr Orthop* 2008;28(7): 747-751.

Five patients with eight affected limb segments with coronal angulation were treated with osteotomy and circular external fixation. There were no major complications, and pin tract infections responded to oral antibiotics. Four of the five patients maintained the alignment achieved at the time of external fixator removal.

6. Thompson GH, Carter JR, Smith CW: Late-onset tibia vara: A comparative analysis. *J Pediatr Orthop* 1984; 4(2):185-194.

7. Feldman MD, Schoenecker PL: Use of the metaphyseal-diaphyseal angle in the evaluation of bowed legs. *J Bone Joint Surg Am* 1993;75(11):1602-1609.

8. Shah HH, Doddabasappa SN, Joseph B: Congenital posteromedial bowing of the tibia: A retrospective analysis of growth abnormalities in the leg. *J Pediatr Orthop B* 2009;18(3):120-128.

Serial radiographs of 20 patients with posteromedial bowing of the tibia were reviewed. The angulatory deformity improved rapidly during the first year of life and much more slowly after that. Remodeling appeared to come from a combination of diaphyseal remodeling and physeal realignment. Shortening of 40% was noted in one patient.

9. Lavelle WF, Shovlin J, Drvaric DM: Reliability of the metaphyseal-diaphyseal angle in tibia vara as measured on digital images by pediatric orthopaedic surgeons. *J Pediatr Orthop* 2008;28(6):695-698.

Digital radiographs of 21 patients including 42 lower extremities were reviewed by 27 pediatric orthopaedic surgeons to determine the intraobserver and interobserver reliability of the metaphyseal-diaphyseal angle. Alternative methods of drawing the angle using either the lateral border of the tibia or the center of the tibial shaft were used. There was excellent reliability of the method and no significant variability was seen using either method of drawing the angle.

10. Langenskiöld A: Tibia vara. *J Pediatr Orthop* 1994; 14(2):141-142.

11. Gordon JE, King DJ, Luhmann SJ, Dobbs MB, Schoenecker PL: Femoral deformity in tibia vara. *J Bone Joint Surg Am* 2006;88(2):380-386.

12. Park SS, Gordon JE, Luhmann SJ, Dobbs MB, Schoenecker PL: Outcome of hemiepiphyseal stapling for late-onset tibia vara. *J Bone Joint Surg Am* 2005;87(10): 2259-2266.

13. Bushnell BD, May R, Campion ER, Schmale GA, Henderson RC: Hemiepiphyseodesis for late-onset tibia vara. *J Pediatr Orthop* 2009;29(3):285-289.

The authors treated 53 patients with 67 limbs with adolescent tibia vara by hemiepiphysiodesis using staples at either the distal femur, proximal tibia or both. This procedure was successful in restoring the mechanical axis in 38 patients. Although younger age and lesser deformity were weakly predictive of correction, neither weight or any other factor was a statistically significant predictor of correction.

14. Gilbody J, Thomas G, Ho K: Acute versus gradual correction of idiopathic tibia vara in children: A systematic review. *J Pediatr Orthop* 2009;29(2):110-114.

A systematic review of the literature revealed only one comparative study that provided weak evidence that correction with computerized ring fixation resulted in improved outcomes. Other series failed to provide evidence of any advantage of either acute or gradual correction of the deformity.

15. Clarke SE, McCarthy JJ, Davidson RS: Treatment of Blount disease: a comparison between the multiaxial correction system and other external fixators. *J Pediatr Orthop* 2009;29(2):103-109.

The multiaxial correction external fixator was compared to correction using traditional circular fixation and monolateral fixation in 58 extremities with tibia vara. There was no difference in accuracy of correction or complications with any of the methods.

16. Feldman DS, Madan SS, Ruchelsman DE, Sala DA, Lehman WB: Accuracy of correction of tibia vara: Acute versus gradual correction. *J Pediatr Orthop* 2006;26(6): 794-798.

17. Gordon JE, Heidenreich FP, Carpenter CJ, Kelly-Hahn J, Schoenecker PL: Comprehensive treatment of late-onset tibia vara. *J Bone Joint Surg Am* 2005;87(7): 1561-1570.

18. Eidelman M, Bialik V, Katzman A: The use of the Taylor spatial frame in adolescent Blount's disease: Is fibular osteotomy necessary? *J Child Orthop* 2008;2(3): 199-204.

The authors reviewed 10 extremities in patients with tibia vara corrected with computer-driven circular fixation without fibular osteotomy. They concluded that placement of the origin at the level of the proximal tibial-fibular joint obviates the need for fibular osteotomy in patients with mild to moderate tibia vara.

19. Cho TJ, Choi IH, Lee KS, et al: Proximal tibial lengthening by distraction osteogenesis in congenital pseudarthrosis of the tibia. *J Pediatr Orthop* 2007;27(8):915-920.

The authors review 27 cases of distraction osteogenesis in 22 patients with congenital pseudarthrosis of the tibia. Patients who had dysplastic proximal tibiae or who were being lengthened for the second time were much more likely to require bone grafting or other procedures to achieve union of the lengthened segment.

20. Wada A, Fujii T, Takamura K, Yanagida H, Surijamorn P: Congenital dislocation of the patella. *J Child Orthop* 2008;2(2):119-123.

   The authors treated seven knees in six patients with congenital dislocation of the patella at ages ranging from 0.6 years to 3.9 years. Genu valgus and external tibial torsion improved after medial transfer of the patellar tendon with posterior knee release and V-Y quadricepsplasty.

21. Peterson HA: The treatment of congenital pseudarthrosis of the tibia with ipsilateral fibular transfer to make a one-bone lower leg: A review of the literature and case report with a 23-year follow-up. *J Pediatr Orthop* 2008;28(4):478-482.

   The author reports a single case with 23-year follow-up and a review of the literature on nonvascularized ipsilateral fibular transfer to repair a congenital pseudarthrosis of the tibia.

22. Ofluoglu O, Davidson RS, Dormans JP: Prophylactic bypass grafting and long-term bracing in the management of anterolateral bowing of the tibia and neurofibromatosis-1. *J Bone Joint Surg Am* 2008; 90(10):2126-2134.

   The authors report a series of 10 patients with dysplastic but intact tibiae treated with allograft fibular grafting. Although several complications occurred, no patient developed a fracture of the dysplastic tibia following allograft placement.

23. Anticevic D, Jelic M, Vukicevic S: Treatment of a congenital pseudarthrosis of the tibia by osteogenic protein-1 (bone morphogenetic protein-7): A case report. *J Pediatr Orthop B* 2006;15(3):220-221.

24. Johnston CE, Birch JG: A tale of two tibias: A review of treatment options for congenital pseudarthrosis of the tibia. *J Child Orthop* 2008;2(2):133-149.

   The authors compare two common treatment options for congenital pseudarthrosis of the tibia and emphasize the importance of careful surgical technique in carrying out intramedullary fixation of the tibia. The use of bone morphogenetic protein–2 is described as an aid to obtain union in a single patient.

25. Lee FY, Sinicropi SM, Lee FS, Vitale MG, Roye DP Jr, Choi IH: Treatment of congenital pseudarthrosis of the tibia with recombinant human bone morphogenetic protein-7 (rhBMP-7). A report of five cases. *J Bone Joint Surg Am* 2006;88(3):627-633.

26. Gordon JE, Pappademos PC, Schoenecker PL, Dobbs MB, Luhmann SJ: Diaphyseal derotational osteotomy with intramedullary fixation for correction of excessive femoral anteversion in children. *J Pediatr Orthop* 2005; 25(4):548-553.

27. Stevens PM, Anderson D: Correction of anteversion in skeletally immature patients: Percutaneous osteotomy and transtrochanteric intramedullary rod. *J Pediatr Orthop* 2008;28(3):277-283.

   Forty percutaneous diaphyseal derotational femoral os-teotomies were performed for anteversion. No immobilization was used. All healed without evidence of femoral growth disturbance or osteonecrosis.

28. Ryan DD, Rethlefsen SA, Skaggs DL, Kay RM: Results of tibial rotational osteotomy without concomitant fibular osteotomy in children with cerebral palsy. *J Pediatr Orthop* 2005;25(1):84-88.

29. Savva N, Ramesh R, Richards RH: Supramalleolar osteotomy for unilateral tibial torsion. *J Pediatr Orthop B* 2006;15(3):190-193.

30. Inan M, Chan G, Littleton AG, Kubiak P, Bowen JR: Efficacy and safety of percutaneous epiphysiodesis. *J Pediatr Orthop* 2008;28(6):648-651.

   The authors report 97 cases of percutaneous epiphysiodesis followed until skeletal maturity. Complications included two knee effusions, one superficial wound infection, and three instances of exostosis formation. Failure of the epiphysiodesis to stop physeal growth occurred in three patients. Complications are infrequent and correction is accurate when the straight-line Mosley graph is used to plan surgical intervention.

31. Gurnett CA, Alaee F, Kruse LM, et al: Asymmetric lower-limb malformations in individuals with homeobox PITX1 gene mutation. *Am J Hum Genet* 2008; 83(5):616-622.

32. Babbs C, Heller R, Everman DB, et al: A new locus for split hand/foot malformation with long bone deficiency (SHFLD) at 2q14.2 identified from a chromosome translocation. *Hum Genet* 2007;122(2):191-199.

   The authors report a sporadic patient with tibial aplasia and a chromosome 2;18 translocation.

33. De Maio F, Corsi A, Roggini M, Riminucci M, Bianco P, Ippolito E: Congenital unilateral posteromedial bowing of the tibia and fibula: Insights regarding pathogenesis from prenatal pathology. A case report. *J Bone Joint Surg Am* 2005;87(7):1601-1605.

34. Dobbs MB, Purcell DB, Nunley R, Morcuende JA: Early results of a new method of treatment for idiopathic congenital vertical talus. *J Bone Joint Surg Am* 2006;88(6): 1192-1200.

35. Alaee F, Boehm S, Dobbs MB: A new approach to the treatment of congenital vertical talus. *J Child Orthop* 2007;1(3):165-174.

   The authors describe a minimally invasive approach to congenital vertical talus that has shown good short-terms results while avoiding the need for more extensive soft-tissue release surgery.

36. Bhaskar A: Congenital vertical talus: Treatment by reverse Ponseti technique. *Indian J Orthop* 2008;42(3): 347-350.

   The authors report on four patients (eight vertical talus feet) treated with the new minimally invasive approach with excellent short-term results and no patient requiring more extensive surgery.

37. Kruse LM, Dobbs MB, Gurnett CA: Polygenic threshold model with sex dimorphism in clubfoot inheritance: The Carter effect. *J Bone Joint Surg Am* 2008;90(12):2688-2694.

   The authors demonstrate that idiopathic clubfoot is a polygenic disorder, with females as the less affected sex, requiring a higher genetic load to be affected.

38. Boehm S, Limpaphayom N, Alaee F, Sinclair MF, Dobbs MB: Early results of the Ponseti method for the treatment of clubfoot in distal arthrogryposis. *J Bone Joint Surg Am* 2008;90(7):1501-1507.

   The authors report the successful correction of 12 consecutive clubfoot patients (24 clubfeet) with the diagnosis of distal arthrogryposis using the Ponseti method. The minimum follow-up was 2 years.

39. Gerlach DJ, Gurnett CA, Limpaphayom N, et al: Early results of the Ponseti method for the treatment of clubfoot associated with myelomeningocele. *J Bone Joint Surg Am* 2009;91(6):1350-1359.

   The authors report the successful use of the Ponseti method of clubfoot correction in 16 consecutive patients with clubfoot and myelomeningocele and 20 patients with idiopathic clubfoot.

40. Gurnett CA, Boehm S, Connolly A, Reimschisel T, Dobbs MB: Impact of congenital talipes equinovarus etiology on treatment outcomes. *Dev Med Child Neurol* 2008;50(7):498-502.

   The authors evaluated 357 consecutive clubfoot patients treated by one physician and found 24% of patients had nonidiopathic clubfoot. Most patients with nonidiopathic clubfoot had disorders affecting the nervous system.

41. Garg S, Dobbs MB: Use of the Ponseti method for recurrent clubfoot following posteromedial release. *Indian J Orthop* 2008;42(1):68-72.

   The authors report 11 consecutive clubfoot patients (17 clubfeet) that had been previously treated with extensive soft-tissue release operations for idiopathic clubfoot and presented with full relapses. The patients were all treated successfully using the Ponseti method of casting followed by tibialis anterior tendon transfer and percutaneous heel cord lengthening.

42. Migues A, Slullitel GA, Suárez E, Galán HL: Case reports: Symptomatic bilateral talonavicular coalition. *Clin Orthop Relat Res* 2009;467(1):288-292.

   The authors report results in a 24-year-old woman with symptomatic talonavicular coalitions bilaterally who underwent successful resections.

43. George HL, Casaletto J, Unnikrishnan PN, et al: Outcome of the scarf osteotomy in adolescent hallux valgus. *J Child Orthop* 2009;3(3):185-190.

   The authors report 13 adolescent patients (19 feet) treated with the scarf osteotomy for symptomatic hallux valgus deformities. Patients were followed for a mean of 37.6 months and had good radiographic and clinical outcomes.

44. Davids JR, McBrayer D, Blackhurst DW: Juvenile hallux valgus deformity: Surgical management by lateral hemiepiphyseodesis of the great toe metatarsal. *J Pediatr Orthop* 2007;27(7):826-830.

   Authors present a series of 7 patients (11 feet) treated with lateral hemiepiphysiodesis of the great toe metatarsal of juvenile hallux valgus. The procedure was effective in halting progression of the deformity in all cases and allowed significant correction of the deformity in 50% of cases. This procedure provides an alternative to osteotomy procedures in this patient population.

45. Weiner DS, Morscher M, Junko JT, Jacoby J, Weiner B: The Akron dome midfoot osteotomy as a salvage procedure for the treatment of rigid pes cavus: A retrospective review. *J Pediatr Orthop* 2008;28(1):68-80.

   A retrospective review of 89 patients (139 feet) treated with a salvage procedure for significant pes cavus deformity is presented. A satisfactory result was reported in 76% of cases.

Chapter 61

Injuries and Conditions of the Pediatric and Adolescent Athlete

Kevin Shea, MD   Theodore J. Ganley, MD

Introduction

The popularity of youth sports continues to grow, with increasing participation of children at younger ages. The benefits of sports participation at a young age are numerous, including the potential for the development of a lifetime of fitness habits, exposure to healthy competition, and psychosocial integration with peers and coaches. The risk of injury increases as children mature and participate in collision sports. This is due in part to increased speed, strength, and contact in older athletes. Medical personnel charged with providing care to these young athletes must be familiar with the unique, age-related anatomy and the injuries specific to this population.

Epidemiology of Athletic Injuries in Youth Sports

The numbers of young athletes participating in sports continues to increase, and recent estimates suggest that 30 million preadolescents and adolescents are involved in organized sports. As society faces increasing numbers of children with obesity, participation in sports should be encouraged to improve overall health. This participation is beneficial to the overall health of these children but is not without risk. In a survey of children and adolescents age 5 to 17 years, the estimated annual number of injuries resulting from participation in sports and recreational activities was 4,379,000, with 1,363,000 classified as serious (requiring hospitaliza-

tion, surgical treatment, missed school, or a half day or more in bed). Up to 36% of injuries may be directly related to sports participation in patients in these age groups.[1] As sports participation continues to increase, the number of young athletes sustaining injury will probably increase. Title IX legislation, enacted in 1972, has dramatically increased the number of female athletes participating in youth sports. For adult patients, females appear to have higher rates of knee injuries than male athletes for sports that involve running, jumping, and pivoting activities. A study by the American Academy of Pediatrics suggested that female athletes have higher rates of injury when compared with male athletes.[2] In a recent study of injury claims from an insurance company providing coverage for youth soccer leagues, knee and anterior cruciate ligament (ACL) injuries in female youth soccer players age 12 through 15 years were more common than ACL injuries in males of the same age.[3]

Training in the Pediatric Population

Historically, strength training in young athletes was discouraged, although investigations have shown that these training programs can be implemented safely.[4] Strength training in young athletes has become more common in the past 10 years. The American Academy of Pediatrics has endorsed resistance/exercise strengthening programs in children. The National Strength and Conditioning Association (NSCA) supports strength training in children, provided that appropriate training and safety guidelines are met. The NSCA published guidelines on proper resistance training in children in 1985, 1996, and 2009 (http://www.nsca-lift.org/youth positionpaper/Youth_Pos_Paper_200902.pdf). With supervision, the implementation of youth strengthening/resistance programs can improve conditioning, power, motor skills, and habits of lifetime fitness. Similar to injury prevention programs advocated for older athletes, injury prevention programs may also play a role in reducing injury risk in pediatric athletes. These injury prevention programs may reduce both traumatic and overuse injuries.[5]

6: Pediatrics

Rehabilitation

As a general rule, young athletes seem to recover from injuries faster than older patients. Prolonged stiffness and weakness are unusual in younger athletes. Because of these differences in healing, younger children seem to return to sports earlier and require less physical therapy supervision in many types of injuries. Arthrofibrosis is less common in younger athletes. Return to recreational play may be one of the best forms of therapy for many young athletes. Even though injury recovery is faster in younger athletes, some injuries, including ankle sprain or distal tibia/fibula fractures, require significant recovery time. Return to throwing programs may be beneficial for those who have undergone surgical or nonsurgical treatment of osteochondritis dissecans (OCD) of the elbow. A close working relationship with a physical therapist who specializes in sports medicine and has experience with young athletes can be very helpful for returning these athletes to sports as soon as possible.

Anatomic Considerations in the Young Athlete

The physis is composed of cartilage, which is less durable than bone; therefore, it is considered a 'weak link' in the pediatric skeleton. These regions are more prone to injury in traumatic or overuse environments. The physeal cartilage is more viscoelastic than bone, adding unique biomechanical features to the pediatric skeleton. In many types of pediatric injuries, the physeal cartilage will fail before the surrounding ligaments or osseous tissues, especially under conditions of high-energy transfer. As the child becomes older, the physis becomes stiffer and may make the incidence of ligament injury more likely than a physeal injury. The weakest area of the physis is believed to be the zone of hypertrophy, although fractures can occur in other regions. Growth plate fractures are complicated by the susceptibility to growth disturbance after injury. In addition to acute traumatic injuries of the physis, overuse injuries of the physeal areas also can occur. This includes overloading conditions of the proximal humerus, olecranon, and medial epicondyle in throwers and distal radius physis in gymnasts.

Acute Injuries

Patellar Dislocation

Acute patellar dislocation is one of the most common causes of acute hemarthrosis in young athletes. When comparing patellar dislocation in male and female patients, some studies have suggested similar rates,[6] and others have demonstrated the highest rates of dislocation in females younger than 18 years.[7]

Patellar dislocations occur in otherwise normal individuals, although soft-tissue laxity may be a significant risk factor. Other risk factors for patella dislocation,

both chronic and acute, include increased genu valgum, patella alta, lower extremity version abnormalities such as femoral anteversion and external tibial torsion, trochlear dysplasia, increased quadriceps angle, foot pronation, and patellar tilt.[6] Recent studies of trochlear dysplasia have attempted to define the relationship between trochlear morphology and patellar dislocation. Some of these studies have suggested that trochlear dysplasia may have a genetic basis,[8] and other studies have suggested that the risk of dislocation may be higher in some families.[7]

Both the medial retinaculum and medial patellofemoral ligament (MPFL) are primary restraints to patellar dislocation. Injury to both of these structures can occur during dislocation. The MPFL originates from the adductor tubercle and attaches to the upper two thirds of the medial patellar border.[9] The MPFL is a primary soft-tissue structure preventing lateral dislocations of the patella. Osteochondral fractures and contusion occur during patellar dislocation, and these contusions are seen in up to 40% to 50% of patients. These injuries most commonly occur on the medial facet of the patella and the distal lateral trochlea of the lateral femoral condyle (**Figure 1**).

Many patients with patellar dislocation will not have another dislocation, but some groups of athletes appear to have a higher probability of repeat dislocation or subluxation symptoms. In a well-designed prospective cohort study, 189 patients were followed for 2 to 5 years.[7] The group with the highest risk of dislocations was females age 10 to 17 years; 61% of dislocations occurred during sports, and 9% during dancing. The risk of recurrent patellar instability/dislocation appeared to be significantly higher in females. Young age at the time of the first dislocation was also a significant risk factor for future dislocation/subluxation events. Soft-tissue laxity, which may be more common in female patients, may increase the risk of primary and recurrent patello-femoral subluxation or dislocation events.[7] Genu recurvatum, hyperextension of the elbows, and soft-tissue laxity of the wrist, thumbs, and fingers are findings associated with increased laxity, which suggest a higher risk of secondary dislocation.

Standard three- or four-view knee series that include AP, lateral, Merchant, and notch views allow for the evaluation of injuries, including osteochondral fragments, avulsion of the soft-tissue attachments and bone from the medial aspect of the patella, as well as other factors such as patella alta, patella tilt, or trochlea dysplasia.[8] MRI may also play a role in the evaluation of these injuries because it may provide significant information about soft-tissue injuries, which are more difficult or impossible to identify with plain radiographs.

The initial treatment option for dislocations may consist of brief periods of immobilization followed by early rehabilitation with range of motion and strengthening activities.[8] The indications for surgical treatment continue to evolve. A recent prospective, randomized study of surgical treatment (repair of the medial retinacular structures) for first-time dislocation of the patella in children/adolescents did not demonstrate better

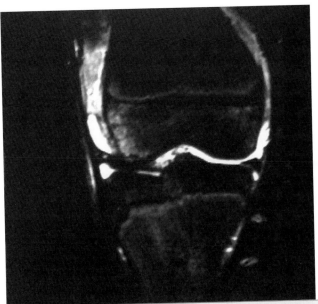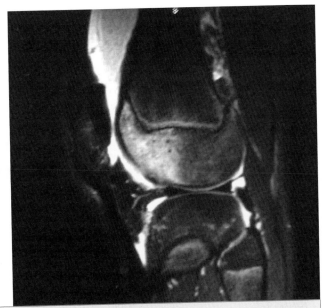

| Figure 1 | MRI findings demonstrating increased signal intensity on T2-weighted images of the lateral femoral condyle consistent with contusion after patella dislocation. (Copyright Intermountain Orthopaedics, Boise, ID.) |

outcomes compared with nonsurgical management.[10] For patients with recurrent symptomatic instability episodes, surgical intervention may be beneficial. The main indications for surgery in young athletes have been outlined in the literature, and it is believed that these surgical indications are appropriate for most patients.[6] The relative indications for surgery include failure to improve with nonsurgical care, concurrent osteochondral injury, continued gross instability, palpable disruption of the MPFL and the vastus medialis obliquus, and high-level athletic demands coupled with mechanical risk factors. The optimal surgical regimen for recurrent patellar dislocation is still evolving; however, soft-tissue procedures that do not involve surgery at the level of the physis are preferred in younger patients to reduce the risk of physeal growth complications.

Meniscal Injuries in Children

Injuries to the meniscus are less common in children than adults. In younger patients, they are more likely to occur in the setting of ACL or other significant knee injuries. Interpretation of MRI meniscal signals can be challenging in children. The MRI signal may suggest a meniscus tear in a young patient, but no tear will be found at arthroscopy. It has been shown that the meniscal signals on MRI in younger patients can appear to be meniscal tears, and these signal variations in young patients are frequently seen during the normal development of the meniscus.[11] MRI meniscal signals that do not clearly show a tear that communicates with the surface of the meniscus, or that do not show a displaced flap, should be interpreted with caution. Because of concerns about meniscectomy and the development of osteoarthritis, many physicians have advocated that meniscal repair be attempted in young patients. Menis-

cus repairs in young patients may have better potential for healing. Some studies show high healing rates in young patients,[12] whereas others show lower healing rates.[13]

Tibial Eminence Fractures

Tibial eminence fractures, also known as tibial spine fractures or avulsions, occur predominantly in skeletally immature patients. The mechanism of injury may be similar to that seen in adult ACL injury. These injuries have been classified into three types: type I, minimal displacement of the tibial eminence; type II, displacement of the anterior third to one half of the tibial eminence, producing a beaklike deformity on the lateral radiograph; and type III, the avulsed tibial eminence is completely lifted from the underlying bone[14] (**Figure 2**). A rare fourth type of tibial eminence fracture is characterized by complete rotation of the fragment, such that the articular cartilage surface faces the donor-site bone. Entrapment of the intermeniscal ligament or anterior meniscus tissue is possible, which may be an impediment to reduction of these fractures[15] (**Figure 3**). These fractures may also be associated with other soft-tissue injury, including bone contusions, ligament injury, and meniscus tears.[16] Treatment options include cast immobilization for nondisplaced fractures, closed reduction for minimally displaced fractures, and surgical treatment of displaced fractures. Both open and arthroscopic techniques have been described for these injuries. Arthroscopic techniques using sutures, wires, and screws have been studied.[17-19] Because arthrofibrosis is a significant complication that has been associated with the treatment of more severe forms of tibial eminence fractures, secure fixation and early motion are recommended for patients treated with surgery.

6: Pediatrics

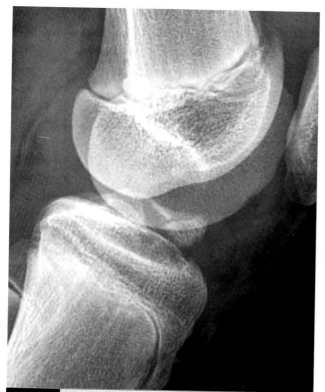

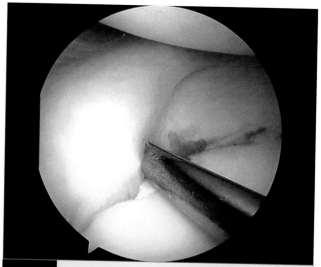

Figure 3 Arthroscopic imaging of entrapped anterior horn of the medial meniscus after a displaced tibial spine fracture. (Copyright Intermountain Orthopaedics, Boise, ID.)

Figure 2 Lateral radiograph of a type III tibial spine fracture. (Copyright Intermountain Orthopaedics, Boise, ID.)

ACL Injury

Treatment of ACL injury in the skeletally immature athlete remains controversial, although clinical studies continue to provide more guidance about the treatment options and avoidance of complications. Recent studies suggest that the incidence of this injury may be increasing, and young female athletes start sustaining these injuries in significant numbers at approximately age 12 to 13 years. These patients may also have a higher risk of ACL injury when compared with age-matched male athletes. Nonsurgical treatment produces poor outcomes in patients with complete tears because of instability and the potential for additional injury, including meniscal tears and chondral damage.[20,21]

Surgical treatment carries the risk of physeal injury, leading to growth disturbance in some cases.[22] A comprehensive understanding of the physeal anatomy about the knee, as well as the impact of fixation and drilling, should be considered before attempting ACL reconstruction in patients with an open physis.[23] Techniques have been described to reduce the risks of physeal injury from ACL reconstruction. A physeal sparing technique using an autogenous iliotibial band graft has been described for patients with significant remaining growth. This procedure has demonstrated excellent results, without growth plate arrest.[24] For older patients, different techniques have been described, although the risk of physeal arrest may still be a concern in those with significant growth remaining. A recent study of

patients at Tanner stage 3 or 4, who underwent ACL reconstruction using a transphyseal technique demonstrated no physeal complications, with excellent clinical outcomes.[25] In these patients, several technical aspects were of importance: metaphyseal fixation was used without injury to the physis; autogenous hamstrings were used, rather than patellar bone-tendon-bone grafts; and Tanner/skeletal maturity staging was used as an important part of the decision process to match the appropriate surgical procedure for each patient.

Another technique for the skeletally immature patient is transepiphyseal ACL reconstruction, which avoids the femoral and tibial physis. Although this is a technically demanding procedure with a small margin of error, results in a small population were excellent and physeal growth disturbance was absent[26] (**Figure 4**).

The risk of physeal complications is still present, and a survey demonstrated significant physeal complications in some surgically treated patients with open physes.[22] The risks, benefits, and alternatives to surgery should be thoroughly discussed with patients and their families.

Quadriceps Contusion

These injuries are relatively common in young athletes, especially in those involved in contact and collision sports. Most of these injuries respond well to rest and activity modifications, followed by a progressive return to sports activities. Physical therapy, including stretching, early motion, and lower impact exercise initially, may be of benefit to these patients. In some cases, a thigh contusion may lead to heterotopic ossification or myositis ossificans. In rare instances, a thigh compartment syndrome can occur.

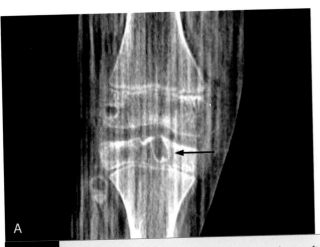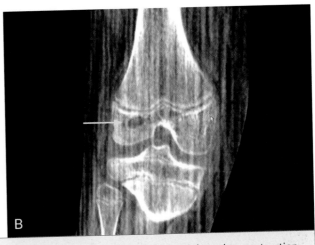

| Figure 4 | **A** and **B,** CT scans of a skeletally immature knee after ACL reconstruction using the transepiphyseal reconstruction technique. The black arrow denotes the tibia tunnel and the yellow arrow indicates the femoral tunnel. (Copyright Intermountain Orthopaedics, Boise, ID.) |

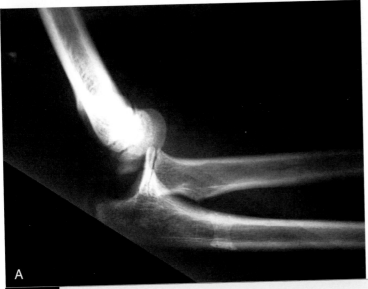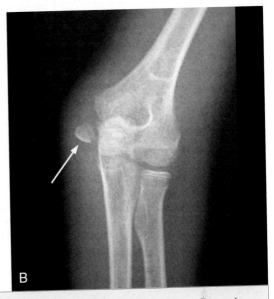

| Figure 5 | **A** and **B,** Radiographs of posterior elbow dislocation with medial epicondyle avulsion. Postreduction radiographs demonstrate a displaced fragment (*arrow*). (Copyright Intermountain Orthopaedics, Boise, ID.) |

Ankle Sprains

Ankle sprains remain one of the most common injuries in skeletally immature athletes. In patients presenting with an ankle sprain, the clinician should strongly consider the possibility of a physeal injury of the distal fibula or tibia. The physis in these patients may be more likely to be injured than the ligaments. If examination demonstrates localized pain over the physis, treatment with several weeks of immobilization may be warranted. The indications for therapy after these injuries are not fully defined. Further study will be necessary to determine which injuries in skeletally immature patients derive benefit from formal physical therapy. A recent evidence-based medicine review from the Cochrane group demonstrated that the use of ankle braces may be effective in reducing the risk of both primary

and secondary sprains in athletes involved in higher-risk sports.[27]

Medial Epicondyle Avulsion

Fractures of the medial epicondyle are more common than dislocations and account for about 10% of elbow fractures in children. The ulnar collateral ligament may avulse the medial epicondyle during elbow trauma (**Figure 5**). Nearly 50% of medial epicondyle fractures are associated with dislocation of the elbow; the displaced fragment can become incarcerated in the joint, preventing a concentric reduction.

Acute medial epicondyle fractures and dislocations of the elbow can occur in young gymnasts[28] and isolated medial epicondyle fractures are occasionally seen in adolescent pitchers. Treatment of medial epicondyle

6: Pediatrics

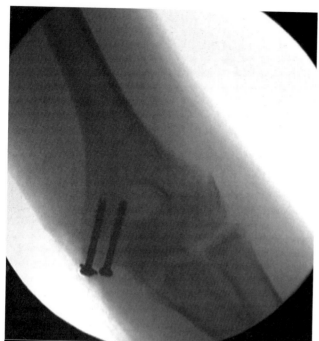

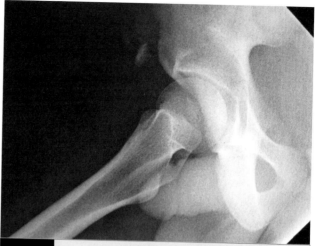

Figure 7 | AP pelvis radiograph in a 16-year-old male athlete demonstrates avulsion fractures in the pelvis anterior inferior iliac spine region. (Copyright Intermountain Orthopaedics, Boise, ID.)

Figure 6 | Intraoperative fluoroscopic view of the arm of a 14-year-old girl involved in gymnastics who had a displaced medial epicondyle fracture. Because of the high demands placed on her arm, open reduction and internal fixation was recommended and performed. (Copyright Intermountain Orthopaedics, Boise, ID.)

fractures is controversial, especially for minimally displaced fractures. Nondisplaced fractures are typically treated with casting, but displaced fractures may require surgery. In athletes such as throwers, gymnasts, and wrestlers who place high physical demands on the elbow, anatomic reduction of medial epicondyle fractures may be important for future athletic performance (**Figure 6**).

Shoulder Dislocations

Traumatic shoulder dislocations primarily occur in collision/contact sports in young athletes. It has been estimated that 40% of shoulder dislocations occur in patients younger than 22 years. Athletes with a history of a pediatric dislocation had more than a 90% chance of recurrent dislocation.[29-31] Pediatric dislocations are believed to stretch the capsule more than adult dislocations and diminish the capsule's ability to provide the support needed for proper function. Surgical treatment of instability is generally successful in young patients.[32]

Physical examination and diagnostic testing may demonstrate the concomitant injuries of anterior bony labrum or labral lesions (Bankart injury, superior labral anterior and posterior tear, Hill-Sachs lesions [posterolateral humeral head compression fracture]) rotator cuff muscle tears, and subscapularis or lesser tubercle avulsions. Three-view radiograph series that include AP, lateral, and axillary views can detect bone injuries of the labrum or Hill-Sachs lesions of the proximal hu-

merus. MRI arthrograms provide detailed information about the capsule and labral tissues.

In the acute setting, dislocated shoulders should be treated with closed reduction. Initial treatment may consist of a supervised physical therapy program to recover strength and range of motion. Several recent studies have suggested an advantage to immobilization in external rotation in adult patients, because this may provide better alignment of the labrum injury during healing.[33,34] Other studies have suggested that immobilization in this position does not improve the outcome for shoulder dislocations.[35] Treatment of first-time dislocation in high-risk athletes remains controversial,[33] and there is some evidence that early surgery may play a role in reducing the risk of secondary dislocation. Families should be counseled about the high risk of recurrent instability episodes and associated symptoms. If nonsurgical treatment is unsuccessful, surgery (open or arthroscopic) will be required to treat the capsular and glenoid injuries to create a stable glenohumeral joint. Historically, open methods may have provided lower redislocation rates, but recent studies in adult patients suggest excellent outcomes with arthroscopic stabilization procedures.[36] With improving surgical experience and technology, some recent literature suggests that arthroscopic surgery can have at least equal outcomes.[36]

Apophyseal Avulsions of the Pelvis

Among the acute injuries of the pelvic region, apophyseal avulsions are the most common and are usually caused by sudden muscle contractions. These injuries can occur at the ischial tuberosity (hamstring), anterior superior iliac spine (tensor fascia lata), lesser trochanter (iliopsoas), pubis (adductors), anterior inferior iliac spine (rectus femoris), and iliac crest (gluteus medius) (**Figure 7**). The athlete may report a sudden "pop," followed immediately by weakness and pain. These symptoms may mimic acute muscle strain. Walking with a

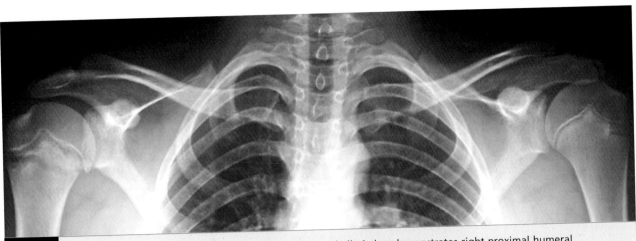

Figure 8 AP radiograph of both shoulders in an adolescent baseball pitcher demonstrates right proximal humeral epiphyseolysis. (Copyright Intermountain Orthopaedics, Boise, ID.)

limp indicates a more severe injury. Radiographic evaluation confirms the diagnosis; however, this injury can be difficult to detect because of the small size and location of the bony fragment. Initial treatment consists of rest, ice, and therapy emphasizing range of motion and gentle strengthening. Surgical intervention is infrequently required because most injuries involve minimal displacement of the avulsed fragment.[37] However, recent literature suggests that surgery may be necessary to ensure the best outcomes for some of these injuries, especially for large, displaced fragments.[38]

Overuse Injuries

Little Leaguer's Shoulder

Patients with little leaguer's shoulder usually present with vague reports of shoulder and proximal arm pain that is usually aggravated by throwing and improved with rest. The condition is common in pitchers, especially those who are throwing on a regular basis or who participate in extended-season baseball programs. The examination findings may be very subtle and in many cases unremarkable. Radiographs may show subtle widening of the physis or changes in the metaphyseal bone (**Figure 8**). This syndrome represents an overuse condition of the proximal humeral physis. Treatment consists of rest until symptoms resolve, followed by a graded return to a throwing program. Treatment is individualized; however, primary areas for improvement include stretches for the posterior shoulder capsule, as well as rotator cuff strengthening, capsular stabilizing, and core strengthening exercises. These exercises as well as lower extremity flexibility training, hip strengthening, and proprioceptive balance training may also provide these young athletes with the added benefit of improved performance.

These patients may benefit from working with a therapist experienced with treating throwing athletes. Pitching coaches may also evaluate the throwing mechanics of these young athletes. Counseling for the family and coaches about this condition, and its relationship to excessive throwing is important. Information about appropriate pitch counts is available from the Little League Baseball and the American Orthopaedic Society for Sports Medicine Websites (http//:www.sportsmed.org/tabs/resources/youthbaseballdetails.aspx?DID=231).

Shoulder injuries in the adolescent athlete are often caused by subtle, atraumatic instability, especially in sports with overhead movements, such as swimming, volleyball, gymnastics, tennis, and baseball. These conditions are more common in female athletes. Repeated overhead motions can stress the joint capsule and allow excessive motion of the humeral head, and these symptoms may be more likely in those with evidence of increased soft-tissue laxity. A comprehensive shoulder therapy program is essential. Many patients will improve significantly, but 6 to 9 months of therapy may be necessary. Only in very rare instances is surgical treatment required for patients with persistent multidirectional instability. This surgery is reserved for patients with persistent instability with activities of daily living despite a prolonged period of intensive nonsurgical treatment.

Elbow Conditions in the Throwing Athlete

Thrower's elbow is a generic term used to describe a variety of overuse syndromes. The common etiology of these injuries is repetitive microtrauma of the immature elbow.[39] Pain at the medial side of the elbow may occur in conjunction with medial epicondyle apophysitis or an avulsion fracture. Radiographs will usually demonstrate physeal widening in an apophysis, but may also demonstrate fragmentation of the ossification center. It may appear to have a growth disturbance represented by a delayed ossification, or conversely, an accelerated growth marked by premature physeal closure. In older adolescents, there may be an injury to the ulnar collateral ligament; the incidence of this injury may be increasing.[40] Differentiating between ulnar collateral ligament tear versus medial epicondyle apophysitis, fragmentation, or avulsion is important (**Figure 9**).

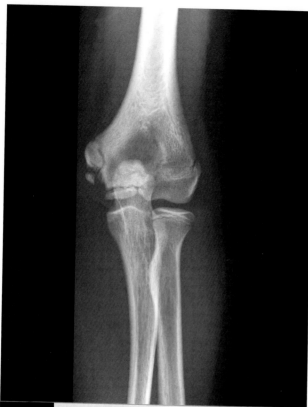

Figure 9 Radiograph of the arm of an adolescent pitcher showing a medial epicondyle partial avulsion. (Copyright Intermountain Orthopaedics, Boise, ID.)

The lateral aspect of the elbow is subject to repetitive compression loading, which can lead to OCD of the capitellum, or more rarely, in the radial head. In some cases, MRI may be necessary to make the diagnosis if no radiolucencies or osteochondral fragments are noted on plain radiographs.

Posterior elbow pain may represent an injury to the olecranon apophysis, an avulsion fracture, or delay of apophyseal closure.[41] Comparison of contralateral radiographs and possibly a bone scan might be required to confirm the diagnosis. With valgus extension overload, the compression stress on the posteromedial olecranon can create osteophytes, which may lead to bony extension contracture. It is important to realize that the osteophytes are a secondary process or a by-product of the pathology and not the primary pathologic process. Loose bodies inside the joint may also require surgical removal and evaluation of the chondral pathology that leads to this condition.[42] For most young athletes, nonsurgical treatment is the appropriate first step. In athletes involved in high-demand sports and who do not respond to therapy, surgical reconstruction may be indicated.

Prevention of injury is important; pitchers, coaches, and families should be aware of the recommendations about limitations involving the number and types of pitches thrown.

Wrist and Hand Injuries

Wrist pain in gymnasts is believed to be caused by the repetitive tension and compressive loads, well beyond those seen in most other sports.[43] The wrist pain can be vague and poorly localized. These loads may lead to increased or decreased growth of the physis. Radiographic findings include physeal widening, changes in metaphyseal bone density, and distortion of the epiphysis.[44] Premature physeal closure of the distal radius has been reported.

Treatment includes activity modification. Many gymnasts can continue to compete, but may need to decrease training in the routines that aggravate symptoms. Ice and the use of protective wrist braces may also play a role in recovery from these overuse injuries. In more severe cases, surgery may be necessary to address symptoms, and continued competition at a high level may be difficult.

Other stress injuries can occur about the wrist in young athletes, including repetitive stress and acute injuries of the scaphoid and the triangular fibrocartilage complex.[45,46]

Anterior Knee Pain

Anterior knee pain is common in adolescents but can be challenging to evaluate and treat. Symptoms are usually aggravated by activities, and patients may report pain with sports, ascending or descending stairs, kneeling, or placing the knee in a bent position for an extended period of time. In most cases, the symptoms will be present bilaterally, although one side may be less symptomatic than the other. Patients will localize pain to the anterior aspect of the patella.

The physical examination should evaluate gait, rotation alignment, patellar tracking, foot alignment, and hip motion. It is important that symmetric hip motion is documented, because a loss of internal rotation may signify hip pathology presenting with referred knee pain (slipped capital femoral epiphysis). The knee should be evaluated for warmth and effusion, the presence of symptomatic plica, atrophy, patellar tracking/alignment, and patellar mobility. These patients will localize discomfort to the inferior pole of the patella, the patellar tendon, and perhaps the medial and/or lateral patellar retinacular tissues. Focal tenderness over the femoral condyle or joint line may suggest osteochondritis, plica, or meniscal pathology. If pain is localized to other areas (such as the hip), plain radiographs or MRI may be necessary to rule out other causes of anterior knee pain. If muscle atrophy, skin abnormalities, or allodynia are present, a diagnosis of reflex sympathetic dystrophy should be considered. In most cases, the radiographic evaluation will be normal.

In many patients, the natural history of this condition will demonstrate significant improvement over time, and many will have resolution of symptoms. Referral to a physical therapist with expertise in this area may be beneficial to these patients.[47] The role of patellofemoral rehabilitation has been studied in terms of expanding the activities that can be performed in a pain-free manner, normalizing the "envelope of function" of the patellofemoral joint.[48] Although adult patients have been the focus of studies, the rehabilitation principles also apply to pediatric and adolescent patients. Therapeutic modalities include activity modifications; flexibility and stretching exercises of the thigh and leg; progressive strengthening programs that do not irritate the patellofemoral joint; intermittent use of ice, massage, and heat; ultrasound; and patellar mobilization exercises.

Osteochondritis Dissecans of the Knee

OCD is an acquired idiopathic lesion of the subchondral bone that affects the overlying cartilage secondarily. Although this condition is potentially reversible, progression may result in articular cartilage instability. In the knee, the most common location is within the lateral aspect of the medial femoral condyle. Juvenile OCD lesions are defined in patients with widely open growth plates and have a better prognosis in terms of healing than in older adolescents with OCD.

Males are more commonly affected than females, with a ratio between 2:1 and 3:1. As females and younger children participate in sports in greater numbers there has been an increased prevalence among girls and a younger mean age of onset for this condition. In the largest study to date, the prevalence was 18 in 100,000 in females and 29 in 100,000 in males.[49]

Although repetitive trauma, inflammation, accessory centers of ossification, ischemia, and genetic factors have all been implicated as causative factors in OCD, no body of evidence exists that is sufficient to currently support any single theory. Although some familial tendencies exist, it is commonly believed that the most prevalent form of OCD is not a familial condition. It has been theorized that acute trauma was the causative factor and that the tibial spine violently impacted the inner condyle of the femur.[50] This theory does not account for the multitude of OCD lesions noted at other sites. Chronic repetitive microtrauma has been suggested to lead to a stress reaction within the subchondral bone, and in more advanced forms it may lead to subchondral bone necrosis. Fragment dissection and separation may ensue. Contributing factors to these repetitive stresses in young athletes may include year-round sports, early sports specialization, multiple sports in a single season, or multiple teams in a single sport, as well as increased training intensity.

Patients with OCD of the knee initially have nonspecific symptoms, with anterior knee pain and variable amounts of intermittent swelling. With progression of the disease, patients may report more persistent swelling or effusion, catching, locking, and/or giving way. Unfortunately, pain and swelling are not good indicators of dissection. Physical findings may include a positive Wilson test, which reproduces the pain by internally rotating the tibia during extension of the knee between 90° and 30°, then relieving the pain with tibial external rotation. The sensitivity of this test has been questioned.

Standard weight-bearing radiographs of both knees are helpful for initially characterizing the lesion type and status of the growth plate. The lateral view helps identify anteroposterior lesion location and normal, benign accessory ossification centers in the skeletally immature knee. An axial view is helpful if a lesion of the patella or trochlea is suspected, and a notch view in 30° to 50° of knee flexion may help identify the lesions of the posterior femoral condyle.

MRI findings may define the ability of OCD lesions to heal following nonsurgical treatment. One study described MRI criteria and noted that a high signal line on T2-weighted images behind the fragment was most predictive and was found in 72% of unstable lesions.[51] Authors of another study attempted to predict the success of nonsurgical treatment using MRI and clinical criteria[52] and found the high signal line the most common sign in patients in whom nonsurgical treatment failed. In a comparison of MRI and arthroscopic findings, staging accuracy improved from 45% to 85% when the authors interpreted a high signal line on T2-weighted images as a predictor of instability when accompanied by a breach in articular cartilage seen on T1-weighted images.[53] Additional research to determine if MRI can identify stability and healing potential of OCD lesions will be necessary. Recent research suggests that the presence of multiple factors associated with instability, including a high T2 signal intensity rim, surrounding cysts, high T2 signal intensity cartilage fracture line, and a fluid-filled osteochondral defect, can collectively improve the sensitivity and specificity of predicting lesion stability.[54]

Nonsurgical treatment is often regarded as the treatment of choice for small, stable lesions in skeletally immature patients. Nonsurgical management focuses on significant activity modification by limiting high-impact activities. Short-term immobilization and protected weight bearing may be helpful. Alternatively, bracing and range-of-motion knee exercises may be beneficial. Typically, a period of 3 to 9 months of nonsurgical treatment is initiated, with success rates from 50% to 94%. Skeletally immature patients with wide, open physes and no signs of instability on MRI are more likely to respond to nonsurgical measures. The prognosis for OCD lesions is worse in patients who have reached skeletal maturity.

Authors of a 2008 study evaluated 42 skeletally immature patients and 47 knees with stable lesions and used a multivariable logistic regression model to determine potential predictors of healing status from the independent variables. After 6 months of nonsurgical treatment, 16 of 47 stable lesions (34%) did not progress to healing. It was found that the size of the lesion determined by MRI was the strongest prognostic variable.[55]

Surgical treatment should be considered for patients with unstable or detached lesions, for patients with persistently symptomatic lesions despite nonsurgical measures, and in those with persistent lesions who are approaching skeletal maturity. The goals of surgical treatment are to promote healing of subchondral bone,

6: Pediatrics

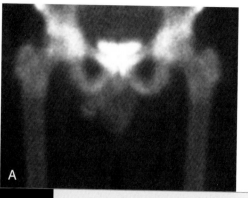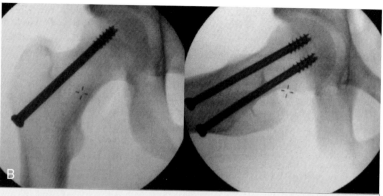

Figure 10 **A,** Bone scan showing stress fracture in the superior femoral neck region. **B,** Screw fixation for a superior femoral neck stress fracture. (Copyright Intermountain Orthopaedics, Boise, ID.)

to maintain joint congruity, to fix rigidly unstable fragments, and to replace osteochondral defects with cells that can replace and grow cartilage.[56] Surgical treatment of stable lesions with intact articular cartilage involves drilling the subchondral bone with the intention of stimulating vascular ingrowth and subchondral bone healing. In one study, 11 knees in 10 children treated with arthroscopic drilling were reviewed. In 1 year there was evidence of healing in 9 of 11 knees.[57] In another study of 23 patients (30 knees) who failed to heal with 6 months of nonsurgical treatment and who also subsequently underwent arthroscopic transarticular drilling, radiographic healing was achieved at an average of 4.4 months after drilling.[58]

When the lesion is unstable and hinged, fixation is indicated to fix the osseous portion of the fragment to allow healing and stabilization of the overlying articular surface. Arthroscopic or open reduction and internal fixation can be performed with a variety of implants. Osteochondral plugs have recently been presented as a biologic alternative to the use of implant fixation of the lesion.[59] In a series of 20 patients treated for unstable OCD lesions of the knee using osteochondral plugs, 19 were reported to meet the criteria of normal and 1 patient met the criteria of nearly normal at 2 years after surgery.[59]

Stress Fractures

Stress fractures are more common in adolescents and older high school-age athletes; however, they can also occur in the preadolescent athlete.[60] These injuries are more common in sports that require a significant volume of running for practice and competition. Stress fractures in both male and female athletes may be associated with osteopenia or osteoporosis, especially in endurance athletes. Athletes with recurrent stress fractures and with a history of amenorrhea, menstrual irregularities, or eating disorders may need formal evaluation for management of underlying metabolic bone disorders. Repetitive loads that exceed the threshold of intrinsic bone healing are believed to lead to the development of stress fractures.

Pain from stress fractures occurs insidiously, may worsen with activity, and improve with rest. The clinical examination, radiographs, and other imaging modalities (bone scan and MRI) are used to make the diagnosis. Treatment in most cases is activity modification; training errors are believed to be the main cause of these injuries in many patients. In addition to reducing their running mileage, athletes may incorporate more cross-training into their training program. This may include weight training, exercise bike training, swimming, or a pool-based running program. These types of training modifications will allow the athletes to maintain some of their aerobic conditioning, while allowing for healing of the stress fracture.

The tibia is the most common location for lower extremity stress fractures; other locations include the lumbar spine, pelvis, femoral neck or shaft, patella, tibia, medial malleolus, talus, tarsals, metatarsals, and sesamoids. In the upper extremity, stress fracture can be found in the distal radius, clavicle, and olecranon, especially in those who participate in throwing and upper extremity weight-bearing sports such as baseball and gymnastics.[41] Stress injury or fracture can occur in the diaphysis, metaphysis, physis, and epiphysis in the long bones of skeletally immature patients.

Femoral neck stress fractures have been rare in younger patients, although this entity has been seen in the skeletally immature patient.[61] Patients present with groin or anterior thigh pain, although specific areas of tenderness may not be identified on physical examination. Plain radiographs may not identify the lesion, and bone scans or MRIs may be necessary (**Figure 10, A**). Femoral neck stress fractures should be treated with great caution because of the possibility of a displaced femoral neck fracture that can lead to osteonecrosis. The risk of fracture progression and displacement is higher for tension-side than compression-side fractures.[62] It is, therefore, prudent to have a lower threshold for prophylactic fixation to prevent progression and/or displacement of the fracture in tension-side fractures (**Figure 10, B**). Other high-risk stress fractures include patella, medial malleolus, talus, navicular, fifth metatarsal, and great toe sesamoids fractures.[63]

Shin splints, or medial tibial stress syndrome, is characterized by pain along the posteromedial border of the tibia. This condition is common in young, running athletes. Treatment of this condition is challenging because definitive treatment is still not defined.[64] In patients with more significant symptoms, radiographic and/or MRI evaluation may be necessary to rule out a tibial stress fracture.[65]

Physeal Stress Reactions/Avulsions

Because the physis is composed of cartilage, it may be prone to overuse injury or even small acute fracture/avulsion in some cases. Sever disease, Osgood-Schlatter disease, Sinding-Larsen-Johansson syndrome, and pelvic apophysites are examples of physeal stress injury in different regions.

Sever disease is characterized by pain in the area of the calcaneal apophysis. It is common in athletes who participate in running and jumping sports, and it occurs frequently before or during peak growth in both males and females. The diagnosis can be based on a tight Achilles tendon and a positive squeeze test as well as pain over the calcaneal apophysis. Treatment includes activity modification, Achilles tendon stretching, and the application of ice before and after activities. In rare cases, calcaneal cysts may present with findings similar to those of Sever disease, and radiographs may be helpful in some cases to rule out this diagnosis. In young athletes, treatment usually consists of activity modification, stretching, use of heel cups, and other local measures. In most cases, the symptoms resolve within 1 to 2 years.

Osgood-Schlatter disease is associated with anterior knee pain with involvement of the proximal tibial apophyseal region. Sinding-Larsen-Johansson syndrome is a chronic apophysitis or minor avulsion injury from the inferior pole of the patella. Although nonsurgical management is indicated in most patients, older patients with significant symptoms and proximal tubercle anomalies may benefit from surgery.[66]

Pelvic apophyses can occur at the ischial tuberosity and the iliac crest. In most cases, the symptoms will resolve with time and activity modifications. In rare cases, surgical treatment to produce a fusion of the apophyses may be necessary.[67]

Treatment of these different disorders includes activity modification and reduction in training that overloads these regions. Local measures, including ice application and strapping/sleeves to decrease tension on the apophysis, may also provide some benefit.

Annotated References

1. Bijur PE, Trumble A, Harel Y, Overpeck MD, Jones D, Scheidt PC: Sports and recreation injuries in US children and adolescents. *Arch Pediatr Adolesc Med* 1995; 149(9):1009-1016.

2. Injuries in youth soccer: A subject review. American Academy of Pediatrics. Committee on Sports Medicine and Fitness. *Pediatrics* 2000;105(3, pt 1):659-661.

3. Shea KG, Pfeiffer R, Wang JH, Curtin M, Apel PJ: Anterior cruciate ligament injury in pediatric and adolescent soccer players: An analysis of insurance data. *J Pediatr Orthop* 2004;24(6):623-628.

4. Faigenbaum AD, Micheli LJ: Preseason conditioning for the preadolescent athlete. *Pediatr Ann* 2000;29(3):156-161.

5. Hewett TE, Myer GD, Ford KR: Reducing knee and anterior cruciate ligament injuries among female athletes: A systematic review of neuromuscular training interventions. *J Knee Surg* 2005;18(1):82-88.

6. Hinton RY, Sharma KM: Acute and recurrent patellar instability in the young athlete. *Orthop Clin North Am* 2003;34(3):385-396.

7. Fithian DC, Paxton EW, Stone ML, et al: Epidemiology and natural history of acute patellar dislocation. *Am J Sports Med* 2004;32(5):1114-1121.

8. Fucentese SF, von Roll A, Koch PP, Epari DR, Fuchs B, Schottle PB: The patella morphology in trochlear dysplasia: A comparative MRI study. *Knee* 2006;13(2):145-150.

9. Desio SM, Burks RT, Bachus KN: Soft tissue restraints to lateral patellar translation in the human knee. *Am J Sports Med* 1998;26(1):59-65.

10. Palmu S, Kallio PE, Donell ST, Helenius I, Nietosvaara Y: Acute patellar dislocation in children and adolescents: A randomized clinical trial. *J Bone Joint Surg Am* 2008;90(3):463-470.

   This randomized prospective study evaluated the outcomes of surgical and nonsurgical treatment of traumatic patellar dislocation in patients younger than 16 years. Family history of patellar dislocation was identified as a significant factor for recurrence of dislocation, and surgery did not affect the long-term functional outcome.

11. Takeda Y, Ikata T, Yoshida S, Takai H, Kashiwaguchi S: MRI high-signal intensity in the menisci of asymptomatic children. *J Bone Joint Surg Br* 1998; 80(3):463-467.

12. Noyes FR, Barber-Westin SD: Arthroscopic repair of meniscal tears extending into the avascular zone in patients younger than twenty years of age. *Am J Sports Med* 2002;30(4):589-600.

13. Accadbled F, Cassard X, Sales de Gauzy J, Cahuzac JP: Meniscal tears in children and adolescents: Results of operative treatment. *J Pediatr Orthop B* 2007;16(1):56-60.

   This retrospective case series of 12 patients demonstrated relatively poor healing rates for surgically repaired meniscus tears in children at an average follow-up of 3 years. Although this was a small series, the healing rate for meniscus repair in children was lower than previous studies have suggested.

14. Meyers MH, McKeever FM: Fracture of the intercondylar eminence of the tibia. *J Bone Joint Surg Am* 1970; 52(8):1677-1684.

15. Kocher MS, Micheli LJ, Gerbino P, Hresko MT: Tibial eminence fractures in children: Prevalence of meniscal entrapment. *Am J Sports Med* 2003;31(3):404-407.

16. Monto RR, Cameron-Donaldson ML, Close MA, Ho CP, Hawkins RJ: Magnetic resonance imaging in the evaluation of tibial eminence fractures in adults. *J Knee Surg* 2006;19(3):187-190.

17. Ahn JH, Lee YS, Lee DH, Ha HC: Arthroscopic physeal sparing all inside repair of the tibial avulsion fracture in the anterior cruciate ligament: Technical note. *Arch Orthop Trauma Surg* 2008;128(11):1309-1312.

    This paper describes an arthroscopy suture technique for fixing tibial spine or eminence fractures. It may be useful for smaller or comminuted injuries.

18. Bonin N, Jeunet L, Obert L, Dejour D: Adult tibial eminence fracture fixation: Arthroscopic procedure using K-wire folded fixation. *Knee Surg Sports Traumatol Arthrosc* 2007;15(7):857-862.

    The retrospective case series reports the outcomes of arthroscopic Bankart repair in a group of pediatric and adolescent patients with traumatic anterior shoulder instability.

19. Eggers AK, Becker C, Weimann A, et al: Biomechanical evaluation of different fixation methods for tibial eminence fractures. *Am J Sports Med* 2007;35(3):404-410.

    The authors reported that suture fixation of tibial eminence fractures provided more fixation strength than screw fixation based on biomechanical data.

20. Graf BK, Lange RH, Fujisaki CK, Landry GL, Saluja RK: Anterior cruciate ligament tears in skeletally immature patients: Meniscal pathology at presentation and after attempted conservative treatment. *Arthroscopy* 1992;8(2):229-233.

21. McCarroll JR, Shelbourne KD, Porter DA, Rettig AC, Murray S: Patellar tendon graft reconstruction for midsubstance anterior cruciate ligament rupture in junior high school athletes: An algorithm for management. *Am J Sports Med* 1994;22(4):478-484.

22. Kocher MS, Saxon HS, Hovis WD, Hawkins RJ: Management and complications of anterior cruciate ligament injuries in skeletally immature patients: Survey of the Herodicus Society and The ACL Study Group. *J Pediatr Orthop* 2002;22(4):452-457.

23. Shea KG, Belzer J, Apel PJ, Nilsson K, Grimm NL, Pfeiffer RP: Volumetric injury of the physis during single bundle anterior cruciate ligament reconstruction in chil-

dren: A 3-dimensional study using magnetic resonance imaging. *Arthroscopy* 2009;245(12):1415-1422.

    The authors determined the volume of injury to the physis during ACL reconstruction in children and concluded that a better understanding of the relationship of the ACL and physis may help guide drill-hole placement and lead to a lower risk of physeal arrest.

24. Kocher MS, Garg S, Micheli LJ: Physeal sparing reconstruction of the anterior cruciate ligament in skeletally immature prepubescent children and adolescents. *J Bone Joint Surg Am* 2005;87(11):2371-2379.

25. Kocher MS, Smith JT, Zoric BJ, Lee B, Micheli LJ: Transphyseal anterior cruciate ligament reconstruction in skeletally immature pubescent adolescents. *J Bone Joint Surg Am* 2007;89(12):2632-2639.

    This retrospective study reports a series of skeletally immature pubescent adolescents who underwent transphyseal reconstruction of the ACL with use of an autogenous quadrupled hamstrings-tendon graft with metaphyseal fixation. This group demonstrated excellent functional outcome with a low revision rate and a minimal risk of growth disturbance.

26. Anderson AF: Transepiphyseal replacement of the anterior cruciate ligament using quadruple hamstring grafts in skeletally immature patients. *J Bone Joint Surg Am* 2004;86(pt 2, suppl 1):201-209.

27. Handoll HH, Rowe BH, Quinn KM, de Bie R: Interventions for preventing ankle ligament injuries. *Cochrane Database Syst Rev* 2001;3:CD0000018.

28. Caine DJ, Nassar L: Gymnastics injuries. *Med Sport Sci* 2005;48:18-58.

29. Bishop JY, Flatow EL: Pediatric shoulder trauma. *Clin Orthop Relat Res* 2005;432:41-48.

30. Deitch J, Mehlman CT, Foad SL, Obbehat A, Mallory M: Traumatic anterior shoulder dislocation in adolescents. *Am J Sports Med* 2003;31(5):758-763.

31. Rowe CR: Prognosis in dislocations of the shoulder. *J Bone Joint Surg Am* 1956;38(5):957-977.

32. Chen FS, Diaz VA, Loebenberg M, Rosen JE: Shoulder and elbow injuries in the skeletally immature athlete. *J Am Acad Orthop Surg* 2005;13:172-185.

33. Bedi A, Ryu RK: The treatment of primary anterior shoulder dislocations. *Instr Course Lect* 2009;58:293-304.

    The authors present a systematic review of the literature on the treatment of traumatic anterior instability of the shoulder. The evidence comparing the outcomes of nonsurgical and surgical treatment based on open and arthroscopic surgery is provided.

34. Itoi E, Sashi R, Minagawa H, Shimizu T, Wakabayashi I, Sato K: Position of immobilization after dislocation of the glenohumeral joint: A study with use of magnetic

resonance imaging. *J Bone Joint Surg Am* 2001;83(5): 661-667.

35. Finestone A, Milgrom C, Radeva-Petrova DR, et al: Bracing in external rotation for traumatic anterior dislocation of the shoulder. *J Bone Joint Surg Br* 2009;91(7): 918-921.

    This randomized prospective study compared bracing in internal and external rotation for the treatment of primary anterior shoulder dislocation. The differences in dislocation rates were statistically significant, suggesting that external rotation bracing may not be as effective as previously reported.

36. Brophy RH, Marx RG: The treatment of traumatic anterior instability of the shoulder: Nonoperative and surgical treatment. *Arthroscopy* 2009;25(3):298-304.

    This case series reviewed the outcomes of patients with unstable OCD lesions treated with mosaicplasty. At short term follow-up, the clinical results and MRI evaluation showed evidence of significant healing.

37. Micheli LJ: *Pediatric and Adolescent Sports Medicine.* Boston, MA, Little, Brown, 1984, p 218.

38. Rajasekhar C, Kumar KS, Bhamra MS: Avulsion fractures of the anterior inferior iliac spine: The case for surgical intervention. *Int Orthop* 2001;24(6):364-365.

39. Klingele KE, Kocher MS: Little league elbow: Valgus overload injury in the paediatric athlete. *Sports Med* 2002;32(15):1005-1015.

40. Petty DH, Andrews JR, Fleisig GS, Cain EL: Ulnar collateral ligament reconstruction in high school baseball players: Clinical results and injury risk factors. *Am J Sports Med* 2004;32(5):1158-1164.

41. Rettig AC, Wurth TR, Mieling P: Nonunion of olecranon stress fractures in adolescent baseball pitchers: A case series of 5 athletes. *Am J Sports Med* 2006;34(4): 653-656.

42. Cain EL Jr, Dugas JR, Wolf RS, Andrews JR: Elbow injuries in throwing athletes: A current concepts review. *Am J Sports Med* 2003;31(4):621-635.

43. DiFiori JP, Caine DJ, Malina RM: Wrist pain, distal radial physeal injury, and ulnar variance in the young gymnast. *Am J Sports Med* 2006;34(5):840-849.

44. Mandelbaum BR, Bartolozzi AR, Davis CA, Teurlings L, Bragonier B: Wrist pain syndrome in the gymnast: Pathogenetic, diagnostic, and therapeutic considerations. *Am J Sports Med* 1989;17(3):305-317.

45. Bae DS, Waters PM: Pediatric distal radius fractures and triangular fibrocartilage complex injuries. *Hand Clin* 2006;22(1):43-53.

46. Waters PM: Operative carpal and hand injuries in children. *J Bone Joint Surg Am* 2007;89(9):2064-2074.

    This article presents a comprehensive summary of hand trauma in children.

47. Bhave A, Baker E: Prescribing quality patellofemoral rehabilitation before advocating operative care. *Orthop Clin North Am* 2008;39(3):275-285, v.

    This is an evidence-based review of the literature for the treatment of medial tibial stress syndrome, a common problem in young athletes. This study confirms that there is insignificant evidence to recommend any specific treatment of this condition.

48. Dye SF, Stäubli HU, Biedert RM, Vaupel GL: The mosaic of pathophysiology causing patellofemoral pain: Therapeutic implications. *Op Tech Sports* 1999;7(2): 46-54.

    This study compares the fixation strength of screws and sutures for the repair of tibial spine/tibial eminence fractures.

49. Lindén B, Telhag H: Osteochondritis dissecans: A histologic and autoradiographic study in man. *Acta Orthop Scand* 1977;48(6):682-686.

50. Fairbanks H: Osteochondritis dissecans. *J Bone Joint Surg Br* 1933;21:67-82.

51. De Smet AA, Ilahi OA, Graf BK: Untreated osteochondritis dissecans of the femoral condyles: Prediction of patient outcome using radiographic and MR findings. *Skeletal Radiol* 1997;26(8):463-467.

52. Pill SG, Ganley TJ, Milam RA, Lou JE, Meyer JS, Flynn JM: Role of magnetic resonance imaging and clinical criteria in predicting successful nonoperative treatment of osteochondritis dissecans in children. *J Pediatr Orthop* 2003;23(1):102-108.

53. O'Connor MA, Palaniappan M, Khan N, Bruce CE: Osteochondritis dissecans of the knee in children. A comparison of MRI and arthroscopic findings. *J Bone Joint Surg Br* 2002;84(2):258-262.

54. Kijowski R, Blankenbaker DJ, Shinki K, Fine JP, Graf BK, De Smet AA: Juvenile versus adult osteochondritis dissecans of the knee: Appropriate MR imaging criteria for instability. *Radiology* 2008;248(2):571-578.

    In a retrospective study, the authors compared the sensitivity and specificity of MRI criteria in the detection of instability in patients with OCD of the knee. Results indicated that MRI criteria for OCD instability have high specificity for adult but not juvenile lesions of the knee.

55. Wall EJ, Vourazeris J, Myer GD, et al: The healing potential of stable juvenile osteochondritis dissecans knee lesions. *J Bone Joint Surg Am* 2008;90(12):2655-2664.

    This study identified factors that predicted healing potential in stable OCD lesions. Smaller size lesions and those without mechanical symptoms at presentation are more likely to heal with nonsurgical treatment protocols.

56. Smillie IS: Treatment of osteochondritis dissecans. *J Bone Joint Surg Br* 1957;39(2):248-260.

6: Pediatrics

57.   Bradley J, Dandy DJ: Results of drilling osteochondritis dissecans before skeletal maturity. *J Bone Joint Surg Br* 1989;71(4):642-644.

58.   Kocher MS, Micheli LJ, Yaniv M, Zurakowski D, Ames A, Adrignolo AA: Functional and radiographic outcome of juvenile osteochondritis dissecans of the knee treated with transarticular arthroscopic drilling. *Am J Sports Med* 2001;29(5):562-566.

59.   Miniaci A, Tytherleigh-Strong G: Fixation of unstable osteochondritis dissecans lesions of the knee using arthroscopic autogenous osteochondral grafting (mosaicplasty). *Arthroscopy* 2007;23(8):845-851.

      This case series reviewed the outcomes of patients with unstable OCD lesions treated with mosaicplasty. At short-term follow-up, the clinical results and MRI evaluation showed evidence of significant healing.

60.   Maezawa K, Nozawa M, Sugimoto M, Sano M, Shitoto K, Kurosawa H: Stress fractures of the femoral neck in child with open capital femoral epiphysis. *J Pediatr Orthop B* 2004;13(6):407-411.

61.   Maezawa K, Nozawa M, Sugimoto M, Sano M, Shitoto K, Kurosawa H: Stress fractures of the femoral neck in child with open capital femoral epiphysis. *J Pediatr Orthop B* 2004;13(6):407-411.

62.   Lehman RA Jr, Shah SA: Tension-sided femoral neck stress fracture in a skeletally immature patient: A case report. *J Bone Joint Surg Am* 2004;86(6):1292-1295.

63.   Boden BP, Osbahr DC: High-risk stress fractures: Evaluation and treatment. *J Am Acad Orthop Surg* 2000;8(6):344-353.

64.   Craig DI: Medial tibial stress syndrome: Evidence-based prevention. *J Athl Train* 2008;43(3):316-318.

      This is an evidence-based review of the literature for the treatment of medial tibial stress syndrome, a common condition in young athletes. This study confirms that there is insignificant evidence to recommend any specific treatment for this condition.

65.   Aoki Y, Yasuda K, Tohyama H, Ito H, Minami A: Magnetic resonance imaging in stress fractures and shin splints. *Clin Orthop Relat Res* 2004;421:260-267.

66.   Weiss JM, Jordan SS, Andersen JS, Lee BM, Kocher M: Surgical treatment of unresolved Osgood-Schlatter disease: Ossicle resection with tibial tubercleplasty. *J Pediatr Orthop* 2007;27(7):844-847.

      The authors evaluated the functional outcome of ossicle excision and tibial tubercleplasty for unresolved Osgood-Schlatter disease.

67.   Holmstrom MC, Greis PE, Horwitz DS: Chronic ischial apophysitis in a gymnast treated with transapophyseal drilling to effect "apophysiodesis": A case report. *Am J Sports Med* 2003;31(2):294-296.

Chapter 62

Skeletal Dysplasias, Connective Tissue Diseases, and Other Genetic Disorders

Jose A. Morcuende, MD, PhD   Benjamin A. Alman, MD

Introduction

Musculoskeletal syndromes can be broadly categorized into groups by the function of the causative gene encoding a protein that is structural, regulates developmentally important signaling pathways, is implicated in neoplasia, has a role in processing molecules (such as an enzyme), or has a role in nerve or muscle function. The syndromes within each broad group have a similar mode of inheritance and similar clinical behavior.

Disorders Caused by Structural Genes

A variety of proteins play an important role in the structure of connective tissues, including the bones, articular cartilage, ligaments, and skin. A mutation in such a gene disrupts the structural integrity of the connective tissue in which it is expressed. The phenotype evolves with time as the abnormal structural components slowly fail or wear out during the individual's growth. The deformity often recurs after surgery because the structural components are abnormal and will wear out again. If the structural abnormality involves cartilage, a growth abnormality may be caused by physeal mechanical failure, or an early degenerative disease of the joints may be caused by articular cartilage failure. If the affected protein is important for lig-

ament or tendon strength, joint subluxation often occurs; Marfan syndrome and osteogenesis imperfecta are two of the most common such disorders. Other disorders are caused by mutations in a gene that encodes structural proteins, such as spondyloepiphyseal dysplasia.

Marfan Syndrome

Marfan syndrome is associated with long limbs and involvement of the cardiovascular, ocular, and skeletal systems.[1] In a patient with Marfan syndrome, scoliosis is sometimes diagnosed first. It is important for the orthopaedist to recognize the underlying condition, as a referral for appropriate prophylactic management of the cardiovascular abnormities can be life saving.

Marfan syndrome is caused by a mutation in the gene encoding for the fibrillin protein, which has a role in maintaining the normal mechanical properties of the soft tissues, especially in resistance to cyclic stress.[2] The clinical findings of laxity and subluxation of the joints, as well as the weakening of arterial walls with resultant aortic dilatation, are easily understood based on the function of fibrillin. The tall stature and arachnodactyly associated with the syndrome are more difficult to attribute to the fibrillin mutation; the explanation is that the extracellular matrix contains growth factors that are bound to extracellular matrix proteins. Fibrillin mutations cause some of these extracellular growth factors, such as transforming growth factor–β, to become more readily accessible to cell receptors.[3] The increased availability of growth factors probably increases cellular growth and rapid longitudinal bone growth, leading to the development of tall stature as well as long, thin fingers and toes. The increased availability of growth factors also may be partly responsible for many of the changes in the mechanical properties of the soft tissues (**Figure 1**). It is possible that growth factor activity modulation could be used to treat some of the sequelae of Marfan syndrome, and studies of such an approach are under way.[3]

Hyperlaxity is responsible for many clinical aspects of Marfan syndrome, including subluxation of joints, a

6: Pediatrics

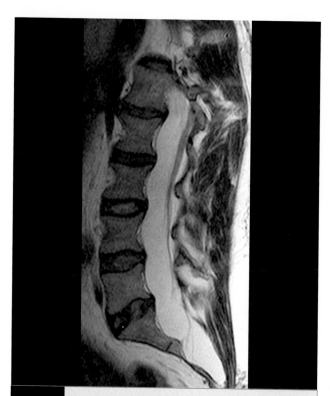

Figure 1 MRI of the lumbar spine of a patient with Marfan syndrome. Dural ectasia and scalloping of the posterior vertebral bodies can be seen.

predisposition to sprains, and scoliosis. Mild scoliosis can be managed in a manner similar to that of idiopathic scoliosis, although bracing appears to be less effective in a patient with Marfan syndrome.[4] Surgery is considered for a rapidly progressing curve in a skeletally immature patient or a large curve in a skeletally mature patient. The complication rate in scoliosis surgery is higher for patients with Marfan syndrome than for those with idiopathic scoliosis. Infection, instrumentation failure, pseudarthrosis, or coronal and sagittal curve decompensation occurs in 10% to 20% of patients.[5] Overcorrection can cause cardiovascular complications; reducing the amount of correction in a patient treated with a growing rod was found to reverse cardiac failure in a case report.[6] Other unusual spine deformities can occur, such as subluxation of vertebrae. Traction should be used with caution, as it can worsen the subluxation, especially if the patient has underlying kyphosis.[7] Infection often is associated with a dural tear. Perioperative death from valvular insufficiency has been reported.

Marfan syndrome is associated with mild osteopenia. Patients do not seem to be especially susceptible to fracture, however, and it is not clear whether intervention is warranted.[8,9] Protrusio acetabula is present in a third of patients with Marfan syndrome, but it is not related to bone mineral density and usually is asymptomatic.[10] Prophylactic fusion of the triradiate cartilage can be used for protrusio acetabula but is not warranted for most patients.

Osteogenesis Imperfecta

Osteogenesis imperfecta (OI), often called brittle bone disease, is a spectrum of disorders characterized by abnormal bone fragility. The incidence is 1 in 20,000 children. OI occurs from mutations in the genes that code for type I collagen (*COL1A1* and *COL1A2*). Type I collagen has a complex structure in which a triple helix is composed of three tightly packed procollagen chains; abnormality in one of these chains affects the structural properties of the molecule. Two different types of collagen abnormalities can cause OI. One type is a quantitative defect in collagen production, usually as the result of a premature stop codon that leads to abnormal messenger RNA and, therefore, to less protein production. The second type is the production of abnormal types of collagen, usually as the result of the substitution of glycine by another amino acid, leading to abnormal structural properties in the collagen molecule. Histologic examination of bone affected by OI reveals a decreased number of trabeculae and decreased cortical thickness, with an increased number of osteoblasts and osteoclasts. Although fractures in patients with OI occur frequently during childhood, they heal at the normal rate. The phenotype of OI is quite variable. Some individuals are only mildly affected, with no skeletal deformity. Others have short stature, extensive bone fragility, and multiple fractures. The most severe form of OI is fatal during the perinatal period.

The Silence classification is most commonly used clinical classification of OI and has been modified to include biochemical and genetic information.[11,12] Type I is a mild disorder characterized by normal or low-normal height and blue sclerae; multiple bone fractures occur during childhood but are less common after puberty. Fifty percent of patients have deafness. Type II is the lethal perinatal form of OI, in which the child has short, crumpled femurs and ribs as well as hypoplastic lungs. Central nervous system malformations and hemorrhage are common. Type III is the most severe of the survivable types of OI. The patient has a large skull and a characteristic underdeveloped triangular appearance of the facial bones; pale blue sclerae, which become normal at puberty; and multiple long bone and vertebral fractures, which lead to kyphosis and severe scoliosis. Many patients with type III OI use a wheelchair for mobility. Muscle weakness and ligament hyperlaxity may be present. Type IV is a moderate form of OI characterized by short stature. Many patients with type IV OI have bowing bones and vertebra fractures but are less severely affected than in type III (**Figure 2**). The sclera typically is white. Most patients with type IV OI are ambulatory. Type V OI has a characteristic hypertrophic callus after fracture, with ossification of the interosseous membrane between the tibia and fibula and the radius and ulna.[13] Type VI is moderate and similar to type IV, but there are abnormalities of mineralization rather than collagen.[14] In type VII OI, the patient has rhizomelia and coxa vara.[15]

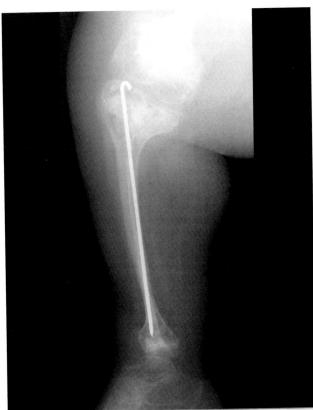

Figure 2 AP radiograph of the tibia of a patient with osteogenesis imperfecta, showing stabilization of the tibia with solid nonexpansile rods. The thin, gracile diaphysis and enlarged epiphyses with popcorn calcifications in the marrow space can be seen.

Table 1
The Cardinal Clinical Findings for the Diagnosis of Neurofibromatosis
Six or more café-au-lait spots (larger than 5 mm in diameter in a child or 15 mm in an adult)
Two neurofibromas or a single plexiform neurofibroma
Freckling in the axilla or inguinal region
An optic glioma
Two or more Lisch nodules (hamartoma of the iris)
A distinctive osseous lesion such as vertebral scalloping or cortical thinning
A first-degree relative with neurofibromatosis type 1

Disorders Caused by Tumor-Related Genes and Overgrowth Syndromes

A variety of cellular proteins and signaling pathways are important in regulating cell reproduction or proliferation. A mutation that results in the dysregulation of such a pathway can cause overgrowth of a cell type or organ. These pathways are commonly dysregulated in a neoplasia.

Neurofibromatosis

Neurofibromatosis (NF) is the most common single-gene disorder in humans. NF has several forms. Orthopaedic manifestations are common in type 1 (NF1). The typical findings are not present at birth. The diagnosis is made as the child grows, based on at least two of the seven cardinal clinical findings (**Table 1**).

NF is caused by a mutation in the *NF1* gene. Its protein product, neurofibromin, acts as a tumor suppressor, stimulating the conversion of Ras-GTP to Ras-GDP, activating the RAt Sarcoma (Ras) signaling system, which is involved in the control of cell growth. Tumors in affected individuals have only the mutated gene because of loss of the normal copy. The gene defect provides a clue to potential therapies; pharmacologic agents that block Ras signaling could be used to treat the disorder. Farnesyl transferase inhibitors block the downstream effects of Ras signaling activation and, thus, have potential use in the treatment of some neoplastic manifestations of NF1. Statin inhibitors such as lovastatin, which regulates Ras signaling by interfering with its membrane binding, also could be used.[16,17] Clinical studies of these agents are ongoing.

The orthopaedic manifestations of NF include scoliosis, overgrowth of the limbs, and pseudarthrosis. A scoliotic curve is categorized as idiopathic or dystrophic. A dystrophic curve is a short, sharp, single curve that is kyphotic and typically involves four to six segments. The onset of a dystrophic curve is early in childhood, and it is relentlessly progressive. A curve that initially appears in a child younger than 7 years has a nearly 70% likelihood of becoming dystrophic. The most important risk factors for progression are early age of onset; a high Cobb angle; and an apical vertebra that is severely rotated, scalloped (with concave loss of bone), and located in the middle to lower thoracic area (**Figure 3**). Dystrophic curves are refractory to brace treatment. Sagittal plane deformities may occur, including an angular kyphosis and a scoliosis that has so much rotation that curve progression is more obvious on a lateral radiograph than on an AP radiograph. The risk of paraplegia is high in patients with an angular kyphosis.

Pseudarthrosis of a long bone typically is associated with NF. The pseudarthrosis usually affects the tibia, with a characteristic anterolateral bow that is obvious in infancy. There is a hamartoma of undifferentiated mesenchymal cells at the pseudarthrosis site, which in some patients is associated with loss of the normal allele of the *NF1* gene.[18,19] A study using a mouse model suggested that lovastatin could be used as a treatment, but clinical studies of this approach are needed.[16] Direct installation of bone morphogenetic protein into the pseudarthrosis site during reconstruction could help in achieving union. Variable results have been reported, however, and it is not known whether the use of bone

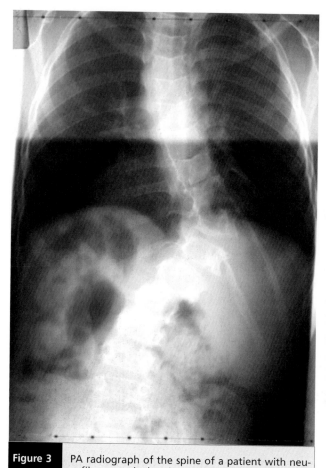

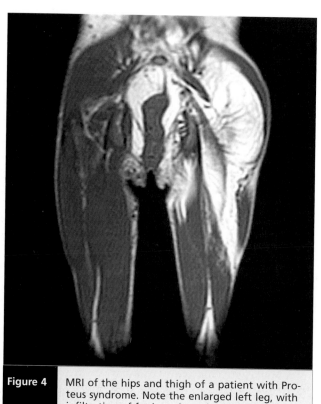

Figure 4 | MRI of the hips and thigh of a patient with Proteus syndrome. Note the enlarged left leg, with infiltration of fat into the pelvis and fascial planes.

Figure 3 | PA radiograph of the spine of a patient with neurofibromatosis showing a thoracic scoliosis with dysplastic ribs and a short, sharply angulated curve. MRI is required to rule out paraspinal plexiform neurofibroma or another intraspinal lesion.

morphogenetic protein in patients with an inherited premalignant condition could have long-term harmful consequences.[20]

The reported incidence of malignancy in patients with NF ranges from less than 1% to more than 20%.[5] There is a risk of malignant degeneration of a neurofibroma into a neurofibrosarcoma. Distinguishing a malignant lesion from a benign lesion can be difficult, and the use of positron emission tomography holds promise for identifying malignancy. Children with neurofibroma have a propensity to develop other malignancies, such as Wilms tumor or rhabdomyosarcoma.

Beckwith-Wiedemann Syndrome

Beckwith-Wiedemann syndrome is linked to the insulin-like growth factor gene. Paternal genomic imprinting plays a role in the inheritance. The child's initial symptom often is hemihypertrophy. Beckwith-Wiedemann syndrome is characterized by organomegaly, omphalocele, and a large tongue that regresses in size as the child ages. Pancreatic islet cell hyperplasia causes hypoglycemia, and neonatal hypoglycemic episodes can cause symptoms resembling those of cerebral palsy. There is a

10% risk of a benign or malignant tumor; the most common is Wilms tumor. Screening for Wilms tumor with abdominal ultrasonography and α-fetoprotein levels should be done at regular intervals until the child reaches age 6 to 8 years. Some other types of tumors, such as alveolar rhabdomyosarcoma, may be present at birth.[21]

Russell-Silver Syndrome

Patients with Russell-Silver syndrome have low birth weight and a triangular face shape, with an average head circumference. Hemihypertrophy is present in 80% of affected individuals.[5] The patient's growth curve may not follow the normal predictive charts, and managing leg-length equality can be difficult. Growth hormone has been administered in an attempt to increase stature. Although growth hormone does increase growth velocity, whether ultimate height is increased has not yet been determined. A case report of Wilms tumor in a patient with Russell-Silver syndrome led to a recommendation that patients with Wilms tumor be screened, like other patients with hemihypertrophy.[22]

Proteus Syndrome

Proteus syndrome is characterized by hemihypertrophy, macrodactyly, and partial giantism of the hands, feet, or both (Figure 4). The characteristic appearance of the plantar surface of the feet often is described as resembling the surface of the brain. The symptoms worsen over time, and new symptoms appear. Unlike other overgrowth syndromes, Proteus syndrome is not associated with an increased incidence of malignancy. The skeletal deformities include focal and regional gigantism, scoliosis, and kyphosis. The patient has relatively large vertebral bodies (megaspondylodysplasia). Angular malformations of the lower extremities, especially genu valgum, are common. Recurrence after surgical intervention is very common. Although osteotomies can correct angular malformations, the decision to undertake surgical correction must take into account the possibility of a rapid recurrence of the deformity. Guided growth is a promising approach to managing limb angular deformity, but data on its results are lacking.[23] Nerve compression can be managed using decompression, but spinal cord compression is difficult or impossible to successfully treat surgically because of the vertebral overgrowth. Scoliosis apparently is caused by overgrowth of one side of the spine.

Disorders Caused by Developmentally Important Signaling Pathways

Cell signaling systems are activated in a coordinated manner during embryonic development to cause cells to proliferate, move, and undergo programmed cell death, so that the organism will develop into adulthood in a normal pattern. The normal patterning is altered by mutations in the genes that encode proteins having a role in these pathways. Environmental events such as exposure to a teratogen also can dysregulate these pathways, resulting in a phenotype similar to that of a gene mutation. A musculoskeletal malformation can result if such an event occurs in a pathway important for skeletal development. Surgery to correct such a malalignment usually is successful.

Achondroplasia and Related Disorders

A mutation in the fibroblast growth factor receptor-3 (FGFR-3) gene can cause skeletal dysplasias of varying severity, including achondroplasia, hypochondroplasia, and thanatophoric dysplasia. Achondroplasia is the most common skeletal dysplasia. This disorder can be inherited as an autosomal dominant trait, although it results from a sporadic mutation in at least 80% of patients. The risk increases with paternal age. The mutation results in uncontrolled activation of the FGFR-3 receptor that leads to an impaired growth in the proliferative zone of the physis.[24-27] Achondroplasia is clinically characterized by rhizomelic shortening with normal trunk length (the proximal bones are most affected), frontal bossing, and trident hands. Spine deformities include foramen magnum and upper cervical stenosis, which results in spinal cord compression as early as the first 2 years of life. Thoracolumbar junction kyphosis and lumbar spinal stenosis also are common (**Figure 5**). The lower extremity malalignment typically involves genu varum with associated tibial torsion. Ligamentous laxity at the knee and ankles is common. In the upper extremities, flexion contractures

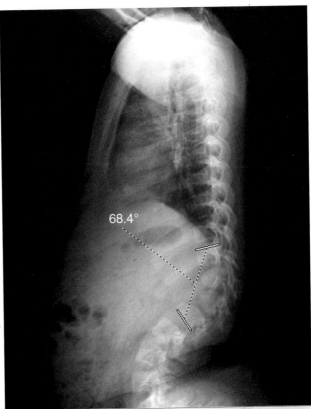

Figure 5 Lateral radiograph of the spine of a 5-year-old boy with achondroplasia showing thoracolumbar kyphosis with symptoms consistent with spinal stenosis.

of the elbows and subluxation of the radial heads are present. The nonorthopaedic manifestations include difficulty with weight control, sleep apnea, recurrent otitis media, and hydrocephalus. The patient has normal intelligence, and life expectancy is not significantly diminished.

The manifestations of hypochondroplasia are similar to those of achondroplasia but are less severe. The gene mutation is in a different location than in achondroplasia and, thus, there is more variability in the phenotype. The clinical features may not be apparent at birth, and mild features may remain undiagnosed until puberty. The features of hypochondroplasia include short stature, small hands, lumbar stenosis, and genu varum.[28]

Thanatophoric dysplasia is severe and almost always is fatal before the patient reaches age 2 years. It is characterized by severe rhizomelic shortening, platyspondyly, a protuberant abdomen, and a small thoracic cavity that is responsible for cardiorespiratory failure.

Camptomelic Dysplasia

The term camptomelic refers to a bowing of the long bones, primarily the tibia and femur. Camptomelic dysplasia appears to be caused by an abnormality in the formation of the cartilage anlagen during fetal development. The endochondral ossification is normal, but the diaphyseal cylinderization is markedly abnormal. Clin-

6: Pediatrics

ically, camptomelic dysplasia is a severe form of short-limbed dwarfism that sometimes is fatal. The defective tracheal cartilage and lower respiratory tract may cause respiratory failure during the neonatal period. Bowing of the long bones and early, progressive spine deformity (kyphosis and scoliosis) are common. The spine deformity further compromises pulmonary function.[29] Hydromyelia and diastematomyelia have been reported, and neurologic complications and pseudarthrosis are common after spine treatment.[30] The other clinical features of camptomelic dysplasia include a flattened head, a cleft palate, micrognathia, defects of the heart and kidneys, and sex reversal (a female has an XY karyotype).

Cleidocranial Dysplasia

Cleidocranial dysplasia is characterized by abnormality of the bones formed by intramembranous ossification (primarily the clavicles, cranium, and pelvis). This disorder is inherited as an autosomal dominant trait. The gene mutation is in runt-related transcription factor 2 (*RUNX2*), an osteoblast-specific transcription factor that regulates osteoblast differentiation.[31] Clinically, the characteristic finding is hypoplasia or absence of the clavicles. If the disorder is bilateral, the child can touch the shoulders together in front of the chest. Mild short stature, a high palate, and abnormal permanent teeth development also are present. Widening of the symphysis pubis, coxa vara (which may require treatment), and a short femoral neck are common, with lumbar spondylolysis occurring in 24% of patients.[32]

Nail-Patella Syndrome

The gene mutation in nail-patella syndrome is in the LIM homeobox transcription factor 1–β (*LMX1B*), which is involved in patterning of the dorsoventral axis of the limbs and early morphogenesis of the glomerular basement membrane. The disorder is inherited as an autosomal dominant trait, but there is marked intrafamilial and interfamilial variation in its clinical features.[33] The characteristic features are dystrophy of the nails, an absent or hypoplastic patella, and iliac horns. Femoral condyle dysplasia and genu valgum are common. Cubitus valgus (hypoplasia of the lateral side of the humerus) of varying severity may occur, with radial head posterior subluxation or dislocation.[34,35] Abnormal pigmentation of the iris occurs in 50% of patients, with glaucoma and nephropathy leading to renal failure in the third or fourth decade of life.

Cornelia de Lange Syndrome

Heterozygous mutations in the nipped-B homolog (*NIPBL*) gene have been documented in 47% of unrelated individuals with Cornelia de Lange syndrome. The familial inheritance is autosomal dominant. *NIPBL* encodes delangin, a protein that is important to chromosome function and DNA repair.[36] The orthopaedic manifestations vary widely in severity and can include short thumbs, clinodactyly of the fifth finger, flexion contractures of the elbow with radial head dis-

location, and radial hemimelia with ray deficiency. In the lower extremities, hip dysplasia, syndactyly of the second and third toes, and hallux valgus can occur.[37] Patients have short stature, microcephaly, mental retardation, cleft palate, and distinctive facial features, including bushy eyebrows, a small nose, and full eyelashes. Approximately 30% of patients have a congenital heart malformation.

Disorders Caused by Multiple Genes and Chromosome Abnormalities

Down Syndrome

Down syndrome (trisomy 21) is the most common and most readily recognizable trisomy disorder. Down syndrome is clinically characterized by hypotonia with joint hyperlaxity, specifically of the upper cervical spine (atlantoaxial and occipitoatlantal instability), relatively short stature, a flat face, and mental retardation to a varying extent. Orthopaedists and pediatricians often are asked to confirm a child's eligibility for participation in the Special Olympics, and, therefore, knowledge of the guidelines for athletic participation by patients with Down syndrome is important.[38-40] In particular, tumbling activities should be avoided. The routine use of radiographs for surveillance of a child with Down syndrome is controversial. Surgical intervention probably should be reserved for children with symptoms because the rate of surgical complications is high. Acetabular dysplasia or hip dislocation is not congenital but occurs between age 2 to 10 years; it is found in 5% of patients. Slipped capital femoral epiphysis and osteonecrosis also can occur. A patient with Down syndrome and slipped capital femoral epiphysis should undergo bilateral pinning of both the symptomatic and the contralateral hip (**Figure 6**). All children with Down syndrome should undergo testing for thyroid dysfunction. Short and broad hands, patellofemoral instability, flatfoot and hallux valgus, a congenital heart defect, and thyroid dysfunction are common in patients with Down syndrome.

Turner Syndrome

Turner syndrome is a complete or partial absence of one of the X chromosomes. Cell mosaicism, in which some cells have the normal two pairs of X chromosomes, is common.[41] The effects of the chromosomal abnormality probably are caused by imprinting and may depend on whether the abnormality is derived from the father or the mother. The clinical features of Turner syndrome include short stature, a wide and webbed neck, low-set ears and hairline, cubitus and genu valgum, swollen hands and feet, scoliosis, and a chest that is broad, flat, and shield shaped.[42] Patients typically have gonadal dysfunction, which results in inadequate production of estrogen, leading to absent or incomplete development at puberty, infertility, diabetes, weight gain, osteoporosis, and a high incidence of fractures. Congenital heart disease and kidney abnormalities are common, as are cognitive deficits related to memory, mathematics, and visuospatial discrimination. The life expectancy is normal.

Noonan Syndrome

Noonan syndrome is a relatively common congenital disorder that affects girls and boys equally. Often it is confused with Turner syndrome because the two conditions share several clinical characteristics. Several causative genes have been identified (*PTPN11*, *SOS1*, and *KRAS*, *NRAS*, *RAF*, *BRAF* and *SHOC2*), although as-yet-undiscovered genes also may cause this disorder.[43] Noonan syndrome is one of the most common syndromes associated with a congenital heart defect. Other clinical features include short stature, cervical spine fusion, low-set ears and hairline, scoliosis, pectus carinatum or excavatum, impaired blood clotting, hypotonia, and learning disabilities. Some patients have severe joint or muscle pain, often with no identifiable cause. Type I Arnold-Chiari malformation is found in some patients.[44,45]

Prader-Willi Syndrome

Prader-Willi syndrome is a disorder caused by a deletion of a small part of chromosome 15 of paternal origin. The distinction of chromosome by paternal origin results from imprinting, and Prader Willi syndrome thus has a sister syndrome, Angelman syndrome, that affects maternally imprinted genes in the region. Prader-Willi syndrome is characterized by hypotonia, hypogonadism, mild mental retardation, short stature that responds well to growth hormone therapy, and a failure to thrive during the early years that is followed by an extreme and insatiable appetite (often leading to morbid obesity). The orthopaedic manifestations include scoliosis in as many as 90% of patients, small hands and feet, hip dysplasia, and joint hyperlaxity.[46-48] Patients with Prader-Willi syndrome have increased morbidity after surgery because of an abnormal physiologic response to hypercapnia and hypoxia, obstructive sleep apnea, thick secretions, obesity, a prolonged and exaggerated response to sedatives, and an increased risk of aspiration. Growth hormone therapy leads to improvement in weight and behavior.[49] The effect of growth hormone therapy on skeletal deformity is unclear, but a recent randomized study suggested that it does not have a negative effect on the sequelae of spine deformity.[50]

Trichorhinophalangeal Syndrome

There are two relatively distinct types of trichorhinophalangeal syndrome (TRPS), with some overlapping of clinical features. Both types are caused by mutation or loss of the *TRPS1* gene. TRPS type II also has a loss of the adjacent exostosin (*EXT-1)* gene, which is responsible for hereditary multiple exostoses and explains the exostoses associated with TRPS type II. Patients with TRPS type I have a bulbous and pear-shaped nose, prominent ears, sparse hair, cone epiphyses, and short fourth and fifth metacarpals. They

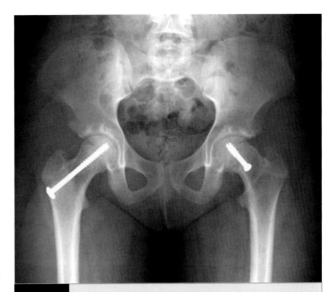

Figure 6 AP radiograph of the pelvis in a 13-year-old girl with Down syndrome showing pinning of both hips after slipped capital femoral epiphysis developed in the left hip. Pinning of the contralateral hip is recommended in children with Down syndrome because of the association of thyroid disorders and contralateral slipped capital femoral epiphysis.

have mild mental retardation. Their hips are radiographically and symptomatically similar to hips with Legg-Calvé-Perthes disease. The key distinguishing feature of TRPS type II is the presence of multiple exostoses, especially in the lower extremities.[51,52] Patients with TRPS type II also have microcephaly and mental retardation. Marked ligamentous laxity and redundant, loose skin may be as severe as in Ehlers-Danlos syndrome.

Disorders Caused by Protein-Processing Genes (Enzymes)

Enzymes modify molecules or other proteins. They often modify substances for degradation, and mutations cause cell dysfunction as these substances accumulate. Mutations in genes that encode for enzymes can have a wide variety of effects on cells, resulting in a broad range of abnormalities in cell function and a wide range of clinical findings. In many disorders, there is an excess accumulation of proteins in cells. The cells become abnormally large, leading to increased pressure in the bones, osteonecrosis, and increased extradural material in the spine that can cause paralysis. Medical treatments have been developed to replace the defective enzyme in many of these disorders. Such treatments often can arrest but not reverse the skeletal manifestations of the disorder. Orthopaedists are treating a slowly decreasing number of patients with these disorders because of early diagnosis and appropriate medical treatment.

Table 2

The Mucopolysaccharidoses

Designation	Syndrome	Enzyme Defect	Stored Substance	Inheritance Pattern
MPS I	Hurler Scheie	A-l-iduronidase	HS + DS	Autosomal recessive
MPS II	Hunter	Iduronidase-2-sulfatase	HS + DS	X-linked recessive
MPS IIIA	Sanfilippo A	Heparin-sulfatase (sulfamidase)	HS	Autosomal recessive
MPS IIIB	Sanfilippo B	A-N-acetylglucosamidase	HS	Autosomal recessive
MPS IIIC	Sanfilippo C	Acetyl-CoA: α-glucosaminide-N-acetyltransferase	HS	Autosomal recessive
MPS IIID	Sanfilippo D	Glucosamine-6-sulfatase	HS	Autosomal recessive
MPS IVA	Morquio A	N-acetyl galactosamine-6-sulfate sulfatase	KS, CS	Autosomal recessive
MPS IVB	Morquio B	B-d-galactosidase	KS	Autosomal recessive
MPS IVC	Morquio C	Unknown	KS	Autosomal recessive
MPS V	Formerly called Scheie disease			
MPS VI	Moroteux-Lamy	Arylsulfatase B, N-acetylgalactosamine-4-sulfatase	DS, CS	Autosomal recessive
MPS VII	Sly	B-d-glucuronidase	CS, HS, DS	Autosomal recessive
MPS VIII		Glucosamine-6-sulfatase	CS, HS	Autosomal recessive

CS = chondroitin sulfate, DS = dermatan sulfate, HS = heparan sulfate, KS = keratan sulfate, MPS = mucopolysaccharidosis.

Mucopolysaccharidoses

The mucopolysaccharidoses are characterized by excretion of mucopolysaccharide in the urine. There are at least 13 types of mucopolysaccharidosis (MPS), all of which are autosomal recessive, except for mucopolysaccharidosis type II (Hunter syndrome), which is X linked (**Table 2**). The most common mucopolysaccharidoses are type I (Hurler syndrome) and type IV (Morquio syndrome). The mucopolysaccharidoses can be diagnosed by urine screening using a toluidine blue-spot test.

Each type of MPS has a deficiency of a specific lysosomal enzyme. The incomplete degradation product accumulates in lysozymes in tissues such as the brain, viscera, and joints. This accumulation is responsible for osteonecrosis, which presumably develops because of too much material in the intramedullary space, and it contributes to symptoms of spinal cord compression caused by accumulation of material in the spinal canal.

Mucopolysaccharidosis Type I

The Hurler and Scheie forms represent the severe and mild ends of the clinical spectrum in MPS type I. Children with the Hurler form have progressive mental retardation, multiple severe skeletal deformities, and organ and soft-tissue deformities. These children die before age 10 years. The Scheie form is characterized by stiffness of the joints and corneal clouding but not by mental retardation. The diagnosis usually is made during the teen years, and patients have a normal life expectancy. Marrow transplantation is used to treat the more severe forms, but its effect on the bones varies. Most children develop the typical skeletal phenotypic features despite the success of the bone marrow transplant.[53] Musculoskeletal deformities that persist after marrow transplantation require further treatment.[54] Malalignment of the limbs can occur, and guided growth or osteotomies may be necessary to treat genu valgum. Approximately one fourth of the patients have an abnormality of the upper cervical spine. The accumulation of degradation products in closed anatomic spaces, such as the carpal tunnel, causes finger triggering and carpal tunnel syndrome.

Mucopolysaccharidosis Type IV

The three types of Morquio syndrome are classified as subtypes of MPS IV. All are caused by enzyme defects involved in the degradation of keratan sulfate. An affected child has a short trunk and ligamentous laxity. There is significant genu valgus, aggravated by the lax ligaments. Realignment osteotomies can restore plumb alignment, but recurrence is common, and osteotomies may not control the instability during ambulation. Guided growth is an attractive alternative to osteotomies because it avoids a possible recurrence, but comparative studies are lacking. Early arthritis develops in the hips and knee. The hips develop progressive acetabular dysplasia. Radiographs may reveal a small femoral ossific nucleus, but MRI or arthrography will show a much larger cartilaginous femoral head. Patients may require total joint arthroplasty.[55] Odontoid hypoplasia or aplasia is common, with resulting C1-C2 instability. A soft-tissue mass in the spinal canal contributes to cord compression. The upper and lower extremities often are flaccid rather than spastic. C1-C2 fusion before the onset of symptoms is controversial; some authors recommend it, but others prefer to reserve surgical intervention for symptomatic patients.[5] No comparative studies have evaluated the outcomes of different management approaches. Elsewhere in the spine, the vertebrae show a progressive platyspondia with a thoracic kyphosis. A progressive deformity should be surgically stabilized. Despite the severity of the disorder, many patients with Morquio syndrome live for decades. Cardiorespiratory disease is common, but the upper cervical spine accounts for most of the disabilities.

Contracture Syndromes

Contractures are common in a variety of orthopaedic conditions, and they are the most prominent phenotypic feature of several disorders. These syndromes have a wide variety of etiologies, including mutations that cause developmental problems, mutations that dysregulate muscle function, and fetal environmental causes. Many of these syndromes are associated with muscle dysfunction. For example, distal arthrogryposis is caused by mutations that disrupt fast-twitch muscle fiber activity. There is some overlap in phenotype between these conditions and some of the myopathies. Despite their different etiologies, these disorders have similar management guidelines.

Arthrogryposis is a physical finding, not a diagnosis, in a large group of disorders characterized by joint contractures present at birth. These disorders can be considered as contracture syndromes and grouped into three general categories, each of which can be represented by a prototypic disease.

Contracture Syndromes Involving All Four Extremities

Arthrogryposis Multiplex Congenita

Arthrogryposis multiplex congenita is the best known of the multiple congenital contracture syndromes. The etiology of arthrogryposis multiplex congenita is unknown. Some mothers of children with arthrogryposis have serum antibodies that inhibit fetal acetylcholine receptor function. The number of anterior horn cells in the spinal cord is decreased. The child's shoulders typically are adducted and internally rotated, the elbow is more often extended rather than flexed, and the wrist is severely flexed, with ulnar deviation. In the lower extremities, the hips are flexed, abducted, and externally rotated; the knees are typically in extension, although flexion is possible; and clubfeet are typical (**Figure 7**). Joint motion is restricted. At least 25% of affected patients are nonambulatory, and many others are limited to household ambulation. Among adults, the level of dependency appears to be more related to educational

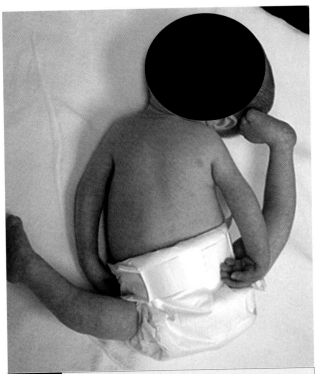

Figure 7 Photograph of a newborn boy with arthrogryposis multiplex congenita, showing hyperflexion of the hips, extended knees, and the typical extended elbows with wrist deformity.

level and coping skills than to the magnitude of the joint contractures.

The overall goals of managing arthrogryposis multiplex congenita are lower limb alignment and stability for ambulation and upper extremity motion for self-care. The outcome appears to be improved if surgery on joints is done when the child is younger than 4 to 6 years, when adaptive intra-articular changes begin to occur. Approximately two thirds of patients have developmental dysplasia of the hip or frank dislocation, and there is considerable controversy about the management of the hips in these children. Closed reduction is rarely or never successful. There is significant variability in the functionality of these children because of the underlying severity of the disease. The range of motion of the hips may be important for functioning. Hip contractures, especially those that cause flexion deformity, adversely affect the gait pattern. Surgery to correct a dislocated hip therefore can lead to worse functioning if it results in significant contracture. A unilateral dislocation generally is treated surgically. Bilateral dislocation management is more controversial. Because of the relatively good results of early surgery, at least one early attempt at surgical relocation of bilaterally dislocated hips may be worthwhile.

Although the knees in arthrogryposis multiplex congenita are classically described as hyperextended, most are in flexion. Ambulation is difficult if the flexion deformity is greater than 30° because of the associated relative weakness of the quadriceps. A posterior soft-

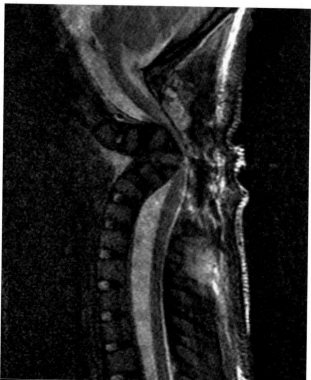

Figure 8 MRI of the cervical spine of a 2-year-old girl with severe cervical kyphosis secondary to Larsen syndrome. She was treated with anterior and posterior decompression and fusion.

tissue procedure initially improves the range of motion and function, but the contractures usually recur, along with a loss of motion.[56-58] Soft-tissue releases may need to be repeated later, before skeletal maturity. Supracondylar osteotomies of the femur are recommended toward the end of growth to correct residual deformity. Femoral shortening is a useful addition to the osteotomies. A guided growth approach at the distal femoral growth plate may correct flexion deformity of the knee, although its effectiveness for correcting the quadriceps mechanism is unclear.[59]

A severe clubfoot is characteristic of arthrogryposis multiplex congenita. Traditionally it was believed that extensive surgery was necessary to correct the deformity. However, the Ponseti method, with minor modifications, has good results in many patients.[60-62]

Most patients do not require upper extremity surgical procedures. It is ideal to achieve elbow flexion to 90° from the fixed extended position. If both elbows are involved, surgery to increase flexion should be done only on one side.[63]

Approximately one third of patients develop scoliosis. The curve usually has a C-shaped neuromuscular pattern. Surgery is indicated for a progressive curve that interferes with balance or function. Some patients have regained their ability to ambulate after surgical correction of a large, rigid curve and surgery should be considered for a patient who loses the ability to ambulate as such a curve develops.[5]

Larsen Syndrome

The essential features of Larsen syndrome are multiple congenital dislocations of large joints, a characteristic flat face, and ligamentous laxity. Kyphosis and abnormal cervical spine segmentation with instability are typical. Kyphosis often is associated with myelopathy. Both autosomal dominant and recessive inheritance patterns have been reported.[5] Mutations in the gene encoding filamin B sometimes causes autosomal dominant inheritance, and a deficiency of carbohydrate sulfotransferase 3 is responsible for some incidences of autosomal recessive inheritance.[64] A phenotype has been reported in which only one side of the body is affected by Larsen syndrome; this pattern suggests a somatic, or mosaic, mutation.[65]

Although knee stability is important for ambulation, knee stability in extension is even more important because it allows optimal quadriceps function. The knee may remain unstable after reduction because of the lack of normal function in the stabilizing ligaments, such as the anterior cruciate ligament. Extra-articular reconstruction of the anterior cruciate ligament may be required.[66]

The hips are dislocated in a patient with Larsen syndrome, often despite a relatively normal-appearing acetabulum. There is a good range of motion, although the hip may prove to be irreducible. The evolution of hip management in Larsen syndrome mirrors that of arthrogryposis multiplex congenita, with a trend toward earlier treatment. The major concern involving the spine is structural abnormality in the cervical vertebrae. This manifestation may occur more frequently than has been recognized, and cervical spine radiographs should be used during the first year of life to identify it. Kyphosis often results from hypoplasia of the vertebral bodies. A combination of cervical kyphosis and forward subluxation may result in quadriplegia and death (**Figure 8**). Posterior stabilization within the first 18 months of life may prevent significant problems associated with complications of treatment after myelopathy has developed and allow a kyphotic deformity to be corrected with growth. In a patient with severe kyphosis or a patient with myelopathy, anterior and posterior decompression and fusion may be required.[67,68]

Contracture Syndromes Primarily Involving the Hands and Feet: Distal Arthrogryposis

Distal arthrogryposis is characterized by fixed hand contractures and foot deformities, but the large joints of the arms and legs are spared. Type I and type II distal arthrogryposis are distinguished by the absence or presence, respectively, of facial features.

In some patients, distal arthrogryposis type I is caused by mutations in the *TPM2* gene, which encodes β-tropomyosin, a protein important in fast-twitch muscle fibers. Type II distal arthrogryposis (Freeman-Sheldon syndrome) is caused by mutations in an isoform of troponin I that is specific to the troponin-tropomyosin complex of fast-twitch myofibers. Both mutations result in abnormal activity of fast-twitch muscle fibers, and dysregulation of these muscle fibers may be the common pathophysiologic cause of distal arthrogryposis.

Children with distal arthrogryposis have overall good function. The hands function well because the shoulders, elbows, and wrists are normal. The most common hand surgery is to lengthen the flexor pollicis longus and rebalance the extensor of the thumb. The feet more frequently require surgery. Some clubfeet can be corrected with manipulation and serial casts, but most are treated with circumferential releases. The outcome of treatment of clubfoot is better in distal arthrogryposis than in other arthrogrypotic syndromes.

Contracture Syndromes With Skin Webs: Pterygia Syndromes

The term pterygium refers to a web and is derived from a Greek word meaning "little wing." The two most common pterygia syndromes are multiple pterygia syndrome and popliteal pterygia syndrome. Multiple pterygia syndrome, also called Escobar syndrome, is characterized by a web across every flexion crease in the extremities, most prominently across the popliteal space, the elbow, and the axilla. Webbing across the neck laterally and anteriorly from sternum to chin draws the facial features downward. The fingers are webbed. There is almost always a vertical talus in multiple pterygium syndrome. Often there is a significant spine deformity, which may interfere with trunk and chest growth and lead to death from respiratory failure during the first or second year of life. The patient's mobility largely depends on the magnitude of the lower extremity webs and the residual motion of the joints. Many patients must use a wheelchair for locomotion.

Popliteal pterygium syndrome is caused by mutations in the gene encoding interferon regulatory factor-6. Patients have a cleft lip and palate, lip pits, intraoral adhesions, and sometimes a fibrous band that crosses the perineum and distorts the genitalia. A popliteal web usually is present bilaterally, running from ischium to calcaneus and resulting in a severe knee flexion deformity. Within the popliteal web is a superficial fibrous band, over which lies a tent of muscle running from the os calcis to the ischium; this feature formerly was referred to as a calcaneoischiadicus muscle. The popliteal artery and vein are usually deep, but the sciatic nerve is superficial in the web, just underneath the fibrous band. Early popliteal web surgery is recommended before further vascular shortening or the onset of adaptive changes in the articular surfaces. Femoral shortening with an extension osteotomy often is required.

Annotated References

1. Pyeritz RE, McKusick VA: The Marfan syndrome: Diagnosis and management. *N Engl J Med* 1979;300(14): 772-777.

2. Doman I, Kövér F, Illés T, Dóczi T: Subluxation of a lumbar vertebra in a patient with Marfan syndrome: Case report. *J Neurosurg* 2001;94(1, suppl):154-157.

3. Pearson GD, Devereux R, Loeys B, et al; National Heart, Lung, and Blood Institute and National Marfan Foundation Working Group: Report of the National Heart, Lung, and Blood Institute and National Marfan Foundation Working Group on research in Marfan syndrome and related disorders. *Circulation* 2008;118(7): 785-791.

   The work group discussed Marfan syndrome and other conditions.

4. Ahn NU, Sponseller PD, Ahn UM, Nallamshetty L, Kuszyk BS, Zinreich SJ: Dural ectasia is associated with back pain in Marfan syndrome. *Spine (Phila Pa 1976)* 2000;25(12):1562-1568.

5. Alman BA, Goldberg MJ: Syndromes of orthopaedic importance, in Morrissy RT, Weisntein SL, eds: *Lovell and Winter's Pediatric Orthopaedics*, ed 6. Philadelphia, PA, Lippincott Williams and Wilkins, 2006, pp 251-313.

6. Skaggs DL, Bushman G, Grunander T, Wong PC, Sankar WN, Tolo VT: Shortening of growing-rod spinal instrumentation reverses cardiac failure in child with Marfan syndrome and scoliosis: A case report. *J Bone Joint Surg Am* 2008;90(12):2745-2750.

   The authors present a case report on the use of growing-rod spinal instrumentation in patients with Marfan syndrome and scoliosis.

7. Yang JS, Sponseller PD: Severe cervical kyphosis complicating halo traction in a patient with Marfan syndrome. *Spine (Phila Pa 1976)* 2009;34(1):E66-E69.

   The authors concluded that cervical kyphosis occurs because of laxity of the connective tissue in patients with Marfan syndrome, and halo gravity traction should be used with caution.

8. Beighton P, De Paepe A, Steinmann B, Tsipouras P, Wenstrup RJ; Ehlers-Danlos National Foundation (USA) and Ehlers-Danlos Support Group (UK): Ehlers-Danlos syndromes: Revised nosology, Villefranche, 1997. *Am J Med Genet* 1998;77(1):31-37.

9. Burrows NP, Nicholls AC, Yates JR, et al: The gene encoding collagen alpha1(V)(COL5A1) is linked to mixed Ehlers-Danlos syndrome type I/II. *J Invest Dermatol* 1996;106(6):1273-1276.

10. Wenstrup RJ, Langland GT, Willing MC, D'Souza VN, Cole WG: A splice-junction mutation in the region of COL5A1 that codes for the carboxyl propeptide of pro alpha 1(V) chains results in the gravis form of the Ehlers-Danlos syndrome (type I). *Hum Mol Genet* 1996;5(11):1733-1736.

11. Sillence DO, Senn A, Danks DM: Genetic heterogeneity in osteogenesis imperfecta. *J Med Genet* 1979;16(2): 101-116.

12. Cole WG: The molecular pathology of osteogenesis imperfecta. *Clin Orthop Relat Res* 1997;343(343):235-248.

13. Glorieux FH, Rauch F, Plotkin H, et al: Type V osteogenesis imperfecta: A new form of brittle bone disease. *J Bone Miner Res* 2000;15(9):1650-1658.

14. Glorieux FH, Ward LM, Rauch F, Lalic L, Roughley PJ, Travers R: Osteogenesis imperfecta type VI: A form of brittle bone disease with a mineralization defect. *J Bone Miner Res* 2002;17(1):30-38.

15. Ward LM, Rauch F, Travers R, et al: Osteogenesis imperfecta type VII: An autosomal recessive form of brittle bone disease. *Bone* 2002;31(1):12-18.

16. Kolanczyk M, Kühnisch J, Kossler N, et al: Modelling neurofibromatosis type 1 tibial dysplasia and its treatment with lovastatin. *BMC Med* 2008;6:21.

    Lovastatin is potentially useful in the treatment of NF1-related fracture healing abnormalities.

17. Korf BR: Statins, bone, and neurofibromatosis type 1. *BMC Med* 2008;6:22.

    The author discusses the major features of NF1.

18. Cho TJ, Seo JB, Lee HR, Yoo WJ, Chung CY, Choi IH: Biologic characteristics of fibrous hamartoma from congenital pseudarthrosis of the tibia associated with neurofibromatosis type 1. *J Bone Joint Surg Am* 2008;90(12):2735-2744.

    The authors studied the biologic characteristics of fibrous hamartoma cells to understand the pathogenesis of this disease. These cells maintain some of the mesenchymal lineage cell phenotypes but do not undergo osteoblastic differentiation in response to bone morphogenetic protein.

19. Stevenson DA, Moyer-Mileur LJ, Murray M, et al: Bone mineral density in children and adolescents with neurofibromatosis type 1. *J Pediatr* 2007;150(1):83-88.

    This study suggests that patients with NF1 have a unique generalized skeletal dysplasia, which makes them more likely to have localized osseous defects.

20. Senta H, Park H, Bergeron E, et al: Cell responses to bone morphogenetic proteins and peptides derived from them: Biomedical applications and limitations. *Cytokine Growth Factor Rev* 2009;20(3):213-222.

    The authors discuss the use of bone morphogenetic proteins and their derived peptides in biomedical delivery systems and gene therapy.

21. Kuroiwa M, Sakamoto J, Shimada A, et al: Manifestation of alveolar rhabdomyosarcoma as primary cutaneous lesions in a neonate with Beckwith-Wiedemann syndrome. *J Pediatr Surg* 2009;44(3):e31-e35.

    The authors determine that neonatal alveolar rhabdomyosarcoma with Beckwith-Wiedemann syndrome may result from an alternative molecular pathway.

22. Bruckheimer E, Abrahamov A: Russell-Silver syndrome and Wilm Tumor. *J Pediatr* 1993;122:165.

23. Stevens PM, Klatt JB: Guided growth for pathological physes: Radiographic improvement during realignment. *J Pediatr Orthop* 2008;28(6):632-639.

    In children with rickets, early intervention, via guided growth, to restore and preserve a neutral axis while maximizing the growth potential of the physes is recommended. Level of evidence: IV.

24. Hall JG: The natural history of achondroplasia. *Basic Life Sci* 1988;48:3-9.

25. Horton WA: Fibroblast growth factor receptor 3 and the human chondrodysplasias. *Curr Opin Pediatr* 1997;9(4):437-442.

26. Maynard JA, Ippolito EG, Ponseti IV, Mickelson MR: Histochemistry and ultrastructure of the growth plate in achondroplasia. *J Bone Joint Surg Am* 1981;63(6):969-979.

27. Yamanaka Y, Ueda K, Seino Y, Tanaka H: Molecular basis for the treatment of achondroplasia. *Horm Res* 2003;60(suppl 3):60-64.

28. Rousseau F, Bonaventure J, Legeai-Mallet L, et al: Clinical and genetic heterogeneity of hypochondroplasia. *J Med Genet* 1996;33(9):749-752.

29. Coscia MF, Bassett GS, Bowen JR, Ogilvie JW, Winter RB, Simonton SC: Spinal abnormalities in camptomelic dysplasia. *J Pediatr Orthop* 1989;9(1):6-14.

30. Thomas S, Winter RB, Lonstein JE: The treatment of progressive kyphoscoliosis in camptomelic dysplasia. *Spine (Phila Pa 1976)* 1997;22(12):1330-1337.

31. Lee B, Thirunavukkarasu K, Zhou L, et al: Missense mutations abolishing DNA binding of the osteoblast-specific transcription factor OSF2/CBFA1 in cleidocranial dysplasia. *Nat Genet* 1997;16(3):307-310.

32. Richie MF, Johnston CE II: Management of developmental coxa vara in cleidocranial dysostosis. *Orthopedics* 1989;12(7):1001-1004.

33. Bongers EM, Gubler MC, Knoers NV: Nail-patella syndrome: Overview of clinical and molecular findings. *Pediatr Nephrol* 2002;17(9):703-712.

34. Guidera KJ, Satterwhite Y, Ogden JA, Pugh L, Ganey T: Nail patella syndrome: A review of 44 orthopaedic patients. *J Pediatr Orthop* 1991;11(6):737-742.

35. Beguiristáin JL, de Rada PD, Barriga A: Nail-patella syndrome: Long term evolution. *J Pediatr Orthop B* 2003;12(1):13-16.

36. Gillis LA, McCallum J, Kaur M, et al: NIPBL mutational analysis in 120 individuals with Cornelia de

Lange syndrome and evaluation of genotype-phenotype correlations. *Am J Hum Genet* 2004;75(4):610-623.

37. Joubin J, Pettrone CF, Pettrone FA: Cornelia de Lange's syndrome: A review article (with emphasis on orthopedic significance). *Clin Orthop Relat Res* 1982;171(171): 180-185.

38. Winell J, Burke SW: Sports participation of children with Down syndrome. *Orthop Clin North Am* 2003; 34(3):439-443.

39. Pizzutillo PD, Herman MJ: Cervical spine issues in Down syndrome. *J Pediatr Orthop* 2005;25(2):253-259.

40. Doyle JS, Lauerman WC, Wood KB, Krause DR: Complications and long-term outcome of upper cervical spine arthrodesis in patients with Down syndrome. *Spine (Phila Pa 1976)* 1996;21(10):1223-1231.

41. Gicquel C, Cabrol S, Schneid H, Girard F, Le Bouc Y: Molecular diagnosis of Turner's syndrome. *J Med Genet* 1992;29(8):547-551.

42. Kim JY, Rosenfeld SR, Keyak JH: Increased prevalence of scoliosis in Turner syndrome. *J Pediatr Orthop* 2001; 21(6):765-766.

43. Tartaglia M, Kalidas K, Shaw A, et al: PTPN11 mutations in Noonan syndrome: Molecular spectrum, genotype-phenotype correlation, and phenotypic heterogeneity. *Am J Hum Genet* 2002;70(6):1555-1563.

44. Wedge JH, Khalifa MM, Shokeir MH: Skeletal anomalies in 40 patients with Noonan's syndrome. *Orthop Trans* 1987;11:40-41.

45. Lee CK, Chang BS, Hong YM, Yang SW, Lee CS, Seo JB: Spinal deformities in Noonan syndrome: A clinical review of sixty cases. *J Bone Joint Surg Am* 2001; 83(10):1495-1502.

46. Holm VA, Cassidy SB, Butler MG, et al: Prader-Willi syndrome: Consensus diagnostic criteria. *Pediatrics* 1993;91(2):398-402.

47. Soriano RM, Weisz I, Houghton GR: Scoliosis in the Prader-Willi syndrome. *Spine (Phila Pa 1976)* 1988; 13(2):209-211.

48. Rees D, Jones MW, Owen R, Dorgan JC: Scoliosis surgery in the Prader-Willi syndrome. *J Bone Joint Surg Br* 1989;71(4):685-688.

49. Festen DA, de Lind van Wijngaarden R, van Eekelen M, et al: Randomized controlled GH trial: Effects on anthropometry, body composition and body proportions in a large group of children with Prader-Willi syndrome. *Clin Endocrinol (Oxf)* 2008;69(3):443-451.

The authors concluded that growth hormone treatment in children with Prader-Willi syndrome improves height, body mass index, head circumference, body composition, and body proportions.

50. de Lind van Wijngaarden RF, de Klerk LW, Festen DA, Duivenvoorden HJ, Otten BJ, Hokken-Koelega AC: Randomized controlled trial to investigate the effects of growth hormone treatment on scoliosis in children with Prader-Willi syndrome. *J Clin Endocrinol Metab* 2009; 94(4):1274-1280.

The authors determined that scoliosis should not be considered a contraindication for growth hormone treatment in children with Prader-Willi syndrome.

51. Bauermeister S, Letts M: The orthopaedic manifestations of the Langer-Giedion syndrome. *Orthop Rev* 1992;21(1):31-35.

52. Minguella I, Ubierna M, Escola J, Roca A, Prats J, Pintos-Morell G: Trichorhinophalangeal syndrome, type I, with avascular necrosis of the femoral head. *Acta Paediatr* 1993;82(3):329-330.

53. Taylor C, Brady P, O'Meara A, Moore D, Dowling F, Fogarty E: Mobility in Hurler syndrome. *J Pediatr Orthop* 2008;28(2):163-168.

The authors studied mobility in 23 patients at a mean of 8.5 years after hematopoietic stem cell transplant for the treatment of Hurler syndrome. All patients had independent mobility, with restriction of internal hip rotation as the most significant clinical finding.

54. Malm G, Gustafsson B, Berglund G, et al: Outcome in six children with mucopolysaccharidosis type IH, Hurler syndrome, after haematopoietic stem cell transplantation (HSCT). *Acta Paediatr* 2008;97(8):1108-1112.

Early hematopoietic stem cell transplantation in patients with mucopolysaccharidosis type I, Hurler syndrome, preserves mental ability.

55. Tassinari E, Boriani L, Traina F, Dallari D, Toni A, Giunti A: Bilateral total hip arthroplasty in Morquio-Brailsford's syndrome: A report of two cases. *Chir Organi Mov* 2008;92(2):123-126.

Young age, severe dysplasia, and joint size are the main technical problems associated with total hip arthroplasty in patients with Morquio-Brailsford syndrome.

56. Ho CA, Karol LA: The utility of knee releases in arthrogryposis. *J Pediatr Orthop* 2008;28(3):307-313.

Although knee releases may improve short-term function in patients with arthrogryposis, function and outcome worsen with age.

57. Devalia KL, Fernandes JA, Moras P, Pagdin J, Jones S, Bell MJ: Joint distraction and reconstruction in complex knee contractures. *J Pediatr Orthop* 2007;27(4):402-407.

A retrospective review of joint distraction and reconstruction in complex knee contractures in six patients (nine knees) found that all patients were able to move with or without an orthosis, and four patients were satisfied with the results of surgery.

6: Pediatrics

58. van Bosse HJ, Feldman DS, Anavian J, Sala DA: Treatment of knee flexion contractures in patients with arthrogryposis. *J Pediatr Orthop* 2007;27(8):930-937.

    Posterior knee releases and flexion contracture distraction by Ilizarov fixation were effective in improving mobility in patients with arthrogryposis.

59. Klatt J, Stevens PM: Guided growth for fixed knee flexion deformity. *J Pediatr Orthop* 2008;28(6):626-631.

    Guided growth is an effective and safe alternative to posterior capsulotomy or supracondylar extension osteotomy in the treatment of fixed knee flexion deformity in children. Level of evidence: IV.

60. Boehm S, Limpaphayom N, Alaee F, Sinclair MF, Dobbs MB: Early results of the Ponseti method for the treatment of clubfoot in distal arthrogryposis. *J Bone Joint Surg Am* 2008;90(7):1501-1507.

    The authors' early results support the use of the Ponseti method to treat distal arthrogrypotic clubfoot. Additional studies are needed to determine the risk of recurrence and the potential need for corrective surgery.

61. van Bosse HJ, Marangoz S, Lehman WB, Sala DA: Correction of arthrogrypotic clubfoot with a modified Ponseti technique. *Clin Orthop Relat Res* 2009;467(5):1283-1293.

    Arthrogrypotic clubfoot can be corrected without extensive surgery in infants and young children.

62. Morcuende JA, Dobbs MB, Frick SL: Results of the Ponseti method in patients with clubfoot associated with arthrogryposis. *Iowa Orthop J* 2008;28:22-26.

    The Ponseti method is effective for correcting clubfoot associated with arthrogryposis, especially during the first few weeks after birth.

63. Van Heest A, James MA, Lewica A, Anderson KA: Posterior elbow capsulotomy with triceps lengthening for treatment of elbow extension contracture in children with arthrogryposis. *J Bone Joint Surg Am* 2008;90(7):1517-1523.

    Elbow capsulotomy with triceps lengthening successfully increased passive elbow flexion and the arc of elbow motion in children with arthrogryposis. None of the children in this study underwent subsequent tendon transfer surgery.

64. Hermanns P, Unger S, Rossi A, et al: Congenital joint dislocations caused by carbohydrate sulfotransferase 3 deficiency in recessive Larsen syndrome and humerospinal dysostosis. *Am J Hum Genet* 2008;82(6):1368-1374.

    The authors studied six patients with congenital joint dislocations who had carbohydrate sulfotransferase 3 deficiency.

65. Debeer P, De Borre L, De Smert L, et al: Asymetrical Larsen syndrome in a young girl: A second example of somatic mosaicism in the syndrome. *Genet Couns* 2003;14:95-100.

66. Johnston CE II, Birch JG, Daniels JL: Cervical kyphosis in patients who have Larsen syndrome. *J Bone Joint Surg Am* 1996;78(4):538-545.

67. Madera M, Crawford A, Mangano FT: Management of severe cervical kyphosis in a patient with Larsen syndrome: Case report. *J Neurosurg Pediatr* 2008;1(4):320-324.

    The authors discuss the first report of a child with Larsen syndrome in whom an asymptomatic cervical instability was treated before neurologic deterioration with synchronous anterior decompression and fixation, posterior fusion and fixation, and halo placement.

68. Sakaura H, Matsuoka T, Iwasaki M, Yonenobu K, Yoshikawa H: Surgical treatment of cervical kyphosis in Larsen syndrome: Report of 3 cases and review of the literature. *Spine (Phila Pa 1976)* 2007;32(1):E39-E44.

    Posterior spinal fusion is indicated in patients with mild and flexible cervical kyphosis. Anterior decompression and circumferential arthrodesis is indicated in patients with severe kyphosis.

Chapter 63

Neuromuscular Disorders in Children

Michael D. Aiona, MD   Arabella I. Leet, MD

Introduction

Cerebral palsy and neuromuscular disorders have many common developments, including an increased awareness that the health risks from obesity in childhood impact children with neuromuscular disorders as well as unaffected children. Obesity may be less well tolerated in patients with muscle weakness than in children with normal muscles. Muscle weakness may also be harder to diagnose because the loss of muscle volume may be replaced with adipose tissue, giving a more normal-looking contour to the limbs and a normal prediction of weight on standard growth curves.

Another common development in the treatment of neuromuscular scoliosis includes increased strength of segmental fixation to include pedicle and sacral screws, which have allowed for increased correction of large neuromuscular curves from a posterior approach. In neuromuscular disorders, where proximal muscle weakness can affect the chest wall musculature and diaphragm, a posterior-only approach can both achieve desired correction and decrease some of the risks associated with an anterior approach.

Some genetic and molecular derangements causing neuromuscular conditions are becoming better understood (**Table 1**); as such there may be new therapies to treat patients. Ongoing clinical trials of medical treatments of neuromuscular disorders include deflazacort for the treatment of Duchenne muscular dystrophy (DMD) or idebenone for the treatment of Friedreich ataxia. Deflazacort has been shown to have an effect on scoliosis and ambulation in DMD. Whether deflazacort effectively stops curve progression or delays progression until later in life is still unknown.[1] The impact of these new medical treatments on the development of

orthopaedic sequelae still requires further clinical research. Gene therapy, which has great potential for curing many neuromuscular disorders, remains an elusive treatment because the packaging of many large gene sequences–such as the gene for dystrophin–into a virus is a challenge yet to be overcome.[1]

Cerebral Palsy

Cerebral palsy (CP) is a group of developmental disorders of movement and posture causing activity restriction or disability, which is attributed to disturbances occurring in the fetal or infant brain. The motor impairment varies in severity and may be accompanied by a seizure disorder or impairment of sensation, cognition, communication and/or behavior. Although the encephalopathy is static, the affected musculoskeletal system changes with growth and development. Orthopaedic management addresses the altered biomechanics of the musculoskeletal system. Though technical success (such as the ability to straighten limbs) can be achieved, correlation to functional outcomes continues to be a challenge.[2] To meet patient and family goals, therapists, pediatricians, physiatrists, orthotists, and social workers provide valuable input in determining a treatment plan.

The incidence of CP has not changed dramatically over the past decade, remaining at approximately 2 in 1,000 births. Improved perinatal care has reduced hypoxic insult at the time of birth as the predominant etiologic factor, along with premature birth, intrauterine exposure to infection, and congenital malformations, depending on the clinical subtype more commonly associated with the development of CP.[3] A genetic-based vulnerability may be elucidated with the identification of common single nucleotide polymorphism. Decreasing the incidence of CP would have a significant economic impact, as the lifetime cost of one patient is a significant social and economic burden, rapidly approaching $1 million,[4] with the social and medical care costs greatest in childhood because of neonatal care and specialized schooling.

Patients are classified descriptively by the tone abnormality present and the anatomic distribution, for example, spastic (velocity-dependent tone) quadriplegia

Dr. Aiona or an immediate family member serves as a board member, owner, officer, or committee member of the American Academy for Cerebral Palsy and Developmental Medicine and the Pediatric Orthopaedic Society of North America. Neither Dr. Leet nor any immediate family member has received anything of value from or owns stock in a commercial company or institution related directly or indirectly to the subject of this chapter.

6: Pediatrics

Table 1

Neuromuscular Conditions

Disease	Prevalence	Gene	Inheritance	Molecular Defect	Clinical Features	Orthopaedic Features
Duchenne muscular dystrophy	2-3/10,000	Xp21.2	X-linked	Dystrophin	Elevated C-reactive protein level Calf hypertrophy Cardiomyopathy	Scoliosis contractures Gait abnormalities
Spinal muscular atrophy	1/6-10,000	5q.13	Autosomal recessive	Survival motor neuron protein	Proximal muscle weakness Tongue fasiculations	Scoliosis Hip dysplasia
Charcot-Marie-Tooth disease	36/100,000	17p11.2	Autosomal recessive, autosomal dominant X-linked	Peripheral myelin protein	Loss of sensation including vibration, light touch, and proprioception Absent deep tendon reflexes	Cavovarus feet Scoliosis Hip dysplasia Hand clawing
Friedreich ataxia	1/50,000	9q13	Autosomal recessive	Mitochondrial protein frataxin	Cardiomyopathy	Scoliosis Cavovarus feet Ataxic gait

(four-limb involvement). Although most patients have spasticity, many have a mixed pattern with varying degrees of dystonia, a movement disorder manifested by involuntary twisting movements and poor motor control. Orthopaedic procedures generally are more successful in treating those patients with pure spasticity and less predictable and at times not indicated in other patients when dystonic or extrapyramidal tone patterns predominate.

The Gross Motor Function Classification Scale (GMFCS) categorizes patients based on function, not on geographic distribution or tone. Level I and II patients are independent ambulators, level III patients are dependent ambulators, level IV patients walk very short distances but use a wheelchair for community mobility, and level V patients are nonambulatory with global involvement with the lowest function and largest disease burden. The usefulness of this classification goes beyond description as each level has differing risks of developing hip subluxation as well as response to surgical intervention, with the greatest risk in GMFCS level V.

Medical Management of CP

Intrathecal Baclofen

Intrathecal baclofen (ITB) is more effective than oral baclofen for reduction of tone without diminishing cognitive capacity. Patients using ITB must have a fairly stable social situation so the pump can be maintained, as sudden withdrawal from ITB can induce seizures. Increasing use of ITB for tone management adds another element of complexity to scoliosis management. Its influence on the progression of deformity is unpredictable as studies in the literature report differing findings. In comparative studies, patients with and without ITB

showed no statistical difference in curve progression,[5] pelvic obliquity, or the incidence of scoliosis.[6] In contrast, a review of 19 consecutive patients with spastic quadriplegia showed a sixfold increase of curve progression (11° per year) after pump placement. A smaller review described four patients with rapid progression of scoliosis after ITB.[7] Because ITB is a tone management tool, the surgeon and family must weigh the benefits of tone reduction separately from its potential influence on spinal deformity in light of this conflicting information. When patients with pumps require subsequent spine surgery, pump- and catheter-related complications resulted in greater re-operation and hospitalization rates.[8,9] There is a reported trend toward more wound infections in patients with pumps.

Botulinum Toxin

Botulinum toxin, when injected into muscle, blocks the release of acetylcholine from vesicles at the neuromuscular junction, allowing muscle relaxation. The drug is not FDA approved for the treatment cerebral palsy and is used off label. Botulinum toxin can be useful to help delay surgical intervention until children are at an age where the risk of recurrence of muscle contractures has decreased.[10] A recent review of the literature by the American Academy of Neurology found enough level I evidence to prove botulinum toxin efficacious in the gastrocnemius-soleus complex, with still undetermined success at other muscles sites.[11] A randomized controlled study of botulinum toxin injection into the hip adductors demonstrated no evidence that the natural history of hip instability was altered when children were treated with botulinum toxin and hip abduction bracing.[12]

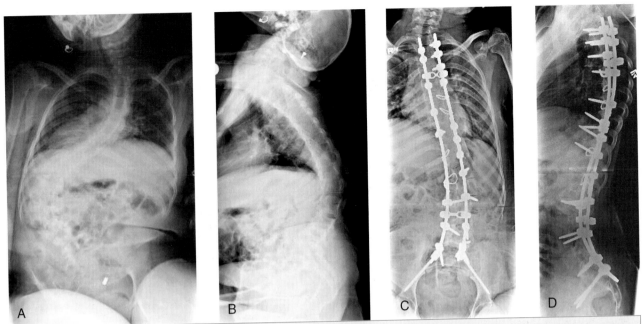

Figure 1 A through **D**, Preoperative and postoperative images after posterior spinal fusion in a premenarchal child with CP. Both frontal and sagittal curves are corrected, allowing for better positioning for sitting, while stopping curve progression.

Obesity

There is a 17% increased prevalence of obesity in the ambulatory patient with CP over a 10-year span, which is similar to that of the general pediatric population.[13] The ambulatory patients (GMFCS level I and II) showed a greater tendency toward being overweight than nonambulatory patients (22.7% versus 9.6%).[14] Because children with CP have associated muscle weakness, the extra weight that they carry may reduce ambulatory efficiency.

Nutrition in patients with CP remains complicated and nutritional status needs to be monitored on an individual basis. Children with extensive neurologic involvement (GMFCS level IV and V) tend to have a greater incidence of gastrointestinal disorders, with feeding problems leading to malnutrition. Level III patients have a lower body mass index than level I and II patients as malnutrition may be present in this select group of dependent ambulatory patients.[15] Although there are some questions about the validity of body mass index in some neuromuscular disorders, nutritional assessment and counseling can play an important role in the overall treatment plan. Individualized care of patients with CP should include a strategy to make sure all children have adequate nutrition while maintaining an appropriate weight to maximize ambulation potential.

Presurgical Medical Management

Surgical risks for elective cases can be significant, especially in patients with GMFCS level V involvement. Careful preoperative evaluation assuring seizures are well controlled, respiratory function is maximized, and nutrition and gastrointestinal function are optimal can help decrease medical complications after surgery. Poor nutrition or uncontrolled seizures are modifiable risk factors in patients with CP and should be addressed before elective orthopaedic intervention.[16]

Scoliosis

The incidence of scoliosis varies with the severity of involvement, with the highest incidence in nonambulatory patients. Although muscle imbalance causes many lower extremity deformities, the cause of scoliosis remains elusive. Bracing does not effectively alter the natural history of scoliosis, but may be used to delay surgery for patients who are too young to consider definitive surgical treatment. Braces can be prescribed in children with trunk hypotonia to assist in positioning and provide comfort.

Surgical indications vary and are dependent on the curve magnitude and family contextual factors. The risks of spinal surgery in children with CP are much higher than for children with adolescent idiopathic scoliosis and include increased risk of bleeding and infection as well as medical complications. These greater risks need to be factored into the clinical decision making process and discussed with the family as part of the informed consent process.

With the advent of more powerful instrumentation, it appears that a posterior approach and fusion alone is sufficient in most cases.[17] In severe curves, osteotomies may be performed posteriorly to achieve similar corrections.[18] Although the trend is toward more pedicle and pelvic screw fixation (**Figure 1**), the use of a unit rod with segmental wire fixation can achieve the same curve correction more economically.[19] More studies comparing screw constructs with other constructs are necessary to demonstrate that pedicle screw fixation is able to achieve better results than other constructs while being cost-effective. Thus, the specific indications for pedicle screw use in CP are still being developed.

Infection rates after spine fusion are higher in children with CP than in children with adolescent idiopathic scoliosis.[20] The complication rate, including infection, is reportedly higher in one series with the use of a unit rod compared to a custom rod,[20] yet at another single institution, the infection rate was as low as 3.9% with the use of gentamicin-soaked allograft.[21] Although caretaker satisfaction, as assessed through surveys, can be as high as 96% with spinal fusion, the presence of infection adversely affected patients' functional status with a trend toward greater persistence of pain. Intraoperative blood loss, a major concern, can be significantly reduced by the use of antifibrinolytic agents such as aminocaproic acid with resultant decreased transfusion requirements.[22]

Hip

A dislocated or significantly subluxated hip with femoral head deformity can impact patient function. The etiology of hip subluxation is thought to be muscle force imbalance as the hip flexors and adductors dominate the hip abductors and extensors. In the nonambulatory patient this condition can affect sitting position, make hygiene difficult, and lead to windswept deformity and discomfort. In the ambulatory patient, progressive subluxation is less common and may affect lever arm function in gait and can cause pain. Dislocated hips are not always painful, but there is no way to predict which significantly subluxated hips will go on to dislocate without pain. As salvage procedures for a dislocated hip are less satisfying than reconstructive procedures, prevention of hip deformity is the goal of treatment.

The rate of hip subluxation is correlated with GMFCS level, minimal in level I and increasing to 90% in level V. Ataxic tone appears to be protective for the hips.[23] Sequential measures of migration percentage, a measure of the percentage of the femoral head that has no acetabular coverage, provides the most accurate method of identifying and monitoring hip stability. Most surgeons would recommend surgery with a migration percentage of 40% to 50% as natural history studies have shown that at migration percentages of greater than 60% to 70% the hip will dislocate in the absence of treatment.[24]

The goal of surgical management is to balance the muscle forces and to treat any significant bony deformities. Adductor and psoas releases through a medial incision with use of an abduction pillow have encouraging initial results in younger children with mild subluxation. Although soft-tissue surgical management alone may provide initial stabilization, it is insufficient to maintain hip stability until skeletal maturity in many cases. Monitoring hip development until skeletal maturity is recommended. Hip monitoring includes clinical assessment of hip abduction in extension with follow-up radiographs if a hip fails to abduct adequately given the patient's clinical picture. Greater deformity usually requires a combination of a proximal femoral varus rotational osteotomy and occasionally a periacetabular osteotomy.[25] Acetabular remodeling is not reliable in the older patient population and thus correction of acetabular dysplasia should be done in the older patient to best protect the reconstruction.[26]

Salvage procedures may necessitate removal of the femoral head with the complications of heterotopic ossification, migration of the femoral shaft superiorly, or incomplete pain relief. The combination of femoral head resection and derotational and valgus osteotomy helps to position the lower extremity for sitting (**Figure 2**).

Knee

Excessive stance-phase knee flexion increases patellofemoral pressure, increases demand on the quadriceps to maintain upright gait, and causes greater energy demands. As in all lower extremity management, understanding the interplay of joints is crucial in distinguishing primary and secondary deformities. Primary deformities need to be addressed, whereas secondary compensatory deformities will improve spontaneously with treatment of the primary deformity at an adjacent joint. Sagittal gait patterns in diplegia have been classified to assist identification of the level of the deformity and recommend treatment.[27] A similar study describes the gait patterns in hemiplegia.[28]

The aggressive management of the fixed flexion contracture and quadriceps insufficiency has significantly improved technical and functional outcomes. Although a 10° improvement of the knee flexion contracture with soft-tissue release and casting can be achieved, a fixed contracture of 20° or more could be treated with a distal femoral extension osteotomy in the ambulatory adolescent. The Koshina Index can quantify patella alta in the immature skeleton.[29] Correction of patella alta addresses the quadriceps insufficiency and improves knee extension in gait.[30] Aggressive rehabilitation and ground reaction ankle-foot orthoses are recommended to assist knee extension during stance phase. However, correction of knee flexion carries the risk of sciatic nerve stretch (9.2%), which results in a dysesthetic foot. When the ability to bear weight and perform therapy is affected, recovery becomes prolonged. Early recognition by careful postoperative examinations with immediate increased knee flexion in response to reports of foot pain can reduce tension across the nerve and help avoid this complication.[31]

In nonambulatory children, identification of knee flexion contractures signals hamstring dysfunction that can interfere with sitting. Attaching at the pelvis, the hamstrings can cause extension of the pelvis out of the seating system with strapping of the feet to the foot plate of the wheelchair. Thus, hamstring lengthening alone may be indicated to improve sitting tolerance and wheelchair mobility in children with significant knee flexion contractures (popliteal angle greater than 90°)

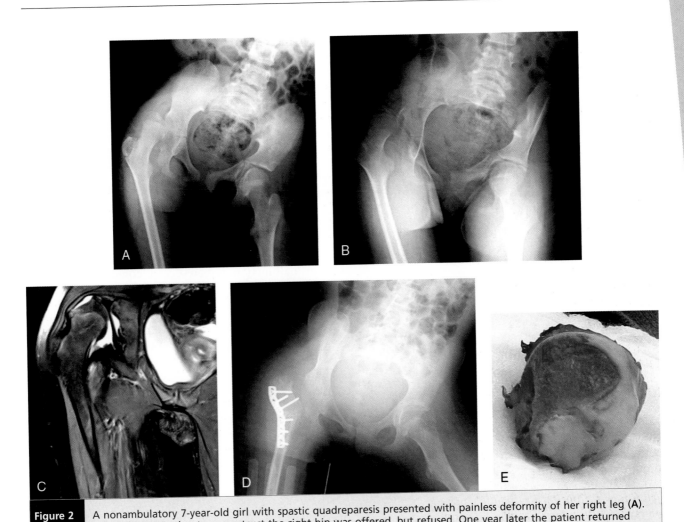

Figure 2 A nonambulatory 7-year-old girl with spastic quadreparesis presented with painless deformity of her right leg (**A**). Surgical intervention to reconstruct the right hip was offered, but refused. One year later the patient returned with reports of new onset of hip pain. Plain films (**B**) demonstrated flattening of the femoral head not seen in the previous radiographs; loss of the cartilage surface was confirmed with MRI (**C**). The patient underwent a femoral head resection and valgus osteotomy (**D**). The femoral head demonstrated an extensive cartilage defect (**E**).

when other medical modalities such as ITB cannot be used.

Foot and Ankle

The goal of foot management is a plantigrade, painless, braceable foot. Fixed deformities require more aggressive intervention, whereas flexible deformities are generally treated with bracing.[32] Though equinus remains the most common ankle deformity, it cannot be overemphasized that a dynamic toe-toe gait does not necessarily mean an equinus deformity requiring surgery. Brace-intolerant dynamic deformities are best treated with casting and adjuvant botulinum toxin injections to the gastrocnemius-soleus complex to reduce tone. Surgical management of equinus should be reserved for fixed contractures and to prevent recurrence. Surgery is most successful in patients at least 6 to 7 years of age. At the time of surgery, the ankle should be reexamined because the physical examination can change under anesthesia. The trend is to perform less traditional Z lengthening (zone 3), as isolated gastrocnemius lengthening (Strayer) (zone 1) or intramuscular fascial length-ening (Vulpius) (zone 2) have lesser chance of postoperative weakness when soleus muscle power is preserved (**Figure 3**). Despite concerns that lengthening procedures could produce significant weakness, the use of ultrasound demonstrates increased volume of the medial gastrocnemius 1 year after Vulpius lengthening.[33] Similar increases in volume (17%) were documented 3 months after plantar flexion strengthening resistive exercises.[34] Ultrasound may prove an excellent tool for investigations on muscle architecture after a variety of interventions.

Equinovalgus deformity, common in the diplegic patient, is a combination of midfoot abduction and heel valgus. This instability and loss of leverage can affect ankle rocker function. In symptomatic patients surgery can include calcaneal neck lengthening, which theoretically preserves motion. Calcaneal cuboid subluxation[35] or the use of allograft[36] do not compromise the results of os calcis lengthening. Subtalar fusion or calcaneal sliding osteotomy is reserved for severe, rigid deformities. Midfoot osteotomy may be needed to correct residual supination, which was noted in a subtalar fusion

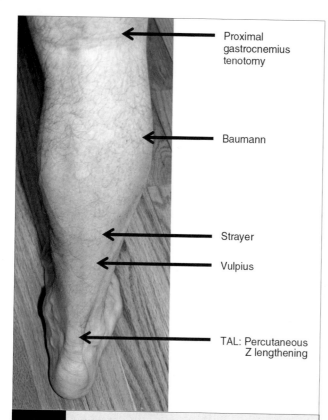

Proximal gastrocnemius tenotomy

Baumann

Strayer

Vulpius

TAL: Percutaneous Z lengthening

Figure 3 Surface anatomy of the calf showing the location of popular sites of muscle releases for equinus. An Achilles tendon lengthening, or a lengthening of the conjoined gastrocnemius and soleus fascia (Vulpius) lengthens both gastrocnemius and soleus muscles. If the soleus is not contracted, these more distal lengthening procedures will result in significant loss of ankle power. Thus, more proximal lengthening procedures are indicated, particularly in diplegic patients, if the ankle can be dorsiflexed past neutral with the knee flexed (Silfverskoid sign). (Reproduced with permission from Professor H. Kerr Graham, MD, Melbourne, Australia.)

group using foot pressure studies.[37] Calf muscle lengthening and other soft-tissue rebalancing is necessary when performing either procedure.

Equinovarus foot causes significant lateral foot pressure with the tendency to lead to significant inversion strain. Varus positioning can result from imbalance due to overpull of the anterior or posterior tibialis. Which muscle to treat via combinations of transfer or lengthening is hard to assess clinically; fine-wire electromyography has not been as helpful as had been hoped. A recent study has shown physical examination tests such as the confusion test to be imperfect, and by electromyography and gait analysis, rebalancing of the varus foot would need to address both the anterior and posterior tibialis in two thirds of feet.[38] Tendon transfers or lengthening are useful in the flexible varus foot whereas calcaneal osteotomy or midfoot osteotomies should also be considered if the foot deformity is rigid.

Myelomeningocele

Myelomeningocele includes the spectrum of spine and spinal cord defects resulting from failure of closure of the neural tube. A multicenter clinical trial sponsored by the National Institutes of Health is currently comparing outcome of fetal surgery to close the defect with postnatal surgical closure of exposed neural tissues.

Spine

Spinal deformities (including scoliosis, kyphosis, and lordosis) are commonly seen in children with myelomeningocele and many result from muscle imbalance and weakness as well as structural vertebral anomalies. Other factors that affect curve progression include shunt malfunction, tethered cord, compensatory pelvic obliquity, and/or hip deformity. The prevalence of scoliosis ranges between 50% to 90%, with curve progression determined by the age of the patient, location of the dysraphism, ambulation potential, and curve size.[39] Curve progression tends to occur before age 15 years. A patient with a curve of 40° or greater can be expected to experience curve progression at a rate of approximately 5° per year.[39]

Bracing can be used to provide support and delay surgical intervention until the child is older, but bracing is not effective in preventing curve progression. Surgical intervention carries a high complication rate, including surgical blood loss measured in liters, poor wound healing, and loss of curve correction over time. In a recent retrospective study of 84 patients undergoing spinal stabilization, the cohort was divided into three groups for comparison: (1) posterior spinal fusion and instrumentation, (2) posterior and anterior spinal fusion with posterior-only instrumentation, and (3) anterior and posterior spinal fusion and instrumentation. The patients in the third group maintained curve correction better than those in group 1; hence, the authors recommend anterior and posterior fusion.[40] Complications related to hardware were found in one third of patients, and loss of correction was directly related to hardware failure.[40]

The goal of spinal surgery is to improve sitting balance as well as stop curve progression. Pressure mapping has been studied as a tool to assess spinal surgery outcome. In 19 wheelchair ambulators undergoing spinal surgery, Cobb angles and pelvic obliquity were significantly corrected radiographically and pressure skin ulcers resolved after surgery, but sitting pressure mapping did not show a significant improvement. Because the patients appeared to achieve curve correction and relief of pressure at the apex of the kyphosis, the authors wondered if pressure mapping was a useful outcomes tool in children with myelomeningocele.[41]

Timing of spinal correction remains controversial. In a small series of 12 patients undergoing neonatal kyphectomy at a single institution and with surgery performed by a single surgeon, surgery was found to be safe with no reported complications. Although the initial correction of kyphosis was almost 80°, the average loss of correction after an average of almost 7 years was 55°. However, the authors noted that the resultant kyphotic deformity was different from the natural history of kyphosis in myelomeningocele; the recurrent kyphosis was noted to occur over more levels with a sagittal contour that was more rounded and technically less difficult to manage surgically.[42]

In a second retrospective study, nine children at an average age of 10.8 years undergoing multilevel spinal fusion and cord transaction achieved an average correction of 81.9° of kyphosis, but had a complication rate of 89%. Most of the reported complications were wound issues; however, an additional 22% of children had shunt revision within 6 weeks of surgery, suggesting alterations in cerebrospinal fluid dynamics with cord transaction in this age group. The authors propose careful preoperative shunt assessment and even suggest temporarily externalizing the shunt to better monitor shunt function in the acute postoperative period.[42-44]

Hip

Hip dysplasia is commonly seen in myelomeningocele with treatment individualized for the level of function. Anterior soft-tissue releases including iliopsoas, rectus femoris, tensor fascia lata, and the hip capsule can be performed for hip flexion contractures greater than 20° to facilitate standing in children who do not have active motor control about the hip. For children with lower-level lesions and who have the potential to ambulate independently, surgical reduction of the hip is indicated for unilateral dislocations in children who have good quadriceps function (L3 motor level).[40] Children with bilateral hip dislocations rarely show functional loss and may, therefore, benefit from surgical release of hip flexion contractures while the hips are left dislocated. In patients with sacral level injury, surgical reduction of the hips is usually indicated. Ambulatory patients with lower-level lesions can have excessive lumbar lordosis as compensation for hip flexion contractures as demonstrated by the correlation between hip flexion contracture angle as measured by the Thomas test with the sagittal Cobb angle.[43]

Foot

Foot deformities in myelomeningocele include clubfeet, calcaneovalgus deformity, metatarsus adductus, and congenital vertical talus; the level of the cord lesion is not predictive of foot deformity, thus suggesting a multifactorial etiology.[45] Traditionally clubfoot deformities have been managed by surgical release. In a retrospective review of 167 clubfeet managed with peritalar release, a plantigrade corrected foot was achieved in 83% of the cohort, with 17% of children requiring reoperation. The authors concede that the results of surgical release were much better than those previously reported in the literature.[40] Recently the trend to use the Ponseti method for treatment of clubfoot deformity has been reported with some success in patients with myelomeningocele. In a prospective 2-year study comparing 28 clubfeet in children with myelomeningocele with

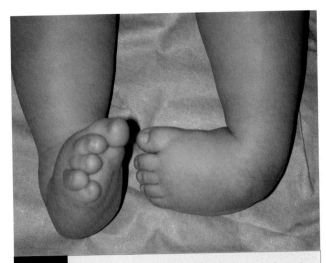

Figure 4 Lumbar level spina bifida in a 2-year-old boy. On his right foot there is L4-level calcaneus deformity due to unopposed pull of the anterior tibialis. On the left foot he has L3 level paralysis and a rigid clubfoot.

35 idiopathic clubfeet, the recurrence rate was 68% in the myelomeningocele group compared with 26% in the idiopathic group. Feet that were insensate had more complications with casting when compared to sensate feet. In addition, two children in the myelomeningocele group sustained nondisplaced fractures. Bracing resulted in more blistering of the feet in the myelomeningocele group.[45] Yet despite the fact that the Ponseti approach does not have the same ultimate success rate as seen in idiopathic clubfeet, partial correction, which decreases the extent of required surgery, can be achieved in children with spina bifida.

Calcaneovalgus feet develop secondary to plantar flexion weakness and can cause loss of toe-off, crouch gait, and heel pad ulcers (**Figure 4**). Early treatment includes bracing, release of foot and toe dorsiflexors, or transfer of the anterior tibialis to the gastrocnemius-soleus complex; late treatment may include osteotomy and arthrodesis. Gait analysis and dynamic foot pressure measurements were used to study the results of anterior tibialis tendon transfer combined with correction of osseous deformity in 18 patients with low lumbar or sacral lesions and calcaneal deformity. Patients with excessive coronal or transverse plane pelvic movement or with loss of knee extension in stance phase did not show improvement in pressure transfer from the hindfoot to the midfoot and forefoot after surgery compared with the more normalized foot pressures seen in patients without pelvic and knee dyskinetic movements.[46]

Fractures

The long bones in patients with myelomeningocele are often gracile and extremely osteoporotic. The fracture rate reportedly is close to 70% in children who have high thoracic lesions. Diagnosis of fractures can be complex because a fracture can easily mimic an infec-

6: Pediatrics

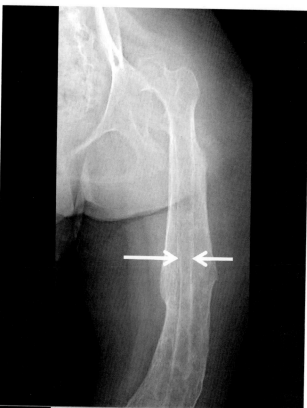

Figure 5 Radiograph showing a thoracic-level myelomeningocele in a patient who sustained a femur fracture. Note the prolific amount of callus formation. Arrows point to the gracile femoral cortices. Fractures in this patient population can be suspicious for infectious process, with a red, swollen knee the presenting complaint.

tious process with leukocytosis, fever, increased erythrocyte sedimentation rate, and a warm, swollen limb (**Figure 5**). In a recent study, no relationship was found between bone mineral density as determined by dual-energy x-ray absorptiometry scan, and the incidence of fracture in children with myelomeningocele.[47] Thus, identification of children at risk for fracture can only be approximated based on the level of the cord lesion. Fractures heal well in this population, but the rate of refracture after immobilization has been reported to be as high as 50%. Thus, patients need to be immobilized for a minimum amount of time and returned to baseline weight bearing as quickly as possible in an attempt to lessen the risk of a refracture.

Skin Ulcers

Skin breakdown often occurs on areas of bone prominence. The combination of loss of sensation and other deformities such as contractures, hip dislocations, and kyphosis commonly lead to ulceration. Iatrogenic causes of skin ulceration must also be considered. In a recent study of 415 patients admitted to the hospital for skin ulcer management, the use of medical devices was found to cause 51% of ulcers; cast application was

responsible for another 22% of clinically significant ulcers. In comparison, only 7% of skin ulcers in the study were caused by a wheelchair cushion or a mattress.[40]

Duchenne Muscular Dystrophy

DMD has an X-linked pattern of inheritance, although one third of all cases are caused by a spontaneous mutation. Because DMD is caused by a single frame shift gene defect encoding the dystrophin protein (Xp21), great hope exists for a cure with gene therapy. Without functioning dystrophin there is poor muscle fiber regeneration, and thus there is a progressive replacement of muscle tissue with fat and fibrous tissues. Over time, skeletal and cardiac muscle undergo loss of elasticity and strength. Clinically, boys present between ages 3 to 6 years with complaints such as delayed walking or toe walking. Often a history is given of difficulty climbing stairs, hopping, or jumping. The first symptoms of DMD can be subtle, with weakness often being attributed to lack of effort, and the child is deemed lazy instead of weak. Clinical features include pseudohypertrophy of the calf and the presence of a positive Gower sign or Trendelenburg sign. Proximal muscle weakness is greater than weakness in distal musculature; lumbar lordosis is a common compensation for gluteal weakness, whereas circumduction of the limb compensates for weakness in the hip flexors. Other orthopaedic concerns include joint contractures and scoliosis.

Diagnosis of DMD can be suspected when serum creatine phosphokinase level is significantly elevated above normal early in the disease course. Dystrophin gene anomalies can be detected in more than half of cases, and muscle biopsy with dystrophin staining can often be helpful in making the diagnosis of DMD if other tests are inconclusive. Becker muscular dystrophy occurs with a less disruptive gene mutation than DMD and has a more benign course. Abnormal dystrophin is produced and, unlike in DMD, can be detected on muscle biopsy.

Glucocorticoids have been found to improve muscle strength, prolong walking, and reduce scoliosis. Prednisone has been found effective but has side effects including weight gain, loss of bone density, and behavioral changes that frequently necessitate tapering of the drug. Deflazacort (available in Canada and Europe) has been shown to have the same benefits as prednisone with fewer side effects.

Scoliosis in DMD begins when patients lose ambulatory capacity; thus, screening for curve progression should commence when children become wheelchair dependent. Scoliosis in DMD is associated with increased kyphosis in the thoracolumbar or lumbar spine as well as pelvic obliquity. Patients are best managed surgically for curves between 20° and 30° to avoid complications. Patients with DMD are at increased risk for malignant hyperthermia and intraoperative cardiac events. A careful preoperative assessment should include studies of cardiac function (such as with an echocardiogram) as well as lung function depending on the needs of the patient. Fusion is usually carried to the pelvis to treat pelvic obliquity, which if left uncorrected may interfere with sitting balance. Pelvic obliquity may be difficult to treat later because of worsening cardiac and pulmonary function.[48]

Spinal Muscular Atrophy

Spinal muscular atrophy (SMA) is an autosomal recessive disorder with proximal muscle weakness caused by primary degeneration of the anterior horn cells in the spinal cord. The incidence of SMA is 1 in 6,000, but SMA is among the most lethal genetic childhood disorders. The gene defect has been identified in chromosome 5q, which codes for the survival motor neuron proteins SMN 1 and SMN 2–the disorder occurs with loss of SMN 1, whereas the severity is predicted by the copy number of SMN 2. The higher the copy number of SMN 2, the milder the phenotype.

SMA is classified into three types; type 1 is often identified at birth—the infant is floppy and has loss of deep tendon reflexes and tongue fasciculation. Although the diaphragm is spared, the clearing of airway secretions is diminished due to intercostal weakness in patients with type 1 SMA, leading to atelectasis and pneumonia. Type 2 SMA has a milder course and presents later in life, between age 6 months and 2 years. Muscle weakness is greater in the lower extremities than the upper extremities, making ambulation difficult. Type 3 SMA is characterized by later presentation and a normal life expectancy.

Progressive scoliosis is the most common orthopaedic concern (**Figure 6**). Bracing is ineffectual in halting curve progression and can exacerbate respiratory difficulties, and thus should be avoided. Children with SMA are more likely to experience increased survival rates,[49] believed to be secondary to better nutritional management and advances in pulmonary care; as a result, spinal deformity management should not be withheld under the assumption that the child with type 1 SMA will not survive. Posterior spinal fusion down to the pelvis for curves greater than 40° should be considered before the curve gets large enough to become a contributing factor to diminished respiratory function. An anterior approach to the spine should be avoided whenever possible.

Other orthopaedic sequelae of SMA include hip dysplasia and joint contractures. Hip dysplasia may require treatment after taking into account walking potential as well as unilateral versus bilateral hip involvement. Contractures can be managed with stretching or surgical releases.

As with CP, patients with SMA have been found to be at risk for obesity with increased fat mass and reduced lean mass despite low body mass index.[50] Increased weight can impede function in children with weakness and should be of concern in this patient population. Awareness of the potential for obesity and referral for dietary management may help optimize function.[50]

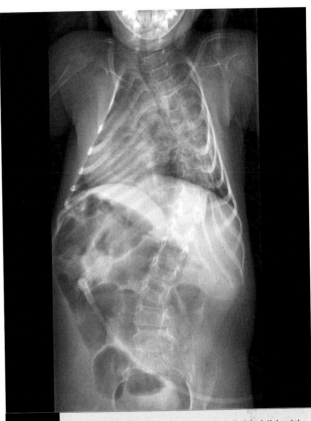

Figure 6 AP scoliosis radiograph of a 4-year-old child with type 1 SMA. Note the long C-shaped curve consistent with paralytic scoliosis and the particular bell-shaped thorax, which is a result of intercostal paralysis and is characteristic of SMA.

Hereditary Motor Sensory Neuropathies

Hereditary motor sensory neuropathies are a group of disorders characterized by sensory neuropathies and progressive wasting of distal musculature caused by degeneration of the peripheral nerves. Charcot-Marie-Tooth (CMT) disease is the most common of the hereditary motor sensory neuropathies that is part of a heterogeneous group of genetic disorders with more than 30 known gene mutations involving many different nerve functional pathways such as myelination, axonal transport, Schwann cell differentiation, and nerve cell function.

There is a wide clinical spectrum to this disease, including all forms of mendelian inheritance patterns, variable age of onset, and of disease progression. Although hip dysplasia is seen in less than 10% of all patients with CMT, a recent study documented hip dysplasia occurring after age 8 years in four patients[51] (**Figure 7**). Hip dysplasia presenting later in childhood is a possible presenting clinical feature in CMT. In children who have late dysplasia and a broad-based gait, a work-up for CMT should be performed.[51] Common orthopaedic findings include cavovarus feet, wasting of the intrinsic muscles of the hand, and clawing of the toes. Patients can also have loss of sensation, including

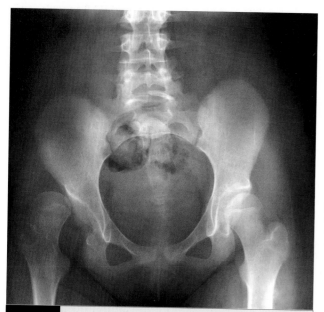

Figure 7 Radiograph of the pelvis of a 12-year-old girl with bilateral foot deformities and left hip pain. She had a history of CMT disease and bilateral hip dysplasia that was worse on the left side.

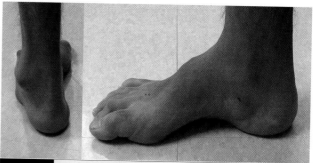

Figure 8 Posterior and side radiographic view of the foot of a boy with Friedreich ataxia and a cavovarus foot. On the posterior view his heel is in marked varus positioning. On the lateral view he has a high arch consistent with cavus deformity and with obvious clawing of the toes.

vibration, light touch, and proprioception, as well as absent deep tendon reflexes.

Analysis of gait patterns in patients with CMT shows that the hip flexors compensate for weakness in ankle plantar flexion by taking over the task of initiation of swing phase. When patients develop hip flexor fatigue, walking velocity and duration are reduced. With fatigue, trunk flexion increases as a secondary compensation. The gait analysis data cause one to wonder whether possible selective proximal muscle strengthening of hips and trunk might help patients improve walking stamina by helping to maintain gait compensations.

Although high-dose ascorbic acid was shown to have a beneficial effect in a mouse model of CMT where remyelination was demonstrated after drug use, initial clinical trials in children did not reproduce the same results seen in the mice but no toxicity was reported as a result of the dosing regimen.[52]

Friedreich Ataxia

Friedreich ataxia is the most common of the spinocerebellar degenerative disorders.[53] The condition is an autosomal recessive disorder caused by a defect on chromosome 9 that causes a loss of the mitochondrial protein fraxatin. The lack of fraxatin causes iron to accumulate in mitochondria, causing oxidative stress–particularly in nerve and muscle tissues. The disorder is progressive with development of an ataxic gait, areflexia, dysarthria, muscle weakness, and loss of vibratory sense and proprioception. Orthopaedic concerns include scoliosis, pes cavovarus, and gait devia-

tions (**Figure 8**). In general, patients lose ambulation in the second or third decade of life, and succumb to cardiomyopathy or respiratory sequelae in the fourth or fifth decades.[53] Treatment of pes cavovarus includes tenotomy, or transfer of either the anterior or posterior tibialis tendon in a supple foot, reserving triple arthrodesis for a rigid foot deformity.

Scoliotic curves can occur in more than 60% of patients and may be difficult to characterize as neuromuscular curves because no real defined curve pattern exists for Friedreich ataxia. Bracing has recently been shown to be of only limited use in slowing curve progression. Bracing is poorly tolerated as it restricts compensatory trunk movement that helps with balance for walking. Curve progression is related to age of disease presentation, and some patients require spinal fusion. The results of spinal fusion using segmental fixation have been outstanding.[54]

Promising medical management with the short chain benzoquinone, idebenone, is in current clinical trials to work out optimal dosing and patient selection. Idebenone was developed for cognitive disorders such as Alzheimer disease and is similar in structure to coenzyme Q 10. Idebenone allows reversible redux reactions to occur. Already idebenone has proved helpful both for improving cardiac hypertrophy as seen on echocardiogram and for improving neurologic function.[55] However, the effect of the drug on the orthopaedic aspects of Friedreich ataxia such as scoliosis curve progression and pes cavovarus are not yet known.

Annotated References

1. Wagner KR: Approaching a new age in Duchenne muscular dystrophy treatment. *Neurotherapeutics* 2008; 5(4):583-591.

   The author reviews novel and emerging therapeutic strategies for the treatment of DMD.

2. Oeffinger D, Bagley A, Rogers S, et al: Outcome tools used for ambulatory children with cerebral palsy: Re-

sponsiveness and minimum clinically important differences. *Dev Med Child Neurol* 2008;50(12):918-925.

The authors evaluate the minimal change needed in outcome measures to be associated with clinical impact.

3. Nelson KB: Causative factors in cerebral palsy. *Clin Obstet Gynecol* 2008;51(4):749-762.

    A review article on the causes of cerebral palsy is presented.

4. Kruse M, Michelsen SI, Flachs EM, Brønnum-Hansen H, Madsen M, Uldall P: Lifetime costs of cerebral palsy. *Dev Med Child Neurol* 2009;51(8):622-628.

    Studies performed in Europe have findings similar to those from earlier studies in the United States.

5. Thompson GH, Florentino-Pineda I, Poe-Kochert C, Armstrong DG, Son-Hing J: Role of Amicar in surgery for neuromuscular scoliosis. *Spine (Phila Pa 1976)* 2008;33(24):2623-2629.

    The authors discuss a group of studies on outcomes of spine surgery and ways to decrease the morbidity of bleeding and infection.

6. Shilt JS, Lai LP, Cabrera MN, Frino J, Smith BP: The impact of intrathecal baclofen on the natural history of scoliosis in cerebral palsy. *J Pediatr Orthop* 2008;28(6):684-687.

    The authors determined that the progression of scoliosis in patients with CP who received ITB treatment is not significantly different from that in patients not treated with ITB.

7. Senaran H, Shah SA, Presedo A, Dabney KW, Glutting JW, Miller F: The risk of progression of scoliosis in cerebral palsy patients after intrathecal baclofen therapy. *Spine (Phila Pa 1976)* 2007;32(21):2348-2354.

8. Ginsburg GM, Lauder AJ: Progression of scoliosis in patients with spastic quadriplegia after the insertion of an intrathecal baclofen pump. *Spine (Phila Pa 1976)* 2007;32(24):2745-2750.

9. Sansone JM, Mann D, Noonan K, Mcleish D, Ward M, Iskandar BJ: Rapid progression of scoliosis following insertion of intrathecal baclofen pump. *J Pediatr Orthop* 2006;26(1):125-128.

    Clinical studies with differing conclusions about the influence of ITB on scoliosis are discussed.

10. Molenaers G, Desloovere K, Fabry G, De Cock P: The effects of quantitative gait assessment and botulinum toxin A on musculoskeletal surgery in children with cerebral palsy. *J Bone Joint Surg Am* 2006;88(1):161-170.

11. Simpson DM, Gracies J-M, Graham H-K, et al; Therapeutics and Technology Assessment Subcommittee of the American Academy of Neurology: Assessment: Botulinum neurotoxin for the treatment of spasticity (an evidence-based review). Report of the Therapeutics and Technology Assessment Subcommittee of the American Academy of Neurology. *Neurology* 2008;70(19):1691-1698.

An analysis of the current literature from the American Academy of Neurology indicates that there is level I evidence to support the efficacy of botulinum-toxin administration for treatment of equinus; other areas of botulinum-toxin administration do not yet have enough information in the literature to assess the outcome of botulinum-toxin treatment.

12. Graham HK, Boyd R, Carlin JB, et al: Does botulinum toxin A combined with bracing prevent hip displacement in children with cerebral palsy and "hips at risk"? A randomized, controlled trial. *J Bone Joint Surg Am* 2008;90(1):23-33.

    This study design demonstrates no effect of botulinum toxin combined with hip abduction bracing for prevention of hip subluxation.

13. Rogozinski BM, Davids JR, Davis RB, et al: Prevalence of obesity in ambulatory children with cerebral palsy. *J Bone Joint Surg Am* 2007;89(11):2421-2426.

14. Hurvitz EA, Green LB, Hornyak JE, Khurana SR, Koch LG: Body mass index measures in children with cerebral palsy related to gross motor function classification: A clinic-based study. *Am J Phys Med Rehabil* 2008;87(5):395-403.

    Analysis of body mass index suggests that patients with CP are more likely to be overweight.

15. Feeley BT, Gollapudi K, Otsuka NY: Body mass index in ambulatory cerebral palsy patients. *J Pediatr Orthop B* 2007;16(3):165-169.

    Counterintuitive findings regarding the presence of obesity in a group of cerebral palsy patients are presented. Confounding variables of malnutrition and mobility affect the findings.

16. Murphy NA, Hoff C, Jorgensen T, Norlin C, Young PC: Costs and complications of hospitalizations for children with cerebral palsy. *Pediatr Rehabil* 2006;9(1):47-52.

17. Modi HN, Hong JY, Mehta SS, et al: Surgical correction and fusion using posterior-only pedicle screw construct for neuropathic scoliosis in patients with cerebral palsy: A three-year follow-up study. *Spine (Phila Pa 1976)* 2009;34(11):1167-1175.

    In a retrospective study of 52 patients with neuromuscular scoliosis and CP, posterior-only pedicle screw fixation resulted in satisfactory coronal and sagittal correction without higher complication rates.

18. Suh SW, Modi HN, Yang J, Song HR, Jang KM: Posterior multilevel vertebral osteotomy for correction of severe and rigid neuromuscular scoliosis: A preliminary study. *Spine (Phila Pa 1976)* 2009;34(12):1315-1320.

    The authors studied the effectiveness of posterior multilevel vertebral osteotomy in patients with severe and rigid neuromuscular scoliosis and determined that one reason the technique should be recommended is because it provides release of the anterior column without an anterior approach.

6: Pediatrics

19. Tsirikos AI, Lipton G, Chang WN, Dabney KW, Miller F: Surgical correction of scoliosis in pediatric patients with cerebral palsy using the unit rod instrumentation. *Spine (Phila Pa 1976)* 2008;33(10):1133-1140.

   In a retrospective clinical and radiographic consecutive case series, it was determined that unit rod instrumentation in the treatment of children with CP is easy to use, less expensive than other systems, and can achieve good deformity correction with low prevalence of associated complications.

20. Sponseller PD, Shah SA, Abel MF, et al; Harms Study Group: Scoliosis surgery in cerebral palsy: Differences between unit rod and custom rods. *Spine (Phila Pa 1976)* 2009;34(8):840-844.

   The outcomes and varying techniques in the management of neuromuscular scoliosis are discussed. It is suggested that correction can be achieved with posterior instrumentation and fusion alone though the choice of instrumentation varies with some discussion of the cost differences between the unit rod and pedicular screws.

21. Borkhuu B, Borowski A, Shah SA, Littleton AG, Dabney KW, Miller F: Antibiotic-loaded allograft decreases the rate of acute deep wound infection after spinal fusion in cerebral palsy. *Spine (Phila Pa 1976)* 2008;33(21):2300-2304.

   This study reports a decrease in the incidence of deep wound infection after spinal fusion in 220 children with CP scoliosis from 15% to 4% with the use of prophylactic antibiotics in the corticocancellous allograft bone.

22. Caird MS, Palanca AA, Garton H, et al: Outcomes of posterior spinal fusion and instrumentation in patients with continuous intrathecal baclofen infusion pumps. *Spine (Phila Pa 1976)* 2008;33(4):E94-E99.

   A descriptive study of complications in patients with continuous ITB pumps is presented.

23. Soo B, Howard JJ, Boyd RN, et al: Hip displacement in cerebral palsy. *J Bone Joint Surg Am* 2006;88(1):121-129.

24. Miller F, Bagg MR: Age and migration percentage as risk factors for progression in spastic hip disease. *Dev Med Child Neurol* 1995;37(5):449-455.

25. Chung CY, Choi IH, Cho TJ, Yoo WJ, Lee SH, Park MS: Morphometric changes in the acetabulum after Dega osteotomy in patients with cerebral palsy. *J Bone Joint Surg Br* 2008;90(1):88-91.

   This study reports an increase in mean acetabular volume of 68% with anterosuperior, superolateral, and posterosuperior coverage improvement after Dega osteotomy in 17 hips in 12 patients as measured by CT scan.

26. Schmale GA, Eilert RE, Chang F, Seidel K: High reoperation rates after early treatment of the subluxating hip in children with spastic cerebral palsy. *J Pediatr Orthop* 2006;26(5):617-623.

27. Rodda JM, Graham HK, Carson L, Galea MP, Wolfe R: Sagittal gait patterns in spastic diplegia. *J Bone Joint Surg Br* 2004;86(2):251-258.

28. Riad J, Haglund-Akerlind Y, Miller F: Classification of spastic hemiplegic cerebral palsy in children. *J Pediatr Orthop* 2007;27(7):758-764.

   Refinement of the classification of Winters of patterns of hemiplegic gait is discussed.

29. Koshino T, Sugimoto K: New measurement of patellar height in the knees of children using the epiphyseal line midpoint. *J Pediatr Orthop* 1989;9(2):216-218.

30. Stout JL, Gage JR, Schwartz MH, Novacheck TF: Distal femoral extension osteotomy and patellar tendon advancement to treat persistent crouch gait in cerebral palsy. *J Bone Joint Surg Am* 2008;90(11):2470-2484.

   A series of patients reviewed showed that patella advancement improves knee extension over extension osteotomy alone. Level of evidence: IV.

31. Karol LA, Chambers C, Popejoy D, Birch JG: Nerve palsy after hamstring lengthening in patients with cerebral palsy. *J Pediatr Orthop* 2008;28(7):773-776.

   The authors present a descriptive series on a complication that is underrecognized.

32. Westberry DE, Davids JR, Shaver JC, Tanner SL, Blackhurst DW, Davis RB: Impact of ankle-foot orthoses on static foot alignment in children with cerebral palsy. *J Bone Joint Surg Am* 2007;89(4):806-813.

   A study using a reproducible standardized radiographic measure shows clinically insignificant improvement in deformity with the use of an orthosis.

33. Fry NR, Gough M, McNee AE, Shortland AP: Changes in the volume and length of the medial gastrocnemius after surgical recession in children with spastic diplegic cerebral palsy. *J Pediatr Orthop* 2007;27(7):769-774.

   The application of a "new" technology to evaluate anatomic outcome in a small series of patients is discussed.

34. McNee AE, Gough M, Morrissey MC, Shortland AP: Increases in muscle volume after plantarflexor strength training in children with spastic cerebral palsy. *Dev Med Child Neurol* 2009;51(6):429-435.

   This study, using ultrasound, demonstrated that muscle volume increased significantly between 7 weeks and 1 year after Vulpius calf surgery in a group of seven patients.

35. Adams SB Jr, Simpson AW, Pugh LI, Stasikelis PJ: Calcaneocuboid joint subluxation after calcaneal lengthening for planovalgus foot deformity in children with cerebral palsy. *J Pediatr Orthop* 2009;29(2):170-174.

   Stabilization of the calcaneocuboid joint at the time of lateral column lengthening did not significantly reduce the incidence or magnitude of subluxation when compared with nonstabilized lengthening and had no significant influence on radiographic outcome or osteoarthritic changes at the calcaneocuboid joint.

6: Pediatrics

36. Templin D, Jones K, Weiner DS: The incorporation of allogeneic and autogenous bone graft in healing of lateral column lengthening of the calcaneus. *J Foot Ankle Surg* 2008;47(4):283-287.

Thirty-five lateral column lengthenings in 26 patients were reviewed, 30 of which used allograft bone and 5 autograft. Ninety-seven percent of the allograft cases and 80% of the autograft cases were incorporated at final follow-up. The authors recommend the use of allograft as outcome was not adversely affected and donor site morbidity can be avoided.

37. Park KB, Park HW, Lee KS, Joo SY, Kim HW: Changes in dynamic foot pressure after surgical treatment of valgus deformity of the hindfoot in cerebral palsy. *J Bone Joint Surg Am* 2008;90(8):1712-1721.

This study demonstrates, through the use of dynamic foot pressure measurement, that both extra-articular subtalar arthrodesis and calcaneal neck lengthening correct the valgus hindfoot deformity in patients with cerebral palsy. However, residual supination deformity with abnormal forefoot pressure was present after fusion with postoperative foot pressure distribution more closely approximates the normal foot pressure distribution after neck lengthening.

38. Michlitsch MG, Rethlefsen SA, Kay RM: The contributions of anterior and posterior tibialis dysfunction to varus foot deformity in patients with cerebral palsy. *J Bone Joint Surg Am* 2006;88(8):1764-1768.

39. Müller EB, Nordwall A, Odén A: Progression of scoliosis in children with myelomeningocele. *Spine (Phila Pa 1976)* 1994;19(2):147-150.

40. Akbar M, Bresch B, Seyler TM, et al: Management of orthopaedic sequelae of congenital spinal disorders. *J Bone Joint Surg Am* 2009;91(suppl 6):87-100.

The authors discuss congenital spinal disorders and their treatment.

41. Ouellet JA, Geller L, Strydom WS, et al: Pressure mapping as an outcome measure for spinal surgery in patients with myelomeningocele. *Spine (Phila Pa 1976)* 2009;34(24):2679-2685.

The authors studied the effect of improved pressure distribution on patients with myelomeningocele and found that pressure mapping may not be useful in predicting outcome of spinal surgery.

42. Crawford AH, Strub WM, Lewis R, et al: Neonatal kyphectomy in the patient with myelomeningocele. *Spine (Phila Pa 1976)* 2003;28(3):260-266.

43. Ko AL, Song K, Ellenbogen RG, Avellino AM: Retrospective review of multilevel spinal fusion combined with spinal cord transection for treatment of kyphoscoliosis in pediatric myelomeningocele patients. *Spine (Phila Pa 1976)* 2007;32(22):2493-2501.

The authors performed a retrospective review of surgical experience, complications, and insights on nine patients with myelomeningocele and kyphoscoliosis treated with spinal cord transection and spinal fusion.

This treatment allowed an average correction of kyphosis of 81.9°.

44. Glard Y, Launay F, Viehweger E, Guillaume JM, Jouve JL, Bollini G: Hip flexion contracture and lumbar spine lordosis in myelomeningocele. *J Pediatr Orthop* 2005;25(4):476-478.

45. Gerlach DJ, Gurnett CA, Limpaphayom N, et al: Early results of the Ponseti method for the treatment of clubfoot associated with myelomeningocele. *J Bone Joint Surg Am* 2009;91(6):1350-1359.

The authors support the use of the Ponseti method to treat clubfoot deformity associated with myelomeningocele. Attention to detail is important to avoid complications.

46. Park KB, Park HW, Joo SY, Kim HW: Surgical treatment of calcaneal deformity in a select group of patients with myelomeningocele. *J Bone Joint Surg Am* 2008;90(10):2149-2159.

The authors studied 31 feet in 18 patients and found that surgical treatment of calcaneal deformity in patients with myelomeningocele can reduce pressure on the calcaneus, increase pressures in the forefoot and midfoot, and prevent recurrence of calcaneal deformity. Level of evidence: IV.

47. Apkon SD, Fenton L, Coll JR: Bone mineral density in children with myelomeningocele. *Dev Med Child Neurol* 2009;51(1):63-67.

In a study of 24 children with myelomeningocele, the authors found that reduced bone mineral density is a major complication.

48. Karol LA: Scoliosis in patients with Duchenne muscular dystrophy. *J Bone Joint Surg Am* 2007;89(suppl 1):155-162.

A comprehensive review of the management of scoliosis in DMD is presented.

49. Mannaa MM, Kalra M, Wong B, Cohen AP, Amin RS: Survival probabilities of patients with childhood spinal muscle atrophy. *J Clin Neuromuscul Dis* 2009;10(3):85-89.

This study reviews two decades of data on children with SMA and finds significantly improved life expectancy in patients with type 1 SMA. The positive trend toward improved survival is thought to be attributable to better nutritional support and pulmonary care.

50. Sproule DM, Montes JM, Montgomery M, et al: Increased fat mass and high incidence of overweight despite low body mass index in patients with spinal muscular atrophy. *Neuromuscul Disord* 2009;19(6):391-396.

Obesity is identified in children with SMA as a potential source of modifiable morbidity. Body mass index was not as predictive of obesity in this patient population as in normal children.

51. Bamford NS, White KK, Robinett SA, Otto RK, Gospe SM Jr: Neuromuscular hip dysplasia in Charcot-Marie-

6: Pediatrics

Tooth disease type 1A. *Dev Med Child Neurol* 2009; 51(5):408-411.

Four patients present with late-onset hip dysplasia. The diagnosis of CMT disease is entertained and peripheral neuropathies are found clinically followed by a formal diagnosis of CMT disease. Thus, hip dysplasia can be a presenting sign of CMT disease, which has a wide spectrum of disease severity and presentation.

52. Burns J, Ouvrier RA, Yiu EM, et al: Ascorbic acid for Charcot-Marie-Tooth disease type 1A in children: A randomised, double-blind, placebo-controlled, safety and efficacy trial. *Lancet Neurol* 2009;8(6):537-544.

High-dose ascorbic acid was well tolerated in children with CMT disease; however, no expected improvements in function, strength, or quality of life could be demonstrated.

53. Bernard G, Shevell M: The wobbly child: An approach to inherited ataxias. *Semin Pediatr Neurol* 2008;15(4): 194-208.

Using three case histories, including one child with Friedreich ataxia, the authors present a systematic approach to diagnosis and genetic evaluation of children with ataxia.

54. Milbrandt TA, Kunes JR, Karol LA: Friedreich's ataxia and scoliosis: The experience at two institutions. *J Pediatr Orthop* 2008;28(2):234-238.

A review of patients with Friedreich ataxia with scoliosis is presented. For those needing surgery, somatosensory-evoked potentials were not reliably obtained during surgery.

55. Meier T, Buyse G: Idebenone: An emerging therapy for Friedreich ataxia. *J Neurol* 2009;256(suppl 1):25-30.

The development of idebenone and the evidence of cardiac and neurologic improvement are reviewed.

Chapter 64

Pediatric Tumors and Hematologic Diseases

Todd Milbrandt, MD, MS   Henry J. Iwinski, Jr, MD   Vishwas R. Talwalkar, MD

Benign Bone Tumors

Children with benign tumors may present with a palpable mass, pain with activities, a pathologic fracture, or an incidental finding on radiographs. History may reveal pain with activities, which may be indicative of weakened bone or sudden onset of pain with minimal trauma as a result of a pathologic fracture. The age of the patient, history, physical examination, and radiographic features are frequently enough to make a diagnosis. Treatment may range from observation for the asymptomatic small lesion with a benign clinical course to resection for locally aggressive lesions.

Osteoid Osteoma

Osteoid osteoma is a benign but painful (often at night) lesion that occurs in all age groups. It is most frequently found in the cortex of the femur and tibia where patients typically present with pain that is progressive and well localized. In the limb they may have surrounding muscle atrophy and/or gait disturbance, depending on location. The tumors also have a predilection for the posterior elements of the spine, and a mild scoliosis may develop as a result of painful paraspinal muscle spasm. Nonsteroidal anti-inflammatory drugs (NSAIDs) are particularly effective in relieving symptoms and can assist in making the diagnosis. The lesion is apparent on plain radiographs as a fusiform cortical thickening with a small radiolucent central nidus less than 1 cm in diameter. The lesion displays markedly increased uptake on bone scan. Because of the width of image slices, MRI of the involved area may only show widespread inflammatory signal change and soft-tissue edema without re-

Dr. Milbrandt or an immediate family member serves as a board member, owner, officer, or committee member of the Pediatric Orthopaedic Society of North America and the Scoliosis Research Society and has received research or institutional support from DePuy, a Johnson & Johnson Company and DJ Orthopaedics. Neither of the following authors or any immediate family member has received anything of value from or owns stock in a commercial company or institution related directly or indirectly to the subject of this chapter: Dr. Iwinski, Dr. Talwalkar.

vealing the nidus. In these cases and especially in the spine, fine-cut CT is effective in outlining the lesion and planning treatment. Treatment of the lesion depends on the location and symptoms. Some lesions will "burn out" and require only observation.[1] Medical treatment with NSAIDs has also been effective, but typically requires several years of management. Minimally invasive ablation using radiofrequency or laser energy has the least morbidity and is the most effective treatment method, particularly for periarticular lesions.[2] Surgical treatment is rarely necessary except to obtain tissue for diagnosis or for lesions that cannot be safely approached with minimally invasive techniques.

Osteoblastoma

Osteoblastoma is a benign bone-forming tumor that is similar to osteoid osteoma in several ways. It is found primarily in the long bones of the lower limbs and the posterior spine. Spinal deformity is often apparent in patients with spinal lesions. Patients present with pain at the lesion and/or signs of disuse. The pain is described as dull and aching but is not relieved by anti-inflammatory medications. Bone scan reveals increased uptake and may be helpful to localize axial lesions. This tumor is less common and is larger in size than osteoid osteoma, occurring chiefly in the second decade and twice as frequently in males. Osteoblastoma is classically described as a fusiform radiodense cortical lesion with a central nidus greater than 1.5 cm in diameter. However, in a large series of appendicular lesions, less than 50% displayed a characteristic radiographic appearance, and 10% were initially thought to be malignant.[3] The lesion may appear locally destructive with cortical resorption, soft-tissue invasion, and periosteal new bone formation. Thus, the diagnosis may be difficult and is delayed on average by 6 months.[4] CT reveals specific location, size, and differentiating characteristics most clearly. MRI assists in defining surrounding soft-tissue involvement and proximity to neurovascular structures. Osteoblastoma can display locally aggressive growth that requires surgical treatment. Intralesional resection has yielded a recurrence rate in patients of all ages of 15% to 30%. A four-step method of complete excision has been described with a 6% recurrence rate.[4]

6: Pediatrics

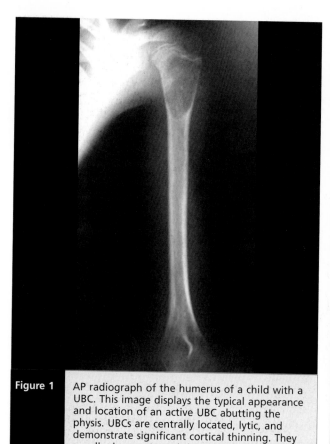

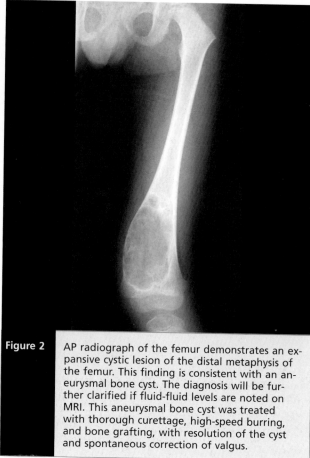

Figure 1 AP radiograph of the humerus of a child with a UBC. This image displays the typical appearance and location of an active UBC abutting the physis. UBCs are centrally located, lytic, and demonstrate significant cortical thinning. They usually do not expand the bone beyond the width of the physis.

Figure 2 AP radiograph of the femur demonstrates an expansive cystic lesion of the distal metaphysis of the femur. This finding is consistent with an aneurysmal bone cyst. The diagnosis will be further clarified if fluid-fluid levels are noted on MRI. This aneurysmal bone cyst was treated with thorough curettage, high-speed burring, and bone grafting, with resolution of the cyst and spontaneous correction of valgus.

Benign Cystic Lesions of Bone

Unicameral Bone Cysts

Simple or unicameral bone cysts (UBCs) are benign bone lesions commonly seen in pediatric patients. They are fluid-filled cysts often located in the proximal femur and proximal humerus. Most are asymptomatic unless pathologic fracture occurs. Fracture healing usually does not stimulate cyst resolution. Radiographs reveal a centrally located, lytic, well-demarcated metaphyseal lesion with cortical thinning (**Figure 1**). Biopsy is usually indicated for questionable diagnosis based on history or atypical imaging. Treatment is usually recommended for large lesions in weight-bearing bones, as these are more likely to be painful or lead to fracture with resultant deformity and functional disability. In the upper extremity, treatment may be recommended because of the risk of recurrent pathologic fractures. A variety of techniques have been used to induce cyst resolution including injection with steroid, bone marrow aspirate, demineralized bone matrix, and calcium sulfate, as well as needle, flexible nail, or cannulated screw decompression.[5] All have reported some success but no single approach has proved to be most advantageous.[6,7] Open treatment with curettage and bone grafting is reserved for lesions with questionable diagnosis, displaced pathologic fractures that require open reduc-

tion (commonly of the proximal femur), very large lesions, or those that have recurred multiple times. The cysts usually resolve as the patient approaches skeletal maturity. Many of these lesions abut the physis, which can make complete removal difficult and result in higher recurrence rates; it should be noted that growth arrest occurs, albeit rarely, as a result of the cyst itself as well as too-aggressive curettage near the growth plate.

Aneurysmal Bone Cysts

Aneurysmal bone cysts are benign, cystic lesions composed of blood-filled spaces with thin fibrous septae. Radiographs demonstrate an eccentric, lytic, expansile metaphyseal lesion with very thin cortical margins. The most common location is the metaphyseal region around the knee. They are less common and more locally aggressive than UBCs. Aneurysmal bone cyts may be considered primary or be secondarily seen in association with other lesions. Primary lesions are associated with a rearrangement of chromosome band 17p13. Approximately 75% of patients are younger than 20 years. Symptoms depend on the location and size of the lesion and include increasing pain, warmth, and a palpable bony mass. Spinal lesions usually are in the posterior elements and may present with neurologic signs and symptoms (**Figure 2**). Differential diagnosis in-

6: Pediatrics

cludes UBC and telangiectatic osteosarcoma.

Because the lesions are locally aggressive, most require open curettage, adjuvant therapy (phenol, cryotherapy, or high-speed burr) and bone grafting. The recurrence rate is approximately 20% but may be higher in young children. Percutaneous injection with a variety of substances (steroids, demineralized bone matrix, bioglass calcium sulfate, and sclerosing agents) has been performed with variable success for lesions that are difficult to approach surgically.[8]

Malignant Bone Tumors

The evaluation of children with suspected musculoskeletal malignancy is similar to that for adults. A thorough assessment of symptoms and the effect of these symptoms on function (along with a skillful physical examination) guides imaging and/or laboratory evaluation to localize and characterize the process. If additional staging studies and biopsy are necessary, they should be performed in consultation with the local musculoskeletal tumor center.

Osteosarcoma

Osteosarcoma is a highly malignant bone-producing tumor composed of spindle cells that produce malignant osteoid and bone. Its peak incidence is in males in the second decade of life. This tumor occurs most often in the appendicular skeleton in the metaphyses of the femur and tibia and is usually painful. Pain that occurs at night, is worsening, causes limping, changes activity, and consistently occurs in the same location is particularly worrisome for a locally destructive process. Initial radiographs of the entire bone are taken and usually show mixed areas of increased bone density and destruction, poorly defined margins and periosteal reaction described as onion-skinning, sunbursting, and Codman triangles (**Figure 3**). MRI of the entire bone should also be performed to evaluate for extent of tumor, skip lesions, soft-tissue involvement, and neurovascular invasion. The role of positron emission tomography in the staging and surveillance of patients with sarcomas is still being refined.[9] Chest CT and bone scan are also vital staging studies to assess for metastatic disease. Although gross metastases are evident in 10% to 20% of cases, all patients should be assumed to have micrometastasis. Biopsy and treatment should be performed at a center with experience caring for musculoskeletal malignancy to optimize diagnostic accuracy and appropriate treatment. Surgical resection and reconstruction typically occurs after two to three cycles of chemotherapy. Neoadjuvant chemotherapeutic protocols have increased 5-year survival rates to almost 80% at multiple centers in patients with nonmetastatic disease and 10% to 20% with metastatic disease.[10] Poor prognostic factors include metastatic disease at presentation, poor response to chemotherapy (less than 90% necrosis of resected tumor), axial location, large tumor size, pathologic fracture, and elevated alkaline

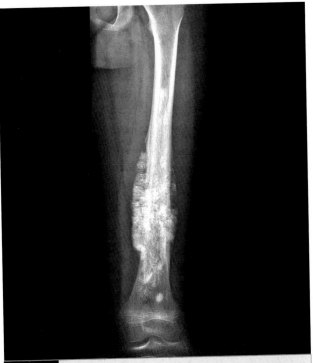

| Figure 3 | AP radiograph from a 12-year-old girl shows characteristic radiographic findings of femoral osteosarcoma: a large metaphyseal lesion with poorly defined margins, blastic expansion into the soft tissues, and periosteal sunbursting. |

phosphatase and lactate dehydrogenase levels. Overall 5-year survival rates are 60% to 80%.

Ewing Sarcoma

Ewing sarcoma is the second most common malignant bone tumor in skeletally immature patients age 5 to 30 years and is most frequently seen in Caucasian males. The particular cell type involved has not been completely characterized, but may be of neuronal origin. Cytogenetic evaluation has revealed a reciprocal translocation of t(11;22) that ultimately results in the production of transcription factor EWS/FLI1 that may have mechanistic importance.[11] The tumor may involve the axial or appendicular skeleton and is usually painful. The tumor is usually seen as a permeative process on plain films with a large soft-tissue mass evident on MRI (**Figure 4**). Prior to surgical treatment, most patients will undergo neoadjuvant chemotherapy to allow for tumor shrinkage, increase the chance of clear surgical margins, and facilitate limb salvage. Systemic chemotherapy is essential and has had a dramatic improvement in 5-year survival rates, which are currently 60% to 80%.[12] Local disease control is obtained surgically in most cases, but in rare cases requires radiation therapy. It primarily metastasizes to the lungs and other bones, but may also involve the bone marrow, thus requiring bone marrow aspirate in addition to standard staging studies. Poor prognostic signs include metastatic disease at presentation, persistently high serum lactate de-

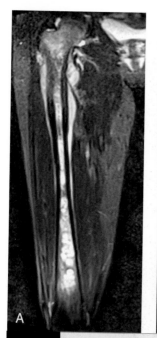
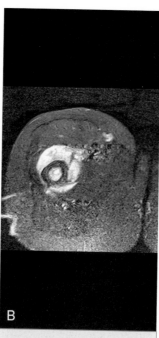

Figure 4   **A,** Coronal T2-weighted MRI of the femur of a 13-year-old girl with thigh pain, illustrating Ewing sarcoma involving the entire femur. The patient was noted to have metastatic disease at presentation, which worsens her prognosis. **B,** Short-tau inversion recovery sequence MRI of the same patient showing a large soft-tissue mass characteristic of patients with Ewing sarcoma.

is performed at the base with resection of the periosteum and perichondrium.[13] Care of shortened and deformed limbs in some patients with multiple hereditary exostosis may require osteotomy, growth arrest, guided growth, or limb lengthening. It is important that patients are aware of the risk of malignant transformation (less than 1% for solitary lesions and 3% for multiple lesions). This occurs in mature patients, and signs include worsening pain, continued growth after skeletal maturity, and a thickened cartilage cap (>1.5 cm).

Enchondroma

Enchondroma is a benign tumor of hyaline cartilage that typically involves the diaphysis of the long bones and is commonly seen in the hand. These can be solitary lesions or multiple enchondromatosis in two genetic conditions. Ollier disease presents with multiple enchondromas in the metaphyses of multiple bones in the upper and lower extremities. Affected individuals can have limb deformity, shortening, intracranial lesions, and overall short stature. Maffucci syndrome consists of similar findings as well as cutaneous hemangioma. Histologically, biopsied tissue is similar to hyaline cartilage except slightly more cellular with atypia and pleomorphism. Limb deformities may require similar procedures used in multiple hereditary exostosis. The risk of malignant transformation is 1% to 3% in Ollier disease, but increased in Maffucci syndrome, with an increased incidence of nonskeletal malignancy.

Chondroblastoma

Chondroblastoma is a rare epiphyseal tumor in the knee, shoulder, and hip seen in the second decade of life. Radiographs show a well-circumscribed epiphyseal lesion possibly with stippled calcification. MRI reveals significant reactive edema, and bone scan shows increased uptake. Complete resection is difficult, and intralesional resection is often unsuccessful, resulting in a 20% rate of recurrence. Significant joint deformity and pain may result from the tumor as well as the treatment. Rarely, pulmonary metastasis may occur.

hydrogenase despite treatment, large tumor size, and pelvic location.

Cartilage Tumors

Osteochondroma

Osteochondroma (exostosis) is a benign tumor most commonly occurring in the metaphyses of the tibia and femur around the knee. However, the lesions are seen in almost any bone and two patterns of involvement, solitary and multiple, are seen. The lesions may limit range of motion depending on location or cause pain by mechanical irritation of the overlying soft tissues, or rarely, compression of adjacent neurovascular structures. Multiple hereditary exostosis is an autosomal dominant condition with variable penetrance. In addition to the presence of multiple exostoses, affected patients may have short stature, limb-length discrepancy, limb angulation, or bowing. The multiple form is linked to mutations in the *EXT 1* and *EXT 2* tumor suppressor genes that code for glycoproteins involved in the regulation of endochondral ossification. The true incidence of spinal lesions that impinge on neural structures is unknown. Certainly any patient with neurologic signs or symptoms should be evaluated with advanced imaging. Surgical treatment of patients may include complete excision of symptomatic lesions; this

Fibrous Lesions

Fibrous Dysplasia

Fibrous dysplasia is a benign fibro-osseous process that can occur in one (monostotic) or multiple (polyostotic) bones. The polyostotic form usually involves half of the skeleton and may be associated with McCune-Albright syndrome (fibrous dysplasia, pigmented skin lesions, and endocrinopathy). It is usually caused by a postzygotic mutation in the gene *GNAS1* (guanine nucleotide-binding protein, alpha stimulating activity polypeptide) on chromosome 20q13.[14] This results in osteoblastic differentiation defects and increased bone resorption. Radiographs reveal mild expansion of the bone, thinning of the cortex, endosteal scalloping, and a "ground glass" appearance of the matrix. Progressive deformity can be seen with large lesions, particularly proximal

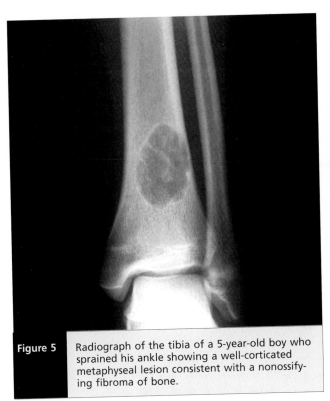

Figure 5 Radiograph of the tibia of a 5-year-old boy who sprained his ankle showing a well-corticated metaphyseal lesion consistent with a nonossifying fibroma of bone.

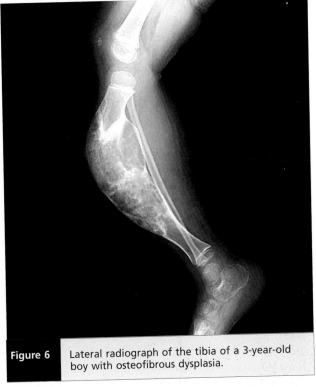

Figure 6 Lateral radiograph of the tibia of a 3-year-old boy with osteofibrous dysplasia.

femoral varus or shepherd's crook deformity. Larger lesions at risk for fracture are best treated with curettage, bone grafting, and prophylactic fixation. Bisphosphonates have been used in the treatment of polyostotic fibrous dysplasia to relieve bone pain, improve lytic lesions, reduce fracture rates, and increase radiographic healing.[15] Calcium, vitamin D, and phosphorus supplements may be useful in some patients.

Nonossifying Fibroma

Nonossifying fibroma of bone is a common incidental finding. The most common locations are the distal femoral metaphysis followed by the proximal tibial and distal tibial metaphyses (**Figure 5**). Radiographs characterize the lesions as metaphyseal, eccentric, lytic, and septated. The cortex can be thinned and there is a rim of bone outlining the lesion. The disorder is benign and most often asymptomatic. Larger lesions may result in pain or a fracture requiring treatment. Treatment is usually observation because most go on to spontaneous regression starting at the end of adolescence. Curettage and prophylactic fixation may be necessary for large symptomatic lesions at risk for fracture. Children who present with nonossifying fibromas at numerous sites may have Jaffe-Campanacci syndrome.[16] These patients may have systemic and dermal findings similar to neurofibromatosis 1.

Osteofibrous Dysplasia

Osteofibrous dysplasia (Campanacci disease) is a fibroosseous condition of the anterior tibial diaphysis that is usually diagnosed before age 10 years. Multiple lesions in the tibia may cause progressive bowing (**Figure 6**),

pathologic fracture, and/or pain. Radiographs reveal the cortex to be focally expanded with a radiolucent lobular pattern and a reactive rim of bone around the periphery. Because of the high rate of recurrence, en bloc resection of a segment of bone is required with reconstruction.[17] The aggressive form is difficult to differentiate from malignant adamantinoma, and requires surgical treatment. This malignant tumor presents with a larger, more painful lesion that is usually found in adults, in whom it can metastasize to the lungs. It usually has soft-tissue extension, intramedullary involvement, and a periosteal reaction in the absence of pathologic fracture.[18]

Eosinophilic Granuloma

Isolated eosinophilic granuloma is the most benign form of histiocytosis X and commonly occurs in children but can occur at any age. Letterer-Siwe disease is a fulminant form that occurs in children younger than 3 years; it usually is lethal. Hand-Christian-Schüller disease is usually seen in children older than 3 years with disseminated histiocytosis X and presents with the triad of exopthalmos, diabetes insipidus, and skull lesions. The most common sites of location for all eosinophilic granulomas are the skull, mandible, pelvis, spine, ribs, and long bones. Pathologic fractures can occur through the lesions. The radiographic appearance differs by location, is nonspecific, and simulates other lesions such as osteomyelitis, leukemia, lymphoma, fibrous dysplasia, or Ewing sarcoma. Commonly, diaphyseal lesions have a lytic, punched-out appearance with periosteal new bone formation or intracortical tunneling. Metaphyseal lesions extend up to but not through the

6: Pediatrics

growth plate. In the spine, the vertebral body is affected, resulting in the characteristic vertebra plana or coin-on-end appearance. Treatment can include observation for the isolated small lesion or vertebral lesions without neurologic involvement. Intralesional treatment with steroids, curettage, radiofrequency ablation,[19] or low-dose radiation has been reported.

Soft-Tissue Tumors

Vascular Malformations

This highly variable group of lesions is the most common type of benign soft-tissue tumor. They vary in size, depth, and type of vascular involvement. Large arterial, venous, or lymphatic malformations continue to grow with the patient. They may be treated by resection, embolization, or sclerotherapy if they become symptomatic. Surgery is often challenging with the potential for large amounts of blood loss and a high rate of recurrence. Local morbidity is also seen from resection of lesions that are infiltrative.

Lipoma

Although very common overall, these lesions are less often seen in children. Lipoblastoma must be considered in the differential diagnosis for infantile fatty tumors. These lesions have an increased recurrence rate and cellularity compared to lipoma. Treatment options include observation for asymptomatic lesions and marginal excision.

Rhabdomyosarcoma

Embryonal and alveolar subtypes of rhabdomyosarcoma occur in the extremities and are the most common soft-tissue malignancy in children. Patients with the embryonal subtype are usually younger than 10 years, whereas those with the alveolar type are adolescents. Alveolar rhabdomyosarcoma has chromosomal translocations: t:(2;13) or t:(1;13). Those with translocation from chromosome 2 usually have a worse prognosis. Patients typically present with a history of a growing soft-tissue mass seen on MRI with increased signal with gadolinium infusion. Ultrasound may be helpful to discern solid from cystic lesions and also to evaluate for blood flow. Positron emission tomography for staging and surveillance is being used more frequently. Staging by chest CT, bone marrow biopsy, and bone scan is also necessary because 20% of patients present with gross metastatic disease (lung, bone marrow, lymphatic tissue, and skeletal tissue). Sentinel lymph node sampling is often necessary. Effective chemotherapeutic regimens have improved overall survival rates from 25% to 70%. Neoadjuvant chemotherapy is used in both subtypes, with the addition of radiation for the alveolar subtype. The 5-year survival is worse overall in alveolar rhabdomyosarcoma (60% survival for nonmetastatic and 30% for metastatic disease). Within this subtype, large tumor size, incomplete resec-

tion, and regional lymph node involvement are all poor prognostic signs.[20]

Synovial Sarcoma

Synovial sarcoma is the second most common pediatric soft-tissue malignancy. It is a lesion that is rarely intra-articular, and the actual tissue of origin is unclear. The tumor may grow undetected for many years and present with an indolent course. Pulmonary metastases and nodal spread are common. A specific translocation, t:(X;18), has been identified that results in several gene products, including the SYT-SSX1 fusion protein, which also is a poor prognostic sign. Treatment is wide excision with adjuvant radiation. The efficacy and role of chemotherapy is still being evaluated.[21]

Infantile Fibrosarcoma

Infantile fibrosarcoma is a very rare but unique tumor of children. It frequently has a striking presentation at birth and is locally aggressive but rarely metastatic. It also has a specific translocation: t:(12;15). Neoadjuvant chemotherapy has been helpful. Complete surgical excision can be curative, but some nonresectable masses may be successfully treated with chemotherapy alone.

Hematologic Diseases

Hemophilia

Hemophilia comprises a group of bleeding disorders in which the most common forms are due to a deficiency in factor VIII (hemophilia A) or factor IX (hemophilia B) and are inherited in a sex-linked recessive pattern. The role of the orthopaedist is to assist the hematologist in the management of muscular hematomas, hemarthroses, and hemophilic joint disease.

Muscular hematomas are treated with clotting factor replacement, prevention of contractures, and rehabilitation. Patients may present with hip pain and a femoral nerve palsy indicative of an iliopsoas hematoma. Diagnosis can be confirmed with MRI, CT, or ultrasonography. Pseudotumors can develop from recurrent bleeding into the muscle or bone and are managed with a combination of factor replacement, radiation therapy, and/or surgical excision.

Hemarthroses are managed conservatively with immediate factor replacement up to 100% for a week to 10 days. Aspiration is only necessary for patients with vascular compromise or severe pain. Factor replacement is required before any invasive procedure. Affected joints are splinted for 1 to 2 days, after which therapy is started to prevent contractures. Recurrent hemarthroses can lead to hemophilic joint disease. Iron perpetuates a chronic inflammatory state via changes at the molecular level and release of cytokines.[22] MRI can be used to identify the early changes seen with hemophilic joint disease.[23] Isotopic, surgical, or chemical synovectomy can provide relief from repeated joint bleeds.[24]

Sickle Cell Disease

Sickle cell disease is a genetic disorder with an abnormal β globin chain of hemoglobin resulting in deformation of red blood cells under low oxygen tension. About 2 million Americans (or 1 in 12 African Americans) carry the sickle cell gene. Sickle cell anemia is seen when two alleles of the abnormal hemoglobin S gene are present. Patients with only a single copy of the gene (HbAS) have sickle cell trait and are generally asymptomatic but may carry a higher risk of exercise-related sudden death.[25] Rarer forms of sickle cell disease include sickle-hemoglobin C disease (HbSC), sickle β-plus-thalassemia (HbS/β+) and sickle β-zero-thalassemia (HbS/β0).

The first manifestation of the disease may be dactylitis (hand-foot syndrome) occurring around age 6 months as fetal hemoglobin is diminishing and hemoglobin S reaches pathologic significance. Early presentation (before age 6 months) may predict a more severe clinical course.[26] Patients with sickle cell anemia are susceptible to infections due to hyposplenia, intestinal infarcts, poor opsonization of polysaccharide antigens due to impaired complement activity, and sluggish microcirculation. Patients with sickle cell anemia frequently present with bone and/or joint pain with signs that may be confused with osteoarticular infection.

Bone infarction (much more common) and infections are similar in presentation consisting of fever, tenderness to palpation, bone pain, swelling, and an elevated erythrocyte sedimentation rate (ESR) and C-reactive protein (CRP) level. Osteomyelitis should be suspected in patients who appear to have sepsis with fever higher than 38.2°C and a white blood cell count greater than 15,000 cells/mm³ or who do not respond after 24 to 48 hours to proper hydration and pain management.[27] Bone scan, bone marrow scan, and MRI may help differentiate between these two conditions. Staphylococcus aureus is the most common organism overall, although Salmonella is also very common and may be more prevalent in certain areas. Treatment consists of prompt abscess drainage followed by prolonged antibiotic treatment.

Osteonecrosis of the femoral epiphysis can occur and frequently is bilateral (50%). Initial treatment consists of crutch ambulation, partial weight bearing, and range of motion. Outcome is dependent on the level of involvement and age of the patient.

Leukemia

Acute lymphoblastic leukemia represents 80% of all leukemias in children and is the most common cancer seen; half of these patients present initially with musculoskeletal complaints. Symptoms include multiple joint complaints, migratory bone pain, limp, back pain, fatigue, flu-like illness, fever, and easy bruising.[28] Early diagnosis is essential and significantly decreases morbidity and mortality. Although early in the disease course laboratory values may be normal, later abnormalities include anemia, thrombocytopenia, increased lymphoblasts, and an elevated ESR. Radiographic changes, seen in 40% of patients, include osteolysis, metaphyseal bands, osteopenia, osteosclerosis, a permeative pattern, pathologic fractures, and periosteal reaction.[29] The diagnosis is made via peripheral smear and/or bone marrow biopsy. Patients are treated with chemotherapy.

In patients with acute lymphoblastic leukemia, the incidence of skeletal complications is approximately 30% over a 5-year period during maintenance therapy. Patients may present with chemotherapy-induced neuropathy that can be treated with gabapentin and bracing. Patients treated with high-dose steroids may present to the orthopaedist with secondary osteonecrosis. Vertebral compression fractures and other pathologic fractures can occur as a result of the disease or due to the osteopenia associated with treatment. Bisphosphonate use has shown some promise in the management of the diffuse bone loss and the pain associated with vertebral compression fractures.

Pediatric Musculoskeletal Infections

Musculoskeletal infections in children are potentially life-threatening processes if left untreated. The sequelae of untreated infection include joint destruction, dislocation, growth arrest, and fracture.[30-32] Many children ultimately diagnosed with a musculoskeletal infection will present with a history of an upper respiratory illness or trauma. Thus, a high index of suspicion is necessary to properly evaluate and treat these infections in a timely manner.

Resistant Bacteria

Methicillin-resistant S aureus (MRSA) has changed the landscape of pediatric musculoskeletal infections. In recent reports, 37% to 74% of community-acquired S aureus infections are MRSA (CA-MRSA).[33,34] CA-MRSA infections are associated with longer hospital stays, a higher rate of subperiosteal abscess formation, more surgical procedures, and the need for prolonged antibiotics. In addition, isolates with the Panton-Valentine-Leukocidin gene cause more destructive, life-threatening infections with septic thromboemboli, venous thrombosis, and necrotic pneumonia.[35]

The local prevalence of CA-MRSA must not be overlooked because many of the musculoskeletal infections are culture negative; thus, empiric coverage for MRSA might be appropriate. Treatment of hospital-acquired MRSA and CA-MRSA also differ. Therapy for hospital-acquired MRSA may include vancomycin, daptomycin, or linezolid; for CA-MRSA, the antibiotics trimethoprim-sulfamethoxazole and clindamycin are effective.

Osteomyelitis

The frequency of osteomyelitis is dependent on geographic location. Some reports in colder climates reveal a rate of 13 cases per 100,000, whereas in warmer climates the rate is closer to 1 case in 5,000 and has been increasing.[36,37] Acute hematogenous infection is the most common type of osteomyelitis. The most frequent

6: Pediatrics

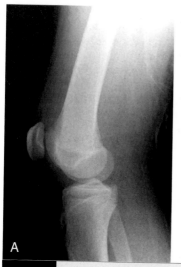
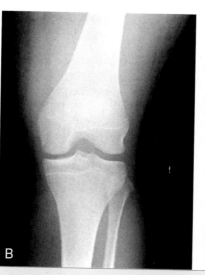
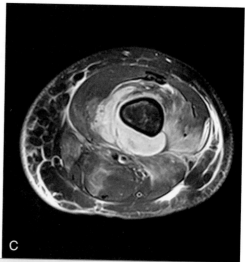

Figure 7 AP (**A**) and lateral (**B**) radiographs of the femur of a 14-year-old boy with fever and leg pain. No radiographic evidence of infection is present. **C,** Axial T2-weighted MRI of the femur of the same child showing a subperiosteal abscess that was surgically drained. Cultures subsequently grew MRSA.

locations, in descending order, are the distal femur, pelvis, tibia, calcaneus, and humerus. *S aureus* is the most common infecting organism, followed by group A streptococcus and *Streptococcus pneumoniae.*

Many families will report a traumatic event before the onset of pain. A history of fever and inability to bear weight are common. In preambulatory children, pseudoparalysis may occur. Laboratory studies should include measurement of white blood cell count, CRP (peaks within a few days), and ESR (peaks at 3 to 5 days). Blood cultures may be helpful, but are only positive in one third of patients. Imaging of the suspected area is crucial in confirming this diagnosis. Plain radiographs may show periosteal reaction and bone changes but lag behind the clinical findings. MRI (**Figure 7**) is the gold standard because it not only confirms the intraosseous infection but also delineates abscess formation, thus guiding surgical intervention in difficult areas such as the pelvis.[38] Additional studies such as color power Doppler sonography may assist in diagnosing deep venous thrombosis, found in older children with CA-MRSA.[35]

Identification of an organism and its antibiotic sensitivity are the mainstays of treatment with parenteral antibiotic therapy. In cases where no bacteria are isolated, local prevalence of resistant bacteria may influence antibiotic choice. The decision to switch to oral antibiotics should be based on clinical and laboratory improvement of the CRP and ESR. Surgical débridement is indicated if abscess or sequestrum is noted. Persistently elevated CRP and continued fevers or symptoms despite treatment require evaluation for septic joint or repeat MRI to rule out reformation of abscess.

Septic Arthritis

Septic arthritis in children presents in a manner similar to that of acute osteomyelitis. The patient can be febrile and be unable to bear weight on the affected extremity. Physical examination reveals a tender, erythematous, swollen joint that is painful to range of motion. Septic arthritis is common in the knee (35%), the hip (35%), the shoulder/elbow/wrist (15%), or ankle (10%). If the hip is affected, the process must be differentiated from other primary hip conditions such as transient synovitis. Ultrasound examination can confirm the presence of effusion at the hip.

Diagnostic testing should evaluate CRP, ESR, and white blood cell count. Specifically, if a child is febrile, is not bearing weight, and has an ESR greater than 40 mm/h, a white blood cell count greater than 12,000 cells/mm³, and a CRP greater than 2 mg/dL, the likelihood of septic arthritis is 98%.[39,40]

Other laboratory tests to consider include a rapid strep test, antistreptolysin O, Lyme antibodies, gonococcal swabs of mucosal surfaces, and a tuberculosis test. Radiographs may delineate the presence of associated osteomyelitis. However, aspiration of the affected joint for fluid examination and culture is the gold standard.

Unfortunately, culture-negative aspirations are common. Placing the aspirate into blood culture bottles may increase the diagnostic yield by allowing growth of both common bacteria (such as *S aureus*) and uncommon bacteria (such as *Kingella kingae*).

Timely surgical drainage of pus followed by parenteral antibiotics is essential to avoid joint destruction because of the presence of proteolytic enzymes in both the synovium and bacterium. Arthroscopic and open lavage techniques are equally effective in cases of early joint infection. Drainage tubes are essential following either technique. Antibiotic duration is generally 3 to 4 weeks but may be longer if concomitant osteomyelitis is present (found in 21% of patients).[41]

Pyomyositis

Recent attention has been paid to CA-MRSA causing nontropical pyomyositis in immunocompetent children.[42,43] Compartment syndrome, septic pulmonary emboli, and toxic shock have all been reported. Intensive medical management including respiratory support may also be required. MRI will confirm the diagnosis. If abscess formation is present, surgical or CT-guided drainage coupled with parenteral antibiotics is suggested.

Annotated References

1. Kneisl JS, Simon MA: Medical management compared with operative treatment for osteoid-osteoma. *J Bone Joint Surg Am* 1992;74(2):179-185.

2. Moser T, Giacomelli MC, Clavert JM, Buy X, Dietemann JL, Gangi A: Image-guided laser ablation of osteoid osteoma in pediatric patients. *J Pediatr Orthop* 2008;28(2):265-270.

   This article is a retrospective review of 68 pediatric patients with osteoid osteoma treated by image-guided laser ablation. The overall success rate was 98%, reported at mean follow-up of 83 months. Seven patients required two procedures. Level of evidence: IV.

3. Lucas DR, Unni KK, McLeod RA, O'Connor MI, Sim FH: Osteoblastoma: clinicopathologic study of 306 cases. *Hum Pathol* 1994;25(2):117-134.

4. Arkader A, Dormans JP: Osteoblastoma in the skeletally immature. *J Pediatr Orthop* 2008;28(5):555-560.

   The authors present the first report of osteoblastoma in children. Also included is a four-step approach to treatment: curettage, high-speed burring, electrocautery, and phenol, a regimen noted to be successful in 16 of 17 patients. Level of evidence: IV.

5. Thawrani D, Thai CC, Welch RD, Copley L, Johnston CE: Successful treatment of unicameral bone cyst by single percutaneous injection of alpha-BSM. *J Pediatr Orthop* 2009;29(5):511-517.

   This article evaluated a single injection of α-BSM for UBC.

6. Sung AD, Anderson ME, Zurakowski D, Hornicek FJ, Gebhardt MC: Unicameral bone cyst: A retrospective study of three surgical treatments. *Clin Orthop Relat Res* 2008;466(10):2519-2526.

   This article evaluated three different treatments (steroids, curettage and bone grafting, or a combination of steroids, demineralized bone matrix and bone marrow aspirate) and found that curettage was associated with the lowest rate of posttreatment pathologic fractures and the highest rate of pain and other complications.

7. Wright JG, Yandow S, Donaldson S, Marley L; Simple Bone Cyst Trial Group: A randomized clinical trial comparing intralesional bone marrow and steroid injections for simple bone cysts. *J Bone Joint Surg Am* 2008;90(4):722-730.

   The authors concluded that the rate of healing of simple bone cysts was low following injection of either bone marrow (23%) or methylprednisolone (42%). Healing rates were superior following injection of methylprednisone.

8. Docquier PL, Delloye C: Treatment of aneurysmal bone cysts by introduction of demineralized bone and autogenous bone marrow. *J Bone Joint Surg Am* 2005;87(10):2253-2258.

9. Völker T, Denecke T, Steffen I, et al: Positron emission tomography for staging of pediatric sarcoma patients: Results of a prospective multicenter trial. *J Clin Oncol* 2007;25(34):5435-5441.

   This prospective multicenter study compares the efficacy of positron emission tomographic scanning and conventional imaging modalities (MRI, CT, bone scan, and ultrasound) in 46 pediatric patients with histologically proven sarcoma.

10. Bacci G, Longhi A, Bertoni F, et al: Bone metastases in osteosarcoma patients treated with neoadjuvant or adjuvant chemotherapy: The Rizzoli experience in 52 patients. *Acta Orthop* 2006;77(6):938-943.

11. Gulley ML, Kaiser-Rogers KA: A rational approach to genetic testing for sarcoma. *Diagn Mol Pathol* 2009;18(1):1-10.

    This article is a summary of the current state of the clinical use of molecular testing in the evaluation of skeletal sarcoma.

12. Bacci G, Longhi A, Ferrari S, Mercuri M, Versari M, Bertoni F: Prognostic factors in non-metastatic Ewing's sarcoma tumor of bone: An analysis of 579 patients treated at a single institution with adjuvant or neoadjuvant chemotherapy between 1972 and 1998. *Acta Oncol* 2006;45(4):469-475.

13. Stieber JR, Dormans JP: Manifestations of hereditary multiple exostoses. *J Am Acad Orthop Surg* 2005;13(2):110-120.

14. Weinstein LS: G(s)alpha mutations in fibrous dysplasia and McCune-Albright syndrome. *J Bone Miner Res* 2006;21(suppl 2):120-124.

15. Chapurlat R: Current pharmacological treatment for fibrous dysplasia and perspectives for the future. *Joint Bone Spine* 2005;72(3):196-198.

16. Mankin HJ, Trahan CA, Fondren G, Mankin CJ: Nonossifying fibroma, fibrous cortical defect and Jaffe-Campanacci syndrome: A biologic and clinical review. *Chir Organi Mov* 2009;93(1):1-7.

    The authors present a review of nonossifying fibroma and differential diagnosis.

17. Lee RS, Weitzel S, Eastwood DM, et al: Osteofibrous dysplasia of the tibia: Is there a need for a radical surgical approach? *J Bone Joint Surg Br* 2006;88(5):658-664.

18. Khanna M, Delaney D, Tirabosco R, Saifuddin A: Osteofibrous dysplasia, osteofibrous dysplasia-like adamantinoma and adamantinoma: Correlation of radiological imaging features with surgical histology and assessment of the use of radiology in contributing to needle biopsy diagnosis. *Skeletal Radiol* 2008;37(12): 1077-1084.

   The aim of this study was to correlate the imaging features with surgical histology for tibial osteofibrous dysplasia, osteofibrous dysplasia-like adamantinoma, and classic adamantinoma.

19. Corby RR, Stacy GS, Peabody TD, Dixon LB: Radiofrequency ablation of solitary eosinophilic granuloma of bone. *AJR Am J Roentgenol* 2008;190(6):1492-1494.

   This article describes the novel application of radiofrequency ablation for the treatment of two cases of solitary eosinophilic granuloma of the bone.

20. Ferrari A, Miceli R, Meazza C, et al: Soft tissue sarcomas of childhood and adolescence: The prognostic role of tumor size in relation to patient body size. *J Clin Oncol* 2009;27(3):371-376.

   This case series of 553 pediatric patients with soft-tissue sarcoma explores the relationship of tumor size relative to patient size in staging and prognosis.

21. Palmerini E, Staals EL, Alberghini M, et al: Synovial sarcoma: Retrospective analysis of 250 patients treated at a single institution. *Cancer* 2009;115(13):2988-2998.

   This review of 30 years of experience at the Rizzoli Institute includes pediatric patients and describes prognostic factors as well as results of treatment.

22. Valentino LA, Hakobyan N, Rodriguez N, Hoots WK: Pathogenesis of haemophilic synovitis: Experimental studies on blood-induced joint damage. *Haemophilia* 2007;13(suppl 3):10-13.

   This article discusses three cellular regulators (p53, p21 and TRAIL) induced in synovial tissue that are important for iron metabolism.

23. Bossard D, Carrillon Y, Stieltjes N, et al: Management of haemophilic arthropathy. *Haemophilia* 2008; 14(suppl 4):11-19.

   The treatment options for patients with hemophilic arthropathy are reviewed.

24. Rodriguez-Merchan EC, Quintana M, De la Corte-Rodriguez H, Coya J: Radioactive synoviorthesis for the treatment of haemophilic synovitis. *Haemophilia* 2007; 13(suppl 3):32-37.

   The procedure should be performed as soon as possible to minimize the degree of articular cartilage damage, which based on many studies is irreversible.

25. Kark JA, Posey DM, Schumacher HR, Ruehle CJ: Sickle-cell trait as a risk factor for sudden death in physical training. *N Engl J Med* 1987;317(13):781-787.

26. Foucan L, Ekouevi D, Etienne-Julan M, Salmi LR, Diara JP; Paediatric Cohort of Guadeloupe: Early onset dactylitis associated with the occurrence of severe events in children with sickle cell anaemia. The Paediatric Cohort of Guadeloupe (1984-99). *Paediatr Perinat Epidemiol* 2006;20(1):59-66.

27. Berger E, Saunders N, Wang L, Friedman JN: Sickle cell disease in children: Differentiating osteomyelitis from vaso-occlusive crisis. *Arch Pediatr Adolesc Med* 2009; 163(3):251-255.

   Multivariate logistic regression showed that the significant predictors of osteomyelitis in sickle cell disease were duration of fever (odds ratio, 1.8; 95% confidence interval, 1.2-2.6) and pain (1.2; 1.0-1.4) before presentation and swelling of the affected limb (8.4; 3.5-20.0).

28. Sinigaglia R, Gigante C, Bisinella G, Varotto S, Zanesco L, Turra S: Musculoskeletal manifestations in pediatric acute leukemia. *J Pediatr Orthop* 2008;28(1):20-28.

   This article emphasizes the frequent clinical (38.3%) and radiologic (40.2%) musculoskeletal manifestations of leukemia in children.

29. Halton J, Gaboury I, Grant R, et al; Canadian STOPP Consortium: Advanced vertebral fracture among newly diagnosed children with acute lymphoblastic leukemia: Results of the Canadian Steroid-Associated Osteoporosis in the Pediatric Population (STOPP) research program. *J Bone Miner Res* 2009;24(7):1326-1334.

   The authors state that vertebral compression is an underrecognized complication of newly diagnosed acute lymphoblastic leukemia (found in 16%).

30. Saisu T, Kawashima A, Kamegaya M, Mikasa M, Moriishi J, Moriya H: Humeral shortening and inferior subluxation as sequelae of septic arthritis of the shoulder in neonates and infants. *J Bone Joint Surg Am* 2007;89(8): 1784-1793.

   The consequences of delayed treatment of septic shoulder are discussed.

31. Forlin E, Milani C: Sequelae of septic arthritis of the hip in children: A new classification and a review of 41 hips. *J Pediatr Orthop* 2008;28(5):524-528.

   The sequelae of septic hip are discussed.

32. Wada A, Fujii T, Takamura K, Yanagida H, Urano N, Surijamorn P: Operative reconstruction of the severe sequelae of infantile septic arthritis of the hip. *J Pediatr Orthop* 2007;27(8):910-914.

   This article focuses on what can be done once the hip has been altered by the sepsis.

33. Mongkolrattanothai K, Aldag JC, Mankin P, Gray BM: Epidemiology of community-onset Staphylococcus aureus infections in pediatric patients: An experience at a Children's Hospital in central Illinois. *BMC Infect Dis* 2009;9:112.

   The changing epidemiology of CA-MRSA is reviewed.

34. Deresinski S: Methicillin-resistant Staphylococcus aureus: An evolutionary, epidemiologic, and therapeutic odyssey. *Clin Infect Dis* 2005;40(4):562-573.

35. Hollmig ST, Copley LA, Browne RH, Grande LM, Wilson PL: Deep venous thrombosis associated with osteomyelitis in children. *J Bone Joint Surg Am* 2007;89(7): 1517-1523.

    A sequela of MRSA infections is summarized.

36. Gafur OA, Copley LA, Hollmig ST, Browne RH, Thornton LA, Crawford SE: The impact of the current epidemiology of pediatric musculoskeletal infection on evaluation and treatment guidelines. *J Pediatr Orthop* 2008;28(7):777-785.

    The authors present an overall review of pediatric infections and MRSA management.

37. Riise OR, Kirkhus E, Handeland KS, et al: Childhood osteomyelitis-incidence and differentiation from other acute onset musculoskeletal features in a population-based study. *BMC Pediatr* 2008;8:45-55.

    The focus of this article is the epidemiology of osteomyelitis.

38. Klein JD, Leach KA: Pediatric pelvic osteomyelitis. *Clin Pediatr (Phila)* 2007;46(9):787-790.

    The sometimes-hidden diagnosis of pediatric pelvic osteomyelitis is discussed.

39. Caird MS, Flynn JM, Leung YL, Millman JE, D'Italia JG, Dormans JP: Factors distinguishing septic arthritis from transient synovitis of the hip in children: A prospective study. *J Bone Joint Surg Am* 2006;88(6):1251-1257.

40. Kocher MS, Mandiga R, Zurakowski D, Barnewolt C, Kasser JR: Validation of a clinical prediction rule for the differentiation between septic arthritis and transient synovitis of the hip in children. *J Bone Joint Surg Am* 2004;86(8):1629-1635.

41. Lavy CB, Thyoka M: For how long should antibiotics be given in acute paediatric septic arthritis? A prospective audit of 96 cases. *Trop Doct* 2007;37(4):195-197.

    This is a larger study regarding the duration of antibiotics in osteomyelitis.

42. Block AA, Marshall C, Ratcliffe A, Athan E: Staphylococcal pyomyositis in a temperate region: Epidemiology and modern management. *Med J Aust* 2008;189(6): 323-325.

    This is a review of staphylococcal pyomyositis, a now-frequent occurrence in nontropical climates.

43. Ovadia D, Ezra E, Ben-Sira L, et al: Primary pyomyositis in children: A retrospective analysis of 11 cases. *J Pediatr Orthop B* 2007;16(2):153-159.

    This is a small retrospective analysis of pyomyositis.

Index

Index

Index

Index